Tables for the Use of Range and Studentized Range in Tests of Hypotheses

H. Leon Harter
Champaign, Illinois

N. Balakrishnan
Department of Mathematics and Statistics
McMaster University
Hamilton, Ontario, Canada

CRC Press
Boca Raton New York

Library of Congress Cataloging-in-Publication Data

Harter, H. Leon (Harman Leon), 1919-
Tables for the use of range and studentized range in tests of hypotheses / H. Leon Harter, N. Balakrishnan.
p. cm.
"A revision of the first author's Order statistics and their use in testing and estimation, volume 1: Tests based on range and studentized range of samples from a normal population ... 1970"–
–Pref.
Includes bibliographical references and indexes.
ISBN 0-8493-3114-5 (alk. paper)
1. Order statistics. I. Balakrishnan, N., 1956– II. Harter, H. Leon (Harman Leon), 1919– Order statistics and their use in testing and estimation. III. Title.
QA278.7.H375 1997
519.5--dc21

97-31075
CIP

International Standard Book Number 0-8493-3114-5
Printed in the United States of America 1 2 3 4 5 6 7 8 9 0
Printed on acid-free paper

To Alice Lauretta

To Priya and Prakash Ramachandran

Preface

This Handbook is a revision of the first author's *Order Statistics and their Use in Testing and Estimation*, Volume 1: *Tests Based on Range and Studentized Range of Samples from a Normal Population* (published in 1970 through the U.S. Government Printing Office) and referred to hereafter as Harter (1970a), of which the Preface reads as follows:

Early in 1954 the author became concerned with the problem of multiple comparisons, and especially with the conflicting claims that were being made by proponents of one or another of the multiple comparison tests that had been proposed during a period of only a few years immediately preceding that time. He approached the problem with the idea, not of proposing a new test, since the number available was already more than adequate, but of comparing the existing tests as to their error rates and the sample sizes required for prescribed error rates. Armed with weapons no more formidable than a desk calculator and tables of the probability integral of the t-distribution, the incomplete Beta function, and Lagrangian interpolation coefficients, he set out to compute tables of error rates and sample sizes for multiple comparison tests, especially those based on the studentized range, which were eventually published in 1957 in a technical journal. Observing certain irregularities in these tables, he became convinced as early as 1955 that published tables of critical values for some of these tests, notably Duncan's new multiple range test, were in error. It soon became evident that correction of the errors in these tables would be impossible without first computing a more accurate table of the probability integral of the studentized range and that this in turn would require the computation of a more accurate table of the probability integral of the range. At this point the author enlisted the aid of a numerical analyst, Dr. Gertrude Blanch, and a computer programmer, Donald S. Clemm; a second programmer, Eugene H. Guthrie, was added to the team later. Further progress would not have been possible without their help. Valuable assistance was also rendered by Professors David B. Duncan, H. O. Hartley, Daniel Teichroew, and John W. Tukey, who offered helpful suggestions and made available unpublished manuscripts and tables, and by Major (now Col.) John V. Armitage, who suggested the iterative interpolation procedure used in determining percentage points. The results of the expenditure of several man-years of effort and several hundred hours of time on a high-speed electronic computer were tables, more extensive and more accurate than any previously computed, of the probability integrals and percentage points of the range and of the studentized range, as well as of moments of the range, which were published in 1959 in a two-volume Air Force technical report. Excerpts, in the form of tables of moments of the range, percentage points of the range and the studentized range (at the most common levels of significance), and critical values for Duncan's new multiple range test, were later published in technical journals. The tables of the probability integrals and the unabridged tables of percentage points have not, to date, appeared in the open literature, though so many requests have been received for copies of the report containing them that it has had to be reprinted two or three times.

Early in the present decade, the author became interested in the F' test, based on the ratio of two ranges, as a substitute for the F test, based on the ratio of two variances. Though this test had been proposed over a decade earlier, no really satisfactory table of percentage points of the ratio of two ranges, without which the test could not be properly implemented, had been computed. This time the author discovered that it was necessary to move not just two, but three, steps backward before taking the first step forward. Computation of a table of percentage points of the ratio of two ranges required a table of the cumulative distribution function of the ratio of two ranges, for which one needed a table of the probability density function of the ratio of two ranges, for which in turn a table of the probability density function of the range itself was a prerequisite. In none of these cases was a sufficiently accurate and extensive table available, so the author found it necessary to compute each of them in turn, this time doing his own programming, which was made easier because of the fact that, by that time, FORTRAN had become available. The resulting tables, together with one comparing the power of the F' and F tests, were published in 1962 in an Air Force technical report. An excerpt of the latter table and the complete table of percentage points of the ratio of two ranges were later published in a technical journal, but the longer antecedent tables have not appeared in the open literature.

As long ago as 1960, the author began making preparations to write a book on order statistics and mentioned his plans to colleagues. While this announcement was greeted with some initial enthusiasm, as time went by his friends began to doubt whether the project would ever be brought to fruition, and the author must admit that he sometimes shared their skepticism. During the intervening years, many ideas as to the title and format of the proposed work have been considered and discarded, and so much material has been collected that plans for a single volume have been expanded to two and then to three. Volume 1 will deal with tests based on range and studentized range of samples from a normal population and Volume 2 with estimates based on order statistics of samples from various populations, on which the author began investigation as early as 1957 and to which he has devoted most of his research effort during the past several years. In these two volumes, the author makes no attempt at exhaustive or even broad coverage, preferring to concentrate almost entirely on his own contributions to theory and tables, with heavy emphasis on the latter, giving just enough references to the related work of others to place his own in perspective. Volume 3 will be devoted to a chronological annotated bibliography, with a brief summary of the contents of each article, together with lists of references to earlier work and citations by later authors.

As the reader is undoubtedly aware after perusing the preceding paragraphs, most of the material to be included in this volume is not new. The text of all of Chapter 1 and the first section of Chapter 2 represents only a minor revision of that which first appeared in Air Force technical reports, while the second section of Chapter 2 is the result of a somewhat more extensive revision of material first published in a technical journal over a decade ago. Tables A1–B3 are exactly as they first appeared in the above-mentioned reports. Tables A4, A7, and A8, as well as portions of Tables A5, B2, and B3 have also appeared in technical journals, and some of them have been reproduced in numerous handbooks of statistical tables and textbooks in statistics and in various subject-matter fields in which statistical methods are applied. Earlier versions of Tables B4–B6, computed on a desk calculator, also appeared in a journal article, but these tables have been entirely recomputed on an electronic computer, programmed by Donald S. Clemm. In Tables B5 and B6, the type II error rate is based on the population standard deviation, σ, not on the square root, s, of the error mean square, the approximation which was used in the earlier version so as to make it possible to employ the central t-distribution in the computations instead of the noncentral t-distribution, with which the author did not feel prepared to cope with the tools then available to him. Even though these latter tables and the discussion of the method of computing them represent the only really new material in this volume, the author believes it is worthwhile to bring all of the tables and the related theory together in a single hard-cover volume so as to make them more readily and permanently accessible.

In case there are any lingering doubts, the author wishes to make it quite clear that this is intended as a reference work, not a textbook. While there is undoubtedly a need for a textbook on the subject, the author, who left university teaching in 1952, does not feel qualified to undertake the task of writing one, which must therefore be left to a university colleague actively engaged in teaching.

In concluding this preface, the author wishes to express his thanks to all those persons whose assistance has been acknowledged above, and also to Miss Eva Brandenburg for typing the manuscript, as well as to Mr. Donald S. Clemm and MSgt John E. Mathis for ruling the tables and preparing overlays.

WRIGHT-PATTERSON AIR FORCE BASE

FEBRUARY, 1969

In addition to the initial distribution of 400 copies by the Aerospace Research Laboratories, 690 copies of the Harter (1970a) volume were sold during the period from 1970 to 1976. Requests for that volume are still being received, even though it has been out of print since 1976. Since that time there have been several developments, some of them due to the second author, which merit attention. In view of these facts, we decided to collaborate on a revision of the Harter (1970a) volume, the proposal for which was accepted by CRC Press, which already published a revision by Harter and Balakrishnan (1996) of the second 1970 volume [Harter (1970b)]. The bibliography, originally planned as the third volume of the series, was expanded to eight volumes and published by American Sciences Press.

We thank Mr. Robert Stern and Mr. Tim Pletscher (both of CRC Press, Boca Raton) for supporting this project and Ms. Nora Konopka and Ms. Andrea Demby (both of CRC Press, Boca Raton) for assisting in the production of this volume. Our sincere thanks also goes to Mrs. Debbie Iscoe (Hamilton, Canada) for the excellent typesetting of the manuscript.

CHAMPAIGN, ILLINOIS, USA
HAMILTON, ONTARIO, CANADA

JUNE 1997

Contents

Preface v

List of Tables xi

Introduction 1

1. The Range of Samples From a Normal Population 3

1.1 Percentage Points of the Ratio of Two Ranges and Related Tables, 3
1.1.1 Introduction, 3
1.1.2 Method of Computation of the Tables, 4
1.1.3 Example of the Use of the Tables, 11
1.1.4 References, 12
1.2 Probability Integral, Percentage Points, and Moments of the Range, 14
1.2.1 History and Introduction, 14
1.2.2 Method of Computation of the Tables, 15
1.2.3 Examples of the Use of the Tables, 17
1.2.4 References, 18
1.3 Applications to Control Charts, 20
1.3.1 Reference, 21
1.4 Applications to Tests of Homogeneity in Multinomial and Multivariate Hypergeometric Distributions, 22
1.4.1 References, 24

2. The Studentized Range of Samples From a Normal Population 25

2.1 Probability Integral and Percentage Points of the Studentized Range; Critical Values for Duncan's Multiple Range Test, 25
2.1.1 History and Introduction, 25
2.1.2 Method of Computation of the Tables, 27
2.1.3 Examples of the Use of the Tables, 31
2.1.4 References, 33
2.2 Error Rates and Sample Sizes for Multiple Comparison Tests Based on the Studentized Range, 35
2.2.1 Introduction, 35
2.2.2 Significance *vs.* Confidence, 35
2.2.3 The Fixed Range Tests, 36
2.2.4 The Multiple Range Tests, 37
2.2.5 Example, 37

2.2.6 Type I Error Rates, 39
2.2.7 Type II and Type III Error Rates, 40
2.2.8 Required Sample Sizes, 42
2.2.9 Computation of the Tables, 43
2.2.10 Monte Carlo Studies, 45
2.2.11 References, 45
2.3 Analysis of Variance Based on the (Studentized) Range, 48
2.3.1 Introduction, 48
2.3.2 Analysis for Single Classification, 48
2.3.3 Analysis for Double Classification, 49
2.3.4 References, 51
2.4 Applications to Outlier-Testing, 52
2.4.1 References, 53

Appendix A Tables Based on the Range **55**

Appendix B Tables Based on the Studentized Range **271**

Author Index **659**

Subject Index **661**

List of Tables

A1 Cumulative distribution function $F(F', n_1, n_2)$ of the ratio F' of the ranges of samples of sizes n_1 and n_2 from $N(\mu, \sigma)$ $(i = 1, 2)$ **57**

A2 Percentage points, corresponding to cumulative probability P, of the ratio F' of the ranges of samples of sizes n_1 and n_2 from $N(\mu_i, \sigma)$ $(i = 1, 2)$ **109**

A3 Power of the F' and F tests (size α) of $H_0 : \sigma_1 = \sigma_2$ vs. $H_1 : \sigma_1 = k\sigma_2$ **115**

A4 Probability integral $P(W, n)$ of the range W for samples of size n from $N(\mu, 1)$ **125**

A5 Percentage points of the range **257**

A6 Moments of the range W for samples of size n from $N(\mu, 1)$ **261**

A7 Constants for constructing $\bar{X}$ and R charts **265**

A8 Approximate upper 5% critical values of the distribution of V **267**

A9 Approximate upper 1% critical values of the distribution of V **269**

B1 Probability integral $P(Q, \nu, n)$ of the studentized range $Q = w/s$ for samples of size n from a normal population with ν degrees of freedom for the independent estimate s^2 of the population variance **273**

B2 Percentage points of the studentized range **515**

B3 Critical values for Duncan's multiple range test **555**

B4 Comparison of type I error rates for multiple comparison tests (Single-classification experiments) **567**

B5 Comparison of type II-III error rates for multiple comparison tests (Single-classification experiments) $[\delta = 0.5(0.5)3.0]$ **575**

B6 Sample size for multiple comparison tests with prescribed error rates (Single-classification experiments) $[\delta = 0.5(0.5)3.0]$ **645**

B7 Tables for analysis of variance based on (studentized) range **655**

B8 5% and 1% critical values for the discordancy test of a lower and upper outlier-pair based on the internally studentized T for a sample of size n **657**

Introduction

Consider a sample consisting of n observations drawn at random from some specified or unspecified population. If the sample values are arranged in order from the smallest, x_1, to the largest, x_n, so that $x_1 \leq x_2 \leq \cdots \leq x_n$, then x_1 is called the *first order statistic*, x_2 the *second order statistic*, ..., and x_n the *nth order statistic* of the sample. The difference, $w = x_n - x_1$, between the nth (largest) and first (smallest) order statistics is called the sample *range*. The ratio, w/s, of the range to an independent root-mean-square estimate, s, of the population standard deviation, σ, is called a *studentized range*. Other functions of order statistics, such as the median, the mid-range, the quasi-ranges, and the studentized maximum modulus, are in common use, but they will not be defined here, since this volume will deal only with the range and the studentized range. More specifically, we shall deal with tests of hypotheses based on the range or the studentized range of samples from a normal population, so unless it is otherwise stated, it will be assumed that the sampled population is normally distributed. The sophisticated reader may protest that the testing of hypotheses, or significance testing, as it is often called, is really inseparable from confidence procedures; nevertheless, the statements made in this volume will be couched in the language of significance, which the reader who is so inclined can easily translate into the language of confidence.

The sample range is often used, for the sake of simplicity, as a substitute for the standard deviation (or the variance) as a measure of dispersion. This is especially true in situations, such as the plotting of statistical quality control charts, in which it is necessary to calculate quickly, without the aid of a computer, a measure of the dispersion of a large number of small samples. One of the topics to be considered in this volume will be the use of the F' test, based on the ratio of two ranges, as a substitute for the conventional F test, based on the ratio of two variances, in testing the hypothesis that two populations, assumed to be normal, have equal dispersion. Computation of a table of critical values for the F' test, which are percentage points of the ratio of two ranges, will require prior computation of tables of the probability density function of the range, the probability density function of the ratio of two ranges, and the cumulative distribution function of the ratio of two ranges. The critical values will then be determined by inverse interpolation in the table of the cumulative distribution function, and they, in turn, will be used to compute the power of the F' test, which will be compared with that of the F test. Also discussed in Chapter 1 will be tables of the cumulative distribution function (probability integral) of the range, percentage points of the range, and moments of the range. The first of these is needed to compute the second, but it is of even greater interest because of the role it will play in connection with the computation of tables of the probability integral and percentage points of the studentized range in Chapter 2.

The studentized range arises quite naturally in connection with the analysis of replicated experiments. To make things as simple as possible, we shall consider a single-classification experiment with k classes and r replications (r observations in each class), though the studentized range is equally applicable in the analysis of more complex experimental designs. There are thus kr observations, and one degree of freedom is lost for the calculation of the grand mean, leaving $kr - 1$ degrees of freedom for the total sum of squares, which is partitioned into a sum of squares between classes, with $k - 1$ degrees of freedom, and a sum of squares within classes (error sum of squares), with $k(r - 1)$ degrees of freedom. The sums of squares are calculated and divided by their respective numbers of degrees of freedom to determine the mean squares, and the ratio of the mean square between classes to the mean square for error is compared with the critical value, at some chosen level of significance, for the F distribution with $k - 1$ and $k(r - 1)$ degrees of freedom for numerator and denominator, respectively. Alternatively, the ratio of the range of the class means to the standard error of the mean, $s_{\bar{x}} = s/\sqrt{r}$, where s^2 is the error mean square, might be compared with the critical value for the studentized range with $k(r - 1)$ degrees of freedom. Most experimenters use the F test of overall significance. If the hypothesis that all the class means are equal is not rejected, no further tests are made; if, however, the class means are found, by the F test, to differ significantly, the experimenter is usually interested in knowing which class means differ significantly from which others. The most convenient tests available for answering that question are the multiple comparison tests based on the studentized range. If the F test shows significance, the test based on the studentized range of all the class means usually shows significance at about the same level. If the studentized range of all the k class means is significant, the studentized ranges of the $k - 1$ largest and the $k - 1$ smallest class means, $(x_n - x_2)/s_{\bar{x}}$ and $(x_{n-1} - x_1)/s_{\bar{x}}$, are then tested for significance, and so on for $k - 2, k - 3, \ldots, 2$ class means. This process continues only as long as the studentized ranges are found to be significant; once the studentized range of a group of ordered means is found to be non-significant, no further tests are made on subgroups of that group. The critical values for testing the significance of the studentized range of ordered subgroups of means depend on the choice of the kind of control the experimenter wishes to exercise over type I error (rejecting the null hypothesis when it is true). This question will be discussed in detail in Chapter 2, along with the computation of tables of the probability integral and percentage points of the studentized range, critical values for Duncan's multiple range test, and error rates and sample sizes for multiple comparison tests.

Tables based on the range will be given in Appendix A, while those based on the studentized range will be given in Appendix B.

1

The Range of Samples From a Normal Population

1.1 Percentage Points of the Ratio of Two Ranges and Related Tables [1]

1.1.1 Introduction

Since Mosteller (1946) pointed out that many inefficient statistics are quite useful because of their simplicity, simple though inefficient substitutes have been proposed for many of the standard statistical tests. Link (1950) suggested the use of a test based on the ratio F' of the ranges of two samples in place of the usual F test of the hypothesis that the samples have been drawn from populations having equal variances. He gave expressions for the cumulative distribution function of F' (R in his notation) for samples from rectangular, exponential and normal populations. In the case of the normal population, results in closed form were given only for samples sizes n_1 and n_2 both equal to 2 and for one sample size equal to 2 and the other equal to 3. In the same paper, Link tabulated the lower percentage points (two-significant-figure values computed by numerical integration) corresponding to cumulative probabilities $P = .005,\ .01,\ .025,\ .05,\ .10$ for samples of sizes $n_1 = 2(1)10$ and $n_2 = 2(1)10$ from normal populations. Dixon and Massey (1951), pp. 243 and 317-318, in the first textbook treatment of the subject known to the authors, gave a brief discussion of the use of the F' test as a substitute for the F test, together with a table of upper percentage points of F' obtained by taking reciprocals of Link's corresponding lower percentage points with n_1 and n_2 interchanged.

The expression mentioned in the preceding paragraph for the cumulative distribution function of F' for samples from a rectangular population was incorrect. The correct expression was given by Rider (1951) and also by Link (1952). Rider also tabulated the upper 10, 5 and 1 percent points of F' for samples from a rectangular population, giving three-significant-figure values for $n_1 = 2(1)10$ and $n_2 = 2(1)10$.

Pillai (1951) showed that the probability density function of F' may be written as the sum of an infinite double series, from which an expression involving incomplete Beta functions may be derived for the cumulative distribution function of F'. Using this method, Pillai (1951, 1957) tabulated upper 5 and 1 percent points of F' for samples of sizes n_1, n_2 ranging up to 8 from normal populations having the same variance. By considering more terms in the expansion, Buenaventura (1959) and Pillai and Buenaventura (1961) obtained somewhat more accurate percentage points for values of n_1, n_2 varying from 2 to 10. These results were given to three significant figures, but there seemed to be reason to question the accuracy of the third digit. There appeared to be little hope either of

[1] Reproduced, with minor changes, from ARL 62-378 (same title). A portion of this material was also published in *Biometrika* **50** (1963), 187-194.

improving the accuracy or of extending the tables to larger sample sizes by considering still more terms in the expansion. The first author, wishing to accomplish both of these objectives and also to increase the number of values of α, the size of the test, decided to return to the approach, first used by Link, based on numerical integration. Here too he encountered difficulties, though not insurmountable ones; in particular, he found it necessary to compute three auxiliary tables, each several times as long as the table of percentage points itself, before proceeding to the main task. The details of the method of computation are given in subsection 1.1.2.

Since the principal use of the percentage points of the ratio of two ranges is as critical values for the F' test, which is a substitute for the F test of the hypothesis that two populations have equal variances, it seemed desirable to compare the power of the F' test with that of the F test against various alternatives. The method of computation is described in subsection 1.1.2 and an example is given in subsection 1.1.3 to illustrate the use of the tables.

1.1.2 Method of Computation of the Tables

Probability Density Function of the Range

The probability density function of the standardized range $W = w/\sigma$ of a sample of size n is known [see Kendall (1948), p. 223], to be

$$f(W,n) = n(n-1)\int_{-\infty}^{\infty}[\Phi(x+W)-\Phi(x)]^{n-2}\phi(x+W)\phi(x)\,dx, \tag{1.1.1}$$

where $\Phi(x) = \int_0^x \phi(x)\,dx$ and where, for the case under consideration, that of sampling from a normal population, $\phi(x) = (2\pi)^{-1/2}e^{-x^2/2}$.

It was decided to tabulate $f(W,n)$ to 8 decimal places, accurate to within a unit in the last place, for $W = 0(0.01)W_{\max}$, where W_{max} is the largest value of W such that $f(W,n) \geq 5 \times 10^{-9}$. A method of computation was devised which made it possible to do this and also to obtain the required accuracy in subsequent tables dependent upon the table of $f(W,n)$. Since single-precision arithmetic on the IBM 7090, the machine used for all the computations, provides only approximately 8 significant decimal digits (27 binary bits), with the last one or two digits affected by rounding error, it was necessary to use double-precision arithmetic to obtain the required accuracy. The program was written in FORTRAN with double-precision input and internal arithmetic and single-precision output, the latter being sufficient to give $f(W,n)$ to 8 decimal places, which is no more than 8 significant digits, since the maximum value of $f(W,n)$ is less than 1, at least for $n = 2(1)16$, the only values of n for which $f(W,n)$ was computed. The input consisted of 15-decimal-place values of $\phi(x)$ and $\Phi(x)$ for $x = 0.(0.01)5.99$ and 7-significant-digit values (15 or more decimal places) of $\phi(x)$ and $1-2\Phi(x)$ for $x = 6.00(0.01)8.00$, all obtained from tables prepared by the WPA Mathematical Tables Project (1942). The values of $f(W,n)$ were obtained from Equation (1.1.1) by numerical integration, using the trapezoidal rule, which Fettis (1955, 1958) has shown to be superior to Simpson's rule or any other integration formula based on equally spaced values of the argument for a class of integrals which includes the integral involved here. It is known that $f(0,2) = \pi^{-1/2} = 0.56418958$ and $f(0,n) = 0$ for $n > 2$. These known values were included in the program, and values of $f(W,n)$ for $W = 0.01(0.01)10.99$ and $n = 2(1)16$ were computed by numerical integration, preliminary computations having shown that $W_{\max} < 10.99$. For each combination of W and n, results were first computed by using intervals $h(x) = 0.32,\ 0.16$. If these results differed by no more than 10^{-8}, the result computed at the smaller interval was taken as $f(W, n)$. Otherwise the numerical integration was repeated using $h(x) = 0.08$, and the result was compared with that obtained at $h(x) = 0.16$. If the difference still did not meet the tolerance of 10^{-8}, the interval was halved again, and this process was continued until the tolerance was met. Since the interval of the input data was $h(x) = 0.01$, nothing further could have been done if the tolerance had not been met by the time $h(x)$ had been cut to 0.01 for the numerical integration. This never happened for $n = 2(1)16$; it did happen for $n = 17$. Since the main justification for computing the table of the probability density function of the range was its use in computing tables of the probability density function, cumulative distribution function, and percentage points of the ratio of two ranges, and since it was not intended to carry these beyond $n = 15$, it was decided to terminate the table of $f(W, n)$ at $n = 16$.

The table of $f(W, n)$ which resulted from these computations was stored on magnetic tape in single-precision, binary form. The results were also converted to decimal form (8 decimal places, accurate to within a unit in the last place), edited, punched on IBM cards, checked by differencing on the IBM 7090, and printed on the IBM 407 tabulator [see Harter (1970a), pp. 37-97].

Probability Density Function of the Ratio of Two Ranges

Let $F' = w_1/w_2$, where w_1 and w_2 are ranges of independent samples of sizes n_1 and n_2, respectively, taken from normal populations having the same variance, σ^2. Since the standardized ranges are $W_1 = w_1/\sigma$ and $W_2 = w_2/\sigma$, respectively, one may write $F' = W_1/W_2$. Since the samples are independent, the joint probability density of W_1 and W_2 may be written as the product of the probability densities of W_1 and W_2. If one makes the change of variable $F' = W_1/W_2$ and integrates over the range of definition of W_2, the result is the probability density function of the ratio of two ranges [see Link (1950)], which is given by

$$f(F', n_1, n_2) = \int_0^\infty W_2\ f_2(W_2, n_2)\ f_1(W_2 F', n_1)\ dW_2, \tag{1.1.2}$$

where f_1 is the probability density function of W_1 and f_2 is the probability density function of W_2. These probability density functions are defined by Equation (1.1.1).

It was decided to tabulate $f(F', n_1, n_2)$ to 6 decimal places, accurate to within a unit in the last place, for $n_1 = 2(1)15$, $n_2 = 2(1)15$, and values of F' at appropriate intervals from 0 up through F'_{max}, where F'_{max} is the largest value of F' such that $f(F', n_1, n_2) \geq 5\times10^{-7}$. A method of computation was devised which made it possible to do this and also to obtain the required accuracy in subsequent tables dependent upon the table of $f(F', n_1, n_2)$. Since F'_{max} is less than 700 except when $n_2 = 2$, and since accurate values of the cumulative distribution function $F(F', n_1, 2)$ can be obtained from a table and an asymptotic formula for the cumulative distribution function $P(Q, 1, n_1)$ of the studentized range given by Harter, Clemm, and Guthrie (1959) by letting $F' = Q/\sqrt{2}$, it was decided for the sake of uniformity to compute $f(F', n_1, n_2)$ for F' up through 700, though the results were tabulated only for F' up through $\min(F'_{\text{max}}, 600)$.

The input to this phase of the problem was the binary form of the table of $f(W, n)$ previously stored on magnetic tape. The tabular values of $f(F', n_1, n_2)$ were obtained by numerical integration in Equation (1.1.2) on the IBM 7090 computer, by use of the seven-point formula

$$y = \frac{h}{120960}[36799(f_1 + f_s) + 176648(f_2 + f_{s-1}) + 54851(f_3 + f_{s-2}) + 177984(f_4 + f_{s-3}) + 89437(f_5 + f_{s-4}) + 130936(f_6 + f_{s-5}) + 119585(f_7 + f_{s-6})] + h(f_8 + f_9 + \cdots + f_{s-7}), \quad (1.1.3)$$

where s is the number of values of the integrand, for arguments at interval h.

The interval for W_2 had to be small enough that numerical integration in Equation (1.1.2) would yield the required accuracy in $f(F', n_1, n_2)$ and the interval in F' had to be small enough that numerical integration of $f(F', n_1, n_2)$, to be discussed in the next subsection, would yield the required accuracy in the cumulative distribution function $F(F', n_1, n_2)$. However, the product of the two intervals had to be 0.01 or a multiple thereof, since the product W_2F' appears as an argument of f_1, and values of f_1, the probability density function of the range, were computed, as noted in the last subsection, only at intervals of 0.01 in this argument. Preliminary computations showed that for small values of F', small values of $h(F')$ were necessary but fairly large values of $h(W_2)$ would suffice, while for large values of F', the reverse was true. Hence the following intervals were decided upon:

Values of F'	$h(F')$	$h(W_2)$
0.00–1.40	0.05	0.2
1.50–4.00	0.1	0.1
4.20–7.00	0.2	0.05
7.50–14.00	0.5	0.02
15.00–40.00	1	0.01
42.00–70.00	2	0.005
75.00–140.00	5	0.002
150.00–300.00	10	0.001
320.00–700.00	20	0.0005

Some refinement of this procedure was required for $F' \le 7$, since the values of $h(F')$ had to be as small as those shown above, but the values of $h(W_2)$ shown above were not small enough to yield the required accuracy in $f(F', n_1, n_2)$. Hence $f(F', n_1, n_2)$ was computed for $F' = 0.00(0.10)1.40$ with $h(W_2) = 0.1$, for $F' = 1.40(0.20)4.00$ with $h(W_2) = 0.05$, and for $F' = 4.00(0.50)7.00$ with $h(W_2) = 0.02$. These values were inserted in place of the less accurate values previously computed, and the intermediate values were adjusted by an amount found by interpolating linearly in the discrepancy between the results at two intervals. For example, the following adjustments were made (the second and third arguments, n_1 and n_2, have been dropped for simplicity):

$$f(0.05) = f(0.05)_{h(W_2)=0.2} + 0.5[f(0.00)_{h(W_2)=0.1} - f(0.00)_{h(W_2)=0.2}] + 0.5[f(0.10)_{h(W_2)=0.1} - f(0.10)_{h(W_2)=0.2}],$$

$$f(1.50) = f(1.50)_{h(W_2)=0.1} + 0.5[f(1.40)_{h(W_2)=0.05} - f(1.40)_{h(W_2)=0.1}] + 0.5[f(1.60)_{h(W_2)=0.05} - f(1.60)_{h(W_2)=0.1}],$$

$$f(4.20) = f(4.20)_{h(W_2)=0.05} + 0.8[f(4.00)_{h(W_2)=0.02} - f(4.00)_{h(W_2)=0.05}] + 0.2[f(5.00)_{h(W_2)=0.02} - f(5.00)_{h(W_2)=0.05}].$$

The use of values of $h(W_2)$ less than 0.01 for $F' > 40$ required subtabulation of the probability density function of the range, since W_2 is an argument of f_2, which was tabulated only at intervals of 0.01, as noted in subsection 1.2.1. This subtabulation was necessary only for small values of W_2 ($W_2 \le 0.39$), since for larger values of W_2, the factor $f_1(W_2F', n_1)$ in Equation (1.1.2) goes to 0. When the $h(F')$ was changed and the new value of $h(F')$ was not a multiple of the old one, values of $f(F', n_1, n_2)$ for some additional values of F' were needed in integrating $f(F', n_1, n_2)$ to obtain $F(F', n_1, n_2)$, as described later in this subsection. Hence the values of $f(F', n_1, n_2)$ mentioned above as having been computed for $F' = 4.00(0.50)7.00$ with $h(W_2) = 0.02$ were retained, and values of $f(F', n_1, n_2)$ for $F' = 40.00(5.00)70.00$ were computed with $h(W_2) = 0.002$ and retained.

The table of $f(F', n_1, n_2)$ which resulted from these computations was stored on magnetic tape in binary form. The results were also converted to decimal form (6 decimal places, accurate to within a unit in the last place), edited, punched on IBM cards, checked by differencing on the IBM 7090, and printed on the IBM 407 tabulator [see Harter (1970a), pp. 99-169].

Cumulative Distribution Function of the Ratio of Two Ranges

The cumulative distribution function of the ratio of two ranges is given by

$$F(F', n_1, n_2) = \int_0^{F'} f(F', n_1, n_2)\, dF', \tag{1.1.4}$$

where $f(F', n_1, n_2)$ is the probability density function of the ratio of two ranges, which is defined by Equation (1.1.2).

It was decided to tabulate $F(F', n_1, n_2)$ to 5 decimal places, accurate to within a unit in the last place, for $n_1 = 2(1)15$, $n_2 = 2(1)15$, and values of F' at appropriate intervals from 1 up through F'_{max} where F'_{max} is the largest value of F' such that $F(F', n_1, n_2) < 0.999995$. (Note that F'_{max} is defined differently, and may have a different numerical value, here than earlier in this subsection.) It was not necessary to tabulate $F(F', n_1, n_2)$ for F' less than 1, since here one can make use of the relation

$$F(F', n_1, n_2) = 1 - F(1/F', n_2, n_1). \tag{1.1.5}$$

Otherwise, $F(F', n_1, n_2)$ was computed for the same values of F' as those for which $f(F', n_1, n_2)$ had previously been computed, with the computations extending up through $F' = 700$, though the results were tabulated only for F' up through $\min(F'_{\text{max}}, 600)$. As explained earlier in this subsection, computations for $n_2 = 2$ were also cut off at this point, even though in this case $F'_{\text{max}} > 700$, since values of $F(F', n_1, n_2)$ for $700 < F' < 1000\sqrt{2}$ can easily be obtained from a table and those for $F' > 1000\sqrt{2}$ from an asymptotic formula, both of which have been given by Harter, Clemm, and Guthrie (1959). [See Table B1 and subsection 2.1.2 of Chapter 2 of the present volume.]

The input to this phase of the problem was the binary form of the table of $f(F', n_1, n_2)$ previously stored on magnetic tape. The tabular values of $F(F', n_1, n_2)$ were obtained by numerical integration in Equation (1.1.4) on the IBM 7090 computer by means of a chain of 7-point formulas.

For $F' = 1.00(0.05)1.40$ one may write simply

$$\begin{aligned} F(1.00) = 0.05[&C_1 f(0.00) + C_2 f(0.05) + \cdots + C_7 f(0.30) + f(0.35) + f(0.40) + \cdots \\ &+ f(0.65) + C_7 f(0.70) + C_6(0.75) + \cdots + C_1 f(1.00)], \end{aligned} \tag{1.1.6}$$

$$F(1.05) = F(1.00) + 0.05[D_1 f(0.70) + D_2 f(0.75) + \cdots + D_8 f(1.05)], \quad (1.1.7)$$

$$\vdots$$

$$F(1.40) = F(1.35) + 0.05[D_1 f(1.05) + D_2 f(1.10) + \cdots + D_8 f(1.40)], \quad (1.1.8)$$

where

$$\begin{array}{ll} C_1 = 36799/120960 & D_1 = 1 - C_7 \\ C_2 = 176648/120960 & D_2 = C_7 - C_6 \\ C_3 = 54851/120960 & D_3 = C_6 - C_5 \\ C_4 = 177984/120960 & D_4 = C_5 - C_4 \\ C_5 = 89437/120960 & D_5 = C_4 - C_3 \\ C_6 = 130936/120960 & D_6 = C_3 - C_2 \\ C_7 = 119585/120960 & D_7 = C_2 - C_1 \\ & D_8 = C_1 \end{array}$$

Now the interval changes from 0.05 to 0.10. One may write

$$\begin{aligned} F(1.40) = {} & 0.10[C_1 f(0.00) + C_2 f(0.10) + \cdots + C_7 f(0.60) + f(0.70) \\ & + C_7 f(0.80) + C_6 f(0.90) + \cdots + C_1 f(1.40)], \end{aligned} \quad (1.1.9)$$

$$F(1.50) = F(1.40) + 0.10[D_1 f(0.80) + D_2 f(0.90) + \cdots + D_8 f(1.50)], \quad (1.1.10)$$

$$\vdots$$

$$F(4.00) = F(3.90) + 0.10[D_1 f(3.30) + D_2 f(3.40) + \cdots + D_8 f(4.00)]. \quad (1.1.11)$$

Of the two formulas for $F(1.40)$, Equation (1.1.8) has a smaller truncation error than Equation (1.1.9). Hence the value substituted for $F(1.40)$ in Equation (1.1.10) was that obtained from Equation (1.1.8) rather than that obtained from Equation (1.1.9). Similarly, one may write

$$\begin{aligned} F(4.00) = {} & 0.20[C_1 f(0.00) + C_2 f(0.20) + \cdots + C_7 f(1.20) + f(1.40) + f(1.60) + \cdots \\ & + f(2.60) + C_7 f(2.80) + C_6 f(3.00) + \cdots + C_1 f(4.00)], \end{aligned} \quad (1.1.12)$$

$$F(4.20) = F(4.00) + 0.20[D_1 f(2.80) + D_2 f(3.00) + \cdots + D_8 f(4.20)], \quad (1.1.13)$$

$$\vdots$$

$$F(7.00) = F(6.80) + 0.20[D_1 f(5.60) + D_2 f(5.80) + \cdots + D_8 f(7.00)]. \quad (1.1.14)$$

Of the two formulas for $F(4.00)$, Equation (1.1.11) has a smaller truncation error than Equation (1.1.12). Hence the value substituted for $F(4.00)$ in Equation (1.1.13) was that obtained from Equation (1.1.11) rather than that obtained from Equation (1.1.12). This process of chaining together 7-point integration formulas can be continued as far as required—in this example, as far as $F' = 700.00$. For each value of F' at which the interval changes, there are two formulas for $F(F')$, one based on a chain of 7-point formulas involving all the intervals up through the old one, and one based on a 7-point formula involving the new interval. The first of these two formulas is based on smaller intervals and hence has a smaller truncation error, so it was the one used to obtain the value of $F(F')$ to be substituted in the next formula.

The values of $F(F', n_1, n_2)$ for $n_2 = 2$ were replaced by somewhat more accurate ones obtained by subtabulation in the previously mentioned table given by Harter, Clemm, and Guthrie (1959), and those for $n_2 \geq 3$ were adjusted so as to make the maximum value 1 for each combination of n_1 and n_2 (the maximum adjustment was 10^{-5}). The adjusted results were stored on magnetic tape in binary form. They were also converted to decimal form (5 decimal places, accurate to within a unit in the last place), edited, punched on IBM cards, checked by differencing on the IBM 7090, and printed on the IBM 407 tabulator as shown in Table A1.

Percentage Points of the Ratio of Two Ranges

After computation of three auxiliary tables, as described earlier in this subsection, it was at last possible to proceed with the computation of a table of percentage points of the ratio of two ranges, which was the main purpose of the investigation.

It was decided that percentage points should be computed for $n_1 = 2(1)15$ and $n_2 = 2(1)15$, corresponding to cumulative probabilities $P = 0.5$, 0.75, 0.9, 0.95, 0.975, 0.99, 0.995, 0.999. It was hoped that the results would be accurate to within a unit in the fourth significant digit. This objective was achieved in all cases except those for which $n_2 = 3$ and $P = .999$; there the most that can be guaranteed is that the values are accurate to within 3 units in the fourth significant digit.

The input to this phase of the problem was the binary form of the table of $F(F', n_1, n_2)$ previously stored on magnetic tape. The method employed was inverse interpolation by Aitken's method on the IBM 7090 computer. Provision was made for carrying the computations up through ninth-degree interpolation if the tolerance of 5 units in the fifth significant digit had not been sooner met. In the case of percentage points whose value is less than 1, Equation (1.1.5) was utilized. For those whose value is greater than 700, which occurs only for $n_2 = 2$, $P = .999$, the percentage points were obtained by dividing by $\sqrt{2}$ the corresponding percentage points of the studentized range given by Harter, Clemm, and Guthrie (1959). [See Table B2.]

The results were converted to decimal form (4 significant digits, accurate to within a unit in the last digit, except as noted above), edited, punched on IBM cards, checked by differencing on the IBM 7090, and printed on the IBM 407 tabulator as shown in Table A2.

Power of the F' and F Tests

The principal use of the percentage points of the ratio F' of two ranges is as critical values of the F' test, which may be used as a substitute for the usual F test, based on sample variances, of the hypothesis that the variances (or the standard deviations) of the two populations are equal. Suppose one has samples of n_1 and n_2 observations, respectively, from populations Π_1 and Π_2, and that the sample ranges are w_1 and w_2, respectively, and the sample variances s_1^2 and s_2^2, respectively. Now, suppose that one wishes to test, at significance level α (also called the size of the test), the null hypothesis $H_0 : \sigma_1^2 = \sigma_2^2$, which may be written more simply as $H_0 : \sigma_1 = \sigma_2$. For this purpose one may use either a test based on the ratio of the sample ranges or one based on the ratio of the sample variances, with test statistics $F' = w_1/w_2$ and $F = s_1^2/s_2^2$, respectively. Critical values of these test statistics may be obtained from tables of the percentage points of F' and F, respectively. Tables of the percentage points of F have been widely used for many years, and are available in almost every textbook on statistics; one of the most extensive and most accurate tables is the one by Merrington and Thompson (1943). Tables of the percentage points of F' have been used very little and are available in only a few places, some of which were mentioned earlier; the most extensive and most accurate one is Table A2 of this volume. For one-sided tests (size α) of H_0 against alternatives specifying $\sigma_1 > \sigma_2$, the critical values of the test statistics F' and F are the percentage points of F' and F, respectively, corresponding to cumulative probability $P = 1 - \alpha$. For two-sided tests with equal tails, the critical values are those corresponding to $P = \alpha/2$ and $P = 1 - \alpha/2$.

It is known that when Π_1 and Π_2 are normally distributed the F test is a uniformly most powerful test of the hypothesis H_0. For small samples, however, the efficiency of the estimator of population variance based on the range is high (nearly 100%) relative to that of the most efficient estimator based on the sample variance. Therefore it is reasonable to believe that the power of the F' test, based on the ratio of two ranges, is almost as great for small samples as that of the F test, based on the ratio of two sample variances. In particular, for n_1 and n_2 both equal to 2, the tests are identical, and hence have the same power. In order to determine how much power is lost by using the F' test as a substitute for the F test, it was decided to compute the power of the two tests against the alternative hypothesis $H_1 : \sigma_1 = k\sigma_2$ for $k = 2(1)10$ and $\alpha = .5, .25, .1, .05, .025, .01, .005, .001$. This was done for equal sample sizes $n_1 = n_2 = 2(1)15$, and to show the maximum effect of unequal sample sizes, for $n_1 = 15$, $n_2 = 2$ and for $n_1 = 2$, $n_2 = 15$. Thus the power was computed for only 16 of 196 possible combinations of n_1 and n_2, but the results are sufficient to give a good comparison of the power of the two tests.

The power of the F' test against the alternative hypothesis $H_1 : \sigma_1 = k\sigma_2$ is the probability that, under the alternative hypothesis, the ratio $F' = w_1/w_2$ of the two ranges exceeds the critical value $F'_{1-\alpha}$, which is equal to the probability that, under the null hypothesis, F' exceeds $F'_{1-\alpha}/k$. Thus the power P' of F' against H_1 is given by

$$P'(n_1, n_2, k, \alpha) = 1 - F(F'_{1-\alpha}/k, n_1, n_2), \qquad (1.1.15)$$

where $F(F'_{1-\alpha}/k, n_1, n_2)$ can be found by interpolation in Table A1.

The power of the F test against the alternative hypothesis $H_1 : \sigma_1 = k\sigma_2$ is the probability that, under the alternative hypothesis, the ratio $F = s_1^2/s_2^2$ of the two sample variances exceeds the critical value $F_{1-\alpha}$, which is equal to the probability that, under the null hypothesis, F exceeds $F_{1-\alpha}/k^2$. Thus the power P of F against H_1 is given by

$$P(n_1, n_2, k, \alpha) = 1 - F(F_{1-\alpha}/k^2, \nu_1, \nu_2), \qquad (1.1.16)$$

where $F(F, \nu_1, \nu_2)$ is the cumulative distribution function of F for $\nu_1 = n_1 - 1$ and $\nu_2 = n_2 - 1$ degrees of freedom. Tables of this function are not available as such, but the required value can be expressed [see Pearson and Hartley (1954), p. 33] in the form

$$P(n_1, n_2, k, \alpha) = I_{x_0}(\nu_2/2, \nu_1/2), \qquad (1.1.17)$$

where $x_0 = \nu_2/(\nu_2 + \nu_1 F_{1-\alpha}/k^2)$ and $I_x(a, b)$ is the incomplete Beta-function ratio. Thus P can be found by interpolation in a table of the incomplete Beta-function ratio.

The input to this phase of the problem consisted of the binary form of the table of $F(F', n_1, n_2)$ previously stored on magnetic tape, values in decimal form of the incomplete

Beta-function ratio for $\nu_1 = \nu_2 = 1(1)14$; $\nu_1 = 14$, $\nu_2 = 1$; and $\nu_1 = 1$, $\nu_2 = 14$ from a table by Pearson (1934), and values in decimal form of the required percentage points of F' and F, the former from Table A2 of this volume and the latter mainly from a table by Merrington and Thompson (1943). The percentage points of F for $\nu_2 = 11, 13, 14$ had to be determined by harmonic interpolation in the Merrington-Thompson table and those for $\alpha = 0.001$ were taken from Pearson and Hartley (1954), Table 18. In cases in which the latter table gives only 3 significant figures, a fourth significant figure was found by interpolation in Pearson's table of the incomplete Beta-function ratio, using Equation (1.1.17) with $k = 1$.

The computations were performed on the IBM 7090 computer. The power P' of the F' test was found by the use of Equation (1.1.15), which required interpolation in the table of the cumulative distribution function of the ratio of two ranges. The power P of the F test was determined from Equation (1.1.17), which required interpolation in the table of the incomplete Beta-function ratio. In both cases the interpolation was performed by Aitken's method with tolerance of 5×10^{-5}. Provision was made for carrying the computations up through sixteenth-degree interpolation if the tolerance had not been sooner met. In some cases difficulty was encountered in interpolation in the table of the incomplete Beta-function ratio, in that the differences of the function at one end of the table (near $x = 0$ or near $x = 1$) behaved so badly that the tolerance could not be met, even with sixteenth-degree interpolation. This difficulty was overcome by squaring either the functional values or their differences from 1 before performing the interpolation.

The results were converted to decimal form (3 decimal places, accurate to within a unit in the last place), edited, punched on IBM cards, checked by differencing on the IBM 7090, and printed on the IBM 407 tabulator as shown in Table A3.

It can be seen from Table A3 that for n_1 and n_2 both equal to 2 the power of the two tests is the same (occasional differences of a unit in the third decimal place of the tabular values are due to rounding errors), but that as either or both of the sample sizes increase, the loss of power by using the F' test in place of the F test tends to increase, though of course values near 0.5 tend to differ more than those near 0 or 1. Differences in power tend to be greater for $n_2 > n_1$ than for $n_1 > n_2$.

1.1.3 Example of the Use of the Tables

The principal use of Table A1 is in the computation of subsequent tables. Undoubtedly other uses will be found now that the tables are available, but no examples of other uses will be given here.

The following example illustrates the use of Tables A2 and A3. Given samples, of 15 observations each, from populations Π_1, Π_2, Φ_1, and Φ_2, one wishes to test, at the 5 percent level of significance for each i $(i = 1, 2)$, the null hypothesis $H_{0i} : \sigma_{\Phi_i} = \sigma_{\Pi_i}$ against the alternative hypothesis $H_{1i} : \sigma_{\Phi_i} = 2\sigma_{\Pi_i}$. Suppose that the samples are as follows:

Sample from Π_1	Sample from Π_2	Sample from Φ_1	Sample from Φ_2
−0.323	−0.288	1.700	−0.540
−0.194	0.187	1.263	−2.816
0.697	0.785	2.299	0.418
3.521	0.194	1.322	1.345
0.321	−0.258	2.017	0.794
0.595	1.579	2.412	−2.111
0.769	1.090	2.224	−1.369
−0.136	0.448	5.177	0.607
−0.345	0.457	1.578	3.024
0.761	0.960	2.990	1.234
−1.229	−0.491	4.116	−1.936
−0.561	0.219	1.876	1.049
1.598	−0.169	1.790	1.869
−0.725	1.096	3.106	0.595
1.231	1.239	1.474	−1.574

The ranges of these samples are 4.750, 2.070, 3.914, and 4.893, respectively, and their variances are 1.345, 0.4569, 1.199, and 2.671, respectively. Thus, for testing H_{01} against H_{11}, one has $F' = 3.914/4.750 = 0.824$ and $F = 1.199/1.345 = 0.891$, which are less than the critical values $F'_{.95} = 1.673$ (from Table A2) and $F_{.95} = 2.483$, respectively, so one accepts H_{01}. For testing H_{02} against H_{12}, one has $F' = 4.893/2.070 = 2.364$ and $F = 2.671/0.4569 = 5.846$, which exceed the respective critical values, so one rejects H_{02} (accepts H_{12}). In all four cases, the conclusions are correct, since $\Pi_1 = \Pi_2 = N(\mu = 0, \sigma = 1)$, $\Phi_1 = N(\mu = 2, \sigma = 1)$, and $\Phi_2 = N(\mu = 0, \sigma = 2)$, the samples having been drawn at random from Rand Corporation tables reproduced by Dixon and Massey (1959), pp. 371, 452, and 457.

The dependence of the conclusions upon the particular samples drawn is realized if one consideres what would have happened if the samples designated as coming from Π_1 and Π_2 had been reversed, which could have occurred just as well as not, since Π_1 and Π_2 are actually the same population. The reader can easily verify that in this event all four conclusions would have been incorrect. If the impression gained from the original tests was slightly too optimistic, as it was, that gained from this reversal would be decidedly too pessimistic. The probability of an error of type I is $\alpha = 0.05$ and the probability of an error of type II is $\beta' = 1 - P' = 0.283$ for the F' test and $\beta = 1 - P = 0.192$ for the F test when $\alpha = 0.05$, $n_1 = n_2 = 15$ (see Table A3).

Referring again to Table A3, one notices that for every α and every k included in the table, one has (where $n' = n + c$ and $c = 0$, 1, 2, 3 for $n = 2$, 3-8, 9-10, 11-12 respectively)

$$P'(n', n', k, \alpha) \geq P(n, n, k, \alpha). \tag{1.1.18}$$

In cases in which the cost of each observation is low as compared with computing costs, it may well be cheaper to take a few more observations and use the F' test in place of the F test, since ranges are easier to compute than variances. Even for samples of the same size, the loss in power is not great if one uses the F' test in place of the F test, especially when the samples are small.

1.1.4 References

1. Buenaventura, A. R. (1959). On a Substitute F-ratio Using Ranges. Unpublished Master's thesis, University of the Philippines.
2. Dixon, Wilfrid J. and Massey, Frank J., Jr. (1951). *Introduction to Statistical Analysis.* McGraw-Hill Book Company, Inc., New York.

3. Dixon, Wilfrid J. and Massey, Frank J., Jr. (1959). *Introduction to Statistical Analysis*, Second edition. McGraw-Hill Book Company, Inc., New York.

4. Fettis, Henry E. (1955). Numerical calculation of certain definite integrals by Poisson's summation formula. *Mathematical Tables and Other Aids to Computation* **9**, 85-92.

5. Fettis, Henry E. (1958). Further remarks concerning the relative accuracy of Simpson's and the trapezoidal rule for a certain class of functions. *Zeitschrift für Angewandte Mathematik und Mechanik* **38**, 159-160.

6. Harter, H. Leon (1970a). *Order Statistics and their Use in Testing and Estimation*, Volume 1: *Tests Based on Range and Studentized Range of Samples from a Normal Population.* U.S. Government Printing Office, Washington.

7. Harter, H. Leon, Clemm, Donald S., and Guthrie, Eugene H. (1959). The Probability Integrals of the Range and of the Studentized Range: Probability Integral and Percentage Points of the Studentized Range; Critical Values for Duncan's New Multiple Range Test. WADC Technical Report 58-484, Volume II. Wright Air Development Center, Wright-Patterson Air Force Base, Ohio. [Reprinted, with minor changes, as Chapter 2, Section 2.1, and Tables B1-B3 of present volume.]

8. Kendall, Maurice G. (1948). *The Advanced Theory of Statistics*, Volume I. (Fourth Edition). Charles Griffin & Company Limited, London.

9. Link, Richard F. (1950). The sampling distribution of the ratio of two ranges from independent samples. *Annals of Mathematical Statistics* **21**, 112-116.

10. Link, Richard F. (1952). Correction to "The sampling distribution of the ratio of two ranges from independent samples." *Annals of Mathematical Statistics* **23**, 298-299.

11. Merrington, Maxine and Thompson, Catherine M. (1943). Table of percentage points of the inverted Beta (F) distribution. *Biometrika* **33**, 73-88.

12. Mosteller, Frederick (1946). On some useful "inefficient" statistics. *Annals of Mathematical Statistics* **17**, 377-408.

13. Pearson, E. S. and Hartley, H. O. (Eds.) (1954). *Biometrika Tables for Statisticians*, Volume 1. Cambridge University Press for the Biometrika Trustees, Cambridge, England.

14. Pearson, Karl (1934). *Tables of the Incomplete B-function.* Cambridge University Press for the Biometrika Trustees, Cambridge, England.

15. Pillai, K. C. S. (1951). Some notes on ordered samples from a normal population. *Sankhyā* **11**, 23-28.

16. Pillai, K. C. S. (1957). *Concise Tables for Statisticians.* The Statistical Center, University of the Philippines, Manila.

17. Pillai, K. C. Sreedharan and Buenaventura, Angeles R. (1961). Upper percentage points of a substitute F-ratio using ranges. *Biometrika* **48**, 195-196.

18. Rider, Paul R. (1951). The distribution of the quotient of ranges in samples from a rectangular population. *Journal of the American Statistical Association* **46**, 502-507.

19. WPA Mathematical Tables Project (1942). *Tables of Probability Functions*, Volume II. WPA New Reading Materials Project for the National Bureau of Standards, New York.

1.2 Probability Integral, Percentage Points, and Moments of the Range [2]

1.2.1 History and Introduction

Theory and Tables

One of the earliest writers to give serious consideration to the use of the sample range as a measure of dispersion was Tippett (1925). Tippett tabulated (to five decimal places) the mean range (in terms of the population standard deviation) of samples of size n taken from a normal population, for $n = 2(1)1000$. He also calculated a few values of the standard deviation σ_W and of $\beta_{1:W} = \alpha^2_{3:W}$ and $\beta_{2:W} = \alpha_{4:W}$, where $\alpha_{3:W}$ and $\alpha_{4:W}$ are the standard third and fourth moments. This work was extended by E. S. Pearson (1926), who computed somewhat more accurate values of β_1 and β_2 for $n = 60$ and 100. "Student" (1927) fitted Pearson curves to the first four theoretical moments of the range for several values of n. Using "Student's" results with modifications, E. S. Pearson (1932) computed lower and upper 0.5, 1, 5, and 10 percent points (to two decimal places) for $n = 2(1)30(5)100$. McKay and Pearson (1933) found the exact distribution of the range for samples of size 3 from a normal population, and gave certain new results regarding the form of the range curve at its terminals.

The probability integral of the range, $P(W, n)$, was first tabulated by Pearson and Hartley (1942) for $n = 2(1)20$, $W = 0.00(0.05)7.25$. Values were computed to five decimal places, but only four decimal places were published. Included in the same paper was a table of lower and upper 0.1, 0.5, 1, 2.5, 5, and 10 percent points for $n = 2(1)12$. The theoretical basis for these computations was outlined by Hartley (1942) in another paper. Grubbs and Weaver (1947) tabulated approximate values of $\mu'_{1:W}$, σ_W, $\alpha_{3:W}$, $\alpha_{4:W}$ and related moment constants for $n = 2(1)12$. Hartley and Pearson (1951) tabulated somewhat more accurate values of the moment constants: μ'_1, σ, μ_2, β_1, β_2, μ_3 and μ_4 for $n = 2(1)20$ and μ_5, μ_6, κ_4, κ_5 and κ_6 for $n = 2(1)12$, where μ'_1 is the mean, the unprimed μ's are the moments about the mean, and the κ's are the cumulants.

Applications

One of the earliest applications of the sample range was in statistical quality control. Shewhart (1931), the father of statistical quality control, considered and tentatively rejected the use of range as a measure of dispersion, but E. S. Pearson (1935) justified its use and tabulated factors for calculation of control limits for range. Due to the greater ease in calculating the range, it soon replaced the standard deviation in most applications of quality control. For further information, see Section 1.3.

E. S. Pearson (1932) showed that if the population standard deviation is to be estimated from the mean range of a number of subgroups, the optimum subgroup size is 8, but it remained for Grubbs and Weaver (1947) to make an extensive study of the use of this method. See Section 1.4 of Harter (1970b) or subsection 1.1.4 of Harter and Balakrishnan

[2] Reproduced, with minor changes, from WADC TR 58-484, Vol. I, The Probability Integrals of the Range and of the Studentized Range (subtitle as above; by H. Leon Harter, with coauthor Donald S. Clemm). Portions of this material were also published in the *Annals of Mathematical Statistics* **31** (1960), 1122-1147 and *Technometrics* **3** (1961), 407-411.

(1996).

The use of range in estimating all the variances involved in the analysis of variance was explored by Rodgers (1944), who credited W. J. Jennett with suggesting this procedure. Further work on the use of range in the analysis of variance was done by Patnaik (1950), Hartley (1950) and David (1951), but the use of range in the overall analysis (as contrasted with the use of studentized range in multiple comparison procedures) has never met with wide acceptance. See, however, Section 2.3 of Chapter 2.

Motivation for the Present Tables

The tables of the probability integral of the range published by Pearson and Hartley (1942) are sufficiently accurate for most direct applications. The basic motivation for the present tables was the desire for more accurate tables of the probability integral of the studentized range, which are needed to obtain more accurate critical values for various multiple comparison tests based on the range.

1.2.2 Method of Computation of the Tables

Probability Integral

The probability integral of the range W for samples of size n from $N(\mu, 1)$ may be written [see Pearson and Hartley (1954), p. 43] in the form

$$P(W,n) = n\int_0^\infty (2\pi)^{-1/2}e^{-X^2/2}\{[G(W,X)^{n-1} + [G(W,-X)]^{n-1}\}dX, \qquad (1.2.1)$$

where the auxiliary functions $G(W, X)$ and $G(W, -X)$ are defined by the equations

$$G(W,X) = P(W+X) - P(X)$$

and

$$G(W,-X) = P(W-X) + P(X),$$

in which

$$P(X) = \int_0^X f(t)dt,$$

where

$$f(t) = (2\pi)^{-1/2}e^{-t^2/2}.$$

The first step in the computation of the probability integral $P(W, n)$ at intervals of $2^{-6} = 1/64$ was the computation of $P(X)$ for $X = 0(2^{-6})7$ on the ERA 1103 (Univac Scientific) computer. The following values were taken from tables and read into the computer to be used as base points:

$$P(0), P(h); P(1), P(1+h); \ldots; P(6), P(6+h);$$

where $h = 2^{-6}$. The expression

$$P(X_0 + 2nh) = P(X_0) + \int_{X_0}^{X_0+2h} f(t)dt + \int_{X_0+2h}^{X_0+4h} f(t)dt + \cdots + \int_{X_0+2(n-1)h}^{X_0+2nh} f(t)dt$$

was computed for $n = 1(1)32$, where $P(X_0)$ is the value of the function at an appropriate base point. This was accomplished by evaluating the integrals in the above expression by a five-point formula of the form

$$\int_{a-h}^{a+h} f(t)dt = h\{b_0 f(a) + b_1[f(a-h) + f(a+h)] + b_2[f(a-2h) + f(a+2h)]\} + R$$

where $b_0 = 19/15$, $b_1 = 17/45$ and $b_2 = -1/90$. It can be shown that the remainder R is given by

$$R = \frac{20h^7 f^{(6)}(\xi)}{21 \cdot 6!}, \qquad a - 2h \le \xi \le a + 2h.$$

In the case under consideration, $h = 2^{-6}$ and $f^{(6)}(\xi) < 6$; hence $R < 1.81 \times 10^{-15}$. Since the integration was performed 32 times before changing to the next base point, the maximum error due to truncation was less than 6×10^{-14}, which is negligible in comparison with the rounding error, whose maximum value is $2^{-35} = 10^{-11}$, since results were rounded to 34 binary bits. The rounding errors were held to a minimum by multiplying by h just before the final rounding, after summing the values of the integrands. The values of $P(X)$ were stored on bioctal paper tape for later use.

The probability integral $P(W, n)$ was computed at intervals $2^{-6} = 1/64$ in W for $n = 2(1)20(2)40(10)100$ by reading the stored values of $P(X)$ into the machine and applying the seven-point Lagrangian integration formula (see [9], p. xxxiv) to Equation (1.2.1). Ten-decimal-place values (with uncertainty in the last two places) were punched on cards. These cards were then fed into the ERA 1103A computer and the tables was subtabulated at intervals of 0.01 in W by the use of Aitken's method of interpolation with a tolerance of 2^{-30}. The resulting tabular values were converted to decimal form and rounded to eight decimal places, with error not exceeding a unit in the last place, then punched on cards and printed on the IBM 407 tabulator. The results are shown in Table A4.

Percentage Points

The values of the range, for samples of size n from $N(\mu, 1)$, corresponding to certain cumulative probabilities P were computed by inverse interpolation, by use of Aitken's method with a tolerance of 5×10^{-7}, in the table of the probability integral of the range with interval 2^{-6}. Values of n were the same as those for which the probability integral was computed, that is, $n = 2(1)10(2)40(10)100$. The cumulative probabilities P involved were .0001, .0005, .001, .005, .01, .025, .05; .1(.1).9; .95, .975, .99, .995, .999, .9995 and .9999. The interpolation was performed on the ERA 1103A computer. In some cases it was necessary to divide each of three intervals in the relevant portion of the table into eight subintervals and subtabulate the probability integral in order to meet the tolerance on the inverse interpolation. This happened especially for small values of P and for values of n near 4. The resulting percentage points were converted to decimal form and rounded to six decimal places, modified as noted under "Sources of Tables," then punched on cards and printed on the IBM 407 tabulator. The results are given in Table A5.

Moments

The expected value of the kth power of the range W, for samples of size n from $N(\mu, 1)$, is given by the equation

$$E(W^k) = n(n-1)\int_{-\infty}^{\infty}\left\{\int_0^{\infty} W^k[\Phi(X+W)-\Phi(X)]^{n-2}\phi(X+W)dW\right\}\phi(X)dX, \tag{1.2.2}$$

with

$$\phi(X) = (2\pi)^{-1/2}e^{-X^2/2}; \quad \Phi(X) = \int_0^X \phi(X)dX.$$

For $n = 2$, the double integration on the right-hand side of Equation (1.2.2) can be performed in closed form, giving the results $E(W) = 2/\sqrt{\pi}$, $E(W^2) = 2$, $E(W^3) = 8/\sqrt{\pi}$, $E(W^4) = 12$, etc. For $n \geq 3$, it is necessary to resort to numerical integration; this was done for $n = 3(1)100$, $k = 1(1)4$, with double precision arithmetic on the ERA 1103A computer, by use of the seven-point Lagrangian integration formula for the inner integral and the trapezoidal rule for the outer integral (since the integrand tends strongly to zero at both limits). From the values of $E(W^k)$, values of the variance σ_W^2, the standard deviation σ_W, and the third and fourth moments about the mean, $\mu_{3:W}$ and $\mu_{4:W}$, were computed. From these in turn the standard third and fourth moments, $\alpha_{3:W}$ and $\alpha_{4:W}$, were computed. For $n = 3(1)15$, intervals $h = .05$ and $2h = .10$ were used for the numerical integration; for $n = 16(1)100$, intervals $h = .10$ and $2h = .20$ were used. Agreement between the results for h and $2h$ is such as to guarantee that results for $E(W)$ can be published to 10 decimal places (11 significant figures), for σ_W^2 to 10 decimal places (10 significant figures), for $\alpha_{3:W}$ to 8 decimal places (8 significant figures), and for $\alpha_{4:W}$ to 7 decimal places (8 significant figures). The error does not exceed a unit in the last place, except possibly in the case of σ_W^2 for $n = 5(1)11$, where the error may be as much as three units in the last place. Corrections were made in the mean and the variance for sample sizes up through 20 when necessary to make them agree with values computed from an unpublished 20-decimal-place version (ten decimal places were published) of tables of the expected values of order statistics and products of order statistics edited by Teichroew (1956). Hence, after correction, all values are accurate to within a unit in the last place. The results were printed on the IBM 407 tabulator, and are shown in Table A6.

1.2.3 Examples of the Use of the Tables

Computation of Probability Integral and Percentage Points of Studentized Range

As mentioned in subsection 1.2.1, the principal reason for the computation of the present tables, especially Table A4, was the desire for more accurate tables of the probability integral of the studentized range, whose percentage points are needed for multiple comparison tests. Appendix B of this volume includes extensive tables of the probability integral of the studentized range and of the percentage points of the studentized range (Tables B1 and B2).

Tests of Hypotheses Concerning the Standard Deviation of a Normal Population

Suppose one wishes to test the hypothesis $H_0 : \sigma = 1$ against the class of alternatives specifying $\sigma > 1$ for a sample of size n from a population which is known or assumed to be normal, using a test having Type I error rate α. If one takes $n = 10$ and $\alpha = .10$, one finds in Table A5 that the critical region for the test based on the sample range w is $w > 4.129$. Consider now the following two samples: Sample (1): −2.015, −0.623, −0.699, 0.481, −0.586, −0.579, −0.120, 0.191, 0.071, −3.001; Sample (2): −0.172, 0.655, 3.345, −1.677, 1.030, −0.912, −0.004, 0.560, −1.568, 0.303. The ranges of these two samples are respectively $w_1 = 3.482$ and $w_2 = 5.022$; hence one accepts H_0 for Sample (1) and rejects H_0 for Sample (2). The conclusion is correct in each case, since both samples were drawn from tables of random normal numbers given by Dixon and Massey (1951), pp. 295 and 355, Sample (1) from a table for $\mu = 0$, $\sigma = 1$ and Sample (2) from a table for $\mu = 0$, $\sigma = 2$. The test based on the range is less powerful than the test based on the sample variance s^2, which is performed by comparing the ratio ns^2/σ^2 with a critical value read from a table of percentage points of the χ^2 distribution. The range test is, however, much simpler to apply, and often one chooses the simpler of two tests rather than the more powerful one, especially when the difference in power is not great.

1.2.4 References

1. David, Herbert A. (1951). Further applications of range to the analysis of variance. *Biometrika* **38**, 393-407.

2. Dixon, Wilfrid J. and Massey, Frank J., Jr. (1951). *Introduction to Statistical Analysis.* McGraw-Hill Book Company, Inc., New York.

3. Grubbs, Frank E. and Weaver, Chalmers L. (1947). The best unbiased estimate of population standard deviation based on group ranges. *Journal of the American Statistical Association* **42**, 224-241.

4. Harter, H. Leon (1970b). *Order Statistics and their Use in Testing and Estimation,* Volume 2: *Estimates Based on Order Statistics of Samples from Various Populations.* U.S. Government Printing Office, Washington.

5. Harter, H. Leon and Balakrishnan, N. (1996). *CRC Handbook of Tables for the Use of Order Statistics in Estimation.* CRC Press, Boca Raton, Florida.

6. Hartley, H. O. (1942). The range in random samples. *Biometrika* **32**, 334-348.

7. Hartley, H. O. (1950). Use of range in analysis of variance. *Biometrika* **37**, 271-280.

8. Hartley, H. O. and Pearson, E. S. (1951). Moment constants for the distribution of the range in normal samples. *Biometrika* **38**, 463-464.

9. Mathematical Tables Project, National Bureau of Standards (1944). *Tables of Lagrangian Interpolation Coefficients.* Columbia University Press, New York.

10. McKay, A. T. and Pearson, E. S. (1933). A note on the distribution of range in samples of n. *Biometrika* **25**, 415-420.

11. Patnaik, P. B. (1950). The use of mean range in statistical tests. *Biometrika* **37**, 78-87.

12. Pearson, Egon S. (1926). A further note on the distribution of range in samples taken from a normal population. *Biometrika* **18**, 173-194.

13. Pearson, Egon S. (1932). The percentage limits for the distribution of range in samples from a normal population ($n \leq 100$). *Biometrika* **24**, 404-417.

14. Pearson, E. S. (1935). *The Application of Statistical Methods to Industrial Standardisation and Quality Control*, British Standards Institution No. 600, London.

15. Pearson, E. S. and Hartley, H. O. (1942). The probability integral of the range in samples of n observations from a normal population. *Biometrika* **32**, 301-310.

16. Pearson, E. S. and Hartley, H. O. (Eds.) (1954). *Biometrika Tables for Statisticians*, Volume 1. Cambridge University Press for the Biometrika Trustees, Cambridge, England.

17. Rodgers, J. W. (1944). Associated statistical techniques. *Symposium on Statistical Quality Control.* Ministry of Production, Birmingham, England.

18. Shewhart, W. A. (1931). *Economic Control of Quality of Manufactured Product.* D. Van Nostrand Company, Inc., New York.

19. "Student" (1927). Errors of routine analysis. *Biometrika* **19**, 151-164.

20. Teichroew, D. (Ed.) (1956). Tables of expected values of order statistics and products of order statistics for samples of size twenty and less from the normal distribution. *Annals of Mathematical Statistics* **27**, 410-426.

21. Tippett, L. H. C. (1925). On the extreme individuals and the range of samples taken from a normal population. *Biometrika* **17**, 364-387.

1.3 Applications to Control Charts

When dealing with quality characteristics that are measurable, it is a common practice to monitor the mean of the quality characteristic and its variability. Control over the average quality of the product is carried out usually by the $\overline{X}$ chart, a control chart for averages. Process variability is commonly controlled by an R chart, a range chart. As an alternative to it, a standard deviation chart is also used in practice.

Suppose the quality measurements were assumed to come from a Normal(μ, σ^2) population. If the parameters μ and σ were known, then in the usage of the $\overline{X}$ chart, we could use μ as the center line and

$$\text{LCL} = \mu - \frac{3\sigma}{\sqrt{n}} \quad \text{and} \quad \text{UCL} = \mu + \frac{3\sigma}{\sqrt{n}}$$

as the lower and upper 3σ control limits, respectively. If the parameters μ and σ were unknown, on the other hand, and if we have k preliminary samples each of size n, we could use

$$\overline{\overline{X}} = \frac{1}{k}\sum_{i=1}^{k} \overline{X}_i \quad \text{and} \quad \overline{w} = \frac{1}{k}\sum_{i=1}^{k} w_i$$

in the construction of the $\overline{X}$ chart. Here, $\overline{X}_i$ and w_i are the mean and range obtained from the ith sample for $i = 1, 2, \ldots, k$. While we may use $\overline{\overline{X}}$ as a pooled unbiased estimate of μ, we have to consider

$$\hat{\sigma} = \frac{1}{k}\sum_{i=1}^{k}(w_i/d_2) = \frac{\overline{w}}{d_2}$$

as a pooled unbiased estimate of σ, where d_2 is the expected value of the sample range in a sample of size n from the standard normal distribution; see Table A6 in this volume and also the tables in Harter and Balakrishnan (1996). By making use of these pooled unbiased estimates, in the implementation of the $\overline{X}$ chart in this case, we may place the center line at $\overline{\overline{X}}$ and use

$$\text{LCL} = \overline{\overline{X}} - A_2\overline{w} \quad \text{and} \quad \text{UCL} = \overline{\overline{X}} + A_2\overline{w},$$

where $A_2 = \frac{3}{d_2\sqrt{n}}$, as the lower and upper control limits, respectively. Values of the constant A_2 for various sample sizes are presented in Table A7.

The constant needed for the construction of the range chart can also be determined similarly. Of course, the center line of the R chart will be at $\overline{w}$. For the determination of the lower and upper control limits of this chart, we first write

$$w = W\,\sigma,$$

where W is the sample range in a sample of size n from the standard normal distribution. Then, the standard deviation of w can be written as

$$\sigma_w = \sigma_W\,\sigma,$$

where σ_W denotes the standard deviation of the sample range in a sample of size n from the standard normal distribution; see Table A6 in this volume and also the tables in Harter and Balakrishnan (1996). Since σ is unknown and may be estimated (as mentioned earlier) by

$$\hat{\sigma} = \frac{\overline{w}}{d_2},$$

we can estimate σ_w by

$$\hat{\sigma}_w = \sigma_W \, \frac{\overline{w}}{d_2}$$

using which we obtain the lower and upper control limits on the range chart as

$$\mathrm{LCL} = \overline{w} - \frac{3\,\sigma_W}{d_2}\,\overline{w} = D_3\,\overline{w}$$

and

$$\mathrm{UCL} = \overline{w} + \frac{3\,\sigma_W}{d_2}\,\overline{w} = D_4\,\overline{w},$$

respectively, where $D_3 = 1 - \frac{3\,\sigma_W}{d_2}$ and $D_4 = 1 + \frac{3\,\sigma_W}{d_2}$. Values of the constants D_3 and D_4 for various sample sizes are presented in Table A7. Note that for some values of n, D_3 may turn out to be negative in which case it may be taken to be 0 for obvious reasons.

1.3.1 Reference

1. Harter, H. Leon and Balakrishnan, N. (1996). *CRC Handbook of Tables for the Use of Order Statistics in Estimation.* CRC Press, Boca Raton, Florida.

1.4 Applications to Tests of Homogeneity in Multinomial and Multivariate Hypergeometric Distributions

Let $\boldsymbol{X} = (X_1, X_2, \ldots, X_k)'$ be a k-dimensional random variable having a Multinomial$(n; p_1, p_2, \ldots, p_k)$ distribution with probability mass function

$$\begin{aligned}
\Pr(\boldsymbol{X} = \boldsymbol{x}) &= \Pr\left(\bigcap_{i=1}^{k}(X_i = x_i)\right) \\
&= \frac{n!}{x_1!\,x_2!\,\cdots\,x_k!}\,p_1^{x_1}\,p_2^{x_2}\,\cdots\,p_k^{x_k} \\
&= n!\prod_{i=1}^{k}\left(p_i^{x_i}/x_i!\right), \qquad 0 \le x_i \le n, \quad \sum_{i=1}^{k} x_i = n, \\
&\qquad\qquad 0 \le p_i \le 1, \quad \sum_{i=1}^{k} p_i = 1.
\end{aligned}$$

For a detailed discussion on various issues concerning multinomial distributions, we refer the readers to Johnson, Kotz and Balakrishnan (1997). One of the problems that has received considerable attention over the years is the testing of the homogeneity hypothesis, viz., $H_0 : p_1 = p_2 = \cdots = p_k = \frac{1}{k}$. A test statistic that has been used for testing this hypothesis is based on the sample range and is given by

$$V = \frac{x_{(k)} - x_{(1)}}{n},$$

where $x_{(1)} \le x_{(2)} \le \cdots \le x_{(k)}$ are the order statistics obtained by arranging the k x_i's in increasing order of magnitude. Interested readers may refer to the papers by Johnson and Young (1960), Johnson (1960) and Young (1962). It is important to note here that

$$\begin{aligned}
E(X_i) &= np_i, \qquad i = 1, 2, \ldots, k, \\
\text{Var}(X_i) &= np_i(1 - p_i), \qquad i = 1, 2, \ldots, k,
\end{aligned}$$

and

$$\text{Cov}(X_i, X_j) = -np_ip_j, \qquad 1 \le i, j \le k \text{ and } i \ne j.$$

Next, let us consider the case when $\boldsymbol{X} = (X_1, X_2, \ldots, X_k)'$ has a multivariate hypergeometric $(n; N_1, N_2, \ldots, N_k)$ distribution with probability mass function

$$\begin{aligned}
\Pr(\boldsymbol{X} = \boldsymbol{x}) &= \Pr\left(\bigcap_{i=1}^{k}(X_i = x_i)\right) \\
&= \frac{\binom{N_1}{x_1}\binom{N_2}{x_2}\cdots\binom{N_k}{x_k}}{\binom{kN}{n}} \\
&= \frac{1}{\binom{kN}{n}}\prod_{i=1}^{k}\binom{N_i}{x_i}, \\
&\qquad 0 \le x_i \le N_i, \quad \sum_{i=1}^{k} x_i = n, \quad \sum_{i=1}^{k} N_i = kN.
\end{aligned}$$

For a detailed discussion on various properties and applications of multivariate hypergeometric distributions, one may refer to Johnson, Kotz and Balakrishnan (1997). Once again, if one is interested in testing for the homogeneity, viz., $H_0 : N_1 = N_2 = \cdots = N_k = N$, one could use the test statistic based on the sample range given by

$$V = \frac{x_{(k)} - x_{(1)}}{n} ,$$

where $x_{(1)} \le x_{(2)} \le \cdots \le x_{(k)}$ are the order statistics obtained by arranging the k x_i's in increasing order of magnitude; see, for example, Childs and Balakrishnan (1997). Note in this case that

$$E(X_i) = \frac{nN_i}{kN} , \quad i = 1, 2, \ldots, k,$$

$$\text{Var}(X_i) = \frac{nN_i}{kN} \left(1 - \frac{N_i}{kN}\right) \left(\frac{kN - n}{kN - 1}\right), \quad i = 1, 2, \ldots, k,$$

and

$$\text{Cov}(X_i, X_j) = -\frac{nN_iN_j}{(kN)^2} \frac{kN - n}{kN - 1} , \quad 1 \le i, j \le k \text{ and } i \ne j.$$

It may be noted here that, as $N_i \to \infty$, $N \to \infty$ and $\frac{N_i}{kN} \to p_i$ for $i = 1, 2, \ldots, k$, the above formulae reduce to the corresponding formulae of the multinomial distribution presented earlier.

A normal approximation to the distribution of $\boldsymbol{X}$ may be obtained by considering the standardized multivariate hypergeometric random variable $\boldsymbol{U} = (U_1, U_2, \ldots, U_k)'$, where

$$U_i = \frac{X_i - \frac{nN_i}{kN}}{\sqrt{\frac{nN_i}{kN}\left(1 - \frac{N_i}{kN}\right)\left(\frac{kN-n}{kN-1}\right)}} , \quad i = 1, 2, \ldots, k,$$

with

$$\text{Cov}(U_i, U_j) = -\frac{1}{kN} \sqrt{\frac{N_iN_j}{\left(1 - \frac{N_i}{kN}\right)\left(1 - \frac{N_j}{kN}\right)}} , \quad i \ne j.$$

Under the null hypothesis of homogeneity, viz., $H_0 : N_1 = N_2 = \cdots = N_k = N$, note that

$$\text{Cov}(U_i, U_j) = -\frac{1}{k - 1} , \quad i \ne j.$$

It is well-known that if $Z_1, Z_2, \ldots, Z_k$ are k i.i.d. standard normal variables, then

$$\sqrt{\frac{k}{k - 1}}\,(Z_1 - \overline{Z}),\ \sqrt{\frac{k}{k - 1}}\,(Z_2 - \overline{Z}), \ldots,\ \sqrt{\frac{k}{k - 1}}\,(Z_k - \overline{Z}),$$

where $\overline{Z} = \frac{1}{k}\sum_{i=1}^{k} Z_i$, follow a multivariate normal distribution with all means as 0, all variances as 1, and all covariances as $-\frac{1}{k-1}$. This, incidentally, suggests that, under the null hypothesis $H_0 : N_1 = N_2 = \cdots = N_k = N$, the distribution of $\boldsymbol{U}$ may be approximated by means of the k variables defined above in terms of the k i.i.d. standard normal variables $Z_1, Z_2, \ldots, Z_k$. Using this approximation, we have

$$V = \frac{x_{(k)} - x_{(1)}}{n} \approx \sqrt{\frac{1}{nk}\left(\frac{kN - n}{kN - 1}\right)}\,(Z_{(k)} - Z_{(1)})$$

under the null hypothesis. Therefore, under the null hypothesis, upper percentage points of the test statistic V can be approximated by using the upper percentage points of the sample range of k i.i.d. standard normal variables tabulated in Table A5.

By making use of this approximation, Childs and Balakrishnan (1997) determined approximations to the upper 5% and 1% critical values of V for $k = 2(1)6$, $n = 25(25)100$, and values of kN as close as possible to $\frac{4}{3}n$, $2n$, $4n$, $20n$ and ∞. These values are reported in Tables A8 and A9. The values corresponding to the case $kN = \infty$ are precisely those for the multinomial distribution given by Johnson and Young (1960). The exact significance levels corresponding to the approximate critical values were also computed, wherever possible. These exact significance levels are presented within brackets below the critical values. Since the exact significance levels do not correspond exactly to the nominal significance level, the exact significance levels for the next possible value of V which could possibly give a significance level that is closer to the nominal one are also presented within brackets below the exact significance levels.

From Tables A8 and A9, just as Childs and Balakrishnan (1997) observed, we see that this approximation gives very close results for almost all the choices of k, n and N. In almost all cases considered, the approximate critical values give procedures with significance levels that are as close as possible to the nominal significance levels.

1.4.1 References

1. Childs, Aaron and Balakrishnan, N. (1997). Some approximations to the multivariate hypergeometric distribution with applications to hypothesis testing. *Submitted for publication.*
2. Johnson, Norman L. (1960). An approximation to the multinomial distribution: some properties and applications. *Biometrika* **47**, 93-102.
3. Johnson, Norman L., Kotz, Samuel and Balakrishnan, N. (1997). *Discrete Multivariate Distributions.* John Wiley & Sons, New York.
4. Johnson, Norman L. and Young, D. H. (1960). Some applications of two approximations to the multinomial distribution. *Biometrika* **47**, 463-469.
5. Young, D. H. (1962). Two alternatives to the standard χ^2 test of the hypothesis of equal cell frequencies. *Biometrika* **49**, 107-116.

2

The Studentized Range of Samples From a Normal Population

2.1 Probability Integral and Percentage Points of the Range; Critical Values for Duncan's Multiple Range Test [1]

2.1.1 History and Introduction

Theory and Tables

The idea of using the ratio of the range w to an independent estimate s of the population standard deviation (studentized range) was first proposed by "Student" in a letter written to and later published by E. S. Pearson (1939). Newman (1939) developed this notion further, and tabulated a number of 5 percent and 1 percent points of $Q = w/s$, which he obtained by quadrature from the approximate probability law of $W = w/\sigma$ given by E. S. Pearson (1932), except for $n = 3$, where the exact distribution of W obtained by McKay and Pearson (1933) was used. Pearson and Hartley (1943) tabulated the probability integral of the studentized range, which they wrote in the form

$$_{\nu}P_n(Q) = P_n(Q) + \nu^{-1}a_n(Q) + \nu^{-2}b_n(Q), \tag{2.1.1}$$

where ν is the number of degrees of freedom for the independent estimate s of the population standard deviation and $P_n(Q)$ is the probability integral of the range. The tables gave values (to four, two, and one decimal places, respectively) of $P_n(Q)$, $a_n(Q)$, and $b_n(Q)$ for $Q = 0.00(0.25)6.50$ and $n = 3(1)20$, with the observation that the results were somewhat inaccurate for small values of ν (< 10) and for large values of Q (> 6). Lower and upper 5 and 1 percent points were given for $n = 2(1)20$, $\nu = 10(1)20$, 24, 30, 40, 60, 120 and ∞, the results for $n = 2$ being obtained by multiplying by $\sqrt{2}$ the corresponding percentage points of the Student t distribution. Upper 5 percent and 1 percent points for $n = 3(1)20$ and $\nu = 10(1)19$ were tabulated to only one decimal place, with two decimal places for the other tabular values. May (1952) published extended and corrected tables of the upper percentage points. Values were given to two decimal places down through $\nu = 2$ and to one decimal place for $\nu = 1$. Values were based on exact quadrature for

[1] Reproduced, with minor changes, from WADC TR 58–484, Vol. II, The Probability Integrals of the Range and of the Studentized Range (subtitle as above; by H. Leon Harter, with coauthors Donald S. Clemm and Eugene H. Guthrie). Portions of this material were also published in the *Annals of Mathematical Statistics* **31** (1960), 1122-1147, *Biometrics* **16** (1960), 671-685, and *Technometrics* **3** (1961), 407-411.

$\nu = 1(1)4$, 6, 8, 12 and 24 and for 6 to 8 equidistant values of $1/Q$, with other values obtained by Lagrangian and/or harmonic interpolation. Hartley (1953) published further corrections for $\nu = 5$ and $\nu = 7$.

Applications

Newman (1939), following a suggestion by "Student", proposed a systematic method of applying the studentized range to multiple comparisons of treatment means in an experiment, but it was a number of years before any further work on this subject was published. One of the notable occurrences of the early 1950's, however, was the development of a number of multiple comparison procedures, several of which are based on the studentized range. Among these are the Newman-Keuls test [a modification by Keuls (1952) of the test first proposed by Newman (1939)], two tests proposed by Tukey (1952, 1953), and the multiple range test proposed by Duncan (1955). Harter (1957a) made a study of the relation between error rates and sample sizes for a number of multiple comparison tests based on the studentized range.

Motivation for the Present Tables

The tables of the probability integral of the studentized range published by Pearson and Hartley (1943) are inaccurate not only for $\nu < 10$ as stated by them, but also for values of ν up to about 20, and the inaccuracy for high values of Q is much greater than was anticipated. Any effect these inaccuracies had on upper 5 percent and 1 percent points was corrected by May (1952) when she recomputed these upper percentage points by quadrature. The inaccuracies in the Pearson-Hartley tables did cause difficulty, however, in the computation by Beyer (1953) of the critical values for Duncan's multiple range test. Beyer was aware of the difficulty for $\nu < 10$ and attempted to correct it by adding a term of the form $\nu^{-3}c_n(Q)$ to the right-hand side of Equation (2.1.1). This alleviated the difficulty to some extent, but did not remove it, and nothing at all was done to correct the inaccuracies for $\nu \geq 10$. Having first become aware of this situation during the course of his investigation of error rates and sample sizes, in which it became evident that certain tables based upon published critical values for Duncan's test did not have smooth differences, Harter (1957b) reported it in a paper presented to the American Statistical Association. Included in that paper was an outline of plans for computation of the present tables. Also included was a two-decimal-place table of critical values for Duncan's test, computed by inverse interpolation in a fragmentary table of the probability integral of the studentized range obtained by numerical integration. This table of critical values, though known to be much more accurate than published tables, was deliberately withheld from publication in anticipation of the completion of the present tables, which required much longer than expected. To summarize, then, the basic motivation for the computation of the present tables was the desire for more accurate critical values for various multiple comparison tests based on the range, especially Duncan's multiple range test. Attainment of this objective required the computation of the more accurate table of the probability integral of the studentized range included in this volume (Table B1), which in turn required the computation of the more accurate table of the probability integral of the range included in this volume (Table A4).

2.1.2 Method of Computation of the Tables

Probability Integral of the Studentized Range

The probability integral of the studentized range Q for samples of size n from a normal population, with ν degrees of freedom for the independent estimate s of the population standard deviation, may be written [see Pearson and Hartley (1943), p. 51] in the form

$$P(Q,\nu,n) = \int_0^\infty [\Gamma(\nu/2)]^{-1}\, 2^{1-\nu/2}\, \nu^{\nu/2}\, s^{\nu-1}\, e^{-\nu s^2/2}\, P(Qs,n)ds$$

$$= C(\nu)\int_0^\infty s^{\nu-1}\, e^{(\nu/2)(1-s^2)} P(Qs,n)ds,$$

where $P(Qs,n)$ is the probability integral of the range $W = Qs$ for samples of size n from a normal population, which has been tabulated in Table A4, and where

$$C(\nu) = \frac{2(\nu/2)^{\nu/2}e^{-\nu/2}}{\Gamma(\nu/2)} .$$

Replacing s by W/Q and hence ds by dW/Q, and letting $Q = z/5$, one obtains

$$P(z,\nu,n) = \frac{5}{z}\, C(\nu)\int_0^\infty \left(\frac{5W}{z}\right)^{\nu-1} e^{(\nu/2)(1-25W^2/z^2)} P(W,n)dW$$

$$= \frac{5}{z}\, C(\nu)[P_1 + P_2],$$

where

$$P_1 = \int_0^{11} \left(\frac{5W}{z}\right)^{\nu-1} e^{(\nu/2)(1-25W^2/z^2)} P(W,n)dW$$

and

$$P_2 = \int_{11}^\infty \left(\frac{5W}{z}\right)^{\nu-1} e^{(\nu/2)(1-25W^2/z^2)} dW,$$

since $P(W,n) = 1$ for all values of n when $W \geq 11$.

A little algebraic manipulation enables one to write P_1 in the form actually used for computation, which is

$$P_1 = \int_0^{11} \left[\left(\frac{5W}{z}\right) e^{(z^2-25W^2)/2z^2}\right]^{\nu-1} e^{(z^2-25W^2)/2z^2} P(W,n)dW.$$

To put P_2 in the form used for computation, one lets $x = 5W/z$, so that $dW = z\,dx/5$, and one obtains

$$P_2 = \frac{z}{5}\int_{55/z}^\infty x^{\nu-1}e^{(\nu/2)(1-x^2)}dx$$

$$= \frac{z}{5}\int_{55/z}^\infty [x\, e^{(1-x^2)/2}]^{\nu-1}e^{(1-x^2)/2}dx$$

$$= \frac{z}{5}\sum_{i=1}^{j}\int_{55/z_i}^{55/(z_i-1)} [x\, e^{(1-x^2)/2}]^{\nu-1}e^{(1-x^2)/2}dx,$$

where the z_i are the values of z for which $P(z,\nu,n)$ is to be tabulated (starting with $z_0 = 0$) and j is the value such that $z_j = z$. If one lets

$$x = \frac{55}{z_i} + t\,\frac{55(z_i - z_{i-1})}{z_i z_{i-1}} ,$$

so that

$$dx = \frac{55(z_i - z_{i-1})}{z_i z_{i-1}}\, dt,$$

one obtains

$$P_2 = \frac{z}{5}\sum_{i=1}^{j} \frac{55(z_i - z_{i-1})}{z_i z_{i-1}} \int_0^1 [x\, e^{(1-x^2)/2}]^{\nu-1} e^{(1-x^2)/2} dt,$$

with x defined as above. It can be shown that for $z < 8$, $P_2 = 0$ to the accuracy carried in the computations. Seven-point Lagrangian numerical integration was used for both P_1 and P_2, with intervals $h(W) = 2^{-6}$ and $h(t) = 2^{-5}$, respectively.

For $n = 2(1)20(2)38$ and $\nu = 1(1)19$, values of the probability integral were computed for

$$z = 0(1)30(2)50(5)100(10)200(25)900(50)2000(100)5000(500)10000,$$

that is for

$$Q = 0(0.2)6(0.4)10(1)20(2)40(5)180(10)400(20)1000(100)2000.$$

Whenever $n = 40(10)100$ and/or $\nu = 20$, 24, 30, 40, 60, or 120, values were computed for $z = 0(0.5)30$, that is for $Q = 0(0.1)6$, with no change in the interval for $z > 30$ ($Q > 6$). In order to make accurate inverse interpolation possible, it was found necessary to compute the probability integral at a smaller interval for $Q < 1$ when $\nu \leq 19$ and n is small. For $\nu = 1$ and $n = 2(1)20(2)24$ and for $2 \leq \nu \leq 19$ and $n = 2(1)15$, values were computed for $Q = 0(0.1)1$. The results were computed to ten decimal places, but since in some sections of the table one can guarantee accuracy only to within a unit in the sixth place, the values have been rounded to six decimal places (five decimal places for values of the probability greater than 0.999995, which are given as 1.00000). The results are shown in Table B1.

For $\nu \geq 3$, $P(Q, \nu, n) = 1.00000$ for $Q \geq 2000$, for all values of n included in the table. For $\nu = 1$ and $\nu = 2$, values of $P(Q, \nu, n)$ for $Q > 2000$ can be obtained by letting $Q_0 = 2000$ in the approximate formula

$$P(Q, \nu, n) \approx 1 - (Q_0/Q)^{\nu}[1 - P(Q_0, \nu, n)]. \tag{2.1.2}$$

It can be shown that the error involved in this approximation is small enough to cause no difficulty for Q_0 sufficiently large ($Q_0 \geq 2000$).

For a few cases involving high values of ν (≥ 12) and low values of n (≤ 4), the agreement between the results of the numerical integration for $h(W) = 2^{-6}$ and $2h(W) = 2^{-5}$ was not sufficiently close to guarantee that the error in $P(Q, \nu, n)$ would not exceed a unit in the sixth decimal place. This difficulty was overcome by substituting a polynomial approximation for $P(W, n)$ and integrating in closed form, the resulting approximation for $P(Q, \nu, n)$ being

$$P(Q, \nu, n) \approx (2/\nu)^{(n-1)/2} Q^{n-1} \sum_{j=0}^{7} b_j Q^j (2/\nu)^{j/2}\, \frac{\Gamma[(\nu + j + n - 1)/2]}{\Gamma(\nu/2)},$$

where b_j is the coefficient of W^{j+n-1} in the polynomial of degree $(n + 6)$ fitted by the method of least squares to the tabular values of $P(W, n)$, which is given by the equation

$$P(W, n) \approx \sum_{j=0}^{7} b_j W^{j+n-1}.$$

Percentage Points of the Studentized Range

The values of the studentized range corresponding to certain cumulative probabilities P were computed, for samples of size n from a normal distribution with ν degrees of freedom for the independent estimate s of the population standard deviation, by inverse interpolation in the table of the probability integral of the studentized range, and the results, rounded to four decimal places or four significant figures, whichever is less accurate, are shown in Table B2. The values of n and ν are the same as those for which the probability integral was computed. Values for $\nu = \infty$, obtained by rounding values from the table of percentage points of the range in this volume (Table A5), are included for convenience in interpolation (linear harmonic ν-wise interpolation is recommended). The cumulative probabilities P involved are 0.001, 0.005, 0.01, 0.025, 0.05; 0.1(0.1)0.9; 0.95, 0.975, 0.99, 0.995 and 0.999. The interpolation necessary to obtain the values in Table B2 was performed on the ERA 1103A computer, by use of an iterative procedure involving the following steps:

1. In the table of the probability integral of the studentized range for the desired values of n and ν, find the two successive probabilities, y_0 and y_1, between which the required cumulative probability P lies. Call the two corresponding arguments (studentized ranges) x_0 and x_1.
2. Compute the tolerance T for P corresponding to a tolerance $5 \times 10^{u-5}$ for Q by means of the equation $T = (\Delta P/\Delta Q) \times 5 \times 10^{u-5}$, where $\Delta P = y_1 - y_0$, $\Delta Q = x_1 - x_0$, and u is the number of digits before the decimal point in numbers between x_0 and x_1.
3. Perform linear inverse interpolation to find an approximation x to the required Q, using the relation
$$x = \frac{(x_1 - x_0)(P - y_0)}{y_1 - y_0} + x_0.$$
4. Perform direct interpolation, using Aitken's method with a tolerance of 5×10^{-7} and with provision for up to 16-point interpolation if the tolerance is not met for fewer points, to find the cumulative probability y corresponding to the value x of the studentized range.
5. Compare the result y of step (**4**) with the required cumulative probability P, using the tolerance T computed in step (**2**):
   (**a**) If $|y - P| \leq T$, stop and set $Q = x$.
   (**b**) If $(y - P) > T$, replace y_1 by y and x_1 by x, then repeat the procedure, starting with step (**3**).
   (**c**) If $(y - P) < -T$, replace y_0 by y and x_0 by x, then repeat the procedure, starting with step (**3**).

The table of the probability integral of the studentized range, Table B1, is accurate to within a unit in the sixth decimal place (except for $P > 0.999995$), and the interval is small enough to make accurate interpolation possible. The tolerance for the direct interpolation was set at 5×10^{-7}, so that the interpolation error would not add appreciably to the error already present, and hence the interpolated values are substantially as accurate as the values in the input table. Inverse interpolation is, of course, not as accurate as direct interpolation, the error being $\Delta Q/\Delta P$ times as great for inverse interpolation as for direct interpolation. Thus the tolerance for P was found by multiplying the tolerance for $Q(5 \times 10^{u-5})$ by $1/(\Delta Q/\Delta P) = \Delta P/\Delta Q$. Since u is defined as the number of digits before the decimal point in the studentized range interval under consideration, this would guarantee that the error in Q would not exceed 5 units in the fifth significant digit for $Q \geq 0.1$, or in the fifth decimal place for $Q < 1$, if the ratio of the change in P to the change in Q were constant throughout the interval under consideration. This condition (P piecewise linear in Q) is obviously not satisfied in practice, but as long as the weaker condition

$$\max[\Delta P_0/\Delta Q_0,\ \Delta P_1/\Delta Q_1] \leq 2\Delta P/\Delta Q, \tag{2.1.3}$$

where $\Delta P_i = |y - y_i|$ and $\Delta Q_i = |x - x_i|$, $(i = 0, 1)$, is satisfied, the error in Q will not exceed a unit in the fourth significant digit for $Q \geq 0.1$, or in the fourth decimal place for $Q < 1$. The condition (2.1.3) is in fact satisfied, and hence it can be stated that the error in the percentage points given in Table B2 does not exceed a unit in the last place.

For $\nu = 1$ and $n \geq 6$, the value of Q corresponding to cumulative probability $P = 0.999$ exceeds 2000. Since Table B1 extends only to $Q = 2000$, those percentage points which exceed 2000 cannot be found by interpolation. They can be found very easily however, by letting $Q_0 = 2000$ in Equation (2.1.2) and solving for Q.

Critical Values for Duncan's Multiple Range Test

For Duncan's multiple range test applied to p successive values out of an ordered arrangement of m means of samples of size k, where $p = 2, 3, \ldots, m$, the protection level for nominal significance level α is defined to be $P = \gamma_{p,\alpha} = (1-\alpha)^{p-1}$. Hence the critical values for Duncan's test are percentage points of the studentized range of $n = p$ observations corresponding to cumulative probability $P = (1-\alpha)^{p-1}$, and they were obtained in much the same manner as other percentage points. The value of Q found to correspond to cumulative probability $P = (1-\alpha)^{p-1}$, by use of the iterative inverse interpolation procedure of the previous section, was designated by $R(p, \nu, \gamma_{p,\alpha})$. Once $R(p, \nu, \gamma_{p,\alpha})$ had been found, the critical value $Q(p, \nu, \alpha)$ for Duncan's test was determined as follows:

$$Q(p, \nu, \alpha) = R(p, \nu, \gamma_{p,\alpha}) \text{ for } p = 2$$

and

$$Q(p, \nu, \alpha) = \max[R(p, \nu, \gamma_{p,\alpha}), Q(p-1, \nu, \alpha)] \text{ for } p > 2.$$

The results are shown in Table B3.

For $\nu = \infty$, the critical values for Duncan's test were obtained by inverse interpolation in the table of the probability integral of the range, which is given in this volume (Table A4). These values are included for convenience in interpolation; as before, linear harmonic ν-wise interpolation is recommended.

Lund and Lund Algorithm

Lund and Lund (1983) developed an algorithm designed to approximate, to three-decimal-place accuracy, cumulative probabilities for the studentized range and to determine from them values for upper quantiles of the studentized range. The algorithm can be incorporated into computer programs producing simultaneous confidence intervals, making multiple comparisons and calculating achieved significance levels for sample ranges. Generating required tabular values in the computer as needed avoids the necessity for providing extensive tables as input, albeit with some loss of accuracy. Lund and Lund (1985) gave corrections to their 1983 algorithm. Royston (1987) pointed out that the Lund and Lund algorithm can, under certain circumstances, produce a "divide by zero" error, and gave a method of circumventing this error.

2.1.3 Examples of the Use of the Tables

Computation of Percentage Points of Studentized Range and Critical Values for Duncan's Multiple Range Test

As mentioned in subsection 2.1.1, the principal reason for the computation of Table B1 was the desire for more accurate percentage points of the studentized range and critical values for Duncan's multiple range test. Table B1 has already been used for this purpose, as described in subsection 2.1.2, and the results are given in Tables B2 and B3. The reader may find other uses for Table B1 but no others will be given here.

Multiple Comparison Tests on Means of Samples From a Normal Population

Suppose one has performed an analysis of variance and has found that the means of m groups, each of size k, differ significantly overall. Let s^2 be the within-groups variance, based upon $\nu = m(k-1)$ degrees of freedom. Now one wishes to know which group means differ significantly from each other. Various tests have been proposed, of which two are the Newman-Keuls test and Duncan's multiple range test. If either of these is to be used, one computes the standard error of the mean, $s_{\bar{x}} = \sqrt{s^2/k}$. He also arranges the group means in order from the smallest, $\bar{x}_1$, to the largest, $\bar{x}_m$, and determines their range, $\bar{x}_m - \bar{x}_1$. He then compares the range with the critical range obtained by multiplying $s_{\bar{x}}$ by the significant studentized range (critical value) for sample size m and degrees of freedom ν for the test under consideration. If the range exceeds the critical range, he next compares $\bar{x}_m - \bar{x}_2$ and $\bar{x}_{m-1} - \bar{x}_1$ with the critical range obtained by multiplying $s_{\bar{x}}$ by the significant studentized range for sample size $(m-1)$ and degrees of freedom ν for the test under consideration, and so on until no further significant ranges are found. Whenever the range of any group is found to be non-significant, one concludes that the entire group has come from a homogeneous source, and no test is made on the range of any subgroup of that group.

Now consider the analysis of data obtained from an experiment performed in the Aero Medical Laboratory of Wright Air Development Center to test the effect of diet on total water intake (grams) of laboratory rats during a 4-day period. Five diets were studied: no food and 8 calories per rat per day of each of four foods. One hundred rats were divided randomly into five groups of 20 rats each, one group on each diet, and the total water intake in grams of each rat for a 4-day period was determined. An analysis of variance applied to the data gave the following results:

Source of Variation	d.f.	S.S.	M.S.	F
Among diets	4	34761	8690	5.69 **
Within diets (error)	95	144926	1526	
Total	99	179687		

** Significant at the 1% level.

The mean water intake for the various diets was as follows:

Glucose	No Food	Olive Oil	Lab Chow	Casein
80.25	99.95	107.35	121.50	134.90

Having found that the overall effect of diets is significant, the experimenter next wanted to know which diet means differ significantly from each other. The question can be answered by the use of one of the multiple comparison procedures, several of which are based on the studentized range. The first step is the computation of the standard error of the mean, $s_{\bar{x}} = \sqrt{1526/20} = \sqrt{76.30} = 8.735$. Next one multiplies $s_{\bar{x}}$ by the significant studentized range (critical value), for p means ($p = 5, 4, 3, 2$) with 95 degrees of freedom for s^2, for the test under consideration. The significant studentized ranges for the Newman-Keuls test can be read from Table B2 and those for Duncan's multiple range test from Table B3, for various levels of significance α, corresponding to cumulative probability P, where $P = 1 - \alpha$ for the Newman-Keuls test and $P = (1-\alpha)^{p-1}$ for Duncan's test. For purpose of illustration, consider 5 percent and 1 percent level tests ($\alpha = .05$ and $.01$). Since there are no values in the tables for $\nu = 95$, it is necessary to apply linear harmonic interpolation between the tabular values for $\nu = 60$ and $\nu = 120$. Since $1/95$ is 0.7369 of the way from $1/60$ to $1/120$, the values for $\nu = 95$ are 0.7369 of the way from those for $\nu = 60$ to those for $\nu = 120$. As the result of linear harmonic interpolation, one finds the following values for the significant studentized range of p means at significance level α with 95 degrees of freedom for s^2:

	Newman-Keuls test		Duncan's test	
p	$\alpha = .05$	$\alpha = .01$	$\alpha = .05$	$\alpha = .01$
5	3.933	4.738	3.123	4.062
4	3.699	4.523	3.052	3.982
3	3.367	4.222	2.955	3.875
2	2.808	3.718	2.808	3.718

By multiplying each of the above significant studentized ranges by the standard error of the mean, $s_{\bar{x}} = 8.735$, one finds the following values for the significant range of p means at significance level α with 95 degrees of freedom for s^2:

	Newman-Keuls test		Duncan's test	
p	$\alpha = .05$	$\alpha = .01$	$\alpha = .05$	$\alpha = .01$
5	34.35	41.39	27.28	35.48
4	32.31	39.51	26.66	34.78
3	29.41	36.88	25.81	33.85
2	24.53	32.48	24.53	32.48

The results of the test are as follows, where any two means not underscored by the same line differ significantly at the indicated level:

Test	Significance Level *(percent)*	Glucose	No Food	Olive Oil	Lab Chow	Casein
Newman-Keuls	5	80.25	99.95	107.35	121.50	134.90
Newman-Keuls	1	80.25	99.95	107.35	121.50	134.90
Duncan	5	80.25	99.95	107.35	121.50	134.90
Duncan	1	80.25	99.95	107.35	121.50	134.90

2.1.4 References

1. Beyer, William H. (1953). Certain Percentage Points of the Distribution of the Studentized Range of Large Samples. Virginia Polytechnic Institute Technical Report No. 4.
2. Duncan, David B. (1955). Multiple range and multiple F tests. *Biometrics* **11**, 1-42.
3. Harter, H. Leon (1957a). Error rates and sample sizes for range tests in multiple comparisons. *Biometrics* **13**, 511-536. [See Chapter 2, Section 2.2 and Tables B4-B6 of present volume for a revised version.]
4. Harter, H. Leon (1957b). Critical values for Duncan's new multiple range test (abstract). *Journal of the American Statistical Association* **52**, 372.
5. Hartley, H. O. (1953). Corrigenda (1) Tables of percentage points of the "studentized" range. *Biometrika* **40**, 236.
6. Keuls, M. (1952). The use of the "studentized range" in connection with an analysis of variance. *Euphytica* **1**, 112-122.
7. Lund, R. E. and Lund, J. R. (1983). Algorithm AS190: Probabilities and upper quantiles for the studentized range. *Applied Statistics* **32**, 204-210.
8. Lund, R. E. and Lund, J. R. (1985). Corrections to Algorithm AS190: Probabilities and upper quantiles for the studentized range. *Applied Statistics* **34**, 104.
9. May, Joyce M. (1952). Extended and corrected tables of the upper percentage points of the "studentized" range. *Biometrika* **39**, 192-193.
10. McKay, A. T. and Pearson, E. S. (1933). A note on the distribution of range in samples of n. *Biometrika* **25**, 415-420.
11. Newman, D. (1939). The distribution of range in samples from a normal population, expressed in terms of an independent estimate of standard deviation. *Biometrika* **31**, 20-30.
12. Pearson, Egon S. (1932). The percentage limits for the distribution of range in samples from a normal population ($n \leq 100$). *Biometrika* **24**, 404-417.
13. Pearson, E. S. (1939). "Student" as statistician. *Biometrika* **30**, 210-250.
14. Pearson, E. S. and Hartley, H. O. (1943). Tables of the probability integral of the studentized range. *Biometrika* **33**, 89-99.
15. Pearson, E. S. and Hartley, H. O. (Eds.) (1954). *Biometrika Tables for Statisticians*, Vol. 1. Cambridge University Press for the Biometrika Trustees, Cambridge, England.
16. Royston, J. P. (1987). A remark on Algorithm AS190: Probabilities and upper

quantiles for the studentized range. *Applied Statistics* **36**, 119.

17. Tukey, J. W. (1952). Allowances for various types of error rates. Unpublished invited address presented at Blacksburg meeting of the Institute of Mathematical Statistics. [For reminder sheets, see Tukey (1994), pp. 335-345.]

18. Tukey, J. W. (1953). The Problem of Multiple Comparisons. Unpublished memorandum in private circulation. [See Tukey (1994), pp. 1-300.]

19. Tukey, J. W. (1994). *The Collected Works of John W. Tukey, Volume VIII: Multiple Comparisons, 1948-1983* (edited by Henry I. Braun). Chapman & Hall, New York.

2.2 Error Rates and Sample Sizes for Multiple Comparison Tests Based on the Studentized Range [2]

2.2.1 Introduction

The problem of multiple comparisons has aroused a great deal of interest among statisticians. The basic F test in an analysis of variance determines whether there is a significant difference among a group of means, but it cannot tell which means differ significantly from which others. The latter is often what the investigator really wants to know. If an investigator wishes to compare the means of two groups of observations, the standard procedure is to perform a Student t test at an appropriate significance level. Suppose, however, he wishes to compare the means of m (≥ 3) groups. If he were to perform $m(m-1)/2$ t tests, one for each pair of means, each at significance level α, then the probability that a significant difference would be found between the largest and smallest means would be larger than α (much larger for large m), even if the groups all came from populations with equal means. This dilemma was recognized more than a century and a half ago by Cournot (1843). Some protection against too many significant differences is provided by first performing an analysis of variance F test on the m groups and then performing t tests only if the F test shows overall significance of difference among means. This procedure, called the protected LSD (least significant difference) test, has often been used in practice, but it is not clear that it provides sufficient protection. A number of other multiple comparison procedures have been proposed, including the studentized range procedures discussed in this section. A study is made here of the error rates, α and β, and their relation to sample size, N, for three fixed range tests and three multiple range tests. An account of the early history of multiple comparison tests was published by Harter (1980). Volume VIII of the collected works of John W. Tukey (1994) is devoted to his work on multiple comparisons during the period 1948-1983, including his previously unpublished (but well-known and influential) 1953 memorandum on the problem of multiple comparisons [Tukey (1953)]. Also included are a biography and a bibliography of John W. Tukey, and extensive references to the work of other authors. Other books on multiple comparisons include those of Miller (1966), Hochberg and Tamhane (1987), Hoppe (1993), and Hsu (1996).

Let it be required to test the significance of the range of p out of m ordered means of samples of size N, where $p = 2, 3, \ldots, m$. For the fixed range tests, the critical range for a particular Type I error rate, α, depends only on m and N; for the multiple range tests, it depends also on p. In fact, for fixed m and N, it is a non-decreasing function of p. The range of p means is said to be significant or non-significant (at the α level) according as it does or does not exceed the critical range, except that the range of p means is automatically non-significant if these p means constitute a subgroup of a larger group whose range is non-significant. Because of this exception, a multiple range test starts with a test on all m means. If the range of all m means is found to be significant, then tests are performed on the ranges of $(m-1)$ successive means, $(m-2)$ successive means, and so on until significant differences are no longer found.

2.2.2 Significance *vs.* Confidence

Though the emphasis here is upon tests of significance of size α for the difference between sample means, some investigators may prefer to set $100(1-\alpha)$ percent confidence intervals

[2] An earlier version of this material was published in *Biometrics* **13** (1957), 511-536.

on differences between population means. The choice between significance tests and confidence limits depends upon the experimental situation and upon the experimenter's philosophy. Many statisticians, including Tukey (1953) [see also Tukey (1991)], prefer confidence procedures in practically all cases, and the authors are convinced that there is much merit in this position. The results of this section, however, will be stated in terms of significance. This is done because the authors prefer multiple range procedures, which are not adapted to the construction of confidence intervals. It simply does not make any sense to us, when comparing three or more ordered sample means, to use the same measuring stick in comparing two adjacent sample means as in comparing the largest and smallest means. Tukey himself made a concession to this point of view when he proposed his X procedure, which is a compromise between his studentized range test and the Newman-Keuls test.

2.2.3 The Fixed Range Tests

The three fixed range tests which will be considered are the least significant difference (ISD) test based upon the work of "Student" (1908), a modification of this proposed by Fisher (1935), and the studentized range test proposed by Tukey (1952). They will be designated by code letters L, E and W respectively.

The differences ISD, WSD and ESD between any two out of m means of samples of size N required for significance (at the α level) by the ISD test, Tukey's studentized range test, and Fisher's test, respectively, are given by

$$ISD = t(\alpha,\nu)s_{\bar{d}} = q(\alpha,2,\nu)s_{\bar{x}}, \tag{2.2.1}$$

$$WSD = q(\alpha,m,\nu)s_{\bar{x}}, \tag{2.2.2}$$

$$ESD = t(\alpha/C_2^m,\nu)s_{\bar{d}} = q(\alpha/C_2^m,2,\nu)s_{\bar{x}}, \tag{2.2.3}$$

where ν is the number of degrees of freedom for the error mean square, s^2; $t(\alpha,\nu)$ is the 2-tailed α point (upper $\alpha/2$ point) of Student's t with ν degrees of freedom; $q(\alpha,r,\nu)$ is the upper α point of the studentized range of r observations with ν degrees of freedom for s; $s_{\bar{x}}$ is the standard error of the mean $s_{\bar{x}} = \sqrt{s^2/N}$; and $s_{\bar{d}}$ is the standard error of the difference between means, $s_{\bar{d}} = \sqrt{2s^2/N} = \sqrt{2}s_{\bar{x}}$.

Each of these three test procedures has Type I error rate α for an appropriate definition of the error rate. As a result of a test on the means of m samples each of size N, a statement of significance or nonsignificance will be made about each of the C_2^m differences between pairs of means. A wrong statement (Type I error) is a statement that two means are significantly different, when actually they are means of random samples from the same population. The appropriate error rates α_L, α_W and α_E for the respective test types are then defined as follows: α_L is the expected proportion of wrong statements (error rate per comparison); α_W is the expected proportion of experiments with one or more wrong statements (experimentwise error rate); and α_E is the expected number of wrong statements per experiment (error rate per experiment).

In practice, many statisticians (including the authors) use the protected LSD test, in which the individual comparisons are made only if an analysis of variance yields a significant F ratio for the comparison of all m means. The Type I error rate, α_L, which will be considered here, however, is that for the unprotected LSD test, otherwise known as the multiple t test.

2.2.4 The Multiple Range Tests

The three multiple range tests which will be considered are the Newman-Keuls test, Tukey's X procedure, and Duncan's multiple range test. They will be designated by the code letters I, X and S, respectively.

The Newman-Keuls test was first proposed by Newman (1939) and modified slightly by Keuls (1952). The critical range of p out of m ordered means of samples each of size N is based on the studentized range of p observations, instead of on the studentized range of m observations as in Tukey's studentized range test. It can easily be seen that the critical range ISD for the Newman-Keuls test is intermediate between the LSD and the WSD, except that it is the same as the LSD for $p = 2$ and the same as the WSD for $p = m$.

Tukey's X procedure was proposed by Tukey (1953) as a compromise between the Newman-Keuls test and Tukey's studentized range test. The critical range is the arithmetic mean of the critical ranges for those two tests. For fixed m and N, the smallest critical range (a value midway between the LSD and the WSD) occurs for $p = 2$, and the largest critical range (equal to the WSD) occurs for $p = m$.

Duncan's multiple range test, proposed by Duncan (1953, 1955), makes use of special protection levels based upon degrees of freedom. Let $\gamma_{2,\alpha} = 1 - \alpha$ be the protection level for testing the significance of difference between two means, that is, the probability that a significant difference between sample means will not be found if the population means are equal. Duncan reasons that one has $(p - 1)$ degrees of freedom for testing p means, and hence one may make $(p-1)$ independent tests, each with protection level $\gamma_{2,\alpha}$. Hence the joint protection level is

$$\gamma_{p,\alpha} = \gamma_{2,\alpha}^{p-1} = (1 - \alpha)^{p-1}; \tag{2.2.4}$$

that is, the probability that one finds no significant differences in making $(p - 1)$ independent tests, each at protection level $\gamma_{2,\alpha}$, is $\gamma_{2,\alpha}^{p-1}$. Thus Duncan's multiple range test is based upon protection level $\gamma_{p,\alpha}$ for tests on p means. The critical range SSD is a minimum (equal to the LSD) for $p = 2$, and a maximum for $p = m$.

The critical ranges ISD, XSD and SSD for p out of m ordered means of samples of size N required for significance (at the α level) by the Newman-Keuls test, Tukey's X procedure, and Duncan's multiple range test, respectively, are given by

$$ISD = q(\alpha, p, \nu)s_{\bar{x}}, \tag{2.2.5}$$

$$XSD = (1/2)[q(\alpha, p, \nu) + q(\alpha, m, \nu)]s_{\bar{x}}, \tag{2.2.6}$$

$$SSD = Q(p, \nu, \alpha)s_{\bar{x}}, \tag{2.2.7}$$

where $Q(p, \nu, \alpha)$ is the studentized range of p observations with ν degrees of freedom for s and protection level $\gamma_{p,\alpha}$ given by Equation (2.2.4), and where the other symbols are defined as in subsection 2.2.3.

2.2.5 Example

At this point an example will serve to illustrate the various test procedures. For the sake of simplicity, a single-classification experiment involving comparisons of five means will be considered. The data represent the weight loss (grams) in four days of rats on five diets (no food and 8 calories per rat per day for four foods). In order to reduce experimental error, only male rats were used, all rats were of the same strain, and their initial weights were nearly constant. All one hundred rats received water ad libitum, but they were randomly divided into five groups of twenty rats each, one group on each of the five diets.

An analysis of variance of the data yields the following results:

Source of Variation	d.f.	S.S.	M.S.	F
Among diets	4	3012.70	753.18	38.14 **
Between diets (error)	95	1876.30	19.75	
Total	99	4889.00		

** Significant at the 1% level.

Thus there is a highly significant difference among mean weight losses of the rats on the five diets. This information is quite interesting to the experimenter, but what he really wishes to know is which diets are significantly better than which others. In order to obtain this information, it is necessary to apply a multiple comparison test to the means:

Purina Laboratory Chow	Casein	Dextrose	Olive Oil	No Food
23.70	24.90	28.25	29.40	39.25

The standard error of the mean, $s_{\bar{x}}$, and the standard error of the difference between means, $s_{\bar{d}}$, are found to be 0.9937 and 1.405, respectively, based upon the internal estimate of variance, $s^2 = 19.75$, with 95 degrees of freedom. The factors by which these must be multiplied to obtain the critical ranges for significance at the 5 percent and 1 percent levels can be found in tables. Tables of the critical values of the Student t distribution can be found in almost any statistics textbook. The 5 percent and 1 percent points of the studentized range have been tabulated by Pearson and Hartley (1954), and the 5 percent and 1 percent points of $Q(p, \nu, \alpha)$ by Beyer (1953) and Duncan (1955). More accurate percentage points are given in Tables B2 and B3 of this volume. The factors by which $s_{\bar{x}} = 0.9937$ must be multiplied to obtain the critical ranges for the various tests are as follows:

	$\alpha = 0.05$				$\alpha = 0.01$			
Code letter	$p=2$	$p=3$	$p=4$	$p=5$	$p=2$	$p=3$	$p=4$	$p=5$
L	2.808	2.808	2.808	2.808	3.718	3.718	3.718	3.718
S	2.808	2.955	3.052	3.123	3.718	3.875	3.982	4.062
I	2.808	3.367	3.699	3.933	3.718	4.222	4.523	4.738
X	3.370	3.650	3.816	3.933	4.228	4.480	4.630	4.738
W	3.933	3.933	3.933	3.933	4.738	4.738	4.738	4.738
E	4.065	4.065	4.065	4.065	4.803	4.803	4.803	4.803

Multiplying the standard error of the mean $s_{\bar{x}} = 0.9937$ by these factors, one finds that the critical ranges for the various tests are as follows:

	$\alpha = 0.05$				$\alpha = 0.01$			
Code letter	$p=2$	$p=3$	$p=4$	$p=5$	$p=2$	$p=3$	$p=4$	$p=5$
L	2.790	2.790	2.790	2.790	3.695	3.695	3.695	3.695
S	2.790	2.936	3.033	3.103	3.695	3.851	3.957	4.036
I	2.790	3.346	3.676	3.908	3.695	4.195	4.495	4.708
X	3.349	3.627	3.792	3.908	4.201	4.452	4.601	4.708
W	3.908	3.908	3.908	3.908	4.708	4.708	4.708	4.708
E	4.039	4.039	4.039	4.039	4.773	4.773	4.773	4.773

The results of the various tests can be summarized as follows, where two means are or are not significantly different at the level α according as they are not or are underscored by the same line:

Test	$\alpha = 0.05$					$\alpha = 0.01$				
LSD	23.70	24.90	28.25	29.40	39.25	23.70	24.90	28.25	29.40	39.25
SSD	23.70	24.90	28.25	29.40	39.25	23.70	24.90	28.25	29.40	39.25
ISD	23.70	24.90	28.25	29.40	39.25	23.70	24.90	28.25	29.40	39.25
XSD	23.70	24.90	28.25	29.40	39.25	23.70	24.90	28.25	29.40	39.25
WSD	23.70	24.90	28.25	29.40	39.25	23.70	24.90	28.25	29.40	39.25
ESD	23.70	24.90	28.25	29.40	39.25	23.70	24.90	28.25	29.40	39.25

Thus, at the 5 percent level, the only disagreement is as to whether the means for casein and dextrose differ significantly. At the 1 percent level, there are disagreements in regard to the following differences: (1) casein and olive oil and (2) Purina laboratory chow and dextrose. For experiments involving a larger number of means, one would expect a greater number of disagreements.

2.2.6 Type I Error Rates

The Type I error rate, α, is defined differently for the various tests. The Type I error rate (as defined for a particular test) is denoted by α with the code letter for that test as a subscript; for example, α_L is the Type I error rate as defined for the LSD test. A comparison of the error rates is in order.

By comparison of Equations (2.2.1) and (2.2.2), one sees that a WSD with Type I error rate α_W is equivalent to an LSD with Type I error rate α_L, where

$$t(\alpha_L, \nu) \equiv q(\alpha_L, 2, \nu)/\sqrt{2} = q(\alpha_W, m, \nu)/\sqrt{2}. \tag{2.2.8}$$

Similarly, by comparison of Equations (2.2.1) and (2.2.3), one sees that an ESD with Type I error rate α_E is equivalent to an LSD with Type I error rate α_L, where

$$\alpha_L = \alpha_E / C_2^m. \tag{2.2.9}$$

Let $\alpha_L|\alpha_M$ be the value of α_L corresponding to a given α_M, where M may be any one of the letters W, E, I, X, or S. Table B4A gives $\alpha_L|\alpha_W$ corresponding to $\alpha_W = 0.05$, 0.01 for $m = 2(1)20(2)40(10)100$ and $N = 2(1)11$, 13, 16, 21, 25, 31, 41, 61, 121, ∞; also $\alpha_L|\alpha_E$ corresponding to $\alpha_E = 0.05$, 0.01 for the same values of m. (The relation between α_L and α_E is independent of N.) This table, as well as others which will follow, has been computed for a single-classification design, and the results would be slightly different for randomized blocks or other experimental designs, due to a slight reduction in the number of degrees of freedom for the error mean square.

In testing the significance of the range of p out of m ordered means of samples of size N by one of the multiple range tests with Type I error rate α (as defined for that particular test), the critical range is a function of m, N and p. If α, m and N are fixed, the critical range is a function of p only. Each critical range, for fixed m and N, corresponds to a particular value of the Type I error rate α_L; the larger the critical range, the smaller the value of α_L to which it corresponds. Since the critical range is a non-decreasing function of p, the maximum value of α_L corresponding to a fixed α for the multiple range test under consideration, with m and N also fixed, occurs for $p = 2$, and the minimum for $p = m$.

For $p = 2$, the Newman-Keuls test and Duncan's multiple range test have critical ranges equal to the LSD; hence $(\alpha_L)_{\max}|\alpha_I$ is equal to α_I and $(\alpha_L)_{\max}|\alpha_S$ is equal to α_S.

For $p = m$, the Newman-Keuls test and Tukey's X procedure have critical ranges equal to the WSD; hence $(\alpha_L)_{\min}|\alpha_I$ is equal to $\alpha_L|\alpha_W = \alpha_I$, and $(\alpha_L)_{\min}|\alpha_X$ is equal to $\alpha_L|\alpha_W = \alpha_X$. The values of $\alpha_L|\alpha_W = 0.05, 0.01$ have been given in Table B4A.

Table B4B gives $(\alpha_L)_{\max}|\alpha_X$ corresponding to $\alpha_X = 0.05, 0.01$ and Table B4C gives $(\alpha_L)_{\min}|\alpha_S$ corresponding to $\alpha_S = 0.05, 0.01$, for the same values of m and N as in Table B4A.

2.2.7 Type II and Type III Error Rates

Let m_U and m_L be the two extreme values of p out of m ordered means of samples of size N. Le μ_U and μ_L be the population means corresponding to m_U and m_L respectively. Let the subscripts U and L be so assigned that $\mu_U \geq \mu_L$. This does not necessarily imply that $m_U > m_L$. It should be noted that, while exactly $(p-2)$ of the $(m-2)$ other sample means lie between m_U and m_L, the number of other population means lying between μ_U and μ_L may be less than, equal to, or greater than $(p-2)$. Now define δ by the relation

$$\delta = (\mu_U - \mu_L)/\sigma. \tag{2.2.10}$$

where σ is the common population standard deviation.

If the conclusion is drawn that m_U and m_L are not significantly different when actually $\mu_U > \mu_L$ $(\delta > 0)$, this constitutes an error of Type II. If m_L is found to be significantly greater than m_U when actually $\mu_U > \mu_L$ $(\delta > 0)$, this will be called an error of Type III. Figure 2.1 shows how such an error may arise. The sum of the Type II error rate, β, and the Type III error rate, γ, will be denoted by β', that is

$$\beta' = \beta + \gamma. \tag{2.2.11}$$

The Type III error rate, γ, may be sizable when δ and N are both small. Otherwise, $\gamma \doteq 0$ and $\beta' \doteq \beta$.

The code letters for the various tests are used as subscripts on β and β'; for example, β_L denotes the Type II error rate for the LSD test.

The Type II and Type III error rates, β and γ, and their sum, β', depend upon α, m, N and δ. In the case of multiple range tests, they also depend upon p; for a fixed combination of α, m, N and δ, β' is a minimum for $p = 2$ and a maximum for $p = m$. For $p = 2$, the Newman-Keuls test and Duncan's multiple range test have critical ranges equal to the LSD; hence $(\beta'_I)_{\min} = (\beta'_S)_{\min} = \beta'_L$. For $p = m$, the Newman-Keuls test and Tukey's X procedure have critical ranges equal to the WSD; hence $(\beta'_I)_{\max} = (\beta'_X)_{\max} = \beta'_W$. Table B5 gives, for $\alpha = 0.05, 0.01$; $\delta = 0.5(0.5)3.0$; $m = 2(1)20(2)40(10)100$; $N = 2(1)11$, 13, 16, 21, 25, 31, 41, 61, 121, values of β'_L, $(\beta'_S)_{\max}$, $(\beta'_X)_{\min}$ and β'_W. For convenience, these are denoted by β'_1, β'_2, β'_3 and β'_4, respectively. Thus one has the following equations and inequalities:

$$\beta'_L = \beta'_1, \tag{2.2.12}$$

$$\beta'_1 \leq \beta'_S \leq \beta'_2, \tag{2.2.13}$$

$$\beta'_1 \leq \beta'_I \leq \beta'_4, \tag{2.2.14}$$

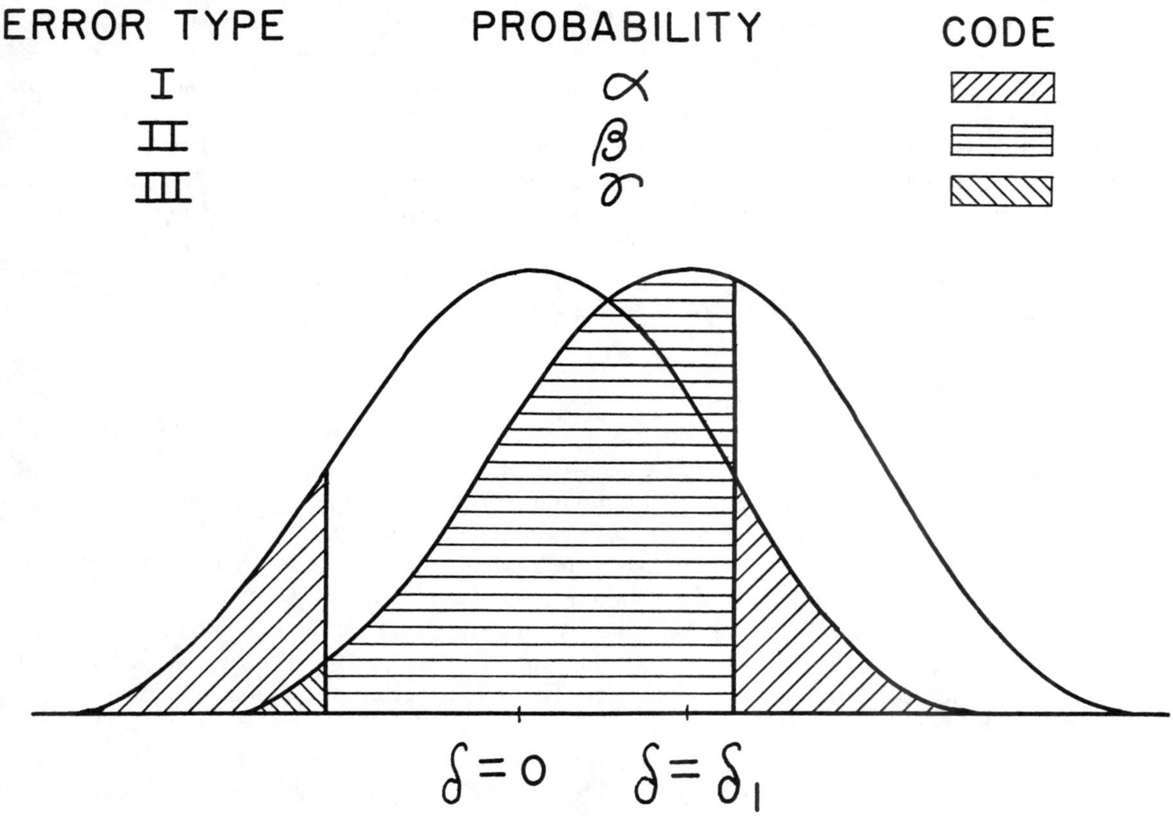

FIGURE 2.1
Graphical Representation of Three Types of Error

$$\beta'_3 \leq \beta'_X \leq \beta'_4, \tag{2.2.15}$$

$$\beta'_W = \beta'_4. \tag{2.2.16}$$

In Inequalities (2.2.13), (2.2.14) and (2.2.15), the left-hand equality holds when $p = 2$ and the right-hand equality when $p = m$. Error rates, β'_E, for Fisher's test have not been computed for $m > 2$, but they are even larger than the corresponding β'_W. Hence one has the inequality

$$\beta'_E \geq \beta'_4, \tag{2.2.17}$$

where the equality holds only for $m = 2$, in which case all six tests are identical.

The values in Table B5, like those in Table B4, were computed for the single-classification case, and the values for randomized blocks and other designs would be slightly different.

No attempt has been made to specify in the hypothesis under test the values or relative values of population means other than μ_U and μ_L. This does not affect the fixed range tests, and leads to no error in the maximum values of β' but produces an upward bias in minimum values of β' for the multiple range tests. This is true since even if the range of two adjacent sample means is significant, the two will be said to differ significantly only if the ranges of all groups containing them are significant. Wine (1955) has made a power study of multiple range tests in which the relative values of all population means are specified. He tabulated the power for tests on 3 and 4 means. For larger values of m, his approach appears forbiddingly difficult and the present approach, though not entirely satisfactory, seems to be the only feasible one.

2.2.8 Required Sample Sizes

If α, β', δ and m are fixed, the required sample size N for each of the fixed range tests can be determined. For multiple range tests, the required sample size N depends upon p. If α, β', δ and m are fixed, the minimum required sample size $N_{\min}$ occurs for $p = 2$, and the maximum required sample size $N_{\max}$ occurs for $p = m$.

The code letters for the various tests are used as subscripts on the required sample size N; for example, N_L denotes the required sample size for the LSD test.

For $p = 2$, the critical ranges for the Newman-Keuls test and Duncan's multiple range test are equal to the LSD; hence $(N_I)_{\min} = (N_S)_{\min} = N_L$. For $p = m$, the critical ranges for the Newman-Keuls test and Tukey's X procedure are equal to the WSD; hence $(N_I)_{\max} = (N_X)_{\max} = N_W$.

Table B6 gives N_L, $(N_S)_{\max}$, $(N_X)_{\min}$ and N_W for $\alpha = 0.05, 0.01$; $\beta' = 0.10, 0.05$; $m = 2(1)20(2)40(10)100$; $\delta = 0.5(0.5)3.0$. The required sample sizes N_E for Fisher's test have not been computed, but they would be slightly larger than the corresponding N_W.

For small values of δ, the required sample size N is approximately inversely proportional to δ^2. Hence, for $\delta < 1$, the approximate value of $N\delta^2$ may be read from the column headed $\delta = 1.0$ in Table B6.

The values in Table B6 have been computed for the single-classification case. To obtain sample sizes which will ensure that α and β' do not exceed the prescribed values for randomized blocks it can be shown that it is sufficient (though not always necessary) to add 2 to the sample sizes for $m = 2$ and to add 1 for $m \geq 3$.

2.2.9 Computation of the Tables

Let the critical range MSD of a range test on p out of m ordered means with significance level α_M be represented by

$$MSD = Q(\alpha_M, p, m, \nu)s_{\bar{x}}, \tag{2.2.18}$$

where M may be I, S, X or W. The equivalent LSD test has significance level α_L such that

$$t(\alpha_L, \nu) = Q(\alpha_M, p, m, \nu)/\sqrt{2}. \tag{2.2.19}$$

It should be noted that Equation (2.2.19) is a generalization of Equation (2.2.8). While Equation (2.2.8) holds only for Tukey's studentized range test, Equation (2.2.19) holds for that test and also for the multiple range tests. The part of Table B4 concerned with α_L corresponding to $\alpha_E = 0.05, 0.01$ was computed directly from Equation (2.2.9). For the remainder of the tables, the critical values for the equivalent LSD tests were computed from Equation (2.2.19). The further computations required were based on the noncentral t distribution, with noncentrality parameter equal to zero for the remainder of Table B4 and greater than zero for Tables B5 and B6.

The cumulative distribution function of the noncentral t distribution with ν degrees of freedom and noncentrality parameter Δ is given [see Owen (1962), p. 108] by

$$\Pr\{T_\mu \leq t \mid \Delta\} = \frac{\sqrt{2\pi}}{\Gamma(\nu/2)2^{(\nu-2)/2}} \int_0^\infty P(tx/\sqrt{\nu} - \Delta)x^{\nu-1}Z(x)\,dx, \tag{2.2.20}$$

where

$$P(y) = (1/\sqrt{2\pi}) \int_{-\infty}^{y} \exp(-u^2/2)\,du \tag{2.2.21}$$

and

$$Z(x) = (1/\sqrt{2\pi})\exp(-x^2/2) \tag{2.2.22}$$

are respectively the cumulative distribution function and the probability density function of the standard normal distribution. After the Gamma function had been converted to integral form, Equation (2.2.20) was rewritten in the form

$$\Pr\{T_\nu \leq t \mid \Delta\} = \frac{\int_0^\infty P(tx/\sqrt{\nu} - \Delta)\exp(-x^2/2)(x^2/2)^{(\nu-1)/2}\,dx}{\int_0^\infty \exp(-x^2/2)(x^2/2)^{(\nu-1)/2}\,dx}, \tag{2.2.23}$$

which was the form actually used in the computations.

For $\delta = 0.0(0.5)3.0$; $N = 2(1)11, 13, 16, 21, 25, 31, 41, 61, 121, \infty$ (for $\delta = 0$ only); $m = 2(1)20(2)40(10)100$; and $\alpha_M = 0.05, 0.01$, where $M = L$, S, X or W (as appropriate), values were computed for

$$P_i = \Pr\{T_\nu \leq t_i \mid \Delta\} - \Pr\{T_\nu \leq -t_i \mid \Delta\}, \quad (i = 1, 2, 3, 4), \tag{2.2.24}$$

where

$$\begin{aligned}
t_1 &= Q(\alpha_L, 2, m, \nu)/\sqrt{2},\\
t_2 &= Q(\alpha_S, m, m, \nu)/\sqrt{2},\\
t_3 &= Q(\alpha_X, 2, m, \nu)/\sqrt{2},\\
t_4 &= Q(\alpha_W, m, m, \nu)/\sqrt{2},\\
\Delta &= \delta\sqrt{N/2},\\
\nu &= m(N-1),
\end{aligned}$$

and where $Q(\alpha_L, 2, m, \nu)$ and $Q(\alpha_W, m, m, \nu)$ are the percentage points of the studentized range of p consecutive values from an ordered group of m, with ν degrees of freedom, for $p = 2$, $P_1 = 1 - \alpha_L$ and $p = m$, $P_4 = 1 - \alpha_W$ respectively; $Q(\alpha_S, m, m, \nu)$ is the critical value for Duncan's multiple range test, with ν degrees of freedom and significance level α_S, applied to m ordered values (out of m); and

$$Q(\alpha_X, 2, m, \nu) = [Q(\alpha_L, 2, m, \nu) + Q(\alpha_W, m, m, \nu)]/2,$$

or, equivalently,

$$t_3 = (t_1 + t_4)/2.$$

The computations were programmed in FORTRAN for the IBM 7094 computer. Values of $Q(\alpha_L, 2, m, \nu)$ and $Q(\alpha_W, m, m, \nu)$ were read in from Table B2 and values of $Q(\alpha_S, 2, m, \nu)$ from Table B3, with those for values of ν not included in Tables B2 and B3 being obtained by linear harmonic interpolation in ν. Values of $P(tx/\sqrt{\nu} - \Delta)$ were computed from Equation (2.2.21) by means of a double-precision subroutine and certain other portions of the computations were also done in double precision so as to avoid any possible loss of accuracy. The values of P_i, as given by Equation (2.2.24), were obtained as the differences between pairs of probabilities obtained from Equation (2.2.23) by numerical integration by the trapezoidal rule [see Fettis (1955, 1958)] in numerator and denominator, using values of the integrands at intervals h of 0.5, 0.2, and 0.1 in x. For $\nu \leq 20$, the numerical integration was performed in a straightforward manner by summing the integrands at $x = 0$, h, $2h$, $\ldots$ until the contribution became negligible with respect to the sum already found. For $\nu > 20$, use was made of the fact that the integrand in the denominator of Equation (2.2.23) attains its maximum value at $x = \sqrt{\nu - 1}$. Let x_0 be the multiple of 0.1 nearest to $\sqrt{\nu - 1}$. Computer time was saved by summing the integrands (in both numerator and denominator) at $x = x_0$, $x_0 \pm h$, $x_0 \pm 2h$, $\ldots$ until the contribution became negligible with respect to the sum already found. There were a few discrepancies between the results for $h = 0.5$ and $h = 0.2$, but the results for $h = 0.2$ and $h = 0.1$ agreed [with an occasional difference of a unit in the last place, due to rounding] when rounded to the desired number of significant figures or decimal places. The results for $h = 0.1$ were tabulated.

The results of the above computations for $\delta = 0$ are given in Table B4 and of those for $\delta > 0$ in Table B5. For $\delta = 0$, Table B4A gives $1 - P_4 = \alpha_L | \alpha_W$ as a function of m, N and α_W, with a column added giving $\alpha_E / \binom{m}{2} = \alpha_L | \alpha_E$ as a function of m and α_E; Table B4B gives $1 - P_3 = (\alpha_L)_{\max} | \alpha_X$ as a function of m, N and α_X; and Table B4C given $1 - P_2 = (\alpha_L)_{\min} | \alpha_S$ as a function of m, N and α_S. Values of $1 - P_1$, all of which were, to within rounding error, equal to α_L, were calculated only as a check, and were not tabulated. The values in Table B4 were rounded to four decimal places, except that those less than .000095 were written in the form $.(X)Y$, where (X) represents X zeros. Tables B5A and B5B give, for $\alpha_M = 0.05$ and $\alpha_M = 0.01$ respectively, the values of P_i $(i = 1, 2, 3, 4)$ for $\delta = 0.5(0.5)3.0$ as a function of m and N. All values in these tables were rounded to three significant figures or five decimal places, whichever is less accurate. Values less than .000005, which round to .00000, were not printed. Five whole pages, which consisted entirely of blanks, have been omitted.

Also, for the same values of δ (excluding zero), m and α_M mentioned above, and with Δ and ν defined as before, the minimum (integer) value of N, N_i, such that

$$P_i \leq \beta_i', \qquad (i = 1, 2, 3, 4), \tag{2.2.25}$$

where $\beta_i' = 0.10$, 0.05 and P_i is defined by Equation (2.2.24), was determined. For $\delta \geq 1.0$, a first approximation to N_i $(i = 1, 2, 3, 4)$ for each combination of m, α_M and

β_i' was found by scanning Table B5, and P_i was computed from Equations (2.2.23) and (2.2.24). If Inequality (2.2.25) was satisfied, the approximate value of N_i was decreased by steps of 1 until Inequality (2.2.25) was no longer satisfied; if Inequality (2.2.25) was not satisfied, the approximate value was increased by steps of 1 until it was satisfied. Then N_i was taken as the smallest (integer) value of N satisfying Inequality (2.2.25). After the value of N_i for $\delta = 1.0$ had been found, this value was multiplied by four to obtain a first approximation to N_i for $\delta = 0.5$, and the exact value of N_i was found as before. The minimum required sample sizes, N_i, are given in Table B6. Tables B6A, B6B, B6C and B6D respectively give N_i $(i = 1, 2, 3, 4)$ as a function of m and δ for $\alpha_M = 0.05$, $\beta_i' = 0.10$; $\alpha_M = 0.05$, $\beta_i' = 0.05$; $\alpha_M = 0.01$, $\beta_i' = 0.10$; and $\alpha_M = 0.01$, $\beta_i' = 0.05$.

Tables B4-B6 are superior to Tables 1-3 given by Harter (1957) in three respects. They are based on more accurate critical values, especially for Duncan's multiple range test, a defect in the 1957 tables which was corrected by Harter (1961). They are also both more extensive and more accurate than the 1957 tables, as corrected in 1961 for inaccuracies in the critical values. The values of error rates and sample sizes given in the earlier tables were, however, much better approximations to the true values than the comments of Miller (1966), p. 107, might lead one to believe.

2.2.10 Monte Carlo Studies

Balaam (1963) reported the results of a large-scale sampling experiment comparing the performance of the *LSD* procedure, the Newman-Keuls procedure, and Duncan's multiple range test. May (1969) reported the results of a Monte Carlo study of those three procedures and Tukey's studentized range procedure applied to data from normal, uniform, double exponential and logistic distributions. Using somewhat different methods of scoring the results, Balaam concluded that the *LSD* procedure is superior to the Duncan procedure, which is in turn superior to the Newman-Keuls procedure, while May eliminated the *LSD* and Tukey procedures at the two extremes and came down to a choice between the Duncan and Newman-Keuls procedures. Other Monte Carlo studies have been performed by Carmer and Swanson (1973) and more recently by Schwertman and Carter (1995). Their results confirm that the *LSD* is best when only the comparisonwise error rate is considered, and indicate that Tukey's test, the Newman-Keuls test, and the restricted (protected) *LSD* have acceptable experimentwise error rates. The choice of procedure ultimately depends upon the type of control the experimenter wishes to exercise over error rates.

2.2.11 References

1. Balaam, L. N. (1963). Multiple comparisons—a sampling experiment. *Australian Journal of Statistics* **5**, 62-84.
2. Beyer, William H. (1953). Certain Percentage Points of the Distribution of the Studentized Range of Large Samples. Virginia Polytechnic Institute Technical Report No. 4 (Sponsored by Office of Ordnance Research, U.S. Army).
3. Carmer, S. G. and Swanson, M. B. (1973). An evaluation of ten pairwise multiple comparison procedures by Monte Carlo methods. *Journal of the American Statistical Association* **68**, 66-74.
4. Cournot, A. A. (1843). *Exposition de la Théorie des Chances et des Probabilités.* Librairie de L. Hachette, Paris. German translation by H. Schnuse, Braunschweig, 1849.

5. Duncan, D. B. (1953). Multiple range tests and the multiple comparisons test (preliminary report). Abstract #220. *Biometrics* **9**, 262.

6. Duncan, David B. (1955). Multiple range and multiple F tests. *Biometrics* **11**, 1-42.

7. Fettis, Henry E. (1955). Numerical calculation of certain definite integrals by Poisson's summation formula. *Mathematical Tables and other Aids to Computation* **9**, 85-92.

8. Fettis, H. E. (1958). Further remarks concerning the relative accuracy of Simpson's and the trapezoidal rule for a certain class of functions. *Zeitschrift für Angewandte Mathematik und Mechanik* **38**, 159-160.

9. Fisher, Ronald A. (1935). *The Design of Experiments.* Oliver and Boyd Ltd., Edinburgh.

10. Harter, H. Leon (1957). Error rates and sample sizes for range tests in multiple comparisons. *Biometrics* **13**, 511-536.

11. Harter, H. Leon (1961). Corrected error rates for Duncan's new multiple range test. *Biometrics* **17**, 321-324.

12. Harter, H. Leon (1980). Early history of multiple comparison tests. In *Handbook of Statistics*, Volume I: *Analysis of Variance* (Ed., P. R. Krishnaiah), pp. 617-622. North-Holland, Amsterdam.

13. Hochberg, Yosef and Tamhane, Ajit C. (1987). *Multiple Comparison Procedures.* John Wiley & Sons, New York.

14. Hoppe, Fred M. (Ed.) (1993). *Multiple Comparisons, Selection and Applications in Biometry (A Festschrift in Honor of Charles W. Dunnett).* Marcel Dekker, Inc., New York.

15. Hsu, J. C. (1996). *Multiple Comparisons: Theory and Methods.* Chapman & Hall, New York.

16. Keuls, M. (1952). The use of the "studentized range" in connection with an analysis of variance, *Euphytica* **1**, 112-122.

17. May, Thomas E. (1969). Monte Carlo Investigation of Duncan and Other Range Tests for Distributional Robustness. M.S. Thesis (GRE/Math/69-6), Air Force Institute of Technology, Wright-Patterson Air Force Base, Ohio.

18. Miller, Rupert G., Jr. (1966). *Simultaneous Statistical Inference.* McGraw-Hill Book Co., New York. Second ed., Springer-Verlag, New York, 1981.

19. Newman, D. (1939). The distribution of range in samples from a normal population, expressed in terms of an independent estimate of standard deviation. *Biometrika* **31**, 20-30.

20. Owen, D. B. (1962). *Handbook of Statistical Tables.* Addison-Wesley Publishing Co., Inc., Reading, Massachusetts.

21. Pearson, E. S. and Hartley, H. O. (Eds.) (1954). *Biometrika Tables for Statisticians*, Volume 1. Cambridge University Press for the Biometrika Trustess, Cambridge, England.

22. "Student" (1908). The probable error of a mean. *Biometrika* **6**, 1-25.

23. Schwertman, Neil C. and Carter, Nancy J. (1995). A more practical Scheffé-type multiple comparison procedure for commonly encountered numbers of comparisons. *Journal of Statistical Computation and Simulation* **53**, 181-196.

24. Tukey, John W. (1952). Allowances for various types of error rates. Unpublished invited address presented at Blacksburg meeting of Institute of Mathematical Statistics and Biometric Society. [For reminder sheets, see Tukey (1994), pp. 335-345.]

25. Tukey, John W. (1953). The Problem of Multiple Comparisons. Unpublished memorandum in private circulation. [see Tukey (1994), pp. 1-300.]

26. Tukey, John W. (1991). The philosophy of multiple comparisons. *Statistical Science* **6**, 100-116.

27. Tukey, John W. (1994). *The Collected Works of John W. Tukey*, Volume VIII: *Multiple Comparisons, 1948-1983.* (Ed., Henry I. Braun). Chapman & Hall, New York.

28. Wine, R. Lowell (1955). A Power Study of Multiple Range and Multiple F Tests. Virginia Polytechnic Institute Technical Report No. 12 (Sponsored by Office of Ordnance Research, U.S. Army).

2.3 Analysis of Variance Based on the (Studentized) Range

2.3.1 Introduction

The analysis of variance is a procedure developed in the 1920s by R. A. Fisher [see Fisher (1925)] for separating the variance of the observations in a randomized experiment into portions due to one or more factors (treatments) and the residual (error) variance. Expressions for the expected values of the variances are used to formulate tests for the significance of the effects of one factor in a simple one-way classification experiment or of two or more factors (and their interactions) in a more sophisticated experiment. Under appropriate null hypotheses, the variances due to the various factors have independent chi-square distributions, and their ratios have F distributions with specified numbers of degrees of freedom for numerator and denominator. Therefore a table of percentage points of the F distribution can be used to test the significance of the factor or factors. While the arithmetic involved in the analysis of variance is not difficult, a somewhat simpler analogue based on the studentized range was worked out in the early 1950s by several authors [Patnaik (1950), Hartley (1950), and David (1951)].

In analysis of variance, the studentized range statistic q may be used as a substitute for the F statistic. The studentized range is defined as the ratio of the range of the k treatment means, each based on n observations, to an independent estimate of the error standard deviation divided by $\sqrt{n}$. This estimate is usually determined from the within-treatment sum of squares. Patnaik (1950) proposed a modified procedure in which both of the variance components are estimated from ranges or mean ranges instead of mean squares. This procedure makes use of the fact that the mean range, $\bar{w}_n$, of k samples, each of size n, from several normal populations having a common variance σ^2, is distributed [see Pearson (1952)] approximately as $c\chi\sigma/\sqrt{\nu}$, where the scale factor c and the equivalent degrees of freedom ν are functions of n and k. Patnaik tabulated the values of c and ν for a single classification experiment and used them in a numerical example. David (1951, p. 408) extended theory and tables to the case of a double classification experiment. He tabulated ν and c for single and double classification experiments, the former for $n = 2(1)10$, $k = 1(1)5, 10$ and the latter for $n = 2(1)9$, $k = 2(1)10, 20$. Pearson and Hartley (1966) summarized the results for single and double classification experiments (pp. 53-55) and reproduced David's tables in their Table 30 (p. 201). We, in turn, have reproduced the tables as our Table B7.

2.3.2 Analysis for Single Classification

For single classification experiments, the procedure is:

(a) Estimate the within-treatment (error) variance from the mean of the k treatment ranges, $\bar{w}_n$;

(b) Estimate the between-treatment variance from the range, $\bar{x}_{\max} - \bar{x}_{\min}$, of the treatment means;

(c) Calculate the ratio

$$q = (\bar{x}_{\max} - \bar{x}_{\min})c\sqrt{n}/\bar{w}_n. \tag{2.3.1}$$

Since the estimates in the numerator and denominator are independent, the expression for q in Equation (2.3.1) is distributed approximately as a studentized range for sample size k, with equivalent degrees of freedom ν, as given in Table B7A, for the estimate of s.

Example 1. Snedecor (1956) gives the following experimental data in his Table 10.4.1, p. 242:

Grams of Fat Absorbed by 6 Batches of Doughnuts in Each of 4 Fats
(100 grams subtracted from each batch)

Fats	Grams Absorbed – 100						Sum	Mean (decoded)
1	64	72	68	77	56	95	432	172
2	78	91	97	82	85	77	510	185
3	75	93	78	71	63	76	456	176
4	55	66	49	64	70	68	372	162

The following calculations are required for the usual analysis of variance:

$$\text{Total } SS = 64^2 + 72^2 + \cdots + 70^2 + 68^2 - \frac{(1,770)^2}{24} = 3,654.5$$

$$SS \text{ for fat means } = \frac{432^2 + \cdots + 372^2}{6} - \frac{(1,770)^2}{24} = 1,636.5$$

$$SS \text{ for batches (within fats) [error] } = 3,654.5 - 1,636.5 = 2,018.0$$

Analysis of variance of Doughnut Data

Source of variation	d.f.	SS	MS	F
Fats	3	1,636.5	545.5	5.41
Error	20	2,018.0	100.9	
Total	23	3,654.5		

Since $F = 5.41$ exceeds the 99% point (upper 1% point) of the F distribution for 3 and 20 degrees of freedom (4.94), the difference between fat means is significant at the 1% level.

For the alternative analysis based on the (studentized) range, we calculate the range w_6 of the 6 observations for each of the four fats, obtaining the values 39, 20, 30 and 21. The mean of these four ranges is $\bar{w}_6 = 27.5$. For sample size $n = 6$ and number of samples $k = 4$, Table B7A gives $\nu = 18.1$, $c = 2.57$. We then use Equation (2.3.1) to calculate

$$q = (185 - 162)2.57\sqrt{6}/27.5 = 5.27.$$

Since $q = 5.27$ exceeds the 99% point (upper 1% point) of the q distribution for 4 means and 18.1 degrees of freedom (5.09) [see Table B2], the difference between fat means is found to be significant at the 1% level, just as in the conventional analysis.

2.3.3 Analysis for Double Classification

Hartley (1950) modified the procedure to make it applicable in the case of a double classification experiment. For a randomized block experiment, it is necessary to calculate the treatment residuals and then their block ranges.

Example 2. Davis (1956) gives the following experimental data in his Table 5.2, pp. 153-154:

Loss of Product in Manufacture of an Organic Chemical

Block	Batch	Blend of Acetanilide	Percent loss
I	1	B	18.2
	2	A	16.9
	3	C	17.0
	4	E	18.3
	5	D	15.1
II	1	A	16.5
	2	E	18.3
	3	B	19.2
	4	C	18.1
	5	D	16.0
III	1	B	17.1
	2	D	17.8
	3	C	17.3
	4	E	19.8
	5	A	17.5

Blend Means: A, 16.97; B = 18.17; C, 17.47; D, 16.30; E, 18.80
Block Means: I, 17.10; II, 17.62; III, 17.90; Grand Mean 17.54

Analysis of Variance

Source of variation	d.f.	SS	MS	F
Between blocks	2	1.65	0.82	0.94
Between blends	4	11.56	2.89	3.32
Error	8	6.99	0.87	
Total	14	20.20		

The difference between blends is significant at the 10% level, but not at the 5% level, since (for 4 and 8 d.f.), the upper 10% point of F is 2.81 and the upper 5% point is 3.84. The difference between blocks is not significant.

For the alternative analysis based on the (studentized) range, we calculate first the blend residuals and their block ranges, as shown in the following table:

Blend Residuals and Their Block Ranges

Block	Blend					Range
	A	B	C	D	E	
I	−0.07	0.03	−0.47	−1.20	−0.50	1.23
II	−0.47	1.03	0.63	−0.30	−0.50	1.53
III	0.53	−1.07	−0.17	1.50	1.00	2.57
Total	–	–	–	–	–	5.33

The mean of the $k = 3$ block ranges of $n = 5$ blend residuals is $\bar{w}_5 = 5.33/3 = 1.78$. Table B7B gives $\nu = 7.4$, $c = 1.96$. For blends, $q = (18.80 - 16.30)1.96\sqrt{3}/1.78 = 4.77$, which is significant at the 10% level, but not at the 5% level, since $q_{.90} = 4.23 < 4.77 < q_{.95} = 4.99$. For blocks, $q = (17.90 - 17.10)1.96\sqrt{5}/1.78 = 2.16$, which is not significant, since $2.16 < q_{.70} = 2.28$. Again, as in Example 1, the results are essentially the same as for the conventional analysis.

2.3.4 References

1. David, Herbert A. (1951). Further applications of range to the analysis of variance. *Biometrika* **38**, 393-409.
2. Davis, Owen L. (Ed.) (1956). *The Design and Analysis of Industrial Experiments*, (2nd edition). Oliver & Boyd, London-Edinburgh; Hafner Publishing Company, New York.
3. Fisher, R. A. (1925). *Statistical Methods for Research Workers.* Oliver and Boyd, London-Edinburgh.
4. Hartley, H. O. (1950). The use of range in analysis of variance. *Biometrika* **37**, 271-280.
5. Patnaik, P. B. (1950). The use of mean range as an estimator of variance in statistical tests. *Biometrika* **37**, 78-87.
6. Pearson, E. S. (1950). Comparison of two approximations to the distribution of the range in small samples from normal populations. *Biometrika* **39**, 130-136.
7. Pearson, E. S. and Hartley, H. O. (Eds.) (1966). *Biometrika Tables for Statisticians*, Volume I (3rd edition). Cambridge University Press for the Biometrika Trustees, Cambridge, England.
8. Snedecor, George W. (1956). *Statistical Methods* (5th edition). Iowa State College Press, Ames.

2.4 Applications to Outlier-Testing

The statistical problem of identification or testing of outliers in a sample historically came first from astronomical data. Since normal distribution was (and still is) commonly assumed as the underlying model for such data sets, it is not surprising that there exists a vast body of literature on issues concerning outliers from normal distributions. Early discussions on this issue can be traced back to the eighteenth century. For an authoritative treatment of this topic of statistical research, we refer the readers to Barnett and Lewis (1994).

Since the normal distribution is commonly used as an all-purpose statistical distribution/model while analyzing data, and since it involves two parameters μ (the mean) and σ (the standard deviation), discordancy tests for outliers proposed in literature deal with different cases arising from the assumptions that one or both of these parameters are unknown. For example, if the population variance σ^2 is assumed to be known, then a discordancy test of a lower and upper outlier-pair, x_1, x_n, can be based on the standardized range

$$W = \frac{w}{\sigma} = \frac{x_n - x_1}{\sigma} .$$

This discordancy test has been discussed by Dixon (1950, 1962) and its performance in the detection of outliers has been discussed by Dixon (1950). The percentage points of the standardized range W presented in Table A5 can, therefore, be used to carry out this discordancy test of a lower and upper outlier-pair.

Next, let us consider the case when the population variance σ^2 is unknown. In this case, a discordancy test of a lower and upper outlier-pair, x_1, x_n, can be based on the internally studentized range

$$T = \frac{w}{s} = \frac{x_n - x_1}{s} ,$$

where $s = \left\{\frac{1}{n-1}\sum_{i=1}^{n}(x_i - \overline{x})^2\right\}^{1/2}$ is the sample standard deviation. The null distribution of this test statistic has been discussed by David, Hartley and Pearson (1954) and Pearson and Stephens (1964), while Pearson and Hartley (1966, Table 29c, p. 200) have presented a table of lower and upper 0.5, 1, 2.5, 5 and 10 percent points for $n = 3(1)20(5)100$, 150, 200, 500, 1000. Table B8 presented in this volume is an abridged version of Pearson and Hartley's Table 29c. Shapiro, Wilk and Chen (1968) have presented values of the power of this discordancy test against 45 different inherent alternatives. From their extensive power study, it appears that as a test against an inherent alternative, the outlier-test based on T has good power properties against a wide variety of symmetric distributions which are alternatives to the normal distribution, but performs poorly against asymmetric alternatives.

Now, let us consider the case when the population variance σ^2 is unknown, and assume that an independent estimator s_ν^2 of σ^2 is available with ν being the associated number of degrees of freedom. Then, a discordancy test of a lower and upper outlier-pair, x_1, x_n, can be based on the externally studentized range

$$A = \frac{w}{s_\nu} = \frac{x_n - x_1}{s_\nu} .$$

This outlier-test and the null distribution of this test statistic have been discussed by a number of authors including Dixon (1950), Thompson (1955), Moore (1957), David (1962), and Fieller (1976). The percentage points of the externally studentized range Q presented in Table B2 can, therefore, be used to carry out this discordancy test of a lower and upper outlier-pair.

In this case, one may also use a discordancy test of a lower and upper outlier-pair, x_1, x_n, based on the externally and internally studentized range

$$T^* = \frac{w}{\tilde{s}} = \frac{x_n - x_1}{\tilde{s}} \,,$$

where $\tilde{s}^2$ is the pooled estimator of σ^2 given by

$$\tilde{s}^2 = \frac{1}{n-1+\nu}\left\{\sum_{i=1}^{n}(x_i - \overline{x})^2 + \nu\, s_\nu^2\right\}.$$

Such an outlier-test has been discussed by Fieller (1976).

2.4.1 References

1. Barnett, Vic and Lewis, Toby (1994). *Outliers in Statistical Data*, Third edition. John Wiley & Sons, Chichester, England.
2. David, Herbert A. (1962). Order statistics in short-cut tests. In *Contributions to Order Statistics* (Eds., Ahmed E. Sarhan and Bernard G. Greenberg), pp. 94-128, John Wiley & Sons, New York.
3. David, Herbert A., Hartley, H. O. and Pearson, Egon S. (1954). The distribution of the ratio, in a single normal sample, of range to standard deviation. *Biometrika* **41**, 482-493.
4. Dixon, Wilfrid J. (1950). Analysis of extreme values. *Annals of Mathematical Statistics* **21**, 488-506.
5. Dixon, Wilfrid J. (1962). Rejection of observations. In *Contributions to Order Statistics* (Eds., Ahmed E. Sarhan and Bernard G. Greenberg), pp. 299-342, John Wiley & Sons, New York.
6. Fieller, N. R. J. (1976). *Some Problems Related to the Rejection of Outlying Observations.* Ph.D. Thesis, University of Hull, Hull, England.
7. Moore, P. G. (1957). The two-sample t-test based on range. *Biometrika* **44**, 482-485.
8. Pearson, Egon S. and Hartley, H. O. (Eds.) (1966). *Biometrika Tables for Statisticians*, Vol. 1, Third edition. Cambridge University Press, London, England.
9. Pearson, Egon S. and Stephens, Michael A. (1964). The ratio of range to standard deviation in the same normal sample. *Biometrika* **51**, 484-487.
10. Shapiro, Samuel S., Wilk, Martin B. and Chen, M. J. (1968). A comparative study of various tests for normality. *Journal of the American Statistical Association* **63**, 1343-1372.
11. Thompson, G. W. (1955). Bounds for the ratio of range to standard deviation. *Biometrika* **42**, 268-269.

Appendix A

Tables Based on the Range

SOURCES OF TABLES

Tables A1–A3	ARL 62-378 (Harter)
Tables A4–A6	WADC TR 58-484, Vol. I (Harter and Clemm) [Table A5 modified to conform with table of percentage points of 0th quasi-range in ARL 31, Part II (Harter).]
Tables A8–A9	Childs and Balakrishnan (1997)

Table A1

CUMULATIVE DISTRIBUTION FUNCTION $F(F', n_1, n_2)$ OF THE RATIO F' OF THE RANGES OF SAMPLES OF SIZES n_1 AND n_2 FROM $N(\mu_i, \sigma)$ $(i = 1, 2)$

$n_2 = 2$

F' \ n_1	2	3	4	5	6	7	8
1.00	.50000	.30984	.21345	.15701	.12083	.09612	.07845
1.05	.51553	.32762	.23064	.17290	.13532	.10930	.09045
1.10	.53029	.34487	.24759	.18881	.15003	.12286	.10293
1.15	.54434	.36157	.26426	.20466	.16487	.13668	.11580
1.20	.55772	.37772	.28059	.22040	.17976	.15068	.12896
1.25	.57045	.39331	.29656	.23595	.19463	.16479	.14232
1.30	.58257	.40835	.31215	.25128	.20941	.17893	.15581
1.35	.59412	.42286	.32733	.26634	.22406	.19305	.16936
1.40	.60514	.43683	.34210	.28112	.23853	.20708	.18292
1.50	.62567	.46326	.37037	.30971	.26680	.23475	.20986
1.60	.64438	.48777	.39697	.33695	.29403	.26166	.23630
1.70	.66149	.51049	.42192	.36278	.32009	.28764	.26202
1.80	.67717	.53156	.44531	.38720	.34494	.31258	.28687
1.90	.69157	.55112	.46721	.41025	.36855	.33642	.31075
2.00	.70483	.56930	.48772	.43198	.39093	.35914	.33363
2.10	.71707	.58621	.50693	.45245	.41212	.38076	.35548
2.20	.72840	.60197	.52494	.47173	.43218	.40128	.37630
2.30	.73890	.61668	.54182	.48990	.45114	.42077	.39612
2.40	.74867	.63042	.55767	.50702	.46907	.43925	.41498
2.50	.75776	.64328	.57257	.52316	.48603	.45677	.43291
2.60	.76625	.65533	.58658	.53839	.50208	.47339	.44994
2.70	.77419	.66665	.59978	.55278	.51728	.48916	.46614
2.80	.78162	.67729	.61223	.56638	.53167	.50413	.48154
2.90	.78860	.68731	.62397	.57924	.54531	.51834	.49618
3.00	.79517	.69675	.63508	.59142	.55825	.53185	.51012
3.10	.80135	.70567	.64558	.60297	.57054	.54469	.52338
3.20	.80718	.71410	.65553	.61393	.58222	.55690	.53602
3.30	.81268	.72208	.66497	.62434	.59332	.56854	.54806
3.40	.81789	.72965	.67393	.63423	.60389	.57962	.55955
3.50	.82283	.73683	.68244	.64365	.61396	.59019	.57051
3.60	.82751	.74365	.69054	.65262	.62357	.60027	.58098
3.70	.83196	.75014	.69826	.66117	.63273	.60991	.59099
3.80	.83618	.75632	.70562	.66933	.64148	.61912	.60057
3.90	.84021	.76220	.71263	.67712	.64984	.62792	.60973
4.00	.84404	.76782	.71934	.68457	.65785	.63635	.61851
4.20	.85119	.77832	.73188	.69852	.67285	.65217	.63499
4.40	.85773	.78793	.74338	.71133	.68664	.66674	.65017
4.60	.86372	.79676	.75396	.72313	.69936	.68017	.66419
4.80	.86924	.80490	.76372	.73404	.71112	.69261	.67718
5.00	.87433	.81242	.77275	.74413	.72202	.70414	.68924
5.20	.87905	.81939	.78114	.75351	.73215	.71487	.70045
5.40	.88343	.82588	.78894	.76224	.74158	.72487	.71091
5.60	.88750	.83191	.79621	.77039	.75039	.73421	.72069
5.80	.89131	.83755	.80300	.77800	.75863	.74295	.72984
6.00	.89486	.84283	.80937	.78514	.76636	.75115	.73843
6.20	.89820	.84778	.81534	.79184	.77362	.75885	.74650
6.40	.90133	.85243	.82095	.79814	.78044	.76610	.75409
6.60	.90427	.85681	.82624	.80407	.78688	.77293	.76126
6.80	.90705	.86094	.83123	.80968	.79295	.77938	.76802
7.00	.90967	.86484	.83594	.81497	.79869	.78548	.77442

$n_2 = 2$

$F' \backslash n_1$	2	3	4	5	6	7	8
7.50	.91561	.87370	.84665	.82702	.81176	.79938	.78900
8.00	.92083	.88148	.85607	.83761	.82326	.81160	.80183
8.50	.92545	.88836	.86440	.84699	.83344	.82244	.81321
9.00	.92955	.89449	.87183	.85535	.84253	.83211	.82337
9.50	.93323	.89999	.87849	.86285	.85068	.84078	.83249
10.00	.93655	.90494	.88449	.86962	.85804	.84862	.84072
10.50	.93955	.90943	.88994	.87575	.86471	.85572	.84818
11.00	.94228	.91352	.89489	.88134	.87078	.86219	.85498
11.50	.94478	.91725	.89942	.88645	.87634	.86811	.86121
12.00	.94707	.92067	.90358	.89113	.88144	.87355	.86692
12.50	.94918	.92383	.90741	.89545	.88614	.87855	.87219
13.00	.95113	.92674	.91095	.89944	.89048	.88318	.87705
13.50	.95293	.92944	.91423	.90314	.89450	.88747	.88156
14.00	.95460	.93195	.91727	.90658	.89824	.89145	.88576
15.00	.95762	.93647	.92276	.91277	.90498	.89864	.89331
16.00	.96026	.94042	.92756	.91819	.91088	.90493	.89993
17.00	.96259	.94392	.93181	.92298	.91610	.91049	.90579
18.00	.96467	.94702	.93558	.92724	.92074	.91544	.91099
19.00	.96652	.94980	.93896	.93106	.92489	.91987	.91565
20.00	.96820	.95231	.94200	.93449	.92863	.92386	.91985
21.00	.96971	.95457	.94476	.93760	.93202	.92747	.92365
22.00	.97108	.95663	.94726	.94043	.93510	.93076	.92711
23.00	.97234	.95852	.94955	.94301	.93792	.93376	.93027
24.00	.97349	.96024	.95165	.94538	.94050	.93651	.93317
25.00	.97455	.96183	.95358	.94756	.94287	.93905	.93583
26.00	.97553	.96330	.95536	.94958	.94506	.94138	.93829
27.00	.97643	.96465	.95701	.95144	.94709	.94355	.94057
28.00	.97727	.96592	.95855	.95317	.94898	.94556	.94269
29.00	.97806	.96709	.95997	.95478	.95074	.94744	.94466
30.00	.97879	.96818	.96131	.95629	.95237	.94919	.94650
31.00	.97947	.96921	.96255	.95770	.95391	.95082	.94823
32.00	.98011	.97017	.96372	.95902	.95535	.95236	.94984
33.00	.98071	.97107	.96482	.96026	.95670	.95380	.95136
34.00	.98128	.97192	.96585	.96143	.95797	.95515	.95279
35.00	.98182	.97273	.96683	.96253	.95917	.95643	.95414
36.00	.98232	.97348	.96775	.96357	.96030	.95764	.95541
37.00	.98280	.97420	.96862	.96455	.96137	.95879	.95661
38.00	.98325	.97488	.96945	.96548	.96239	.95987	.95775
39.00	.98368	.97552	.97023	.96637	.96335	.96090	.95883
40.00	.98409	.97613	.97097	.96721	.96427	.96187	.95986
42.00	.98485	.97727	.97235	.96877	.96597	.96369	.96177
44.00	.98553	.97830	.97361	.97019	.96751	.96534	.96351
46.00	.98616	.97925	.97476	.97148	.96893	.96684	.96509
48.00	.98674	.98011	.97581	.97267	.97022	.96822	.96655
50.00	.98727	.98090	.97677	.97376	.97141	.96949	.96788
52.00	.98776	.98164	.97767	.97477	.97251	.97067	.96912
54.00	.98821	.98232	.97849	.97570	.97353	.97175	.97026
56.00	.98863	.98295	.97926	.97657	.97447	.97276	.97132
58.00	.98902	.98354	.97998	.97738	.97535	.97370	.97231
60.00	.98939	.98409	.98064	.97813	.97617	.97458	.97323

$n_2 = 2$

F \ n_1	2	3	4	5	6	7	8
62.00	.98973	.98460	.98127	.97884	.97694	.97540	.97410
64.00	.99005	.98508	.98185	.97950	.97766	.97616	.97491
66.00	.99036	.98553	.98240	.98012	.97834	.97689	.97567
68.00	.99064	.98596	.98292	.98070	.97898	.97757	.97638
70.00	.99091	.98636	.98341	.98126	.97958	.97821	.97706
75.00	.99151	.98727	.98451	.98251	.98094	.97966	.97859
80.00	.99204	.98806	.98548	.98360	.98213	.98093	.97992
85.00	.99251	.98877	.98634	.98456	.98318	.98205	.98110
90.00	.99293	.98939	.98710	.98542	.98411	.98305	.98215
95.00	.99330	.98995	.98777	.98619	.98495	.98394	.98309
100.00	.99363	.99045	.98838	.98688	.98570	.98474	.98394
105.00	.99394	.99091	.98894	.98750	.98638	.98547	.98470
110.00	.99421	.99132	.98944	.98807	.98700	.98613	.98540
115.00	.99446	.99170	.98990	.98859	.98757	.98673	.98603
120.00	.99469	.99204	.99032	.98907	.98808	.98729	.98661
125.00	.99491	.99236	.99071	.98950	.98856	.98779	.98715
130.00	.99510	.99265	.99107	.98991	.98900	.98826	.98764
135.00	.99528	.99293	.99140	.99028	.98941	.98870	.98810
140.00	.99545	.99318	.99170	.99063	.98979	.98910	.98853
150.00	.99576	.99363	.99226	.99125	.99047	.98983	.98929
160.00	.99602	.99403	.99274	.99180	.99106	.99046	.98996
170.00	.99626	.99438	.99317	.99228	.99159	.99103	.99055
180.00	.99646	.99469	.99355	.99271	.99206	.99152	.99108
190.00	.99665	.99497	.99389	.99309	.99247	.99197	.99155
200.00	.99682	.99523	.99419	.99344	.99285	.99237	.99197
210.00	.99697	.99545	.99447	.99375	.99319	.99273	.99235
220.00	.99711	.99566	.99472	.99404	.99350	.99307	.99270
230.00	.99723	.99585	.99495	.99429	.99378	.99337	.99302
240.00	.99735	.99602	.99516	.99453	.99404	.99364	.99331
250.00	.99745	.99618	.99535	.99475	.99428	.99390	.99357
260.00	.99755	.99633	.99553	.99495	.99450	.99413	.99382
270.00	.99764	.99646	.99570	.99514	.99470	.99435	.99405
280.00	.99773	.99659	.99585	.99531	.99489	.99455	.99426
290.00	.99780	.99671	.99599	.99547	.99507	.99474	.99446
300.00	.99788	.99682	.99613	.99563	.99523	.99491	.99465
320.00	.99801	.99702	.99637	.99590	.99553	.99523	.99498
340.00	.99813	.99719	.99658	.99614	.99579	.99551	.99528
360.00	.99823	.99735	.99677	.99635	.99603	.99576	.99554
380.00	.99832	.99749	.99694	.99655	.99624	.99598	.99577
400.00	.99841	.99761	.99710	.99672	.99643	.99619	.99598
420.00	.99848	.99773	.99723	.99688	.99660	.99637	.99618
440.00	.99855	.99783	.99736	.99702	.99675	.99653	.99635
460.00	.99862	.99792	.99747	.99715	.99689	.99668	.99651
480.00	.99867	.99801	.99758	.99727	.99702	.99682	.99665
500.00	.99873	.99809	.99768	.99738	.99714	.99695	.99679
520.00	.99878	.99816	.99777	.99748	.99725	.99707	.99691
540.00	.99882	.99823	.99785	.99757	.99735	.99717	.99703
560.00	.99886	.99830	.99793	.99766	.99745	.99728	.99713
580.00	.99890	.99835	.99800	.99774	.99753	.99737	.99723
600.00	.99894	.99841	.99806	.99781	.99762	.99746	.99732

$n_2 = 2$

$F' \backslash n_1$	9	10	11	12	13	14	15
1.00	.06534	.05533	.04750	.04126	.03619	.03202	.02855
1.05	.07631	.06538	.05675	.04980	.04411	.03938	.03542
1.10	.08783	.07605	.06666	.05903	.05273	.04747	.04301
1.15	.09982	.08725	.07714	.06887	.06200	.05621	.05128
1.20	.11218	.09888	.08811	.07925	.07182	.06554	.06015
1.25	.12483	.11087	.09950	.09007	.08214	.07538	.06956
1.30	.13769	.12314	.11121	.10127	.09286	.08566	.07944
1.35	.15069	.13561	.12318	.11277	.10392	.09632	.08972
1.40	.16377	.14822	.13534	.12450	.11526	.10728	.10033
1.50	.18994	.17362	.15999	.14843	.13850	.12988	.12230
1.60	.21584	.19895	.18475	.17263	.16216	.15300	.14492
1.70	.24121	.22392	.20931	.19676	.18586	.17629	.16781
1.80	.26586	.24833	.23342	.22057	.20936	.19947	.19068
1.90	.28968	.27201	.25692	.24387	.23243	.22232	.21329
2.00	.31259	.29488	.27970	.26652	.25495	.24467	.23548
2.10	.33455	.31687	.30168	.28845	.27679	.26642	.25712
2.20	.35555	.33797	.32282	.30959	.29791	.28749	.27813
2.30	.37560	.35817	.34311	.32992	.31826	.30784	.29845
2.40	.39472	.37747	.36253	.34944	.33782	.32743	.31806
2.50	.41294	.39589	.38111	.36813	.35660	.34626	.33693
2.60	.43028	.41347	.39887	.38602	.37460	.36434	.35507
2.70	.44680	.43024	.41583	.40314	.39183	.38167	.37248
2.80	.46253	.44623	.43203	.41950	.40833	.39828	.38917
2.90	.47751	.46148	.44749	.43514	.42412	.41419	.40518
3.00	.49178	.47602	.46226	.45009	.43922	.42942	.42052
3.10	.50539	.48990	.47636	.46438	.45367	.44400	.43522
3.20	.51836	.50314	.48983	.47804	.46749	.45797	.44931
3.30	.53073	.51579	.50271	.49111	.48072	.47134	.46281
3.40	.54255	.52787	.51502	.50361	.49339	.48415	.47574
3.50	.55383	.53942	.52679	.51558	.50552	.49643	.48815
3.60	.56462	.55047	.53806	.52704	.51715	.50820	.50004
3.70	.57493	.56104	.54885	.53801	.52829	.51948	.51145
3.80	.58481	.57117	.55919	.54854	.53897	.53031	.52241
3.90	.59426	.58087	.56910	.55863	.54922	.54070	.53293
4.00	.60333	.59017	.57861	.56832	.55907	.55068	.54303
4.20	.62035	.60766	.59650	.58655	.57761	.56950	.56208
4.40	.63606	.62380	.61302	.60340	.59475	.58690	.57972
4.60	.65057	.63873	.62831	.61901	.61063	.60303	.59608
4.80	.66402	.65258	.64249	.63349	.62539	.61802	.61129
5.00	.67651	.66544	.65568	.64697	.63911	.63198	.62544
5.20	.68814	.67742	.66797	.65952	.65191	.64499	.63866
5.40	.69899	.68861	.67944	.67126	.66387	.65716	.65101
5.60	.70913	.69906	.69018	.68223	.67507	.66855	.66258
5.80	.71863	.70886	.70024	.69252	.68557	.67923	.67343
6.00	.72754	.71806	.70968	.70219	.69543	.68928	.68364
6.20	.73592	.72671	.71857	.71129	.70471	.69873	.69324
6.40	.74382	.73486	.72694	.71986	.71346	.70764	.70230
6.60	.75126	.74255	.73484	.72794	.72172	.71605	.71085
6.80	.75829	.74981	.74230	.73559	.72952	.72400	.71893
7.00	.76495	.75668	.74937	.74283	.73691	.73153	.72659

$n_2 = 2$

F \ n_1	9	10	11	12	13	14	15
7.50	.78011	.77234	.76548	.75933	.75377	.74871	.74406
8.00	.79346	.78614	.77967	.77387	.76863	.76386	.75948
8.50	.80530	.79839	.79227	.78679	.78183	.77731	.77317
9.00	.81587	.80932	.80352	.79832	.79362	.78934	.78541
9.50	.82536	.81914	.81363	.80869	.80422	.80015	.79641
10.00	.83393	.82801	.82276	.81805	.81380	.80992	.80635
10.50	.84171	.83606	.83104	.82655	.82249	.81878	.81538
11.00	.84880	.84339	.83859	.83430	.83041	.82686	.82361
11.50	.85528	.85010	.84550	.84139	.83766	.83426	.83114
12.00	.86123	.85626	.85185	.84790	.84432	.84106	.83806
12.50	.86672	.86194	.85770	.85390	.85046	.84733	.84444
13.00	.87179	.86719	.86311	.85945	.85614	.85312	.85034
13.50	.87649	.87205	.86812	.86460	.86140	.85849	.85582
14.00	.88086	.87658	.87278	.86938	.86630	.86349	.86090
15.00	.88874	.88474	.88119	.87800	.87512	.87250	.87008
16.00	.89564	.89188	.88855	.88557	.88286	.88039	.87812
17.00	.90174	.89820	.89506	.89225	.88970	.88737	.88524
18.00	.90717	.90382	.90086	.89819	.89578	.89359	.89156
19.00	.91203	.90886	.90604	.90352	.90124	.89915	.89723
20.00	.91641	.91339	.91072	.90832	.90615	.90416	.90234
21.00	.92037	.91750	.91495	.91266	.91059	.90870	.90697
22.00	.92398	.92123	.91880	.91662	.91464	.91283	.91118
23.00	.92727	.92464	.92232	.92023	.91834	.91661	.91502
24.00	.93029	.92777	.92554	.92354	.92172	.92007	.91855
25.00	.93307	.93065	.92851	.92659	.92484	.92325	.92179
26.00	.93564	.93331	.93125	.92940	.92773	.92620	.92479
27.00	.93802	.93578	.93379	.93201	.93039	.92892	.92757
28.00	.94022	.93806	.93615	.93443	.93287	.93145	.93015
29.00	.94228	.94020	.93835	.93669	.93518	.93381	.93255
30.00	.94420	.94218	.94040	.93879	.93734	.93601	.93479
31.00	.94600	.94405	.94231	.94076	.93935	.93807	.93689
32.00	.94768	.94579	.94411	.94261	.94125	.94000	.93886
33.00	.94926	.94743	.94580	.94434	.94302	.94181	.94071
34.00	.95075	.94897	.94740	.94598	.94469	.94352	.94245
35.00	.95216	.95043	.94890	.94752	.94627	.94513	.94409
36.00	.95349	.95181	.95031	.94897	.94776	.94665	.94564
37.00	.95474	.95311	.95165	.95035	.94917	.94809	.94711
38.00	.95593	.95434	.95292	.95166	.95051	.94946	.94849
39.00	.95706	.95551	.95413	.95289	.95177	.95075	.94981
40.00	.95813	.95662	.95528	.95407	.95298	.95198	.95107
42.00	.96012	.95868	.95740	.95625	.95521	.95427	.95339
44.00	.96193	.96056	.95934	.95824	.95725	.95634	.95551
46.00	.96359	.96227	.96110	.96006	.95910	.95824	.95744
48.00	.96510	.96384	.96272	.96172	.96081	.95998	.95921
50.00	.96650	.96529	.96421	.96325	.96237	.96158	.96084
52.00	.96779	.96662	.96559	.96466	.96382	.96305	.96235
54.00	.96898	.96786	.96686	.96597	.96516	.96442	.96374
56.00	.97009	.96900	.96804	.96718	.96640	.96569	.96503
58.00	.97112	.97007	.96915	.96831	.96756	.96687	.96624
60.00	.97208	.97107	.97017	.96937	.96864	.96798	.96736

$n_2 = 2$

F'\n1	9	10	11	12	13	14	15
62.00	.97298	.97200	.97113	.97036	.96965	.96901	.96842
64.00	.97382	.97288	.97204	.97128	.97060	.96998	.96940
66.00	.97462	.97370	.97288	.97215	.97149	.97088	.97033
68.00	.97536	.97447	.97368	.97297	.97233	.97174	.97120
70.00	.97607	.97520	.97443	.97374	.97312	.97255	.97202
75.00	.97766	.97685	.97614	.97549	.97491	.97438	.97389
80.00	.97906	.97830	.97763	.97702	.97648	.97598	.97552
85.00	.98029	.97958	.97894	.97838	.97786	.97739	.97696
90.00	.98138	.98071	.98011	.97958	.97909	.97865	.97824
95.00	.98236	.98173	.98116	.98065	.98019	.97977	.97938
100.00	.98324	.98264	.98210	.98162	.98118	.98078	.98041
105.00	.98404	.98346	.98295	.98249	.98208	.98170	.98135
110.00	.98477	.98422	.98373	.98329	.98289	.98253	.98219
115.00	.98543	.98490	.98443	.98401	.98364	.98329	.98297
120.00	.98604	.98553	.98508	.98468	.98432	.98398	.98368
125.00	.98660	.98611	.98568	.98529	.98494	.98462	.98433
130.00	.98711	.98664	.98623	.98586	.98552	.98522	.98493
135.00	.98759	.98714	.98674	.98638	.98606	.98576	.98549
140.00	.98803	.98760	.98721	.98687	.98656	.98627	.98601
150.00	.98883	.98843	.98807	.98774	.98745	.98719	.98694
160.00	.98953	.98915	.98881	.98851	.98824	.98799	.98776
170.00	.99014	.98979	.98947	.98919	.98893	.98869	.98848
180.00	.99069	.99035	.99006	.98979	.98954	.98932	.98912
190.00	.99118	.99086	.99058	.99032	.99009	.98988	.98969
200.00	.99162	.99132	.99105	.99081	.99059	.99039	.99021
210.00	.99202	.99173	.99148	.99125	.99104	.99085	.99067
220.00	.99238	.99211	.99186	.99164	.99145	.99126	.99110
230.00	.99271	.99245	.99222	.99201	.99182	.99164	.99148
240.00	.99302	.99277	.99254	.99234	.99216	.99199	.99184
250.00	.99330	.99305	.99284	.99265	.99247	.99231	.99217
260.00	.99355	.99332	.99312	.99293	.99276	.99261	.99247
270.00	.99379	.99357	.99337	.99319	.99303	.99288	.99275
280.00	.99402	.99380	.99361	.99343	.99328	.99314	.99300
290.00	.99422	.99401	.99383	.99366	.99351	.99337	.99325
300.00	.99441	.99421	.99403	.99387	.99373	.99359	.99347
320.00	.99476	.99457	.99441	.99425	.99412	.99399	.99388
340.00	.99507	.99489	.99474	.99459	.99446	.99435	.99424
360.00	.99535	.99518	.99503	.99489	.99477	.99466	.99456
380.00	.99559	.99543	.99529	.99516	.99505	.99494	.99485
400.00	.99581	.99566	.99552	.99540	.99529	.99519	.99510
420.00	.99601	.99587	.99574	.99562	.99552	.99542	.99534
440.00	.99619	.99605	.99593	.99582	.99572	.99563	.99555
460.00	.99636	.99623	.99611	.99600	.99591	.99582	.99574
480.00	.99651	.99638	.99627	.99617	.99608	.99600	.99592
500.00	.99665	.99653	.99642	.99632	.99624	.99616	.99608
520.00	.99678	.99666	.99656	.99646	.99638	.99630	.99623
540.00	.99690	.99678	.99668	.99660	.99651	.99644	.99637
560.00	.99701	.99690	.99680	.99672	.99664	.99657	.99650
580.00	.99711	.99701	.99691	.99683	.99675	.99669	.99662
600.00	.99721	.99711	.99702	.99694	.99686	.99680	.99674

$n_2 = 3$

F \ n_1	2	3	4	5	6	7	8
1.00	.69016	.50000	.37921	.29807	.24092	.19909	.16751
1.05	.70758	.52429	.40566	.32462	.26665	.22363	.19073
1.10	.72379	.54734	.43120	.35065	.29223	.24833	.21436
1.15	.73889	.56918	.45577	.37603	.31748	.27298	.23820
1.20	.75295	.58985	.47934	.40068	.34228	.29744	.26206
1.25	.76605	.60938	.50189	.42452	.36651	.32155	.28578
1.30	.77826	.62782	.52343	.44752	.39008	.34521	.30923
1.35	.78965	.64522	.54396	.46965	.41295	.36832	.33230
1.40	.80027	.66164	.56351	.49089	.43507	.39083	.35490
1.50	.81946	.69172	.59977	.53073	.47695	.43382	.39840
1.60	.83624	.71846	.63249	.56712	.51563	.47393	.43938
1.70	.85096	.74226	.66195	.60024	.55119	.51111	.47765
1.80	.86392	.76346	.68848	.63034	.58374	.54541	.51319
1.90	.87536	.78238	.71236	.65764	.61349	.57693	.54604
2.00	.88550	.79931	.73388	.68241	.64063	.60586	.57632
2.10	.89452	.81447	.75330	.70489	.66539	.63236	.60419
2.20	.90256	.82809	.77085	.72531	.68798	.65664	.62981
2.30	.90975	.84036	.78673	.74387	.70860	.67887	.65335
2.40	.91621	.85143	.80113	.76077	.72743	.69925	.67498
2.50	.92203	.86144	.81421	.77617	.74465	.71793	.69486
2.60	.92728	.87053	.82612	.79024	.76042	.73508	.71315
2.70	.93204	.87879	.83698	.80310	.77488	.75084	.72999
2.80	.93636	.88631	.84690	.81488	.78815	.76533	.74551
2.90	.94029	.89319	.85599	.82570	.80035	.77868	.75982
3.00	.94388	.89948	.86432	.83564	.81159	.79100	.77305
3.10	.94717	.90525	.87199	.84479	.82196	.80237	.78528
3.20	.95018	.91055	.87904	.85324	.83154	.81289	.79661
3.30	.95294	.91543	.88555	.86104	.84039	.82264	.80711
3.40	.95549	.91993	.89156	.86826	.84860	.83168	.81686
3.50	.95784	.92410	.89713	.87495	.85622	.84008	.82592
3.60	.96001	.92795	.90229	.88116	.86330	.84788	.83436
3.70	.96202	.93153	.90709	.88693	.86988	.85516	.84223
3.80	.96389	.93485	.91155	.89231	.87602	.86194	.84957
3.90	.96562	.93794	.91570	.89732	.88175	.86828	.85643
4.00	.96724	.94082	.91958	.90201	.88710	.87420	.86285
4.20	.97015	.94602	.92658	.91048	.89680	.88494	.87450
4.40	.97269	.95058	.93273	.91792	.90533	.89440	.88477
4.60	.97493	.95459	.93815	.92449	.91286	.90277	.89385
4.80	.97690	.95814	.94295	.93032	.91955	.91020	.90193
5.00	.97865	.96129	.94722	.93551	.92552	.91683	.90915
5.20	.98022	.96410	.95103	.94015	.93085	.92276	.91561
5.40	.98161	.96662	.95446	.94431	.93564	.92809	.92141
5.60	.98287	.96889	.95753	.94806	.93996	.93290	.92665
5.80	.98400	.97094	.96031	.95145	.94386	.93725	.93139
6.00	.98503	.97279	.96283	.95452	.94740	.94119	.93569
6.20	.98596	.97447	.96512	.95731	.95062	.94478	.93961
6.40	.98681	.97601	.96721	.95985	.95355	.94805	.94318
6.60	.98758	.97740	.96911	.96218	.95624	.95105	.94645
6.80	.98829	.97869	.97086	.96431	.95870	.95379	.94944
7.00	.98893	.97986	.97246	.96627	.96096	.95632	.95220

$n_2 = 3$

F' \ n_1	2	3	4	5	6	7	8
7.50	.99034	.98241	.97594	.97052	.96586	.96180	.95819
8.00	.99149	.98451	.97880	.97401	.96991	.96631	.96312
8.50	.99245	.98625	.98118	.97693	.97328	.97008	.96724
9.00	.99326	.98772	.98318	.97938	.97611	.97325	.97071
9.50	.99395	.98896	.98489	.98146	.97852	.97595	.97366
10.00	.99453	.99003	.98634	.98325	.98059	.97826	.97619
10.50	.99503	.99095	.98760	.98479	.98237	.98025	.97837
11.00	.99547	.99174	.98869	.98612	.98392	.98198	.98026
11.50	.99586	.99244	.98964	.98729	.98527	.98350	.98192
12.00	.99619	.99305	.99048	.98832	.98646	.98483	.98338
12.50	.99649	.99359	.99122	.98923	.98751	.98601	.98467
13.00	.99675	.99407	.99188	.99003	.98845	.98705	.98582
13.50	.99699	.99450	.99247	.99075	.98928	.98799	.98684
14.00	.99720	.99489	.99299	.99140	.99003	.98882	.98775
15.00	.99756	.99554	.99389	.99250	.99130	.99025	.98932
16.00	.99785	.99608	.99463	.99340	.99235	.99143	.99061
17.00	.99810	.99653	.99524	.99415	.99322	.99240	.99167
18.00	.99830	.99690	.99575	.99478	.99395	.99322	.99257
19.00	.99847	.99722	.99618	.99531	.99457	.99391	.99333
20.00	.99862	.99749	.99655	.99577	.99509	.99450	.99397
21.00	.99875	.99772	.99687	.99616	.99555	.99501	.99453
22.00	.99886	.99792	.99715	.99650	.99594	.99545	.99502
23.00	.99896	.99810	.99739	.99680	.99629	.99584	.99544
24.00	.99904	.99825	.99760	.99706	.99659	.99618	.99581
25.00	.99912	.99839	.99779	.99729	.99686	.99648	.99614
26.00	.99918	.99851	.99796	.99749	.99709	.99674	.99643
27.00	.99924	.99862	.99811	.99767	.99730	.99698	.99669
28.00	.99930	.99871	.99824	.99784	.99749	.99719	.99692
29.00	.99934	.99880	.99836	.99798	.99766	.99738	.99713
30.00	.99939	.99888	.99846	.99812	.99781	.99755	.99731
31.00	.99942	.99895	.99856	.99823	.99795	.99771	.99748
32.00	.99946	.99902	.99865	.99834	.99808	.99785	.99764
33.00	.99949	.99907	.99873	.99844	.99819	.99797	.99778
34.00	.99952	.99913	.99880	.99853	.99830	.99809	.99791
35.00	.99955	.99918	.99887	.99861	.99839	.99820	.99803
36.00	.99957	.99922	.99893	.99869	.99848	.99830	.99813
37.00	.99960	.99926	.99899	.99876	.99856	.99839	.99823
38.00	.99962	.99930	.99904	.99882	.99864	.99847	.99832
39.00	.99964	.99934	.99909	.99888	.99871	.99855	.99841
40.00	.99965	.99937	.99914	.99894	.99877	.99862	.99849
42.00	.99969	.99943	.99922	.99904	.99888	.99875	.99863
44.00	.99971	.99948	.99928	.99912	.99898	.99886	.99875
46.00	.99974	.99952	.99935	.99920	.99907	.99896	.99886
48.00	.99976	.99956	.99940	.99926	.99914	.99904	.99895
50.00	.99978	.99959	.99945	.99932	.99921	.99912	.99903
52.00	.99979	.99963	.99949	.99937	.99927	.99918	.99910
54.00	.99981	.99965	.99952	.99942	.99932	.99924	.99917
56.00	.99982	.99968	.99956	.99946	.99937	.99930	.99923
58.00	.99983	.99970	.99959	.99949	.99941	.99934	.99928
60.00	.99984	.99972	.99961	.99953	.99945	.99939	.99933

$n_2 = 3$

F' \ n_1	2	3	4	5	6	7	8
62.00	.99985	.99974	.99964	.99956	.99949	.99942	.99937
64.00	.99986	.99975	.99966	.99958	.99952	.99946	.99941
66.00	.99987	.99977	.99968	.99961	.99955	.99949	.99944
68.00	.99988	.99978	.99970	.99963	.99957	.99952	.99948
70.00	.99988	.99979	.99972	.99965	.99960	.99955	.99951
75.00	.99990	.99982	.99975	.99970	.99965	.99961	.99957
80.00	.99991	.99984	.99978	.99973	.99969	.99965	.99962
85.00	.99992	.99986	.99981	.99976	.99973	.99969	.99966
90.00	.99993	.99987	.99983	.99979	.99976	.99973	.99970
95.00	.99994	.99989	.99984	.99981	.99978	.99975	.99973
100.00	.99994	.99990	.99986	.99983	.99980	.99978	.99976
105.00	.99995	.99991	.99987	.99984	.99982	.99980	.99978
110.00	.99995	.99991	.99988	.99986	.99984	.99982	.99980
115.00	.99996	.99992	.99989	.99987	.99985	.99983	.99982
120.00	.99996	.99993	.99990	.99988	.99986	.99985	.99983
125.00	.99996	.99993	.99991	.99989	.99987	.99986	.99984
130.00	.99996	.99994	.99992	.99990	.99988	.99987	.99986
135.00	.99997	.99994	.99992	.99991	.99989	.99988	.99987
140.00	.99997	.99995	.99993	.99991	.99990	.99989	.99988
150.00	.99997	.99995	.99994	.99992	.99991	.99990	.99989
160.00	.99998	.99996	.99994	.99993	.99992	.99991	.99990
170.00	.99998	.99996	.99995	.99994	.99993	.99992	.99992
180.00	.99998	.99997	.99996	.99995	.99994	.99993	.99992
190.00	.99998	.99997	.99996	.99995	.99994	.99994	.99993
200.00	.99998	.99997	.99996	.99996	.99995	.99994	.99994
210.00	.99999	.99998	.99997	.99996	.99995	.99995	.99994
220.00	.99999	.99998	.99997	.99996	.99996	.99995	.99995
230.00	.99999	.99998	.99997	.99997	.99996	.99996	.99995
240.00	.99999	.99998	.99997	.99997	.99997	.99996	.99996
250.00	.99999	.99998	.99998	.99997	.99997	.99996	.99996
260.00	.99999	.99998	.99998	.99997	.99997	.99997	.99996
270.00	.99999	.99998	.99998	.99998	.99997	.99997	.99997
280.00	.99999	.99999	.99998	.99998	.99997	.99997	.99997
290.00	.99999	.99999	.99998	.99998	.99998	.99997	.99997
300.00	.99999	.99999	.99998	.99998	.99998	.99998	.99997
320.00	.99999	.99999	.99999	.99998	.99998	.99998	.99998
340.00	.99999	.99999	.99999	.99999	.99998	.99998	.99998
360.00	.99999	.99999	.99999	.99999	.99999	.99998	.99998
380.00	1.00000	.99999	.99999	.99999	.99999	.99999	.99998
400.00		.99999	.99999	.99999	.99999	.99999	.99999
420.00		.99999	.99999	.99999	.99999	.99999	.99999
440.00		.99999	.99999	.99999	.99999	.99999	.99999
460.00		1.00000	.99999	.99999	.99999	.99999	.99999
480.00			.99999	.99999	.99999	.99999	.99999
500.00			1.00000	.99999	.99999	.99999	.99999
520.00				1.00000	.99999	.99999	.99999
540.00					1.00000	1.00000	.99999
560.00							1.00000

$n_2 = 3$

F' \ n_1	9	10	11	12	13	14	15
1.00	.14306	.12372	.10814	.09539	.08482	.07596	.06845
1.05	.16493	.14430	.12750	.11363	.10201	.09219	.08379
1.10	.18744	.16570	.14783	.13293	.12037	.10965	.10042
1.15	.21037	.18768	.16889	.15310	.13968	.12815	.11816
1.20	.23351	.21006	.19047	.17391	.15974	.14749	.13681
1.25	.25670	.23263	.21240	.19518	.18037	.16749	.15620
1.30	.27978	.25524	.23450	.21674	.20138	.18796	.17614
1.35	.30262	.27775	.25661	.23842	.22261	.20874	.19647
1.40	.32512	.30004	.27861	.26010	.24393	.22968	.21704
1.50	.36877	.34357	.32186	.30295	.28631	.27155	.25836
1.60	.41022	.38524	.36357	.34456	.32773	.31271	.29921
1.70	.44922	.42470	.40330	.38442	.36763	.35256	.33896
1.80	.48565	.46176	.44081	.42224	.40564	.39069	.37714
1.90	.51949	.49637	.47599	.45785	.44158	.42687	.41350
2.00	.55083	.52854	.50881	.49120	.47535	.46097	.44786
2.10	.57978	.55836	.53934	.52231	.50694	.49296	.48017
2.20	.60649	.58595	.56767	.55125	.53639	.52286	.51045
2.30	.63109	.61144	.59391	.57812	.56380	.55073	.53873
2.40	.65376	.63498	.61819	.60304	.58927	.57668	.56509
2.50	.67465	.65671	.64065	.62613	.61291	.60080	.58964
2.60	.69390	.67678	.66142	.64752	.63485	.62322	.61249
2.70	.71165	.69533	.68065	.66734	.65520	.64404	.63373
2.80	.72804	.71247	.69844	.68572	.67408	.66339	.65349
2.90	.74318	.72832	.71493	.70276	.69162	.68136	.67187
3.00	.75719	.74301	.73021	.71857	.70791	.69808	.68898
3.10	.77015	.75662	.74439	.73326	.72305	.71363	.70490
3.20	.78218	.76925	.75756	.74691	.73714	.72811	.71974
3.30	.79334	.78099	.76981	.75962	.75025	.74161	.73358
3.40	.80371	.79190	.78121	.77145	.76248	.75419	.74649
3.50	.81336	.80207	.79183	.78248	.77389	.76594	.75855
3.60	.82234	.81154	.80174	.79278	.78454	.77692	.76982
3.70	.83073	.82038	.81099	.80241	.79450	.78718	.78038
3.80	.83856	.82865	.81965	.81141	.80382	.79680	.79026
3.90	.84588	.83638	.82774	.81984	.81256	.80581	.79952
4.00	.85273	.84362	.83533	.82774	.82074	.81426	.80822
4.20	.86518	.85678	.84913	.84212	.83566	.82966	.82407
4.40	.87616	.86839	.86132	.85484	.84885	.84329	.83811
4.60	.88589	.87870	.87214	.86612	.86057	.85540	.85059
4.80	.89454	.88786	.88177	.87618	.87101	.86621	.86173
5.00	.90227	.89606	.89039	.88518	.88036	.87588	.87170
5.20	.90920	.90340	.89811	.89325	.88875	.88457	.88066
5.40	.91543	.91001	.90507	.90052	.89631	.89240	.88874
5.60	.92105	.91598	.91135	.90709	.90314	.89947	.89604
5.80	.92614	.92138	.91704	.91304	.90934	.90589	.90267
6.00	.93076	.92629	.92220	.91844	.91496	.91172	.90869
6.20	.93496	.93076	.92691	.92337	.92009	.91704	.91418
6.40	.93880	.93484	.93121	.92787	.92478	.92189	.91920
6.60	.94232	.93857	.93515	.93199	.92907	.92634	.92379
6.80	.94554	.94200	.93876	.93577	.93301	.93043	.92802
7.00	.94850	.94515	.94208	.93925	.93663	.93419	.93190

$n_2 = 3$

F' \ n_1	9	10	11	12	13	14	15
7.50	.95494	.95200	.94930	.94682	.94452	.94237	.94036
8.00	.96026	.95765	.95527	.95307	.95103	.94913	.94735
8.50	.96469	.96237	.96025	.95829	.95647	.95478	.95319
9.00	.96842	.96635	.96444	.96269	.96106	.95954	.95812
9.50	.97160	.96973	.96801	.96643	.96496	.96360	.96231
10.00	.97432	.97263	.97108	.96964	.96831	.96707	.96591
10.50	.97667	.97513	.97372	.97242	.97121	.97008	.96902
11.00	.97872	.97731	.97602	.97483	.97372	.97269	.97172
11.50	.98050	.97921	.97803	.97694	.97593	.97498	.97409
12.00	.98208	.98089	.97980	.97880	.97786	.97699	.97618
12.50	.98347	.98237	.98137	.98044	.97958	.97877	.97802
13.00	.98470	.98369	.98276	.98190	.98110	.98035	.97966
13.50	.98580	.98486	.98400	.98320	.98246	.98177	.98112
14.00	.98679	.98591	.98511	.98437	.98368	.98303	.98243
15.00	.98848	.98771	.98701	.98636	.98576	.98520	.98467
16.00	.98986	.98919	.98857	.98800	.98747	.98698	.98651
17.00	.99102	.99042	.98987	.98936	.98889	.98845	.98804
18.00	.99198	.99145	.99096	.99051	.99009	.98969	.98933
19.00	.99280	.99232	.99188	.99147	.99110	.99074	.99041
20.00	.99350	.99306	.99267	.99230	.99196	.99164	.99134
21.00	.99410	.99371	.99335	.99301	.99270	.99241	.99214
22.00	.99462	.99426	.99393	.99363	.99335	.99309	.99284
23.00	.99508	.99475	.99445	.99417	.99391	.99367	.99344
24.00	.99548	.99518	.99490	.99464	.99441	.99419	.99398
25.00	.99583	.99555	.99530	.99506	.99484	.99464	.99445
26.00	.99615	.99589	.99565	.99543	.99523	.99504	.99487
27.00	.99642	.99619	.99597	.99577	.99558	.99540	.99524
28.00	.99667	.99645	.99625	.99606	.99589	.99572	.99557
29.00	.99690	.99669	.99650	.99633	.99616	.99601	.99587
30.00	.99710	.99691	.99673	.99657	.99642	.99627	.99614
31.00	.99729	.99710	.99694	.99679	.99664	.99651	.99638
32.00	.99745	.99728	.99713	.99698	.99685	.99672	.99661
33.00	.99760	.99744	.99730	.99716	.99704	.99692	.99681
34.00	.99774	.99759	.99745	.99733	.99721	.99710	.99699
35.00	.99787	.99773	.99760	.99748	.99736	.99726	.99716
36.00	.99799	.99785	.99773	.99761	.99751	.99741	.99732
37.00	.99809	.99797	.99785	.99774	.99764	.99755	.99746
38.00	.99819	.99807	.99796	.99786	.99776	.99767	.99759
39.00	.99828	.99817	.99806	.99797	.99788	.99779	.99771
40.00	.99837	.99826	.99816	.99807	.99798	.99790	.99783
42.00	.99852	.99842	.99833	.99825	.99817	.99810	.99803
44.00	.99865	.99856	.99848	.99840	.99833	.99826	.99820
46.00	.99877	.99868	.99861	.99854	.99847	.99841	.99835
48.00	.99887	.99879	.99872	.99866	.99860	.99854	.99849
50.00	.99895	.99888	.99882	.99876	.99871	.99866	.99861
52.00	.99903	.99897	.99891	.99885	.99880	.99876	.99871
54.00	.99910	.99904	.99899	.99894	.99889	.99885	.99881
56.00	.99917	.99911	.99906	.99901	.99897	.99893	.99889
58.00	.99922	.99917	.99912	.99908	.99904	.99900	.99896
60.00	.99927	.99923	.99918	.99914	.99910	.99907	.99903

$n_2 = 3$

$F' \backslash n_1$	9	10	11	12	13	14	15
62.00	.99932	.99927	.99923	.99919	.99916	.99912	.99909
64.00	.99936	.99932	.99928	.99924	.99921	.99918	.99915
66.00	.99940	.99936	.99932	.99929	.99926	.99923	.99920
68.00	.99943	.99940	.99936	.99933	.99930	.99927	.99925
70.00	.99947	.99943	.99940	.99937	.99934	.99931	.99929
75.00	.99953	.99950	.99947	.99945	.99942	.99940	.99938
80.00	.99959	.99956	.99954	.99951	.99949	.99947	.99945
85.00	.99964	.99961	.99959	.99957	.99955	.99953	.99952
90.00	.99968	.99965	.99963	.99962	.99960	.99958	.99957
95.00	.99971	.99969	.99967	.99966	.99964	.99963	.99961
100.00	.99974	.99972	.99970	.99969	.99968	.99966	.99965
105.00	.99976	.99975	.99973	.99972	.99971	.99969	.99968
110.00	.99978	.99977	.99976	.99974	.99973	.99972	.99971
115.00	.99980	.99979	.99978	.99976	.99975	.99974	.99974
120.00	.99982	.99981	.99979	.99978	.99977	.99977	.99976
125.00	.99983	.99982	.99981	.99980	.99979	.99978	.99978
130.00	.99984	.99983	.99982	.99982	.99981	.99980	.99979
135.00	.99986	.99985	.99984	.99983	.99982	.99981	.99981
140.00	.99987	.99986	.99985	.99984	.99983	.99983	.99982
150.00	.99988	.99988	.99987	.99986	.99986	.99985	.99984
160.00	.99990	.99989	.99988	.99988	.99987	.99987	.99986
170.00	.99991	.99990	.99990	.99989	.99989	.99988	.99988
180.00	.99992	.99991	.99991	.99990	.99990	.99990	.99989
190.00	.99993	.99992	.99992	.99991	.99991	.99991	.99990
200.00	.99993	.99993	.99993	.99992	.99992	.99992	.99991
210.00	.99994	.99994	.99993	.99993	.99993	.99992	.99992
220.00	.99995	.99994	.99994	.99994	.99993	.99993	.99993
230.00	.99995	.99995	.99994	.99994	.99994	.99994	.99993
240.00	.99995	.99995	.99995	.99995	.99994	.99994	.99994
250.00	.99996	.99996	.99995	.99995	.99995	.99995	.99994
260.00	.99996	.99996	.99996	.99995	.99995	.99995	.99995
270.00	.99996	.99996	.99996	.99996	.99996	.99995	.99995
280.00	.99997	.99997	.99996	.99996	.99996	.99996	.99996
290.00	.99997	.99997	.99997	.99996	.99996	.99996	.99996
300.00	.99997	.99997	.99997	.99997	.99996	.99996	.99996
320.00	.99998	.99997	.99997	.99997	.99997	.99997	.99997
340.00	.99998	.99998	.99998	.99997	.99997	.99997	.99997
360.00	.99998	.99998	.99998	.99998	.99998	.99998	.99997
380.00	.99998	.99998	.99998	.99998	.99998	.99998	.99998
400.00	.99999	.99998	.99998	.99998	.99998	.99998	.99998
420.00	.99999	.99999	.99999	.99998	.99998	.99998	.99998
440.00	.99999	.99999	.99999	.99999	.99999	.99999	.99999
460.00	.99999	.99999	.99999	.99999	.99999	.99999	.99999
480.00	.99999	.99999	.99999	.99999	.99999	.99999	.99999
500.00	.99999	.99999	.99999	.99999	.99999	.99999	.99999
520.00	.99999	.99999	.99999	.99999	.99999	.99999	.99999
540.00	.99999	.99999	.99999	.99999	.99999	.99999	.99999
560.00	1.00000	1.00000	.99999	.99999	.99999	.99999	.99999
580.00			1.00000	1.00000	1.00000	1.00000	.99999
600.00							1.00000

$n_2 = 4$

F' \ n_1	2	3	4	5	6	7	8
1.00	.78655	.62079	.50000	.41099	.34393	.29224	.25158
1.05	.80307	.64676	.53066	.44363	.37702	.32495	.28345
1.10	.81816	.67094	.55970	.47502	.40930	.35726	.31529
1.15	.83194	.69341	.58710	.50504	.44056	.38891	.34681
1.20	.84453	.71427	.61288	.53364	.47066	.41970	.37777
1.25	.85603	.73360	.63708	.56078	.49952	.44949	.40796
1.30	.86654	.75150	.65974	.58646	.52707	.47815	.43724
1.35	.87616	.76807	.68093	.61069	.55328	.50563	.46550
1.40	.88496	.78339	.70072	.63350	.57813	.53186	.49265
1.50	.90040	.81068	.73639	.67506	.62388	.58058	.54347
1.60	.91339	.83403	.76735	.71161	.66456	.62434	.58956
1.70	.92437	.85403	.79420	.74365	.70056	.66341	.63102
1.80	.93367	.87120	.81749	.77169	.73232	.69813	.66813
1.90	.94159	.88597	.83771	.79621	.76030	.72891	.70121
2.00	.94836	.89870	.85528	.81768	.78494	.75616	.73064
2.10	.95417	.90972	.87058	.83649	.80664	.78027	.75679
2.20	.95917	.91929	.88394	.85299	.82576	.80161	.78002
2.30	.96350	.92761	.89563	.86749	.84264	.82051	.80066
2.40	.96726	.93488	.90588	.88026	.85755	.83727	.81901
2.50	.97054	.94125	.91490	.89154	.87076	.85215	.83535
2.60	.97341	.94684	.92286	.90152	.88248	.86539	.84992
2.70	.97592	.95177	.92989	.91037	.89290	.87718	.86293
2.80	.97814	.95613	.93613	.91823	.90219	.88771	.87456
2.90	.98010	.96000	.94168	.92524	.91048	.89713	.88499
3.00	.98184	.96344	.94662	.93150	.91789	.90557	.89435
3.10	.98339	.96650	.95104	.93711	.92455	.91316	.90276
3.20	.98477	.96924	.95500	.94214	.93053	.91998	.91035
3.30	.98600	.97170	.95855	.94667	.93591	.92614	.91719
3.40	.98711	.97391	.96175	.95074	.94077	.93170	.92338
3.50	.98810	.97590	.96464	.95443	.94517	.93673	.92900
3.60	.98900	.97770	.96725	.95776	.94915	.94130	.93409
3.70	.98981	.97932	.96961	.96079	.95277	.94545	.93873
3.80	.99054	.98080	.97176	.96354	.95606	.94923	.94295
3.90	.99121	.98214	.97372	.96605	.95906	.95268	.94680
4.00	.99182	.98336	.97550	.96833	.96180	.95583	.95033
4.20	.99287	.98549	.97861	.97233	.96660	.96135	.95651
4.40	.99376	.98727	.98123	.97570	.97065	.96601	.96173
4.60	.99450	.98878	.98344	.97855	.97407	.96996	.96617
4.80	.99513	.99006	.98532	.98098	.97699	.97333	.96995
5.00	.99567	.99116	.98693	.98305	.97950	.97623	.97320
5.20	.99614	.99210	.98832	.98484	.98166	.97872	.97601
5.40	.99654	.99292	.98952	.98639	.98353	.98088	.97844
5.60	.99688	.99362	.99056	.98774	.98515	.98277	.98056
5.80	.99719	.99424	.99147	.98892	.98657	.98441	.98241
6.00	.99745	.99478	.99227	.98995	.98782	.98586	.98404
6.20	.99768	.99525	.99297	.99086	.98892	.98713	.98547
6.40	.99789	.99567	.99359	.99166	.98989	.98826	.98674
6.60	.99807	.99604	.99414	.99238	.99075	.98926	.98787
6.80	.99823	.99638	.99462	.99301	.99152	.99015	.98887
7.00	.99838	.99667	.99506	.99358	.99221	.99094	.98977

$n_2 = 4$

$F' \backslash n_1$	2	3	4	5	6	7	8
7.50	.99868	.99728	.99596	.99475	.99363	.99259	.99163
8.00	.99890	.99775	.99666	.99565	.99472	.99386	.99307
8.50	.99908	.99812	.99721	.99636	.99558	.99486	.99419
9.00	.99923	.99841	.99764	.99693	.99627	.99566	.99509
9.50	.99934	.99865	.99799	.99738	.99682	.99630	.99581
10.00	.99943	.99884	.99827	.99775	.99727	.99682	.99640
10.50	.99951	.99899	.99850	.99805	.99763	.99724	.99688
11.00	.99957	.99912	.99870	.99830	.99794	.99760	.99728
11.50	.99963	.99923	.99886	.99851	.99819	.99789	.99762
12.00	.99967	.99932	.99899	.99869	.99841	.99814	.99790
12.50	.99971	.99940	.99911	.99884	.99859	.99836	.99814
13.00	.99974	.99947	.99921	.99897	.99874	.99854	.99834
13.50	.99977	.99952	.99929	.99908	.99888	.99869	.99852
14.00	.99979	.99957	.99936	.99917	.99899	.99883	.99867
15.00	.99983	.99965	.99948	.99932	.99918	.99904	.99892
16.00	.99986	.99971	.99957	.99944	.99932	.99921	.99911
17.00	.99988	.99976	.99964	.99953	.99943	.99934	.99925
18.00	.99990	.99980	.99970	.99961	.99952	.99944	.99937
19.00	.99992	.99983	.99974	.99967	.99959	.99953	.99947
20.00	.99993	.99985	.99978	.99971	.99965	.99959	.99954
21.00	.99994	.99987	.99981	.99975	.99970	.99965	.99960
22.00	.99994	.99989	.99983	.99978	.99974	.99969	.99965
23.00	.99995	.99990	.99985	.99981	.99977	.99973	.99970
24.00	.99996	.99991	.99987	.99983	.99980	.99976	.99973
25.00	.99996	.99992	.99989	.99985	.99982	.99979	.99976
26.00	.99997	.99993	.99990	.99987	.99984	.99981	.99979
27.00	.99997	.99994	.99991	.99988	.99986	.99983	.99981
28.00	.99997	.99994	.99992	.99989	.99987	.99985	.99983
29.00	.99997	.99995	.99993	.99990	.99988	.99987	.99985
30.00	.99998	.99995	.99993	.99991	.99990	.99988	.99986
31.00	.99998	.99996	.99994	.99992	.99991	.99989	.99988
32.00	.99998	.99996	.99995	.99993	.99991	.99990	.99989
33.00	.99998	.99997	.99995	.99994	.99992	.99991	.99990
34.00	.99998	.99997	.99995	.99994	.99993	.99992	.99991
35.00	.99998	.99997	.99996	.99995	.99993	.99992	.99991
36.00	.99999	.99997	.99996	.99995	.99994	.99993	.99992
37.00	.99999	.99997	.99996	.99995	.99994	.99993	.99993
38.00	.99999	.99998	.99997	.99996	.99995	.99994	.99993
39.00	.99999	.99998	.99997	.99996	.99995	.99994	.99994
40.00	.99999	.99998	.99997	.99996	.99996	.99995	.99994
42.00	.99999	.99998	.99997	.99997	.99996	.99995	.99995
44.00	.99999	.99998	.99998	.99997	.99997	.99996	.99996
46.00	.99999	.99999	.99998	.99998	.99997	.99997	.99996
48.00	.99999	.99999	.99998	.99998	.99997	.99997	.99997
50.00	.99999	.99999	.99998	.99998	.99998	.99997	.99997
52.00	.99999	.99999	.99999	.99998	.99998	.99998	.99997
54.00	.99999	.99999	.99999	.99998	.99998	.99998	.99998
56.00	1.00000	.99999	.99999	.99999	.99998	.99998	.99998
58.00		.99999	.99999	.99999	.99998	.99998	.99998
60.00		.99999	.99999	.99999	.99999	.99998	.99998

$n_2 = 4$

$F' \backslash n_1$	2	3	4	5	6	7	8
62.00		.99999	.99999	.99999	.99999	.99999	.99998
64.00		.99999	.99999	.99999	.99999	.99999	.99998
66.00		.99999	.99999	.99999	.99999	.99999	.99999
68.00		.99999	.99999	.99999	.99999	.99999	.99999
70.00		.99999	.99999	.99999	.99999	.99999	.99999
75.00		1.00000	.99999	.99999	.99999	.99999	.99999
80.00			1.00000	.99999	.99999	.99999	.99999
85.00				1.00000	.99999	.99999	.99999
90.00					.99999	.99999	.99999
95.00					1.00000	1.00000	.99999
100.00							1.00000

$n_2 = 4$

$F \backslash n_1$	9	10	11	12	13	14	15
1.00	.21902	.19252	.17067	.15242	.13702	.12390	.11262
1.05	.24980	.22211	.19902	.17954	.16294	.14867	.13630
1.10	.28089	.25229	.22822	.20773	.19012	.17486	.16152
1.15	.31197	.28274	.25792	.23663	.21819	.20210	.18794
1.20	.34276	.31314	.28781	.26592	.24683	.23007	.21523
1.25	.37302	.34325	.31760	.29529	.27573	.25845	.24308
1.30	.40257	.37283	.34706	.32451	.30463	.28698	.27120
1.35	.43127	.40173	.37599	.35336	.33330	.31541	.29934
1.40	.45901	.42981	.40424	.38166	.36155	.34353	.32729
1.50	.51130	.48313	.45824	.43606	.41617	.39822	.38192
1.60	.55915	.53230	.50840	.48697	.46762	.45004	.43400
1.70	.60250	.57716	.55446	.53398	.51539	.49842	.48285
1.80	.64154	.61778	.59638	.57698	.55929	.54307	.52813
1.90	.67653	.65436	.63431	.61605	.59934	.58396	.56974
2.00	.70779	.68719	.66847	.65138	.63567	.62117	.60772
2.10	.73568	.71658	.69917	.68321	.66851	.65490	.64224
2.20	.76054	.74286	.72670	.71184	.69811	.68538	.67351
2.30	.78270	.76635	.75136	.73755	.72477	.71287	.70177
2.40	.80246	.78734	.77346	.76063	.74874	.73765	.72729
2.50	.82009	.80611	.79325	.78136	.77030	.75998	.75031
2.60	.83583	.82292	.81101	.79997	.78969	.78008	.77107
2.70	.84992	.83797	.82694	.81670	.80715	.79821	.78981
2.80	.86254	.85148	.84126	.83175	.82287	.81455	.80673
2.90	.87387	.86362	.85414	.84531	.83705	.82931	.82202
3.00	.88405	.87455	.86574	.85754	.84986	.84265	.83585
3.10	.89322	.88440	.87622	.86858	.86144	.85472	.84838
3.20	.90149	.89330	.88569	.87858	.87192	.86566	.85974
3.30	.90896	.90134	.89426	.88764	.88143	.87558	.87006
3.40	.91573	.90863	.90203	.89586	.89006	.88460	.87944
3.50	.92186	.91525	.90909	.90333	.89791	.89281	.88798
3.60	.92744	.92127	.91552	.91013	.90507	.90029	.89577
3.70	.93252	.92675	.92137	.91633	.91159	.90712	.90289
3.80	.93714	.93175	.92672	.92200	.91756	.91336	.90939
3.90	.94137	.93632	.93160	.92718	.92301	.91908	.91535
4.00	.94524	.94050	.93608	.93193	.92802	.92432	.92082
4.20	.95203	.94785	.94395	.94028	.93683	.93356	.93046
4.40	.95777	.95407	.95061	.94736	.94430	.94139	.93864
4.60	.96264	.95936	.95628	.95339	.95066	.94807	.94562
4.80	.96681	.96388	.96113	.95855	.95611	.95379	.95160
5.00	.97039	.96777	.96530	.96299	.96080	.95872	.95675
5.20	.97348	.97112	.96891	.96682	.96485	.96299	.96121
5.40	.97616	.97404	.97204	.97016	.96838	.96669	.96509
5.60	.97850	.97658	.97477	.97307	.97146	.96993	.96847
5.80	.98054	.97880	.97716	.97561	.97415	.97276	.97144
6.00	.98234	.98075	.97926	.97785	.97652	.97526	.97406
6.20	.98392	.98248	.98111	.97983	.97862	.97746	.97636
6.40	.98533	.98400	.98276	.98158	.98047	.97941	.97841
6.60	.98657	.98536	.98422	.98314	.98212	.98115	.98023
6.80	.98768	.98656	.98552	.98453	.98359	.98270	.98185
7.00	.98867	.98764	.98668	.98577	.98490	.98408	.98330

$n_2 = 4$

F' \ n_1	9	10	11	12	13	14	15
7.50	.99073	.98989	.98909	.98834	.98763	.98696	.98631
8.00	.99232	.99162	.99096	.99034	.98975	.98919	.98865
8.50	.99357	.99298	.99243	.99190	.99141	.99094	.99049
9.00	.99456	.99406	.99359	.99315	.99273	.99233	.99195
9.50	.99536	.99493	.99453	.99416	.99380	.99345	.99313
10.00	.99601	.99564	.99530	.99497	.99466	.99437	.99409
10.50	.99655	.99623	.99593	.99565	.99538	.99512	.99488
11.00	.99699	.99671	.99645	.99620	.99597	.99575	.99553
11.50	.99736	.99712	.99689	.99667	.99647	.99627	.99608
12.00	.99767	.99746	.99726	.99707	.99688	.99671	.99655
12.50	.99794	.99775	.99757	.99740	.99724	.99709	.99694
13.00	.99816	.99800	.99784	.99768	.99754	.99741	.99727
13.50	.99836	.99821	.99807	.99793	.99780	.99768	.99756
14.00	.99853	.99839	.99826	.99814	.99803	.99792	.99781
15.00	.99880	.99869	.99859	.99849	.99839	.99830	.99822
16.00	.99901	.99892	.99883	.99875	.99867	.99860	.99853
17.00	.99917	.99910	.99903	.99896	.99889	.99883	.99877
18.00	.99930	.99924	.99918	.99912	.99907	.99901	.99896
19.00	.99941	.99935	.99930	.99925	.99920	.99916	.99912
20.00	.99949	.99944	.99940	.99936	.99932	.99928	.99924
21.00	.99956	.99952	.99948	.99944	.99941	.99938	.99934
22.00	.99962	.99958	.99955	.99952	.99949	.99946	.99943
23.00	.99966	.99963	.99960	.99958	.99955	.99952	.99950
24.00	.99970	.99968	.99965	.99963	.99960	.99958	.99956
25.00	.99974	.99971	.99969	.99967	.99965	.99963	.99961
26.00	.99977	.99975	.99973	.99971	.99969	.99967	.99965
27.00	.99979	.99977	.99975	.99974	.99972	.99970	.99969
28.00	.99981	.99980	.99978	.99976	.99975	.99974	.99972
29.00	.99983	.99982	.99980	.99979	.99977	.99976	.99975
30.00	.99985	.99983	.99982	.99981	.99980	.99978	.99977
31.00	.99986	.99985	.99984	.99983	.99981	.99980	.99979
32.00	.99987	.99986	.99985	.99984	.99983	.99982	.99981
33.00	.99989	.99987	.99986	.99986	.99985	.99984	.99983
34.00	.99990	.99989	.99988	.99987	.99986	.99985	.99984
35.00	.99990	.99989	.99989	.99988	.99987	.99986	.99986
36.00	.99991	.99990	.99990	.99989	.99988	.99987	.99987
37.00	.99992	.99991	.99990	.99990	.99989	.99988	.99988
38.00	.99992	.99992	.99991	.99990	.99990	.99989	.99989
39.00	.99993	.99992	.99992	.99991	.99991	.99990	.99990
40.00	.99994	.99993	.99992	.99992	.99991	.99991	.99990
42.00	.99994	.99994	.99993	.99993	.99992	.99992	.99992
44.00	.99995	.99995	.99994	.99994	.99993	.99993	.99993
46.00	.99996	.99995	.99995	.99995	.99994	.99994	.99994
48.00	.99996	.99996	.99995	.99995	.99995	.99995	.99994
50.00	.99997	.99996	.99996	.99996	.99995	.99995	.99995
52.00	.99997	.99997	.99996	.99996	.99996	.99996	.99995
54.00	.99997	.99997	.99997	.99997	.99996	.99996	.99996
56.00	.99998	.99997	.99997	.99997	.99997	.99997	.99996
58.00	.99998	.99998	.99997	.99997	.99997	.99997	.99997
60.00	.99998	.99998	.99998	.99997	.99997	.99997	.99997

$n_2 = 4$

F' \ n_1	9	10	11	12	13	14	15
62.00	.99998	.99998	.99998	.99998	.99998	.99997	.99997
64.00	.99998	.99998	.99998	.99998	.99998	.99998	.99997
66.00	.99998	.99998	.99998	.99998	.99998	.99998	.99998
68.00	.99999	.99998	.99998	.99998	.99998	.99998	.99998
70.00	.99999	.99999	.99998	.99998	.99998	.99998	.99998
75.00	.99999	.99999	.99999	.99999	.99999	.99998	.99998
80.00	.99999	.99999	.99999	.99999	.99999	.99999	.99999
85.00	.99999	.99999	.99999	.99999	.99999	.99999	.99999
90.00	.99999	.99999	.99999	.99999	.99999	.99999	.99999
95.00	.99999	.99999	.99999	.99999	.99999	.99999	.99999
100.00	.99999	.99999	.99999	.99999	.99999	.99999	.99999
105.00	1.00000	.99999	.99999	.99999	.99999	.99999	.99999
110.00		1.00000	1.00000	.99999	.99999	.99999	.99999
115.00				1.00000	1.00000	.99999	.99999
120.00						.99999	.99999
125.00						1.00000	1.00000

$n_2 = 5$

F' \ n_1	2	3	4	5	6	7	8
1.00	.84299	.70193	.58901	.50000	.42941	.37277	.32673
1.05	.85801	.72757	.62111	.53573	.46695	.41095	.36483
1.10	.87150	.75103	.65099	.56950	.50293	.44802	.40225
1.15	.88360	.77246	.67870	.60126	.53718	.48371	.43866
1.20	.89447	.79200	.70432	.63097	.56959	.51783	.47381
1.25	.90422	.80979	.72794	.65868	.60011	.55026	.50749
1.30	.91298	.82598	.74967	.68443	.62873	.58093	.53959
1.35	.92084	.84070	.76964	.70830	.65549	.60981	.57002
1.40	.92792	.85407	.78795	.73037	.68042	.63690	.59875
1.50	.94001	.87726	.82009	.76955	.72510	.68589	.65113
1.60	.94982	.89642	.84703	.80280	.76345	.72838	.69699
1.70	.95783	.91225	.86957	.83093	.79621	.76500	.73683
1.80	.96438	.92538	.88845	.85471	.82413	.79643	.77127
1.90	.96976	.93628	.90429	.87480	.84790	.82336	.80094
2.00	.97421	.94537	.91759	.89180	.86812	.84641	.82646
2.10	.97791	.95298	.92879	.90621	.88535	.86613	.84840
2.20	.98098	.95937	.93826	.91844	.90005	.88303	.86726
2.30	.98356	.96475	.94628	.92885	.91261	.89752	.88350
2.40	.98573	.96931	.95309	.93773	.92337	.90997	.89749
2.50	.98757	.97317	.95891	.94534	.93260	.92070	.90956
2.60	.98912	.97647	.96388	.95186	.94055	.92995	.92001
2.70	.99045	.97929	.96815	.95748	.94741	.93795	.92906
2.80	.99159	.98172	.97183	.96233	.95335	.94489	.93693
2.90	.99256	.98380	.97500	.96654	.95851	.95093	.94378
3.00	.99340	.98561	.97776	.97019	.96299	.95619	.94977
3.10	.99413	.98718	.98015	.97337	.96691	.96079	.95501
3.20	.99476	.98854	.98224	.97615	.97033	.96482	.95960
3.30	.99531	.98973	.98407	.97858	.97334	.96836	.96364
3.40	.99579	.99078	.98568	.98072	.97598	.97148	.96721
3.50	.99622	.99169	.98709	.98261	.97832	.97423	.97036
3.60	.99659	.99250	.98833	.98427	.98038	.97667	.97315
3.70	.99691	.99321	.98943	.98575	.98221	.97884	.97562
3.80	.99720	.99384	.99041	.98706	.98383	.98076	.97783
3.90	.99746	.99441	.99128	.98822	.98528	.98247	.97980
4.00	.99769	.99491	.99205	.98926	.98657	.98400	.98155
4.20	.99808	.99575	.99336	.99102	.98877	.98661	.98454
4.40	.99838	.99643	.99442	.99244	.99053	.98871	.98696
4.60	.99863	.99698	.99527	.99359	.99197	.99042	.98893
4.80	.99884	.99743	.99597	.99454	.99315	.99182	.99054
5.00	.99901	.99780	.99655	.99532	.99412	.99298	.99188
5.20	.99914	.99810	.99702	.99596	.99493	.99394	.99299
5.40	.99926	.99836	.99742	.99650	.99561	.99475	.99392
5.60	.99936	.99857	.99776	.99695	.99617	.99542	.99470
5.80	.99944	.99875	.99804	.99734	.99665	.99599	.99536
6.00	.99951	.99890	.99828	.99766	.99706	.99648	.99592
6.20	.99957	.99903	.99848	.99794	.99741	.99690	.99640
6.40	.99962	.99915	.99866	.99817	.99770	.99725	.99682
6.60	.99966	.99924	.99881	.99838	.99796	.99756	.99717
6.80	.99970	.99932	.99894	.99856	.99818	.99782	.99748
7.00	.99973	.99940	.99905	.99871	.99838	.99805	.99775

$n_2 = 5$

F' \ n_1	2	3	4	5	6	7	8
7.50	.99979	.99954	.99928	.99901	.99876	.99851	.99827
8.00	.99984	.99964	.99944	.99923	.99903	.99884	.99866
8.50	.99987	.99972	.99956	.99939	.99924	.99909	.99894
9.00	.99990	.99977	.99964	.99952	.99939	.99927	.99915
9.50	.99992	.99982	.99971	.99961	.99951	.99941	.99931
10.00	.99993	.99985	.99977	.99968	.99960	.99952	.99944
10.50	.99994	.99988	.99981	.99974	.99967	.99960	.99954
11.00	.99995	.99990	.99984	.99978	.99972	.99967	.99961
11.50	.99996	.99991	.99986	.99982	.99977	.99972	.99968
12.00	.99997	.99993	.99989	.99984	.99980	.99976	.99973
12.50	.99997	.99994	.99990	.99987	.99983	.99980	.99977
13.00	.99998	.99995	.99992	.99989	.99986	.99983	.99980
13.50	.99998	.99995	.99993	.99990	.99988	.99985	.99983
14.00	.99998	.99996	.99994	.99992	.99989	.99987	.99985
15.00	.99999	.99997	.99995	.99994	.99992	.99990	.99989
16.00	.99999	.99998	.99996	.99995	.99994	.99992	.99991
17.00	.99999	.99998	.99997	.99996	.99995	.99994	.99993
18.00	.99999	.99998	.99998	.99997	.99996	.99995	.99995
19.00	.99999	.99999	.99998	.99997	.99997	.99996	.99996
20.00	.99999	.99999	.99998	.99998	.99997	.99997	.99996
21.00	1.00000	.99999	.99999	.99998	.99998	.99997	.99997
22.00		.99999	.99999	.99999	.99998	.99998	.99998
23.00		.99999	.99999	.99999	.99998	.99998	.99998
24.00		.99999	.99999	.99999	.99999	.99998	.99998
25.00		1.00000	.99999	.99999	.99999	.99999	.99999
26.00			.99999	.99999	.99999	.99999	.99999
27.00			.99999	.99999	.99999	.99999	.99999
28.00			1.00000	.99999	.99999	.99999	.99999
29.00				.99999	.99999	.99999	.99999
30.00				1.00000	.99999	.99999	.99999
31.00					1.00000	.99999	.99999
32.00						.99999	.99999
33.00						1.00000	.99999
34.00							1.00000

$n_2 = 5$

F' \ n_1	9	10	11	12	13	14	15
1.00	.28883	.25727	.23072	.20816	.18884	.17214	.15762
1.05	.32638	.29400	.26645	.24281	.22235	.20452	.18887
1.10	.36368	.33085	.30265	.27823	.25691	.23818	.22161
1.15	.40033	.36739	.33886	.31394	.29202	.27262	.25535
1.20	.43600	.40326	.37467	.34952	.32724	.30740	.28961
1.25	.47047	.43816	.40975	.38460	.36219	.34210	.32400
1.30	.50354	.47187	.44385	.41890	.39653	.37638	.35814
1.35	.53510	.50424	.47677	.45217	.43002	.40997	.39173
1.40	.56507	.53513	.50835	.48426	.46246	.44264	.42454
1.50	.62012	.59229	.56717	.54437	.52358	.50454	.48703
1.60	.66874	.64318	.61994	.59870	.57920	.56123	.54459
1.70	.71130	.68804	.66675	.64717	.62910	.61236	.59679
1.80	.74831	.72727	.70791	.69003	.67343	.65799	.64356
1.90	.78037	.76143	.74392	.72767	.71253	.69838	.68513
2.00	.80808	.79108	.77529	.76059	.74684	.73395	.72184
2.10	.83199	.81675	.80256	.78929	.77685	.76516	.75413
2.20	.85262	.83898	.82623	.81428	.80305	.79246	.78246
2.30	.87043	.85822	.84678	.83603	.82590	.81633	.80727
2.40	.88582	.87489	.86462	.85496	.84583	.83718	.82898
2.50	.89913	.88934	.88013	.87143	.86321	.85540	.84799
2.60	.91068	.90190	.89362	.88580	.87838	.87134	.86463
2.70	.92070	.91282	.90538	.89833	.89164	.88528	.87922
2.80	.92943	.92235	.91565	.90929	.90325	.89750	.89201
2.90	.93704	.93067	.92463	.91889	.91343	.90823	.90326
3.00	.94370	.93795	.93250	.92731	.92238	.91766	.91316
3.10	.94953	.94434	.93941	.93472	.93025	.92597	.92188
3.20	.95465	.94996	.94549	.94124	.93719	.93331	.92959
3.30	.95916	.95491	.95086	.94700	.94332	.93979	.93641
3.40	.96315	.95929	.95561	.95210	.94875	.94554	.94246
3.50	.96667	.96316	.95981	.95662	.95356	.95064	.94783
3.60	.96979	.96660	.96355	.96063	.95785	.95517	.95261
3.70	.97257	.96965	.96687	.96421	.96166	.95922	.95687
3.80	.97504	.97237	.96983	.96740	.96507	.96283	.96068
3.90	.97724	.97481	.97248	.97025	.96811	.96606	.96409
4.00	.97922	.97698	.97485	.97280	.97084	.96896	.96714
4.20	.98257	.98069	.97888	.97716	.97550	.97390	.97236
4.40	.98529	.98369	.98216	.98069	.97928	.97792	.97661
4.60	.98750	.98614	.98483	.98357	.98237	.98121	.98009
4.80	.98932	.98815	.98703	.98595	.98491	.98391	.98295
5.00	.99083	.98982	.98885	.98792	.98702	.98616	.98532
5.20	.99208	.99120	.99036	.98956	.98878	.98803	.98731
5.40	.99313	.99237	.99163	.99093	.99025	.98960	.98897
5.60	.99401	.99334	.99270	.99209	.99150	.99092	.99037
5.80	.99475	.99417	.99361	.99307	.99255	.99205	.99156
6.00	.99539	.99487	.99438	.99390	.99344	.99300	.99257
6.20	.99593	.99548	.99504	.99462	.99421	.99382	.99344
6.40	.99640	.99599	.99561	.99523	.99487	.99452	.99419
6.60	.99680	.99644	.99609	.99576	.99544	.99513	.99483
6.80	.99715	.99682	.99652	.99622	.99593	.99565	.99539
7.00	.99745	.99716	.99688	.99662	.99636	.99611	.99587

$n_2 = 5$

F' \ n_1	9	10	11	12	13	14	15
7.50	.99805	.99782	.99761	.99741	.99721	.99702	.99683
8.00	.99848	.99831	.99814	.99798	.99783	.99768	.99753
8.50	.99880	.99866	.99853	.99840	.99828	.99816	.99805
9.00	.99904	.99893	.99883	.99872	.99863	.99853	.99844
9.50	.99922	.99913	.99905	.99897	.99889	.99881	.99874
10.00	.99936	.99929	.99922	.99915	.99909	.99903	.99897
10.50	.99948	.99942	.99936	.99930	.99925	.99920	.99915
11.00	.99956	.99951	.99947	.99942	.99937	.99933	.99929
11.50	.99963	.99959	.99955	.99951	.99947	.99944	.99940
12.00	.99969	.99965	.99962	.99959	.99956	.99952	.99949
12.50	.99974	.99971	.99968	.99965	.99962	.99959	.99957
13.00	.99977	.99975	.99972	.99970	.99968	.99965	.99963
13.50	.99981	.99978	.99976	.99974	.99972	.99970	.99968
14.00	.99983	.99981	.99979	.99978	.99976	.99974	.99972
15.00	.99987	.99986	.99984	.99983	.99982	.99980	.99979
16.00	.99990	.99989	.99988	.99987	.99986	.99985	.99984
17.00	.99992	.99991	.99990	.99990	.99989	.99988	.99987
18.00	.99994	.99993	.99992	.99992	.99991	.99990	.99990
19.00	.99995	.99994	.99994	.99993	.99993	.99992	.99992
20.00	.99996	.99995	.99995	.99995	.99994	.99994	.99993
21.00	.99997	.99996	.99996	.99995	.99995	.99995	.99994
22.00	.99997	.99997	.99997	.99996	.99996	.99996	.99995
23.00	.99998	.99997	.99997	.99997	.99997	.99996	.99996
24.00	.99998	.99998	.99998	.99997	.99997	.99997	.99997
25.00	.99998	.99998	.99998	.99998	.99998	.99997	.99997
26.00	.99999	.99998	.99998	.99998	.99998	.99998	.99998
27.00	.99999	.99999	.99998	.99998	.99998	.99998	.99998
28.00	.99999	.99999	.99999	.99999	.99998	.99998	.99998
29.00	.99999	.99999	.99999	.99999	.99999	.99998	.99998
30.00	.99999	.99999	.99999	.99999	.99999	.99999	.99999
31.00	.99999	.99999	.99999	.99999	.99999	.99999	.99999
32.00	.99999	.99999	.99999	.99999	.99999	.99999	.99999
33.00	.99999	.99999	.99999	.99999	.99999	.99999	.99999
34.00	1.00000	.99999	.99999	.99999	.99999	.99999	.99999
35.00		.99999	.99999	.99999	.99999	.99999	.99999
36.00		1.00000	.99999	.99999	.99999	.99999	.99999
37.00			1.00000	.99999	.99999	.99999	.99999
38.00				1.00000	.99999	.99999	.99999
39.00					1.00000	.99999	.99999
40.00						1.00000	.99999
42.00							1.00000

$n_2 = 6$

F' \ n_1	2	3	4	5	6	7	8
1.00	.87917	.75908	.65607	.57059	.50000	.44148	.39261
1.05	.89267	.78356	.68814	.60756	.53997	.48311	.43498
1.10	.90460	.80562	.71752	.64196	.57767	.52289	.47595
1.15	.91514	.82544	.74434	.67379	.61300	.56058	.51519
1.20	.92445	.84323	.76873	.70310	.64589	.59604	.55246
1.25	.93267	.85917	.79086	.72999	.67637	.62920	.58760
1.30	.93994	.87343	.81089	.75457	.70449	.66005	.62055
1.35	.94636	.88619	.82899	.77698	.73034	.68863	.65128
1.40	.95203	.89759	.84532	.79737	.75403	.71500	.67982
1.50	.96150	.91689	.87329	.83268	.79546	.76153	.73059
1.60	.96894	.93230	.89596	.86166	.82987	.80057	.77360
1.70	.97481	.94463	.91432	.88539	.85831	.83312	.80975
1.80	.97946	.95452	.92919	.90479	.88176	.86017	.84000
1.90	.98316	.96247	.94127	.92067	.90108	.88260	.86522
2.00	.98612	.96889	.95109	.93367	.91700	.90118	.88624
2.10	.98850	.97410	.95911	.94435	.93014	.91659	.90373
2.20	.99042	.97833	.96567	.95313	.94100	.92939	.91832
2.30	.99198	.98179	.97106	.96038	.95000	.94003	.93049
2.40	.99325	.98463	.97550	.96638	.95748	.94890	.94067
2.50	.99430	.98698	.97918	.97137	.96372	.95632	.94920
2.60	.99516	.98891	.98224	.97552	.96893	.96253	.95636
2.70	.99588	.99053	.98479	.97900	.97330	.96776	.96240
2.80	.99647	.99187	.98692	.98192	.97698	.97216	.96750
2.90	.99697	.99300	.98872	.98438	.98008	.97589	.97182
3.00	.99738	.99395	.99023	.98646	.98271	.97905	.97549
3.10	.99773	.99475	.99152	.98822	.98495	.98174	.97862
3.20	.99803	.99543	.99261	.98972	.98685	.98404	.98130
3.30	.99828	.99601	.99354	.99101	.98849	.98601	.98359
3.40	.99850	.99651	.99433	.99211	.98988	.98770	.98556
3.50	.99868	.99693	.99502	.99305	.99109	.98916	.98727
3.60	.99884	.99729	.99560	.99387	.99213	.99042	.98874
3.70	.99897	.99761	.99611	.99457	.99303	.99151	.99002
3.80	.99909	.99788	.99655	.99518	.99381	.99246	.99113
3.90	.99919	.99812	.99694	.99572	.99449	.99328	.99209
4.00	.99928	.99832	.99727	.99618	.99509	.99400	.99294
4.20	.99943	.99866	.99782	.99694	.99606	.99519	.99433
4.40	.99954	.99892	.99824	.99753	.99682	.99611	.99541
4.60	.99963	.99912	.99857	.99799	.99741	.99683	.99626
4.80	.99969	.99928	.99883	.99835	.99787	.99740	.99693
5.00	.99975	.99941	.99903	.99864	.99824	.99785	.99746
5.20	.99979	.99951	.99919	.99887	.99854	.99821	.99788
5.40	.99982	.99959	.99933	.99905	.99878	.99850	.99823
5.60	.99985	.99965	.99943	.99920	.99897	.99874	.99851
5.80	.99988	.99971	.99952	.99933	.99913	.99893	.99874
6.00	.99989	.99975	.99959	.99943	.99926	.99909	.99892
6.20	.99991	.99979	.99965	.99951	.99937	.99922	.99908
6.40	.99992	.99982	.99970	.99958	.99945	.99933	.99921
6.60	.99993	.99984	.99974	.99964	.99953	.99942	.99932
6.80	.99994	.99986	.99978	.99969	.99959	.99950	.99941
7.00	.99995	.99988	.99981	.99973	.99965	.99957	.99949

$n_2 = 6$

F'\ n_1	2	3	4	5	6	7	8
7.50	.99996	.99991	.99986	.99980	.99975	.99969	.99963
8.00	.99997	.99994	.99990	.99986	.99981	.99977	.99973
8.50	.99998	.99995	.99992	.99989	.99986	.99983	.99980
9.00	.99998	.99996	.99994	.99992	.99990	.99987	.99985
9.50	.99999	.99997	.99996	.99994	.99992	.99990	.99988
10.00	.99999	.99998	.99997	.99995	.99994	.99992	.99991
10.50	.99999	.99998	.99997	.99996	.99995	.99994	.99993
11.00	.99999	.99999	.99998	.99997	.99996	.99995	.99994
11.50	.99999	.99999	.99998	.99998	.99997	.99996	.99996
12.00	1.00000	.99999	.99999	.99998	.99997	.99997	.99996
12.50		.99999	.99999	.99998	.99998	.99997	.99997
13.00		.99999	.99999	.99999	.99998	.99998	.99998
13.50		.99999	.99999	.99999	.99999	.99998	.99998
14.00		1.00000	.99999	.99999	.99999	.99999	.99998
15.00			1.00000	.99999	.99999	.99999	.99999
16.00				1.00000	.99999	.99999	.99999
17.00					1.00000	.99999	.99999
18.00						1.00000	1.00000

$n_2 = 6$

$F \backslash n_1$	9	10	11	12	13	14	15
1.00	.35145	.31652	.28661	.26083	.23845	.21889	.20169
1.05	.39394	.35869	.32819	.30161	.27831	.25775	.23952
1.10	.43549	.40036	.36966	.34266	.31879	.29755	.27856
1.15	.47566	.44102	.41049	.38341	.35928	.33765	.31818
1.20	.51416	.48031	.45024	.42338	.39926	.37751	.35781
1.25	.55075	.51793	.48857	.46216	.43831	.41667	.39695
1.30	.58529	.55369	.52523	.49948	.47608	.45474	.43520
1.35	.61772	.58746	.56004	.53510	.51233	.49146	.47225
1.40	.64802	.61917	.59291	.56890	.54687	.52659	.50785
1.50	.70232	.67643	.65264	.63070	.61041	.59159	.57407
1.60	.74874	.72578	.70452	.68477	.66638	.64921	.63314
1.70	.78805	.76786	.74905	.73147	.71500	.69954	.68499
1.80	.82114	.80350	.78696	.77143	.75682	.74303	.73000
1.90	.84889	.83354	.81907	.80543	.79253	.78032	.76873
2.00	.87212	.85878	.84617	.83423	.82290	.81213	.80188
2.10	.89154	.87997	.86900	.85857	.84864	.83918	.83015
2.20	.90778	.89776	.88821	.87911	.87043	.86213	.85419
2.30	.92138	.91269	.90438	.89645	.88886	.88159	.87462
2.40	.93278	.92523	.91801	.91109	.90446	.89809	.89198
2.50	.94236	.93580	.92951	.92347	.91767	.91209	.90673
2.60	.95042	.94471	.93923	.93395	.92888	.92399	.91927
2.70	.95723	.95225	.94746	.94284	.93840	.93411	.92996
2.80	.96299	.95864	.95445	.95040	.94650	.94273	.93909
2.90	.96788	.96407	.96039	.95684	.95341	.95010	.94689
3.00	.97204	.96870	.96547	.96235	.95933	.95640	.95357
3.10	.97559	.97265	.96981	.96706	.96439	.96181	.95931
3.20	.97863	.97604	.97353	.97110	.96875	.96647	.96425
3.30	.98124	.97895	.97674	.97459	.97250	.97048	.96851
3.40	.98348	.98146	.97950	.97759	.97574	.97395	.97220
3.50	.98542	.98363	.98189	.98019	.97855	.97695	.97540
3.60	.98710	.98551	.98396	.98245	.98098	.97956	.97817
3.70	.98856	.98714	.98576	.98441	.98310	.98183	.98059
3.80	.98983	.98856	.98732	.98612	.98495	.98381	.98271
3.90	.99093	.98980	.98869	.98762	.98657	.98555	.98455
4.00	.99190	.99088	.98989	.98893	.98799	.98707	.98618
4.20	.99349	.99267	.99187	.99109	.99033	.98959	.98886
4.40	.99473	.99406	.99341	.99277	.99215	.99154	.99095
4.60	.99570	.99515	.99462	.99409	.99358	.99308	.99260
4.80	.99647	.99601	.99557	.99514	.99472	.99430	.99390
5.00	.99708	.99670	.99633	.99597	.99562	.99528	.99494
5.20	.99756	.99725	.99694	.99664	.99635	.99606	.99578
5.40	.99796	.99770	.99744	.99718	.99694	.99669	.99646
5.60	.99828	.99806	.99784	.99763	.99742	.99721	.99701
5.80	.99854	.99835	.99817	.99799	.99781	.99763	.99746
6.00	.99876	.99860	.99844	.99828	.99813	.99798	.99784
6.20	.99894	.99880	.99866	.99853	.99840	.99827	.99815
6.40	.99909	.99897	.99885	.99874	.99862	.99851	.99841
6.60	.99921	.99911	.99901	.99891	.99881	.99872	.99862
6.80	.99932	.99923	.99914	.99905	.99897	.99889	.99881
7.00	.99941	.99933	.99925	.99918	.99910	.99903	.99896

$n_2 = 6$

F'\ n_1	9	10	11	12	13	14	15
7.50	.99958	.99952	.99946	.99941	.99936	.99930	.99925
8.00	.99969	.99965	.99961	.99957	.99953	.99949	.99945
8.50	.99977	.99974	.99971	.99968	.99965	.99962	.99959
9.00	.99983	.99980	.99978	.99976	.99973	.99971	.99969
9.50	.99987	.99985	.99983	.99981	.99980	.99978	.99976
10.00	.99990	.99988	.99987	.99985	.99984	.99983	.99981
10.50	.99992	.99991	.99990	.99989	.99987	.99986	.99985
11.00	.99994	.99993	.99992	.99991	.99990	.99989	.99988
11.50	.99995	.99994	.99993	.99993	.99992	.99991	.99991
12.00	.99996	.99995	.99995	.99994	.99993	.99993	.99992
12.50	.99997	.99996	.99996	.99995	.99995	.99994	.99994
13.00	.99997	.99997	.99996	.99996	.99996	.99995	.99995
13.50	.99998	.99997	.99997	.99997	.99996	.99996	.99996
14.00	.99998	.99998	.99998	.99997	.99997	.99997	.99996
15.00	.99999	.99998	.99998	.99998	.99998	.99998	.99997
16.00	.99999	.99999	.99999	.99999	.99998	.99998	.99998
17.00	.99999	.99999	.99999	.99999	.99999	.99999	.99999
18.00	.99999	.99999	.99999	.99999	.99999	.99999	.99999
19.00	1.00000	1.00000	.99999	.99999	.99999	.99999	.99999
20.00			1.00000	1.00000	.99999	.99999	.99999
21.00					1.00000	1.00000	.99999
22.00							1.00000

$n_2 = 7$

F'\ n_1	2	3	4	5	6	7	8
1.00	.90388	.80091	.70776	.62723	.55852	.50000	.45001
1.05	.91599	.82393	.73902	.66432	.59957	.54361	.49516
1.10	.92654	.84437	.76725	.69833	.63774	.58469	.53820
1.15	.93573	.86248	.79264	.72934	.67297	.62304	.57880
1.20	.94372	.87849	.81539	.75747	.70529	.65858	.61679
1.25	.95068	.89263	.83572	.78288	.73479	.69132	.65209
1.30	.95673	.90508	.85384	.80577	.76159	.72131	.68467
1.35	.96201	.91605	.86997	.82631	.78585	.74867	.71460
1.40	.96659	.92571	.88430	.84472	.80775	.77353	.74197
1.50	.97408	.94168	.90828	.87587	.84517	.81640	.78955
1.60	.97978	.95405	.92713	.90066	.87529	.85126	.82863
1.70	.98414	.96364	.94192	.92032	.89942	.87944	.86047
1.80	.98749	.97110	.95354	.93592	.91871	.90214	.88629
1.90	.99007	.97691	.96268	.94828	.93412	.92039	.90717
2.00	.99207	.98147	.96990	.95811	.94643	.93505	.92404
2.10	.99364	.98505	.97561	.96593	.95629	.94685	.93767
2.20	.99486	.98787	.98015	.97217	.96420	.95635	.94869
2.30	.99583	.99012	.98377	.97718	.97056	.96403	.95762
2.40	.99660	.99191	.98666	.98120	.97570	.97024	.96487
2.50	.99721	.99334	.98899	.98445	.97986	.97529	.97078
2.60	.99770	.99449	.99088	.98709	.98324	.97940	.97561
2.70	.99809	.99542	.99241	.98923	.98600	.98276	.97956
2.80	.99841	.99618	.99365	.99098	.98825	.98552	.98281
2.90	.99867	.99680	.99467	.99241	.99011	.98779	.98549
3.00	.99888	.99731	.99551	.99360	.99164	.98967	.98771
3.10	.99906	.99772	.99620	.99458	.99291	.99123	.98956
3.20	.99920	.99807	.99677	.99539	.99396	.99253	.99109
3.30	.99932	.99836	.99725	.99606	.99484	.99361	.99238
3.40	.99942	.99860	.99764	.99663	.99558	.99452	.99346
3.50	.99950	.99880	.99798	.99710	.99620	.99528	.99437
3.60	.99957	.99896	.99826	.99750	.99672	.99593	.99513
3.70	.99963	.99910	.99849	.99784	.99716	.99647	.99578
3.80	.99968	.99922	.99870	.99813	.99754	.99694	.99634
3.90	.99972	.99933	.99887	.99837	.99786	.99733	.99681
4.00	.99976	.99941	.99901	.99858	.99813	.99767	.99721
4.20	.99982	.99955	.99924	.99891	.99856	.99821	.99786
4.40	.99986	.99965	.99941	.99916	.99889	.99861	.99834
4.60	.99989	.99973	.99954	.99934	.99913	.99891	.99870
4.80	.99991	.99979	.99964	.99948	.99931	.99914	.99897
5.00	.99993	.99983	.99971	.99958	.99945	.99932	.99918
5.20	.99994	.99986	.99977	.99967	.99956	.99945	.99934
5.40	.99995	.99989	.99981	.99973	.99964	.99956	.99947
5.60	.99996	.99991	.99985	.99978	.99971	.99964	.99957
5.80	.99997	.99993	.99988	.99982	.99976	.99970	.99964
6.00	.99997	.99994	.99990	.99985	.99980	.99976	.99971
6.20	.99998	.99995	.99991	.99988	.99984	.99980	.99976
6.40	.99998	.99996	.99993	.99990	.99986	.99983	.99980
6.60	.99999	.99996	.99994	.99991	.99989	.99986	.99983
6.80	.99999	.99997	.99995	.99993	.99990	.99988	.99986
7.00	.99999	.99997	.99996	.99994	.99992	.99990	.99988

$n_2 = 7$

F' \ n_1	2	3	4	5	6	7	8
7.50	.99999	.99998	.99997	.99996	.99995	.99993	.99992
8.00	.99999	.99999	.99998	.99997	.99996	.99995	.99994
8.50	1.00000	.99999	.99999	.99998	.99997	.99997	.99996
9.00		.99999	.99999	.99999	.99998	.99998	.99997
9.50		1.00000	.99999	.99999	.99999	.99998	.99998
10.00			.99999	.99999	.99999	.99999	.99999
10.50			1.00000	.99999	.99999	.99999	.99999
11.00				1.00000	.99999	.99999	.99999
11.50					1.00000	.99999	.99999
12.00						1.00000	1.00000

$n_2 = 7$

F' \ n_1	9	10	11	12	13	14	15
1.00	.40709	.37004	.33786	.30976	.28507	.26328	.24394
1.05	.45304	.41624	.38392	.35540	.33009	.30754	.28735
1.10	.49732	.46123	.42922	.40070	.37517	.35223	.33152
1.15	.53951	.50450	.47316	.44501	.41961	.39662	.37571
1.20	.57934	.54568	.51532	.48783	.46286	.44010	.41927
1.25	.61664	.58453	.55536	.52878	.50447	.48218	.46167
1.30	.65131	.62090	.59308	.56758	.54413	.52250	.50250
1.35	.68337	.65472	.62836	.60407	.58161	.56079	.54145
1.40	.71286	.68600	.66117	.63815	.61678	.59688	.57832
1.50	.76453	.74121	.71944	.69909	.68004	.66216	.64536
1.60	.80734	.78733	.76851	.75078	.73407	.71829	.70336
1.70	.84248	.82546	.80934	.79407	.77959	.76583	.75275
1.80	.87117	.85677	.84306	.82999	.81755	.80567	.79432
1.90	.89449	.88235	.87074	.85963	.84899	.83880	.82903
2.00	.91342	.90321	.89340	.88398	.87493	.86622	.85785
2.10	.92878	.92020	.91192	.90395	.89626	.88884	.88169
2.20	.94125	.93403	.92706	.92031	.91379	.90748	.90138
2.30	.95138	.94531	.93942	.93372	.92819	.92283	.91763
2.40	.95963	.95452	.94955	.94472	.94003	.93547	.93104
2.50	.96637	.96205	.95785	.95375	.94977	.94589	.94212
2.60	.97188	.96823	.96467	.96119	.95781	.95450	.95128
2.70	.97641	.97332	.97029	.96733	.96445	.96163	.95888
2.80	.98014	.97751	.97494	.97242	.96995	.96754	.96519
2.90	.98322	.98098	.97878	.97663	.97452	.97246	.97044
3.00	.98577	.98386	.98198	.98014	.97833	.97656	.97482
3.10	.98790	.98626	.98465	.98306	.98151	.97999	.97849
3.20	.98967	.98826	.98688	.98552	.98418	.98286	.98157
3.30	.99115	.98994	.98875	.98757	.98642	.98528	.98417
3.40	.99240	.99136	.99032	.98931	.98831	.98732	.98636
3.50	.99345	.99255	.99165	.99077	.98990	.98905	.98821
3.60	.99434	.99356	.99278	.99201	.99126	.99051	.98978
3.70	.99510	.99441	.99373	.99307	.99241	.99176	.99112
3.80	.99574	.99514	.99455	.99397	.99339	.99282	.99226
3.90	.99628	.99576	.99524	.99473	.99423	.99373	.99324
4.00	.99675	.99629	.99584	.99539	.99495	.99451	.99408
4.20	.99750	.99715	.99679	.99645	.99610	.99576	.99543
4.40	.99806	.99778	.99751	.99723	.99696	.99670	.99643
4.60	.99848	.99826	.99804	.99783	.99761	.99740	.99719
4.80	.99880	.99862	.99845	.99828	.99811	.99794	.99777
5.00	.99904	.99890	.99876	.99863	.99849	.99835	.99822
5.20	.99923	.99912	.99900	.99889	.99878	.99868	.99857
5.40	.99938	.99928	.99919	.99910	.99901	.99893	.99884
5.60	.99949	.99942	.99934	.99927	.99920	.99912	.99905
5.80	.99958	.99952	.99946	.99940	.99934	.99928	.99922
6.00	.99966	.99961	.99956	.99950	.99945	.99941	.99936
6.20	.99971	.99967	.99963	.99959	.99955	.99951	.99947
6.40	.99976	.99973	.99969	.99966	.99962	.99959	.99955
6.60	.99980	.99977	.99974	.99971	.99968	.99965	.99962
6.80	.99983	.99981	.99978	.99976	.99973	.99971	.99968
7.00	.99986	.99984	.99982	.99979	.99977	.99975	.99973

$n_2 = 7$

F' \ n_1	9	10	11	12	13	14	15
7.50	.99991	.99989	.99988	.99986	.99985	.99983	.99982
8.00	.99994	.99993	.99992	.99991	.99990	.99989	.99988
8.50	.99995	.99995	.99994	.99993	.99993	.99992	.99991
9.00	.99997	.99996	.99996	.99995	.99995	.99994	.99994
9.50	.99998	.99997	.99997	.99997	.99996	.99996	.99995
10.00	.99998	.99998	.99998	.99997	.99997	.99997	.99997
10.50	.99999	.99999	.99998	.99998	.99998	.99998	.99997
11.00	.99999	.99999	.99999	.99999	.99998	.99998	.99998
11.50	.99999	.99999	.99999	.99999	.99999	.99999	.99998
12.00	.99999	.99999	.99999	.99999	.99999	.99999	.99999
12.50	1.00000	1.00000	.99999	.99999	.99999	.99999	.99999
13.00			1.00000	.99999	.99999	.99999	.99999
13.50				1.00000	1.00000	.99999	.99999
14.00						1.00000	.99999
15.00							1.00000

$n_2 = 8$

F' \ n_1	2	3	4	5	6	7	8
1.00	.92155	.83249	.74842	.67327	.60739	.54999	.50000
1.05	.93244	.85398	.77848	.70981	.64864	.59456	.54682
1.10	.94181	.87282	.80527	.74286	.68647	.63597	.59085
1.15	.94985	.88929	.82903	.77258	.72092	.67410	.63182
1.20	.95676	.90364	.85003	.79916	.75208	.70895	.66962
1.25	.96269	.91614	.86854	.82285	.78011	.74060	.70424
1.30	.96777	.92700	.88480	.84387	.80523	.76918	.73574
1.35	.97214	.93642	.89906	.86248	.82763	.79488	.76427
1.40	.97588	.94460	.91156	.87891	.84756	.81789	.78998
1.50	.98187	.95785	.93203	.90612	.88090	.85673	.83372
1.60	.98629	.96781	.94764	.92714	.90696	.88739	.86860
1.70	.98958	.97531	.95954	.94334	.92722	.91146	.89619
1.80	.99203	.98098	.96862	.95580	.94295	.93028	.91791
1.90	.99387	.98527	.97556	.96540	.95514	.94496	.93497
2.00	.99526	.98853	.98088	.97281	.96461	.95643	.94835
2.10	.99630	.99102	.98496	.97854	.97197	.96539	.95886
2.20	.99710	.99293	.98812	.98299	.97771	.97240	.96711
2.30	.99772	.99441	.99056	.98645	.98220	.97790	.97361
2.40	.99819	.99555	.99247	.98915	.98572	.98223	.97874
2.50	.99856	.99644	.99396	.99128	.98849	.98566	.98281
2.60	.99884	.99714	.99513	.99296	.99069	.98837	.98604
2.70	.99907	.99769	.99606	.99428	.99243	.99053	.98861
2.80	.99924	.99812	.99679	.99534	.99382	.99226	.99068
2.90	.99938	.99847	.99738	.99618	.99493	.99364	.99234
3.00	.99950	.99874	.99784	.99686	.99582	.99476	.99367
3.10	.99959	.99896	.99822	.99741	.99655	.99566	.99476
3.20	.99966	.99914	.99853	.99785	.99713	.99639	.99564
3.30	.99972	.99929	.99877	.99821	.99761	.99699	.99636
3.40	.99976	.99941	.99898	.99850	.99800	.99748	.99695
3.50	.99980	.99950	.99914	.99874	.99832	.99788	.99743
3.60	.99983	.99958	.99928	.99894	.99858	.99821	.99783
3.70	.99986	.99965	.99939	.99911	.99880	.99849	.99817
3.80	.99988	.99970	.99948	.99924	.99898	.99872	.99844
3.90	.99990	.99975	.99956	.99935	.99913	.99891	.99867
4.00	.99991	.99978	.99962	.99945	.99926	.99907	.99887
4.20	.99994	.99984	.99972	.99959	.99946	.99931	.99916
4.40	.99995	.99988	.99979	.99970	.99959	.99949	.99938
4.60	.99996	.99991	.99985	.99977	.99969	.99961	.99953
4.80	.99997	.99993	.99988	.99983	.99977	.99971	.99964
5.00	.99998	.99995	.99991	.99987	.99982	.99977	.99973
5.20	.99998	.99996	.99993	.99990	.99986	.99983	.99979
5.40	.99999	.99997	.99995	.99992	.99989	.99986	.99983
5.60	.99999	.99997	.99996	.99994	.99991	.99989	.99987
5.80	.99999	.99998	.99997	.99995	.99993	.99991	.99990
6.00	.99999	.99998	.99997	.99996	.99995	.99993	.99992
6.20	.99999	.99999	.99998	.99997	.99996	.99995	.99993
6.40	1.00000	.99999	.99998	.99997	.99996	.99996	.99995
6.60		.99999	.99999	.99998	.99997	.99996	.99996
6.80		.99999	.99999	.99998	.99998	.99997	.99996
7.00		.99999	.99999	.99999	.99998	.99998	.99997

$n_2 = 8$

F' \ n_1	2	3	4	5	6	7	8
7.50		1.00000	.99999	.99999	.99999	.99998	.99998
8.00			1.00000	.99999	.99999	.99999	.99999
8.50				1.00000	.99999	.99999	.99999
9.00					1.00000	1.00000	1.00000

$n_2 = 8$

$F' \backslash n_1$	9	10	11	12	13	14	15
1.00	.45636	.41814	.38451	.35480	.32844	.30496	.28394
1.05	.50462	.46721	.43393	.40422	.37758	.35363	.33199
1.10	.55050	.51435	.48188	.45260	.42613	.40211	.38025
1.15	.59362	.55908	.52776	.49930	.47335	.44963	.42788
1.20	.63376	.60106	.57117	.54380	.51867	.49554	.47419
1.25	.67082	.64010	.61183	.58575	.56166	.53935	.51865
1.30	.70479	.67613	.64958	.62495	.60206	.58074	.56086
1.35	.73574	.70916	.68440	.66129	.63970	.61950	.60056
1.40	.76380	.73927	.71630	.69475	.67452	.65550	.63760
1.50	.81191	.79128	.77176	.75329	.73581	.71925	.70354
1.60	.85062	.83346	.81710	.80152	.78666	.77248	.75895
1.70	.88147	.86733	.85375	.84073	.82824	.81627	.80477
1.80	.90592	.89432	.88312	.87233	.86192	.85190	.84223
1.90	.92522	.91574	.90655	.89764	.88902	.88068	.87260
2.00	.94043	.93270	.92517	.91784	.91072	.90381	.89710
2.10	.95242	.94612	.93995	.93394	.92807	.92235	.91679
2.20	.96188	.95674	.95169	.94675	.94192	.93720	.93259
2.30	.96935	.96515	.96101	.95696	.95298	.94908	.94527
2.40	.97527	.97183	.96843	.96510	.96182	.95860	.95544
2.50	.97996	.97714	.97435	.97160	.96890	.96623	.96362
2.60	.98370	.98138	.97909	.97682	.97458	.97237	.97020
2.70	.98669	.98478	.98288	.98100	.97915	.97732	.97551
2.80	.98909	.98751	.98594	.98438	.98284	.98131	.97981
2.90	.99102	.98971	.98840	.98711	.98582	.98455	.98330
3.00	.99258	.99149	.99040	.98932	.98825	.98718	.98613
3.10	.99385	.99294	.99203	.99112	.99022	.98933	.98845
3.20	.99488	.99412	.99335	.99259	.99184	.99109	.99034
3.30	.99572	.99508	.99444	.99380	.99316	.99253	.99190
3.40	.99641	.99587	.99533	.99479	.99425	.99372	.99318
3.50	.99698	.99652	.99606	.99561	.99515	.99470	.99425
3.60	.99745	.99706	.99667	.99628	.99590	.99551	.99513
3.70	.99784	.99751	.99718	.99685	.99652	.99619	.99586
3.80	.99816	.99788	.99760	.99732	.99703	.99675	.99647
3.90	.99843	.99819	.99795	.99771	.99747	.99722	.99698
4.00	.99866	.99845	.99825	.99804	.99783	.99762	.99741
4.20	.99901	.99886	.99870	.99855	.99839	.99824	.99808
4.40	.99926	.99915	.99903	.99892	.99880	.99868	.99857
4.60	.99944	.99936	.99927	.99918	.99909	.99900	.99891
4.80	.99958	.99951	.99944	.99938	.99931	.99924	.99917
5.00	.99968	.99962	.99957	.99952	.99947	.99941	.99936
5.20	.99975	.99971	.99967	.99963	.99959	.99954	.99950
5.40	.99980	.99977	.99974	.99971	.99968	.99964	.99961
5.60	.99985	.99982	.99980	.99977	.99974	.99972	.99969
5.80	.99988	.99986	.99984	.99982	.99980	.99978	.99976
6.00	.99990	.99989	.99987	.99985	.99984	.99982	.99980
6.20	.99992	.99991	.99990	.99988	.99987	.99986	.99984
6.40	.99994	.99993	.99992	.99990	.99989	.99988	.99987
6.60	.99995	.99994	.99993	.99992	.99991	.99990	.99990
6.80	.99996	.99995	.99994	.99994	.99993	.99992	.99991
7.00	.99997	.99996	.99995	.99995	.99994	.99994	.99993

$n_2 = 8$

$F' \backslash n_1$	9	10	11	12	13	14	15
7.50	.99998	.99998	.99997	.99997	.99996	.99996	.99996
8.00	.99999	.99998	.99998	.99998	.99998	.99997	.99997
8.50	.99999	.99999	.99999	.99999	.99998	.99998	.99998
9.00	.99999	.99999	.99999	.99999	.99999	.99999	.99999
9.50	1.00000	1.00000	1.00000	.99999	.99999	.99999	.99999
10.00				1.00000	1.00000	.99999	.99999
10.50						1.00000	1.00000

$n_2 = 9$

F'\ n_1	2	3	4	5	6	7	8
1.00	.93466	.85694	.78098	.71117	.64854	.59291	.54364
1.05	.94449	.87696	.80967	.74675	.68941	.63771	.59131
1.10	.95285	.89429	.83492	.77853	.72641	.67882	.63557
1.15	.95993	.90924	.85703	.80675	.75967	.71618	.67623
1.20	.96594	.92211	.87633	.83166	.78937	.74988	.71325
1.25	.97103	.93317	.89310	.85357	.81574	.78007	.74670
1.30	.97534	.94265	.90765	.87275	.83904	.80698	.77674
1.35	.97899	.95078	.92024	.88950	.85955	.83084	.80357
1.40	.98208	.95773	.93111	.90408	.87754	.85192	.82741
1.50	.98692	.96877	.94858	.92776	.90703	.88677	.86717
1.60	.99040	.97684	.96154	.94555	.92945	.91354	.89800
1.70	.99291	.98276	.97114	.95888	.94640	.93396	.92171
1.80	.99474	.98710	.97827	.96885	.95919	.94948	.93985
1.90	.99607	.99030	.98356	.97632	.96883	.96126	.95371
2.00	.99705	.99266	.98750	.98192	.97611	.97020	.96428
2.10	.99776	.99442	.99045	.98613	.98162	.97700	.97234
2.20	.99830	.99573	.99267	.98931	.98579	.98217	.97850
2.30	.99870	.99671	.99434	.99172	.98896	.98612	.98323
2.40	.99899	.99746	.99561	.99356	.99139	.98914	.98686
2.50	.99922	.99802	.99657	.99496	.99325	.99147	.98966
2.60	.99939	.99845	.99731	.99604	.99468	.99327	.99182
2.70	.99952	.99878	.99788	.99687	.99579	.99466	.99351
2.80	.99962	.99904	.99832	.99751	.99665	.99575	.99482
2.90	.99970	.99923	.99866	.99802	.99732	.99660	.99585
3.00	.99976	.99939	.99893	.99841	.99785	.99726	.99666
3.10	.99981	.99951	.99914	.99872	.99827	.99779	.99730
3.20	.99985	.99960	.99930	.99896	.99859	.99821	.99781
3.30	.99987	.99968	.99943	.99916	.99886	.99854	.99821
3.40	.99990	.99974	.99954	.99931	.99907	.99881	.99854
3.50	.99992	.99978	.99962	.99944	.99923	.99902	.99880
3.60	.99993	.99982	.99969	.99953	.99937	.99919	.99901
3.70	.99994	.99985	.99974	.99962	.99948	.99933	.99918
3.80	.99995	.99988	.99979	.99968	.99957	.99944	.99932
3.90	.99996	.99990	.99982	.99973	.99964	.99954	.99943
4.00	.99997	.99992	.99985	.99978	.99970	.99961	.99952
4.20	.99998	.99994	.99990	.99984	.99979	.99973	.99966
4.40	.99998	.99996	.99993	.99989	.99985	.99980	.99976
4.60	.99999	.99997	.99995	.99992	.99989	.99986	.99983
4.80	.99999	.99998	.99996	.99994	.99992	.99990	.99987
5.00	.99999	.99998	.99997	.99996	.99994	.99992	.99991
5.20	.99999	.99999	.99998	.99997	.99995	.99994	.99993
5.40	1.00000	.99999	.99998	.99998	.99997	.99996	.99995
5.60		.99999	.99999	.99998	.99997	.99997	.99996
5.80		.99999	.99999	.99999	.99998	.99997	.99997
6.00		1.00000	.99999	.99999	.99998	.99998	.99998
6.20			.99999	.99999	.99999	.99998	.99998
6.40			1.00000	.99999	.99999	.99999	.99999
6.60				.99999	.99999	.99999	.99999
6.80				1.00000	.99999	.99999	.99999
7.00					.99999	.99999	.99999

$n_2 = 9$

F' \ n_1	2	3	4	5	6	7	8
7.50					1.00000	1.00000	1.00000

$n_2 = 9$

F' \ n_1	9	10	11	12	13	14	15
1.00	.50000	.46128	.42683	.39609	.36856	.34383	.32154
1.05	.54969	.51232	.47869	.44836	.42093	.39604	.37340
1.10	.59634	.56073	.52837	.49890	.47201	.44740	.42483
1.15	.63961	.60606	.57530	.54705	.52106	.49710	.47495
1.20	.67937	.64806	.61912	.59234	.56752	.54448	.52306
1.25	.71558	.68660	.65962	.63448	.61103	.58912	.56863
1.30	.74833	.72169	.69672	.67332	.65135	.63073	.61133
1.35	.77777	.75343	.73047	.70883	.68842	.66916	.65095
1.40	.80409	.78196	.76098	.74109	.72225	.70438	.68742
1.50	.84832	.83024	.81294	.79640	.78059	.76548	.75103
1.60	.88291	.86832	.85425	.84070	.82765	.81510	.80302
1.70	.90972	.89805	.88671	.87573	.86509	.85479	.84483
1.80	.93037	.92108	.91201	.90317	.89456	.88619	.87806
1.90	.94623	.93886	.93162	.92454	.91761	.91085	.90425
2.00	.95838	.95254	.94678	.94112	.93557	.93013	.92480
2.10	.96769	.96306	.95849	.95397	.94953	.94516	.94087
2.20	.97483	.97116	.96752	.96392	.96037	.95686	.95341
2.30	.98032	.97741	.97451	.97163	.96879	.96597	.96320
2.40	.98455	.98223	.97992	.97762	.97534	.97308	.97084
2.50	.98782	.98597	.98412	.98228	.98045	.97863	.97683
2.60	.99036	.98888	.98739	.98591	.98444	.98297	.98152
2.70	.99233	.99114	.98995	.98876	.98757	.98638	.98520
2.80	.99388	.99292	.99196	.99099	.99003	.98907	.98811
2.90	.99509	.99431	.99353	.99275	.99197	.99119	.99041
3.00	.99604	.99541	.99478	.99415	.99351	.99287	.99223
3.10	.99680	.99629	.99577	.99525	.99473	.99421	.99369
3.20	.99740	.99698	.99656	.99613	.99571	.99528	.99485
3.30	.99788	.99754	.99719	.99684	.99649	.99614	.99578
3.40	.99826	.99798	.99769	.99741	.99712	.99682	.99653
3.50	.99857	.99834	.99810	.99786	.99762	.99738	.99714
3.60	.99882	.99863	.99843	.99823	.99803	.99783	.99763
3.70	.99902	.99886	.99870	.99853	.99837	.99820	.99803
3.80	.99919	.99905	.99892	.99878	.99864	.99850	.99836
3.90	.99932	.99921	.99910	.99898	.99886	.99875	.99863
4.00	.99943	.99934	.99924	.99915	.99905	.99895	.99885
4.20	.99960	.99953	.99946	.99939	.99932	.99925	.99918
4.40	.99971	.99966	.99962	.99957	.99951	.99946	.99941
4.60	.99979	.99976	.99972	.99968	.99965	.99961	.99957
4.80	.99985	.99982	.99980	.99977	.99974	.99971	.99968
5.00	.99989	.99987	.99985	.99983	.99981	.99979	.99977
5.20	.99992	.99990	.99989	.99987	.99986	.99984	.99982
5.40	.99994	.99993	.99991	.99990	.99989	.99988	.99987
5.60	.99995	.99994	.99994	.99993	.99992	.99991	.99990
5.80	.99996	.99996	.99995	.99994	.99994	.99993	.99992
6.00	.99997	.99997	.99996	.99996	.99995	.99994	.99994
6.20	.99998	.99997	.99997	.99997	.99996	.99996	.99995
6.40	.99998	.99998	.99998	.99997	.99997	.99997	.99996
6.60	.99999	.99998	.99998	.99998	.99998	.99997	.99997
6.80	.99999	.99999	.99999	.99998	.99998	.99998	.99998
7.00	.99999	.99999	.99999	.99999	.99999	.99998	.99998

$n_2 = 9$

F' \ n_1	9	10	11	12	13	14	15
7.50	1.00000	1.00000	.99999	.99999	.99999	.99999	.99999
8.00			1.00000	1.00000	1.00000	.99999	.99999
8.50						1.00000	1.00000

$n_2 = 10$

F'\n₁	2	3	4	5	6	7	8
1.00	.94467	.87628	.80748	.74273	.68348	.62996	.58187
1.05	.95359	.89492	.83474	.77713	.72358	.67450	.62979
1.10	.96108	.91086	.85845	.80750	.75947	.71487	.67375
1.15	.96736	.92445	.87898	.83414	.79134	.75113	.71365
1.20	.97261	.93601	.89666	.85738	.81944	.78342	.74952
1.25	.97702	.94582	.91185	.87755	.84408	.81200	.78154
1.30	.98070	.95413	.92486	.89500	.86558	.83714	.80992
1.35	.98378	.96116	.93598	.91003	.88426	.85915	.83494
1.40	.98635	.96711	.94546	.92296	.90044	.87834	.85689
1.50	.99031	.97636	.96039	.94355	.92646	.90947	.89279
1.60	.99309	.98295	.97119	.95862	.94571	.93275	.91990
1.70	.99504	.98766	.97898	.96961	.95988	.95003	.94019
1.80	.99642	.99102	.98461	.97761	.97030	.96283	.95531
1.90	.99740	.99343	.98868	.98345	.97794	.97228	.96654
2.00	.99810	.99517	.99163	.98771	.98355	.97926	.97489
2.10	.99860	.99643	.99378	.99083	.98769	.98442	.98108
2.20	.99896	.99734	.99535	.99313	.99074	.98825	.98569
2.30	.99923	.99801	.99651	.99482	.99300	.99110	.98914
2.40	.99942	.99850	.99736	.99607	.99468	.99322	.99171
2.50	.99956	.99886	.99799	.99701	.99594	.99481	.99365
2.60	.99967	.99913	.99847	.99771	.99688	.99601	.99511
2.70	.99974	.99933	.99882	.99824	.99760	.99692	.99621
2.80	.99980	.99949	.99909	.99863	.99814	.99761	.99706
2.90	.99985	.99960	.99929	.99894	.99855	.99813	.99770
3.00	.99988	.99969	.99945	.99917	.99886	.99854	.99819
3.10	.99991	.99976	.99957	.99935	.99910	.99885	.99858
3.20	.99993	.99981	.99966	.99948	.99929	.99909	.99887
3.30	.99994	.99985	.99973	.99959	.99944	.99927	.99910
3.40	.99995	.99988	.99978	.99967	.99955	.99942	.99928
3.50	.99996	.99990	.99983	.99974	.99964	.99953	.99942
3.60	.99997	.99992	.99986	.99979	.99971	.99962	.99954
3.70	.99998	.99994	.99989	.99983	.99976	.99970	.99962
3.80	.99998	.99995	.99991	.99986	.99981	.99975	.99969
3.90	.99998	.99996	.99993	.99989	.99984	.99980	.99975
4.00	.99999	.99997	.99994	.99991	.99987	.99983	.99980
4.20	.99999	.99998	.99996	.99994	.99991	.99989	.99986
4.40	.99999	.99998	.99997	.99996	.99994	.99992	.99991
4.60	1.00000	.99999	.99998	.99997	.99996	.99995	.99993
4.80		.99999	.99999	.99998	.99997	.99996	.99995
5.00		.99999	.99999	.99998	.99998	.99997	.99997
5.20		1.00000	.99999	.99999	.99998	.99998	.99998
5.40			.99999	.99999	.99999	.99999	.99998
5.60			1.00000	.99999	.99999	.99999	.99999
5.80				1.00000	.99999	.99999	.99999
6.00					1.00000	.99999	.99999
6.20						1.00000	1.00000

$n_2 = 10$

F' \ n_1	9	10	11	12	13	14	15
1.00	.53872	.50000	.46520	.43386	.40557	.37996	.35672
1.05	.58918	.55229	.51876	.48824	.46040	.43496	.41165
1.10	.63597	.60129	.56945	.54018	.51325	.48843	.46550
1.15	.67886	.64662	.61675	.58907	.56339	.53953	.51733
1.20	.71777	.68809	.66037	.63449	.61029	.58766	.56647
1.25	.75277	.72567	.70018	.67621	.65366	.63244	.61245
1.30	.78402	.75945	.73619	.71418	.69336	.67364	.65497
1.35	.81175	.78961	.76853	.74846	.72937	.71122	.69394
1.40	.83622	.81638	.79737	.77919	.76181	.74521	.72933
1.50	.87655	.86079	.84556	.83086	.81669	.80304	.78988
1.60	.90726	.89491	.88287	.87116	.85979	.84877	.83808
1.70	.93044	.92083	.91140	.90218	.89317	.88438	.87582
1.80	.94781	.94038	.93305	.92583	.91875	.91181	.90501
1.90	.96079	.95506	.94938	.94376	.93823	.93277	.92741
2.00	.97048	.96606	.96167	.95731	.95299	.94873	.94452
2.10	.97770	.97430	.97091	.96752	.96416	.96083	.95754
2.20	.98310	.98048	.97785	.97522	.97261	.97001	.96743
2.30	.98714	.98511	.98308	.98104	.97900	.97697	.97495
2.40	.99017	.98860	.98702	.98543	.98384	.98226	.98067
2.50	.99245	.99123	.99000	.98876	.98752	.98628	.98504
2.60	.99418	.99323	.99227	.99130	.99032	.98935	.98837
2.70	.99549	.99475	.99399	.99323	.99246	.99170	.99093
2.80	.99649	.99590	.99531	.99471	.99411	.99350	.99289
2.90	.99725	.99679	.99632	.99585	.99537	.99489	.99441
3.00	.99784	.99748	.99711	.99673	.99635	.99597	.99558
3.10	.99830	.99801	.99771	.99741	.99711	.99680	.99649
3.20	.99865	.99842	.99818	.99794	.99770	.99745	.99721
3.30	.99892	.99874	.99855	.99836	.99816	.99796	.99777
3.40	.99914	.99899	.99884	.99868	.99853	.99837	.99821
3.50	.99931	.99919	.99907	.99894	.99881	.99868	.99855
3.60	.99944	.99934	.99925	.99914	.99904	.99893	.99883
3.70	.99955	.99947	.99939	.99930	.99922	.99913	.99905
3.80	.99963	.99957	.99950	.99943	.99936	.99929	.99922
3.90	.99970	.99965	.99959	.99954	.99948	.99942	.99936
4.00	.99975	.99971	.99967	.99962	.99957	.99953	.99948
4.20	.99983	.99980	.99977	.99974	.99971	.99968	.99964
4.40	.99989	.99987	.99984	.99982	.99980	.99978	.99975
4.60	.99992	.99991	.99989	.99988	.99986	.99984	.99983
4.80	.99994	.99993	.99992	.99991	.99990	.99989	.99988
5.00	.99996	.99995	.99995	.99994	.99993	.99992	.99991
5.20	.99997	.99997	.99996	.99996	.99995	.99994	.99994
5.40	.99998	.99998	.99997	.99997	.99996	.99996	.99995
5.60	.99999	.99998	.99998	.99998	.99997	.99997	.99997
5.80	.99999	.99999	.99999	.99998	.99998	.99998	.99997
6.00	.99999	.99999	.99999	.99999	.99999	.99998	.99998
6.20	.99999	.99999	.99999	.99999	.99999	.99999	.99999
6.40	1.00000	1.00000	.99999	.99999	.99999	.99999	.99999
6.60			1.00000	1.00000	.99999	.99999	.99999
6.80					1.00000	.99999	.99999
7.00						1.00000	1.00000

$n_2 = 11$

F' \ n_1	2	3	4	5	6	7	8
1.00	.95250	.89186	.82933	.76928	.71339	.66214	.61549
1.05	.96062	.90922	.85518	.80240	.75249	.70607	.66324
1.10	.96737	.92390	.87742	.83131	.78710	.74544	.70654
1.15	.97297	.93629	.89645	.85638	.81748	.78039	.74538
1.20	.97760	.94670	.91266	.87800	.84396	.81116	.77990
1.25	.98144	.95544	.92643	.89655	.86690	.83807	.81034
1.30	.98461	.96275	.93807	.91239	.88668	.86145	.83700
1.35	.98723	.96886	.94790	.92589	.90366	.88168	.86022
1.40	.98939	.97396	.95619	.93735	.91818	.89909	.88034
1.50	.99267	.98177	.96901	.95528	.94111	.92683	.91264
1.60	.99490	.98720	.97805	.96807	.95766	.94705	.93641
1.70	.99644	.99098	.98440	.97717	.96954	.96169	.95376
1.80	.99750	.99361	.98888	.98362	.97804	.97225	.96636
1.90	.99823	.99545	.99204	.98821	.98412	.97985	.97548
2.00	.99874	.99674	.99427	.99148	.98847	.98532	.98207
2.10	.99910	.99765	.99585	.99381	.99160	.98926	.98685
2.20	.99935	.99830	.99698	.99548	.99384	.99211	.99032
2.30	.99953	.99876	.99779	.99668	.99547	.99418	.99284
2.40	.99965	.99909	.99837	.99755	.99665	.99568	.99468
2.50	.99974	.99933	.99880	.99818	.99750	.99678	.99602
2.60	.99981	.99950	.99910	.99864	.99813	.99759	.99701
2.70	.99986	.99963	.99933	.99898	.99859	.99818	.99775
2.80	.99989	.99972	.99949	.99923	.99894	.99862	.99829
2.90	.99992	.99979	.99962	.99941	.99919	.99895	.99870
3.00	.99994	.99984	.99971	.99955	.99938	.99920	.99900
3.10	.99995	.99988	.99977	.99966	.99952	.99938	.99923
3.20	.99996	.99990	.99983	.99973	.99963	.99952	.99941
3.30	.99997	.99993	.99987	.99979	.99971	.99963	.99954
3.40	.99998	.99994	.99989	.99984	.99978	.99971	.99964
3.50	.99998	.99995	.99992	.99987	.99982	.99977	.99972
3.60	.99999	.99996	.99994	.99990	.99986	.99982	.99978
3.70	.99999	.99997	.99995	.99992	.99989	.99986	.99982
3.80	.99999	.99998	.99996	.99994	.99991	.99989	.99986
3.90	.99999	.99998	.99997	.99995	.99993	.99991	.99989
4.00	.99999	.99999	.99997	.99996	.99994	.99993	.99991
4.20	1.00000	.99999	.99998	.99997	.99996	.99995	.99994
4.40		.99999	.99999	.99998	.99998	.99997	.99996
4.60		1.00000	.99999	.99999	.99998	.99998	.99998
4.80			.99999	.99999	.99999	.99999	.99998
5.00			1.00000	.99999	.99999	.99999	.99999
5.20				1.00000	.99999	.99999	.99999
5.40					1.00000	1.00000	1.00000

$n_2 = 11$

F' \ n_1	9	10	11	12	13	14	15
1.00	.57317	.53480	.50000	.46840	.43966	.41347	.38955
1.05	.62388	.58777	.55466	.52426	.49633	.47062	.44693
1.10	.67038	.63686	.60580	.57702	.55033	.52556	.50254
1.15	.71251	.68175	.65298	.62610	.60097	.57747	.55546
1.20	.75029	.72233	.69597	.67116	.64779	.62578	.60504
1.25	.78386	.75866	.73474	.71206	.69057	.67019	.65087
1.30	.81347	.79093	.76939	.74884	.72924	.71056	.69276
1.35	.83943	.81938	.80012	.78163	.76391	.74693	.73067
1.40	.86205	.84432	.82719	.81066	.79474	.77942	.76468
1.50	.89865	.88495	.87158	.85858	.84594	.83368	.82180
1.60	.92583	.91537	.90509	.89501	.88515	.87552	.86612
1.70	.94581	.93790	.93007	.92234	.91474	.90727	.89994
1.80	.96041	.95446	.94853	.94265	.93683	.93109	.92543
1.90	.97104	.96657	.96211	.95765	.95322	.94884	.94449
2.00	.97877	.97542	.97206	.96869	.96533	.96199	.95867
2.10	.98438	.98187	.97934	.97680	.97426	.97172	.96919
2.20	.98847	.98659	.98468	.98276	.98083	.97891	.97698
2.30	.99145	.99004	.98860	.98715	.98568	.98422	.98275
2.40	.99363	.99257	.99148	.99038	.98927	.98815	.98703
2.50	.99524	.99443	.99360	.99277	.99192	.99107	.99021
2.60	.99642	.99580	.99518	.99454	.99389	.99324	.99258
2.70	.99729	.99683	.99635	.99586	.99536	.99486	.99435
2.80	.99795	.99759	.99722	.99684	.99646	.99607	.99568
2.90	.99843	.99816	.99787	.99758	.99729	.99699	.99669
3.00	.99880	.99858	.99837	.99814	.99791	.99768	.99744
3.10	.99907	.99891	.99874	.99856	.99838	.99820	.99802
3.20	.99928	.99915	.99902	.99888	.99875	.99860	.99846
3.30	.99944	.99934	.99924	.99913	.99902	.99891	.99880
3.40	.99956	.99948	.99940	.99932	.99923	.99914	.99905
3.50	.99966	.99960	.99953	.99946	.99940	.99933	.99925
3.60	.99973	.99968	.99963	.99958	.99952	.99947	.99941
3.70	.99979	.99975	.99971	.99966	.99962	.99958	.99953
3.80	.99983	.99980	.99977	.99973	.99970	.99966	.99963
3.90	.99987	.99984	.99981	.99979	.99976	.99973	.99970
4.00	.99989	.99987	.99985	.99983	.99981	.99978	.99976
4.20	.99993	.99992	.99990	.99989	.99987	.99986	.99984
4.40	.99995	.99995	.99994	.99993	.99992	.99991	.99990
4.60	.99997	.99996	.99996	.99995	.99994	.99994	.99993
4.80	.99998	.99998	.99997	.99997	.99996	.99996	.99995
5.00	.99999	.99998	.99998	.99998	.99997	.99997	.99997
5.20	.99999	.99999	.99999	.99999	.99998	.99998	.99998
5.40	.99999	.99999	.99999	.99999	.99999	.99999	.99998
5.60	1.00000	1.00000	.99999	.99999	.99999	.99999	.99999
5.80			1.00000	1.00000	.99999	.99999	.99999
6.00					1.00000	1.00000	.99999
6.20							1.00000

$n_2 = 12$

F'\n1	2	3	4	5	6	7	8
1.00	.95874	.90461	.84758	.79184	.73917	.69024	.64520
1.05	.96617	.92079	.87206	.82362	.77714	.73333	.69245
1.10	.97228	.93435	.89291	.85109	.81039	.77154	.73484
1.15	.97730	.94566	.91056	.87465	.83926	.80508	.77246
1.20	.98141	.95507	.92544	.89474	.86414	.83429	.80552
1.25	.98478	.96287	.93792	.91178	.88546	.85954	.83434
1.30	.98753	.96934	.94837	.92618	.90364	.88124	.85929
1.35	.98978	.97468	.95709	.93831	.91906	.89979	.88076
1.40	.99161	.97909	.96436	.94848	.93209	.91557	.89915
1.50	.99434	.98572	.97541	.96413	.95232	.94028	.92817
1.60	.99617	.99022	.98301	.97503	.96657	.95786	.94901
1.70	.99739	.99328	.98824	.98259	.97655	.97028	.96385
1.80	.99821	.99536	.99183	.98783	.98352	.97901	.97436
1.90	.99877	.99678	.99429	.99146	.98839	.98515	.98179
2.00	.99914	.99775	.99600	.99398	.99179	.98945	.98703
2.10	.99940	.99842	.99718	.99574	.99416	.99248	.99072
2.20	.99958	.99888	.99800	.99697	.99583	.99462	.99334
2.30	.99970	.99921	.99857	.99783	.99701	.99613	.99520
2.40	.99979	.99943	.99897	.99844	.99784	.99720	.99652
2.50	.99985	.99959	.99926	.99887	.99843	.99796	.99746
2.60	.99989	.99970	.99946	.99918	.99886	.99851	.99814
2.70	.99992	.99978	.99961	.99940	.99916	.99890	.99863
2.80	.99994	.99984	.99971	.99955	.99938	.99919	.99899
2.90	.99996	.99988	.99978	.99967	.99954	.99940	.99925
3.00	.99997	.99991	.99984	.99975	.99966	.99955	.99944
3.10	.99998	.99993	.99988	.99981	.99974	.99966	.99958
3.20	.99998	.99995	.99991	.99986	.99980	.99974	.99968
3.30	.99999	.99996	.99993	.99989	.99985	.99981	.99976
3.40	.99999	.99997	.99995	.99992	.99989	.99985	.99982
3.50	.99999	.99998	.99996	.99994	.99991	.99989	.99986
3.60	.99999	.99998	.99997	.99995	.99993	.99991	.99989
3.70	.99999	.99999	.99998	.99996	.99995	.99993	.99992
3.80	1.00000	.99999	.99998	.99997	.99996	.99995	.99993
3.90		.99999	.99999	.99998	.99997	.99996	.99995
4.00		.99999	.99999	.99998	.99997	.99997	.99996
4.20		1.00000	.99999	.99999	.99998	.99998	.99998
4.40			1.00000	.99999	.99999	.99999	.99999
4.60				1.00000	.99999	.99999	.99999
4.80					1.00000	.99999	.99999
5.00						1.00000	1.00000

$n_2 = 12$

F' \ n_1	9	10	11	12	13	14	15
1.00	.60391	.56614	.53160	.50000	.47106	.44453	.42016
1.05	.65450	.61937	.58688	.55684	.52904	.50330	.47944
1.10	.70040	.66816	.63805	.60995	.58370	.55919	.53628
1.15	.74152	.71229	.68474	.65881	.63439	.61141	.58977
1.20	.77798	.75174	.72681	.70316	.68074	.65948	.63933
1.25	.81001	.78667	.76432	.74297	.72259	.70316	.68463
1.30	.83795	.81732	.79745	.77834	.76000	.74241	.72554
1.35	.86215	.84403	.82648	.80951	.79314	.77735	.76214
1.40	.88299	.86717	.85176	.83679	.82226	.80820	.79458
1.50	.91612	.90421	.89250	.88101	.86978	.85881	.84812
1.60	.94013	.93128	.92250	.91383	.90529	.89689	.88865
1.70	.95735	.95083	.94432	.93784	.93143	.92509	.91883
1.80	.96963	.96485	.96005	.95525	.95047	.94572	.94101
1.90	.97835	.97485	.97133	.96779	.96425	.96071	.95719
2.00	.98453	.98198	.97939	.97679	.97417	.97155	.96893
2.10	.98891	.98704	.98515	.98323	.98130	.97936	.97742
2.20	.99202	.99065	.98926	.98785	.98643	.98499	.98355
2.30	.99423	.99323	.99221	.99117	.99012	.98905	.98798
2.40	.99581	.99508	.99432	.99355	.99277	.99198	.99119
2.50	.99694	.99640	.99584	.99527	.99469	.99411	.99351
2.60	.99776	.99736	.99694	.99652	.99609	.99565	.99520
2.70	.99835	.99805	.99774	.99742	.99710	.99677	.99644
2.80	.99878	.99855	.99832	.99808	.99784	.99759	.99734
2.90	.99909	.99892	.99875	.99857	.99839	.99820	.99801
3.00	.99932	.99919	.99906	.99892	.99879	.99864	.99850
3.10	.99949	.99939	.99929	.99919	.99908	.99898	.99886
3.20	.99961	.99954	.99946	.99938	.99930	.99922	.99914
3.30	.99971	.99965	.99959	.99953	.99947	.99941	.99934
3.40	.99978	.99973	.99969	.99964	.99959	.99954	.99949
3.50	.99983	.99980	.99976	.99972	.99969	.99965	.99961
3.60	.99987	.99984	.99982	.99979	.99976	.99973	.99970
3.70	.99990	.99988	.99986	.99984	.99981	.99979	.99977
3.80	.99992	.99991	.99989	.99987	.99985	.99984	.99982
3.90	.99994	.99993	.99991	.99990	.99989	.99987	.99986
4.00	.99995	.99994	.99993	.99992	.99991	.99990	.99989
4.20	.99997	.99997	.99996	.99995	.99995	.99994	.99993
4.40	.99998	.99998	.99997	.99997	.99997	.99996	.99996
4.60	.99999	.99999	.99998	.99998	.99998	.99998	.99997
4.80	.99999	.99999	.99999	.99999	.99999	.99998	.99998
5.00	1.00000	1.00000	.99999	.99999	.99999	.99999	.99999
5.20			1.00000	1.00000	1.00000	.99999	.99999
5.40						1.00000	1.00000

$n_2 = 13$

F' \ n_1	2	3	4	5	6	7	8
1.00	.96381	.91518	.86298	.81116	.76155	.71493	.67156
1.05	.97063	.93029	.88617	.84163	.79831	.75702	.71809
1.10	.97619	.94283	.90572	.86768	.83018	.79397	.75942
1.15	.98071	.95319	.92210	.88981	.85756	.82607	.79570
1.20	.98438	.96172	.93577	.90848	.88092	.85373	.82726
1.25	.98735	.96872	.94712	.92415	.90072	.87739	.85447
1.30	.98975	.97446	.95652	.93725	.91741	.89749	.87777
1.35	.99170	.97915	.96428	.94816	.93142	.91448	.89760
1.40	.99327	.98298	.97067	.95721	.94314	.92879	.91439
1.50	.99556	.98865	.98024	.97090	.96101	.95080	.94045
1.60	.99707	.99241	.98668	.98023	.97332	.96611	.95873
1.70	.99805	.99491	.99100	.98655	.98174	.97667	.97145
1.80	.99870	.99657	.99389	.99083	.98748	.98393	.98024
1.90	.99912	.99768	.99584	.99372	.99139	.98891	.98631
2.00	.99941	.99842	.99715	.99568	.99406	.99232	.99048
2.10	.99959	.99892	.99804	.99702	.99588	.99466	.99336
2.20	.99972	.99925	.99864	.99793	.99713	.99627	.99535
2.30	.99981	.99948	.99906	.99855	.99799	.99738	.99673
2.40	.99987	.99964	.99934	.99898	.99858	.99815	.99769
2.50	.99991	.99974	.99953	.99928	.99900	.99869	.99836
2.60	.99993	.99982	.99967	.99949	.99928	.99906	.99883
2.70	.99995	.99987	.99976	.99963	.99949	.99933	.99916
2.80	.99997	.99991	.99983	.99974	.99963	.99951	.99939
2.90	.99998	.99993	.99988	.99981	.99973	.99965	.99956
3.00	.99998	.99995	.99991	.99986	.99980	.99974	.99968
3.10	.99999	.99996	.99993	.99990	.99986	.99981	.99976
3.20	.99999	.99997	.99995	.99992	.99989	.99986	.99982
3.30	.99999	.99998	.99996	.99994	.99992	.99990	.99987
3.40	.99999	.99999	.99997	.99996	.99994	.99992	.99990
3.50	1.00000	.99999	.99998	.99997	.99996	.99994	.99993
3.60		.99999	.99998	.99998	.99997	.99996	.99995
3.70		.99999	.99999	.99998	.99997	.99997	.99996
3.80		.99999	.99999	.99999	.99998	.99997	.99997
3.90		1.00000	.99999	.99999	.99998	.99998	.99998
4.00			.99999	.99999	.99999	.99999	.99998
4.20			1.00000	1.00000	.99999	.99999	.99999
4.40					1.00000	.99999	.99999
4.60						1.00000	1.00000

$n_2 = 13$

F'\ n_1	9	10	11	12	13	14	15
1.00	.63144	.59443	.56034	.52894	.50000	.47331	.44867
1.05	.68163	.64759	.61587	.58635	.55886	.53326	.50940
1.10	.72669	.69581	.66675	.63944	.61378	.58968	.56702
1.15	.76664	.73897	.71268	.68777	.66418	.64184	.62069
1.20	.80169	.77714	.75363	.73118	.70976	.68934	.66987
1.25	.83215	.81056	.78974	.76971	.75048	.73203	.71434
1.30	.85842	.83957	.82128	.80357	.78647	.76997	.75406
1.35	.88093	.86457	.84861	.83308	.81799	.80336	.78919
1.40	.90009	.88598	.87214	.85860	.84538	.83250	.81998
1.50	.93005	.91969	.90942	.89929	.88932	.87953	.86992
1.60	.95126	.94375	.93624	.92879	.92139	.91408	.90687
1.70	.96612	.96072	.95529	.94986	.94445	.93906	.93372
1.80	.97646	.97260	.96870	.96478	.96084	.95692	.95300
1.90	.98362	.98088	.97808	.97526	.97242	.96957	.96672
2.00	.98858	.98663	.98463	.98261	.98056	.97850	.97643
2.10	.99202	.99062	.98920	.98775	.98627	.98479	.98329
2.20	.99440	.99340	.99238	.99134	.99028	.98921	.98812
2.30	.99605	.99534	.99461	.99386	.99309	.99232	.99153
2.40	.99720	.99669	.99617	.99563	.99507	.99451	.99394
2.50	.99801	.99764	.99726	.99687	.99647	.99606	.99565
2.60	.99857	.99831	.99803	.99775	.99746	.99716	.99686
2.70	.99897	.99878	.99858	.99837	.99816	.99794	.99772
2.80	.99926	.99912	.99897	.99882	.99866	.99850	.99834
2.90	.99946	.99936	.99925	.99914	.99902	.99891	.99879
3.00	.99961	.99953	.99945	.99937	.99928	.99920	.99911
3.10	.99971	.99965	.99960	.99954	.99947	.99941	.99934
3.20	.99979	.99975	.99970	.99966	.99961	.99956	.99951
3.30	.99984	.99981	.99978	.99974	.99971	.99967	.99963
3.40	.99988	.99986	.99983	.99981	.99978	.99975	.99973
3.50	.99991	.99989	.99988	.99986	.99984	.99982	.99979
3.60	.99993	.99992	.99991	.99989	.99988	.99986	.99984
3.70	.99995	.99994	.99993	.99992	.99991	.99990	.99988
3.80	.99996	.99996	.99995	.99994	.99993	.99992	.99991
3.90	.99997	.99997	.99996	.99995	.99995	.99994	.99993
4.00	.99998	.99997	.99997	.99996	.99996	.99995	.99995
4.20	.99999	.99999	.99998	.99998	.99998	.99997	.99997
4.40	.99999	.99999	.99999	.99999	.99999	.99998	.99998
4.60	1.00000	1.00000	1.00000	.99999	.99999	.99999	.99999
4.80				1.00000	1.00000	1.00000	.99999
5.00							1.00000

$n_2 = 14$

F' \ n_1	2	3	4	5	6	7	8
1.00	.96798	.92404	.87610	.82786	.78111	.73672	.69504
1.05	.97427	.93818	.89807	.85702	.81663	.77772	.74071
1.10	.97935	.94981	.91642	.88173	.84712	.81337	.78086
1.15	.98344	.95932	.93165	.90250	.87307	.84403	.81578
1.20	.98673	.96708	.94423	.91986	.89499	.87019	.84583
1.25	.98936	97339	.95457	.93429	.91337	.89233	.87147
1.30	.99148	.97850	.96305	.94623	.92871	.91095	.89321
1.35	.99317	.98264	.96998	.95606	.94145	.92652	.91151
1.40	.99452	.98599	.97562	.96414	.95199	.93949	.92684
1.50	.99647	.99087	.98394	.97616	.96782	.95914	.95024
1.60	.99772	.99403	.98942	.98417	.97848	.97249	.96631
1.70	.99852	.99609	.99302	.98948	.98561	.98151	.97723
1.80	.99903	.99743	.99537	.99299	.99037	.98756	.98461
1.90	.99936	.99830	.99692	.99532	.99353	.99161	.98959
2.00	.99958	.99887	.99794	.99686	.99564	.99433	.99294
2.10	.99972	.99924	.99862	.99788	.99705	.99615	.99519
2.20	.99981	.99949	.99907	.99856	.99799	.99737	.99671
2.30	.99987	.99965	.99937	.99902	.99863	.99820	.99774
2.40	.99991	.99976	.99957	.99933	.99906	.99876	.99844
2.50	.99994	.99984	.99970	.99954	.99935	.99914	.99892
2.60	.99996	.99989	.99979	.99968	.99954	.99940	.99924
2.70	.99997	.99992	.99985	.99977	.99968	.99958	.99947
2.80	.99998	.99994	.99990	.99984	.99977	.99970	.99963
2.90	.99999	.99996	.99993	.99989	.99984	.99979	.99973
3.00	.99999	.99997	.99995	.99992	.99989	.99985	.99981
3.10	.99999	.99998	.99996	.99994	.99992	.99989	.99986
3.20	.99999	.99999	.99997	.99996	.99994	.99992	.99990
3.30	1.00000	.99999	.99998	.99997	.99996	.99994	.99993
3.40		.99999	.99999	.99998	.99997	.99996	.99995
3.50		.99999	.99999	.99998	.99998	.99997	.99996
3.60		1.00000	.99999	.99999	.99998	.99998	.99997
3.70			.99999	.99999	.99999	.99998	.99998
3.80			1.00000	.99999	.99999	.99999	.99999
3.90				.99999	.99999	.99999	.99999
4.00				1.00000	.99999	.99999	.99999
4.20					1.00000	1.00000	1.00000

$n_2 = 14$

$F' \backslash n_1$	9	10	11	12	13	14	15
1.00	.65617	.62004	.58653	.55547	.52669	.50000	.47524
1.05	.70574	.67286	.64202	.61312	.58607	.56074	.53702
1.10	.74982	.72031	.69236	.66592	.64094	.61735	.59506
1.15	.78851	.76235	.73735	.71350	.69078	.66915	.64858
1.20	.82211	.79916	.77704	.75579	.73539	.71585	.69713
1.25	.85101	.83105	.81168	.79294	.77483	.75738	.74055
1.30	.87566	.85844	.84162	.82524	.80932	.79389	.77894
1.35	.89656	.88180	.86729	.85308	.83920	.82568	.81251
1.40	.91417	.90158	.88914	.87690	.86489	.85312	.84162
1.50	.94125	.93222	.92321	.91427	.90542	.89669	.88808
1.60	.96000	.95361	.94718	.94076	.93435	.92799	.92168
1.70	.97284	.96835	.96382	.95926	.95468	.95010	.94554
1.80	.98157	.97844	.97526	.97205	.96880	.96554	.96228
1.90	.98748	.98531	.98309	.98083	.97854	.97624	.97392
2.00	.99148	.98997	.98842	.98684	.98524	.98361	.98197
2.10	.99418	.99314	.99206	.99095	.98982	.98868	.98752
2.20	.99601	.99529	.99453	.99376	.99296	.99216	.99134
2.30	.99726	.99675	.99622	.99568	.99512	.99455	.99397
2.40	.99810	.99775	.99738	.99699	.99660	.99620	.99579
2.50	.99868	.99843	.99817	.99790	.99762	.99734	.99705
2.60	.99908	.99890	.99872	.99853	.99833	.99813	.99792
2.70	.99935	.99923	.99910	.99896	.99882	.99867	.99853
2.80	.99954	.99945	.99936	.99926	.99916	.99906	.99895
2.90	.99968	.99961	.99955	.99948	.99940	.99933	.99925
3.00	.99977	.99972	.99968	.99962	.99957	.99952	.99946
3.10	.99983	.99980	.99977	.99973	.99969	.99965	.99961
3.20	.99988	.99986	.99983	.99981	.99978	.99975	.99972
3.30	.99991	.99990	.99988	.99986	.99984	.99982	.99980
3.40	.99994	.99993	.99991	.99990	.99988	.99987	.99985
3.50	.99996	.99995	.99994	.99993	.99991	.99990	.99989
3.60	.99997	.99996	.99995	.99995	.99994	.99993	.99992
3.70	.99998	.99997	.99997	.99996	.99995	.99995	.99994
3.80	.99998	.99998	.99998	.99997	.99997	.99996	.99996
3.90	.99999	.99999	.99998	.99998	.99998	.99997	.99997
4.00	.99999	.99999	.99999	.99998	.99998	.99998	.99998
4.20	1.00000	1.00000	.99999	.99999	.99999	.99999	.99999
4.40			1.00000	1.00000	1.00000	.99999	.99999
4.60						1.00000	1.00000

$n_2 = 15$

F' \ n_1	2	3	4	5	6	7	8
1.00	.97145	.93155	.88738	.84238	.79830	.75605	.71606
1.05	.97727	.94481	.90821	.87028	.83257	.79591	.76074
1.10	.98193	.95562	.92544	.89371	.86173	.83024	.79968
1.15	.98565	.96438	.93962	.91323	.88631	.85950	.83320
1.20	.98861	.97146	.95122	.92939	.90687	.88422	.86178
1.25	.99097	.97716	.96067	.94269	.92395	.90493	.88593
1.30	.99283	.98174	.96834	.95358	.93806	.92218	.90619
1.35	.99432	.98541	.97454	.96247	.94967	.93646	.92308
1.40	.99549	.98835	.97955	.96969	.95916	.94823	.93708
1.50	.99716	.99257	.98682	.98029	.97322	.96579	.95813
1.60	.99820	.99525	.99150	.98720	.98248	.97748	.97227
1.70	.99886	.99696	.99452	.99168	.98855	.98520	.98168
1.80	.99927	.99804	.99645	.99458	.99251	.99027	.98790
1.90	.99953	.99873	.99769	.99646	.99508	.99359	.99200
2.00	.99970	.99918	.99849	.99768	.99676	.99576	.99470
2.10	.99980	.99946	.99901	.99847	.99786	.99719	.99647
2.20	.99987	.99965	.99935	.99899	.99858	.99813	.99764
2.30	.99991	.99977	.99957	.99932	.99905	.99874	.99842
2.40	.99994	.99984	.99971	.99955	.99936	.99915	.99893
2.50	.99996	.99989	.99980	.99969	.99957	.99943	.99928
2.60	.99997	.99993	.99987	.99979	.99970	.99961	.99951
2.70	.99998	.99995	.99991	.99986	.99980	.99973	.99966
2.80	.99999	.99997	.99994	.99990	.99986	.99982	.99977
2.90	.99999	.99998	.99996	.99993	.99990	.99987	.99984
3.00	.99999	.99998	.99997	.99995	.99993	.99991	.99989
3.10	1.00000	.99999	.99998	.99997	.99995	.99994	.99992
3.20		.99999	.99998	.99998	.99997	.99996	.99995
3.30		.99999	.99999	.99998	.99998	.99997	.99996
3.40		1.00000	.99999	.99999	.99998	.99998	.99997
3.50			.99999	.99999	.99999	.99998	.99998
3.60			1.00000	.99999	.99999	.99999	.99999
3.70				1.00000	.99999	.99999	.99999
3.80					.99999	.99999	.99999
3.90					1.00000	1.00000	1.00000

$n_2 = 15$

F' \ n_1	9	10	11	12	13	14	15
1.00	.67846	.64329	.61045	.57984	.55133	.52476	.50000
1.05	.72727	.69558	.66566	.63748	.61095	.58599	.56251
1.10	.77026	.74211	.71528	.68975	.66551	.64251	.62068
1.15	.80764	.78295	.75920	.73641	.71460	.69373	.67379
1.20	.83978	.81835	.79756	.77748	.75811	.73945	.72150
1.25	.86715	.84872	.83071	.81319	.79618	.77970	.76375
1.30	.89027	.87454	.85907	.84393	.82914	.81473	.80070
1.35	.90966	.89632	.88313	.87015	.85740	.84491	.83270
1.40	.92583	.91459	.90341	.89234	.88143	.87069	.86015
1.50	.95033	.94244	.93453	.92663	.91878	.91098	.90327
1.60	.96692	.96147	.95596	.95041	.94486	.93931	.93379
1.70	.97804	.97431	.97050	.96666	.96278	.95889	.95499
1.80	.98544	.98289	.98029	.97764	.97496	.97225	.96953
1.90	.99034	.98861	.98683	.98502	.98317	.98130	.97941
2.00	.99357	.99240	.99119	.98995	.98869	.98740	.98609
2.10	.99571	.99492	.99410	.99325	.99238	.99149	.99059
2.20	.99713	.99659	.99603	.99545	.99485	.99424	.99362
2.30	.99807	.99770	.99732	.99692	.99651	.99609	.99566
2.40	.99870	.99845	.99818	.99791	.99763	.99734	.99704
2.50	.99912	.99894	.99876	.99857	.99838	.99818	.99797
2.60	.99940	.99928	.99915	.99902	.99889	.99875	.99860
2.70	.99959	.99950	.99942	.99933	.99923	.99914	.99903
2.80	.99971	.99966	.99960	.99953	.99947	.99940	.99933
2.90	.99980	.99976	.99972	.99968	.99963	.99958	.99953
3.00	.99986	.99984	.99981	.99977	.99974	.99971	.99967
3.10	.99990	.99989	.99986	.99984	.99982	.99979	.99977
3.20	.99993	.99992	.99990	.99989	.99987	.99986	.99984
3.30	.99995	.99994	.99993	.99992	.99991	.99990	.99988
3.40	.99997	.99996	.99995	.99995	.99994	.99993	.99992
3.50	.99998	.99997	.99997	.99996	.99996	.99995	.99994
3.60	.99998	.99998	.99998	.99997	.99997	.99996	.99996
3.70	.99999	.99999	.99998	.99998	.99998	.99997	.99997
3.80	.99999	.99999	.99999	.99999	.99998	.99998	.99998
3.90	1.00000	.99999	.99999	.99999	.99999	.99999	.99999
4.00		1.00000	1.00000	.99999	.99999	.99999	.99999
4.20				1.00000	1.00000	1.00000	1.00000

Table A2

PERCENTAGE POINTS, CORRESPONDING TO CUMULATIVE PROBABILITY P, OF THE RATIO F' OF THE RANGES OF SAMPLES OF SIZES n_1 AND n_2 FROM $N(\mu_i, \sigma)$ $(i = 1, 2)$

PERCENTAGE POINTS OF THE RATIO OF TWO RANGES

n_1	n_2	P=.500	P=.750	P=.900	P=.950	P=.975	P=.990	P=.995	P=.999
2	2	1.000	2.414	6.314	12.71	25.45	63.66	127.3	636.6
3	2	1.653	3.698	9.501	19.07	38.19	95.49	191.0	955.0
4	2	2.063	4.523	11.57	23.21	46.45	116.1	232.3	1162.
5	2	2.358	5.123	13.07	26.22	52.48	131.2	262.5	1312.
6	2	2.587	5.591	14.25	28.57	57.18	143.0	286.0	1430.
7	2	2.772	5.971	15.21	30.49	61.02	152.6	305.1	1526.
8	2	2.927	6.291	16.01	32.10	64.24	160.6	321.3	1607.
9	2	3.060	6.565	16.70	33.49	67.01	167.6	335.1	1676.
10	2	3.176	6.805	17.31	34.70	69.44	173.6	347.3	1736.
11	2	3.279	7.018	17.85	35.77	71.59	179.0	358.0	1790.
12	2	3.371	7.209	18.33	36.74	73.52	183.8	367.7	1838.
13	2	3.454	7.382	18.76	37.61	75.27	188.2	376.4	1882.
14	2	3.530	7.540	19.16	38.41	76.87	192.2	384.4	1922.
15	2	3.600	7.685	19.53	39.15	78.34	195.9	391.8	1959.
2	3	.6050	1.189	2.167	3.194	4.607	7.370	10.46	23.49
3	3	1.000	1.735	3.009	4.373	6.267	9.986	14.16	31.76
4	3	1.246	2.082	3.555	5.144	7.355	11.71	16.59	37.19
5	3	1.422	2.335	3.956	5.712	8.159	12.98	18.39	41.22
6	3	1.559	2.533	4.272	6.160	8.794	13.98	19.81	44.39
7	3	1.669	2.695	4.531	6.528	9.315	14.81	20.98	47.00
8	3	1.762	2.831	4.750	6.839	9.756	15.50	21.97	49.21
9	3	1.841	2.948	4.939	7.108	10.14	16.11	22.82	51.12
10	3	1.911	3.050	5.105	7.344	10.47	16.64	23.57	52.80
11	3	1.972	3.142	5.252	7.554	10.77	17.11	24.24	54.31
12	3	2.028	3.224	5.385	7.743	11.04	17.54	24.84	55.66
13	3	2.077	3.298	5.505	7.914	11.28	17.92	25.39	56.88
14	3	2.123	3.366	5.616	8.072	11.50	18.28	25.89	58.01
15	3	2.165	3.428	5.717	8.216	11.71	18.60	26.35	59.04
2	4	.4847	.9032	1.497	2.027	2.662	3.725	4.755	8.250
3	4	.8028	1.296	2.011	2.663	3.453	4.789	6.090	10.52
4	4	1.000	1.542	2.341	3.075	3.971	5.489	6.971	12.03
5	4	1.141	1.721	2.584	3.381	4.356	6.010	7.626	13.15
6	4	1.251	1.862	2.775	3.623	4.660	6.424	8.147	14.04
7	4	1.340	1.976	2.933	3.822	4.911	6.765	8.578	14.77
8	4	1.414	2.073	3.066	3.990	5.125	7.056	8.944	15.40
9	4	1.478	2.156	3.181	4.137	5.310	7.307	9.262	15.95
10	4	1.533	2.229	3.283	4.265	5.473	7.529	9.542	16.43
11	4	1.583	2.294	3.373	4.380	5.618	7.728	9.792	16.85
12	4	1.627	2.353	3.454	4.484	5.749	7.906	10.02	17.24
13	4	1.667	2.406	3.528	4.578	5.869	8.069	10.22	17.60
14	4	1.703	2.454	3.596	4.664	5.978	8.218	10.41	17.92
15	4	1.737	2.499	3.658	4.744	6.079	8.356	10.59	18.22
2	5	.4240	.7717	1.228	1.602	2.020	2.664	3.242	4.993
3	5	.7032	1.098	1.621	2.059	2.553	3.324	4.020	6.145
4	5	.8761	1.301	1.871	2.353	2.900	3.757	4.532	6.905
5	5	1.000	1.448	2.055	2.570	3.157	4.079	4.914	7.474
6	5	1.096	1.563	2.200	2.742	3.361	4.335	5.219	7.929
7	5	1.174	1.657	2.319	2.884	3.530	4.547	5.471	8.307
8	5	1.239	1.736	2.420	3.004	3.674	4.728	5.686	8.628

PERCENTAGE POINTS OF THE RATIO OF TWO RANGES

n_1	n_2	P=.500	P=.750	P=.900	P=.950	P=.975	P=.990	P=.995	P=.999
9	5	1.295	1.805	2.507	3.109	3.798	4.885	5.874	8.907
10	5	1.343	1.865	2.584	3.201	3.908	5.024	6.039	9.156
11	5	1.387	1.918	2.653	3.283	4.007	5.149	6.187	9.378
12	5	1.425	1.966	2.714	3.357	4.096	5.261	6.321	9.580
13	5	1.460	2.010	2.771	3.425	4.176	5.363	6.443	9.764
14	5	1.492	2.050	2.822	3.487	4.251	5.457	6.555	9.932
15	5	1.522	2.086	2.870	3.544	4.319	5.544	6.659	10.09
2	6	.3866	.6944	1.080	1.381	1.704	2.176	2.580	3.720
3	6	.6416	.9827	1.411	1.752	2.120	2.665	3.135	4.472
4	6	.7995	1.161	1.620	1.988	2.388	2.983	3.498	4.967
5	6	.9125	1.290	1.773	2.162	2.586	3.220	3.768	5.339
6	6	1.000	1.391	1.894	2.300	2.744	3.409	3.985	5.636
7	6	1.071	1.474	1.993	2.414	2.875	3.565	4.164	5.883
8	6	1.130	1.543	2.077	2.510	2.986	3.699	4.317	6.093
9	6	1.181	1.603	2.150	2.594	3.082	3.815	4.451	6.277
10	6	1.226	1.655	2.214	2.668	3.168	3.918	4.569	6.441
11	6	1.265	1.702	2.271	2.734	3.244	4.010	4.675	6.588
12	6	1.301	1.744	2.323	2.794	3.313	4.093	4.770	6.721
13	6	1.333	1.783	2.370	2.849	3.376	4.169	4.858	6.842
14	6	1.362	1.818	2.413	2.899	3.433	4.238	4.938	6.954
15	6	1.389	1.850	2.452	2.945	3.487	4.303	5.013	7.058
2	7	.3608	.6426	.9853	1.245	1.514	1.897	2.213	3.064
3	7	.5991	.9063	1.279	1.564	1.864	2.294	2.652	3.624
4	7	.7465	1.069	1.463	1.767	2.088	2.551	2.937	3.992
5	7	.8521	1.186	1.597	1.916	2.254	2.742	3.150	4.267
6	7	.9338	1.278	1.703	2.034	2.385	2.894	3.320	4.487
7	7	1.000	1.353	1.790	2.131	2.494	3.020	3.461	4.671
8	7	1.056	1.416	1.863	2.213	2.586	3.127	3.581	4.827
9	7	1.103	1.470	1.927	2.285	2.667	3.221	3.686	4.964
10	7	1.145	1.518	1.983	2.348	2.738	3.304	3.779	5.086
11	7	1.182	1.560	2.033	2.405	2.802	3.378	3.863	5.196
12	7	1.215	1.598	2.079	2.456	2.859	3.445	3.939	5.295
13	7	1.245	1.633	2.120	2.503	2.912	3.507	4.008	5.386
14	7	1.272	1.665	2.157	2.545	2.960	3.563	4.071	5.469
15	7	1.297	1.694	2.192	2.585	3.004	3.615	4.130	5.547
2	8	.3417	.6050	.9188	1.151	1.387	1.715	1.979	2.667
3	8	.5675	.8513	1.187	1.437	1.695	2.056	2.349	3.119
4	8	.7073	1.002	1.354	1.618	1.891	2.275	2.588	3.413
5	8	.8073	1.112	1.475	1.750	2.035	2.437	2.765	3.633
6	8	.8847	1.197	1.571	1.855	2.150	2.566	2.907	3.810
7	8	.9474	1.266	1.649	1.941	2.244	2.673	3.025	3.957
8	8	1.000	1.324	1.716	2.014	2.325	2.765	3.125	4.082
9	8	1.045	1.375	1.773	2.078	2.395	2.844	3.213	4.192
10	8	1.085	1.419	1.824	2.134	2.457	2.915	3.291	4.290
11	8	1.119	1.458	1.870	2.184	2.512	2.978	3.361	4.377
12	8	1.151	1.494	1.911	2.229	2.563	3.035	3.424	4.457
13	8	1.179	1.526	1.948	2.271	2.608	3.088	3.482	4.530
14	8	1.205	1.555	1.982	2.309	2.650	3.136	3.535	4.598
15	8	1.229	1.582	2.013	2.344	2.689	3.180	3.584	4.660

PERCENTAGE POINTS OF THE RATIO OF TWO RANGES

n_1	n_2	P=.500	P=.750	P=.900	P=.950	P=.975	P=.990	P=.995	P=.999
2	9	.3268	.5763	.8690	1.082	1.296	1.587	1.817	2.402
3	9	.5430	.8093	1.118	1.345	1.574	1.889	2.141	2.784
4	9	.6767	.9521	1.273	1.509	1.750	2.083	2.349	3.032
5	9	.7725	1.055	1.385	1.630	1.880	2.226	2.503	3.218
6	9	.8465	1.135	1.474	1.725	1.983	2.339	2.626	3.366
7	9	.9065	1.200	1.546	1.804	2.068	2.434	2.728	3.490
8	9	.9568	1.255	1.607	1.870	2.140	2.514	2.816	3.595
9	9	1.000	1.303	1.661	1.928	2.203	2.584	2.892	3.687
10	9	1.038	1.344	1.707	1.979	2.258	2.646	2.959	3.769
11	9	1.071	1.381	1.749	2.025	2.308	2.702	3.020	3.843
12	9	1.101	1.415	1.787	2.066	2.353	2.753	3.075	3.911
13	9	1.128	1.445	1.821	2.104	2.394	2.799	3.125	3.972
14	9	1.153	1.473	1.853	2.138	2.432	2.841	3.172	4.029
15	9	1.176	1.498	1.882	2.170	2.467	2.880	3.215	4.082
2	10	.3149	.5534	.8301	1.029	1.226	1.491	1.698	2.212
3	10	.5233	.7761	1.065	1.274	1.483	1.766	1.989	2.547
4	10	.6522	.9122	1.210	1.427	1.645	1.941	2.175	2.763
5	10	.7444	1.010	1.316	1.539	1.764	2.070	2.313	2.925
6	10	.8157	1.086	1.399	1.627	1.858	2.173	2.422	3.054
7	10	.8736	1.148	1.466	1.700	1.935	2.258	2.514	3.161
8	10	.9221	1.201	1.524	1.761	2.002	2.330	2.591	3.253
9	10	.9637	1.246	1.574	1.815	2.059	2.394	2.659	3.333
10	10	1.000	1.286	1.617	1.862	2.110	2.450	2.720	3.404
11	10	1.032	1.321	1.657	1.904	2.155	2.500	2.774	3.469
12	10	1.061	1.352	1.692	1.942	2.197	2.545	2.823	3.527
13	10	1.087	1.381	1.724	1.977	2.234	2.587	2.868	3.581
14	10	1.111	1.407	1.754	2.009	2.269	2.625	2.909	3.630
15	10	1.133	1.432	1.781	2.039	2.301	2.661	2.947	3.676
2	11	.3050	.5347	.7986	.9863	1.171	1.416	1.605	2.069
3	11	.5070	.7490	1.023	1.218	1.411	1.670	1.872	2.370
4	11	.6318	.8797	1.160	1.362	1.562	1.831	2.042	2.563
5	11	.7212	.9736	1.260	1.467	1.673	1.950	2.168	2.707
6	11	.7903	1.047	1.339	1.549	1.760	2.045	2.268	2.822
7	11	.8463	1.106	1.403	1.618	1.832	2.123	2.350	2.918
8	11	.8933	1.156	1.457	1.675	1.894	2.189	2.421	2.999
9	11	.9336	1.200	1.504	1.725	1.947	2.247	2.483	3.071
10	11	.9688	1.238	1.546	1.770	1.994	2.299	2.538	3.134
11	11	1.000	1.271	1.583	1.809	2.037	2.345	2.587	3.192
12	11	1.028	1.302	1.616	1.845	2.075	2.387	2.632	3.244
13	11	1.053	1.329	1.646	1.878	2.110	2.425	2.672	3.292
14	11	1.076	1.355	1.674	1.908	2.142	2.460	2.710	3.336
15	11	1.098	1.378	1.700	1.935	2.171	2.492	2.745	3.377
2	12	.2967	.5190	.7726	.9513	1.126	1.356	1.531	1.957
3	12	.4932	.7264	.9872	1.172	1.353	1.594	1.779	2.232
4	12	.6147	.8526	1.119	1.309	1.496	1.744	1.937	2.408
5	12	.7016	.9432	1.215	1.408	1.600	1.855	2.053	2.539
6	12	.7688	1.014	1.289	1.487	1.682	1.943	2.145	2.643
7	12	.8233	1.071	1.351	1.551	1.749	2.015	2.222	2.730
8	12	.8690	1.119	1.403	1.606	1.807	2.077	2.287	2.804

PERCENTAGE POINTS OF THE RATIO OF TWO RANGES

n_1	n_2	P=.500	P=.750	P=.900	P=.950	P=.975	P=.990	P=.995	P=.999
9	12	.9082	1.161	1.447	1.653	1.857	2.131	2.344	2.868
10	12	.9424	1.198	1.487	1.695	1.902	2.179	2.395	2.926
11	12	.9728	1.230	1.522	1.732	1.941	2.222	2.440	2.978
12	12	1.000	1.260	1.554	1.766	1.977	2.261	2.482	3.025
13	12	1.025	1.286	1.583	1.797	2.010	2.296	2.519	3.069
14	12	1.047	1.310	1.609	1.825	2.040	2.329	2.554	3.109
15	12	1.068	1.333	1.634	1.851	2.068	2.359	2.586	3.146
2	13	.2895	.5056	.7505	.9220	1.088	1.306	1.471	1.866
3	13	.4814	.7071	.9576	1.134	1.305	1.531	1.704	2.121
4	13	.5999	.8295	1.084	1.264	1.440	1.673	1.851	2.284
5	13	.6848	.9174	1.176	1.359	1.539	1.777	1.960	2.404
6	13	.7503	.9856	1.248	1.434	1.617	1.860	2.047	2.501
7	13	.8035	1.041	1.307	1.496	1.681	1.928	2.118	2.581
8	13	.8481	1.088	1.357	1.547	1.736	1.986	2.179	2.648
9	13	.8863	1.128	1.400	1.593	1.783	2.037	2.232	2.708
10	13	.9198	1.164	1.438	1.633	1.825	2.082	2.280	2.761
11	13	.9494	1.195	1.471	1.668	1.863	2.122	2.322	2.809
12	13	.9760	1.224	1.502	1.701	1.897	2.158	2.360	2.852
13	13	1.000	1.249	1.530	1.730	1.928	2.192	2.396	2.892
14	13	1.022	1.273	1.555	1.757	1.956	2.222	2.428	2.929
15	13	1.042	1.295	1.579	1.782	1.983	2.250	2.458	2.963
2	14	.2833	.4940	.7316	.8970	1.057	1.264	1.420	1.792
3	14	.4710	.6904	.9322	1.101	1.265	1.479	1.641	2.030
4	14	.5871	.8096	1.055	1.227	1.394	1.613	1.781	2.182
5	14	.6701	.8950	1.144	1.318	1.488	1.712	1.883	2.295
6	14	.7342	.9614	1.213	1.390	1.562	1.791	1.965	2.384
7	14	.7863	1.016	1.270	1.449	1.624	1.855	2.032	2.458
8	14	.8299	1.061	1.318	1.499	1.676	1.910	2.090	2.522
9	14	.8673	1.100	1.359	1.542	1.721	1.958	2.139	2.577
10	14	.9000	1.135	1.396	1.580	1.761	2.001	2.184	2.626
11	14	.9290	1.165	1.428	1.614	1.797	2.038	2.224	2.671
12	14	.9550	1.193	1.458	1.645	1.829	2.073	2.260	2.711
13	14	.9785	1.218	1.484	1.673	1.859	2.105	2.293	2.748
14	14	1.000	1.241	1.509	1.699	1.886	2.133	2.324	2.782
15	14	1.020	1.262	1.532	1.723	1.911	2.160	2.352	2.814
2	15	.2778	.4838	.7151	.8753	1.029	1.228	1.377	1.729
3	15	.4620	.6758	.9101	1.073	1.230	1.434	1.588	1.954
4	15	.5757	.7922	1.029	1.194	1.354	1.562	1.721	2.098
5	15	.6571	.8755	1.115	1.282	1.445	1.657	1.818	2.203
6	15	.7201	.9403	1.182	1.352	1.516	1.731	1.896	2.287
7	15	.7711	.9930	1.237	1.408	1.575	1.793	1.959	2.357
8	15	.8138	1.037	1.284	1.456	1.625	1.845	2.014	2.416
9	15	.8505	1.076	1.324	1.498	1.668	1.892	2.061	2.468
10	15	.8826	1.109	1.359	1.535	1.707	1.932	2.104	2.514
11	15	.9110	1.139	1.391	1.568	1.741	1.968	2.141	2.556
12	15	.9365	1.166	1.419	1.598	1.772	2.001	2.176	2.594
13	15	.9596	1.190	1.445	1.625	1.800	2.031	2.207	2.628
14	15	.9807	1.212	1.469	1.649	1.826	2.058	2.236	2.660
15	15	1.000	1.233	1.491	1.673	1.850	2.084	2.263	2.690

Table A3

POWER OF THE F' AND F TESTS (SIZE α) OF $H_0 : \sigma_1 = \sigma_2$ VS.
$H_1 : \sigma_1 = k\sigma_2$

(The first line of each pair gives the power of the F' test, the second line that of the F test; n_1 and n_2 are sample sizes)

Power of F' and F Tests (Size α) of $H_0: \sigma_1 = \sigma_2$ vs. $H_1: \sigma_1 = k\sigma_2$

(The first line of each pair gives the power of the F' test, the second line that of the F test; n_1 and n_2 are sample sizes)

$\alpha = .5$										
n_1	n_2 \ k	2	3	4	5	6	7	8	9	10
2	2	0.705	0.795	0.844	0.874	0.895	0.910	0.921	0.930	0.937
2	2	0.705	0.795	0.844	0.874	0.895	0.910	0.921	0.929	0.937
3	3	0.799	0.899	0.941	0.961	0.973	0.980	0.985	0.988	0.990
3	3	0.800	0.900	0.941	0.962	0.973	0.980	0.985	0.988	0.990
4	4	0.855	0.947	0.975	0.987	0.992	0.995	0.997	0.998	0.998
4	4	0.858	0.948	0.976	0.987	0.993	0.995	0.997	0.998	0.998
5	5	0.892	0.970	0.989	0.995	0.998	0.999	0.999	1.000	1.000
5	5	0.896	0.972	0.990	0.996	0.998	0.999	0.999	1.000	1.000
6	6	0.917	0.983	0.995	0.998	0.999	1.000	1.000	1.000	1.000
6	6	0.923	0.985	0.996	0.998	0.999	1.000	1.000	1.000	1.000
7	7	0.935	0.990	0.998	0.999	1.000	1.000	1.000	1.000	1.000
7	7	0.942	0.991	0.998	0.999	1.000	1.000	1.000	1.000	1.000
8	8	0.948	0.994	0.999	1.000	1.000	1.000	1.000	1.000	1.000
8	8	0.956	0.995	0.999	1.000	1.000	1.000	1.000	1.000	1.000
9	9	0.958	0.996	0.999	1.000	1.000	1.000	1.000	1.000	1.000
9	9	0.967	0.997	1.000	1.000	1.000	1.000	1.000	1.000	1.000
10	10	0.966	0.997	1.000	1.000	1.000	1.000	1.000	1.000	1.000
10	10	0.974	0.998	1.000	1.000	1.000	1.000	1.000	1.000	1.000
11	11	0.972	0.998	1.000	1.000	1.000	1.000	1.000	1.000	1.000
11	11	0.980	0.999	1.000	1.000	1.000	1.000	1.000	1.000	1.000
12	12	0.977	0.999	1.000	1.000	1.000	1.000	1.000	1.000	1.000
12	12	0.985	0.999	1.000	1.000	1.000	1.000	1.000	1.000	1.000
13	13	0.981	0.999	1.000	1.000	1.000	1.000	1.000	1.000	1.000
13	13	0.988	1.000	1.000	1.000	1.000	1.000	1.000	1.000	1.000
14	14	0.984	1.000	1.000	1.000	1.000	1.000	1.000	1.000	1.000
14	14	0.991	1.000	1.000	1.000	1.000	1.000	1.000	1.000	1.000
15	15	0.986	1.000	1.000	1.000	1.000	1.000	1.000	1.000	1.000
15	15	0.993	1.000	1.000	1.000	1.000	1.000	1.000	1.000	1.000
15	2	0.809	0.940	0.983	0.995	0.999	1.000	1.000	1.000	1.000
15	2	0.812	0.943	0.985	0.996	0.999	1.000	1.000	1.000	1.000
2	15	0.734	0.820	0.865	0.892	0.910	0.922	0.932	0.940	0.946
2	15	0.734	0.821	0.865	0.892	0.910	0.923	0.932	0.940	0.946

Power of F' and F Tests (Size α) of $H_0: \sigma_1 = \sigma_2$ vs. $H_1: \sigma_1 = k\sigma_2$

(The first line of each pair gives the power of the F' test, the second line that of the F test; n_1 and n_2 are sample sizes)

		$\alpha = .25$								
n_1	n_2 \ k	2	3	4	5	6	7	8	9	10
2	2	0.440	0.569	0.654	0.714	0.756	0.789	0.813	0.833	0.849
2	2	0.440	0.569	0.654	0.714	0.756	0.789	0.813	0.833	0.849
3	3	0.570	0.749	0.841	0.892	0.922	0.942	0.955	0.964	0.971
3	3	0.571	0.750	0.842	0.893	0.923	0.942	0.955	0.964	0.971
4	4	0.658	0.846	0.922	0.957	0.974	0.983	0.988	0.992	0.994
4	4	0.663	0.850	0.925	0.958	0.975	0.984	0.989	0.992	0.994
5	5	0.722	0.902	0.961	0.982	0.991	0.995	0.997	0.998	0.999
5	5	0.731	0.909	0.964	0.983	0.991	0.995	0.997	0.998	0.999
6	6	0.771	0.937	0.979	0.992	0.997	0.998	0.999	0.999	1.000
6	6	0.784	0.944	0.982	0.993	0.997	0.999	0.999	1.000	1.000
7	7	0.808	0.958	0.989	0.996	0.999	0.999	1.000	1.000	1.000
7	7	0.826	0.965	0.991	0.997	0.999	1.000	1.000	1.000	1.000
8	8	0.838	0.972	0.994	0.998	0.999	1.000	1.000	1.000	1.000
8	8	0.859	0.979	0.996	0.999	1.000	1.000	1.000	1.000	1.000
9	9	0.861	0.980	0.997	0.999	1.000	1.000	1.000	1.000	1.000
9	9	0.886	0.987	0.998	1.000	1.000	1.000	1.000	1.000	1.000
10	10	0.881	0.986	0.998	1.000	1.000	1.000	1.000	1.000	1.000
10	10	0.907	0.992	0.999	1.000	1.000	1.000	1.000	1.000	1.000
11	11	0.897	0.990	0.999	1.000	1.000	1.000	1.000	1.000	1.000
11	11	0.924	0.995	1.000	1.000	1.000	1.000	1.000	1.000	1.000
12	12	0.910	0.993	0.999	1.000	1.000	1.000	1.000	1.000	1.000
12	12	0.938	0.997	1.000	1.000	1.000	1.000	1.000	1.000	1.000
13	13	0.922	0.995	1.000	1.000	1.000	1.000	1.000	1.000	1.000
13	13	0.950	0.998	1.000	1.000	1.000	1.000	1.000	1.000	1.000
14	14	0.931	0.996	1.000	1.000	1.000	1.000	1.000	1.000	1.000
14	14	0.959	0.999	1.000	1.000	1.000	1.000	1.000	1.000	1.000
15	15	0.939	0.997	1.000	1.000	1.000	1.000	1.000	1.000	1.000
15	15	0.967	0.999	1.000	1.000	1.000	1.000	1.000	1.000	1.000
15	2	0.473	0.652	0.782	0.869	0.924	0.957	0.976	0.987	0.993
15	2	0.474	0.654	0.785	0.874	0.929	0.961	0.979	0.989	0.994
2	15	0.556	0.693	0.767	0.812	0.843	0.865	0.882	0.895	0.905
2	15	0.558	0.695	0.769	0.814	0.844	0.866	0.883	0.896	0.906

Power of F' and F Tests (Size α) of $H_0: \sigma_1 = \sigma_2$ vs. $H_1: \sigma_1 = k\sigma_2$

(The first line of each pair gives the power of the F' test, the second line that of the F test; n_1 and n_2 are sample sizes)

$\alpha = .1$										
n_1	n_2 \ k	2	3	4	5	6	7	8	9	10
2	2	0.195	0.282	0.359	0.426	0.484	0.533	0.575	0.611	0.641
2	2	0.195	0.282	0.360	0.426	0.484	0.533	0.575	0.611	0.641
3	3	0.307	0.499	0.638	0.733	0.798	0.843	0.875	0.899	0.917
3	3	0.308	0.500	0.640	0.735	0.800	0.845	0.877	0.900	0.917
4	4	0.402	0.652	0.796	0.876	0.920	0.946	0.962	0.973	0.980
4	4	0.406	0.658	0.802	0.880	0.923	0.949	0.964	0.974	0.981
5	5	0.480	0.755	0.883	0.940	0.967	0.981	0.988	0.992	0.995
5	5	0.490	0.767	0.892	0.946	0.971	0.983	0.990	0.993	0.995
6	6	0.545	0.825	0.932	0.971	0.986	0.993	0.996	0.998	0.999
6	6	0.562	0.842	0.941	0.976	0.989	0.994	0.997	0.998	0.999
7	7	0.598	0.873	0.959	0.985	0.994	0.997	0.999	0.999	1.000
7	7	0.624	0.893	0.968	0.989	0.996	0.998	0.999	1.000	1.000
8	8	0.644	0.907	0.975	0.993	0.997	0.999	1.000	1.000	1.000
8	8	0.678	0.928	0.983	0.995	0.998	0.999	1.000	1.000	1.000
9	9	0.682	0.931	0.985	0.996	0.999	1.000	1.000	1.000	1.000
9	9	0.724	0.951	0.991	0.998	0.999	1.000	1.000	1.000	1.000
10	10	0.716	0.949	0.991	0.998	0.999	1.000	1.000	1.000	1.000
10	10	0.764	0.967	0.995	0.999	1.000	1.000	1.000	1.000	1.000
11	11	0.744	0.962	0.994	0.999	1.000	1.000	1.000	1.000	1.000
11	11	0.798	0.978	0.997	1.000	1.000	1.000	1.000	1.000	1.000
12	12	0.770	0.971	0.996	0.999	1.000	1.000	1.000	1.000	1.000
12	12	0.827	0.985	0.999	1.000	1.000	1.000	1.000	1.000	1.000
13	13	0.791	0.978	0.998	1.000	1.000	1.000	1.000	1.000	1.000
13	13	0.853	0.990	0.999	1.000	1.000	1.000	1.000	1.000	1.000
14	14	0.811	0.983	0.998	1.000	1.000	1.000	1.000	1.000	1.000
14	14	0.874	0.994	1.000	1.000	1.000	1.000	1.000	1.000	1.000
15	15	0.828	0.987	0.999	1.000	1.000	1.000	1.000	1.000	1.000
15	15	0.893	0.996	1.000	1.000	1.000	1.000	1.000	1.000	1.000
15	2	0.198	0.293	0.383	0.466	0.543	0.612	0.674	0.728	0.775
15	2	0.198	0.293	0.383	0.467	0.545	0.614	0.677	0.731	0.779
2	15	0.389	0.562	0.662	0.726	0.770	0.802	0.827	0.845	0.861
2	15	0.393	0.566	0.666	0.730	0.773	0.805	0.829	0.848	0.863

Power of F' and F Tests (Size α) of $H_0: \sigma_1 = \sigma_2$ vs. $H_1: \sigma_1 = k\sigma_2$

(The first line of each pair gives the power of the F' test, the second line that of the F test; n_1 and n_2 are sample sizes)

$\alpha = .05$										
n_1	n_2 \ k	2	3	4	5	6	7	8	9	10
2	2	0.099	0.148	0.194	0.239	0.281	0.320	0.358	0.392	0.424
2	2	0.099	0.148	0.194	0.239	0.281	0.321	0.358	0.392	0.425
3	3	0.174	0.321	0.456	0.566	0.653	0.719	0.769	0.808	0.839
3	3	0.174	0.321	0.457	0.568	0.655	0.721	0.771	0.810	0.840
4	4	0.251	0.484	0.660	0.775	0.847	0.893	0.923	0.943	0.957
4	4	0.254	0.490	0.667	0.781	0.853	0.897	0.926	0.946	0.959
5	5	0.323	0.612	0.789	0.883	0.932	0.959	0.974	0.983	0.988
5	5	0.331	0.626	0.802	0.893	0.939	0.963	0.977	0.985	0.990
6	6	0.387	0.707	0.868	0.938	0.969	0.984	0.991	0.995	0.997
6	6	0.402	0.729	0.884	0.948	0.975	0.987	0.993	0.996	0.997
7	7	0.443	0.777	0.917	0.967	0.986	0.993	0.997	0.998	0.999
7	7	0.468	0.806	0.933	0.975	0.990	0.995	0.998	0.999	0.999
8	8	0.493	0.830	0.947	0.982	0.993	0.997	0.999	0.999	1.000
8	8	0.528	0.862	0.962	0.988	0.996	0.998	0.999	1.000	1.000
9	9	0.537	0.869	0.966	0.990	0.997	0.999	1.000	1.000	1.000
9	9	0.582	0.902	0.978	0.994	0.998	0.999	1.000	1.000	1.000
10	10	0.576	0.898	0.978	0.995	0.998	1.000	1.000	1.000	1.000
10	10	0.631	0.931	0.988	0.997	0.999	1.000	1.000	1.000	1.000
11	11	0.611	0.921	0.985	0.997	0.999	1.000	1.000	1.000	1.000
11	11	0.675	0.952	0.993	0.999	1.000	1.000	1.000	1.000	1.000
12	12	0.642	0.938	0.990	0.998	1.000	1.000	1.000	1.000	1.000
12	12	0.714	0.967	0.996	0.999	1.000	1.000	1.000	1.000	1.000
13	13	0.670	0.951	0.993	0.999	1.000	1.000	1.000	1.000	1.000
13	13	0.749	0.977	0.998	1.000	1.000	1.000	1.000	1.000	1.000
14	14	0.695	0.961	0.996	0.999	1.000	1.000	1.000	1.000	1.000
14	14	0.781	0.984	0.999	1.000	1.000	1.000	1.000	1.000	1.000
15	15	0.717	0.969	0.997	1.000	1.000	1.000	1.000	1.000	1.000
15	15	0.808	0.989	0.999	1.000	1.000	1.000	1.000	1.000	1.000
15	2	0.100	0.149	0.198	0.246	0.292	0.338	0.382	0.425	0.466
15	2	0.100	0.149	0.198	0.246	0.293	0.338	0.382	0.425	0.466
2	15	0.295	0.479	0.594	0.669	0.721	0.759	0.789	0.812	0.830
2	15	0.302	0.486	0.600	0.674	0.726	0.764	0.793	0.815	0.833

Power of F' and F Tests (Size α) of $H_0: \sigma_1 = \sigma_2$ and $H_1: \sigma_1 = k\sigma_2$

(The first line of each pair gives the power of the F' test, the second line that of the F test; n_1 and n_2 are sample sizes)

$\alpha = .025$										
n_1	n_2 \ k	2	3	4	5	6	7	8	9	10
2	2	0.050	0.075	0.099	0.123	0.147	0.171	0.194	0.216	0.238
2	2	0.050	0.075	0.099	0.123	0.147	0.171	0.194	0.216	0.238
3	3	0.093	0.187	0.290	0.389	0.478	0.555	0.619	0.673	0.717
3	3	0.093	0.187	0.291	0.391	0.480	0.557	0.621	0.675	0.719
4	4	0.147	0.330	0.505	0.641	0.740	0.809	0.858	0.892	0.916
4	4	0.148	0.334	0.511	0.649	0.748	0.816	0.863	0.897	0.920
5	5	0.204	0.463	0.668	0.798	0.875	0.920	0.948	0.965	0.975
5	5	0.209	0.476	0.683	0.812	0.886	0.928	0.953	0.969	0.978
6	6	0.259	0.573	0.779	0.886	0.940	0.966	0.981	0.988	0.993
6	6	0.270	0.597	0.801	0.902	0.950	0.973	0.984	0.991	0.994
7	7	0.311	0.661	0.852	0.936	0.971	0.986	0.993	0.996	0.998
7	7	0.330	0.695	0.878	0.950	0.978	0.990	0.995	0.997	0.998
8	8	0.358	0.730	0.901	0.963	0.985	0.994	0.997	0.999	0.999
8	8	0.388	0.772	0.926	0.975	0.991	0.996	0.998	0.999	1.000
9	9	0.402	0.784	0.933	0.979	0.993	0.997	0.999	1.000	1.000
9	9	0.444	0.832	0.956	0.988	0.996	0.999	0.999	1.000	1.000
10	10	0.443	0.827	0.955	0.988	0.996	0.999	1.000	1.000	1.000
10	10	0.496	0.877	0.974	0.994	0.998	1.000	1.000	1.000	1.000
11	11	0.479	0.861	0.969	0.993	0.998	0.999	1.000	1.000	1.000
11	11	0.545	0.910	0.985	0.997	0.999	1.000	1.000	1.000	1.000
12	12	0.514	0.887	0.978	0.996	0.999	1.000	1.000	1.000	1.000
12	12	0.591	0.935	0.991	0.999	1.000	1.000	1.000	1.000	1.000
13	13	0.544	0.909	0.985	0.997	0.999	1.000	1.000	1.000	1.000
13	13	0.632	0.954	0.995	0.999	1.000	1.000	1.000	1.000	1.000
14	14	0.573	0.926	0.990	0.998	1.000	1.000	1.000	1.000	1.000
14	14	0.671	0.967	0.997	1.000	1.000	1.000	1.000	1.000	1.000
15	15	0.599	0.939	0.993	0.999	1.000	1.000	1.000	1.000	1.000
15	15	0.706	0.976	0.998	1.000	1.000	1.000	1.000	1.000	1.000
15	2	0.050	0.075	0.100	0.124	0.149	0.173	0.198	0.222	0.245
15	2	0.050	0.075	0.100	0.124	0.149	0.173	0.198	0.222	0.246
2	15	0.223	0.408	0.532	0.616	0.675	0.719	0.753	0.779	0.801
2	15	0.230	0.417	0.540	0.624	0.682	0.725	0.758	0.784	0.805

Power of F' and F Tests (Size α) of $H_0 : \sigma_1 = \sigma_2$ vs. $H_1 : \sigma_1 = k\sigma_2$

(The first line of each pair gives the power of the F' test, the second line that of the F test; n_1 and n_2 are sample sizes)

α = .01										
n_1	n_2 \ k	2	3	4	5	6	7	8	9	10
2	2	0.020	0.030	0.040	0.050	0.060	0.070	0.080	0.089	0.099
2	2	0.020	0.030	0.040	0.050	0.060	0.070	0.080	0.089	0.099
3	3	0.039	0.083	0.139	0.201	0.266	0.330	0.391	0.448	0.501
3	3	0.039	0.083	0.139	0.202	0.267	0.331	0.393	0.450	0.503
4	4	0.067	0.176	0.310	0.442	0.556	0.649	0.722	0.778	0.822
4	4	0.068	0.178	0.314	0.448	0.563	0.657	0.730	0.786	0.829
5	5	0.102	0.287	0.486	0.646	0.759	0.835	0.886	0.919	0.942
5	5	0.104	0.296	0.500	0.662	0.775	0.848	0.896	0.927	0.948
6	6	0.141	0.396	0.629	0.783	0.873	0.924	0.954	0.971	0.981
6	6	0.146	0.417	0.656	0.806	0.891	0.937	0.962	0.977	0.985
7	7	0.180	0.494	0.735	0.868	0.933	0.965	0.981	0.989	0.994
7	7	0.192	0.529	0.771	0.893	0.949	0.975	0.987	0.993	0.996
8	8	0.219	0.578	0.812	0.919	0.965	0.984	0.992	0.996	0.998
8	8	0.239	0.626	0.851	0.943	0.977	0.990	0.995	0.998	0.999
9	9	0.257	0.649	0.866	0.951	0.981	0.992	0.997	0.999	0.999
9	9	0.288	0.708	0.905	0.970	0.990	0.996	0.998	0.999	1.000
10	10	0.293	0.707	0.904	0.970	0.990	0.996	0.999	0.999	1.000
10	10	0.336	0.775	0.941	0.984	0.995	0.999	0.999	1.000	1.000
11	11	0.327	0.756	0.931	0.981	0.995	0.998	0.999	1.000	1.000
11	11	0.383	0.828	0.963	0.992	0.998	0.999	1.000	1.000	1.000
12	12	0.360	0.796	0.950	0.988	0.997	0.999	1.000	1.000	1.000
12	12	0.430	0.870	0.978	0.996	0.999	1.000	1.000	1.000	1.000
13	13	0.390	0.829	0.964	0.993	0.998	1.000	1.000	1.000	1.000
13	13	0.474	0.902	0.986	0.998	1.000	1.000	1.000	1.000	1.000
14	14	0.420	0.856	0.974	0.995	0.999	1.000	1.000	1.000	1.000
14	14	0.517	0.927	0.992	0.999	1.000	1.000	1.000	1.000	1.000
15	15	0.447	0.879	0.981	0.997	0.999	1.000	1.000	1.000	1.000
15	15	0.558	0.946	0.995	1.000	1.000	1.000	1.000	1.000	1.000
15	2	0.020	0.030	0.040	0.050	0.060	0.070	0.080	0.090	0.100
15	2	0.020	0.030	0.040	0.050	0.060	0.070	0.080	0.090	0.100
2	15	0.151	0.326	0.457	0.550	0.617	0.668	0.707	0.738	0.764
2	15	0.159	0.338	0.469	0.561	0.627	0.677	0.715	0.746	0.770

Power of F' and F Tests (Size α) of $H_0 : \sigma_1 = \sigma_2$ vs. $H_1 : \sigma_1 = k\sigma_2$

(The first line of each pair gives the power of the F' test, the second line that of the F test; n_1 and n_2 are sample sizes)

α = .005										
n_1	n_2 \ k	2	3	4	5	6	7	8	9	10
2	2	0.010	0.015	0.020	0.025	0.030	0.035	0.040	0.045	0.050
2	2	0.010	0.015	0.020	0.025	0.030	0.035	0.040	0.045	0.050
3	3	0.020	0.043	0.074	0.111	0.153	0.197	0.243	0.288	0.333
3	3	0.020	0.043	0.074	0.112	0.153	0.198	0.243	0.289	0.334
4	4	0.036	0.102	0.195	0.302	0.407	0.503	0.586	0.656	0.714
4	4	0.036	0.103	0.198	0.306	0.413	0.510	0.594	0.664	0.722
5	5	0.058	0.186	0.353	0.513	0.643	0.741	0.811	0.861	0.897
5	5	0.059	0.191	0.364	0.529	0.660	0.757	0.826	0.874	0.907
6	6	0.084	0.281	0.503	0.679	0.798	0.872	0.918	0.946	0.964
6	6	0.087	0.296	0.529	0.707	0.822	0.891	0.932	0.956	0.971
7	7	0.113	0.374	0.627	0.794	0.888	0.938	0.965	0.979	0.988
7	7	0.120	0.404	0.667	0.828	0.911	0.953	0.975	0.986	0.992
8	8	0.144	0.461	0.724	0.869	0.938	0.970	0.985	0.992	0.996
8	8	0.157	0.507	0.772	0.902	0.958	0.981	0.991	0.995	0.998
9	9	0.174	0.537	0.796	0.916	0.966	0.985	0.993	0.997	0.998
9	9	0.196	0.599	0.848	0.946	0.980	0.992	0.997	0.999	0.999
10	10	0.205	0.604	0.849	0.946	0.981	0.993	0.997	0.999	0.999
10	10	0.238	0.679	0.901	0.971	0.991	0.997	0.999	1.000	1.000
11	11	0.235	0.662	0.888	0.966	0.989	0.996	0.999	1.000	1.000
11	11	0.280	0.746	0.936	0.984	0.996	0.999	1.000	1.000	1.000
12	12	0.264	0.710	0.917	0.978	0.994	0.998	0.999	1.000	1.000
12	12	0.322	0.802	0.959	0.992	0.998	1.000	1.000	1.000	1.000
13	13	0.292	0.752	0.938	0.986	0.997	0.999	1.000	1.000	1.000
13	13	0.365	0.847	0.975	0.996	0.999	1.000	1.000	1.000	1.000
14	14	0.319	0.788	0.954	0.991	0.998	1.000	1.000	1.000	1.000
14	14	0.406	0.882	0.984	0.998	1.000	1.000	1.000	1.000	1.000
15	15	0.345	0.818	0.965	0.994	0.999	1.000	1.000	1.000	1.000
15	15	0.447	0.910	0.990	0.999	1.000	1.000	1.000	1.000	1.000
15	2	0.010	0.015	0.020	0.025	0.030	0.035	0.040	0.045	0.050
15	2	0.010	0.015	0.020	0.025	0.030	0.035	0.040	0.045	0.050
2	15	0.112	0.274	0.406	0.504	0.576	0.631	0.674	0.708	0.736
2	15	0.119	0.286	0.420	0.517	0.588	0.642	0.684	0.717	0.744

Power of F' and F Tests (Size α) of $H_0: \sigma_1 = \sigma_2$ vs. $H_1: \sigma_1 = k\sigma_2$

(The first line of each pair gives the power of the F' test, the second line that of the F test; n_1 and n_2 are sample sizes)

α = .001										
n_1	n_2 \ k	2	3	4	5	6	7	8	9	10
2	2	0.002	0.003	0.004	0.005	0.006	0.007	0.008	0.009	0.010
2	2	0.002	0.003	0.004	0.005	0.006	0.007	0.008	0.009	0.010
3	3	0.004	0.009	0.016	0.024	0.035	0.047	0.060	0.075	0.091
3	3	0.004	0.009	0.016	0.024	0.035	0.047	0.060	0.075	0.091
4	4	0.008	0.024	0.053	0.094	0.144	0.201	0.262	0.325	0.386
4	4	0.008	0.024	0.053	0.095	0.146	0.204	0.266	0.330	0.392
5	5	0.014	0.055	0.131	0.232	0.344	0.452	0.550	0.633	0.703
5	5	0.014	0.056	0.135	0.240	0.356	0.468	0.567	0.652	0.721
6	6	0.022	0.103	0.242	0.403	0.551	0.672	0.763	0.829	0.876
6	6	0.023	0.108	0.256	0.427	0.580	0.701	0.790	0.852	0.895
7	7	0.034	0.163	0.364	0.561	0.712	0.816	0.883	0.925	0.951
7	7	0.035	0.177	0.396	0.603	0.753	0.850	0.908	0.943	0.964
8	8	0.047	0.230	0.480	0.687	0.822	0.900	0.943	0.967	0.981
8	8	0.051	0.258	0.532	0.741	0.864	0.929	0.963	0.980	0.989
9	9	0.062	0.299	0.583	0.781	0.891	0.946	0.973	0.986	0.993
9	9	0.070	0.345	0.651	0.839	0.929	0.968	0.985	0.993	0.996
10	10	0.079	0.367	0.668	0.848	0.934	0.971	0.987	0.994	0.997
10	10	0.092	0.433	0.748	0.903	0.964	0.986	0.994	0.998	0.999
11	11	0.096	0.431	0.737	0.895	0.960	0.984	0.994	0.997	0.999
11	11	0.116	0.517	0.822	0.943	0.982	0.994	0.998	0.999	1.000
12	12	0.114	0.490	0.793	0.927	0.976	0.992	0.997	0.999	1.000
12	12	0.143	0.595	0.877	0.968	0.991	0.998	0.999	1.000	1.000
13	13	0.133	0.544	0.837	0.950	0.985	0.995	0.999	0.999	1.000
13	13	0.172	0.664	0.917	0.982	0.996	0.999	1.000	1.000	1.000
14	14	0.152	0.593	0.871	0.965	0.991	0.997	0.999	1.000	1.000
14	14	0.203	0.725	0.944	0.990	0.998	1.000	1.000	1.000	1.000
15	15	0.170	0.637	0.898	0.976	0.994	0.999	1.000	1.000	1.000
15	15	0.235	0.778	0.963	0.995	0.999	1.000	1.000	1.000	1.000
15	2	0.002	0.003	0.004	0.005	0.006	0.007	0.008	0.009	0.010
15	2	0.002	0.003	0.004	0.005	0.006	0.007	0.008	0.009	0.010
2	15	0.052	0.176	0.301	0.404	0.485	0.548	0.598	0.639	0.673
2	15	0.057	0.189	0.318	0.422	0.501	0.564	0.613	0.653	0.685

Table A4

PROBABILITY INTEGRAL $P(W, n)$ OF THE RANGE W FOR SAMPLES OF SIZE n FROM $N(\mu, 1)$

W	P(W,2)	P(W,3)	P(W,4)	P(W,5)	P(W,6)
0.00	.0000 0000	.0000 0000	.0000 0000		
0.01	.0056 4185	.0000 2757	.0000 0013	.0000 0000	
0.02	.0112 8342	.0001 1026	.0000 0102	.0000 0001	
0.03	.0169 2442	.0002 4807	.0000 0343	.0000 0005	
0.04	.0225 6457	.0004 4097	.0000 0812	.0000 0014	.0000 0000
0.05	.0282 0360	.0006 8892	.0000 1587	.0000 0035	.0000 0001
0.06	.0338 4122	.0009 9190	.0000 2741	.0000 0073	.0000 0002
0.07	.0394 7715	.0013 4984	.0000 4352	.0000 0136	.0000 0004
0.08	.0451 1111	.0017 6269	.0000 6494	.0000 0232	.0000 0008
0.09	.0507 4281	.0022 3037	.0000 9243	.0000 0371	.0000 0015
0.10	.0563 7198	.0027 5282	.0001 2675	.0000 0565	.0000 0025
0.11	.0619 9833	.0033 2994	.0001 6864	.0000 0827	.0000 0040
0.12	.0676 2159	.0039 6164	.0002 1884	.0000 1171	.0000 0061
0.13	.0732 4148	.0046 4781	.0002 7811	.0000 1611	.0000 0091
0.14	.0788 5772	.0053 8834	.0003 4718	.0000 2166	.0000 0132
0.15	.0844 7003	.0061 8311	.0004 2678	.0000 2852	.0000 0187
0.16	.0900 7813	.0070 3198	.0005 1765	.0000 3690	.0000 0258
0.17	.0956 8174	.0079 3481	.0006 2052	.0000 4699	.0000 0349
0.18	.1012 8059	.0088 9146	.0007 3611	.0000 5901	.0000 0464
0.19	.1068 7441	.0099 0176	.0008 6513	.0000 7320	.0000 0607
0.20	.1124 6292	.0109 6555	.0010 0831	.0000 8978	.0000 0783
0.21	.1180 4584	.0120 8265	.0011 6635	.0001 0903	.0000 0999
0.22	.1236 2290	.0132 5287	.0013 3996	.0001 3119	.0000 1259
0.23	.1291 9383	.0144 7603	.0015 2982	.0001 5656	.0000 1570
0.24	.1347 5835	.0157 5193	.0017 3664	.0001 8541	.0000 1940
0.25	.1403 1620	.0170 8034	.0019 6109	.0002 1805	.0000 2376
0.26	.1458 6711	.0184 6105	.0022 0386	.0002 5479	.0000 2886
0.27	.1514 1081	.0198 9384	.0024 6561	.0002 9594	.0000 3481
0.28	.1569 4703	.0213 7847	.0027 4701	.0003 4184	.0000 4168
0.29	.1624 7551	.0229 1470	.0030 4872	.0003 9283	.0000 4960
0.30	.1679 9597	.0245 0227	.0033 7139	.0004 4927	.0000 5867
0.31	.1735 0816	.0261 4092	.0037 1565	.0005 1151	.0000 6900
0.32	.1790 1181	.0278 3038	.0040 8215	.0005 7992	.0000 8073
0.33	.1845 0667	.0295 7039	.0044 7151	.0006 5489	.0000 9399
0.34	.1899 9246	.0313 6065	.0048 8434	.0007 3680	.0001 0892
0.35	.1954 6894	.0332 0087	.0053 2125	.0008 2606	.0001 2567
0.36	.2009 3584	.0350 9075	.0057 8285	.0009 2307	.0001 4439
0.37	.2063 9291	.0370 2999	.0062 6972	.0010 2824	.0001 6526
0.38	.2118 3989	.0390 1827	.0067 8245	.0011 4200	.0001 8844
0.39	.2172 7654	.0410 5526	.0073 2161	.0012 6478	.0002 1412
0.40	.2227 0259	.0431 4064	.0078 8775	.0013 9701	.0002 4248
0.41	.2281 1780	.0452 7408	.0084 8144	.0015 3914	.0002 7373
0.42	.2335 2192	.0474 5521	.0091 0322	.0016 9163	.0003 0808
0.43	.2389 1471	.0496 8371	.0097 5361	.0018 5492	.0003 4573
0.44	.2442 9591	.0519 5919	.0104 3313	.0020 2949	.0003 8691
0.45	.2496 6529	.0542 8131	.0111 4231	.0022 1580	.0004 3186
0.46	.2550 2260	.0566 4968	.0118 8164	.0024 1433	.0004 8082
0.47	.2603 6760	.0590 6393	.0126 5161	.0026 2556	.0005 3403
0.48	.2657 0006	.0615 2367	.0134 5270	.0028 4998	.0005 9176
0.49	.2710 1973	.0640 2851	.0142 8537	.0030 8806	.0006 5428

W	P(W,2)	P(W,3)	P(W,4)	P(W,5)	P(W,6)
0.50	.2763 2639	.0665 7805	.0151 5009	.0033 4032	.0007 2185
0.51	.2816 1980	.0691 7189	.0160 4729	.0036 0723	.0007 9477
0.52	.2868 9972	.0718 0961	.0169 7741	.0038 8932	.0008 7332
0.53	.2921 6594	.0744 9079	.0179 4087	.0041 8707	.0009 5782
0.54	.2974 1822	.0772 1502	.0189 3808	.0045 0100	.0010 4856
0.55	.3026 5634	.0799 8186	.0199 6943	.0048 3161	.0011 4588
0.56	.3078 8007	.0827 9088	.0210 3532	.0051 7942	.0012 5009
0.57	.3130 8919	.0856 4163	.0221 3611	.0055 4494	.0013 6153
0.58	.3182 8350	.0885 3367	.0232 7216	.0059 2868	.0014 8054
0.59	.3234 6276	.0914 6655	.0244 4382	.0063 3116	.0016 0748
0.60	.3286 2676	.0944 3981	.0256 5143	.0067 5290	.0017 4271
0.61	.3337 7529	.0974 5299	.0268 9531	.0071 9441	.0018 8658
0.62	.3389 0815	.1005 0562	.0281 7577	.0076 5620	.0020 3949
0.63	.3440 2512	.1035 9723	.0294 9311	.0081 3880	.0022 0180
0.64	.3491 2599	.1067 2734	.0308 4761	.0086 4271	.0023 7391
0.65	.3542 1057	.1098 9547	.0322 3954	.0091 6846	.0025 5621
0.66	.3592 7866	.1131 0113	.0336 6916	.0097 1655	.0027 4912
0.67	.3643 3004	.1163 4383	.0351 3671	.0102 8749	.0029 5303
0.68	.3693 6453	.1196 2307	.0366 4243	.0108 8180	.0031 6837
0.69	.3743 8193	.1229 3837	.0381 8654	.0114 9998	.0033 9555
0.70	.3793 8205	.1262 8920	.0397 6924	.0121 4253	.0036 3502
0.71	.3843 6471	.1296 7507	.0413 9073	.0128 0996	.0038 8720
0.72	.3893 2970	.1330 9547	.0430 5118	.0135 0275	.0041 5253
0.73	.3942 7685	.1365 4987	.0447 5076	.0142 2141	.0044 3146
0.74	.3992 0598	.1400 3776	.0464 8962	.0149 6642	.0047 2445
0.75	.4041 1691	.1435 5862	.0482 6791	.0157 3827	.0050 3195
0.76	.4090 0945	.1471 1193	.0500 8574	.0165 3744	.0053 5442
0.77	.4138 8344	.1506 9714	.0519 4323	.0173 6439	.0056 9232
0.78	.4187 3870	.1543 1374	.0538 4049	.0182 1961	.0060 4614
0.79	.4235 7506	.1579 6118	.0557 7759	.0191 0354	.0064 1634
0.80	.4283 9236	.1616 3894	.0577 5461	.0200 1666	.0068 0339
0.81	.4331 9042	.1653 4646	.0597 7161	.0209 5941	.0072 0779
0.82	.4379 6909	.1690 8321	.0618 2863	.0219 3223	.0076 3001
0.83	.4427 2821	.1728 4865	.0639 2572	.0229 3557	.0080 7055
0.84	.4474 6762	.1766 4222	.0660 6288	.0239 6985	.0085 2988
0.85	.4521 8716	.1804 6338	.0682 4013	.0250 3549	.0090 0851
0.86	.4568 8669	.1843 1157	.0704 5746	.0261 3291	.0095 0692
0.87	.4615 6606	.1881 8624	.0727 1485	.0272 6252	.0100 2562
0.88	.4662 2512	.1920 8684	.0750 1227	.0284 2472	.0105 6509
0.89	.4708 6372	.1960 1281	.0773 4967	.0296 1988	.0111 2583
0.90	.4754 8172	.1999 6360	.0797 2700	.0308 4841	.0117 0835
0.91	.4800 7899	.2039 3864	.0821 4418	.0321 1066	.0123 1313
0.92	.4846 5539	.2079 3737	.0846 0113	.0334 0700	.0129 4068
0.93	.4892 1079	.2119 5923	.0870 9777	.0347 3778	.0135 9150
0.94	.4937 4505	.2160 0366	.0896 3397	.0361 0335	.0142 6607
0.95	.4982 5805	.2200 7010	.0922 0961	.0375 0403	.0149 6489
0.96	.5027 4967	.2241 5798	.0948 2457	.0389 4016	.0156 8847
0.97	.5072 1978	.2282 6674	.0974 7871	.0404 1203	.0164 3728
0.98	.5116 6826	.2323 9582	.1001 7185	.0419 1997	.0172 1182
0.99	.5160 9500	.2365 4464	.1029 0384	.0434 6424	.0180 1257

W	P(W,2)	P(W,3)	P(W,4)	P(W,5)	P(W,6)
1.00	.5204 9988	.2407 1264	.1056 7449	.0450 4514	.0188 4003
1.01	.5248 8279	.2448 9926	.1084 8361	.0466 6294	.0196 9466
1.02	.5292 4362	.2491 0394	.1113 3099	.0483 1788	.0205 7696
1.03	.5335 8227	.2533 2610	.1142 1642	.0500 1022	.0214 8738
1.04	.5378 9863	.2575 6518	.1171 3968	.0517 4018	.0224 2640
1.05	.5421 9261	.2618 2062	.1201 0051	.0535 0800	.0233 9449
1.06	.5464 6410	.2660 9185	.1230 9868	.0553 1387	.0243 9210
1.07	.5507 1301	.2703 7832	.1261 3393	.0571 5800	.0254 1969
1.08	.5549 3925	.2746 7946	.1292 0597	.0590 4057	.0264 7771
1.09	.5591 4273	.2789 9470	.1323 1453	.0609 6176	.0275 6660
1.10	.5633 2337	.2833 2350	.1354 5932	.0629 2172	.0286 8679
1.11	.5674 8107	.2876 6528	.1386 4004	.0649 2059	.0298 3872
1.12	.5716 1576	.2920 1949	.1418 5636	.0669 5853	.0310 2281
1.13	.5757 2737	.2963 8558	.1451 0798	.0690 3564	.0322 3948
1.14	.5798 1581	.3007 6299	.1483 9454	.0711 5203	.0334 8913
1.15	.5838 8101	.3051 5117	.1517 1572	.0733 0781	.0347 7217
1.16	.5879 2290	.3095 4956	.1550 7116	.0755 0305	.0360 8899
1.17	.5919 4142	.3139 5762	.1584 6050	.0777 3782	.0374 3997
1.18	.5959 3650	.3183 7480	.1618 8336	.0800 1218	.0388 2549
1.19	.5999 0807	.3228 0055	.1653 3938	.0823 2617	.0402 4591
1.20	.6038 5609	.3272 3434	.1688 2815	.0846 7982	.0417 0159
1.21	.6077 8049	.3316 7561	.1723 4929	.0870 7315	.0431 9289
1.22	.6116 8122	.3361 2384	.1759 0238	.0895 0615	.0447 2013
1.23	.6155 5823	.3405 7848	.1794 8702	.0919 7883	.0462 8364
1.24	.6194 1146	.3450 3900	.1831 0277	.0944 9115	.0478 8375
1.25	.6232 4088	.3495 0487	.1867 4922	.0970 4308	.0495 2076
1.26	.6270 4644	.3539 7557	.1904 2593	.0996 3456	.0511 9496
1.27	.6308 2811	.3584 5056	.1941 3244	.1022 6554	.0529 0664
1.28	.6345 8583	.3629 2934	.1978 6831	.1049 3594	.0546 5608
1.29	.6383 1958	.3674 1136	.2016 3308	.1076 4566	.0564 4353
1.30	.6420 2933	.3718 9613	.2054 2629	.1103 9460	.0582 6925
1.31	.6457 1504	.3763 8313	.2092 4745	.1131 8264	.0601 3347
1.32	.6493 7669	.3808 7185	.2130 9609	.1160 0966	.0620 3642
1.33	.6530 1425	.3853 6179	.2169 7173	.1188 7551	.0639 7832
1.34	.6566 2770	.3898 5243	.2208 7388	.1217 8003	.0659 5936
1.35	.6602 1703	.3943 4329	.2248 0203	.1247 2306	.0679 7974
1.36	.6637 8220	.3988 3387	.2287 5568	.1277 0441	.0700 3963
1.37	.6673 2322	.4033 2368	.2327 3433	.1307 2389	.0721 3919
1.38	.6708 4006	.4078 1222	.2367 3746	.1337 8129	.0742 7857
1.39	.6743 3272	.4122 9903	.2407 6455	.1368 7639	.0764 5791
1.40	.6778 0119	.4167 8361	.2448 1508	.1400 0895	.0786 7733
1.41	.6812 4547	.4212 6550	.2488 8853	.1431 7874	.0809 3694
1.42	.6846 6555	.4257 4421	.2529 8435	.1463 8549	.0832 3684
1.43	.6880 6143	.4302 1930	.2571 0202	.1496 2894	.0855 7711
1.44	.6914 3312	.4346 9029	.2612 4099	.1529 0881	.0879 5781
1.45	.6947 8062	.4391 5672	.2654 0071	.1562 2479	.0903 7900
1.46	.6981 0394	.4436 1814	.2695 8065	.1595 7659	.0928 4072
1.47	.7014 0309	.4480 7411	.2737 8024	.1629 6389	.0953 4300
1.48	.7046 7808	.4525 2417	.2779 9894	.1663 8636	.0978 8584
1.49	.7079 2892	.4569 6790	.2822 3618	.1698 4367	.1004 6925

W	P(W,2)	P(W,3)	P(W,4)	P(W,5)	P(W,6)
1.50	.7111 5563	.4614 0484	.2864 9141	.1733 3546	.1030 9320
1.51	.7143 5824	.4658 3458	.2907 6407	.1768 6136	.1057 5767
1.52	.7175 3675	.4702 5669	.2950 5358	.1804 2102	.1084 6262
1.53	.7206 9120	.4746 7074	.2993 5939	.1840 1405	.1112 0797
1.54	.7238 2161	.4790 7633	.3036 8092	.1876 4005	.1139 9366
1.55	.7269 2801	.4834 7303	.3080 1760	.1912 9863	.1168 1959
1.56	.7300 1043	.4878 6045	.3123 6886	.1949 8936	.1196 8567
1.57	.7330 6890	.4922 3817	.3167 3413	.1987 1183	.1225 9178
1.58	.7361 0345	.4966 0582	.3211 1283	.2024 6561	.1255 3779
1.59	.7391 1413	.5009 6299	.3255 0439	.2062 5024	.1285 2355
1.60	.7421 0096	.5053 0931	.3299 0823	.2100 6530	.1315 4889
1.61	.7450 6400	.5096 4438	.3343 2377	.2139 1030	.1346 1366
1.62	.7480 0328	.5139 6784	.3387 5044	.2177 8479	.1377 1765
1.63	.7509 1885	.5182 7932	.3431 8766	.2216 8828	.1408 6067
1.64	.7538 1075	.5225 7844	.3476 3486	.2256 2030	.1440 4251
1.65	.7566 7904	.5268 6486	.3520 9145	.2295 8035	.1472 6292
1.66	.7595 2376	.5311 3822	.3565 5686	.2335 6793	.1505 2167
1.67	.7623 4496	.5353 9817	.3610 3052	.2375 8253	.1538 1851
1.68	.7651 4271	.5396 4436	.3655 1185	.2416 2363	.1571 5316
1.69	.7679 1706	.5438 7647	.3700 0028	.2456 9071	.1605 2533
1.70	.7706 6806	.5480 9415	.3744 9522	.2497 8324	.1639 3473
1.71	.7733 9577	.5522 9709	.3789 9612	.2539 0069	.1673 8106
1.72	.7761 0027	.5564 8496	.3835 0241	.2580 4251	.1708 6398
1.73	.7787 8160	.5606 5744	.3880 1351	.2622 0815	.1743 8316
1.74	.7814 3985	.5648 1423	.3925 2885	.2663 9705	.1779 3826
1.75	.7840 7506	.5689 5503	.3970 4788	.2706 0866	.1815 2891
1.76	.7866 8732	.5730 7952	.4015 7003	.2748 4241	.1851 5474
1.77	.7892 7669	.5771 8743	.4060 9475	.2790 9773	.1888 1537
1.78	.7918 4325	.5812 7846	.4106 2147	.2833 7404	.1925 1039
1.79	.7943 8706	.5853 5233	.4151 4964	.2876 7076	.1962 3940
1.80	.7969 0821	.5894 0877	.4196 7871	.2919 8730	.2000 0198
1.81	.7994 0677	.5934 4750	.4242 0813	.2963 2308	.2037 9770
1.82	.8018 8283	.5974 6826	.4287 3736	.3006 7750	.2076 2612
1.83	.8043 3645	.6014 7079	.4332 6585	.3050 4996	.2114 8677
1.84	.8067 6772	.6054 5484	.4377 9306	.3094 3986	.2153 7920
1.85	.8091 7673	.6094 2015	.4423 1846	.3138 4661	.2193 0293
1.86	.8115 6356	.6133 6650	.4468 4152	.3182 6958	.2232 5748
1.87	.8139 2829	.6172 9363	.4513 6171	.3227 0817	.2272 4235
1.88	.8162 7102	.6212 0132	.4558 7850	.3271 6177	.2312 5704
1.89	.8185 9183	.6250 8935	.4603 9138	.3316 2977	.2353 0104
1.90	.8208 9081	.6289 5749	.4648 9983	.3361 1154	.2393 7382
1.91	.8231 6805	.6328 0552	.4694 0334	.3406 0648	.2434 7484
1.92	.8254 2365	.6366 3325	.4739 0140	.3451 1395	.2476 0358
1.93	.8276 5770	.6404 4046	.4783 9352	.3496 3334	.2517 5947
1.94	.8298 7029	.6442 2697	.4828 7919	.3541 6403	.2559 4197
1.95	.8320 6153	.6479 9257	.4873 5792	.3587 0540	.2601 5050
1.96	.8342 3150	.6517 3708	.4918 2922	.3632 5681	.2643 8450
1.97	.8363 8032	.6554 6031	.4962 9261	.3678 1766	.2686 4338
1.98	.8385 0807	.6591 6211	.5007 4762	.3723 8730	.2729 2655
1.99	.8406 1486	.6628 4228	.5051 9377	.3769 6513	.2772 3343

W	P(W,2)	P(W,3)	P(W,4)	P(W,5)	P(W,6)
2.00	.8427 0079	.6665 0067	.5096 3059	.3815 5052	.2815 6340
2.01	.8447 6597	.6701 3713	.5140 5763	.3861 4284	.2859 1588
2.02	.8468 1050	.6737 5148	.5184 7442	.3907 4148	.2902 9023
2.03	.8488 3448	.6773 4360	.5228 8052	.3953 4581	.2946 8584
2.04	.8508 3802	.6809 1332	.5272 7548	.3999 5522	.2991 0210
2.05	.8528 2123	.6844 6052	.5316 5886	.4045 6909	.3035 3836
2.06	.8547 8421	.6879 8507	.5360 3024	.4091 8680	.3079 9400
2.07	.8567 2708	.6914 8682	.5403 8917	.4138 0773	.3124 6837
2.08	.8586 4995	.6949 6567	.5447 3525	.4184 3129	.3169 6084
2.09	.8605 5292	.6984 2149	.5490 6806	.4230 5685	.3214 7076
2.10	.8624 3611	.7018 5418	.5533 8718	.4276 8381	.3259 9747
2.11	.8642 9962	.7052 6362	.5576 9221	.4323 1157	.3305 4033
2.12	.8661 4359	.7086 4971	.5619 8277	.4369 3953	.3350 9867
2.13	.8679 6811	.7120 1236	.5662 5845	.4415 6709	.3396 7184
2.14	.8697 7330	.7153 5148	.5705 1887	.4461 9365	.3442 5918
2.15	.8715 5928	.7186 6697	.5747 6366	.4508 1862	.3488 6001
2.16	.8733 2616	.7219 5876	.5789 9245	.4554 4142	.3534 7368
2.17	.8750 7406	.7252 2677	.5832 0486	.4600 6147	.3580 9952
2.18	.8768 0310	.7284 7093	.5874 0054	.4646 7817	.3627 3685
2.19	.8785 1340	.7316 9116	.5915 7915	.4692 9097	.3673 8501
2.20	.8802 0507	.7348 8741	.5957 4033	.4738 9929	.3720 4332
2.21	.8818 7823	.7380 5961	.5998 8375	.4785 0256	.3767 1112
2.22	.8835 3301	.7412 0772	.6040 0907	.4831 0022	.3813 8773
2.23	.8851 6952	.7443 3169	.6081 1597	.4876 9172	.3860 7248
2.24	.8867 8789	.7474 3146	.6122 0413	.4922 7650	.3907 6470
2.25	.8883 8823	.7505 0701	.6162 7324	.4968 5402	.3954 6372
2.26	.8899 7067	.7535 5829	.6203 2300	.5014 2374	.4001 6886
2.27	.8915 3533	.7565 8528	.6243 5311	.5059 8513	.4048 7946
2.28	.8930 8233	.7595 8794	.6283 6327	.5105 3764	.4095 9485
2.29	.8946 1179	.7625 6626	.6323 5320	.5150 8077	.4143 1436
2.30	.8961 2384	.7655 2022	.6363 2262	.5196 1399	.4190 3733
2.31	.8976 1861	.7684 4980	.6402 7127	.5241 3679	.4237 6310
2.32	.8990 9620	.7713 5499	.6441 9887	.5286 4866	.4284 9101
2.33	.9005 5676	.7742 3580	.6481 0518	.5331 4911	.4332 2040
2.34	.9020 0040	.7770 9221	.6519 8994	.5376 3764	.4379 5061
2.35	.9034 2725	.7799 2423	.6558 5290	.5421 1377	.4426 8100
2.36	.9048 3743	.7827 3187	.6596 9383	.5465 7701	.4474 1091
2.37	.9062 3107	.7855 1513	.6635 1251	.5510 2690	.4521 3970
2.38	.9076 0829	.7882 7403	.6673 0869	.5554 6296	.4568 6673
2.39	.9089 6922	.7910 0860	.6710 8218	.5598 8474	.4615 9137
2.40	.9103 1398	.7937 1884	.6748 3276	.5642 9178	.4663 1298
2.41	.9116 4270	.7964 0479	.6785 6023	.5686 8364	.4710 3093
2.42	.9129 5551	.7990 6647	.6822 6438	.5730 5988	.4757 4461
2.43	.9142 5253	.8017 0393	.6859 4504	.5774 2007	.4804 5338
2.44	.9155 3388	.8043 1718	.6896 0201	.5817 6378	.4851 5664
2.45	.9167 9970	.8069 0628	.6932 3512	.5860 9060	.4898 5378
2.46	.9180 5010	.8094 7127	.6968 4420	.5904 0011	.4945 4419
2.47	.9192 8522	.8120 1219	.7004 2909	.5946 9193	.4992 2728
2.48	.9205 0518	.8145 2909	.7039 8963	.5989 6564	.5039 0246
2.49	.9217 1011	.8170 2203	.7075 2567	.6032 2087	.5085 6914

W	P(W,2)	P(W,3)	P(W,4)	P(W,5)	P(W,6)
2.50	.9229 0013	.8194 9106	.7110 3706	.6074 5724	.5132 2674
2.51	.9240 7536	.8219 3625	.7145 2367	.6116 7437	.5178 7469
2.52	.9252 3594	.8243 5764	.7179 8537	.6158 7190	.5225 1242
2.53	.9263 8199	.8267 5532	.7214 2203	.6200 4947	.5271 3936
2.54	.9275 1363	.8291 2934	.7248 3354	.6242 0675	.5317 5498
2.55	.9286 3099	.8314 7978	.7282 1977	.6283 4338	.5363 5871
2.56	.9297 3419	.8338 0672	.7315 8063	.6324 5903	.5409 5003
2.57	.9308 2337	.8361 1022	.7349 1601	.6365 5338	.5455 2839
2.58	.9318 9863	.8383 9037	.7382 2583	.6406 2611	.5500 9327
2.59	.9329 6012	.8406 4726	.7415 0998	.6446 7692	.5546 4416
2.60	.9340 0795	.8428 8096	.7447 6840	.6487 0549	.5591 8054
2.61	.9350 4224	.8450 9157	.7480 0100	.6527 1155	.5637 0191
2.62	.9360 6312	.8472 7917	.7512 0772	.6566 9480	.5682 0778
2.63	.9370 7072	.8494 4385	.7543 8849	.6606 5496	.5726 9766
2.64	.9380 6516	.8515 8572	.7575 4324	.6645 9177	.5771 7106
2.65	.9390 4655	.8537 0487	.7606 7194	.6685 0496	.5816 2753
2.66	.9400 1503	.8558 0139	.7637 7453	.6723 9428	.5860 6659
2.67	.9409 7071	.8578 7539	.7668 5096	.6762 5949	.5904 8779
2.68	.9419 1372	.8599 2698	.7699 0121	.6801 0035	.5948 9069
2.69	.9428 4417	.8619 5626	.7729 2525	.6839 1662	.5992 7484
2.70	.9437 6220	.8639 6333	.7759 2304	.6877 0808	.6036 3983
2.71	.9446 6791	.8659 4831	.7788 9456	.6914 7453	.6079 8521
2.72	.9455 6144	.8679 1132	.7818 3981	.6952 1574	.6123 1059
2.73	.9464 4289	.8698 5245	.7847 5877	.6989 3153	.6166 1557
2.74	.9473 1240	.8717 7184	.7876 5144	.7026 2170	.6208 9973
2.75	.9481 7007	.8736 6959	.7905 1782	.7062 8607	.6251 6270
2.76	.9490 1604	.8755 4583	.7933 5791	.7099 2447	.6294 0411
2.77	.9498 5040	.8774 0068	.7961 7173	.7135 3671	.6336 2357
2.78	.9506 7330	.8792 3425	.7989 5929	.7171 2265	.6378 2074
2.79	.9514 8483	.8810 4668	.8017 2060	.7206 8213	.6419 9526
2.80	.9522 8512	.8828 3810	.8044 5570	.7242 1500	.6461 4678
2.81	.9530 7428	.8846 0862	.8071 6461	.7277 2112	.6502 7498
2.82	.9538 5244	.8863 5837	.8098 4737	.7312 0037	.6543 7953
2.83	.9546 1970	.8880 8749	.8125 0402	.7346 5262	.6584 6012
2.84	.9553 7618	.8897 9611	.8151 3459	.7380 7774	.6625 1643
2.85	.9561 2199	.8914 8436	.8177 3914	.7414 7565	.6665 4817
2.86	.9568 5725	.8931 5238	.8203 1771	.7448 4622	.6705 5506
2.87	.9575 8207	.8948 0029	.8228 7037	.7481 8936	.6745 3680
2.88	.9582 9657	.8964 2824	.8253 9716	.7515 0500	.6784 9314
2.89	.9590 0085	.8980 3637	.8278 9816	.7547 9303	.6824 2380
2.90	.9596 9503	.8996 2480	.8303 7343	.7580 5340	.6863 2854
2.91	.9603 7921	.9011 9369	.8328 2304	.7612 8603	.6902 0711
2.92	.9610 5351	.9027 4317	.8352 4707	.7644 9085	.6940 5927
2.93	.9617 1804	.9042 7338	.8376 4560	.7676 6783	.6978 8481
2.94	.9623 7290	.9057 8447	.8400 1870	.7708 1690	.7016 8349
2.95	.9630 1821	.9072 7657	.8423 6647	.7739 3803	.7054 5511
2.96	.9636 5407	.9087 4984	.8446 8899	.7770 3118	.7091 9948
2.97	.9642 8058	.9102 0442	.8469 8636	.7800 9632	.7129 1639
2.98	.9648 9786	.9116 4044	.8492 5867	.7831 3343	.7166 0566
2.99	.9655 0602	.9130 5806	.8515 0602	.7861 4249	.7202 6713

W	P(W,2)	P(W,3)	P(W,4)	P(W,5)	P(W,6)
3.00	.9661 0515	.9144 5743	.8537 2852	.7891 2349	.7239 0062
3.01	.9666 9536	.9158 3869	.8559 2626	.7920 7644	.7275 0598
3.02	.9672 7675	.9172 0198	.8580 9937	.7950 0132	.7310 8305
3.03	.9678 4943	.9185 4746	.8602 4794	.7978 9815	.7346 3169
3.04	.9684 1350	.9198 7528	.8623 7210	.8007 6693	.7381 5178
3.05	.9689 6906	.9211 8557	.8644 7196	.8036 0770	.7416 4318
3.06	.9695 1621	.9224 7851	.8665 4764	.8064 2047	.7451 0578
3.07	.9700 5505	.9237 5422	.8685 9926	.8092 0527	.7485 3948
3.08	.9705 8569	.9250 1286	.8706 2695	.8119 6213	.7519 4416
3.09	.9711 0822	.9262 5459	.8726 3084	.8146 9110	.7553 1974
3.10	.9716 2273	.9274 7955	.8746 1105	.8173 9223	.7586 6613
3.11	.9721 2934	.9286 8789	.8765 6773	.8200 6555	.7619 8325
3.12	.9726 2812	.9298 7976	.8785 0099	.8227 1114	.7652 7104
3.13	.9731 1919	.9310 5531	.8804 1099	.8253 2904	.7685 2943
3.14	.9736 0263	.9322 1471	.8822 9785	.8279 1933	.7717 5837
3.15	.9740 7854	.9333 5808	.8841 6173	.8304 8207	.7749 5781
3.16	.9745 4701	.9344 8559	.8860 0276	.8330 1734	.7781 2771
3.17	.9750 0814	.9355 9739	.8878 2108	.8355 2521	.7812 6803
3.18	.9754 6202	.9366 9362	.8896 1686	.8380 0578	.7843 7875
3.19	.9759 0873	.9377 7444	.8913 9022	.8404 5913	.7874 5985
3.20	.9763 4838	.9388 4000	.8931 4133	.8428 8534	.7905 1132
3.21	.9767 8105	.9398 9044	.8948 7033	.8452 8453	.7935 3316
3.22	.9772 0684	.9409 2593	.8965 7739	.8476 5678	.7965 2536
3.23	.9776 2582	.9419 4660	.8982 6265	.8500 0220	.7994 8793
3.24	.9780 3809	.9429 5261	.8999 2627	.8523 2090	.8024 2089
3.25	.9784 4373	.9439 4411	.9015 6841	.8546 1300	.8053 2426
3.26	.9788 4284	.9449 2124	.9031 8922	.8568 7860	.8081 9806
3.27	.9792 3549	.9458 8416	.9047 8888	.8591 1783	.8110 4233
3.28	.9796 2178	.9468 3300	.9063 6754	.8613 3081	.8138 5711
3.29	.9800 0178	.9477 6793	.9079 2536	.8635 1766	.8166 4244
3.30	.9803 7559	.9486 8909	.9094 6250	.8656 7852	.8193 9837
3.31	.9807 4327	.9495 9663	.9109 7914	.8678 1352	.8221 2497
3.32	.9811 0492	.9504 9068	.9124 7544	.8699 2279	.8248 2228
3.33	.9814 6062	.9513 7141	.9139 5156	.8720 0647	.8274 9039
3.34	.9818 1044	.9522 3895	.9154 0768	.8740 6471	.8301 2937
3.35	.9821 5447	.9530 9345	.9168 4395	.8760 9764	.8327 3928
3.36	.9824 9279	.9539 3505	.9182 6056	.8781 0542	.8353 2022
3.37	.9828 2547	.9547 6390	.9196 5766	.8800 8820	.8378 7228
3.38	.9831 5259	.9555 8014	.9210 3544	.8820 4613	.8403 9555
3.39	.9834 7423	.9563 8392	.9223 9405	.8839 7936	.8428 9012
3.40	.9837 9046	.9571 7537	.9237 3368	.8858 8805	.8453 5611
3.41	.9841 0136	.9579 5465	.9250 5450	.8877 7236	.8477 9361
3.42	.9844 0701	.9587 2188	.9263 5667	.8896 3245	.8502 0275
3.43	.9847 0747	.9594 7721	.9276 4037	.8914 6850	.8525 8364
3.44	.9850 0283	.9602 2078	.9289 0577	.8932 8065	.8549 3640
3.45	.9852 9315	.9609 5273	.9301 5305	.8950 6909	.8572 6116
3.46	.9855 7850	.9616 7320	.9313 8238	.8968 3398	.8595 5804
3.47	.9858 5896	.9623 8231	.9325 9393	.8985 7550	.8618 2718
3.48	.9861 3460	.9630 8022	.9337 8788	.9002 9381	.8640 6872
3.49	.9864 0548	.9637 6706	.9349 6440	.9019 8910	.8662 8279

W	P(W,2)	P(W,3)	P(W,4)	P(W,5)	P(W,6)
3.50	.9866 7167	.9644 4296	.9361 2367	.9036 6154	.8684 6955
3.51	.9869 3325	.9651 0805	.9372 6585	.9053 1130	.8706 2914
3.52	.9871 9028	.9657 6247	.9383 9112	.9069 3858	.8727 6172
3.53	.9874 4282	.9664 0636	.9394 9966	.9085 4355	.8748 6743
3.54	.9876 9094	.9670 3984	.9405 9164	.9101 2638	.8769 4643
3.55	.9879 3471	.9676 6304	.9416 6723	.9116 8728	.8789 9890
3.56	.9881 7420	.9682 7610	.9427 2661	.9132 2642	.8810 2499
3.57	.9884 0945	.9688 7914	.9437 6995	.9147 4398	.8830 2487
3.58	.9886 4055	.9694 7229	.9447 9741	.9162 4016	.8849 9870
3.59	.9888 6754	.9700 5568	.9458 0918	.9177 1514	.8869 4667
3.60	.9890 9050	.9706 2944	.9468 0542	.9191 6912	.8888 6895
3.61	.9893 0948	.9711 9369	.9477 8631	.9206 0227	.8907 6571
3.62	.9895 2454	.9717 4855	.9487 5202	.9220 1479	.8926 3714
3.63	.9897 3575	.9722 9416	.9497 0271	.9234 0688	.8944 8342
3.64	.9899 4316	.9728 3063	.9506 3857	.9247 7872	.8963 0473
3.65	.9901 4682	.9733 5808	.9515 5974	.9261 3050	.8981 0126
3.66	.9903 4681	.9738 7664	.9524 6642	.9274 6242	.8998 7320
3.67	.9905 4316	.9743 8642	.9533 5875	.9287 7466	.9016 2074
3.68	.9907 3595	.9748 8755	.9542 3692	.9300 6744	.9033 4407
3.69	.9909 2522	.9753 8014	.9551 0109	.9313 4092	.9050 4339
3.70	.9911 1103	.9758 6431	.9559 5142	.9325 9532	.9067 1889
3.71	.9912 9344	.9763 4017	.9567 8808	.9338 3082	.9083 7077
3.72	.9914 7249	.9768 0784	.9576 1123	.9350 4762	.9099 9923
3.73	.9916 4824	.9772 6744	.9584 2104	.9362 4590	.9116 0446
3.74	.9918 2075	.9777 1907	.9592 1768	.9374 2588	.9131 8668
3.75	.9919 9006	.9781 6285	.9600 0129	.9385 8772	.9147 4609
3.76	.9921 5622	.9785 9889	.9607 7205	.9397 3165	.9162 8287
3.77	.9923 1929	.9790 2730	.9615 3012	.9408 5783	.9177 9726
3.78	.9924 7932	.9794 4819	.9622 7565	.9419 6648	.9192 8944
3.79	.9926 3635	.9798 6167	.9630 0881	.9430 5778	.9207 5962
3.80	.9927 9043	.9802 6784	.9637 2975	.9441 3192	.9222 0802
3.81	.9929 4161	.9806 6681	.9644 3862	.9451 8909	.9236 3483
3.82	.9930 8994	.9810 5868	.9651 3560	.9462 2950	.9250 4028
3.83	.9932 3546	.9814 4356	.9658 2082	.9472 5332	.9264 2456
3.84	.9933 7823	.9818 2155	.9664 9444	.9482 6075	.9277 8790
3.85	.9935 1827	.9821 9276	.9671 5662	.9492 5199	.9291 3049
3.86	.9936 5565	.9825 5727	.9678 0751	.9502 2721	.9304 5255
3.87	.9937 9040	.9829 1520	.9684 4725	.9511 8662	.9317 5429
3.88	.9939 2257	.9832 6664	.9690 7601	.9521 3039	.9330 3592
3.89	.9940 5220	.9836 1169	.9696 9392	.9530 5872	.9342 9766
3.90	.9941 7933	.9839 5045	.9703 0114	.9539 7179	.9355 3970
3.91	.9943 0401	.9842 8300	.9708 9781	.9548 6979	.9367 6228
3.92	.9944 2628	.9846 0945	.9714 8407	.9557 5291	.9379 6559
3.93	.9945 4617	.9849 2990	.9720 6007	.9566 2132	.9391 4985
3.94	.9946 6372	.9852 4442	.9726 2596	.9574 7522	.9403 1527
3.95	.9947 7899	.9855 5312	.9731 8187	.9583 1478	.9414 6205
3.96	.9948 9200	.9858 5608	.9737 2795	.9591 4020	.9425 9042
3.97	.9950 0280	.9861 5339	.9742 6433	.9599 5164	.9437 0058
3.98	.9951 1141	.9864 4515	.9747 9116	.9607 4929	.9447 9273
3.99	.9952 1789	.9867 3144	.9753 0856	.9615 3333	.9458 6710

W	P(W,2)	P(W,3)	P(W,4)	P(W,5)	P(W,6)
4.00	.9953 2226	.9870 1234	.9758 1668	.9623 0393	.9469 2388
4.01	.9954 2457	.9872 8794	.9763 1566	.9630 6128	.9479 6329
4.02	.9955 2485	.9875 5833	.9768 0561	.9638 0555	.9489 8554
4.03	.9956 2313	.9878 2359	.9772 8669	.9645 3691	.9499 9082
4.04	.9957 1945	.9880 8380	.9777 5901	.9652 5553	.9509 7936
4.05	.9958 1385	.9883 3904	.9782 2271	.9659 6160	.9519 5134
4.06	.9959 0635	.9885 8940	.9786 7791	.9666 5528	.9529 0698
4.07	.9959 9699	.9888 3495	.9791 2475	.9673 3674	.9538 4649
4.08	.9960 8581	.9890 7577	.9795 6334	.9680 0614	.9547 7006
4.09	.9961 7283	.9893 1194	.9799 9382	.9686 6367	.9556 7789
4.10	.9962 5810	.9895 4354	.9804 1631	.9693 0948	.9565 7019
4.11	.9963 4163	.9897 7064	.9808 3093	.9699 4373	.9574 4716
4.12	.9964 2346	.9899 9332	.9812 3779	.9705 6660	.9583 0900
4.13	.9965 0363	.9902 1164	.9816 3703	.9711 7824	.9591 5590
4.14	.9965 8215	.9904 2569	.9820 2875	.9717 7882	.9599 8807
4.15	.9966 5907	.9906 3554	.9824 1308	.9723 6849	.9608 0569
4.16	.9967 3441	.9908 4125	.9827 9014	.9729 4742	.9616 0897
4.17	.9968 0820	.9910 4289	.9831 6002	.9735 1576	.9623 9809
4.18	.9968 8046	.9912 4054	.9835 2286	.9740 7366	.9631 7326
4.19	.9969 5123	.9914 3427	.9838 7876	.9746 2129	.9639 3465
4.20	.9970 2053	.9916 2413	.9842 2784	.9751 5878	.9646 8246
4.21	.9970 8840	.9918 1020	.9845 7019	.9756 8631	.9654 1688
4.22	.9971 5485	.9919 9255	.9849 0594	.9762 0401	.9661 3810
4.23	.9972 1991	.9921 7123	.9852 3518	.9767 1203	.9668 4630
4.24	.9972 8361	.9923 4631	.9855 5803	.9772 1052	.9675 4166
4.25	.9973 4597	.9925 1785	.9858 7459	.9776 9963	.9682 2438
4.26	.9974 0702	.9926 8593	.9861 8495	.9781 7950	.9688 9462
4.27	.9974 6679	.9928 5058	.9864 8924	.9786 5028	.9695 5258
4.28	.9975 2529	.9930 1189	.9867 8753	.9791 1210	.9701 9843
4.29	.9975 8256	.9931 6990	.9870 7995	.9795 6511	.9708 3234
4.30	.9976 3861	.9933 2467	.9873 6657	.9800 0944	.9714 5450
4.31	.9976 9346	.9934 7627	.9876 4751	.9804 4523	.9720 6507
4.32	.9977 4715	.9936 2475	.9879 2285	.9808 7262	.9726 6424
4.33	.9977 9969	.9937 7016	.9881 9269	.9812 9174	.9732 5217
4.34	.9978 5111	.9939 1257	.9884 5713	.9817 0273	.9738 2902
4.35	.9979 0142	.9940 5202	.9887 1626	.9821 0571	.9743 9498
4.36	.9979 5065	.9941 8857	.9889 7016	.9825 0081	.9749 5021
4.37	.9979 9882	.9943 2227	.9892 1894	.9828 8817	.9754 9487
4.38	.9980 4594	.9944 5317	.9894 6267	.9832 6791	.9760 2912
4.39	.9980 9205	.9945 8134	.9897 0144	.9836 4015	.9765 5313
4.40	.9981 3715	.9947 0680	.9899 3535	.9840 0503	.9770 6705
4.41	.9981 8128	.9948 2962	.9901 6447	.9843 6266	.9775 7106
4.42	.9982 2444	.9949 4985	.9903 8890	.9847 1316	.9780 6529
4.43	.9982 6666	.9950 6753	.9906 0870	.9850 5665	.9785 4992
4.44	.9983 0795	.9951 8271	.9908 2398	.9853 9325	.9790 2508
4.45	.9983 4833	.9952 9544	.9910 3480	.9857 2308	.9794 9094
4.46	.9983 8783	.9954 0576	.9912 4125	.9860 4626	.9799 4765
4.47	.9984 2646	.9955 1373	.9914 4340	.9863 6289	.9803 9535
4.48	.9984 6423	.9956 1937	.9916 4134	.9866 7309	.9808 3419
4.49	.9985 0117	.9957 2274	.9918 3513	.9869 7697	.9812 6432

W	P(W,2)	P(W,3)	P(W,4)	P(W,5)	P(W,6)
4.50	.9985 3728	.9958 2389	.9920 2486	.9872 7464	.9816 8588
4.51	.9985 7260	.9959 2284	.9922 1060	.9875 6621	.9820 9901
4.52	.9986 0712	.9960 1966	.9923 9242	.9878 5178	.9825 0386
4.53	.9986 4087	.9961 1437	.9925 7039	.9881 3146	.9829 0056
4.54	.9986 7387	.9962 0701	.9927 4458	.9884 0536	.9832 8925
4.55	.9987 0613	.9962 9764	.9929 1507	.9886 7357	.9836 7006
4.56	.9987 3766	.9963 8628	.9930 8193	.9889 3620	.9840 4314
4.57	.9987 6848	.9964 7297	.9932 4521	.9891 9334	.9844 0860
4.58	.9987 9861	.9965 5776	.9934 0499	.9894 4510	.9847 6660
4.59	.9988 2805	.9966 4068	.9935 6133	.9896 9158	.9851 1724
4.60	.9988 5682	.9967 2177	.9937 1431	.9899 3286	.9854 6066
4.61	.9988 8494	.9968 0105	.9938 6397	.9901 6904	.9857 9700
4.62	.9989 1242	.9968 7858	.9940 1039	.9904 0022	.9861 2636
4.63	.9989 3928	.9969 5439	.9941 5363	.9906 2649	.9864 4887
4.64	.9989 6551	.9970 2850	.9942 9375	.9908 4794	.9867 6466
4.65	.9989 9115	.9971 0095	.9944 3080	.9910 6465	.9870 7384
4.66	.9990 1620	.9971 7178	.9945 6485	.9912 7672	.9873 7654
4.67	.9990 4066	.9972 4101	.9946 9595	.9914 8422	.9876 7286
4.68	.9990 6457	.9973 0869	.9948 2417	.9916 8726	.9879 6293
4.69	.9990 8792	.9973 7484	.9949 4955	.9918 8590	.9882 4685
4.70	.9991 1073	.9974 3949	.9950 7216	.9920 8024	.9885 2474
4.71	.9991 3301	.9975 0267	.9951 9205	.9922 7035	.9887 9671
4.72	.9991 5478	.9975 6442	.9953 0926	.9924 5632	.9890 6287
4.73	.9991 7603	.9976 2476	.9954 2386	.9926 3822	.9893 2332
4.74	.9991 9679	.9976 8372	.9955 3590	.9928 1613	.9895 7817
4.75	.9992 1706	.9977 4132	.9956 4543	.9929 9013	.9898 2752
4.76	.9992 3686	.9977 9761	.9957 5249	.9931 6030	.9900 7148
4.77	.9992 5619	.9978 5260	.9958 5714	.9933 2670	.9903 1015
4.78	.9992 7506	.9979 0633	.9959 5942	.9934 8941	.9905 4362
4.79	.9992 9349	.9979 5881	.9960 5939	.9936 4851	.9907 7199
4.80	.9993 1149	.9980 1007	.9961 5708	.9938 0406	.9909 9537
4.81	.9993 2905	.9980 6015	.9962 5255	.9939 5613	.9912 1385
4.82	.9993 4620	.9981 0906	.9963 4584	.9941 0480	.9914 2751
4.83	.9993 6294	.9981 5682	.9964 3700	.9942 5012	.9916 3646
4.84	.9993 7928	.9982 0347	.9965 2606	.9943 9217	.9918 4078
4.85	.9993 9523	.9982 4903	.9966 1308	.9945 3101	.9920 4056
4.86	.9994 1080	.9982 9352	.9966 9808	.9946 6671	.9922 3590
4.87	.9994 2600	.9983 3696	.9967 8113	.9947 9932	.9924 2687
4.88	.9994 4083	.9983 7938	.9968 6225	.9949 2892	.9926 1357
4.89	.9994 5530	.9984 2079	.9969 4149	.9950 5555	.9927 9607
4.90	.9994 6942	.9984 6122	.9970 1888	.9951 7929	.9929 7446
4.91	.9994 8320	.9985 0069	.9970 9447	.9953 0019	.9931 4882
4.92	.9994 9665	.9985 3922	.9971 6828	.9954 1831	.9933 1924
4.93	.9995 0977	.9985 7683	.9972 4037	.9955 3370	.9934 8579
4.94	.9995 2257	.9986 1355	.9973 1076	.9956 4642	.9936 4854
4.95	.9995 3505	.9986 4938	.9973 7950	.9957 5653	.9938 0758
4.96	.9995 4724	.9986 8435	.9974 4661	.9958 6408	.9939 6297
4.97	.9995 5912	.9987 1848	.9975 1213	.9959 6912	.9941 1480
4.98	.9995 7071	.9987 5179	.9975 7609	.9960 7171	.9942 6314
4.99	.9995 8202	.9987 8429	.9976 3854	.9961 7189	.9944 0805

W	P(W,2)	P(W,3)	P(W,4)	P(W,5)	P(W,6)
5.00	.9995 9305	.9988 1601	.9976 9950	.9962 6973	.9945 4960
5.01	.9996 0380	.9988 4695	.9977 5900	.9963 6526	.9946 8788
5.02	.9996 1429	.9988 7715	.9978 1707	.9964 5853	.9948 2293
5.03	.9996 2452	.9989 0660	.9978 7375	.9965 4960	.9949 5483
5.04	.9996 3450	.9989 3534	.9979 2907	.9966 3851	.9950 8365
5.05	.9996 4423	.9989 6337	.9979 8305	.9967 2530	.9952 0945
5.06	.9996 5371	.9989 9072	.9980 3573	.9968 1003	.9953 3230
5.07	.9996 6296	.9990 1739	.9980 8713	.9968 9273	.9954 5224
5.08	.9996 7198	.9990 4340	.9981 3728	.9969 7345	.9955 6935
5.09	.9996 8077	.9990 6878	.9981 8621	.9970 5224	.9956 8369
5.10	.9996 8934	.9990 9352	.9982 3395	.9971 2913	.9957 9531
5.11	.9996 9769	.9991 1765	.9982 8052	.9972 0416	.9959 0427
5.12	.9997 0584	.9991 4118	.9983 2595	.9972 7738	.9960 1063
5.13	.9997 1377	.9991 6413	.9983 7027	.9973 4882	.9961 1445
5.14	.9997 2151	.9991 8650	.9984 1349	.9974 1853	.9962 1577
5.15	.9997 2905	.9992 0831	.9984 5565	.9974 8654	.9963 1466
5.16	.9997 3640	.9992 2958	.9984 9676	.9975 5289	.9964 1116
5.17	.9997 4356	.9992 5031	.9985 3686	.9976 1761	.9965 0533
5.18	.9997 5054	.9992 7052	.9985 7596	.9976 8075	.9965 9721
5.19	.9997 5734	.9992 9022	.9986 1408	.9977 4234	.9966 8686
5.20	.9997 6397	.9993 0943	.9986 5126	.9978 0240	.9967 7433
5.21	.9997 7042	.9993 2815	.9986 8751	.9978 6099	.9968 5967
5.22	.9997 7671	.9993 4639	.9987 2284	.9979 1812	.9969 4291
5.23	.9997 8284	.9993 6417	.9987 5729	.9979 7384	.9970 2412
5.24	.9997 8881	.9993 8149	.9987 9088	.9980 2817	.9971 0332
5.25	.9997 9462	.9993 9837	.9988 2361	.9980 8115	.9971 8057
5.26	.9998 0029	.9994 1483	.9988 5552	.9981 3280	.9972 5592
5.27	.9998 0581	.9994 3086	.9988 8662	.9981 8316	.9973 2939
5.28	.9998 1118	.9994 4647	.9989 1694	.9982 3225	.9974 0104
5.29	.9998 1641	.9994 6169	.9989 4648	.9982 8011	.9974 7091
5.30	.9998 2151	.9994 7651	.9989 7526	.9983 2676	.9975 3904
5.31	.9998 2648	.9994 9095	.9990 0332	.9983 7224	.9976 0546
5.32	.9998 3131	.9995 0502	.9990 3065	.9984 1656	.9976 7021
5.33	.9998 3602	.9995 1872	.9990 5728	.9984 5976	.9977 3334
5.34	.9998 4060	.9995 3207	.9990 8323	.9985 0186	.9977 9488
5.35	.9998 4506	.9995 4507	.9991 0851	.9985 4288	.9978 5487
5.36	.9998 4941	.9995 5773	.9991 3314	.9985 8286	.9979 1333
5.37	.9998 5364	.9995 7006	.9991 5713	.9986 2181	.9979 7032
5.38	.9998 5776	.9995 8206	.9991 8050	.9986 5976	.9980 2585
5.39	.9998 6177	.9995 9375	.9992 0326	.9986 9674	.9980 7998
5.40	.9998 6567	.9996 0513	.9992 2543	.9987 3276	.9981 3271
5.41	.9998 6947	.9996 1622	.9992 4702	.9987 6786	.9981 8410
5.42	.9998 7316	.9996 2701	.9992 6805	.9988 0204	.9982 3417
5.43	.9998 7676	.9996 3751	.9992 8852	.9988 3534	.9982 8296
5.44	.9998 8026	.9996 4774	.9993 0846	.9988 6777	.9983 3048
5.45	.9998 8367	.9996 5769	.9993 2787	.9988 9936	.9983 7678
5.46	.9998 8698	.9996 6738	.9993 4677	.9989 3012	.9984 2188
5.47	.9998 9021	.9996 7681	.9993 6518	.9989 6008	.9984 6581
5.48	.9998 9335	.9996 8599	.9993 8309	.9989 8925	.9985 0860
5.49	.9998 9641	.9996 9493	.9994 0053	.9990 1765	.9985 5027

W	P(W,2)	P(W,3)	P(W,4)	P(W,5)	P(W,6)
5.50	.9998 9938	.9997 0362	.9994 1751	.9990 4531	.9985 9086
5.51	.9999 0227	.9997 1208	.9994 3404	.9990 7224	.9986 3038
5.52	.9999 0508	.9997 2031	.9994 5012	.9990 9845	.9986 6886
5.53	.9999 0782	.9997 2833	.9994 6578	.9991 2397	.9987 0634
5.54	.9999 1048	.9997 3612	.9994 8101	.9991 4881	.9987 4282
5.55	.9999 1307	.9997 4370	.9994 9584	.9991 7299	.9987 7835
5.56	.9999 1559	.9997 5108	.9995 1027	.9991 9653	.9988 1293
5.57	.9999 1804	.9997 5826	.9995 2431	.9992 1944	.9988 4660
5.58	.9999 2042	.9997 6524	.9995 3797	.9992 4173	.9988 7937
5.59	.9999 2273	.9997 7203	.9995 5126	.9992 6343	.9989 1127
5.60	.9999 2499	.9997 7864	.9995 6419	.9992 8454	.9989 4231
5.61	.9999 2718	.9997 8506	.9995 7677	.9993 0508	.9989 7253
5.62	.9999 2931	.9997 9131	.9995 8901	.9993 2507	.9990 0194
5.63	.9999 3138	.9997 9739	.9996 0091	.9993 4452	.9990 3056
5.64	.9999 3339	.9998 0330	.9996 1249	.9993 6344	.9990 5840
5.65	.9999 3535	.9998 0905	.9996 2375	.9993 8185	.9990 8550
5.66	.9999 3725	.9998 1464	.9996 3471	.9993 9975	.9991 1186
5.67	.9999 3910	.9998 2007	.9996 4536	.9994 1717	.9991 3751
5.68	.9999 4090	.9998 2535	.9996 5572	.9994 3411	.9991 6247
5.69	.9999 4265	.9998 3049	.9996 6579	.9994 5059	.9991 8674
5.70	.9999 4434	.9998 3548	.9996 7559	.9994 6662	.9992 1035
5.71	.9999 4599	.9998 4034	.9996 8511	.9994 8220	.9992 3332
5.72	.9999 4760	.9998 4505	.9996 9437	.9994 9736	.9992 5566
5.73	.9999 4916	.9998 4964	.9997 0337	.9995 1209	.9992 7739
5.74	.9999 5067	.9998 5410	.9997 1213	.9995 2642	.9992 9852
5.75	.9999 5215	.9998 5843	.9997 2063	.9995 4036	.9993 1907
5.76	.9999 5358	.9998 6264	.9997 2890	.9995 5390	.9993 3905
5.77	.9999 5497	.9998 6673	.9997 3694	.9995 6707	.9993 5848
5.78	.9999 5632	.9998 7071	.9997 4476	.9995 7988	.9993 7737
5.79	.9999 5763	.9998 7457	.9997 5235	.9995 9232	.9993 9574
5.80	.9999 5890	.9998 7833	.9997 5973	.9996 0442	.9994 1360
5.81	.9999 6014	.9998 8198	.9997 6690	.9996 1617	.9994 3095
5.82	.9999 6134	.9998 8552	.9997 7387	.9996 2760	.9994 4783
5.83	.9999 6251	.9998 8896	.9997 8064	.9996 3871	.9994 6423
5.84	.9999 6365	.9998 9231	.9997 8722	.9996 4950	.9994 8017
5.85	.9999 6475	.9998 9556	.9997 9361	.9996 5999	.9994 9567
5.86	.9999 6582	.9998 9871	.9997 9983	.9996 7018	.9995 1072
5.87	.9999 6686	.9999 0178	.9998 0586	.9996 8008	.9995 2536
5.88	.9999 6787	.9999 0476	.9998 1172	.9996 8970	.9995 3958
5.89	.9999 6885	.9999 0765	.9998 1741	.9996 9905	.9995 5340
5.90	.9999 6980	.9999 1046	.9998 2294	.9997 0813	.9995 6682
5.91	.9999 7072	.9999 1319	.9998 2832	.9997 1695	.9995 7987
5.92	.9999 7162	.9999 1583	.9998 3353	.9997 2552	.9995 9254
5.93	.9999 7249	.9999 1841	.9998 3860	.9997 3384	.9996 0485
5.94	.9999 7333	.9999 2090	.9998 4352	.9997 4193	.9996 1681
5.95	.9999 7415	.9999 2333	.9998 4830	.9997 4978	.9996 2843
5.96	.9999 7495	.9999 2568	.9998 5294	.9997 5740	.9996 3971
5.97	.9999 7572	.9999 2797	.9998 5744	.9997 6481	.9996 5067
5.98	.9999 7647	.9999 3018	.9998 6181	.9997 7200	.9996 6131
5.99	.9999 7720	.9999 3234	.9998 6606	.9997 7898	.9996 7165

W	P(W,2)	P(W,3)	P(W,4)	P(W,5)	P(W,6)
6.00	.9999 7791	.9999 3443	.9998 7018	.9997 8576	.9996 8169
6.01	.9999 7860	.9999 3645	.9998 7418	.9997 9234	.9996 9143
6.02	.9999 7926	.9999 3842	.9998 7807	.9997 9873	.9997 0090
6.03	.9999 7991	.9999 4033	.9998 8184	.9998 0493	.9997 1009
6.04	.9999 8053	.9999 4219	.9998 8550	.9998 1095	.9997 1901
6.05	.9999 8114	.9999 4399	.9998 8905	.9998 1680	.9997 2767
6.06	.9999 8173	.9999 4573	.9998 9250	.9998 2247	.9997 3608
6.07	.9999 8230	.9999 4743	.9998 9584	.9998 2798	.9997 4424
6.08	.9999 8286	.9999 4907	.9998 9909	.9998 3332	.9997 5216
6.09	.9999 8340	.9999 5067	.9999 0224	.9998 3851	.9997 5985
6.10	.9999 8392	.9999 5221	.9999 0529	.9998 4354	.9997 6731
6.11	.9999 8443	.9999 5371	.9999 0826	.9998 4843	.9997 7455
6.12	.9999 8492	.9999 5517	.9999 1114	.9998 5316	.9997 8158
6.13	.9999 8540	.9999 5658	.9999 1393	.9998 5776	.9997 8840
6.14	.9999 8586	.9999 5795	.9999 1663	.9998 6222	.9997 9502
6.15	.9999 8631	.9999 5928	.9999 1926	.9998 6655	.9998 0144
6.16	.9999 8674	.9999 6057	.9999 2181	.9998 7075	.9998 0767
6.17	.9999 8716	.9999 6182	.9999 2428	.9998 7482	.9998 1371
6.18	.9999 8757	.9999 6303	.9999 2668	.9998 7877	.9998 1958
6.19	.9999 8797	.9999 6421	.9999 2900	.9998 8261	.9998 2527
6.20	.9999 8835	.9999 6535	.9999 3125	.9998 8632	.9998 3078
6.21	.9999 8872	.9999 6645	.9999 3344	.9998 8993	.9998 3614
6.22	.9999 8908	.9999 6752	.9999 3556	.9998 9342	.9998 4133
6.23	.9999 8943	.9999 6856	.9999 3761	.9998 9681	.9998 4636
6.24	.9999 8977	.9999 6957	.9999 3961	.9999 0010	.9998 5124
6.25	.9999 9010	.9999 7054	.9999 4154	.9999 0329	.9998 5598
6.26	.9999 9042	.9999 7149	.9999 4341	.9999 0638	.9998 6057
6.27	.9999 9073	.9999 7241	.9999 4523	.9999 0937	.9998 6502
6.28	.9999 9103	.9999 7330	.9999 4699	.9999 1228	.9998 6933
6.29	.9999 9132	.9999 7416	.9999 4869	.9999 1509	.9998 7352
6.30	.9999 9160	.9999 7499	.9999 5035	.9999 1782	.9998 7758
6.31	.9999 9187	.9999 7580	.9999 5195	.9999 2047	.9998 8151
6.32	.9999 9214	.9999 7659	.9999 5350	.9999 2304	.9998 8532
6.33	.9999 9239	.9999 7735	.9999 5501	.9999 2552	.9998 8902
6.34	.9999 9264	.9999 7808	.9999 5647	.9999 2793	.9998 9260
6.35	.9999 9288	.9999 7880	.9999 5788	.9999 3026	.9998 9607
6.36	.9999 9311	.9999 7949	.9999 5925	.9999 3253	.9998 9944
6.37	.9999 9334	.9999 8016	.9999 6058	.9999 3472	.9999 0270
6.38	.9999 9356	.9999 8081	.9999 6186	.9999 3684	.9999 0586
6.39	.9999 9377	.9999 8143	.9999 6311	.9999 3890	.9999 0892
6.40	.9999 9397	.9999 8204	.9999 6432	.9999 4090	.9999 1188
6.41	.9999 9417	.9999 8263	.9999 6548	.9999 4283	.9999 1476
6.42	.9999 9436	.9999 8320	.9999 6662	.9999 4470	.9999 1754
6.43	.9999 9455	.9999 8376	.9999 6771	.9999 4651	.9999 2024
6.44	.9999 9473	.9999 8429	.9999 6878	.9999 4827	.9999 2286
6.45	.9999 9491	.9999 8481	.9999 6980	.9999 4997	.9999 2539
6.46	.9999 9507	.9999 8531	.9999 7080	.9999 5162	.9999 2784
6.47	.9999 9524	.9999 8580	.9999 7177	.9999 5321	.9999 3021
6.48	.9999 9540	.9999 8627	.9999 7270	.9999 5476	.9999 3252
6.49	.9999 9555	.9999 8673	.9999 7361	.9999 5626	.9999 3474

W	P(W,2)	P(W,3)	P(W,4)	P(W,5)	P(W,6)
6.50	.9999 9570	.9999 8717	.9999 7448	.9999 5770	.9999 3690
6.51	.9999 9584	.9999 8759	.9999 7533	.9999 5911	.9999 3899
6.52	.9999 9598	.9999 8801	.9999 7615	.9999 6047	.9999 4101
6.53	.9999 9611	.9999 8841	.9999 7695	.9999 6178	.9999 4297
6.54	.9999 9624	.9999 8880	.9999 7772	.9999 6306	.9999 4487
6.55	.9999 9637	.9999 8917	.9999 7846	.9999 6429	.9999 4671
6.56	.9999 9649	.9999 8954	.9999 7918	.9999 6548	.9999 4848
6.57	.9999 9661	.9999 8989	.9999 7988	.9999 6664	.9999 5021
6.58	.9999 9672	.9999 9023	.9999 8055	.9999 6776	.9999 5187
6.59	.9999 9684	.9999 9056	.9999 8121	.9999 6884	.9999 5348
6.60	.9999 9694	.9999 9087	.9999 8184	.9999 6988	.9999 5505
6.61	.9999 9705	.9999 9118	.9999 8245	.9999 7090	.9999 5656
6.62	.9999 9715	.9999 9148	.9999 8305	.9999 7188	.9999 5802
6.63	.9999 9724	.9999 9177	.9999 8362	.9999 7283	.9999 5943
6.64	.9999 9734	.9999 9205	.9999 8417	.9999 7375	.9999 6080
6.65	.9999 9743	.9999 9232	.9999 8471	.9999 7464	.9999 6213
6.66	.9999 9751	.9999 9258	.9999 8523	.9999 7550	.9999 6341
6.67	.9999 9760	.9999 9283	.9999 8573	.9999 7633	.9999 6465
6.68	.9999 9768	.9999 9308	.9999 8622	.9999 7713	.9999 6585
6.69	.9999 9776	.9999 9331	.9999 8669	.9999 7791	.9999 6701
6.70	.9999 9784	.9999 9354	.9999 8714	.9999 7866	.9999 6813
6.71	.9999 9791	.9999 9376	.9999 8758	.9999 7939	.9999 6922
6.72	.9999 9798	.9999 9398	.9999 8801	.9999 8010	.9999 7027
6.73	.9999 9805	.9999 9418	.9999 8842	.9999 8078	.9999 7129
6.74	.9999 9812	.9999 9438	.9999 8882	.9999 8144	.9999 7227
6.75	.9999 9818	.9999 9458	.9999 8920	.9999 8208	.9999 7322
6.76	.9999 9825	.9999 9476	.9999 8957	.9999 8269	.9999 7414
6.77	.9999 9831	.9999 9495	.9999 8993	.9999 8329	.9999 7503
6.78	.9999 9837	.9999 9512	.9999 9028	.9999 8386	.9999 7589
6.79	.9999 9842	.9999 9529	.9999 9062	.9999 8442	.9999 7672
6.80	.9999 9848	.9999 9545	.9999 9094	.9999 8496	.9999 7753
6.81	.9999 9853	.9999 9561	.9999 9126	.9999 8548	.9999 7830
6.82	.9999 9858	.9999 9576	.9999 9156	.9999 8598	.9999 7905
6.83	.9999 9863	.9999 9591	.9999 9185	.9999 8647	.9999 7978
6.84	.9999 9868	.9999 9605	.9999 9214	.9999 8694	.9999 8048
6.85	.9999 9873	.9999 9619	.9999 9241	.9999 8740	.9999 8116
6.86	.9999 9877	.9999 9632	.9999 9268	.9999 8784	.9999 8182
6.87	.9999 9881	.9999 9645	.9999 9293	.9999 8826	.9999 8245
6.88	.9999 9885	.9999 9658	.9999 9318	.9999 8867	.9999 8306
6.89	.9999 9890	.9999 9670	.9999 9342	.9999 8907	.9999 8366
6.90	.9999 9893	.9999 9681	.9999 9365	.9999 8945	.9999 8423
6.91	.9999 9897	.9999 9693	.9999 9387	.9999 8982	.9999 8478
6.92	.9999 9901	.9999 9703	.9999 9409	.9999 9018	.9999 8532
6.93	.9999 9904	.9999 9714	.9999 9430	.9999 9052	.9999 8583
6.94	.9999 9908	.9999 9724	.9999 9450	.9999 9086	.9999 8633
6.95	.9999 9911	.9999 9734	.9999 9469	.9999 9118	.9999 8681
6.96	.9999 9914	.9999 9743	.9999 9488	.9999 9149	.9999 8728
6.97	.9999 9917	.9999 9752	.9999 9506	.9999 9179	.9999 8773
6.98	.9999 9920	.9999 9761	.9999 9524	.9999 9209	.9999 8816
6.99	.9999 9923	.9999 9770	.9999 9541	.9999 9237	.9999 8858

W	P(W,2)	P(W,3)	P(W,4)	P(W,5)	P(W,6)
7.00	.9999 9926	.9999 9778	.9999 9557	.9999 9264	.9999 8899
7.01	.9999 9928	.9999 9786	.9999 9573	.9999 9290	.9999 8938
7.02	.9999 9931	.9999 9793	.9999 9588	.9999 9315	.9999 8976
7.03	.9999 9933	.9999 9801	.9999 9603	.9999 9340	.9999 9012
7.04	.9999 9936	.9999 9808	.9999 9617	.9999 9363	.9999 9048
7.05	.9999 9938	.9999 9815	.9999 9631	.9999 9386	.9999 9082
7.06	.9999 9940	.9999 9821	.9999 9644	.9999 9408	.9999 9115
7.07	.9999 9942	.9999 9828	.9999 9657	.9999 9429	.9999 9146
7.08	.9999 9945	.9999 9834	.9999 9669	.9999 9450	.9999 9177
7.09	.9999 9947	.9999 9840	.9999 9681	.9999 9470	.9999 9206
7.10	.9999 9948	.9999 9846	.9999 9692	.9999 9489	.9999 9235
7.11	.9999 9950	.9999 9851	.9999 9704	.9999 9507	.9999 9263
7.12	.9999 9952	.9999 9857	.9999 9714	.9999 9525	.9999 9289
7.13	.9999 9954	.9999 9862	.9999 9725	.9999 9542	.9999 9315
7.14	.9999 9956	.9999 9867	.9999 9735	.9999 9559	.9999 9340
7.15	.9999 9957	.9999 9872	.9999 9744	.9999 9575	.9999 9364
7.16	.9999 9959	.9999 9876	.9999 9753	.9999 9590	.9999 9387
7.17	.9999 9960	.9999 9881	.9999 9762	.9999 9605	.9999 9409
7.18	.9999 9962	.9999 9885	.9999 9771	.9999 9619	.9999 9430
7.19	.9999 9963	.9999 9889	.9999 9779	.9999 9633	.9999 9451
7.20	.9999 9964	.9999 9893	.9999 9788	.9999 9647	.9999 9471
7.21	.9999 9966	.9999 9897	.9999 9795	.9999 9660	.9999 9491
7.22	.9999 9967	.9999 9901	.9999 9803	.9999 9672	.9999 9509
7.23	.9999 9968	.9999 9905	.9999 9810	.9999 9684	.9999 9527
7.24	.9999 9969	.9999 9908	.9999 9817	.9999 9696	.9999 9544
7.25	.9999 9970	.9999 9912	.9999 9824	.9999 9707	.9999 9561
7.26	.9999 9972	.9999 9915	.9999 9830	.9999 9718	.9999 9577
7.27	.9999 9973	.9999 9918	.9999 9836	.9999 9728	.9999 9593
7.28	.9999 9974	.9999 9921	.9999 9842	.9999 9738	.9999 9608
7.29	.9999 9975	.9999 9924	.9999 9848	.9999 9748	.9999 9622
7.30	.9999 9976	.9999 9927	.9999 9854	.9999 9757	.9999 9636
7.31	.9999 9976	.9999 9930	.9999 9859	.9999 9766	.9999 9650
7.32	.9999 9977	.9999 9932	.9999 9865	.9999 9775	.9999 9663
7.33	.9999 9978	.9999 9935	.9999 9870	.9999 9783	.9999 9675
7.34	.9999 9979	.9999 9937	.9999 9874	.9999 9791	.9999 9687
7.35	.9999 9980	.9999 9939	.9999 9879	.9999 9799	.9999 9699
7.36	.9999 9981	.9999 9942	.9999 9884	.9999 9806	.9999 9710
7.37	.9999 9981	.9999 9944	.9999 9888	.9999 9814	.9999 9721
7.38	.9999 9982	.9999 9946	.9999 9892	.9999 9821	.9999 9731
7.39	.9999 9983	.9999 9948	.9999 9896	.9999 9827	.9999 9741
7.40	.9999 9983	.9999 9950	.9999 9900	.9999 9834	.9999 9751
7.41	.9999 9984	.9999 9952	.9999 9904	.9999 9840	.9999 9760
7.42	.9999 9985	.9999 9954	.9999 9907	.9999 9846	.9999 9769
7.43	.9999 9985	.9999 9955	.9999 9911	.9999 9852	.9999 9778
7.44	.9999 9986	.9999 9957	.9999 9914	.9999 9857	.9999 9786
7.45	.9999 9986	.9999 9959	.9999 9918	.9999 9863	.9999 9794
7.46	.9999 9987	.9999 9960	.9999 9921	.9999 9868	.9999 9802
7.47	.9999 9987	.9999 9962	.9999 9924	.9999 9873	.9999 9810
7.48	.9999 9988	.9999 9963	.9999 9927	.9999 9878	.9999 9817
7.49	.9999 9988	.9999 9965	.9999 9929	.9999 9882	.9999 9824

W	P(W,2)	P(W,3)	P(W,4)	P(W,5)	P(W,6)
7.50	.9999 9989	.9999 9966	.9999 9932	.9999 9887	.9999 9830
7.51	.9999 9989	.9999 9967	.9999 9935	.9999 9891	.9999 9837
7.52	.9999 9989	.9999 9968	.9999 9937	.9999 9895	.9999 9843
7.53	.9999 9990	.9999 9970	.9999 9939	.9999 9899	.9999 9849
7.54	.9999 9990	.9999 9971	.9999 9942	.9999 9903	.9999 9855
7.55	.9999 9991	.9999 9972	.9999 9944	.9999 9907	.9999 9860
7.56	.9999 9991	.9999 9973	.9999 9946	.9999 9910	.9999 9866
7.57	.9999 9991	.9999 9974	.9999 9948	.9999 9914	.9999 9871
7.58	.9999 9992	.9999 9975	.9999 9950	.9999 9917	.9999 9876
7.59	.9999 9992	.9999 9976	.9999 9952	.9999 9920	.9999 9881
7.60	.9999 9992	.9999 9977	.9999 9954	.9999 9923	.9999 9885
7.61	.9999 9993	.9999 9978	.9999 9956	.9999 9926	.9999 9890
7.62	.9999 9993	.9999 9979	.9999 9957	.9999 9929	.9999 9894
7.63	.9999 9993	.9999 9979	.9999 9959	.9999 9932	.9999 9898
7.64	.9999 9993	.9999 9980	.9999 9961	.9999 9934	.9999 9902
7.65	.9999 9994	.9999 9981	.9999 9962	.9999 9937	.9999 9906
7.66	.9999 9994	.9999 9982	.9999 9964	.9999 9939	.9999 9909
7.67	.9999 9994	.9999 9982	.9999 9965	.9999 9942	.9999 9913
7.68	.9999 9994	.9999 9983	.9999 9966	.9999 9944	.9999 9916
7.69	.9999 9995	.9999 9984	.9999 9968	.9999 9946	.9999 9919
7.70	.9999 9995	.9999 9984	.9999 9969	.9999 9948	.9999 9923
7.71	.9999 9995	.9999 9985	.9999 9970	.9999 9950	.9999 9926
7.72	.9999 9995	.9999 9986	.9999 9971	.9999 9952	.9999 9928
7.73	.9999 9995	.9999 9986	.9999 9972	.9999 9954	.9999 9931
7.74	.9999 9996	.9999 9987	.9999 9974	.9999 9956	.9999 9934
7.75	.9999 9996	.9999 9987	.9999 9975	.9999 9958	.9999 9936
7.76	.9999 9996	.9999 9988	.9999 9976	.9999 9959	.9999 9939
7.77	.9999 9996	.9999 9988	.9999 9977	.9999 9961	.9999 9941
7.78	.9999 9996	.9999 9989	.9999 9977	.9999 9962	.9999 9944
7.79	.9999 9996	.9999 9989	.9999 9978	.9999 9964	.9999 9946
7.80	.9999 9997	.9999 9990	.9999 9979	.9999 9965	.9999 9948
7.81	.9999 9997	.9999 9990	.9999 9980	.9999 9967	.9999 9950
7.82	.9999 9997	.9999 9990	.9999 9981	.9999 9968	.9999 9952
7.83	.9999 9997	.9999 9991	.9999 9982	.9999 9969	.9999 9954
7.84	.9999 9997	.9999 9991	.9999 9982	.9999 9970	.9999 9956
7.85	.9999 9997	.9999 9991	.9999 9983	.9999 9972	.9999 9957
7.86	.9999 9997	.9999 9992	.9999 9984	.9999 9973	.9999 9959
7.87	.9999 9997	.9999 9992	.9999 9984	.9999 9974	.9999 9961
7.88	.9999 9997	.9999 9992	.9999 9985	.9999 9975	.9999 9962
7.89	.9999 9998	.9999 9993	.9999 9986	.9999 9976	.9999 9964
7.90	.9999 9998	.9999 9993	.9999 9986	.9999 9977	.9999 9965
7.91	.9999 9998	.9999 9993	.9999 9987	.9999 9978	.9999 9967
7.92	.9999 9998	.9999 9994	.9999 9987	.9999 9979	.9999 9968
7.93	.9999 9998	.9999 9994	.9999 9988	.9999 9979	.9999 9969
7.94	.9999 9998	.9999 9994	.9999 9988	.9999 9980	.9999 9971
7.95	.9999 9998	.9999 9994	.9999 9989	.9999 9981	.9999 9972
7.96	.9999 9998	.9999 9995	.9999 9989	.9999 9982	.9999 9973
7.97	.9999 9998	.9999 9995	.9999 9990	.9999 9983	.9999 9974
7.98	.9999 9998	.9999 9995	.9999 9990	.9999 9983	.9999 9975
7.99	.9999 9998	.9999 9995	.9999 9990	.9999 9984	.9999 9976

W	P(W,2)	P(W,3)	P(W,4)	P(W,5)	P(W,6)
8.00	.9999 9998	.9999 9995	.9999 9991	.9999 9985	.9999 9977
8.01	.9999 9999	.9999 9996	.9999 9991	.9999 9985	.9999 9978
8.02	.9999 9999	.9999 9996	.9999 9991	.9999 9986	.9999 9979
8.03	.9999 9999	.9999 9996	.9999 9992	.9999 9986	.9999 9980
8.04	.9999 9999	.9999 9996	.9999 9992	.9999 9987	.9999 9980
8.05	.9999 9999	.9999 9996	.9999 9992	.9999 9987	.9999 9981
8.06	.9999 9999	.9999 9996	.9999 9993	.9999 9988	.9999 9982
8.07	.9999 9999	.9999 9997	.9999 9993	.9999 9988	.9999 9983
8.08	.9999 9999	.9999 9997	.9999 9993	.9999 9989	.9999 9983
8.09	.9999 9999	.9999 9997	.9999 9994	.9999 9989	.9999 9984
8.10	.9999 9999	.9999 9997	.9999 9994	.9999 9990	.9999 9985
8.11	.9999 9999	.9999 9997	.9999 9994	.9999 9990	.9999 9985
8.12	.9999 9999	.9999 9997	.9999 9994	.9999 9991	.9999 9986
8.13	.9999 9999	.9999 9997	.9999 9995	.9999 9991	.9999 9987
8.14	.9999 9999	.9999 9997	.9999 9995	.9999 9991	.9999 9987
8.15	.9999 9999	.9999 9998	.9999 9995	.9999 9992	.9999 9988
8.16	.9999 9999	.9999 9998	.9999 9995	.9999 9992	.9999 9988
8.17	.9999 9999	.9999 9998	.9999 9995	.9999 9992	.9999 9989
8.18	.9999 9999	.9999 9998	.9999 9996	.9999 9993	.9999 9989
8.19	.9999 9999	.9999 9998	.9999 9996	.9999 9993	.9999 9990
8.20	.9999 9999	.9999 9998	.9999 9996	.9999 9993	.9999 9990
8.21	.9999 9999	.9999 9998	.9999 9996	.9999 9994	.9999 9990
8.22	.9999 9999	.9999 9998	.9999 9996	.9999 9994	.9999 9991
8.23	.9999 9999	.9999 9998	.9999 9996	.9999 9994	.9999 9991
8.24	.9999 9999	.9999 9998	.9999 9997	.9999 9994	.9999 9992
8.25	.9999 9999	.9999 9998	.9999 9997	.9999 9995	.9999 9992
8.26	.9999 9999	.9999 9998	.9999 9997	.9999 9995	.9999 9992
8.27	.9999 9999	.9999 9998	.9999 9997	.9999 9995	.9999 9993
8.28	1.0000 0000	.9999 9999	.9999 9997	.9999 9995	.9999 9993
8.29		.9999 9999	.9999 9997	.9999 9995	.9999 9993
8.30		.9999 9999	.9999 9997	.9999 9996	.9999 9993
8.31		.9999 9999	.9999 9997	.9999 9996	.9999 9994
8.32		.9999 9999	.9999 9998	.9999 9996	.9999 9994
8.33		.9999 9999	.9999 9998	.9999 9996	.9999 9994
8.34		.9999 9999	.9999 9998	.9999 9996	.9999 9994
8.35		.9999 9999	.9999 9998	.9999 9996	.9999 9995
8.36		.9999 9999	.9999 9998	.9999 9997	.9999 9995
8.37		.9999 9999	.9999 9998	.9999 9997	.9999 9995
8.38		.9999 9999	.9999 9998	.9999 9997	.9999 9995
8.39		.9999 9999	.9999 9998	.9999 9997	.9999 9996
8.40		.9999 9999	.9999 9998	.9999 9997	.9999 9996
8.41		.9999 9999	.9999 9998	.9999 9997	.9999 9996
8.42		.9999 9999	.9999 9998	.9999 9997	.9999 9996
8.43		.9999 9999	.9999 9998	.9999 9997	.9999 9996
8.44		.9999 9999	.9999 9999	.9999 9998	.9999 9996
8.45		.9999 9999	.9999 9999	.9999 9998	.9999 9997
8.46		.9999 9999	.9999 9999	.9999 9998	.9999 9997
8.47		.9999 9999	.9999 9999	.9999 9998	.9999 9997
8.48		.9999 9999	.9999 9999	.9999 9998	.9999 9997
8.49		.9999 9999	.9999 9999	.9999 9998	.9999 9997

W	P(W,2)	P(W,3)	P(W,4)	P(W,5)	P(W,6)
8.50		.9999 9999	.9999 9999	.9999 9998	.9999 9997
8.51		.9999 9999	.9999 9999	.9999 9998	.9999 9997
8.52		.9999 9999	.9999 9999	.9999 9998	.9999 9997
8.53		.9999 9999	.9999 9999	.9999 9998	.9999 9998
8.54		1.0000 0000	.9999 9999	.9999 9998	.9999 9998
8.55			.9999 9999	.9999 9998	.9999 9998
8.56			.9999 9999	.9999 9999	.9999 9998
8.57			.9999 9999	.9999 9999	.9999 9998
8.58			.9999 9999	.9999 9999	.9999 9998
8.59			.9999 9999	.9999 9999	.9999 9998
8.60			.9999 9999	.9999 9999	.9999 9998
8.61			.9999 9999	.9999 9999	.9999 9998
8.62			.9999 9999	.9999 9999	.9999 9998
8.63			.9999 9999	.9999 9999	.9999 9998
8.64			.9999 9999	.9999 9999	.9999 9998
8.65			.9999 9999	.9999 9999	.9999 9999
8.66			.9999 9999	.9999 9999	.9999 9999
8.67			.9999 9999	.9999 9999	.9999 9999
8.68			.9999 9999	.9999 9999	.9999 9999
8.69			1.0000 0000	.9999 9999	.9999 9999
8.70				.9999 9999	.9999 9999
8.71				.9999 9999	.9999 9999
8.72				.9999 9999	.9999 9999
8.73				.9999 9999	.9999 9999
8.74				.9999 9999	.9999 9999
8.75				.9999 9999	.9999 9999
8.76				.9999 9999	.9999 9999
8.77				.9999 9999	.9999 9999
8.78				.9999 9999	.9999 9999
8.79				.9999 9999	.9999 9999
8.80				.9999 9999	.9999 9999
8.81				1.0000 0000	.9999 9999
8.82					.9999 9999
8.83					.9999 9999
8.84					.9999 9999
8.85					.9999 9999
8.86					.9999 9999
8.87					.9999 9999
8.88					.9999 9999
8.89					.9999 9999
8.90					1.0000 0000
8.91					
8.92					
8.93					
8.94					
8.95					
8.96					
8.97					
8.98					
8.99					

W	P(W,7)	P(W,8)	P(W,9)	P(W,10)	P(W,11)
0.00					
0.01					
0.02					
0.03					
0.04					
0.05					
0.06					
0.07					
0.08	.0000 0000				
0.09	.0000 0001				
0.10	.0000 0001				
0.11	.0000 0002				
0.12	.0000 0003				
0.13	.0000 0005				
0.14	.0000 0008	.0000 0000			
0.15	.0000 0012	.0000 0001			
0.16	.0000 0018	.0000 0001			
0.17	.0000 0025	.0000 0002			
0.18	.0000 0036	.0000 0003			
0.19	.0000 0050	.0000 0004			
0.20	.0000 0067	.0000 0006	.0000 0000		
0.21	.0000 0090	.0000 0008	.0000 0001		
0.22	.0000 0119	.0000 0011	.0000 0001		
0.23	.0000 0155	.0000 0015	.0000 0001		
0.24	.0000 0200	.0000 0020	.0000 0002		
0.25	.0000 0255	.0000 0027	.0000 0003		
0.26	.0000 0322	.0000 0036	.0000 0004	.0000 0000	
0.27	.0000 0404	.0000 0046	.0000 0005	.0000 0001	
0.28	.0000 0501	.0000 0060	.0000 0007	.0000 0001	
0.29	.0000 0618	.0000 0076	.0000 0009	.0000 0001	
0.30	.0000 0755	.0000 0096	.0000 0012	.0000 0002	
0.31	.0000 0918	.0000 0121	.0000 0016	.0000 0002	
0.32	.0000 1108	.0000 0151	.0000 0020	.0000 0003	
0.33	.0000 1330	.0000 0186	.0000 0026	.0000 0004	.0000 0000
0.34	.0000 1588	.0000 0229	.0000 0033	.0000 0005	.0000 0001
0.35	.0000 1885	.0000 0280	.0000 0041	.0000 0006	.0000 0001
0.36	.0000 2227	.0000 0340	.0000 0052	.0000 0008	.0000 0001
0.37	.0000 2619	.0000 0411	.0000 0064	.0000 0010	.0000 0002
0.38	.0000 3066	.0000 0494	.0000 0079	.0000 0013	.0000 0002
0.39	.0000 3575	.0000 0591	.0000 0097	.0000 0016	.0000 0003
0.40	.0000 4150	.0000 0703	.0000 0118	.0000 0020	.0000 0003
0.41	.0000 4801	.0000 0833	.0000 0144	.0000 0025	.0000 0004
0.42	.0000 5533	.0000 0984	.0000 0173	.0000 0030	.0000 0005
0.43	.0000 6355	.0000 1156	.0000 0209	.0000 0037	.0000 0007
0.44	.0000 7274	.0000 1354	.0000 0250	.0000 0046	.0000 0008
0.45	.0000 8301	.0000 1579	.0000 0298	.0000 0056	.0000 0010
0.46	.0000 9443	.0000 1836	.0000 0354	.0000 0068	.0000 0013
0.47	.0001 0712	.0000 2127	.0000 0419	.0000 0082	.0000 0016
0.48	.0001 2118	.0000 2456	.0000 0494	.0000 0099	.0000 0020
0.49	.0001 3671	.0000 2828	.0000 0580	.0000 0118	.0000 0024

W	P(W,7)	P(W,8)	P(W,9)	P(W,10)	P(W,11)
0.50	.0001 5384	.0000 3246	.0000 0679	.0000 0141	.0000 0029
0.51	.0001 7270	.0000 3714	.0000 0793	.0000 0168	.0000 0035
0.52	.0001 9340	.0000 4240	.0000 0922	.0000 0199	.0000 0043
0.53	.0002 1609	.0000 4826	.0000 1069	.0000 0235	.0000 0052
0.54	.0002 4092	.0000 5479	.0000 1237	.0000 0277	.0000 0062
0.55	.0002 6802	.0000 6206	.0000 1426	.0000 0326	.0000 0074
0.56	.0002 9757	.0000 7012	.0000 1639	.0000 0381	.0000 0088
0.57	.0003 2972	.0000 7904	.0000 1880	.0000 0445	.0000 0105
0.58	.0003 6466	.0000 8891	.0000 2151	.0000 0517	.0000 0124
0.59	.0004 0254	.0000 9979	.0000 2455	.0000 0600	.0000 0146
0.60	.0004 4357	.0001 1177	.0000 2794	.0000 0694	.0000 0172
0.61	.0004 8794	.0001 2493	.0000 3174	.0000 0801	.0000 0201
0.62	.0005 3585	.0001 3937	.0000 3597	.0000 0923	.0000 0236
0.63	.0005 8751	.0001 5519	.0000 4068	.0000 1060	.0000 0275
0.64	.0006 4314	.0001 7249	.0000 4590	.0000 1214	.0000 0320
0.65	.0007 0296	.0001 9137	.0000 5170	.0000 1388	.0000 0371
0.66	.0007 6720	.0002 1196	.0000 5811	.0000 1583	.0000 0429
0.67	.0008 3612	.0002 3436	.0000 6519	.0000 1802	.0000 0496
0.68	.0009 0995	.0002 5871	.0000 7299	.0000 2047	.0000 0571
0.69	.0009 8895	.0002 8514	.0000 8158	.0000 2320	.0000 0657
0.70	.0010 7339	.0003 1379	.0000 9103	.0000 2625	.0000 0753
0.71	.0011 6355	.0003 4480	.0001 0139	.0000 2963	.0000 0862
0.72	.0012 5970	.0003 7832	.0001 1275	.0000 3340	.0000 0984
0.73	.0013 6214	.0004 1451	.0001 2517	.0000 3757	.0000 1122
0.74	.0014 7116	.0004 5354	.0001 3875	.0000 4219	.0000 1277
0.75	.0015 8707	.0004 9557	.0001 5356	.0000 4729	.0000 1449
0.76	.0017 1018	.0005 4078	.0001 6970	.0000 5293	.0000 1643
0.77	.0018 4082	.0005 8937	.0001 8725	.0000 5913	.0000 1858
0.78	.0019 7931	.0006 4152	.0002 0634	.0000 6596	.0000 2098
0.79	.0021 2600	.0006 9743	.0002 2704	.0000 7347	.0000 2366
0.80	.0022 8123	.0007 5731	.0002 4949	.0000 8170	.0000 2662
0.81	.0024 4534	.0008 2138	.0002 7380	.0000 9072	.0000 2991
0.82	.0026 1871	.0008 8986	.0003 0008	.0001 0058	.0000 3355
0.83	.0028 0171	.0009 6298	.0003 2847	.0001 1137	.0000 3757
0.84	.0029 9470	.0010 4098	.0003 5910	.0001 2313	.0000 4201
0.85	.0031 9807	.0011 2411	.0003 9212	.0001 3596	.0000 4691
0.86	.0034 1222	.0012 1261	.0004 2766	.0001 4992	.0000 5230
0.87	.0036 3754	.0013 0676	.0004 6588	.0001 6510	.0000 5822
0.88	.0038 7443	.0014 0682	.0005 0695	.0001 8158	.0000 6472
0.89	.0041 2331	.0015 1307	.0005 5102	.0001 9947	.0000 7185
0.90	.0043 8459	.0016 2580	.0005 9828	.0002 1884	.0000 7966
0.91	.0046 5871	.0017 4530	.0006 4890	.0002 3982	.0000 8820
0.92	.0049 4608	.0018 7188	.0007 0307	.0002 6249	.0000 9752
0.93	.0052 4715	.0020 0584	.0007 6099	.0002 8698	.0001 0770
0.94	.0055 6236	.0021 4751	.0008 2285	.0003 1341	.0001 1879
0.95	.0058 9215	.0022 9720	.0008 8888	.0003 4189	.0001 3086
0.96	.0062 3699	.0024 5527	.0009 5927	.0003 7255	.0001 4398
0.97	.0065 9733	.0026 2205	.0010 3427	.0004 0554	.0001 5824
0.98	.0069 7363	.0027 9788	.0011 1410	.0004 4099	.0001 7371
0.99	.0073 6636	.0029 8314	.0011 9901	.0004 7905	.0001 9047

W	P(W,7)	P(W,8)	P(W,9)	P(W,10)	P(W,11)
1.00	.0077 7599	.0031 7818	.0012 8923	.0005 1987	.0002 0862
1.01	.0082 0301	.0033 8338	.0013 8504	.0005 6362	.0002 2825
1.02	.0086 4789	.0035 9912	.0014 8669	.0006 1046	.0002 4946
1.03	.0091 1112	.0038 2580	.0015 9446	.0006 6057	.0002 7235
1.04	.0095 9317	.0040 6380	.0017 0862	.0007 1413	.0002 9704
1.05	.0100 9456	.0043 1353	.0018 2948	.0007 7133	.0003 2364
1.06	.0106 1576	.0045 7541	.0019 5731	.0008 3236	.0003 5227
1.07	.0111 5728	.0048 4985	.0020 9244	.0008 9743	.0003 8305
1.08	.0117 1960	.0051 3728	.0022 3517	.0009 6675	.0004 1613
1.09	.0123 0324	.0054 3812	.0023 8583	.0010 4054	.0004 5164
1.10	.0129 0870	.0057 5282	.0025 4474	.0011 1902	.0004 8972
1.11	.0135 3647	.0060 8182	.0027 1225	.0012 0243	.0005 3053
1.12	.0141 8705	.0064 2557	.0028 8870	.0012 9102	.0005 7422
1.13	.0148 6097	.0067 8453	.0030 7445	.0013 8502	.0006 2096
1.14	.0155 5870	.0071 5916	.0032 6987	.0014 8471	.0006 7092
1.15	.0162 8077	.0075 4993	.0034 7531	.0015 9034	.0007 2428
1.16	.0170 2767	.0079 5730	.0036 9117	.0017 0219	.0007 8123
1.17	.0177 9990	.0083 8177	.0039 1782	.0018 2056	.0008 4196
1.18	.0185 9798	.0088 2381	.0041 5567	.0019 4571	.0009 0666
1.19	.0194 2238	.0092 8390	.0044 0511	.0020 7797	.0009 7556
1.20	.0202 7363	.0097 6255	.0046 6657	.0022 1764	.0010 4886
1.21	.0211 5219	.0102 6024	.0049 4045	.0023 6503	.0011 2678
1.22	.0220 5858	.0107 7748	.0052 2717	.0025 2047	.0012 0957
1.23	.0229 9328	.0113 1476	.0055 2719	.0026 8430	.0012 9746
1.24	.0239 5678	.0118 7259	.0058 4092	.0028 5685	.0013 9070
1.25	.0249 4955	.0124 5149	.0061 6882	.0030 3848	.0014 8954
1.26	.0259 7208	.0130 5195	.0065 1135	.0032 2956	.0015 9426
1.27	.0270 2484	.0136 7450	.0068 6896	.0034 3044	.0017 0512
1.28	.0281 0830	.0143 1965	.0072 4211	.0036 4150	.0018 2241
1.29	.0292 2292	.0149 8791	.0076 3129	.0038 6314	.0019 4641
1.30	.0303 6916	.0156 7980	.0080 3697	.0040 9574	.0020 7743
1.31	.0315 4747	.0163 9584	.0084 5962	.0043 3970	.0022 1577
1.32	.0327 5830	.0171 3654	.0088 9975	.0045 9544	.0023 6175
1.33	.0340 0208	.0179 0243	.0093 5784	.0048 6337	.0025 1570
1.34	.0352 7925	.0186 9403	.0098 3440	.0051 4392	.0026 7796
1.35	.0365 9024	.0195 1184	.0103 2993	.0054 3752	.0028 4885
1.36	.0379 3545	.0203 5639	.0108 4494	.0057 4461	.0030 2874
1.37	.0393 1530	.0212 2818	.0113 7993	.0060 6565	.0032 1799
1.38	.0407 3020	.0221 2775	.0119 3543	.0064 0108	.0034 1697
1.39	.0421 8052	.0230 5558	.0125 1195	.0067 5137	.0036 2605
1.40	.0436 6665	.0240 1220	.0131 1003	.0071 1699	.0038 4562
1.41	.0451 8898	.0249 9810	.0137 3017	.0074 9842	.0040 7608
1.42	.0467 4786	.0260 1379	.0143 7292	.0078 9613	.0043 1784
1.43	.0483 4364	.0270 5977	.0150 3880	.0083 1063	.0045 7130
1.44	.0499 7667	.0281 3653	.0157 2834	.0087 4239	.0048 3688
1.45	.0516 4728	.0292 4455	.0164 4208	.0091 9194	.0051 1503
1.46	.0533 5580	.0303 8433	.0171 8056	.0096 5977	.0054 0617
1.47	.0551 0253	.0315 5635	.0179 4429	.0101 4639	.0057 1075
1.48	.0568 8778	.0327 6107	.0187 3384	.0106 5233	.0060 2922
1.49	.0587 1183	.0339 9896	.0195 4972	.0111 7811	.0063 6206

W	P(W,7)	P(W,8)	P(W,9)	P(W,10)	P(W,11)
1.50	.0605 7496	.0352 7049	.0203 9247	.0117 2425	.0067 0972
1.51	.0624 7744	.0365 7610	.0212 6263	.0122 9128	.0070 7268
1.52	.0644 1951	.0379 1625	.0221 6073	.0128 7974	.0074 5143
1.53	.0664 0141	.0392 9138	.0230 8730	.0134 9016	.0078 4646
1.54	.0684 2338	.0407 0191	.0240 4287	.0141 2310	.0082 5827
1.55	.0704 8561	.0421 4826	.0250 2797	.0147 7909	.0086 8736
1.56	.0725 8832	.0436 3086	.0260 4313	.0154 5868	.0091 3425
1.57	.0747 3169	.0451 5011	.0270 8886	.0161 6242	.0095 9945
1.58	.0769 1589	.0467 0640	.0281 6567	.0168 9086	.0100 8349
1.59	.0791 4108	.0483 0012	.0292 7410	.0176 4456	.0105 8689
1.60	.0814 0740	.0499 3164	.0304 1463	.0184 2406	.0111 1018
1.61	.0837 1499	.0516 0133	.0315 8778	.0192 2992	.0116 5392
1.62	.0860 6395	.0533 0954	.0327 9405	.0200 6270	.0122 1864
1.63	.0884 5440	.0550 5662	.0340 3392	.0209 2295	.0128 0490
1.64	.0908 8641	.0568 4290	.0353 0788	.0218 1121	.0134 1323
1.65	.0933 6006	.0586 6870	.0366 1642	.0227 2806	.0140 4421
1.66	.0958 7540	.0605 3433	.0379 6001	.0236 7403	.0146 9839
1.67	.0984 3248	.0624 4008	.0393 3910	.0246 4967	.0153 7634
1.68	.1010 3133	.0643 8623	.0407 5417	.0256 5554	.0160 7861
1.69	.1036 7195	.0663 7306	.0422 0565	.0266 9217	.0168 0578
1.70	.1063 5434	.0684 0082	.0436 9400	.0277 6011	.0175 5842
1.71	.1090 7849	.0704 6975	.0452 1963	.0288 5989	.0183 3710
1.72	.1118 4435	.0725 8009	.0467 8298	.0299 9205	.0191 4239
1.73	.1146 5188	.0747 3205	.0483 8446	.0311 5712	.0199 7486
1.74	.1175 0101	.0769 2583	.0500 2446	.0323 5562	.0208 3509
1.75	.1203 9166	.0791 6161	.0517 0338	.0335 8806	.0217 2365
1.76	.1233 2374	.0814 3958	.0534 2161	.0348 5497	.0226 4111
1.77	.1262 9714	.0837 5989	.0551 7950	.0361 5684	.0235 8805
1.78	.1293 1172	.0861 2267	.0569 7742	.0374 9418	.0245 6503
1.79	.1323 6734	.0885 2807	.0588 1572	.0388 6748	.0255 7262
1.80	.1354 6386	.0909 7618	.0606 9472	.0402 7723	.0266 1140
1.81	.1386 0108	.0934 6710	.0626 1475	.0417 2389	.0276 8191
1.82	.1417 7883	.0960 0092	.0645 7612	.0432 0794	.0287 8472
1.83	.1449 9690	.0985 7770	.0665 7911	.0447 2984	.0299 2038
1.84	.1482 5507	.1011 9748	.0686 2401	.0462 9003	.0310 8945
1.85	.1515 5311	.1038 6031	.0707 1109	.0478 8897	.0322 9247
1.86	.1548 9077	.1065 6619	.0728 4059	.0495 2707	.0335 2999
1.87	.1582 6779	.1093 1513	.0750 1276	.0512 0475	.0348 0253
1.88	.1616 8388	.1121 0710	.0772 2782	.0529 2243	.0361 1063
1.89	.1651 3875	.1149 4208	.0794 8598	.0546 8050	.0374 5481
1.90	.1686 3210	.1178 2002	.0817 8742	.0564 7934	.0388 3558
1.91	.1721 6361	.1207 4085	.0841 3233	.0583 1933	.0402 5346
1.92	.1757 3293	.1237 0448	.0865 2087	.0602 0083	.0417 0894
1.93	.1793 3972	.1267 1083	.0889 5317	.0621 2418	.0432 0250
1.94	.1829 8361	.1297 5976	.0914 2937	.0640 8972	.0447 3465
1.95	.1866 6422	.1328 5116	.0939 4959	.0660 9777	.0463 0583
1.96	.1903 8117	.1359 8486	.0965 1391	.0681 4862	.0479 1653
1.97	.1941 3405	.1391 6071	.0991 2243	.0702 4258	.0495 6718
1.98	.1979 2243	.1423 7852	.1017 7518	.0723 7992	.0512 5824
1.99	.2017 4590	.1456 3810	.1044 7223	.0745 6090	.0529 9012

W	P(W,7)	P(W,8)	P(W,9)	P(W,10)	P(W,11)
2.00	.2056 0401	.1489 3922	.1072 1361	.0767 8576	.0547 6325
2.01	.2094 9629	.1522 8167	.1099 9931	.0790 5474	.0565 7804
2.02	.2134 2229	.1556 6518	.1128 2934	.0813 6805	.0584 3487
2.03	.2173 8151	.1590 8949	.1157 0366	.0837 2589	.0603 3412
2.04	.2213 7348	.1625 5433	.1186 2225	.0861 2843	.0622 7617
2.05	.2253 9768	.1660 5940	.1215 8503	.0885 7585	.0642 6135
2.06	.2294 5361	.1696 0439	.1245 9193	.0910 6829	.0662 9002
2.07	.2335 4073	.1731 8897	.1276 4285	.0936 0588	.0683 6249
2.08	.2376 5851	.1768 1279	.1307 3769	.0961 8874	.0704 7908
2.09	.2418 0640	.1804 7551	.1338 7631	.0988 1695	.0726 4007
2.10	.2459 8384	.1841 7674	.1370 5856	.1014 9060	.0748 4575
2.11	.2501 9028	.1879 1609	.1402 8427	.1042 0975	.0770 9636
2.12	.2544 2512	.1916 9317	.1435 5327	.1069 7443	.0793 9217
2.13	.2586 8779	.1955 0756	.1468 6535	.1097 8468	.0817 3339
2.14	.2629 7769	.1993 5882	.1502 2029	.1126 4049	.0841 2024
2.15	.2672 9421	.2032 4650	.1536 1786	.1155 4184	.0865 5291
2.16	.2716 3674	.2071 7015	.1570 5779	.1184 8872	.0890 3157
2.17	.2760 0467	.2111 2930	.1605 3983	.1214 8107	.0915 5639
2.18	.2803 9737	.2151 2345	.1640 6367	.1245 1881	.0941 2751
2.19	.2848 1419	.2191 5210	.1676 2901	.1276 0186	.0967 4504
2.20	.2892 5450	.2232 1475	.1712 3554	.1307 3011	.0994 0909
2.21	.2937 1765	.2273 1085	.1748 8291	.1339 0343	.1021 1974
2.22	.2982 0297	.2314 3989	.1785 7076	.1371 2168	.1048 7706
2.23	.3027 0982	.2356 0129	.1822 9872	.1403 8470	.1076 8110
2.24	.3072 3751	.2397 9451	.1860 6640	.1436 9230	.1105 3188
2.25	.3117 8538	.2440 1896	.1898 7340	.1470 4427	.1134 2940
2.26	.3163 5275	.2482 7407	.1937 1929	.1504 4040	.1163 7367
2.27	.3209 3893	.2525 5922	.1976 0364	.1538 8046	.1193 6464
2.28	.3255 4323	.2568 7383	.2015 2600	.1573 6417	.1224 0227
2.29	.3301 6496	.2612 1727	.2054 8588	.1608 9126	.1254 8647
2.30	.3348 0343	.2655 8890	.2094 8282	.1644 6144	.1286 1718
2.31	.3394 5793	.2699 8811	.2135 1632	.1680 7440	.1317 9426
2.32	.3441 2776	.2744 1423	.2175 8585	.1717 2979	.1350 1759
2.33	.3488 1221	.2788 6662	.2216 9090	.1754 2728	.1382 8702
2.34	.3535 1058	.2833 4460	.2258 3093	.1791 6650	.1416 0237
2.35	.3582 2215	.2878 4752	.2300 0537	.1829 4706	.1449 6346
2.36	.3629 4621	.2923 7468	.2342 1367	.1867 6855	.1483 7008
2.37	.3676 8204	.2969 2540	.2384 5523	.1906 3056	.1518 2199
2.38	.3724 2892	.3014 9899	.2427 2948	.1945 3265	.1553 1895
2.39	.3771 8615	.3060 9474	.2470 3580	.1984 7436	.1588 6068
2.40	.3819 5300	.3107 1195	.2513 7357	.2024 5523	.1624 4689
2.41	.3867 2875	.3153 4990	.2557 4216	.2064 7477	.1660 7728
2.42	.3915 1268	.3200 0786	.2601 4094	.2105 3248	.1697 5151
2.43	.3963 0408	.3246 8513	.2645 6925	.2146 2782	.1734 6924
2.44	.4011 0223	.3293 8096	.2690 2642	.2187 6028	.1772 3009
2.45	.4059 0641	.3340 9462	.2735 1179	.2229 2930	.1810 3369
2.46	.4107 1590	.3388 2536	.2780 2467	.2271 3432	.1848 7963
2.47	.4155 2999	.3435 7246	.2825 6437	.2313 7476	.1887 6748
2.48	.4203 4797	.3483 3516	.2871 3019	.2356 5002	.1926 9681
2.49	.4251 6912	.3531 1270	.2917 2141	.2399 5949	.1966 6714

W	P(W,7)	P(W,8)	P(W,9)	P(W,10)	P(W,11)
2.50	.4299 9275	.3579 0434	.2963 3732	.2443 0256	.2006 7801
2.51	.4348 1814	.3627 0933	.3009 7718	.2486 7859	.2047 2892
2.52	.4396 4459	.3675 2689	.3056 4028	.2530 8693	.2088 1936
2.53	.4444 7140	.3723 5628	.3103 2585	.2575 2692	.2129 4880
2.54	.4492 9787	.3771 9674	.3150 3316	.2619 9789	.2171 1668
2.55	.4541 2332	.3820 4749	.3197 6144	.2664 9916	.2213 2246
2.56	.4589 4704	.3869 0778	.3245 0994	.2710 3003	.2255 6554
2.57	.4637 6837	.3917 7685	.3292 7789	.2755 8979	.2298 4534
2.58	.4685 8662	.3966 5394	.3340 6451	.2801 7773	.2341 6124
2.59	.4734 0112	.4015 3827	.3388 6904	.2847 9312	.2385 1263
2.60	.4782 1118	.4064 2909	.3436 9068	.2894 3522	.2428 9885
2.61	.4830 1616	.4113 2564	.3485 2865	.2941 0328	.2473 1926
2.62	.4878 1539	.4162 2716	.3533 8216	.2987 9656	.2517 7319
2.63	.4926 0821	.4211 3290	.3582 5042	.3035 1428	.2562 5995
2.64	.4973 9398	.4260 4208	.3631 3263	.3082 5567	.2607 7885
2.65	.5021 7206	.4309 5397	.3680 2800	.3130 1996	.2653 2919
2.66	.5069 4180	.4358 6781	.3729 3572	.3178 0636	.2699 1024
2.67	.5117 0259	.4407 8286	.3778 5500	.3226 1406	.2745 2128
2.68	.5164 5380	.4456 9837	.3827 8502	.3274 4228	.2791 6155
2.69	.5211 9481	.4506 1359	.3877 2499	.3322 9021	.2838 3031
2.70	.5259 2502	.4555 2780	.3926 7410	.3371 5703	.2885 2679
2.71	.5306 4382	.4604 4026	.3976 3154	.3420 4193	.2932 5021
2.72	.5353 5061	.4653 5025	.4025 9652	.3469 4408	.2979 9979
2.73	.5400 4483	.4702 5703	.4075 6823	.3518 6266	.3027 7474
2.74	.5447 2587	.4751 5989	.4125 4586	.3567 9685	.3075 7425
2.75	.5493 9318	.4800 5813	.4175 2862	.3617 4580	.3123 9751
2.76	.5540 4619	.4849 5102	.4225 1570	.3667 0869	.3172 4371
2.77	.5586 8435	.4898 3787	.4275 0631	.3716 8466	.3221 1200
2.78	.5633 0711	.4947 1799	.4324 9966	.3766 7289	.3270 0158
2.79	.5679 1394	.4995 9068	.4374 9494	.3816 7254	.3319 1158
2.80	.5725 0429	.5044 5527	.4424 9138	.3866 8275	.3368 4117
2.81	.5770 7766	.5093 1108	.4474 8819	.3917 0269	.3417 8949
2.82	.5816 3354	.5141 5743	.4524 8459	.3967 3151	.3467 5569
2.83	.5861 7141	.5189 9368	.4574 7979	.4017 6837	.3517 3891
2.84	.5906 9079	.5238 1915	.4624 7303	.4068 1242	.3567 3828
2.85	.5951 9119	.5286 3322	.4674 6355	.4118 6283	.3617 5294
2.86	.5996 7214	.5334 3524	.4724 5057	.4169 1875	.3667 8200
2.87	.6041 3317	.5382 2458	.4774 3334	.4219 7933	.3718 2460
2.88	.6085 7382	.5430 0062	.4824 1111	.4270 4376	.3768 7986
2.89	.6129 9365	.5477 6274	.4873 8313	.4321 1119	.3819 4691
2.90	.6173 9222	.5525 1035	.4923 4867	.4371 8078	.3870 2485
2.91	.6217 6911	.5572 4284	.4973 0699	.4422 5172	.3921 1281
2.92	.6261 2388	.5619 5963	.5022 5738	.4473 2317	.3972 0991
2.93	.6304 5614	.5666 6014	.5071 9910	.4523 9431	.4023 1527
2.94	.6347 6549	.5713 4381	.5121 3145	.4574 6434	.4074 2800
2.95	.6390 5153	.5760 1007	.5170 5373	.4625 3244	.4125 4724
2.96	.6433 1389	.5806 5837	.5219 6524	.4675 9780	.4176 7209
2.97	.6475 5219	.5852 8818	.5268 6529	.4726 5962	.4228 0169
2.98	.6517 6609	.5898 9897	.5317 5321	.4777 1710	.4279 3516
2.99	.6559 5522	.5944 9020	.5366 2833	.4827 6947	.4330 7162

W	P(W,7)	P(W,8)	P(W,9)	P(W,10)	P(W,11)
3.00	.6601 1925	.5990 6139	.5414 8998	.4878 1593	.4382 1022
3.01	.6642 5784	.6036 1201	.5463 3751	.4928 5570	.4433 5008
3.02	.6683 7069	.6081 4160	.5511 7029	.4978 8804	.4484 9035
3.03	.6724 5747	.6126 4965	.5559 8767	.5029 1216	.4536 3017
3.04	.6765 1788	.6171 3572	.5607 8904	.5079 2731	.4587 6868
3.05	.6805 5165	.6215 9933	.5655 7378	.5129 3276	.4639 0505
3.06	.6845 5848	.6260 4003	.5703 4128	.5179 2776	.4690 3842
3.07	.6885 3810	.6304 5740	.5750 9095	.5229 1159	.4741 6797
3.08	.6924 9025	.6348 5100	.5798 2220	.5278 8352	.4792 9287
3.09	.6964 1469	.6392 2042	.5845 3448	.5328 4284	.4844 1229
3.10	.7003 1116	.6435 6526	.5892 2720	.5377 8886	.4895 2542
3.11	.7041 7945	.6478 8510	.5938 9982	.5427 2087	.4946 3145
3.12	.7080 1932	.6521 7958	.5985 5179	.5476 3820	.4997 2958
3.13	.7118 3056	.6564 4832	.6031 8259	.5525 4018	.5048 1902
3.14	.7156 1297	.6606 9095	.6077 9170	.5574 2613	.5098 9898
3.15	.7193 6635	.6649 0712	.6123 7861	.5622 9541	.5149 6869
3.16	.7230 9053	.6690 9649	.6169 4281	.5671 4738	.5200 2738
3.17	.7267 8532	.6732 5874	.6214 8383	.5719 8140	.5250 7429
3.18	.7304 5056	.6773 9353	.6260 0118	.5767 9685	.5301 0867
3.19	.7340 8610	.6815 0057	.6304 9441	.5815 9312	.5351 2979
3.20	.7376 9179	.6855 7955	.6349 6306	.5863 6962	.5401 3692
3.21	.7412 6748	.6896 3019	.6394 0669	.5911 2576	.5451 2933
3.22	.7448 1305	.6936 5220	.6438 2487	.5958 6096	.5501 0632
3.23	.7483 2838	.6976 4533	.6482 1718	.6005 7465	.5550 6720
3.24	.7518 1336	.7016 0931	.6525 8323	.6052 6629	.5600 1126
3.25	.7552 6788	.7055 4391	.6569 2260	.6099 3533	.5649 3784
3.26	.7586 9186	.7094 4888	.6612 3492	.6145 8125	.5698 4627
3.27	.7620 8520	.7133 2400	.6655 1983	.6192 0352	.5747 3591
3.28	.7654 4782	.7171 6906	.6697 7695	.6238 0165	.5796 0609
3.29	.7687 7967	.7209 8386	.6740 0594	.6283 7513	.5844 5621
3.30	.7720 8068	.7247 6820	.6782 0646	.6329 2349	.5892 8563
3.31	.7753 5079	.7285 2190	.6823 7819	.6374 4626	.5940 9375
3.32	.7785 8997	.7322 4478	.6865 2082	.6419 4298	.5988 7998
3.33	.7817 9817	.7359 3669	.6906 3404	.6464 1321	.6036 4374
3.34	.7849 7538	.7395 9746	.6947 1756	.6508 5651	.6083 8445
3.35	.7881 2156	.7432 2697	.6987 7111	.6552 7248	.6131 0156
3.36	.7912 3671	.7468 2507	.7027 9441	.6596 6069	.6177 9452
3.37	.7943 2081	.7503 9163	.7067 8721	.6640 2076	.6224 6281
3.38	.7973 7388	.7539 2656	.7107 4927	.6683 5230	.6271 0591
3.39	.8003 9592	.7574 2974	.7146 8035	.6726 5494	.6317 2330
3.40	.8033 8694	.7609 0107	.7185 8023	.6769 2834	.6363 1450
3.41	.8063 4698	.7643 4047	.7224 4870	.6811 7213	.6408 7903
3.42	.8092 7606	.7677 4787	.7262 8556	.6853 8599	.6454 1641
3.43	.8121 7421	.7711 2320	.7300 9061	.6895 6961	.6499 2621
3.44	.8150 4149	.7744 6639	.7338 6369	.6937 2266	.6544 0797
3.45	.8178 7794	.7777 7740	.7376 0462	.6978 4486	.6588 6127
3.46	.8206 8362	.7810 5619	.7413 1324	.7019 3593	.6632 8569
3.47	.8234 5860	.7843 0272	.7449 8942	.7059 9558	.6676 8084
3.48	.8262 0293	.7875 1698	.7486 3301	.7100 2357	.6720 4632
3.49	.8289 1670	.7906 9894	.7522 4389	.7140 1964	.6763 8177

W	P(W,7)	P(W,8)	P(W,9)	P(W,10)	P(W,11)
3.50	.8315 9999	.7938 4860	.7558 2194	.7179 8356	.6806 8682
3.51	.8342 5289	.7969 6595	.7593 6706	.7219 1511	.6849 6112
3.52	.8368 7549	.8000 5101	.7628 7916	.7258 1408	.6892 0433
3.53	.8394 6788	.8031 0380	.7663 5814	.7296 8026	.6934 1615
3.54	.8420 3017	.8061 2433	.7698 0394	.7335 1347	.6975 9625
3.55	.8445 6248	.8091 1264	.7732 1649	.7373 1353	.7017 4434
3.56	.8470 6491	.8120 6877	.7765 9573	.7410 8028	.7058 6013
3.57	.8495 3758	.8149 9277	.7799 4161	.7448 1357	.7099 4337
3.58	.8519 8062	.8178 8468	.7832 5411	.7485 1324	.7139 9378
3.59	.8543 9415	.8207 4457	.7865 3319	.7521 7917	.7180 1113
3.60	.8567 7832	.8235 7250	.7897 7882	.7558 1124	.7219 9519
3.61	.8591 3326	.8263 6856	.7929 9102	.7594 0935	.7259 4572
3.62	.8614 5911	.8291 3282	.7961 6976	.7629 7338	.7298 6253
3.63	.8637 5601	.8318 6536	.7993 1506	.7665 0325	.7337 4543
3.64	.8660 2413	.8345 6629	.8024 2694	.7699 9889	.7375 9422
3.65	.8682 6361	.8372 3570	.8055 0541	.7734 6023	.7414 0874
3.66	.8704 7462	.8398 7369	.8085 5052	.7768 8721	.7451 8883
3.67	.8726 5731	.8424 8039	.8115 6229	.7802 7978	.7489 3434
3.68	.8748 1185	.8450 5590	.8145 4078	.7836 3790	.7526 4514
3.69	.8769 3842	.8476 0034	.8174 8605	.7869 6156	.7563 2110
3.70	.8790 3719	.8501 1386	.8203 9816	.7902 5072	.7599 6211
3.71	.8811 0833	.8525 9657	.8232 7718	.7935 0539	.7635 6808
3.72	.8831 5202	.8550 4863	.8261 2318	.7967 2556	.7671 3891
3.73	.8851 6846	.8574 7017	.8289 3625	.7999 1124	.7706 7453
3.74	.8871 5781	.8598 6134	.8317 1649	.8030 6245	.7741 7486
3.75	.8891 2028	.8622 2230	.8344 6400	.8061 7923	.7776 3985
3.76	.8910 5605	.8645 5320	.8371 7887	.8092 6160	.7810 6946
3.77	.8929 6532	.8668 5420	.8398 6122	.8123 0961	.7844 6365
3.78	.8948 4828	.8691 2548	.8425 1117	.8153 2332	.7878 2239
3.79	.8967 0514	.8713 6721	.8451 2885	.8183 0278	.7911 4567
3.80	.8985 3609	.8735 7955	.8477 1437	.8212 4807	.7944 3348
3.81	.9003 4134	.8757 6270	.8502 6789	.8241 5926	.7976 8584
3.82	.9021 2110	.8779 1682	.8527 8954	.8270 3644	.8009 0274
3.83	.9038 7557	.8800 4212	.8552 7947	.8298 7969	.8040 8422
3.84	.9056 0496	.8821 3877	.8577 3784	.8326 8913	.8072 3031
3.85	.9073 0948	.8842 0698	.8601 6479	.8354 6486	.8103 4106
3.86	.9089 8936	.8862 4693	.8625 6050	.8382 0698	.8134 1650
3.87	.9106 4479	.8882 5883	.8649 2513	.8409 1563	.8164 5671
3.88	.9122 7599	.8902 4289	.8672 5885	.8435 9093	.8194 6175
3.89	.9138 8320	.8921 9930	.8695 6185	.8462 3301	.8224 3169
3.90	.9154 6661	.8941 2828	.8718 3430	.8488 4202	.8253 6663
3.91	.9170 2646	.8960 3003	.8740 7640	.8514 1809	.8282 6665
3.92	.9185 6296	.8979 0478	.8762 8832	.8539 6139	.8311 3186
3.93	.9200 7633	.8997 5273	.8784 7027	.8564 7206	.8339 6237
3.94	.9215 6680	.9015 7411	.8806 2245	.8589 5028	.8367 5828
3.95	.9230 3459	.9033 6913	.8827 4505	.8613 9622	.8395 1973
3.96	.9244 7993	.9051 3803	.8848 3828	.8638 1004	.8422 4684
3.97	.9259 0304	.9068 8101	.8869 0235	.8661 9193	.8449 3976
3.98	.9273 0414	.9085 9831	.8889 3748	.8685 4207	.8475 9861
3.99	.9286 8346	.9102 9016	.8909 4388	.8708 6065	.8502 2357

W	P(W,7)	P(W,8)	P(W,9)	P(W,10)	P(W,11)
4.00	.9300 4123	.9119 5679	.8929 2176	.8731 4787	.8528 1477
4.01	.9313 7768	.9135 9842	.8948 7135	.8754 0392	.8553 7240
4.02	.9326 9302	.9152 1529	.8967 9287	.8776 2901	.8578 9660
4.03	.9339 8750	.9168 0764	.8986 8656	.8798 2334	.8603 8757
4.04	.9352 6133	.9183 7569	.9005 5263	.8819 8712	.8628 4548
4.05	.9365 1473	.9199 1969	.9023 9133	.8841 2058	.8652 7051
4.06	.9377 4795	.9214 3987	.9042 0288	.8862 2392	.8676 6286
4.07	.9389 6121	.9229 3646	.9059 8752	.8882 9738	.8700 2273
4.08	.9401 5472	.9244 0971	.9077 4548	.8903 4117	.8723 5031
4.09	.9413 2873	.9258 5986	.9094 7702	.8923 5552	.8746 4581
4.10	.9424 8344	.9272 8714	.9111 8237	.8943 4067	.8769 0945
4.11	.9436 1910	.9286 9180	.9128 6176	.8962 9685	.8791 4143
4.12	.9447 3593	.9300 7407	.9145 1546	.8982 2429	.8813 4198
4.13	.9458 3414	.9314 3420	.9161 4370	.9001 2325	.8835 1132
4.14	.9469 1397	.9327 7242	.9177 4673	.9019 9396	.8856 4968
4.15	.9479 7563	.9340 8899	.9193 2480	.9038 3666	.8877 5729
4.16	.9490 1936	.9353 8413	.9208 7815	.9056 5160	.8898 3438
4.17	.9500 4537	.9366 5810	.9224 0705	.9074 3904	.8918 8119
4.18	.9510 5388	.9379 1112	.9239 1174	.9091 9922	.8938 9797
4.19	.9520 4512	.9391 4345	.9253 9246	.9109 3239	.8958 8495
4.20	.9530 1930	.9403 5533	.9268 4948	.9126 3882	.8978 4239
4.21	.9539 7664	.9415 4699	.9282 8305	.9143 1876	.8997 7053
4.22	.9549 1736	.9427 1867	.9296 9342	.9159 7246	.9016 6963
4.23	.9558 4168	.9438 7061	.9310 8085	.9176 0018	.9035 3995
4.24	.9567 4981	.9450 0306	.9324 4558	.9192 0219	.9053 8174
4.25	.9576 4197	.9461 1625	.9337 8788	.9207 7874	.9071 9526
4.26	.9585 1837	.9472 1042	.9351 0799	.9223 3011	.9089 8077
4.27	.9593 7922	.9482 8580	.9364 0617	.9238 5654	.9107 3854
4.28	.9602 2473	.9493 4264	.9376 8268	.9253 5831	.9124 6884
4.29	.9610 5512	.9503 8116	.9389 3777	.9268 3568	.9141 7192
4.30	.9618 7058	.9514 0160	.9401 7169	.9282 8892	.9158 4806
4.31	.9626 7134	.9524 0420	.9413 8470	.9297 1829	.9174 9754
4.32	.9634 5758	.9533 8919	.9425 7704	.9311 2405	.9191 2061
4.33	.9642 2953	.9543 5680	.9437 4898	.9325 0648	.9207 1756
4.34	.9649 8737	.9553 0725	.9449 0076	.9338 6583	.9222 8865
4.35	.9657 3132	.9562 4079	.9460 3264	.9352 0238	.9238 3417
4.36	.9664 6157	.9571 5763	.9471 4485	.9365 1640	.9253 5438
4.37	.9671 7831	.9580 5801	.9482 3767	.9378 0814	.9268 4957
4.38	.9678 8176	.9589 4214	.9493 1132	.9390 7787	.9283 2000
4.39	.9685 7209	.9598 1026	.9503 6607	.9403 2586	.9297 6596
4.40	.9692 4951	.9606 6259	.9514 0215	.9415 5237	.9311 8772
4.41	.9699 1421	.9614 9934	.9524 1981	.9427 5768	.9325 8557
4.42	.9705 6638	.9623 2074	.9534 1931	.9439 4203	.9339 5977
4.43	.9712 0620	.9631 2701	.9544 0087	.9451 0570	.9353 1060
4.44	.9718 3387	.9639 1836	.9553 6475	.9462 4895	.9366 3835
4.45	.9724 4957	.9646 9501	.9563 1118	.9473 7204	.9379 4329
4.46	.9730 5348	.9654 5717	.9572 4040	.9484 7523	.9392 2569
4.47	.9736 4579	.9662 0506	.9581 5266	.9495 5878	.9404 8584
4.48	.9742 2667	.9669 3888	.9590 4819	.9506 2295	.9417 2400
4.49	.9747 9631	.9676 5885	.9599 2722	.9516 6799	.9429 4046

W	P(W,7)	P(W,8)	P(W,9)	P(W,10)	P(W,11)
4.50	.9753 5488	.9683 6516	.9607 8999	.9526 9417	.9441 3549
4.51	.9759 0256	.9690 5804	.9616 3673	.9537 0174	.9453 0935
4.52	.9764 3951	.9697 3767	.9624 6767	.9546 9095	.9464 6234
4.53	.9769 6592	.9704 0427	.9632 8305	.9556 6206	.9475 9471
4.54	.9774 8195	.9710 5803	.9640 8309	.9566 1532	.9487 0674
4.55	.9779 8777	.9716 9916	.9648 6801	.9575 5097	.9497 9870
4.56	.9784 8355	.9723 2784	.9656 3804	.9584 6927	.9508 7086
4.57	.9789 6944	.9729 4427	.9663 9340	.9593 7046	.9519 2348
4.58	.9794 4563	.9735 4865	.9671 3432	.9602 5479	.9529 5684
4.59	.9799 1225	.9741 4117	.9678 6100	.9611 2251	.9539 7120
4.60	.9803 6948	.9747 2202	.9685 7368	.9619 7385	.9549 6682
4.61	.9808 1747	.9752 9137	.9692 7256	.9628 0905	.9559 4396
4.62	.9812 5637	.9758 4943	.9699 5786	.9636 2836	.9569 0289
4.63	.9816 8635	.9763 9637	.9706 2979	.9644 3202	.9578 4386
4.64	.9821 0755	.9769 3238	.9712 8856	.9652 2024	.9587 6714
4.65	.9825 2012	.9774 5762	.9719 3437	.9659 9328	.9596 7298
4.66	.9829 2421	.9779 7229	.9725 6744	.9667 5136	.9605 6163
4.67	.9833 1996	.9784 7656	.9731 8796	.9674 9471	.9614 3335
4.68	.9837 0753	.9789 7060	.9737 9614	.9682 2356	.9622 8839
4.69	.9840 8705	.9794 5459	.9743 9218	.9689 3813	.9631 2700
4.70	.9844 5867	.9799 2868	.9749 7627	.9696 3865	.9639 4942
4.71	.9848 2252	.9803 9306	.9755 4861	.9703 2534	.9647 5591
4.72	.9851 7875	.9808 4788	.9761 0940	.9709 9842	.9655 4669
4.73	.9855 2748	.9812 9332	.9766 5882	.9716 5811	.9663 2203
4.74	.9858 6885	.9817 2953	.9771 9707	.9723 0461	.9670 8215
4.75	.9862 0300	.9821 5667	.9777 2433	.9729 3815	.9678 2729
4.76	.9865 3005	.9825 7491	.9782 4079	.9735 5894	.9685 5769
4.77	.9868 5013	.9829 8439	.9787 4663	.9741 6719	.9692 7358
4.78	.9871 6338	.9833 8528	.9792 4203	.9747 6309	.9699 7520
4.79	.9874 6990	.9837 7772	.9797 2717	.9753 4687	.9706 6276
4.80	.9877 6984	.9841 6186	.9802 0223	.9759 1871	.9713 3651
4.81	.9880 6331	.9845 3786	.9806 6738	.9764 7882	.9719 9666
4.82	.9883 5042	.9849 0586	.9811 2280	.9770 2740	.9726 4344
4.83	.9886 3131	.9852 6601	.9815 6866	.9775 6465	.9732 7706
4.84	.9889 0607	.9856 1844	.9820 0512	.9780 9075	.9738 9775
4.85	.9891 7484	.9859 6330	.9824 3235	.9786 0590	.9745 0571
4.86	.9894 3772	.9863 0072	.9828 5052	.9791 1029	.9751 0118
4.87	.9896 9483	.9866 3085	.9832 5978	.9796 0411	.9756 8434
4.88	.9899 4627	.9869 5382	.9836 6030	.9800 8754	.9762 5542
4.89	.9901 9215	.9872 6976	.9840 5224	.9805 6076	.9768 1462
4.90	.9904 3258	.9875 7880	.9844 3575	.9810 2395	.9773 6214
4.91	.9906 6767	.9878 8108	.9848 1099	.9814 7730	.9778 9819
4.92	.9908 9751	.9881 7671	.9851 7810	.9819 2098	.9784 2296
4.93	.9911 2222	.9884 6584	.9855 3725	.9823 5515	.9789 3666
4.94	.9913 4188	.9887 4857	.9858 8856	.9827 8000	.9794 3948
4.95	.9915 5660	.9890 2503	.9862 3220	.9831 9570	.9799 3160
4.96	.9917 6648	.9892 9535	.9865 6830	.9836 0240	.9804 1322
4.97	.9919 7161	.9895 5963	.9868 9701	.9840 0027	.9808 8454
4.98	.9921 7209	.9898 1800	.9872 1847	.9843 8949	.9813 4572
4.99	.9923 6800	.9900 7058	.9875 3281	.9847 7020	.9817 9696

W	P(W,7)	P(W,8)	P(W,9)	P(W,10)	P(W,11)
5.00	.9925 5944	.9903 1747	.9878 4016	.9851 4256	.9822 3844
5.01	.9927 4651	.9905 5878	.9881 4067	.9855 0674	.9826 7034
5.02	.9929 2928	.9907 9464	.9884 3447	.9858 6288	.9830 9282
5.03	.9931 0784	.9910 2513	.9887 2168	.9862 1114	.9835 0607
5.04	.9932 8228	.9912 5038	.9890 0243	.9865 5167	.9839 1026
5.05	.9934 5269	.9914 7048	.9892 7685	.9868 8461	.9843 0555
5.06	.9936 1915	.9916 8554	.9895 4506	.9872 1011	.9846 9211
5.07	.9937 8173	.9918 9566	.9898 0718	.9875 2831	.9850 7011
5.08	.9939 4051	.9921 0094	.9900 6334	.9878 3936	.9854 3971
5.09	.9940 9559	.9923 0147	.9903 1365	.9881 4339	.9858 0106
5.10	.9942 4702	.9924 9736	.9905 5823	.9884 4054	.9861 5433
5.11	.9943 9490	.9926 8870	.9907 9719	.9887 3094	.9864 9967
5.12	.9945 3928	.9928 7557	.9910 3065	.9890 1474	.9868 3724
5.13	.9946 8026	.9930 5808	.9912 5872	.9892 9204	.9871 6718
5.14	.9948 1789	.9932 3632	.9914 8150	.9895 6300	.9874 8964
5.15	.9949 5224	.9934 1036	.9916 9911	.9898 2773	.9878 0478
5.16	.9950 8340	.9935 8031	.9919 1164	.9900 8636	.9881 1272
5.17	.9952 1142	.9937 4624	.9921 1921	.9903 3900	.9884 1362
5.18	.9953 3637	.9939 0823	.9923 2191	.9905 8579	.9887 0762
5.19	.9954 5833	.9940 6638	.9925 1985	.9908 2684	.9889 9485
5.20	.9955 7734	.9942 2076	.9927 1312	.9910 6227	.9892 7545
5.21	.9956 9348	.9943 7146	.9929 0183	.9912 9218	.9895 4954
5.22	.9958 0681	.9945 1854	.9930 8606	.9915 1671	.9898 1727
5.23	.9959 1739	.9946 6209	.9932 6591	.9917 3595	.9900 7877
5.24	.9960 2528	.9948 0219	.9934 4148	.9919 5001	.9903 3415
5.25	.9961 3054	.9949 3890	.9936 1284	.9921 5901	.9905 8354
5.26	.9962 3322	.9950 7230	.9937 8011	.9923 6305	.9908 2707
5.27	.9963 3339	.9952 0247	.9939 4335	.9925 6223	.9910 6486
5.28	.9964 3109	.9953 2946	.9941 0266	.9927 5666	.9912 9702
5.29	.9965 2639	.9954 5336	.9942 5811	.9929 4643	.9915 2367
5.30	.9966 1933	.9955 7423	.9944 0981	.9931 3164	.9917 4494
5.31	.9967 0997	.9956 9213	.9945 5781	.9933 1240	.9919 6092
5.32	.9967 9836	.9958 0714	.9947 0221	.9934 8879	.9921 7174
5.33	.9968 8455	.9959 1931	.9948 4308	.9936 6092	.9923 7750
5.34	.9969 6859	.9960 2871	.9949 8051	.9938 2886	.9925 7830
5.35	.9970 5053	.9961 3540	.9951 1456	.9939 9272	.9927 7426
5.36	.9971 3041	.9962 3943	.9952 4530	.9941 5258	.9929 6548
5.37	.9972 0829	.9963 4088	.9953 7283	.9943 0852	.9931 5206
5.38	.9972 8421	.9964 3979	.9954 9719	.9944 6064	.9933 3409
5.39	.9973 5821	.9965 3623	.9956 1847	.9946 0902	.9935 1168
5.40	.9974 3033	.9966 3025	.9957 3673	.9947 5373	.9936 8493
5.41	.9975 0063	.9967 2191	.9958 5204	.9948 9486	.9938 5392
5.42	.9975 6914	.9968 1125	.9959 6447	.9950 3250	.9940 1876
5.43	.9976 3590	.9968 9833	.9960 7408	.9951 6671	.9941 7953
5.44	.9977 0096	.9969 8321	.9961 8094	.9952 9757	.9943 3632
5.45	.9977 6435	.9970 6594	.9962 8510	.9954 2517	.9944 8922
5.46	.9978 2612	.9971 4655	.9963 8664	.9955 4956	.9946 3832
5.47	.9978 8629	.9972 2511	.9964 8560	.9956 7083	.9947 8370
5.48	.9979 4492	.9973 0166	.9965 8205	.9957 8904	.9949 2544
5.49	.9980 0202	.9973 7625	.9966 7604	.9959 0427	.9950 6362

W	P(W,7)	P(W,8)	P(W,9)	P(W,10)	P(W,11)
5.50	.9980 5765	.9974 4892	.9967 6764	.9960 1658	.9951 9834
5.51	.9981 1184	.9975 1972	.9968 5689	.9961 2604	.9953 2966
5.52	.9981 6461	.9975 8868	.9969 4386	.9962 3271	.9954 5765
5.53	.9982 1601	.9976 5587	.9970 2859	.9963 3666	.9955 8241
5.54	.9982 6606	.9977 2131	.9971 1114	.9964 3795	.9957 0399
5.55	.9983 1480	.9977 8505	.9971 9155	.9965 3664	.9958 2248
5.56	.9983 6227	.9978 4712	.9972 6989	.9966 3280	.9959 3795
5.57	.9984 0848	.9979 0757	.9973 4619	.9967 2648	.9960 5045
5.58	.9984 5347	.9979 6645	.9974 2051	.9968 1773	.9961 6007
5.59	.9984 9728	.9980 2377	.9974 9289	.9969 0663	.9962 6687
5.60	.9985 3992	.9980 7959	.9975 6337	.9969 9321	.9963 7091
5.61	.9985 8143	.9981 3393	.9976 3202	.9970 7755	.9964 7227
5.62	.9986 2184	.9981 8684	.9976 9885	.9971 5968	.9965 7099
5.63	.9986 6117	.9982 3835	.9977 6393	.9972 3966	.9966 6715
5.64	.9986 9945	.9982 8848	.9978 2730	.9973 1755	.9967 6080
5.65	.9987 3670	.9983 3729	.9978 8898	.9973 9339	.9968 5201
5.66	.9987 7295	.9983 8479	.9979 4904	.9974 6723	.9969 4083
5.67	.9988 0823	.9984 3103	.9980 0749	.9975 3913	.9970 2732
5.68	.9988 4255	.9984 7602	.9980 6440	.9976 0912	.9971 1153
5.69	.9988 7595	.9985 1981	.9981 1978	.9976 7725	.9971 9352
5.70	.9989 0845	.9985 6241	.9981 7368	.9977 4357	.9972 7334
5.71	.9989 4006	.9986 0387	.9982 2614	.9978 0813	.9973 5105
5.72	.9989 7081	.9986 4421	.9982 7718	.9978 7096	.9974 2670
5.73	.9990 0073	.9986 8346	.9983 2685	.9979 3210	.9975 0032
5.74	.9990 2982	.9987 2164	.9983 7519	.9979 9161	.9975 7199
5.75	.9990 5813	.9987 5878	.9984 2221	.9980 4951	.9976 4174
5.76	.9990 8565	.9987 9491	.9984 6796	.9981 0586	.9977 0961
5.77	.9991 1242	.9988 3005	.9985 1247	.9981 6068	.9977 7566
5.78	.9991 3845	.9988 6423	.9985 5576	.9982 1402	.9978 3994
5.79	.9991 6377	.9988 9747	.9985 9787	.9982 6591	.9979 0247
5.80	.9991 8838	.9989 2980	.9986 3883	.9983 1639	.9979 6332
5.81	.9992 1231	.9989 6124	.9986 7867	.9983 6549	.9980 2251
5.82	.9992 3558	.9989 9181	.9987 1742	.9984 1325	.9980 8009
5.83	.9992 5820	.9990 2153	.9987 5509	.9984 5970	.9981 3611
5.84	.9992 8019	.9990 5043	.9987 9173	.9985 0487	.9981 9059
5.85	.9993 0156	.9990 7853	.9988 2736	.9985 4881	.9982 4358
5.86	.9993 2234	.9991 0584	.9988 6199	.9985 9153	.9982 9512
5.87	.9993 4253	.9991 3239	.9988 9567	.9986 3307	.9983 4524
5.88	.9993 6216	.9991 5820	.9989 2841	.9986 7346	.9983 9398
5.89	.9993 8123	.9991 8328	.9989 6024	.9987 1273	.9984 4138
5.90	.9993 9977	.9992 0767	.9989 9117	.9987 5091	.9984 8746
5.91	.9994 1778	.9992 3136	.9990 2124	.9987 8802	.9985 3226
5.92	.9994 3528	.9992 5439	.9990 5047	.9988 2410	.9985 7582
5.93	.9994 5228	.9992 7676	.9990 7888	.9988 5917	.9986 1816
5.94	.9994 6880	.9992 9851	.9991 0648	.9988 9325	.9986 5932
5.95	.9994 8485	.9993 1963	.9991 3331	.9989 2638	.9986 9933
5.96	.9995 0045	.9993 4016	.9991 5937	.9989 5857	.9987 3821
5.97	.9995 1559	.9993 6010	.9991 8470	.9989 8985	.9987 7600
5.98	.9995 3030	.9993 7947	.9992 0931	.9990 2025	.9988 1273
5.99	.9995 4459	.9993 9829	.9992 3321	.9990 4979	.9988 4842

W	P(W,7)	P(W,8)	P(W,9)	P(W,10)	P(W,11)
6.00	.9995 5847	.9994 1657	.9992 5644	.9990 7848	.9988 8310
6.01	.9995 7195	.9994 3433	.9992 7900	.9991 0636	.9989 1680
6.02	.9995 8503	.9994 5157	.9993 0091	.9991 3345	.9989 4954
6.03	.9995 9774	.9994 6832	.9993 2220	.9991 5976	.9989 8135
6.04	.9996 1008	.9994 8458	.9993 4287	.9991 8532	.9990 1225
6.05	.9996 2207	.9995 0037	.9993 6295	.9992 1014	.9990 4227
6.06	.9996 3370	.9995 1571	.9993 8245	.9992 3425	.9990 7143
6.07	.9996 4499	.9995 3060	.9994 0138	.9992 5767	.9990 9975
6.08	.9996 5596	.9995 4505	.9994 1977	.9992 8041	.9991 2725
6.09	.9996 6660	.9995 5909	.9994 3762	.9993 0249	.9991 5396
6.10	.9996 7693	.9995 7271	.9994 5495	.9993 2393	.9991 7990
6.11	.9996 8696	.9995 8594	.9994 7178	.9993 4475	.9992 0509
6.12	.9996 9669	.9995 9878	.9994 8811	.9993 6496	.9992 2955
6.13	.9997 0613	.9996 1124	.9995 0397	.9993 8458	.9992 5330
6.14	.9997 1530	.9996 2333	.9995 1936	.9994 0363	.9992 7636
6.15	.9997 2419	.9996 3507	.9995 3430	.9994 2212	.9992 9874
6.16	.9997 3283	.9996 4646	.9995 4880	.9994 4007	.9993 2047
6.17	.9997 4120	.9996 5751	.9995 6287	.9994 5749	.9993 4156
6.18	.9997 4932	.9996 6824	.9995 7653	.9994 7439	.9993 6203
6.19	.9997 5721	.9996 7864	.9995 8978	.9994 9080	.9993 8190
6.20	.9997 6485	.9996 8874	.9996 0264	.9995 0673	.9994 0119
6.21	.9997 7227	.9996 9854	.9996 1511	.9995 2218	.9994 1990
6.22	.9997 7947	.9997 0804	.9996 2722	.9995 3717	.9994 3806
6.23	.9997 8645	.9997 1726	.9996 3896	.9995 5172	.9994 5569
6.24	.9997 9322	.9997 2620	.9996 5035	.9995 6583	.9994 7278
6.25	.9997 9978	.9997 3487	.9996 6140	.9995 7952	.9994 8937
6.26	.9998 0615	.9997 4328	.9996 7212	.9995 9280	.9995 0547
6.27	.9998 1232	.9997 5144	.9996 8252	.9996 0569	.9995 2108
6.28	.9998 1831	.9997 5935	.9996 9260	.9996 1818	.9995 3623
6.29	.9998 2412	.9997 6702	.9997 0238	.9996 3030	.9995 5092
6.30	.9998 2974	.9997 7446	.9997 1186	.9996 4206	.9995 6517
6.31	.9998 3520	.9997 8168	.9997 2106	.9996 5346	.9995 7900
6.32	.9998 4049	.9997 8867	.9997 2997	.9996 6452	.9995 9240
6.33	.9998 4562	.9997 9545	.9997 3862	.9996 7524	.9996 0540
6.34	.9998 5059	.9998 0203	.9997 4700	.9996 8563	.9996 1800
6.35	.9998 5541	.9998 0840	.9997 5513	.9996 9571	.9996 3023
6.36	.9998 6008	.9998 1457	.9997 6301	.9997 0548	.9996 4208
6.37	.9998 6461	.9998 2056	.9997 7065	.9997 1495	.9996 5357
6.38	.9998 6900	.9998 2636	.9997 7805	.9997 2414	.9996 6471
6.39	.9998 7325	.9998 3199	.9997 8522	.9997 3304	.9996 7551
6.40	.9998 7737	.9998 3744	.9997 9218	.9997 4167	.9996 8598
6.41	.9998 8136	.9998 4272	.9997 9892	.9997 5003	.9996 9612
6.42	.9998 8523	.9998 4784	.9998 0545	.9997 5813	.9997 0596
6.43	.9998 8898	.9998 5280	.9998 1178	.9997 6599	.9997 1549
6.44	.9998 9261	.9998 5760	.9998 1791	.9997 7360	.9997 2473
6.45	.9998 9613	.9998 6226	.9998 2386	.9997 8098	.9997 3368
6.46	.9998 9953	.9998 6677	.9998 2961	.9997 8812	.9997 4236
6.47	.9999 0284	.9998 7114	.9998 3519	.9997 9505	.9997 5076
6.48	.9999 0603	.9998 7537	.9998 4060	.9998 0176	.9997 5891
6.49	.9999 0913	.9998 7947	.9998 4583	.9998 0826	.9997 6680

W	P(W,7)	P(W,8)	P(W,9)	P(W,10)	P(W,11)
6.50	.9999 1213	.9998 8344	.9998 5090	.9998 1455	.9997 7445
6.51	.9999 1503	.9998 8729	.9998 5581	.9998 2065	.9997 8185
6.52	.9999 1785	.9998 9102	.9998 6057	.9998 2656	.9997 8903
6.53	.9999 2057	.9998 9462	.9998 6518	.9998 3228	.9997 9598
6.54	.9999 2321	.9998 9812	.9998 6964	.9998 3782	.9998 0271
6.55	.9999 2576	.9999 0150	.9998 7396	.9998 4319	.9998 0923
6.56	.9999 2823	.9999 0477	.9998 7815	.9998 4839	.9998 1554
6.57	.9999 3063	.9999 0794	.9998 8220	.9998 5342	.9998 2166
6.58	.9999 3294	.9999 1102	.9998 8612	.9998 5830	.9998 2758
6.59	.9999 3519	.9999 1399	.9998 8992	.9998 6301	.9998 3331
6.60	.9999 3736	.9999 1686	.9998 9359	.9998 6758	.9998 3886
6.61	.9999 3946	.9999 1965	.9998 9715	.9998 7201	.9998 4424
6.62	.9999 4150	.9999 2235	.9999 0060	.9998 7629	.9998 4944
6.63	.9999 4346	.9999 2495	.9999 0393	.9998 8043	.9998 5448
6.64	.9999 4537	.9999 2748	.9999 0716	.9998 8444	.9998 5935
6.65	.9999 4721	.9999 2992	.9999 1029	.9998 8833	.9998 6407
6.66	.9999 4900	.9999 3229	.9999 1331	.9998 9209	.9998 6864
6.67	.9999 5072	.9999 3458	.9999 1624	.9998 9572	.9998 7306
6.68	.9999 5239	.9999 3679	.9999 1907	.9998 9924	.9998 7734
6.69	.9999 5401	.9999 3894	.9999 2181	.9999 0265	.9998 8149
6.70	.9999 5557	.9999 4101	.9999 2446	.9999 0595	.9998 8549
6.71	.9999 5709	.9999 4301	.9999 2702	.9999 0914	.9998 8937
6.72	.9999 5855	.9999 4496	.9999 2951	.9999 1222	.9998 9312
6.73	.9999 5997	.9999 4683	.9999 3191	.9999 1521	.9998 9675
6.74	.9999 6133	.9999 4865	.9999 3423	.9999 1810	.9999 0027
6.75	.9999 6266	.9999 5040	.9999 3648	.9999 2089	.9999 0367
6.76	.9999 6394	.9999 5210	.9999 3865	.9999 2359	.9999 0695
6.77	.9999 6518	.9999 5375	.9999 4075	.9999 2621	.9999 1013
6.78	.9999 6638	.9999 5533	.9999 4278	.9999 2874	.9999 1321
6.79	.9999 6753	.9999 5687	.9999 4475	.9999 3118	.9999 1618
6.80	.9999 6865	.9999 5836	.9999 4665	.9999 3355	.9999 1906
6.81	.9999 6974	.9999 5979	.9999 4849	.9999 3583	.9999 2184
6.82	.9999 7078	.9999 6118	.9999 5027	.9999 3805	.9999 2453
6.83	.9999 7179	.9999 6253	.9999 5198	.9999 4018	.9999 2714
6.84	.9999 7277	.9999 6382	.9999 5365	.9999 4225	.9999 2965
6.85	.9999 7372	.9999 6508	.9999 5525	.9999 4425	.9999 3209
6.86	.9999 7463	.9999 6629	.9999 5681	.9999 4618	.9999 3444
6.87	.9999 7552	.9999 6747	.9999 5831	.9999 4805	.9999 3671
6.88	.9999 7637	.9999 6860	.9999 5976	.9999 4986	.9999 3891
6.89	.9999 7720	.9999 6969	.9999 6116	.9999 5160	.9999 4103
6.90	.9999 7799	.9999 7075	.9999 6252	.9999 5329	.9999 4309
6.91	.9999 7876	.9999 7178	.9999 6383	.9999 5492	.9999 4507
6.92	.9999 7951	.9999 7277	.9999 6509	.9999 5650	.9999 4699
6.93	.9999 8023	.9999 7372	.9999 6632	.9999 5802	.9999 4885
6.94	.9999 8093	.9999 7464	.9999 6750	.9999 5950	.9999 5064
6.95	.9999 8160	.9999 7554	.9999 6864	.9999 6092	.9999 5237
6.96	.9999 8225	.9999 7640	.9999 6975	.9999 6229	.9999 5404
6.97	.9999 8287	.9999 7723	.9999 7081	.9999 6362	.9999 5566
6.98	.9999 8348	.9999 7804	.9999 7184	.9999 6490	.9999 5722
6.99	.9999 8406	.9999 7881	.9999 7284	.9999 6614	.9999 5873

W	P(W,7)	P(W,8)	P(W,9)	P(W,10)	P(W,11)
7.00	.9999 8463	.9999 7956	.9999 7380	.9999 6734	.9999 6019
7.01	.9999 8518	.9999 8029	.9999 7473	.9999 6850	.9999 6160
7.02	.9999 8570	.9999 8099	.9999 7563	.9999 6961	.9999 6296
7.03	.9999 8621	.9999 8167	.9999 7649	.9999 7069	.9999 6428
7.04	.9999 8670	.9999 8232	.9999 7733	.9999 7174	.9999 6555
7.05	.9999 8718	.9999 8295	.9999 7814	.9999 7274	.9999 6677
7.06	.9999 8764	.9999 8356	.9999 7892	.9999 7371	.9999 6796
7.07	.9999 8808	.9999 8415	.9999 7967	.9999 7465	.9999 6910
7.08	.9999 8851	.9999 8472	.9999 8040	.9999 7556	.9999 7020
7.09	.9999 8892	.9999 8526	.9999 8110	.9999 7644	.9999 7127
7.10	.9999 8932	.9999 8579	.9999 8178	.9999 7728	.9999 7230
7.11	.9999 8970	.9999 8630	.9999 8243	.9999 7810	.9999 7329
7.12	.9999 9007	.9999 8680	.9999 8307	.9999 7888	.9999 7425
7.13	.9999 9043	.9999 8727	.9999 8368	.9999 7965	.9999 7518
7.14	.9999 9078	.9999 8773	.9999 8427	.9999 8038	.9999 7607
7.15	.9999 9111	.9999 8818	.9999 8484	.9999 8109	.9999 7694
7.16	.9999 9143	.9999 8861	.9999 8538	.9999 8177	.9999 7777
7.17	.9999 9174	.9999 8902	.9999 8591	.9999 8243	.9999 7857
7.18	.9999 9204	.9999 8942	.9999 8642	.9999 8307	.9999 7935
7.19	.9999 9233	.9999 8980	.9999 8692	.9999 8368	.9999 8010
7.20	.9999 9261	.9999 9017	.9999 8739	.9999 8428	.9999 8082
7.21	.9999 9288	.9999 9053	.9999 8785	.9999 8485	.9999 8152
7.22	.9999 9314	.9999 9088	.9999 8830	.9999 8540	.9999 8219
7.23	.9999 9339	.9999 9121	.9999 8872	.9999 8593	.9999 8284
7.24	.9999 9364	.9999 9153	.9999 8914	.9999 8645	.9999 8347
7.25	.9999 9387	.9999 9184	.9999 8953	.9999 8694	.9999 8408
7.26	.9999 9409	.9999 9214	.9999 8992	.9999 8742	.9999 8466
7.27	.9999 9431	.9999 9243	.9999 9029	.9999 8788	.9999 8522
7.28	.9999 9452	.9999 9271	.9999 9065	.9999 8833	.9999 8576
7.29	.9999 9472	.9999 9298	.9999 9099	.9999 8876	.9999 8629
7.30	.9999 9492	.9999 9324	.9999 9132	.9999 8917	.9999 8679
7.31	.9999 9511	.9999 9349	.9999 9164	.9999 8957	.9999 8728
7.32	.9999 9529	.9999 9373	.9999 9195	.9999 8996	.9999 8775
7.33	.9999 9546	.9999 9396	.9999 9225	.9999 9033	.9999 8820
7.34	.9999 9563	.9999 9418	.9999 9254	.9999 9069	.9999 8864
7.35	.9999 9579	.9999 9440	.9999 9281	.9999 9103	.9999 8906
7.36	.9999 9595	.9999 9461	.9999 9308	.9999 9137	.9999 8947
7.37	.9999 9610	.9999 9481	.9999 9334	.9999 9169	.9999 8986
7.38	.9999 9625	.9999 9500	.9999 9359	.9999 9200	.9999 9024
7.39	.9999 9639	.9999 9519	.9999 9383	.9999 9230	.9999 9060
7.40	.9999 9652	.9999 9537	.9999 9406	.9999 9258	.9999 9095
7.41	.9999 9665	.9999 9554	.9999 9428	.9999 9286	.9999 9129
7.42	.9999 9678	.9999 9571	.9999 9449	.9999 9313	.9999 9161
7.43	.9999 9690	.9999 9587	.9999 9470	.9999 9339	.9999 9193
7.44	.9999 9701	.9999 9603	.9999 9490	.9999 9363	.9999 9223
7.45	.9999 9713	.9999 9618	.9999 9509	.9999 9387	.9999 9252
7.46	.9999 9724	.9999 9632	.9999 9528	.9999 9410	.9999 9280
7.47	.9999 9734	.9999 9646	.9999 9545	.9999 9433	.9999 9308
7.48	.9999 9744	.9999 9659	.9999 9563	.9999 9454	.9999 9334
7.49	.9999 9754	.9999 9672	.9999 9579	.9999 9475	.9999 9359

W	P(W,7)	P(W,8)	P(W,9)	P(W,10)	P(W,11)
7.50	.9999 9763	.9999 9685	.9999 9595	.9999 9494	.9999 9383
7.51	.9999 9772	.9999 9696	.9999 9610	.9999 9514	.9999 9406
7.52	.9999 9781	.9999 9708	.9999 9625	.9999 9532	.9999 9429
7.53	.9999 9789	.9999 9719	.9999 9639	.9999 9550	.9999 9451
7.54	.9999 9797	.9999 9730	.9999 9653	.9999 9567	.9999 9471
7.55	.9999 9805	.9999 9740	.9999 9666	.9999 9583	.9999 9492
7.56	.9999 9812	.9999 9750	.9999 9679	.9999 9599	.9999 9511
7.57	.9999 9819	.9999 9760	.9999 9691	.9999 9615	.9999 9530
7.58	.9999 9826	.9999 9769	.9999 9703	.9999 9629	.9999 9548
7.59	.9999 9833	.9999 9778	.9999 9714	.9999 9644	.9999 9565
7.60	.9999 9839	.9999 9786	.9999 9725	.9999 9657	.9999 9582
7.61	.9999 9846	.9999 9794	.9999 9736	.9999 9670	.9999 9598
7.62	.9999 9851	.9999 9802	.9999 9746	.9999 9683	.9999 9613
7.63	.9999 9857	.9999 9810	.9999 9756	.9999 9695	.9999 9628
7.64	.9999 9863	.9999 9817	.9999 9765	.9999 9707	.9999 9642
7.65	.9999 9868	.9999 9824	.9999 9774	.9999 9718	.9999 9656
7.66	.9999 9873	.9999 9831	.9999 9783	.9999 9729	.9999 9669
7.67	.9999 9878	.9999 9838	.9999 9791	.9999 9740	.9999 9682
7.68	.9999 9883	.9999 9844	.9999 9799	.9999 9750	.9999 9694
7.69	.9999 9887	.9999 9850	.9999 9807	.9999 9759	.9999 9706
7.70	.9999 9892	.9999 9856	.9999 9815	.9999 9769	.9999 9718
7.71	.9999 9896	.9999 9861	.9999 9822	.9999 9778	.9999 9729
7.72	.9999 9900	.9999 9867	.9999 9829	.9999 9786	.9999 9739
7.73	.9999 9904	.9999 9872	.9999 9836	.9999 9795	.9999 9749
7.74	.9999 9908	.9999 9877	.9999 9842	.9999 9803	.9999 9759
7.75	.9999 9911	.9999 9882	.9999 9848	.9999 9810	.9999 9768
7.76	.9999 9915	.9999 9886	.9999 9854	.9999 9818	.9999 9777
7.77	.9999 9918	.9999 9891	.9999 9860	.9999 9825	.9999 9786
7.78	.9999 9921	.9999 9895	.9999 9865	.9999 9832	.9999 9795
7.79	.9999 9924	.9999 9899	.9999 9871	.9999 9838	.9999 9803
7.80	.9999 9927	.9999 9903	.9999 9876	.9999 9845	.9999 9810
7.81	.9999 9930	.9999 9907	.9999 9881	.9999 9851	.9999 9818
7.82	.9999 9933	.9999 9911	.9999 9885	.9999 9857	.9999 9825
7.83	.9999 9936	.9999 9914	.9999 9890	.9999 9862	.9999 9832
7.84	.9999 9938	.9999 9918	.9999 9894	.9999 9868	.9999 9839
7.85	.9999 9941	.9999 9921	.9999 9898	.9999 9873	.9999 9845
7.86	.9999 9943	.9999 9924	.9999 9902	.9999 9878	.9999 9851
7.87	.9999 9945	.9999 9927	.9999 9906	.9999 9883	.9999 9857
7.88	.9999 9947	.9999 9930	.9999 9910	.9999 9887	.9999 9863
7.89	.9999 9949	.9999 9933	.9999 9913	.9999 9892	.9999 9868
7.90	.9999 9951	.9999 9935	.9999 9917	.9999 9896	.9999 9873
7.91	.9999 9953	.9999 9938	.9999 9920	.9999 9900	.9999 9878
7.92	.9999 9955	.9999 9940	.9999 9923	.9999 9904	.9999 9883
7.93	.9999 9957	.9999 9943	.9999 9926	.9999 9908	.9999 9888
7.94	.9999 9959	.9999 9945	.9999 9929	.9999 9912	.9999 9892
7.95	.9999 9960	.9999 9947	.9999 9932	.9999 9915	.9999 9897
7.96	.9999 9962	.9999 9949	.9999 9935	.9999 9919	.9999 9901
7.97	.9999 9963	.9999 9951	.9999 9938	.9999 9922	.9999 9905
7.98	.9999 9965	.9999 9953	.9999 9940	.9999 9925	.9999 9909
7.99	.9999 9966	.9999 9955	.9999 9942	.9999 9928	.9999 9912

W	P(W,7)	P(W,8)	P(W,9)	P(W,10)	P(W,11)
8.00	.9999 9968	.9999 9957	.9999 9945	.9999 9931	.9999 9916
8.01	.9999 9969	.9999 9959	.9999 9947	.9999 9934	.9999 9919
8.02	.9999 9970	.9999 9960	.9999 9949	.9999 9936	.9999 9922
8.03	.9999 9971	.9999 9962	.9999 9951	.9999 9939	.9999 9926
8.04	.9999 9973	.9999 9964	.9999 9953	.9999 9941	.9999 9929
8.05	.9999 9974	.9999 9965	.9999 9955	.9999 9944	.9999 9931
8.06	.9999 9975	.9999 9966	.9999 9957	.9999 9946	.9999 9934
8.07	.9999 9976	.9999 9968	.9999 9959	.9999 9948	.9999 9937
8.08	.9999 9977	.9999 9969	.9999 9960	.9999 9950	.9999 9939
8.09	.9999 9978	.9999 9970	.9999 9962	.9999 9952	.9999 9942
8.10	.9999 9979	.9999 9972	.9999 9963	.9999 9954	.9999 9944
8.11	.9999 9980	.9999 9973	.9999 9965	.9999 9956	.9999 9947
8.12	.9999 9980	.9999 9974	.9999 9966	.9999 9958	.9999 9949
8.13	.9999 9981	.9999 9975	.9999 9968	.9999 9960	.9999 9951
8.14	.9999 9982	.9999 9976	.9999 9969	.9999 9961	.9999 9953
8.15	.9999 9983	.9999 9977	.9999 9970	.9999 9963	.9999 9955
8.16	.9999 9983	.9999 9978	.9999 9972	.9999 9964	.9999 9957
8.17	.9999 9984	.9999 9979	.9999 9973	.9999 9966	.9999 9958
8.18	.9999 9985	.9999 9980	.9999 9974	.9999 9967	.9999 9960
8.19	.9999 9985	.9999 9980	.9999 9975	.9999 9969	.9999 9962
8.20	.9999 9986	.9999 9981	.9999 9976	.9999 9970	.9999 9963
8.21	.9999 9987	.9999 9982	.9999 9977	.9999 9971	.9999 9965
8.22	.9999 9987	.9999 9983	.9999 9978	.9999 9972	.9999 9966
8.23	.9999 9988	.9999 9984	.9999 9979	.9999 9974	.9999 9968
8.24	.9999 9988	.9999 9984	.9999 9980	.9999 9975	.9999 9969
8.25	.9999 9989	.9999 9985	.9999 9981	.9999 9976	.9999 9970
8.26	.9999 9989	.9999 9985	.9999 9981	.9999 9977	.9999 9972
8.27	.9999 9990	.9999 9986	.9999 9982	.9999 9978	.9999 9973
8.28	.9999 9990	.9999 9987	.9999 9983	.9999 9979	.9999 9974
8.29	.9999 9990	.9999 9987	.9999 9984	.9999 9979	.9999 9975
8.30	.9999 9991	.9999 9988	.9999 9984	.9999 9980	.9999 9976
8.31	.9999 9991	.9999 9988	.9999 9985	.9999 9981	.9999 9977
8.32	.9999 9992	.9999 9989	.9999 9986	.9999 9982	.9999 9978
8.33	.9999 9992	.9999 9989	.9999 9986	.9999 9983	.9999 9979
8.34	.9999 9992	.9999 9990	.9999 9987	.9999 9983	.9999 9980
8.35	.9999 9993	.9999 9990	.9999 9987	.9999 9984	.9999 9981
8.36	.9999 9993	.9999 9990	.9999 9988	.9999 9985	.9999 9981
8.37	.9999 9993	.9999 9991	.9999 9988	.9999 9985	.9999 9982
8.38	.9999 9993	.9999 9991	.9999 9989	.9999 9986	.9999 9983
8.39	.9999 9994	.9999 9992	.9999 9989	.9999 9987	.9999 9984
8.40	.9999 9994	.9999 9992	.9999 9990	.9999 9987	.9999 9984
8.41	.9999 9994	.9999 9992	.9999 9990	.9999 9988	.9999 9985
8.42	.9999 9994	.9999 9993	.9999 9991	.9999 9988	.9999 9986
8.43	.9999 9995	.9999 9993	.9999 9991	.9999 9989	.9999 9986
8.44	.9999 9995	.9999 9993	.9999 9991	.9999 9989	.9999 9987
8.45	.9999 9995	.9999 9994	.9999 9992	.9999 9990	.9999 9987
8.46	.9999 9995	.9999 9994	.9999 9992	.9999 9990	.9999 9988
8.47	.9999 9996	.9999 9994	.9999 9992	.9999 9990	.9999 9988
8.48	.9999 9996	.9999 9994	.9999 9993	.9999 9991	.9999 9989
8.49	.9999 9996	.9999 9995	.9999 9993	.9999 9991	.9999 9989

W	P(W,7)	P(W,8)	P(W,9)	P(W,10)	P(W,11)
8.50	.9999 9996	.9999 9995	.9999 9993	.9999 9992	.9999 9990
8.51	.9999 9996	.9999 9995	.9999 9994	.9999 9992	.9999 9990
8.52	.9999 9996	.9999 9995	.9999 9994	.9999 9992	.9999 9991
8.53	.9999 9997	.9999 9995	.9999 9994	.9999 9993	.9999 9991
8.54	.9999 9997	.9999 9996	.9999 9994	.9999 9993	.9999 9991
8.55	.9999 9997	.9999 9996	.9999 9995	.9999 9993	.9999 9992
8.56	.9999 9997	.9999 9996	.9999 9995	.9999 9994	.9999 9992
8.57	.9999 9997	.9999 9996	.9999 9995	.9999 9994	.9999 9992
8.58	.9999 9997	.9999 9996	.9999 9995	.9999 9994	.9999 9993
8.59	.9999 9997	.9999 9996	.9999 9995	.9999 9994	.9999 9993
8.60	.9999 9997	.9999 9997	.9999 9996	.9999 9995	.9999 9993
8.61	.9999 9998	.9999 9997	.9999 9996	.9999 9995	.9999 9994
8.62	.9999 9998	.9999 9997	.9999 9996	.9999 9995	.9999 9994
8.63	.9999 9998	.9999 9997	.9999 9996	.9999 9995	.9999 9994
8.64	.9999 9998	.9999 9997	.9999 9996	.9999 9995	.9999 9994
8.65	.9999 9998	.9999 9997	.9999 9997	.9999 9996	.9999 9995
8.66	.9999 9998	.9999 9997	.9999 9997	.9999 9996	.9999 9995
8.67	.9999 9998	.9999 9998	.9999 9997	.9999 9996	.9999 9995
8.68	.9999 9998	.9999 9998	.9999 9997	.9999 9996	.9999 9995
8.69	.9999 9998	.9999 9998	.9999 9997	.9999 9996	.9999 9996
8.70	.9999 9998	.9999 9998	.9999 9997	.9999 9997	.9999 9996
8.71	.9999 9998	.9999 9998	.9999 9997	.9999 9997	.9999 9996
8.72	.9999 9998	.9999 9998	.9999 9997	.9999 9997	.9999 9996
8.73	.9999 9999	.9999 9998	.9999 9998	.9999 9997	.9999 9996
8.74	.9999 9999	.9999 9998	.9999 9998	.9999 9997	.9999 9996
8.75	.9999 9999	.9999 9998	.9999 9998	.9999 9997	.9999 9997
8.76	.9999 9999	.9999 9998	.9999 9998	.9999 9997	.9999 9997
8.77	.9999 9999	.9999 9998	.9999 9998	.9999 9997	.9999 9997
8.78	.9999 9999	.9999 9998	.9999 9998	.9999 9998	.9999 9997
8.79	.9999 9999	.9999 9999	.9999 9998	.9999 9998	.9999 9997
8.80	.9999 9999	.9999 9999	.9999 9998	.9999 9998	.9999 9997
8.81	.9999 9999	.9999 9999	.9999 9998	.9999 9998	.9999 9997
8.82	.9999 9999	.9999 9999	.9999 9998	.9999 9998	.9999 9997
8.83	.9999 9999	.9999 9999	.9999 9998	.9999 9998	.9999 9998
8.84	.9999 9999	.9999 9999	.9999 9998	.9999 9998	.9999 9998
8.85	.9999 9999	.9999 9999	.9999 9999	.9999 9998	.9999 9998
8.86	.9999 9999	.9999 9999	.9999 9999	.9999 9998	.9999 9998
8.87	.9999 9999	.9999 9999	.9999 9999	.9999 9998	.9999 9998
8.88	.9999 9999	.9999 9999	.9999 9999	.9999 9998	.9999 9998
8.89	.9999 9999	.9999 9999	.9999 9999	.9999 9999	.9999 9998
8.90	.9999 9999	.9999 9999	.9999 9999	.9999 9999	.9999 9998
8.91	.9999 9999	.9999 9999	.9999 9999	.9999 9999	.9999 9998
8.92	.9999 9999	.9999 9999	.9999 9999	.9999 9999	.9999 9998
8.93	.9999 9999	.9999 9999	.9999 9999	.9999 9999	.9999 9998
8.94	.9999 9999	.9999 9999	.9999 9999	.9999 9999	.9999 9999
8.95	.9999 9999	.9999 9999	.9999 9999	.9999 9999	.9999 9999
8.96	.9999 9999	.9999 9999	.9999 9999	.9999 9999	.9999 9999
8.97	.9999 9999	.9999 9999	.9999 9999	.9999 9999	.9999 9999
8.98	1.0000 0000	.9999 9999	.9999 9999	.9999 9999	.9999 9999
8.99		.9999 9999	.9999 9999	.9999 9999	.9999 9999

W	P(W,7)	P(W,8)	P(W,9)	P(W,10)	P(W,11)
9.00		.9999 9999	.9999 9999	.9999 9999	.9999 9999
9.01		.9999 9999	.9999 9999	.9999 9999	.9999 9999
9.02		.9999 9999	.9999 9999	.9999 9999	.9999 9999
9.03		.9999 9999	.9999 9999	.9999 9999	.9999 9999
9.04		1.0000 0000	.9999 9999	.9999 9999	.9999 9999
9.05			.9999 9999	.9999 9999	.9999 9999
9.06			.9999 9999	.9999 9999	.9999 9999
9.07			.9999 9999	.9999 9999	.9999 9999
9.08			.9999 9999	.9999 9999	.9999 9999
9.09			.9999 9999	.9999 9999	.9999 9999
9.10			1.0000 0000	.9999 9999	.9999 9999
9.11				.9999 9999	.9999 9999
9.12				.9999 9999	.9999 9999
9.13				.9999 9999	.9999 9999
9.14				.9999 9999	.9999 9999
9.15				1.0000 0000	.9999 9999
9.16					.9999 9999
9.17					.9999 9999
9.18					.9999 9999
9.19					1.0000 0000
9.20					
9.21					
9.22					
9.23					
9.24					
9.25					
9.26					
9.27					
9.28					
9.29					
9.30					
9.31					
9.32					
9.33					
9.34					
9.35					
9.36					
9.37					
9.38					
9.39					
9.40					
9.41					
9.42					
9.43					
9.44					
9.45					
9.46					
9.47					
9.48					
9.49					

W	P(W,7)	P(W,8)	P(W,9)	P(W,10)	P(W,11)
9.50					
9.51					
9.52					
9.53					
9.54					
9.55					
9.56					
9.57					
9.58					
9.59					
9.60					
9.61					
9.62					
9.63					
9.64					
9.65					
9.66					
9.67					
9.68					
9.69					
9.70					
9.71					
9.72					
9.73					
9.74					
9.75					
9.76					
9.77					
9.78					
9.79					
9.80					
9.81					
9.82					
9.83					
9.84					
9.85					
9.86					
9.87					
9.88					
9.89					
9.90					
9.91					
9.92					
9.93					
9.94					
9.95					
9.96					
9.97					
9.98					
9.99					

W	P(W,12)	P(W,13)	P(W,14)	P(W,15)	P(W,16)
0.00					
0.01					
0.02					
0.03					
0.04					
0.05					
0.06					
0.07					
0.08					
0.09					
0.10					
0.11					
0.12					
0.13					
0.14					
0.15					
0.16					
0.17					
0.18					
0.19					
0.20					
0.21					
0.22					
0.23					
0.24					
0.25					
0.26					
0.27					
0.28					
0.29					
0.30					
0.31					
0.32					
0.33					
0.34					
0.35					
0.36					
0.37					
0.38					
0.39	.0000 0000				
0.40	.0000 0001				
0.41	.0000 0001				
0.42	.0000 0001				
0.43	.0000 0001				
0.44	.0000 0002				
0.45	.0000 0002				
0.46	.0000 0002	.0000 0000			
0.47	.0000 0003	.0000 0001			
0.48	.0000 0004	.0000 0001			
0.49	.0000 0005	.0000 0001			

W	P(W,12)	P(W,13)	P(W,14)	P(W,15)	P(W,16)
0.50	.0000 0006	.0000 0001			
0.51	.0000 0007	.0000 0002			
0.52	.0000 0009	.0000 0002	.0000 0000		
0.53	.0000 0011	.0000 0002	.0000 0001		
0.54	.0000 0014	.0000 0003	.0000 0001		
0.55	.0000 0017	.0000 0004	.0000 0001		
0.56	.0000 0020	.0000 0005	.0000 0001		
0.57	.0000 0024	.0000 0006	.0000 0001		
0.58	.0000 0029	.0000 0007	.0000 0002		
0.59	.0000 0035	.0000 0009	.0000 0002	.0000 0000	
0.60	.0000 0042	.0000 0010	.0000 0003	.0000 0001	
0.61	.0000 0050	.0000 0013	.0000 0003	.0000 0001	
0.62	.0000 0060	.0000 0015	.0000 0004	.0000 0001	
0.63	.0000 0071	.0000 0018	.0000 0005	.0000 0001	
0.64	.0000 0084	.0000 0022	.0000 0006	.0000 0001	
0.65	.0000 0099	.0000 0026	.0000 0007	.0000 0002	.0000 0000
0.66	.0000 0116	.0000 0031	.0000 0008	.0000 0002	.0000 0001
0.67	.0000 0136	.0000 0037	.0000 0010	.0000 0003	.0000 0001
0.68	.0000 0159	.0000 0044	.0000 0012	.0000 0003	.0000 0001
0.69	.0000 0185	.0000 0052	.0000 0015	.0000 0004	.0000 0001
0.70	.0000 0215	.0000 0061	.0000 0017	.0000 0005	.0000 0001
0.71	.0000 0250	.0000 0072	.0000 0021	.0000 0006	.0000 0002
0.72	.0000 0289	.0000 0085	.0000 0025	.0000 0007	.0000 0002
0.73	.0000 0334	.0000 0099	.0000 0029	.0000 0009	.0000 0003
0.74	.0000 0385	.0000 0116	.0000 0035	.0000 0010	.0000 0003
0.75	.0000 0442	.0000 0135	.0000 0041	.0000 0012	.0000 0004
0.76	.0000 0508	.0000 0156	.0000 0048	.0000 0015	.0000 0004
0.77	.0000 0582	.0000 0181	.0000 0056	.0000 0017	.0000 0005
0.78	.0000 0665	.0000 0210	.0000 0066	.0000 0021	.0000 0006
0.79	.0000 0759	.0000 0242	.0000 0077	.0000 0025	.0000 0008
0.80	.0000 0864	.0000 0279	.0000 0090	.0000 0029	.0000 0009
0.81	.0000 0982	.0000 0321	.0000 0105	.0000 0034	.0000 0011
0.82	.0000 1114	.0000 0369	.0000 0122	.0000 0040	.0000 0013
0.83	.0000 1262	.0000 0423	.0000 0141	.0000 0047	.0000 0016
0.84	.0000 1428	.0000 0484	.0000 0163	.0000 0055	.0000 0018
0.85	.0000 1612	.0000 0552	.0000 0189	.0000 0064	.0000 0022
0.86	.0000 1817	.0000 0629	.0000 0217	.0000 0075	.0000 0026
0.87	.0000 2045	.0000 0716	.0000 0250	.0000 0087	.0000 0030
0.88	.0000 2298	.0000 0813	.0000 0287	.0000 0101	.0000 0035
0.89	.0000 2578	.0000 0922	.0000 0329	.0000 0117	.0000 0041
0.90	.0000 2888	.0000 1043	.0000 0376	.0000 0135	.0000 0048
0.91	.0000 3231	.0000 1179	.0000 0429	.0000 0156	.0000 0056
0.92	.0000 3609	.0000 1331	.0000 0489	.0000 0179	.0000 0066
0.93	.0000 4026	.0000 1500	.0000 0557	.0000 0206	.0000 0076
0.94	.0000 4484	.0000 1687	.0000 0633	.0000 0237	.0000 0088
0.95	.0000 4989	.0000 1895	.0000 0718	.0000 0271	.0000 0102
0.96	.0000 5542	.0000 2126	.0000 0813	.0000 0310	.0000 0118
0.97	.0000 6150	.0000 2382	.0000 0920	.0000 0354	.0000 0136
0.98	.0000 6815	.0000 2665	.0000 1039	.0000 0404	.0000 0157
0.99	.0000 7543	.0000 2977	.0000 1171	.0000 0460	.0000 0180

W	P(W,12)	P(W,13)	P(W,14)	P(W,15)	P(W,16)
1.00	.0000 8338	.0000 3321	.0000 1319	.0000 0523	.0000 0207
1.01	.0000 9206	.0000 3701	.0000 1483	.0000 0593	.0000 0237
1.02	.0001 0153	.0000 4118	.0000 1666	.0000 0672	.0000 0271
1.03	.0001 1184	.0000 4577	.0000 1868	.0000 0760	.0000 0309
1.04	.0001 2306	.0000 5081	.0000 2092	.0000 0859	.0000 0352
1.05	.0001 3525	.0000 5633	.0000 2339	.0000 0969	.0000 0401
1.06	.0001 4849	.0000 6238	.0000 2613	.0000 1092	.0000 0455
1.07	.0001 6285	.0000 6900	.0000 2915	.0000 1229	.0000 0517
1.08	.0001 7841	.0000 7623	.0000 3248	.0000 1380	.0000 0585
1.09	.0001 9525	.0000 8413	.0000 3614	.0000 1549	.0000 0662
1.10	.0002 1346	.0000 9273	.0000 4017	.0000 1736	.0000 0748
1.11	.0002 3314	.0001 0211	.0000 4460	.0000 1943	.0000 0845
1.12	.0002 5439	.0001 1232	.0000 4945	.0000 2172	.0000 0952
1.13	.0002 7730	.0001 2342	.0000 5477	.0000 2425	.0000 1071
1.14	.0003 0198	.0001 3547	.0000 6060	.0000 2704	.0000 1204
1.15	.0003 2855	.0001 4854	.0000 6696	.0000 3011	.0000 1351
1.16	.0003 5713	.0001 6271	.0000 7392	.0000 3350	.0000 1515
1.17	.0003 8784	.0001 7806	.0000 8152	.0000 3723	.0000 1696
1.18	.0004 2082	.0001 9467	.0000 8979	.0000 4132	.0000 1897
1.19	.0004 5619	.0002 1262	.0000 9881	.0000 4581	.0000 2119
1.20	.0004 9411	.0002 3200	.0001 0862	.0000 5073	.0000 2364
1.21	.0005 3472	.0002 5291	.0001 1928	.0000 5612	.0000 2635
1.22	.0005 7819	.0002 7546	.0001 3086	.0000 6202	.0000 2933
1.23	.0006 2467	.0002 9975	.0001 4343	.0000 6846	.0000 3261
1.24	.0006 7433	.0003 2589	.0001 5705	.0000 7550	.0000 3622
1.25	.0007 2735	.0003 5399	.0001 7179	.0000 8317	.0000 4018
1.26	.0007 8392	.0003 8418	.0001 8775	.0000 9153	.0000 4452
1.27	.0008 4422	.0004 1660	.0002 0500	.0001 0063	.0000 4929
1.28	.0009 0846	.0004 5137	.0002 2363	.0001 1053	.0000 5451
1.29	.0009 7685	.0004 8863	.0002 4373	.0001 2128	.0000 6022
1.30	.0010 4959	.0005 2854	.0002 6541	.0001 3295	.0000 6646
1.31	.0011 2692	.0005 7125	.0002 8876	.0001 4561	.0000 7327
1.32	.0012 0906	.0006 1692	.0003 1389	.0001 5932	.0000 8070
1.33	.0012 9625	.0006 6571	.0003 4093	.0001 7417	.0000 8879
1.34	.0013 8874	.0007 1781	.0003 6998	.0001 9023	.0000 9760
1.35	.0014 8678	.0007 7339	.0004 0117	.0002 0759	.0001 0719
1.36	.0015 9065	.0008 3265	.0004 3464	.0002 2633	.0001 1761
1.37	.0017 0061	.0008 9578	.0004 7052	.0002 4655	.0001 2892
1.38	.0018 1695	.0009 6299	.0005 0896	.0002 6835	.0001 4118
1.39	.0019 3996	.0010 3450	.0005 5011	.0002 9182	.0001 5448
1.40	.0020 6993	.0011 1052	.0005 9413	.0003 1709	.0001 6887
1.41	.0022 0718	.0011 9128	.0006 4117	.0003 4426	.0001 8445
1.42	.0023 5202	.0012 7702	.0006 9142	.0003 7345	.0002 0129
1.43	.0025 0478	.0013 6799	.0007 4505	.0004 0480	.0002 1947
1.44	.0026 6580	.0014 6445	.0008 0226	.0004 3843	.0002 3910
1.45	.0028 3542	.0015 6666	.0008 6322	.0004 7449	.0002 6026
1.46	.0030 1400	.0016 7489	.0009 2815	.0005 1311	.0002 8306
1.47	.0032 0189	.0017 8942	.0009 9726	.0005 5445	.0003 0761
1.48	.0033 9948	.0019 1054	.0010 7077	.0005 9867	.0003 3402
1.49	.0036 0714	.0020 3856	.0011 4889	.0006 4594	.0003 6240

W	P(W,12)	P(W,13)	P(W,14)	P(W,15)	P(W,16)
1.50	.0038 2527	.0021 7378	.0012 3187	.0006 9643	.0003 9289
1.51	.0040 5426	.0023 1652	.0013 1996	.0007 5031	.0004 2561
1.52	.0042 9453	.0024 6712	.0014 1340	.0008 0779	.0004 6071
1.53	.0045 4648	.0026 2590	.0015 1245	.0008 6905	.0004 9831
1.54	.0048 1056	.0027 9321	.0016 1739	.0009 3431	.0005 3859
1.55	.0050 8719	.0029 6942	.0017 2850	.0010 0376	.0005 8168
1.56	.0053 7682	.0031 5488	.0018 4606	.0010 7764	.0006 2776
1.57	.0056 7989	.0033 4998	.0019 7038	.0011 5618	.0006 7701
1.58	.0059 9689	.0035 5509	.0021 0176	.0012 3960	.0007 2959
1.59	.0063 2826	.0037 7061	.0022 4051	.0013 2817	.0007 8570
1.60	.0066 7449	.0039 9694	.0023 8698	.0014 2213	.0008 4552
1.61	.0070 3607	.0042 3450	.0025 4148	.0015 2175	.0009 0928
1.62	.0074 1348	.0044 8371	.0027 0438	.0016 2730	.0009 7717
1.63	.0078 0723	.0047 4500	.0028 7602	.0017 3908	.0010 4942
1.64	.0082 1784	.0050 1882	.0030 5677	.0018 5737	.0011 2625
1.65	.0086 4580	.0053 0561	.0032 4701	.0019 8247	.0012 0790
1.66	.0090 9165	.0056 0582	.0034 4712	.0021 1470	.0012 9463
1.67	.0095 5591	.0059 1994	.0036 5750	.0022 5438	.0013 8668
1.68	.0100 3913	.0062 4843	.0038 7855	.0024 0185	.0014 8433
1.69	.0105 4183	.0065 9179	.0041 1069	.0025 5745	.0015 8783
1.70	.0110 6457	.0069 5050	.0043 5435	.0027 2152	.0016 9749
1.71	.0116 0791	.0073 2506	.0046 0995	.0028 9443	.0018 1359
1.72	.0121 7240	.0077 1599	.0048 7794	.0030 7656	.0019 3644
1.73	.0127 5859	.0081 2381	.0051 5878	.0032 6829	.0020 6635
1.74	.0133 6707	.0085 4904	.0054 5294	.0034 7001	.0022 0365
1.75	.0139 9840	.0089 9221	.0057 6087	.0036 8212	.0023 4866
1.76	.0146 5316	.0094 5386	.0060 8306	.0039 0504	.0025 0174
1.77	.0153 3193	.0099 3454	.0064 2001	.0041 3919	.0026 6323
1.78	.0160 3529	.0104 3481	.0067 7222	.0043 8500	.0028 3351
1.79	.0167 6382	.0109 5522	.0071 4019	.0046 4293	.0030 1295
1.80	.0175 1811	.0114 9633	.0075 2443	.0049 1341	.0032 0193
1.81	.0182 9875	.0120 5873	.0079 2549	.0051 9693	.0034 0085
1.82	.0191 0634	.0126 4299	.0083 4388	.0054 9394	.0036 1011
1.83	.0199 4146	.0132 4969	.0087 8015	.0058 0494	.0038 3015
1.84	.0208 0470	.0138 7941	.0092 3485	.0061 3041	.0040 6137
1.85	.0216 9666	.0145 3275	.0097 0854	.0064 7086	.0043 0423
1.86	.0226 1792	.0152 1030	.0102 0178	.0068 2681	.0045 5916
1.87	.0235 6909	.0159 1267	.0107 1514	.0071 9876	.0048 2664
1.88	.0245 5075	.0166 4044	.0112 4920	.0075 8726	.0051 0712
1.89	.0255 6349	.0173 9423	.0118 0454	.0079 9283	.0054 0110
1.90	.0266 0789	.0181 7465	.0123 8175	.0084 1603	.0057 0905
1.91	.0276 8453	.0189 8229	.0129 8142	.0088 5741	.0060 3148
1.92	.0287 9401	.0198 1777	.0136 0416	.0093 1754	.0063 6890
1.93	.0299 3688	.0206 8171	.0142 5058	.0097 9699	.0067 2183
1.94	.0311 1374	.0215 7471	.0149 2127	.0102 9633	.0070 9079
1.95	.0323 2513	.0224 9738	.0156 1685	.0108 1614	.0074 7634
1.96	.0335 7163	.0234 5033	.0163 3795	.0113 5704	.0078 7900
1.97	.0348 5379	.0244 3418	.0170 8518	.0119 1960	.0082 9935
1.98	.0361 7216	.0254 4952	.0178 5915	.0125 0444	.0087 3794
1.99	.0375 2728	.0264 9697	.0186 6051	.0131 1217	.0091 9535

W	P(W,12)	P(W,13)	P(W,14)	P(W,15)	P(W,16)
2.00	.0389 1969	.0275 7713	.0194 8987	.0137 4340	.0096 7216
2.01	.0403 4992	.0286 9060	.0203 4786	.0143 9876	.0101 6896
2.02	.0418 1849	.0298 3798	.0212 3512	.0150 7887	.0106 8635
2.03	.0433 2591	.0310 1985	.0221 5226	.0157 8436	.0112 2494
2.04	.0448 7268	.0322 3682	.0230 9993	.0165 1587	.0117 8533
2.05	.0464 5929	.0334 8944	.0240 7874	.0172 7403	.0123 6814
2.06	.0480 8623	.0347 7832	.0250 8933	.0180 5948	.0129 7401
2.07	.0497 5396	.0361 0401	.0261 3233	.0188 7288	.0136 0355
2.08	.0514 6295	.0374 6708	.0272 0834	.0197 1485	.0142 5740
2.09	.0532 1364	.0388 6809	.0283 1800	.0205 8605	.0149 3621
2.10	.0550 0648	.0403 0759	.0294 6193	.0214 8713	.0156 4062
2.11	.0568 4187	.0417 8611	.0306 4073	.0224 1872	.0163 7128
2.12	.0587 2024	.0433 0418	.0318 5501	.0233 8149	.0171 2884
2.13	.0606 4198	.0448 6234	.0331 0538	.0243 7607	.0179 1396
2.14	.0626 0747	.0464 6109	.0343 9244	.0254 0310	.0187 2730
2.15	.0646 1709	.0481 0092	.0357 1678	.0264 6325	.0195 6952
2.16	.0666 7117	.0497 8235	.0370 7898	.0275 5713	.0204 4128
2.17	.0687 7006	.0515 0583	.0384 7962	.0286 8540	.0213 4324
2.18	.0709 1409	.0532 7183	.0399 1927	.0298 4869	.0222 7608
2.19	.0731 0356	.0550 8082	.0413 9849	.0310 4762	.0232 4045
2.20	.0753 3876	.0569 3324	.0429 1784	.0322 8282	.0242 3702
2.21	.0776 1996	.0588 2950	.0444 7786	.0335 5492	.0252 6645
2.22	.0799 4741	.0607 7002	.0460 7908	.0348 6453	.0263 2941
2.23	.0823 2136	.0627 5520	.0477 2202	.0362 1225	.0274 2655
2.24	.0847 4203	.0647 8543	.0494 0720	.0375 9869	.0285 5853
2.25	.0872 0961	.0668 6107	.0511 3511	.0390 2444	.0297 2601
2.26	.0897 2429	.0689 8248	.0529 0624	.0404 9009	.0309 2962
2.27	.0922 8625	.0711 4998	.0547 2106	.0419 9621	.0321 7002
2.28	.0948 9561	.0733 6391	.0565 8004	.0435 4336	.0334 4785
2.29	.0975 5251	.0756 2456	.0584 8362	.0451 3212	.0347 6373
2.30	.1002 5705	.0779 3221	.0604 3224	.0467 6301	.0361 1830
2.31	.1030 0933	.0802 8714	.0624 2630	.0484 3658	.0375 1217
2.32	.1058 0941	.0826 8959	.0644 6622	.0501 5335	.0389 4595
2.33	.1086 5734	.0851 3979	.0665 5237	.0519 1384	.0404 2026
2.34	.1115 5314	.0876 3795	.0686 8514	.0537 1853	.0419 3567
2.35	.1144 9682	.0901 8426	.0708 6486	.0555 6791	.0434 9279
2.36	.1174 8836	.0927 7890	.0730 9188	.0574 6246	.0450 9217
2.37	.1205 2774	.0954 2201	.0753 6651	.0594 0262	.0467 3439
2.38	.1236 1490	.0981 1373	.0776 8905	.0613 8884	.0484 1999
2.39	.1267 4976	.1008 5417	.0800 5978	.0634 2155	.0501 4952
2.40	.1299 3222	.1036 4342	.0824 7897	.0655 0115	.0519 2350
2.41	.1331 6216	.1064 8155	.0849 4685	.0676 2803	.0537 4245
2.42	.1364 3945	.1093 6861	.0874 6365	.0698 0256	.0556 0686
2.43	.1397 6393	.1123 0462	.0900 2958	.0720 2512	.0575 1722
2.44	.1431 3540	.1152 8959	.0926 4480	.0742 9602	.0594 7400
2.45	.1465 5368	.1183 2351	.0953 0949	.0766 1559	.0614 7765
2.46	.1500 1853	.1214 0634	.0980 2379	.0789 8414	.0635 2862
2.47	.1535 2972	.1245 3801	.1007 8781	.0814 0195	.0656 2732
2.48	.1570 8697	.1277 1845	.1036 0165	.0838 6927	.0677 7415
2.49	.1606 9000	.1309 4755	.1064 6539	.0863 8634	.0699 6951

W	P(W,12)	P(W,13)	P(W,14)	P(W,15)	P(W,16)
2.50	.1643 3851	.1342 2520	.1093 7908	.0889 5339	.0722 1376
2.51	.1680 3216	.1375 5123	.1123 4276	.0915 7062	.0745 0724
2.52	.1717 7062	.1409 2549	.1153 5642	.0942 3820	.0768 5029
2.53	.1755 5350	.1443 4778	.1184 2007	.0969 5630	.0792 4322
2.54	.1793 8042	.1478 1788	.1215 3366	.0997 2503	.0816 8632
2.55	.1832 5098	.1513 3557	.1246 9713	.1025 4453	.0841 7985
2.56	.1871 6474	.1549 0058	.1279 1041	.1054 1486	.0867 2406
2.57	.1911 2127	.1585 1263	.1311 7338	.1083 3612	.0893 1918
2.58	.1951 2008	.1621 7143	.1344 8592	.1113 0832	.0919 6542
2.59	.1991 6071	.1658 7665	.1378 4789	.1143 3150	.0946 6294
2.60	.2032 4264	.1696 2794	.1412 5910	.1174 0566	.0974 1192
2.61	.2073 6534	.1734 2494	.1447 1936	.1205 3076	.1002 1249
2.62	.2115 2829	.1772 6727	.1482 2844	.1237 0676	.1030 6477
2.63	.2157 3092	.1811 5451	.1517 8612	.1269 3358	.1059 6883
2.64	.2199 7266	.1850 8623	.1553 9211	.1302 1112	.1089 2476
2.65	.2242 5291	.1890 6199	.1590 4613	.1335 3926	.1119 3259
2.66	.2285 7106	.1930 8132	.1627 4787	.1369 1786	.1149 9233
2.67	.2329 2648	.1971 4372	.1664 9700	.1403 4674	.1181 0399
2.68	.2373 1854	.2012 4869	.1702 9315	.1438 2571	.1212 6753
2.69	.2417 4658	.2053 9570	.1741 3595	.1473 5456	.1244 8290
2.70	.2462 0992	.2095 8420	.1780 2500	.1509 3303	.1277 5001
2.71	.2507 0787	.2138 1361	.1819 5987	.1545 6087	.1310 6876
2.72	.2552 3973	.2180 8336	.1859 4012	.1582 3778	.1344 3903
2.73	.2598 0478	.2223 9284	.1899 6527	.1619 6345	.1378 6064
2.74	.2644 0230	.2267 4143	.1940 3485	.1657 3754	.1413 3344
2.75	.2690 3154	.2311 2848	.1981 4835	.1695 5969	.1448 5720
2.76	.2736 9173	.2355 5335	.2023 0523	.1734 2951	.1484 3171
2.77	.2783 8213	.2400 1535	.2065 0494	.1773 4660	.1520 5669
2.78	.2831 0193	.2445 1380	.2107 4691	.1813 1053	.1557 3188
2.79	.2878 5036	.2490 4799	.2150 3056	.1853 2084	.1594 5698
2.80	.2926 2660	.2536 1720	.2193 5527	.1893 7705	.1632 3164
2.81	.2974 2985	.2582 2070	.2237 2042	.1934 7867	.1670 5551
2.82	.3022 5928	.2628 5773	.2281 2535	.1976 2518	.1709 2822
2.83	.3071 1405	.2675 2752	.2325 6940	.2018 1603	.1748 4937
2.84	.3119 9334	.2722 2931	.2370 5190	.2060 5066	.1788 1852
2.85	.3168 9628	.2769 6229	.2415 7213	.2103 2849	.1828 3523
2.86	.3218 2201	.2817 2567	.2461 2939	.2146 4891	.1868 9902
2.87	.3267 6969	.2865 1862	.2507 2293	.2190 1130	.1910 0939
2.88	.3317 3842	.2913 4032	.2553 5200	.2234 1501	.1951 6582
2.89	.3367 2733	.2961 8993	.2600 1585	.2278 5937	.1993 6778
2.90	.3417 3554	.3010 6660	.2647 1369	.2323 4371	.2036 1468
2.91	.3467 6216	.3059 6947	.2694 4472	.2368 6732	.2079 0595
2.92	.3518 0628	.3108 9767	.2742 0814	.2414 2947	.2122 4098
2.93	.3568 6702	.3158 5032	.2790 0312	.2460 2943	.2166 1912
2.94	.3619 4347	.3208 2653	.2838 2883	.2506 6645	.2210 3974
2.95	.3670 3473	.3258 2542	.2886 8441	.2553 3975	.2255 0216
2.96	.3721 3987	.3308 4607	.2935 6902	.2600 4854	.2300 0569
2.97	.3772 5799	.3358 8758	.2984 8176	.2647 9203	.2345 4961
2.98	.3823 8818	.3409 4903	.3034 2177	.2695 6938	.2391 3319
2.99	.3875 2953	.3460 2950	.3083 8815	.2743 7976	.2437 5568

W	P(W,12)	P(W,13)	P(W,14)	P(W,15)	P(W,16)
3.00	.3926 8111	.3511 2806	.3133 7999	.2792 2233	.2484 1632
3.01	.3978 4200	.3562 4379	.3183 9639	.2840 9622	.2531 1431
3.02	.4030 1130	.3613 7574	.3234 3642	.2890 0057	.2578 4886
3.03	.4081 8809	.3665 2298	.3284 9915	.2939 3447	.2626 1914
3.04	.4133 7145	.3716 8456	.3335 8366	.2988 9703	.2674 2432
3.05	.4185 6047	.3768 5954	.3386 8898	.3038 8734	.2722 6355
3.06	.4237 5424	.3820 4698	.3438 1418	.3089 0448	.2771 3596
3.07	.4289 5185	.3872 4591	.3489 5830	.3139 4751	.2820 4066
3.08	.4341 5239	.3924 5541	.3541 2037	.3190 1550	.2869 7677
3.09	.4393 5496	.3976 7450	.3592 9944	.3241 0749	.2919 4338
3.10	.4445 5866	.4029 0225	.3644 9453	.3292 2253	.2969 3955
3.11	.4497 6261	.4081 3771	.3697 0467	.3343 5964	.3019 6437
3.12	.4549 6590	.4133 7992	.3749 2889	.3395 1786	.3070 1689
3.13	.4601 6766	.4186 2794	.3801 6620	.3446 9620	.3120 9615
3.14	.4653 6700	.4238 8083	.3854 1563	.3498 9368	.3172 0119
3.15	.4705 6305	.4291 3764	.3906 7619	.3551 0931	.3223 3103
3.16	.4757 5495	.4343 9743	.3959 4690	.3603 4209	.3274 8469
3.17	.4809 4183	.4396 5927	.4012 2679	.3655 9101	.3326 6118
3.18	.4861 2284	.4449 2223	.4065 1486	.3708 5508	.3378 5949
3.19	.4912 9714	.4501 8538	.4118 1014	.3761 3329	.3430 7863
3.20	.4964 6389	.4554 4780	.4171 1165	.3814 2463	.3483 1757
3.21	.5016 2225	.4607 0858	.4224 1842	.3867 2809	.3535 7530
3.22	.5067 7141	.4659 6679	.4277 2946	.3920 4265	.3588 5079
3.23	.5119 1056	.4712 2154	.4330 4380	.3973 6731	.3641 4303
3.24	.5170 3888	.4764 7193	.4383 6049	.4027 0105	.3694 5096
3.25	.5221 5559	.4817 1706	.4436 7855	.4080 4286	.3747 7357
3.26	.5272 5990	.4869 5606	.4489 9702	.4133 9172	.3801 0980
3.27	.5323 5104	.4921 8805	.4543 1496	.4187 4664	.3854 5863
3.28	.5374 2824	.4974 1216	.4596 3141	.4241 0660	.3908 1901
3.29	.5424 9074	.5026 2754	.4649 4542	.4294 7059	.3961 8989
3.30	.5475 3782	.5078 3333	.4702 5607	.4348 3763	.4015 7025
3.31	.5525 6873	.5130 2869	.4755 6243	.4402 0670	.4069 5902
3.32	.5575 8275	.5182 1279	.4808 6356	.4455 7683	.4123 5518
3.33	.5625 7918	.5233 8481	.4861 5857	.4509 4702	.4177 5769
3.34	.5675 5731	.5285 4394	.4914 4653	.4563 1628	.4231 6550
3.35	.5725 1647	.5336 8938	.4967 2656	.4616 8365	.4285 7760
3.36	.5774 5597	.5388 2035	.5019 9776	.4670 4816	.4339 9293
3.37	.5823 7517	.5439 3605	.5072 5926	.4724 0884	.4394 1049
3.38	.5872 7340	.5490 3574	.5125 1019	.4777 6473	.4448 2925
3.39	.5921 5004	.5541 1864	.5177 4968	.4831 1490	.4502 4819
3.40	.5970 0446	.5591 8403	.5229 7689	.4884 5840	.4556 6630
3.41	.6018 3606	.5642 3116	.5281 9098	.4937 9430	.4610 8257
3.42	.6066 4422	.5692 5932	.5333 9112	.4991 2168	.4664 9602
3.43	.6114 2838	.5742 6781	.5385 7649	.5044 3962	.4719 0564
3.44	.6161 8796	.5792 5593	.5437 4630	.5097 4724	.4773 1046
3.45	.6209 2240	.5842 2300	.5488 9975	.5150 4362	.4827 0950
3.46	.6256 3117	.5891 6835	.5540 3606	.5203 2791	.4881 0179
3.47	.6303 1372	.5940 9134	.5591 5446	.5255 9922	.4934 8638
3.48	.6349 6955	.5989 9132	.5642 5419	.5308 5669	.4988 6232
3.49	.6395 9815	.6038 6766	.5693 3452	.5360 9949	.5042 2866

W	P(W,12)	P(W,13)	P(W,14)	P(W,15)	P(W,16)
3.50	.6441 9904	.6087 1976	.5743 9472	.5413 2677	.5095 8450
3.51	.6487 7173	.6135 4702	.5794 3407	.5465 3771	.5149 2889
3.52	.6533 1577	.6183 4884	.5844 5187	.5517 3151	.5202 6095
3.53	.6578 3072	.6231 2467	.5894 4744	.5569 0737	.5255 7977
3.54	.6623 1613	.6278 7394	.5944 2009	.5620 6450	.5308 8448
3.55	.6667 7159	.6325 9612	.5993 6917	.5672 0214	.5361 7420
3.56	.6711 9670	.6372 9067	.6042 9404	.5723 1953	.5414 4808
3.57	.6755 9105	.6419 5708	.6091 9406	.5774 1592	.5467 0527
3.58	.6799 5429	.6465 9486	.6140 6862	.5824 9059	.5519 4494
3.59	.6842 8603	.6512 0353	.6189 1711	.5875 4283	.5571 6627
3.60	.6885 8594	.6557 8260	.6237 3896	.5925 7193	.5623 6846
3.61	.6928 5367	.6603 3164	.6285 3358	.5975 7722	.5675 5071
3.62	.6970 8890	.6648 5019	.6333 0042	.6025 5802	.5727 1226
3.63	.7012 9133	.6693 3784	.6380 3895	.6075 1367	.5778 5234
3.64	.7054 6066	.6737 9417	.6427 4863	.6124 4354	.5829 7020
3.65	.7095 9661	.6782 1878	.6474 2895	.6173 4701	.5880 6511
3.66	.7136 9891	.6826 1131	.6520 7942	.6222 2346	.5931 3636
3.67	.7177 6730	.6869 7137	.6566 9955	.6270 7231	.5981 8324
3.68	.7218 0155	.6912 9861	.6612 8888	.6318 9297	.6032 0506
3.69	.7258 0143	.6955 9271	.6658 4697	.6366 8488	.6082 0117
3.70	.7297 6672	.6998 5332	.6703 7336	.6414 4751	.6131 7090
3.71	.7336 9722	.7040 8016	.6748 6766	.6461 8030	.6181 1361
3.72	.7375 9275	.7082 7291	.6793 2944	.6508 8277	.6230 2869
3.73	.7414 5311	.7124 3130	.6837 5833	.6555 5439	.6279 1552
3.74	.7452 7816	.7165 5507	.6881 5395	.6601 9470	.6327 7352
3.75	.7490 6774	.7206 4395	.6925 1593	.6648 0323	.6376 0212
3.76	.7528 2171	.7246 9772	.6968 4394	.6693 7952	.6424 0074
3.77	.7565 3995	.7287 1614	.7011 3765	.6739 2314	.6471 6887
3.78	.7602 2233	.7326 9900	.7053 9674	.6784 3368	.6519 0596
3.79	.7638 6877	.7366 4611	.7096 2091	.6829 1072	.6566 1152
3.80	.7674 7916	.7405 5728	.7138 0989	.6873 5389	.6612 8506
3.81	.7710 5343	.7444 3234	.7179 6339	.6917 6280	.6659 2608
3.82	.7745 9152	.7482 7114	.7220 8117	.6961 3711	.6705 3415
3.83	.7780 9335	.7520 7352	.7261 6299	.7004 7648	.6751 0882
3.84	.7815 5890	.7558 3935	.7302 0861	.7047 8057	.6796 4966
3.85	.7849 8812	.7595 6852	.7342 1783	.7090 4909	.6841 5626
3.86	.7883 8099	.7632 6091	.7381 9045	.7132 8173	.6886 2824
3.87	.7917 3751	.7669 1644	.7421 2629	.7174 7823	.6930 6521
3.88	.7950 5766	.7705 3502	.7460 2517	.7216 3831	.6974 6682
3.89	.7983 4145	.7741 1658	.7498 8694	.7257 6173	.7018 3273
3.90	.8015 8891	.7776 6106	.7537 1145	.7298 4826	.7061 6260
3.91	.8048 0005	.7811 6842	.7574 9858	.7338 9768	.7104 5612
3.92	.8079 7493	.7846 3861	.7612 4821	.7379 0978	.7147 1301
3.93	.8111 1358	.7880 7162	.7649 6024	.7418 8437	.7189 3298
3.94	.8142 1606	.7914 6743	.7686 3457	.7458 2128	.7231 1576
3.95	.8172 8244	.7948 2604	.7722 7113	.7497 2036	.7272 6112
3.96	.8203 1279	.7981 4746	.7758 6985	.7535 8144	.7313 6881
3.97	.8233 0719	.8014 3171	.7794 3068	.7574 0441	.7354 3863
3.98	.8262 6574	.8046 7881	.7829 5358	.7611 8914	.7394 7036
3.99	.8291 8854	.8078 8882	.7864 3852	.7649 3553	.7434 6382

W	P(W,12)	P(W,13)	P(W,14)	P(W,15)	P(W,16)
4.00	.8320 7570	.8110 6176	.7898 8547	.7686 4348	.7474 1884
4.01	.8349 2732	.8141 9772	.7932 9445	.7723 1291	.7513 3526
4.02	.8377 4354	.8172 9674	.7966 6544	.7759 4377	.7552 1294
4.03	.8405 2449	.8203 5893	.7999 9847	.7795 3599	.7590 5174
4.04	.8432 7030	.8233 8435	.8032 9356	.7830 8954	.7628 5156
4.05	.8459 8113	.8263 7311	.8065 5075	.7866 0438	.7666 1230
4.06	.8486 5712	.8293 2531	.8097 7010	.7900 8051	.7703 3385
4.07	.8512 9844	.8322 4107	.8129 5165	.7935 1791	.7740 1617
4.08	.8539 0525	.8351 2051	.8160 9547	.7969 1660	.7776 5917
4.09	.8564 7773	.8379 6376	.8192 0166	.8002 7659	.7812 6282
4.10	.8590 1605	.8407 7095	.8222 7028	.8035 9791	.7848 2708
4.11	.8615 2040	.8435 4223	.8253 0145	.8068 8061	.7883 5193
4.12	.8639 9097	.8462 7776	.8282 9526	.8101 2473	.7918 3735
4.13	.8664 2796	.8489 7769	.8312 5183	.8133 3034	.7952 8337
4.14	.8688 3157	.8516 4220	.8341 7129	.8164 9752	.7986 8998
4.15	.8712 0200	.8542 7145	.8370 5377	.8196 2634	.8020 5721
4.16	.8735 3948	.8568 6564	.8398 9941	.8227 1690	.8053 8511
4.17	.8758 4421	.8594 2493	.8427 0836	.8257 6930	.8086 7372
4.18	.8781 1642	.8619 4954	.8454 8077	.8287 8366	.8119 2311
4.19	.8803 5633	.8644 3965	.8482 1682	.8317 6009	.8151 3334
4.20	.8825 6418	.8668 9548	.8509 1666	.8346 9872	.8183 0450
4.21	.8847 4021	.8693 1723	.8535 8049	.8375 9970	.8214 3668
4.22	.8868 8464	.8717 0513	.8562 0848	.8404 6318	.8245 2998
4.23	.8889 9772	.8740 5939	.8588 0083	.8432 8930	.8275 8452
4.24	.8910 7971	.8763 8024	.8613 5774	.8460 7823	.8306 0042
4.25	.8931 3084	.8786 6791	.8638 7941	.8488 3015	.8335 7780
4.26	.8951 5138	.8809 2264	.8663 6606	.8515 4524	.8365 1682
4.27	.8971 4158	.8831 4466	.8688 1790	.8542 2367	.8394 1762
4.28	.8991 0169	.8853 3424	.8712 3516	.8568 6565	.8422 8035
4.29	.9010 3199	.8874 9160	.8736 1806	.8594 7138	.8451 0519
4.30	.9029 3273	.8896 1701	.8759 6684	.8620 4106	.8478 9231
4.31	.9048 0418	.8917 1072	.8782 8174	.8645 7490	.8506 4189
4.32	.9066 4661	.8937 7300	.8805 6299	.8670 7314	.8533 5413
4.33	.9084 6030	.8958 0410	.8828 1086	.8695 3599	.8560 2921
4.34	.9102 4552	.8978 0430	.8850 2559	.8719 6368	.8586 6735
4.35	.9120 0254	.8997 7385	.8872 0743	.8743 5646	.8612 6876
4.36	.9137 3163	.9017 1305	.8893 5666	.8767 1457	.8638 3366
4.37	.9154 3309	.9036 2215	.8914 7353	.8790 3826	.8663 6226
4.38	.9171 0719	.9055 0144	.8935 5832	.8813 2777	.8688 5482
4.39	.9187 5421	.9073 5120	.8956 1129	.8835 8337	.8713 1155
4.40	.9203 7443	.9091 7171	.8976 3272	.8858 0531	.8737 3271
4.41	.9219 6814	.9109 6326	.8996 2289	.8879 9387	.8761 1854
4.42	.9235 3563	.9127 2613	.9015 8209	.8901 4932	.8784 6930
4.43	.9250 7717	.9144 6061	.9035 1058	.8922 7193	.8807 8524
4.44	.9265 9306	.9161 6698	.9054 0867	.8943 6198	.8830 6664
4.45	.9280 8358	.9178 4555	.9072 7664	.8964 1975	.8853 1376
4.46	.9295 4901	.9194 9660	.9091 1479	.8984 4553	.8875 2687
4.47	.9309 8966	.9211 2042	.9109 2340	.9004 3960	.8897 0626
4.48	.9324 0580	.9227 1731	.9127 0277	.9024 0226	.8918 5219
4.49	.9337 9772	.9242 8757	.9144 5320	.9043 3379	.8939 6497

W	P(W,12)	P(W,13)	P(W,14)	P(W,15)	P(W,16)
4.50	.9351 6571	.9258 3148	.9161 7499	.9062 3451	.8960 4488
4.51	.9365 1006	.9273 4936	.9178 6843	.9081 0470	.8980 9221
4.52	.9378 3105	.9288 4148	.9195 3384	.9099 4466	.9001 0725
4.53	.9391 2898	.9303 0816	.9211 7151	.9117 5471	.9020 9031
4.54	.9404 0412	.9317 4969	.9227 8174	.9135 3514	.9040 4169
4.55	.9416 5677	.9331 6636	.9243 6484	.9152 8626	.9059 6170
4.56	.9428 8721	.9345 5847	.9259 2112	.9170 0838	.9078 5063
4.57	.9440 9572	.9359 2633	.9274 5088	.9187 0182	.9097 0880
4.58	.9452 8260	.9372 7023	.9289 5443	.9203 6687	.9115 3652
4.59	.9464 4812	.9385 9046	.9304 3207	.9220 0386	.9133 3411
4.60	.9475 9256	.9398 8732	.9318 8412	.9236 1309	.9151 0187
4.61	.9487 1621	.9411 6112	.9333 1087	.9251 9488	.9168 4013
4.62	.9498 1934	.9424 1213	.9347 1264	.9267 4955	.9185 4920
4.63	.9509 0224	.9436 4066	.9360 8973	.9282 7741	.9202 2941
4.64	.9519 6518	.9448 4701	.9374 4244	.9297 7877	.9218 8107
4.65	.9530 0844	.9460 3146	.9387 7109	.9312 5395	.9235 0450
4.66	.9540 3229	.9471 9431	.9400 7598	.9327 0327	.9251 0003
4.67	.9550 3701	.9483 3584	.9413 5742	.9341 2704	.9266 6798
4.68	.9560 2287	.9494 5635	.9426 1570	.9355 2558	.9282 0868
4.69	.9569 9014	.9505 5613	.9438 5114	.9368 9920	.9297 2244
4.70	.9579 3908	.9516 3546	.9450 6403	.9382 4821	.9312 0959
4.71	.9588 6998	.9526 9463	.9462 5468	.9395 7294	.9326 7046
4.72	.9597 8308	.9537 3392	.9474 2338	.9408 7369	.9341 0536
4.73	.9606 7865	.9547 5362	.9485 7044	.9421 5079	.9355 1463
4.74	.9615 5696	.9557 5400	.9496 9616	.9434 0453	.9368 9859
4.75	.9624 1826	.9567 3535	.9508 0083	.9446 3523	.9382 5755
4.76	.9632 6282	.9576 9794	.9518 8474	.9458 4321	.9395 9185
4.77	.9640 9088	.9586 4205	.9529 4819	.9470 2877	.9409 0180
4.78	.9649 0271	.9595 6796	.9539 9148	.9481 9222	.9421 8772
4.79	.9656 9855	.9604 7593	.9550 1489	.9493 3386	.9434 4994
4.80	.9664 7865	.9613 6624	.9560 1871	.9504 5401	.9446 8877
4.81	.9672 4327	.9622 3916	.9570 0323	.9515 5296	.9459 0454
4.82	.9679 9264	.9630 9494	.9579 6874	.9526 3102	.9470 9755
4.83	.9687 2700	.9639 3387	.9589 1552	.9536 8849	.9482 6814
4.84	.9694 4661	.9647 5618	.9598 4384	.9547 2567	.9494 1660
4.85	.9701 5170	.9655 6216	.9607 5400	.9557 4285	.9505 4325
4.86	.9708 4250	.9663 5205	.9616 4626	.9567 4033	.9516 4841
4.87	.9715 1925	.9671 2612	.9625 2090	.9577 1841	.9527 3238
4.88	.9721 8218	.9678 8460	.9633 7820	.9586 7737	.9537 9548
4.89	.9728 3152	.9686 2776	.9642 1843	.9596 1751	.9548 3800
4.90	.9734 6749	.9693 5585	.9650 4186	.9605 3911	.9558 6026
4.91	.9740 9033	.9700 6911	.9658 4874	.9614 4246	.9568 6255
4.92	.9747 0025	.9707 6778	.9666 3936	.9623 2784	.9578 4518
4.93	.9752 9748	.9714 5210	.9674 1396	.9631 9553	.9588 0844
4.94	.9758 8222	.9721 2232	.9681 7281	.9640 4581	.9597 5263
4.95	.9764 5471	.9727 7867	.9689 1617	.9648 7896	.9606 7805
4.96	.9770 1514	.9734 2139	.9696 4428	.9656 9526	.9615 8499
4.97	.9775 6372	.9740 5070	.9703 5741	.9664 9496	.9624 7374
4.98	.9781 0068	.9746 6684	.9710 5580	.9672 7835	.9633 4458
4.99	.9786 2620	.9752 7003	.9717 3970	.9680 4569	.9641 9780

W	P(W,12)	P(W,13)	P(W,14)	P(W,15)	P(W,16)
5.00	.9791 4050	.9758 6050	.9724 0936	.9687 9725	.9650 3368
5.01	.9796 4378	.9764 3847	.9730 6501	.9695 3327	.9658 5251
5.02	.9801 3622	.9770 0415	.9737 0689	.9702 5404	.9666 5456
5.03	.9806 1804	.9775 5777	.9743 3525	.9709 5979	.9674 4010
5.04	.9810 8941	.9780 9954	.9749 5032	.9716 5079	.9682 0941
5.05	.9815 5053	.9786 2966	.9755 5232	.9723 2728	.9689 6276
5.06	.9820 0160	.9791 4835	.9761 4149	.9729 8952	.9697 0042
5.07	.9824 4278	.9796 5582	.9767 1806	.9736 3775	.9704 2264
5.08	.9828 7428	.9801 5226	.9772 8224	.9742 7222	.9711 2970
5.09	.9832 9626	.9806 3789	.9778 3426	.9748 9316	.9718 2185
5.10	.9837 0890	.9811 1289	.9783 7434	.9755 0081	.9724 9935
5.11	.9841 1239	.9815 7746	.9789 0269	.9760 9541	.9731 6245
5.12	.9845 0689	.9820 3180	.9794 1953	.9766 7718	.9738 1141
5.13	.9848 9258	.9824 7609	.9799 2507	.9772 4637	.9744 4646
5.14	.9852 6962	.9829 1053	.9804 1950	.9778 0319	.9750 6787
5.15	.9856 3818	.9833 3530	.9809 0305	.9783 4788	.9756 7586
5.16	.9859 9842	.9837 5058	.9813 7590	.9788 8064	.9762 7068
5.17	.9863 5050	.9841 5656	.9818 3827	.9794 0170	.9768 5256
5.18	.9866 9459	.9845 5341	.9822 9035	.9799 1128	.9774 2175
5.19	.9870 3084	.9849 4131	.9827 3232	.9804 0959	.9779 7846
5.20	.9873 5940	.9853 2042	.9831 6439	.9808 9683	.9785 2294
5.21	.9876 8043	.9856 9093	.9835 8674	.9813 7322	.9790 5540
5.22	.9879 9407	.9860 5300	.9839 9956	.9818 3896	.9795 7606
5.23	.9883 0048	.9864 0678	.9844 0303	.9822 9424	.9800 8515
5.24	.9885 9979	.9867 5246	.9847 9734	.9827 3928	.9805 8288
5.25	.9888 9215	.9870 9018	.9851 8265	.9831 7427	.9810 6947
5.26	.9891 7770	.9874 2011	.9855 5916	.9835 9939	.9815 4513
5.27	.9894 5658	.9877 4240	.9859 2702	.9840 1485	.9820 1006
5.28	.9897 2892	.9880 5720	.9862 8641	.9844 2082	.9824 6448
5.29	.9899 9486	.9883 6467	.9866 3751	.9848 1750	.9829 0857
5.30	.9902 5453	.9886 6495	.9869 8046	.9852 0507	.9833 4255
5.31	.9905 0806	.9889 5820	.9873 1545	.9855 8370	.9837 6661
5.32	.9907 5557	.9892 4454	.9876 4262	.9859 5357	.9841 8094
5.33	.9909 9720	.9895 2413	.9879 6214	.9863 1486	.9845 8573
5.34	.9912 3306	.9897 9710	.9882 7416	.9866 6774	.9849 8118
5.35	.9914 6328	.9900 6360	.9885 7883	.9870 1238	.9853 6746
5.36	.9916 8797	.9903 2375	.9888 7631	.9873 4894	.9857 4476
5.37	.9919 0725	.9905 7769	.9891 6674	.9876 7760	.9861 1327
5.38	.9921 2124	.9908 2554	.9894 5027	.9879 9850	.9864 7315
5.39	.9923 3004	.9910 6745	.9897 2704	.9883 1181	.9868 2458
5.40	.9925 3378	.9913 0352	.9899 9720	.9886 1769	.9871 6773
5.41	.9927 3256	.9915 3389	.9902 6087	.9889 1629	.9875 0278
5.42	.9929 2648	.9917 5868	.9905 1821	.9892 0776	.9878 2989
5.43	.9931 1565	.9919 7800	.9907 6933	.9894 9225	.9881 4921
5.44	.9933 0018	.9921 9198	.9910 1438	.9897 6990	.9884 6092
5.45	.9934 8017	.9924 0073	.9912 5348	.9900 4086	.9887 6517
5.46	.9936 5571	.9926 0436	.9914 8677	.9903 0528	.9890 6212
5.47	.9938 2690	.9928 0298	.9917 1435	.9905 6328	.9893 5192
5.48	.9939 9384	.9929 9671	.9919 3637	.9908 1501	.9896 3472
5.49	.9941 5663	.9931 8565	.9921 5293	.9910 6060	.9899 1066

W	P(W,12)	P(W,13)	P(W,14)	P(W,15)	P(W,16)
5.50	.9943 1535	.9933 6990	.9923 6416	.9913 0018	.9901 7991
5.51	.9944 7010	.9935 4957	.9925 7017	.9915 3389	.9904 4259
5.52	.9946 2096	.9937 2476	.9927 7109	.9917 6184	.9906 9885
5.53	.9947 6803	.9938 9558	.9929 6701	.9919 8417	.9909 4882
5.54	.9949 1138	.9940 6211	.9931 5805	.9922 0100	.9911 9265
5.55	.9950 5111	.9942 2445	.9933 4432	.9924 1244	.9914 3046
5.56	.9951 8730	.9943 8270	.9935 2593	.9926 1863	.9916 6239
5.57	.9953 2002	.9945 3696	.9937 0297	.9928 1966	.9918 8857
5.58	.9954 4935	.9946 8730	.9938 7555	.9930 1567	.9921 0912
5.59	.9955 7538	.9948 3382	.9940 4378	.9932 0675	.9923 2416
5.60	.9956 9818	.9949 7661	.9942 0775	.9933 9302	.9925 3382
5.61	.9958 1782	.9951 1576	.9943 6755	.9935 7459	.9927 3822
5.62	.9959 3438	.9952 5133	.9945 2328	.9937 5157	.9929 3748
5.63	.9960 4792	.9953 8343	.9946 7504	.9939 2405	.9931 3170
5.64	.9961 5853	.9955 1213	.9948 2291	.9940 9214	.9933 2101
5.65	.9962 6627	.9956 3750	.9949 6699	.9942 5594	.9935 0552
5.66	.9963 7120	.9957 5963	.9951 0736	.9944 1555	.9936 8533
5.67	.9964 7339	.9958 7859	.9952 4411	.9945 7107	.9938 6055
5.68	.9965 7291	.9959 9446	.9953 7732	.9947 2258	.9940 3128
5.69	.9966 6982	.9961 0730	.9955 0707	.9948 7018	.9941 9763
5.70	.9967 6418	.9962 1719	.9956 3345	.9950 1397	.9943 5971
5.71	.9968 5605	.9963 2420	.9957 5654	.9951 5402	.9945 1760
5.72	.9969 4550	.9964 2840	.9958 7640	.9952 9044	.9946 7140
5.73	.9970 3258	.9965 2986	.9959 9313	.9954 2329	.9948 2121
5.74	.9971 1734	.9966 2864	.9961 0679	.9955 5268	.9949 6713
5.75	.9971 9985	.9967 2480	.9962 1745	.9956 7867	.9951 0924
5.76	.9972 8016	.9968 1840	.9963 2520	.9958 0135	.9952 4764
5.77	.9973 5832	.9969 0952	.9964 3009	.9959 2080	.9953 8241
5.78	.9974 3439	.9969 9821	.9965 3219	.9960 3709	.9955 1363
5.79	.9975 0841	.9970 8453	.9966 3158	.9961 5031	.9956 4139
5.80	.9975 8044	.9971 6853	.9967 2832	.9962 6052	.9957 6578
5.81	.9976 5052	.9972 5028	.9968 2247	.9963 6779	.9958 8688
5.82	.9977 1871	.9973 2982	.9969 1410	.9964 7221	.9960 0476
5.83	.9977 8505	.9974 0722	.9970 0327	.9965 7383	.9961 1949
5.84	.9978 4959	.9974 8252	.9970 9003	.9966 7272	.9962 3117
5.85	.9979 1236	.9975 5578	.9971 7446	.9967 6896	.9963 3986
5.86	.9979 7342	.9976 2705	.9972 5659	.9968 6260	.9964 4563
5.87	.9980 3282	.9976 9638	.9973 3650	.9969 5372	.9965 4855
5.88	.9980 9058	.9977 6381	.9974 1424	.9970 4237	.9966 4870
5.89	.9981 4675	.9978 2940	.9974 8985	.9971 2861	.9967 4615
5.90	.9982 0137	.9978 9319	.9975 6340	.9972 1250	.9968 4095
5.91	.9982 5449	.9979 5522	.9976 3494	.9972 9411	.9969 3318
5.92	.9983 0613	.9980 1554	.9977 0451	.9973 7348	.9970 2289
5.93	.9983 5634	.9980 7420	.9977 7217	.9974 5068	.9971 1016
5.94	.9984 0516	.9981 3123	.9978 3796	.9975 2576	.9971 9504
5.95	.9984 5261	.9981 8668	.9979 0193	.9975 9877	.9972 7759
5.96	.9984 9874	.9982 4058	.9979 6413	.9976 6977	.9973 5787
5.97	.9985 4358	.9982 9299	.9980 2460	.9977 3880	.9974 3594
5.98	.9985 8716	.9983 4392	.9980 8339	.9978 0592	.9975 1185
5.99	.9986 2952	.9983 9344	.9981 4054	.9978 7117	.9975 8566

W	P(W,12)	P(W,13)	P(W,14)	P(W,15)	P(W,16)
6.00	.9986 7068	.9984 4156	.9981 9609	.9979 3461	.9976 5742
6.01	.9987 1067	.9984 8832	.9982 5008	.9979 9627	.9977 2719
6.02	.9987 4954	.9985 3377	.9983 0256	.9980 5621	.9977 9500
6.03	.9987 8730	.9985 7794	.9983 5356	.9981 1446	.9978 6093
6.04	.9988 2399	.9986 2085	.9984 0312	.9981 7108	.9979 2500
6.05	.9988 5964	.9986 6255	.9984 5128	.9982 2610	.9979 8728
6.06	.9988 9427	.9987 0306	.9984 9807	.9982 7957	.9980 4780
6.07	.9989 2790	.9987 4242	.9985 4354	.9983 3153	.9981 0662
6.08	.9989 6058	.9987 8065	.9985 8771	.9983 8201	.9981 6378
6.09	.9989 9231	.9988 1778	.9986 3062	.9984 3106	.9982 1931
6.10	.9990 2313	.9988 5386	.9986 7231	.9984 7870	.9982 7327
6.11	.9990 5306	.9988 8889	.9987 1279	.9985 2499	.9983 2569
6.12	.9990 8213	.9989 2292	.9987 5212	.9985 6996	.9983 7661
6.13	.9991 1035	.9989 5596	.9987 9032	.9986 1363	.9984 2608
6.14	.9991 3776	.9989 8805	.9988 2741	.9986 5605	.9984 7413
6.15	.9991 6437	.9990 1920	.9988 6343	.9986 9724	.9985 2081
6.16	.9991 9020	.9990 4945	.9988 9841	.9987 3725	.9985 6614
6.17	.9992 1528	.9990 7882	.9989 3238	.9987 7610	.9986 1016
6.18	.9992 3962	.9991 0734	.9989 6535	.9988 1382	.9986 5290
6.19	.9992 6325	.9991 3502	.9989 9737	.9988 5045	.9986 9441
6.20	.9992 8619	.9991 6189	.9990 2845	.9988 8601	.9987 3472
6.21	.9993 0845	.9991 8797	.9990 5862	.9989 2053	.9987 7385
6.22	.9993 3005	.9992 1328	.9990 8790	.9989 5404	.9988 1184
6.23	.9993 5102	.9992 3785	.9991 1633	.9989 8658	.9988 4872
6.24	.9993 7136	.9992 6169	.9991 4391	.9990 1815	.9988 8453
6.25	.9993 9110	.9992 8483	.9991 7069	.9990 4880	.9989 1928
6.26	.9994 1025	.9993 0728	.9991 9667	.9990 7854	.9989 5300
6.27	.9994 2884	.9993 2906	.9992 2188	.9991 0740	.9989 8574
6.28	.9994 4686	.9993 5020	.9992 4635	.9991 3541	.9990 1751
6.29	.9994 6435	.9993 7070	.9992 7008	.9991 6259	.9990 4834
6.30	.9994 8132	.9993 9059	.9992 9311	.9991 8896	.9990 7825
6.31	.9994 9777	.9994 0989	.9993 1545	.9992 1455	.9991 0728
6.32	.9995 1373	.9994 2861	.9993 3712	.9992 3937	.9991 3544
6.33	.9995 2921	.9994 4676	.9993 5814	.9992 6345	.9991 6276
6.34	.9995 4422	.9994 6437	.9993 7854	.9992 8681	.9991 8926
6.35	.9995 5878	.9994 8144	.9993 9831	.9993 0946	.9992 1497
6.36	.9995 7289	.9994 9800	.9994 1749	.9993 3143	.9992 3991
6.37	.9995 8658	.9995 1406	.9994 3609	.9993 5275	.9992 6410
6.38	.9995 9985	.9995 2963	.9994 5413	.9993 7341	.9992 8756
6.39	.9996 1271	.9995 4473	.9994 7162	.9993 9346	.9993 1031
6.40	.9996 2519	.9995 5936	.9994 8858	.9994 1289	.9993 3237
6.41	.9996 3728	.9995 7355	.9995 0502	.9994 3173	.9993 5376
6.42	.9996 4900	.9995 8731	.9995 2096	.9994 5000	.9993 7450
6.43	.9996 6036	.9996 0064	.9995 3641	.9994 6771	.9993 9462
6.44	.9996 7137	.9996 1357	.9995 5139	.9994 8489	.9994 1411
6.45	.9996 8204	.9996 2609	.9995 6591	.9995 0153	.9994 3302
6.46	.9996 9238	.9996 3823	.9995 7998	.9995 1766	.9994 5134
6.47	.9997 0240	.9996 5000	.9995 9362	.9995 3330	.9994 6910
6.48	.9997 1211	.9996 6140	.9996 0683	.9995 4846	.9994 8632
6.49	.9997 2152	.9996 7245	.9996 1964	.9995 6315	.9995 0300

W	P(W,12)	P(W,13)	P(W,14)	P(W,15)	P(W,16)
6.50	.9997 3063	.9996 8315	.9996 3206	.9995 7738	.9995 1917
6.51	.9997 3946	.9996 9352	.9996 4408	.9995 9117	.9995 3484
6.52	.9997 4802	.9997 0357	.9996 5573	.9996 0454	.9995 5003
6.53	.9997 5631	.9997 1331	.9996 6702	.9996 1749	.9995 6474
6.54	.9997 6433	.9997 2274	.9996 7796	.9996 3004	.9995 7900
6.55	.9997 7211	.9997 3187	.9996 8856	.9996 4219	.9995 9281
6.56	.9997 7964	.9997 4072	.9996 9882	.9996 5396	.9996 0619
6.57	.9997 8693	.9997 4929	.9997 0876	.9996 6537	.9996 1915
6.58	.9997 9400	.9997 5759	.9997 1839	.9996 7642	.9996 3171
6.59	.9998 0084	.9997 6563	.9997 2771	.9996 8712	.9996 4387
6.60	.9998 0746	.9997 7341	.9997 3674	.9996 9748	.9996 5565
6.61	.9998 1387	.9997 8095	.9997 4549	.9997 0752	.9996 6706
6.62	.9998 2008	.9997 8825	.9997 5396	.9997 1723	.9996 7811
6.63	.9998 2610	.9997 9531	.9997 6215	.9997 2664	.9996 8881
6.64	.9998 3191	.9998 0215	.9997 7009	.9997 3576	.9996 9917
6.65	.9998 3755	.9998 0878	.9997 7778	.9997 4458	.9997 0920
6.66	.9998 4300	.9998 1519	.9997 8522	.9997 5312	.9997 1891
6.67	.9998 4828	.9998 2139	.9997 9242	.9997 6139	.9997 2832
6.68	.9998 5339	.9998 2740	.9997 9939	.9997 6939	.9997 3742
6.69	.9998 5833	.9998 3321	.9998 0614	.9997 7714	.9997 4623
6.70	.9998 6312	.9998 3884	.9998 1267	.9997 8464	.9997 5476
6.71	.9998 6775	.9998 4428	.9998 1899	.9997 9190	.9997 6302
6.72	.9998 7223	.9998 4955	.9998 2511	.9997 9893	.9997 7101
6.73	.9998 7656	.9998 5465	.9998 3103	.9998 0572	.9997 7874
6.74	.9998 8076	.9998 5958	.9998 3676	.9998 1230	.9997 8623
6.75	.9998 8482	.9998 6436	.9998 4230	.9998 1867	.9997 9347
6.76	.9998 8874	.9998 6897	.9998 4767	.9998 2483	.9998 0048
6.77	.9998 9254	.9998 7344	.9998 5285	.9998 3079	.9998 0726
6.78	.9998 9621	.9998 7776	.9998 5787	.9998 3655	.9998 1382
6.79	.9998 9977	.9998 8194	.9998 6273	.9998 4213	.9998 2016
6.80	.9999 0320	.9998 8599	.9998 6742	.9998 4753	.9998 2630
6.81	.9999 0653	.9998 8990	.9998 7197	.9998 5275	.9998 3224
6.82	.9999 0974	.9998 9368	.9998 7636	.9998 5779	.9998 3799
6.83	.9999 1285	.9998 9734	.9998 8061	.9998 6268	.9998 4355
6.84	.9999 1586	.9999 0088	.9998 8472	.9998 6740	.9998 4892
6.85	.9999 1876	.9999 0430	.9998 8869	.9998 7197	.9998 5412
6.86	.9999 2157	.9999 0760	.9998 9254	.9998 7638	.9998 5915
6.87	.9999 2429	.9999 1080	.9998 9625	.9998 8065	.9998 6401
6.88	.9999 2692	.9999 1389	.9998 9985	.9998 8478	.9998 6871
6.89	.9999 2946	.9999 1688	.9999 0332	.9998 8877	.9998 7325
6.90	.9999 3191	.9999 1977	.9999 0668	.9998 9263	.9998 7765
6.91	.9999 3429	.9999 2257	.9999 0992	.9998 9636	.9998 8189
6.92	.9999 3658	.9999 2527	.9999 1306	.9998 9997	.9998 8600
6.93	.9999 3880	.9999 2788	.9999 1609	.9999 0346	.9998 8997
6.94	.9999 4094	.9999 3040	.9999 1903	.9999 0683	.9998 9381
6.95	.9999 4301	.9999 3284	.9999 2186	.9999 1008	.9998 9752
6.96	.9999 4501	.9999 3519	.9999 2460	.9999 1323	.9999 0110
6.97	.9999 4694	.9999 3747	.9999 2724	.9999 1627	.9999 0457
6.98	.9999 4881	.9999 3967	.9999 2980	.9999 1921	.9999 0791
6.99	.9999 5061	.9999 4179	.9999 3227	.9999 2205	.9999 1115

W	P(W,12)	P(W,13)	P(W,14)	P(W,15)	P(W,16)
7.00	.9999 5236	.9999 4385	.9999 3466	.9999 2480	.9999 1428
7.01	.9999 5404	.9999 4583	.9999 3696	.9999 2745	.9999 1730
7.02	.9999 5567	.9999 4775	.9999 3919	.9999 3001	.9999 2021
7.03	.9999 5724	.9999 4960	.9999 4134	.9999 3249	.9999 2303
7.04	.9999 5876	.9999 5139	.9999 4342	.9999 3488	.9999 2576
7.05	.9999 6023	.9999 5311	.9999 4543	.9999 3719	.9999 2839
7.06	.9999 6164	.9999 5478	.9999 4737	.9999 3942	.9999 3093
7.07	.9999 6301	.9999 5639	.9999 4925	.9999 4158	.9999 3339
7.08	.9999 6433	.9999 5795	.9999 5106	.9999 4366	.9999 3576
7.09	.9999 6561	.9999 5945	.9999 5280	.9999 4567	.9999 3805
7.10	.9999 6684	.9999 6090	.9999 5449	.9999 4761	.9999 4026
7.11	.9999 6803	.9999 6230	.9999 5612	.9999 4948	.9999 4240
7.12	.9999 6918	.9999 6365	.9999 5769	.9999 5129	.9999 4446
7.13	.9999 7028	.9999 6496	.9999 5921	.9999 5304	.9999 4645
7.14	.9999 7135	.9999 6622	.9999 6068	.9999 5473	.9999 4837
7.15	.9999 7239	.9999 6744	.9999 6209	.9999 5636	.9999 5023
7.16	.9999 7338	.9999 6861	.9999 6346	.9999 5793	.9999 5202
7.17	.9999 7435	.9999 6975	.9999 6478	.9999 5945	.9999 5375
7.18	.9999 7528	.9999 7084	.9999 6605	.9999 6091	.9999 5542
7.19	.9999 7617	.9999 7190	.9999 6728	.9999 6233	.9999 5703
7.20	.9999 7704	.9999 7292	.9999 6847	.9999 6369	.9999 5859
7.21	.9999 7787	.9999 7390	.9999 6961	.9999 6501	.9999 6009
7.22	.9999 7868	.9999 7485	.9999 7072	.9999 6628	.9999 6154
7.23	.9999 7945	.9999 7577	.9999 7179	.9999 6751	.9999 6294
7.24	.9999 8020	.9999 7665	.9999 7281	.9999 6869	.9999 6429
7.25	.9999 8093	.9999 7751	.9999 7381	.9999 6983	.9999 6559
7.26	.9999 8163	.9999 7833	.9999 7476	.9999 7094	.9999 6685
7.27	.9999 8230	.9999 7912	.9999 7569	.9999 7200	.9999 6806
7.28	.9999 8295	.9999 7989	.9999 7658	.9999 7303	.9999 6923
7.29	.9999 8358	.9999 8063	.9999 7744	.9999 7402	.9999 7036
7.30	.9999 8418	.9999 8134	.9999 7827	.9999 7497	.9999 7145
7.31	.9999 8476	.9999 8203	.9999 7907	.9999 7589	.9999 7250
7.32	.9999 8533	.9999 8269	.9999 7984	.9999 7678	.9999 7351
7.33	.9999 8587	.9999 8333	.9999 8058	.9999 7764	.9999 7449
7.34	.9999 8639	.9999 8395	.9999 8130	.9999 7846	.9999 7543
7.35	.9999 8690	.9999 8454	.9999 8199	.9999 7926	.9999 7634
7.36	.9999 8738	.9999 8511	.9999 8266	.9999 8003	.9999 7721
7.37	.9999 8785	.9999 8567	.9999 8330	.9999 8077	.9999 7806
7.38	.9999 8830	.9999 8620	.9999 8393	.9999 8148	.9999 7887
7.39	.9999 8874	.9999 8671	.9999 8452	.9999 8217	.9999 7966
7.40	.9999 8916	.9999 8721	.9999 8510	.9999 8283	.9999 8041
7.41	.9999 8956	.9999 8769	.9999 8566	.9999 8348	.9999 8114
7.42	.9999 8995	.9999 8815	.9999 8619	.9999 8409	.9999 8185
7.43	.9999 9033	.9999 8859	.9999 8671	.9999 8469	.9999 8253
7.44	.9999 9069	.9999 8902	.9999 8721	.9999 8526	.9999 8318
7.45	.9999 9104	.9999 8943	.9999 8769	.9999 8581	.9999 8381
7.46	.9999 9138	.9999 8983	.9999 8815	.9999 8635	.9999 8442
7.47	.9999 9170	.9999 9021	.9999 8859	.9999 8686	.9999 8500
7.48	.9999 9202	.9999 9058	.9999 8902	.9999 8735	.9999 8557
7.49	.9999 9232	.9999 9093	.9999 8944	.9999 8783	.9999 8611

W	P(W,12)	P(W,13)	P(W,14)	P(W,15)	P(W,16)
7.50	.9999 9261	.9999 9128	.9999 8984	.9999 8829	.9999 8663
7.51	.9999 9289	.9999 9161	.9999 9022	.9999 8873	.9999 8714
7.52	.9999 9316	.9999 9192	.9999 9059	.9999 8916	.9999 8763
7.53	.9999 9342	.9999 9223	.9999 9095	.9999 8957	.9999 8809
7.54	.9999 9367	.9999 9252	.9999 9129	.9999 8996	.9999 8855
7.55	.9999 9391	.9999 9281	.9999 9162	.9999 9035	.9999 8898
7.56	.9999 9414	.9999 9308	.9999 9194	.9999 9071	.9999 8940
7.57	.9999 9436	.9999 9335	.9999 9225	.9999 9107	.9999 8980
7.58	.9999 9458	.9999 9360	.9999 9254	.9999 9141	.9999 9019
7.59	.9999 9479	.9999 9384	.9999 9283	.9999 9174	.9999 9057
7.60	.9999 9498	.9999 9408	.9999 9310	.9999 9205	.9999 9093
7.61	.9999 9518	.9999 9431	.9999 9337	.9999 9236	.9999 9127
7.62	.9999 9536	.9999 9453	.9999 9362	.9999 9265	.9999 9161
7.63	.9999 9554	.9999 9474	.9999 9387	.9999 9293	.9999 9193
7.64	.9999 9571	.9999 9494	.9999 9410	.9999 9320	.9999 9224
7.65	.9999 9588	.9999 9513	.9999 9433	.9999 9346	.9999 9254
7.66	.9999 9604	.9999 9532	.9999 9455	.9999 9372	.9999 9283
7.67	.9999 9619	.9999 9550	.9999 9476	.9999 9396	.9999 9310
7.68	.9999 9634	.9999 9568	.9999 9496	.9999 9419	.9999 9337
7.69	.9999 9648	.9999 9584	.9999 9516	.9999 9442	.9999 9363
7.70	.9999 9661	.9999 9600	.9999 9534	.9999 9463	.9999 9387
7.71	.9999 9675	.9999 9616	.9999 9552	.9999 9484	.9999 9411
7.72	.9999 9687	.9999 9631	.9999 9570	.9999 9504	.9999 9434
7.73	.9999 9699	.9999 9645	.9999 9586	.9999 9523	.9999 9456
7.74	.9999 9711	.9999 9659	.9999 9603	.9999 9542	.9999 9477
7.75	.9999 9722	.9999 9672	.9999 9618	.9999 9560	.9999 9497
7.76	.9999 9733	.9999 9685	.9999 9633	.9999 9577	.9999 9517
7.77	.9999 9744	.9999 9697	.9999 9647	.9999 9593	.9999 9536
7.78	.9999 9754	.9999 9709	.9999 9661	.9999 9609	.9999 9554
7.79	.9999 9763	.9999 9721	.9999 9674	.9999 9625	.9999 9571
7.80	.9999 9773	.9999 9732	.9999 9687	.9999 9639	.9999 9588
7.81	.9999 9782	.9999 9742	.9999 9699	.9999 9654	.9999 9604
7.82	.9999 9790	.9999 9752	.9999 9711	.9999 9667	.9999 9620
7.83	.9999 9798	.9999 9762	.9999 9723	.9999 9680	.9999 9635
7.84	.9999 9806	.9999 9771	.9999 9734	.9999 9693	.9999 9649
7.85	.9999 9814	.9999 9780	.9999 9744	.9999 9705	.9999 9663
7.86	.9999 9821	.9999 9789	.9999 9754	.9999 9717	.9999 9676
7.87	.9999 9828	.9999 9797	.9999 9764	.9999 9728	.9999 9689
7.88	.9999 9835	.9999 9805	.9999 9773	.9999 9739	.9999 9702
7.89	.9999 9842	.9999 9813	.9999 9782	.9999 9749	.9999 9713
7.90	.9999 9848	.9999 9821	.9999 9791	.9999 9759	.9999 9725
7.91	.9999 9854	.9999 9828	.9999 9799	.9999 9768	.9999 9736
7.92	.9999 9860	.9999 9835	.9999 9807	.9999 9778	.9999 9746
7.93	.9999 9866	.9999 9841	.9999 9815	.9999 9787	.9999 9756
7.94	.9999 9871	.9999 9848	.9999 9822	.9999 9795	.9999 9766
7.95	.9999 9876	.9999 9854	.9999 9829	.9999 9803	.9999 9775
7.96	.9999 9881	.9999 9859	.9999 9836	.9999 9811	.9999 9784
7.97	.9999 9886	.9999 9865	.9999 9843	.9999 9819	.9999 9793
7.98	.9999 9890	.9999 9871	.9999 9849	.9999 9826	.9999 9801
7.99	.9999 9895	.9999 9876	.9999 9855	.9999 9833	.9999 9809

W	P(W,12)	P(W,13)	P(W,14)	P(W,15)	P(W,16)
8.00	.9999 9899	.9999 9881	.9999 9861	.9999 9840	.9999 9817
8.01	.9999 9903	.9999 9886	.9999 9867	.9999 9846	.9999 9824
8.02	.9999 9907	.9999 9890	.9999 9872	.9999 9852	.9999 9831
8.03	.9999 9911	.9999 9895	.9999 9877	.9999 9858	.9999 9838
8.04	.9999 9914	.9999 9899	.9999 9882	.9999 9864	.9999 9845
8.05	.9999 9918	.9999 9903	.9999 9887	.9999 9869	.9999 9851
8.06	.9999 9921	.9999 9907	.9999 9891	.9999 9875	.9999 9857
8.07	.9999 9924	.9999 9911	.9999 9896	.9999 9880	.9999 9863
8.08	.9999 9927	.9999 9914	.9999 9900	.9999 9885	.9999 9868
8.09	.9999 9930	.9999 9918	.9999 9904	.9999 9889	.9999 9874
8.10	.9999 9933	.9999 9921	.9999 9908	.9999 9894	.9999 9879
8.11	.9999 9936	.9999 9924	.9999 9912	.9999 9898	.9999 9884
8.12	.9999 9938	.9999 9927	.9999 9915	.9999 9902	.9999 9888
8.13	.9999 9941	.9999 9930	.9999 9919	.9999 9906	.9999 9893
8.14	.9999 9943	.9999 9933	.9999 9922	.9999 9910	.9999 9897
8.15	.9999 9946	.9999 9936	.9999 9925	.9999 9914	.9999 9902
8.16	.9999 9948	.9999 9939	.9999 9928	.9999 9917	.9999 9906
8.17	.9999 9950	.9999 9941	.9999 9931	.9999 9921	.9999 9909
8.18	.9999 9952	.9999 9943	.9999 9934	.9999 9924	.9999 9913
8.19	.9999 9954	.9999 9946	.9999 9937	.9999 9927	.9999 9917
8.20	.9999 9956	.9999 9948	.9999 9939	.9999 9930	.9999 9920
8.21	.9999 9958	.9999 9950	.9999 9942	.9999 9933	.9999 9923
8.22	.9999 9960	.9999 9952	.9999 9944	.9999 9936	.9999 9927
8.23	.9999 9961	.9999 9954	.9999 9947	.9999 9938	.9999 9930
8.24	.9999 9963	.9999 9956	.9999 9949	.9999 9941	.9999 9933
8.25	.9999 9964	.9999 9958	.9999 9951	.9999 9943	.9999 9935
8.26	.9999 9966	.9999 9960	.9999 9953	.9999 9946	.9999 9938
8.27	.9999 9967	.9999 9961	.9999 9955	.9999 9948	.9999 9941
8.28	.9999 9969	.9999 9963	.9999 9957	.9999 9950	.9999 9943
8.29	.9999 9970	.9999 9964	.9999 9959	.9999 9952	.9999 9945
8.30	.9999 9971	.9999 9966	.9999 9960	.9999 9954	.9999 9948
8.31	.9999 9972	.9999 9967	.9999 9962	.9999 9956	.9999 9950
8.32	.9999 9974	.9999 9969	.9999 9964	.9999 9958	.9999 9952
8.33	.9999 9975	.9999 9970	.9999 9965	.9999 9960	.9999 9954
8.34	.9999 9976	.9999 9971	.9999 9967	.9999 9961	.9999 9956
8.35	.9999 9977	.9999 9972	.9999 9968	.9999 9963	.9999 9958
8.36	.9999 9978	.9999 9974	.9999 9969	.9999 9965	.9999 9959
8.37	.9999 9979	.9999 9975	.9999 9971	.9999 9966	.9999 9961
8.38	.9999 9980	.9999 9976	.9999 9972	.9999 9967	.9999 9963
8.39	.9999 9980	.9999 9977	.9999 9973	.9999 9969	.9999 9964
8.40	.9999 9981	.9999 9978	.9999 9974	.9999 9970	.9999 9966
8.41	.9999 9982	.9999 9979	.9999 9975	.9999 9971	.9999 9967
8.42	.9999 9983	.9999 9980	.9999 9976	.9999 9973	.9999 9969
8.43	.9999 9983	.9999 9980	.9999 9977	.9999 9974	.9999 9970
8.44	.9999 9984	.9999 9981	.9999 9978	.9999 9975	.9999 9971
8.45	.9999 9985	.9999 9982	.9999 9979	.9999 9976	.9999 9972
8.46	.9999 9985	.9999 9983	.9999 9980	.9999 9977	.9999 9974
8.47	.9999 9986	.9999 9984	.9999 9981	.9999 9978	.9999 9975
8.48	.9999 9987	.9999 9984	.9999 9982	.9999 9979	.9999 9976
8.49	.9999 9987	.9999 9985	.9999 9982	.9999 9980	.9999 9977

W	P(W,12)	P(W,13)	P(W,14)	P(W,15)	P(W,16)
8.50	.9999 9988	.9999 9986	.9999 9983	.9999 9981	.9999 9978
8.51	.9999 9988	.9999 9986	.9999 9984	.9999 9981	.9999 9979
8.52	.9999 9989	.9999 9987	.9999 9985	.9999 9982	.9999 9980
8.53	.9999 9989	.9999 9987	.9999 9985	.9999 9983	.9999 9981
8.54	.9999 9990	.9999 9988	.9999 9986	.9999 9984	.9999 9981
8.55	.9999 9990	.9999 9988	.9999 9986	.9999 9984	.9999 9982
8.56	.9999 9991	.9999 9989	.9999 9987	.9999 9985	.9999 9983
8.57	.9999 9991	.9999 9989	.9999 9988	.9999 9986	.9999 9984
8.58	.9999 9991	.9999 9990	.9999 9988	.9999 9986	.9999 9984
8.59	.9999 9992	.9999 9990	.9999 9989	.9999 9987	.9999 9985
8.60	.9999 9992	.9999 9991	.9999 9989	.9999 9987	.9999 9986
8.61	.9999 9992	.9999 9991	.9999 9990	.9999 9988	.9999 9986
8.62	.9999 9993	.9999 9991	.9999 9990	.9999 9989	.9999 9987
8.63	.9999 9993	.9999 9992	.9999 9990	.9999 9989	.9999 9987
8.64	.9999 9993	.9999 9992	.9999 9991	.9999 9989	.9999 9988
8.65	.9999 9994	.9999 9993	.9999 9991	.9999 9990	.9999 9989
8.66	.9999 9994	.9999 9993	.9999 9992	.9999 9990	.9999 9989
8.67	.9999 9994	.9999 9993	.9999 9992	.9999 9991	.9999 9989
8.68	.9999 9994	.9999 9993	.9999 9992	.9999 9991	.9999 9990
8.69	.9999 9995	.9999 9994	.9999 9993	.9999 9992	.9999 9990
8.70	.9999 9995	.9999 9994	.9999 9993	.9999 9992	.9999 9991
8.71	.9999 9995	.9999 9994	.9999 9993	.9999 9992	.9999 9991
8.72	.9999 9995	.9999 9994	.9999 9994	.9999 9993	.9999 9992
8.73	.9999 9996	.9999 9995	.9999 9994	.9999 9993	.9999 9992
8.74	.9999 9996	.9999 9995	.9999 9994	.9999 9993	.9999 9992
8.75	.9999 9996	.9999 9995	.9999 9994	.9999 9994	.9999 9993
8.76	.9999 9996	.9999 9995	.9999 9995	.9999 9994	.9999 9993
8.77	.9999 9996	.9999 9996	.9999 9995	.9999 9994	.9999 9993
8.78	.9999 9996	.9999 9996	.9999 9995	.9999 9994	.9999 9994
8.79	.9999 9997	.9999 9996	.9999 9995	.9999 9995	.9999 9994
8.80	.9999 9997	.9999 9996	.9999 9995	.9999 9995	.9999 9994
8.81	.9999 9997	.9999 9996	.9999 9996	.9999 9995	.9999 9994
8.82	.9999 9997	.9999 9996	.9999 9996	.9999 9995	.9999 9995
8.83	.9999 9997	.9999 9997	.9999 9996	.9999 9995	.9999 9995
8.84	.9999 9997	.9999 9997	.9999 9996	.9999 9996	.9999 9995
8.85	.9999 9997	.9999 9997	.9999 9996	.9999 9996	.9999 9995
8.86	.9999 9997	.9999 9997	.9999 9997	.9999 9996	.9999 9995
8.87	.9999 9998	.9999 9997	.9999 9997	.9999 9996	.9999 9996
8.88	.9999 9998	.9999 9997	.9999 9997	.9999 9996	.9999 9996
8.89	.9999 9998	.9999 9997	.9999 9997	.9999 9997	.9999 9996
8.90	.9999 9998	.9999 9998	.9999 9997	.9999 9997	.9999 9996
8.91	.9999 9998	.9999 9998	.9999 9997	.9999 9997	.9999 9996
8.92	.9999 9998	.9999 9998	.9999 9997	.9999 9997	.9999 9997
8.93	.9999 9998	.9999 9998	.9999 9997	.9999 9997	.9999 9997
8.94	.9999 9998	.9999 9998	.9999 9998	.9999 9997	.9999 9997
8.95	.9999 9998	.9999 9998	.9999 9998	.9999 9997	.9999 9997
8.96	.9999 9998	.9999 9998	.9999 9998	.9999 9997	.9999 9997
8.97	.9999 9998	.9999 9998	.9999 9998	.9999 9998	.9999 9997
8.98	.9999 9999	.9999 9998	.9999 9998	.9999 9998	.9999 9997
8.99	.9999 9999	.9999 9998	.9999 9998	.9999 9998	.9999 9997

W	P(W,12)	P(W,13)	P(W,14)	P(W,15)	P(W,16)
9.00	.9999 9999	.9999 9998	.9999 9998	.9999 9998	.9999 9998
9.01	.9999 9999	.9999 9998	.9999 9998	.9999 9998	.9999 9998
9.02	.9999 9999	.9999 9999	.9999 9998	.9999 9998	.9999 9998
9.03	.9999 9999	.9999 9999	.9999 9998	.9999 9998	.9999 9998
9.04	.9999 9999	.9999 9999	.9999 9998	.9999 9998	.9999 9998
9.05	.9999 9999	.9999 9999	.9999 9999	.9999 9998	.9999 9998
9.06	.9999 9999	.9999 9999	.9999 9999	.9999 9998	.9999 9998
9.07	.9999 9999	.9999 9999	.9999 9999	.9999 9998	.9999 9998
9.08	.9999 9999	.9999 9999	.9999 9999	.9999 9999	.9999 9998
9.09	.9999 9999	.9999 9999	.9999 9999	.9999 9999	.9999 9998
9.10	.9999 9999	.9999 9999	.9999 9999	.9999 9999	.9999 9998
9.11	.9999 9999	.9999 9999	.9999 9999	.9999 9999	.9999 9999
9.12	.9999 9999	.9999 9999	.9999 9999	.9999 9999	.9999 9999
9.13	.9999 9999	.9999 9999	.9999 9999	.9999 9999	.9999 9999
9.14	.9999 9999	.9999 9999	.9999 9999	.9999 9999	.9999 9999
9.15	.9999 9999	.9999 9999	.9999 9999	.9999 9999	.9999 9999
9.16	.9999 9999	.9999 9999	.9999 9999	.9999 9999	.9999 9999
9.17	.9999 9999	.9999 9999	.9999 9999	.9999 9999	.9999 9999
9.18	.9999 9999	.9999 9999	.9999 9999	.9999 9999	.9999 9999
9.19	.9999 9999	.9999 9999	.9999 9999	.9999 9999	.9999 9999
9.20	.9999 9999	.9999 9999	.9999 9999	.9999 9999	.9999 9999
9.21	.9999 9999	.9999 9999	.9999 9999	.9999 9999	.9999 9999
9.22	.9999 9999	.9999 9999	.9999 9999	.9999 9999	.9999 9999
9.23	.9999 9999	.9999 9999	.9999 9999	.9999 9999	.9999 9999
9.24	1.0000 0000	.9999 9999	.9999 9999	.9999 9999	.9999 9999
9.25		.9999 9999	.9999 9999	.9999 9999	.9999 9999
9.26		.9999 9999	.9999 9999	.9999 9999	.9999 9999
9.27		1.0000 0000	.9999 9999	.9999 9999	.9999 9999
9.28			.9999 9999	.9999 9999	.9999 9999
9.29			.9999 9999	.9999 9999	.9999 9999
9.30			.9999 9999	.9999 9999	.9999 9999
9.31			1.0000 0000	.9999 9999	.9999 9999
9.32				.9999 9999	.9999 9999
9.33				1.0000 0000	.9999 9999
9.34					.9999 9999
9.35					.9999 9999
9.36					1.0000 0000
9.37					
9.38					
9.39					
9.40					
9.41					
9.42					
9.43					
9.44					
9.45					
9.46					
9.47					
9.48					
9.49					

W	P(W,12)	P(W,13)	P(W,14)	P(W,15)	P(W,16)
9.50					
9.51					
9.52					
9.53					
9.54					
9.55					
9.56					
9.57					
9.58					
9.59					
9.60					
9.61					
9.62					
9.63					
9.64					
9.65					
9.66					
9.67					
9.68					
9.69					
9.70					
9.71					
9.72					
9.73					
9.74					
9.75					
9.76					
9.77					
9.78					
9.79					
9.80					
9.81					
9.82					
9.83					
9.84					
9.85					
9.86					
9.87					
9.88					
9.89					
9.90					
9.91					
9.92					
9.93					
9.94					
9.95					
9.96					
9.97					
9.98					
9.99					

W	P(W,17)	P(W,18)	P(W,19)	P(W,20)	P(W,22)
0.00					
0.01					
0.02					
0.03					
0.04					
0.05					
0.06					
0.07					
0.08					
0.09					
0.10					
0.11					
0.12					
0.13					
0.14					
0.15					
0.16					
0.17					
0.18					
0.19					
0.20					
0.21					
0.22					
0.23					
0.24					
0.25					
0.26					
0.27					
0.28					
0.29					
0.30					
0.31					
0.32					
0.33					
0.34					
0.35					
0.36					
0.37					
0.38					
0.39					
0.40					
0.41					
0.42					
0.43					
0.44					
0.45					
0.46					
0.47					
0.48					
0.49					

W	P(W,17)	P(W,18)	P(W,19)	P(W,20)	P(W,22)
0.50					
0.51					
0.52					
0.53					
0.54					
0.55					
0.56					
0.57					
0.58					
0.59					
0.60					
0.61					
0.62					
0.63					
0.64					
0.65					
0.66					
0.67					
0.68					
0.69					
0.70					
0.71	.0000 0000				
0.72	.0000 0001				
0.73	.0000 0001				
0.74	.0000 0001				
0.75	.0000 0001				
0.76	.0000 0001	.0000 0000			
0.77	.0000 0002	.0000 0001			
0.78	.0000 0002	.0000 0001			
0.79	.0000 0002	.0000 0001			
0.80	.0000 0003	.0000 0001			
0.81	.0000 0004	.0000 0001			
0.82	.0000 0004	.0000 0001	.0000 0000		
0.83	.0000 0005	.0000 0002	.0000 0001		
0.84	.0000 0006	.0000 0002	.0000 0001		
0.85	.0000 0007	.0000 0002	.0000 0001		
0.86	.0000 0009	.0000 0003	.0000 0001		
0.87	.0000 0010	.0000 0004	.0000 0001	.0000 0000	
0.88	.0000 0012	.0000 0004	.0000 0001	.0000 0001	
0.89	.0000 0015	.0000 0005	.0000 0002	.0000 0001	
0.90	.0000 0017	.0000 0006	.0000 0002	.0000 0001	
0.91	.0000 0020	.0000 0007	.0000 0003	.0000 0001	
0.92	.0000 0024	.0000 0009	.0000 0003	.0000 0001	
0.93	.0000 0028	.0000 0010	.0000 0004	.0000 0001	
0.94	.0000 0033	.0000 0012	.0000 0005	.0000 0002	
0.95	.0000 0038	.0000 0014	.0000 0005	.0000 0002	
0.96	.0000 0045	.0000 0017	.0000 0006	.0000 0002	
0.97	.0000 0052	.0000 0020	.0000 0008	.0000 0003	
0.98	.0000 0061	.0000 0023	.0000 0009	.0000 0003	.0000 0000
0.99	.0000 0070	.0000 0027	.0000 0011	.0000 0004	.0000 0001

W	P(W,17)	P(W,18)	P(W,19)	P(W,20)	P(W,22)
1.00	.0000 0081	.0000 0032	.0000 0013	.0000 0005	.0000 0001
1.01	.0000 0094	.0000 0037	.0000 0015	.0000 0006	.0000 0001
1.02	.0000 0109	.0000 0044	.0000 0017	.0000 0007	.0000 0001
1.03	.0000 0125	.0000 0051	.0000 0020	.0000 0008	.0000 0001
1.04	.0000 0144	.0000 0059	.0000 0024	.0000 0010	.0000 0002
1.05	.0000 0165	.0000 0068	.0000 0028	.0000 0011	.0000 0002
1.06	.0000 0189	.0000 0079	.0000 0033	.0000 0014	.0000 0002
1.07	.0000 0217	.0000 0091	.0000 0038	.0000 0016	.0000 0003
1.08	.0000 0248	.0000 0105	.0000 0044	.0000 0019	.0000 0003
1.09	.0000 0283	.0000 0120	.0000 0051	.0000 0022	.0000 0004
1.10	.0000 0322	.0000 0138	.0000 0059	.0000 0025	.0000 0005
1.11	.0000 0366	.0000 0159	.0000 0069	.0000 0030	.0000 0005
1.12	.0000 0416	.0000 0182	.0000 0079	.0000 0034	.0000 0007
1.13	.0000 0472	.0000 0208	.0000 0091	.0000 0040	.0000 0008
1.14	.0000 0535	.0000 0237	.0000 0105	.0000 0046	.0000 0009
1.15	.0000 0605	.0000 0271	.0000 0121	.0000 0054	.0000 0011
1.16	.0000 0684	.0000 0308	.0000 0139	.0000 0062	.0000 0013
1.17	.0000 0772	.0000 0350	.0000 0159	.0000 0072	.0000 0015
1.18	.0000 0869	.0000 0398	.0000 0182	.0000 0083	.0000 0017
1.19	.0000 0978	.0000 0451	.0000 0208	.0000 0095	.0000 0020
1.20	.0000 1100	.0000 0511	.0000 0237	.0000 0110	.0000 0023
1.21	.0000 1235	.0000 0578	.0000 0270	.0000 0126	.0000 0027
1.22	.0000 1384	.0000 0652	.0000 0307	.0000 0144	.0000 0032
1.23	.0000 1550	.0000 0736	.0000 0349	.0000 0165	.0000 0037
1.24	.0000 1734	.0000 0829	.0000 0396	.0000 0189	.0000 0043
1.25	.0000 1937	.0000 0932	.0000 0448	.0000 0215	.0000 0049
1.26	.0000 2162	.0000 1048	.0000 0507	.0000 0245	.0000 0057
1.27	.0000 2410	.0000 1176	.0000 0573	.0000 0279	.0000 0066
1.28	.0000 2683	.0000 1319	.0000 0647	.0000 0317	.0000 0076
1.29	.0000 2984	.0000 1477	.0000 0729	.0000 0360	.0000 0087
1.30	.0000 3316	.0000 1651	.0000 0821	.0000 0408	.0000 0100
1.31	.0000 3680	.0000 1845	.0000 0924	.0000 0462	.0000 0115
1.32	.0000 4079	.0000 2059	.0000 1038	.0000 0522	.0000 0132
1.33	.0000 4518	.0000 2295	.0000 1164	.0000 0590	.0000 0151
1.34	.0000 4998	.0000 2556	.0000 1305	.0000 0665	.0000 0172
1.35	.0000 5524	.0000 2843	.0000 1460	.0000 0749	.0000 0197
1.36	.0000 6100	.0000 3158	.0000 1633	.0000 0843	.0000 0224
1.37	.0000 6728	.0000 3506	.0000 1824	.0000 0948	.0000 0255
1.38	.0000 7414	.0000 3887	.0000 2035	.0000 1064	.0000 0290
1.39	.0000 8162	.0000 4305	.0000 2268	.0000 1193	.0000 0329
1.40	.0000 8977	.0000 4764	.0000 2525	.0000 1336	.0000 0373
1.41	.0000 9864	.0000 5267	.0000 2808	.0000 1495	.0000 0422
1.42	.0001 0829	.0000 5816	.0000 3119	.0000 1671	.0000 0478
1.43	.0001 1877	.0000 6417	.0000 3462	.0000 1865	.0000 0539
1.44	.0001 3015	.0000 7073	.0000 3838	.0000 2080	.0000 0609
1.45	.0001 4249	.0000 7788	.0000 4251	.0000 2317	.0000 0686
1.46	.0001 5587	.0000 8568	.0000 4703	.0000 2578	.0000 0772
1.47	.0001 7035	.0000 9418	.0000 5199	.0000 2866	.0000 0868
1.48	.0001 8601	.0001 0342	.0000 5742	.0000 3183	.0000 0975
1.49	.0002 0295	.0001 1347	.0000 6335	.0000 3532	.0000 1094

W	P(W,17)	P(W,18)	P(W,19)	P(W,20)	P(W,22)
1.50	.0002 2124	.0001 2438	.0000 6982	.0000 3914	.0000 1226
1.51	.0002 4098	.0001 3622	.0000 7689	.0000 4334	.0000 1372
1.52	.0002 6227	.0001 4906	.0000 8459	.0000 4794	.0000 1535
1.53	.0002 8521	.0001 6297	.0000 9298	.0000 5298	.0000 1714
1.54	.0003 0990	.0001 7802	.0001 0212	.0000 5850	.0000 1913
1.55	.0003 3647	.0001 9431	.0001 1205	.0000 6453	.0000 2133
1.56	.0003 6502	.0002 1190	.0001 2283	.0000 7111	.0000 2375
1.57	.0003 9570	.0002 3090	.0001 3454	.0000 7829	.0000 2642
1.58	.0004 2862	.0002 5140	.0001 4724	.0000 8612	.0000 2936
1.59	.0004 6394	.0002 7350	.0001 6100	.0000 9465	.0000 3260
1.60	.0005 0179	.0002 9731	.0001 7590	.0001 0393	.0000 3616
1.61	.0005 4232	.0003 2293	.0001 9201	.0001 1402	.0000 4007
1.62	.0005 8570	.0003 5049	.0002 0943	.0001 2498	.0000 4436
1.63	.0006 3210	.0003 8011	.0002 2825	.0001 3688	.0000 4906
1.64	.0006 8168	.0004 1192	.0002 4856	.0001 4978	.0000 5421
1.65	.0007 3463	.0004 4606	.0002 7046	.0001 6377	.0000 5984
1.66	.0007 9114	.0004 8267	.0002 9405	.0001 7891	.0000 6600
1.67	.0008 5140	.0005 2191	.0003 1946	.0001 9529	.0000 7273
1.68	.0009 1564	.0005 6392	.0003 4680	.0002 1300	.0000 8007
1.69	.0009 8405	.0006 0887	.0003 7619	.0002 3212	.0000 8808
1.70	.0010 5686	.0006 5694	.0004 0776	.0002 5277	.0000 9680
1.71	.0011 3431	.0007 0830	.0004 4165	.0002 7503	.0001 0629
1.72	.0012 1663	.0007 6315	.0004 7801	.0002 9902	.0001 1661
1.73	.0013 0408	.0008 2168	.0005 1699	.0003 2486	.0001 2783
1.74	.0013 9692	.0008 8410	.0005 5874	.0003 5265	.0001 4001
1.75	.0014 9541	.0009 5061	.0006 0342	.0003 8254	.0001 5322
1.76	.0015 9984	.0010 2145	.0006 5122	.0004 1465	.0001 6754
1.77	.0017 1050	.0010 9683	.0007 0232	.0004 4913	.0001 8305
1.78	.0018 2768	.0011 7701	.0007 5690	.0004 8611	.0001 9983
1.79	.0019 5170	.0012 6223	.0008 1516	.0005 2576	.0002 1797
1.80	.0020 8287	.0013 5275	.0008 7731	.0005 6824	.0002 3758
1.81	.0022 2152	.0014 4884	.0009 4357	.0006 1371	.0002 5875
1.82	.0023 6800	.0015 5078	.0010 1415	.0006 6236	.0002 8158
1.83	.0025 2265	.0016 5886	.0010 8929	.0007 1436	.0003 0620
1.84	.0026 8585	.0017 7337	.0011 6923	.0007 6992	.0003 3271
1.85	.0028 5795	.0018 9463	.0012 5423	.0008 2923	.0003 6125
1.86	.0030 3935	.0020 2296	.0013 4455	.0008 9251	.0003 9194
1.87	.0032 3043	.0021 5868	.0014 4046	.0009 5997	.0004 2492
1.88	.0034 3161	.0023 0214	.0015 4224	.0010 3185	.0004 6035
1.89	.0036 4329	.0024 5369	.0016 5018	.0011 0838	.0004 9836
1.90	.0038 6591	.0026 1369	.0017 6459	.0011 8982	.0005 3913
1.91	.0040 9990	.0027 8252	.0018 8578	.0012 7642	.0005 8282
1.92	.0043 4571	.0029 6057	.0020 1408	.0013 6844	.0006 2961
1.93	.0046 0381	.0031 4822	.0021 4981	.0014 6617	.0006 7968
1.94	.0048 7465	.0033 4588	.0022 9333	.0015 6990	.0007 3322
1.95	.0051 5872	.0035 5398	.0024 4500	.0016 7993	.0007 9044
1.96	.0054 5651	.0037 7294	.0026 0517	.0017 9656	.0008 5154
1.97	.0057 6853	.0040 0321	.0027 7423	.0019 2012	.0009 1676
1.98	.0060 9528	.0042 4523	.0029 5258	.0020 5094	.0009 8631
1.99	.0064 3729	.0044 9947	.0031 4061	.0021 8937	.0010 6044

W	P(W,17)	P(W,18)	P(W,19)	P(W,20)	P(W,22)
2.00	.0067 9509	.0047 6641	.0033 3874	.0023 3575	.0011 3939
2.01	.0071 6922	.0050 4653	.0035 4739	.0024 9045	.0012 2343
2.02	.0075 6023	.0053 4032	.0037 6700	.0026 5386	.0013 1282
2.03	.0079 6869	.0056 4830	.0039 9802	.0028 2636	.0014 0785
2.04	.0083 9517	.0059 7098	.0042 4091	.0030 0835	.0015 0881
2.05	.0088 4023	.0063 0888	.0044 9614	.0032 0025	.0016 1599
2.06	.0093 0448	.0066 6256	.0047 6419	.0034 0248	.0017 2972
2.07	.0097 8852	.0070 3256	.0050 4556	.0036 1547	.0018 5031
2.08	.0102 9293	.0074 1943	.0053 4076	.0038 3968	.0019 7811
2.09	.0108 1835	.0078 2375	.0056 5030	.0040 7556	.0021 1346
2.10	.0113 6538	.0082 4610	.0059 7470	.0043 2359	.0022 5672
2.11	.0119 3466	.0086 8707	.0063 1451	.0045 8425	.0024 0826
2.12	.0125 2681	.0091 4724	.0066 7028	.0048 5804	.0025 6847
2.13	.0131 4249	.0096 2724	.0070 4257	.0051 4546	.0027 3774
2.14	.0137 8234	.0101 2767	.0074 3195	.0054 4704	.0029 1648
2.15	.0144 4700	.0106 4917	.0078 3900	.0057 6330	.0031 0511
2.16	.0151 3715	.0111 9235	.0082 6431	.0060 9478	.0033 0406
2.17	.0158 5343	.0117 5786	.0087 0849	.0064 4204	.0035 1379
2.18	.0165 9652	.0123 4635	.0091 7214	.0068 0565	.0037 3474
2.19	.0173 6708	.0129 5847	.0096 5588	.0071 8618	.0039 6739
2.20	.0181 6579	.0135 9488	.0101 6034	.0075 8421	.0042 1221
2.21	.0189 9333	.0142 5624	.0106 8616	.0080 0034	.0044 6972
2.22	.0198 5037	.0149 4322	.0112 3399	.0084 3518	.0047 4041
2.23	.0207 3760	.0156 5651	.0118 0448	.0088 8935	.0050 2480
2.24	.0216 5569	.0163 9678	.0123 9828	.0093 6346	.0053 2343
2.25	.0226 0533	.0171 6472	.0130 1607	.0098 5817	.0056 3684
2.26	.0235 8720	.0179 6101	.0136 5852	.0103 7410	.0059 6559
2.27	.0246 0197	.0187 8636	.0143 2631	.0109 1192	.0063 1025
2.28	.0256 5034	.0196 4144	.0150 2013	.0114 7229	.0066 7139
2.29	.0267 3297	.0205 2696	.0157 4067	.0120 5588	.0070 4962
2.30	.0278 5055	.0214 4361	.0164 8863	.0126 6336	.0074 4553
2.31	.0290 0374	.0223 9210	.0172 6470	.0132 9542	.0078 5974
2.32	.0301 9321	.0233 7311	.0180 6959	.0139 5275	.0082 9288
2.33	.0314 1963	.0243 8736	.0189 0401	.0146 3605	.0087 4558
2.34	.0326 8367	.0254 3553	.0197 6867	.0153 4602	.0092 1849
2.35	.0339 8596	.0265 1832	.0206 6429	.0160 8338	.0097 1227
2.36	.0353 2716	.0276 3643	.0215 9156	.0168 4882	.0102 2758
2.37	.0367 0792	.0287 9054	.0225 5121	.0176 4308	.0107 6510
2.38	.0381 2886	.0299 8134	.0235 4396	.0184 6687	.0113 2552
2.39	.0395 9060	.0312 0951	.0245 7051	.0193 2092	.0119 0953
2.40	.0410 9377	.0324 7573	.0256 3158	.0202 0595	.0125 1783
2.41	.0426 3898	.0337 8067	.0267 2788	.0211 2269	.0131 5113
2.42	.0442 2681	.0351 2500	.0278 6013	.0220 7187	.0138 1015
2.43	.0458 5785	.0365 0938	.0290 2901	.0230 5423	.0144 9562
2.44	.0475 3268	.0379 3445	.0302 3525	.0240 7048	.0152 0826
2.45	.0492 5185	.0394 0085	.0314 7953	.0251 2137	.0159 4881
2.46	.0510 1593	.0409 0923	.0327 6254	.0262 0761	.0167 1801
2.47	.0528 2543	.0424 6020	.0340 8498	.0273 2994	.0175 1660
2.48	.0546 8089	.0440 5439	.0354 4752	.0284 8907	.0183 4535
2.49	.0565 8281	.0456 9238	.0368 5084	.0296 8573	.0192 0499

W	P(W,17)	P(W,18)	P(W,19)	P(W,20)	P(W,22)
2.50	.0585 3169	.0473 7477	.0382 9560	.0309 2064	.0200 9629
2.51	.0605 2799	.0491 0214	.0397 8245	.0321 9450	.0210 2000
2.52	.0625 7217	.0508 7505	.0413 1205	.0335 0801	.0219 7688
2.53	.0646 6469	.0526 9406	.0428 8502	.0348 6188	.0229 6770
2.54	.0668 0595	.0545 5970	.0445 0200	.0362 5680	.0239 9321
2.55	.0689 9638	.0564 7249	.0461 6360	.0376 9344	.0250 5418
2.56	.0712 3635	.0584 3294	.0478 7042	.0391 7250	.0261 5136
2.57	.0735 2624	.0604 4153	.0496 2304	.0406 9462	.0272 8550
2.58	.0758 6638	.0624 9875	.0514 2205	.0422 6047	.0284 5737
2.59	.0782 5712	.0646 0504	.0532 6800	.0438 7069	.0296 6771
2.60	.0806 9876	.0667 6085	.0551 6145	.0455 2591	.0309 1727
2.61	.0831 9158	.0689 6658	.0571 0291	.0472 2676	.0322 0679
2.62	.0857 3584	.0712 2264	.0590 9290	.0489 7383	.0335 3700
2.63	.0883 3180	.0735 2941	.0611 3192	.0507 6774	.0349 0863
2.64	.0909 7967	.0758 8725	.0632 2045	.0526 0904	.0363 2240
2.65	.0936 7965	.0782 9649	.0653 5895	.0544 9832	.0377 7903
2.66	.0964 3190	.0807 5745	.0675 4786	.0564 3611	.0392 7921
2.67	.0992 3659	.0832 7042	.0697 8760	.0584 2295	.0408 2365
2.68	.1020 9383	.0858 3567	.0720 7858	.0604 5936	.0424 1301
2.69	.1050 0374	.0884 5347	.0744 2117	.0625 4582	.0440 4798
2.70	.1079 6638	.0911 2402	.0768 1573	.0646 8282	.0457 2922
2.71	.1109 8181	.0938 4753	.0792 6260	.0668 7081	.0474 5736
2.72	.1140 5006	.0966 2418	.0817 6211	.0691 1023	.0492 3305
2.73	.1171 7112	.0994 5412	.0843 1453	.0714 0151	.0510 5689
2.74	.1203 4499	.1023 3749	.0869 2015	.0737 4504	.0529 2950
2.75	.1235 7160	.1052 7438	.0895 7920	.0761 4118	.0548 5146
2.76	.1268 5090	.1082 6488	.0922 9191	.0785 9031	.0568 2333
2.77	.1301 8276	.1113 0904	.0950 5848	.0810 9274	.0588 4567
2.78	.1335 6708	.1144 0687	.0978 7908	.0836 4878	.0609 1901
2.79	.1370 0370	.1175 5840	.1007 5385	.0862 5872	.0630 4387
2.80	.1404 9244	.1207 6358	.1036 8292	.0889 2281	.0652 2073
2.81	.1440 3310	.1240 2237	.1066 6638	.0916 4129	.0674 5008
2.82	.1476 2544	.1273 3469	.1097 0431	.0944 1436	.0697 3237
2.83	.1512 6922	.1307 0044	.1127 9673	.0972 4222	.0720 6802
2.84	.1549 6416	.1341 1948	.1159 4368	.1001 2501	.0744 5745
2.85	.1587 0994	.1375 9165	.1191 4514	.1030 6287	.0769 0104
2.86	.1625 0624	.1411 1678	.1224 0106	.1060 5589	.0793 9915
2.87	.1663 5269	.1446 9464	.1257 1139	.1091 0417	.0819 5212
2.88	.1702 4891	.1483 2500	.1290 7603	.1122 0774	.0845 6026
2.89	.1741 9450	.1520 0759	.1324 9486	.1153 6662	.0872 2386
2.90	.1781 8902	.1557 4213	.1359 6772	.1185 8083	.0899 4317
2.91	.1822 3201	.1595 2828	.1394 9446	.1218 5030	.0927 1844
2.92	.1863 2299	.1633 6571	.1430 7485	.1251 7500	.0955 4988
2.93	.1904 6145	.1672 5403	.1467 0868	.1285 5482	.0984 3765
2.94	.1946 4686	.1711 9287	.1503 9567	.1319 8965	.1013 8192
2.95	.1988 7867	.1751 8178	.1541 3555	.1354 7934	.1043 8281
2.96	.2031 5629	.1792 2032	.1579 2799	.1390 2372	.1074 4041
2.97	.2074 7914	.1833 0801	.1617 7266	.1426 2257	.1105 5481
2.98	.2118 4658	.1874 4436	.1656 6919	.1462 7567	.1137 2602
2.99	.2162 5796	.1916 2883	.1696 1717	.1499 8275	.1169 5406

W	P(W,17)	P(W,18)	P(W,19)	P(W,20)	P(W,22)
3.00	.2207 1263	.1958 6088	.1736 1619	.1537 4353	.1202 3892
3.01	.2252 0988	.2001 3992	.1776 6579	.1575 5769	.1235 8054
3.02	.2297 4902	.2044 6536	.1817 6550	.1614 2487	.1269 7885
3.03	.2343 2931	.2088 3659	.1859 1482	.1653 4471	.1304 3373
3.04	.2389 5000	.2132 5294	.1901 1321	.1693 1680	.1339 4504
3.05	.2436 1032	.2177 1375	.1943 6012	.1733 4071	.1375 1262
3.06	.2483 0949	.2222 1833	.1986 5497	.1774 1598	.1411 3626
3.07	.2530 4669	.2267 6597	.2029 9716	.1815 4212	.1448 1573
3.08	.2578 2111	.2313 5593	.2073 8605	.1857 1862	.1485 5077
3.09	.2626 3189	.2359 8745	.2118 2099	.1899 4495	.1523 4110
3.10	.2674 7819	.2406 5977	.2163 0131	.1942 2053	.1561 8639
3.11	.2723 5912	.2453 7207	.2208 2630	.1985 4478	.1600 8629
3.12	.2772 7380	.2501 2356	.2253 9524	.2029 1707	.1640 4041
3.13	.2822 2132	.2549 1338	.2300 0738	.2073 3676	.1680 4835
3.14	.2872 0076	.2597 4070	.2346 6196	.2118 0318	.1721 0967
3.15	.2922 1118	.2646 0464	.2393 5819	.2163 1564	.1762 2390
3.16	.2972 5165	.2695 0431	.2440 9525	.2208 7342	.1803 9054
3.17	.3023 2120	.2744 3881	.2488 7232	.2254 7579	.1846 0905
3.18	.3074 1887	.2794 0721	.2536 8854	.2301 2198	.1888 7890
3.19	.3125 4366	.2844 0859	.2585 4306	.2348 1120	.1931 9949
3.20	.3176 9459	.2894 4200	.2634 3497	.2395 4264	.1975 7020
3.21	.3228 7066	.2945 0647	.2683 6339	.2443 1548	.2019 9041
3.22	.3280 7085	.2996 0102	.2733 2738	.2491 2887	.2064 5945
3.23	.3332 9414	.3047 2467	.2783 2601	.2539 8193	.2109 7662
3.24	.3385 3951	.3098 7642	.2833 5832	.2588 7378	.2155 4121
3.25	.3438 0593	.3150 5524	.2884 2334	.2638 0351	.2201 5246
3.26	.3490 9234	.3202 6013	.2935 2009	.2687 7019	.2248 0963
3.27	.3543 9770	.3254 9005	.2986 4758	.2737 7287	.2295 1190
3.28	.3597 2097	.3307 4395	.3038 0479	.2788 1060	.2342 5847
3.29	.3650 6108	.3360 2078	.3089 9070	.2838 8241	.2390 4849
3.30	.3704 1697	.3413 1950	.3142 0428	.2889 8728	.2438 8111
3.31	.3757 8758	.3466 3903	.3194 4447	.2941 2423	.2487 5543
3.32	.3811 7185	.3519 7830	.3247 1023	.2992 9222	.2536 7056
3.33	.3865 6870	.3573 3624	.3300 0048	.3044 9022	.2586 2556
3.34	.3919 7706	.3627 1175	.3353 1416	.3097 1719	.2636 1949
3.35	.3973 9587	.3681 0377	.3406 5018	.3149 7206	.2686 5138
3.36	.4028 2405	.3735 1119	.3460 0745	.3202 5376	.2737 2025
3.37	.4082 6054	.3789 3293	.3513 8488	.3255 6121	.2788 2510
3.38	.4137 0426	.3843 6789	.3567 8136	.3308 9332	.2839 6491
3.39	.4191 5415	.3898 1498	.3621 9578	.3362 4900	.2891 3864
3.40	.4246 0916	.3952 7309	.3676 2705	.3416 2712	.2943 4524
3.41	.4300 6821	.4007 4113	.3730 7403	.3470 2658	.2995 8364
3.42	.4355 3025	.4062 1800	.3785 3561	.3524 4625	.3048 5277
3.43	.4409 9422	.4117 0261	.3840 1067	.3578 8501	.3101 5152
3.44	.4464 5909	.4171 9386	.3894 9809	.3633 4172	.3154 7881
3.45	.4519 2381	.4226 9067	.3949 9675	.3688 1524	.3208 3350
3.46	.4573 8734	.4281 9194	.4005 0551	.3743 0444	.3262 1446
3.47	.4628 4866	.4336 9659	.4060 2327	.3798 0817	.3316 2057
3.48	.4683 0674	.4392 0354	.4115 4889	.3853 2528	.3370 5067
3.49	.4737 6056	.4447 1171	.4170 8125	.3908 5462	.3425 0361

W	P(W,17)	P(W,18)	P(W,19)	P(W,20)	P(W,22)
3.50	.4792 0913	.4502 2004	.4226 1925	.3963 9505	.3479 7822
3.51	.4846 5143	.4557 2746	.4281 6177	.4019 4542	.3534 7333
3.52	.4900 8650	.4612 3291	.4337 0769	.4075 0458	.3589 8776
3.53	.4955 1334	.4667 3535	.4392 5591	.4130 7139	.3645 2034
3.54	.5009 3098	.4722 3373	.4448 0533	.4186 4469	.3700 6987
3.55	.5063 3847	.4777 2701	.4503 5486	.4242 2336	.3756 3517
3.56	.5117 3487	.4832 1418	.4559 0340	.4298 0624	.3812 1504
3.57	.5171 1922	.4886 9422	.4614 4988	.4353 9221	.3868 0830
3.58	.5224 9062	.4941 6612	.4669 9322	.4409 8015	.3924 1373
3.59	.5278 4814	.4996 2888	.4725 3235	.4465 6892	.3980 3015
3.60	.5331 9089	.5050 8153	.4780 6623	.4521 5741	.4036 5636
3.61	.5385 1798	.5105 2309	.4835 9379	.4577 4451	.4092 9117
3.62	.5438 2854	.5159 5259	.4891 1401	.4633 2911	.4149 3338
3.63	.5491 2170	.5213 6909	.4946 2584	.4689 1013	.4205 8180
3.64	.5543 9662	.5267 7165	.5001 2829	.4744 8647	.4262 3524
3.65	.5596 5246	.5321 5934	.5056 2033	.4800 5706	.4318 9253
3.66	.5648 8841	.5375 3126	.5111 0098	.4856 2084	.4375 5248
3.67	.5701 0367	.5428 8650	.5165 6926	.4911 7673	.4432 1392
3.68	.5752 9745	.5482 2419	.5220 2418	.4967 2371	.4488 7569
3.69	.5804 6896	.5535 4344	.5274 6480	.5022 6073	.4545 3662
3.70	.5856 1747	.5588 4342	.5328 9018	.5077 8677	.4601 9557
3.71	.5907 4221	.5641 2328	.5382 9937	.5133 0081	.4658 5138
3.72	.5958 4247	.5693 8219	.5436 9147	.5188 0187	.4715 0293
3.73	.6009 1754	.5746 1934	.5490 6558	.5242 8894	.4771 4908
3.74	.6059 6672	.5798 3394	.5544 2080	.5297 6108	.4827 8872
3.75	.6109 8933	.5850 2522	.5597 5627	.5352 1730	.4884 2076
3.76	.6159 8472	.5901 9241	.5650 7113	.5406 5668	.4940 4408
3.77	.6209 5224	.5953 3477	.5703 6455	.5460 7827	.4996 5761
3.78	.6258 9125	.6004 5156	.5756 3568	.5514 8118	.5052 6029
3.79	.6308 0115	.6055 4208	.5808 8374	.5568 6450	.5108 5104
3.80	.6356 8135	.6106 0563	.5861 0793	.5622 2734	.5164 2884
3.81	.6405 3127	.6156 4154	.5913 0746	.5675 6885	.5219 9264
3.82	.6453 5034	.6206 4913	.5964 8159	.5728 8817	.5275 4144
3.83	.6501 3802	.6256 2778	.6016 2958	.5781 8446	.5330 7422
3.84	.6548 9379	.6305 7685	.6067 5070	.5834 5692	.5385 9001
3.85	.6596 1714	.6354 9574	.6118 4424	.5887 0473	.5440 8783
3.86	.6643 0758	.6403 8384	.6169 0952	.5939 2713	.5495 6673
3.87	.6689 6463	.6452 4060	.6219 4586	.5991 2335	.5550 2577
3.88	.6735 8783	.6500 6545	.6269 5262	.6042 9263	.5604 6403
3.89	.6781 7675	.6548 5786	.6319 2916	.6094 3425	.5658 8059
3.90	.6827 3095	.6596 1730	.6368 7486	.6145 4751	.5712 7458
3.91	.6872 5004	.6643 4328	.6417 8912	.6196 3170	.5766 4512
3.92	.6917 3363	.6690 3531	.6466 7137	.6246 8616	.5819 9137
3.93	.6961 8133	.6736 9292	.6515 2104	.6297 1022	.5873 1247
3.94	.7005 9280	.6783 1565	.6563 3759	.6347 0325	.5926 0763
3.95	.7049 6770	.6829 0309	.6611 2050	.6396 6464	.5978 7604
3.96	.7093 0571	.6874 5482	.6658 6925	.6445 9378	.6031 1692
3.97	.7136 0651	.6919 7043	.6705 8336	.6494 9010	.6083 2951
3.98	.7178 6983	.6964 4955	.6752 6235	.6543 5302	.6135 1307
3.99	.7220 9538	.7008 9183	.6799 0578	.6591 8201	.6186 6688

W	P(W,17)	P(W,18)	P(W,19)	P(W,20)	P(W,22)
4.00	.7262 8291	.7052 9690	.6845 1321	.6639 7655	.6237 9024
4.01	.7304 3218	.7096 6445	.6890 8423	.6687 3612	.6288 8246
4.02	.7345 4296	.7139 9416	.6936 1843	.6734 6025	.6339 4288
4.03	.7386 1505	.7182 8575	.6981 1544	.6781 4846	.6389 7086
4.04	.7426 4824	.7225 3893	.7025 7489	.6828 0030	.6439 6578
4.05	.7466 4237	.7267 5345	.7069 9645	.6874 1535	.6489 2702
4.06	.7505 9727	.7309 2906	.7113 7978	.6919 9319	.6538 5401
4.07	.7545 1279	.7350 6554	.7157 2457	.6965 3342	.6587 4618
4.08	.7583 8880	.7391 6266	.7200 3053	.7010 3569	.6636 0298
4.09	.7622 2518	.7432 2025	.7242 9740	.7054 9962	.6684 2390
4.10	.7660 2182	.7472 3812	.7285 2490	.7099 2488	.6732 0843
4.11	.7697 7863	.7512 1610	.7327 1280	.7143 1114	.6779 5608
4.12	.7734 9554	.7551 5405	.7368 6088	.7186 5812	.6826 6638
4.13	.7771 7249	.7590 5184	.7409 6893	.7229 6551	.6873 3890
4.14	.7808 0943	.7629 0934	.7450 3676	.7272 3306	.6919 7321
4.15	.7844 0631	.7667 2646	.7490 6420	.7314 6052	.6965 6889
4.16	.7879 6313	.7705 0311	.7530 5108	.7356 4765	.7011 2557
4.17	.7914 7986	.7742 3921	.7569 9726	.7397 9424	.7056 4288
4.18	.7949 5652	.7779 3470	.7609 0262	.7439 0008	.7101 2046
4.19	.7983 9312	.7815 8954	.7647 6704	.7479 6501	.7145 5800
4.20	.8017 8968	.7852 0370	.7685 9044	.7519 8885	.7189 5517
4.21	.8051 4625	.7887 7715	.7723 7272	.7559 7146	.7233 1168
4.22	.8084 6288	.7923 0990	.7761 1382	.7599 1270	.7276 2727
4.23	.8117 3963	.7958 0195	.7798 1368	.7638 1245	.7319 0168
4.24	.8149 7657	.7992 5331	.7834 7228	.7676 7063	.7361 3467
4.25	.8181 7379	.8026 6403	.7870 8958	.7714 8713	.7403 2603
4.26	.8213 3139	.8060 3415	.7906 6558	.7752 6189	.7444 7555
4.27	.8244 4946	.8093 6372	.7942 0027	.7789 9485	.7485 8304
4.28	.8275 2814	.8126 5282	.7976 9368	.7826 8598	.7526 4835
4.29	.8305 6754	.8159 0152	.8011 4583	.7863 3525	.7566 7133
4.30	.8335 6780	.8191 0992	.8045 5677	.7899 4264	.7606 5184
4.31	.8365 2907	.8222 7811	.8079 2654	.7935 0816	.7645 8976
4.32	.8394 5149	.8254 0622	.8112 5523	.7970 3181	.7684 8500
4.33	.8423 3524	.8284 9436	.8145 4289	.8005 1364	.7723 3748
4.34	.8451 8049	.8315 4267	.8177 8963	.8039 5368	.7761 4713
4.35	.8479 8741	.8345 5129	.8209 9555	.8073 5199	.7799 1390
4.36	.8507 5619	.8375 2037	.8241 6075	.8107 0863	.7836 3775
4.37	.8534 8704	.8404 5008	.8272 8536	.8140 2368	.7873 1865
4.38	.8561 8015	.8433 4059	.8303 6952	.8172 9724	.7909 5662
4.39	.8588 3574	.8461 9208	.8334 1337	.8205 2940	.7945 5164
4.40	.8614 5402	.8490 0473	.8364 1705	.8237 2028	.7981 0375
4.41	.8640 3523	.8517 7875	.8393 8074	.8268 7001	.8016 1299
4.42	.8665 7959	.8545 1434	.8423 0462	.8299 7872	.8050 7939
4.43	.8690 8734	.8572 1171	.8451 8885	.8330 4655	.8085 0303
4.44	.8715 5873	.8598 7108	.8480 3363	.8360 7368	.8118 8398
4.45	.8739 9401	.8624 9269	.8508 3916	.8390 6025	.8152 2233
4.46	.8763 9343	.8650 7676	.8536 0565	.8420 0645	.8185 1818
4.47	.8787 5726	.8676 2353	.8563 3331	.8449 1247	.8217 7164
4.48	.8810 8576	.8701 3326	.8590 2238	.8477 7849	.8249 8285
4.49	.8833 7921	.8726 0619	.8616 7307	.8506 0473	.8281 5193

W	P(W,17)	P(W,18)	P(W,19)	P(W,20)	P(W,22)
4.50	.8856 3789	.8750 4260	.8642 8563	.8533 9139	.8312 7904
4.51	.8878 6207	.8774 4273	.8668 6030	.8561 3870	.8343 6433
4.52	.8900 5204	.8798 0688	.8693 9733	.8588 4688	.8374 0798
4.53	.8922 0809	.8821 3530	.8718 9699	.8615 1618	.8404 1016
4.54	.8943 3051	.8844 2829	.8743 5954	.8641 4683	.8433 7106
4.55	.8964 1961	.8866 8612	.8767 8524	.8667 3908	.8462 9088
4.56	.8984 7568	.8889 0910	.8791 7438	.8692 9319	.8491 6983
4.57	.9004 9903	.8910 9751	.8815 2723	.8718 0943	.8520 0813
4.58	.9024 8997	.8932 5165	.8838 4409	.8742 8807	.8548 0601
4.59	.9044 4880	.8953 7183	.8861 2525	.8767 2939	.8575 6370
4.60	.9063 7584	.8974 5836	.8883 7099	.8791 3366	.8602 8144
4.61	.9082 7140	.8995 1154	.8905 8163	.8815 0117	.8629 5948
4.62	.9101 3581	.9015 3169	.8927 5747	.8838 3222	.8655 9809
4.63	.9119 6938	.9035 1912	.8948 9881	.8861 2711	.8681 9753
4.64	.9137 7243	.9054 7416	.8970 0598	.8883 8614	.8707 5807
4.65	.9155 4529	.9073 9712	.8990 7928	.8906 0962	.8732 7999
4.66	.9172 8828	.9092 8834	.9011 1904	.8927 9786	.8757 6357
4.67	.9190 0173	.9111 4813	.9031 2558	.8949 5117	.8782 0912
4.68	.9206 8597	.9129 7683	.9050 9923	.8970 6988	.8806 1693
4.69	.9223 4132	.9147 7476	.9070 4032	.8991 5431	.8829 8729
4.70	.9239 6811	.9165 4226	.9089 4917	.9012 0479	.8853 2053
4.71	.9255 6669	.9182 7966	.9108 2612	.9032 2164	.8876 1695
4.72	.9271 3737	.9199 8730	.9126 7151	.9052 0521	.8898 7688
4.73	.9286 8049	.9216 6551	.9144 8567	.9071 5582	.8921 0063
4.74	.9301 9637	.9233 1463	.9162 6894	.9090 7381	.8942 8854
4.75	.9316 8536	.9249 3500	.9180 2167	.9109 5954	.8964 4093
4.76	.9331 4779	.9265 2696	.9197 4419	.9128 1333	.8985 5815
4.77	.9345 8397	.9280 9084	.9214 3686	.9146 3553	.9006 4053
4.78	.9359 9426	.9296 2698	.9231 0000	.9164 2649	.9026 8841
4.79	.9373 7898	.9311 3573	.9247 3398	.9181 8657	.9047 0214
4.80	.9387 3845	.9326 1743	.9263 3913	.9199 1609	.9066 8208
4.81	.9400 7301	.9340 7240	.9279 1580	.9216 1543	.9086 2856
4.82	.9413 8299	.9355 0100	.9294 6433	.9232 8493	.9105 4194
4.83	.9426 6872	.9369 0356	.9309 8509	.9249 2493	.9124 2259
4.84	.9439 3053	.9382 8042	.9324 7840	.9265 3581	.9142 7085
4.85	.9451 6873	.9396 3192	.9339 4462	.9281 1790	.9160 8709
4.86	.9463 8366	.9409 5839	.9353 8409	.9296 7156	.9178 7166
4.87	.9475 7565	.9422 6017	.9367 9717	.9311 9714	.9196 2494
4.88	.9487 4500	.9435 3760	.9381 8419	.9326 9501	.9213 4728
4.89	.9498 9205	.9447 9101	.9395 4550	.9341 6551	.9230 3905
4.90	.9510 1711	.9460 2073	.9408 8145	.9356 0899	.9247 0061
4.91	.9521 2051	.9472 2709	.9421 9237	.9370 2582	.9263 3234
4.92	.9532 0255	.9484 1043	.9434 7862	.9384 1633	.9279 3459
4.93	.9542 6356	.9495 7107	.9447 4052	.9397 8089	.9295 0773
4.94	.9553 0385	.9507 0935	.9459 7843	.9411 1985	.9310 5214
4.95	.9563 2371	.9518 2557	.9471 9268	.9424 3354	.9325 6817
4.96	.9573 2348	.9529 2008	.9483 8360	.9437 2233	.9340 5620
4.97	.9583 0344	.9539 9319	.9495 5154	.9449 8656	.9355 1659
4.98	.9592 6391	.9550 4522	.9506 9682	.9462 2657	.9369 4971
4.99	.9602 0519	.9560 7649	.9518 1979	.9474 4272	.9383 5592

W	P(W,17)	P(W,18)	P(W,19)	P(W,20)	P(W,22)
5.00	.9611 2758	.9570 8731	.9529 2075	.9486 3534	.9397 3558
5.01	.9620 3137	.9580 7800	.9540 0006	.9498 0477	.9410 8907
5.02	.9629 1687	.9590 4887	.9550 5803	.9509 5136	.9424 1674
5.03	.9637 8435	.9600 0023	.9560 9499	.9520 7544	.9437 1895
5.04	.9646 3412	.9609 3239	.9571 1125	.9531 7735	.9449 9607
5.05	.9654 6646	.9618 4565	.9581 0715	.9542 5743	.9462 4845
5.06	.9662 8166	.9627 4030	.9590 8299	.9553 1600	.9474 7645
5.07	.9670 8000	.9636 1666	.9600 3910	.9563 5340	.9486 8043
5.08	.9678 6175	.9644 7502	.9609 7577	.9573 6995	.9498 6073
5.09	.9686 2721	.9653 1567	.9618 9334	.9583 6598	.9510 1772
5.10	.9693 7663	.9661 3890	.9627 9209	.9593 4180	.9521 5174
5.11	.9701 1029	.9669 4501	.9636 7235	.9602 9775	.9532 6313
5.12	.9708 2847	.9677 3427	.9645 3440	.9612 3414	.9543 5225
5.13	.9715 3142	.9685 0698	.9653 7856	.9621 5129	.9554 1944
5.14	.9722 1942	.9692 6341	.9662 0511	.9630 4950	.9564 6503
5.15	.9728 9271	.9700 0384	.9670 1435	.9639 2909	.9574 8938
5.16	.9735 5157	.9707 2855	.9678 0658	.9647 9036	.9584 9280
5.17	.9741 9624	.9714 3780	.9685 8208	.9656 3362	.9594 7564
5.18	.9748 2697	.9721 3187	.9693 4113	.9664 5918	.9604 3824
5.19	.9754 4402	.9728 1103	.9700 8403	.9672 6732	.9613 8090
5.20	.9760 4762	.9734 7553	.9708 1104	.9680 5834	.9623 0397
5.21	.9766 3803	.9741 2563	.9715 2246	.9688 3255	.9632 0777
5.22	.9772 1549	.9747 6160	.9722 1854	.9695 9022	.9640 9261
5.23	.9777 8022	.9753 8369	.9728 9956	.9703 3165	.9649 5881
5.24	.9783 3247	.9759 9214	.9735 6579	.9710 5712	.9658 0669
5.25	.9788 7246	.9765 8721	.9742 1750	.9717 6690	.9666 3656
5.26	.9794 0043	.9771 6915	.9748 5494	.9724 6129	.9674 4872
5.27	.9799 1660	.9777 3819	.9754 7838	.9731 4054	.9682 4349
5.28	.9804 2118	.9782 9457	.9760 8806	.9738 0494	.9690 2115
5.29	.9809 1441	.9788 3853	.9766 8425	.9744 5475	.9697 8202
5.30	.9813 9649	.9793 7030	.9772 6718	.9750 9023	.9705 2639
5.31	.9818 6765	.9798 9011	.9778 3712	.9757 1166	.9712 5454
5.32	.9823 2808	.9803 9819	.9783 9429	.9763 1928	.9719 6678
5.33	.9827 7800	.9808 9476	.9789 3894	.9769 1335	.9726 6337
5.34	.9832 1761	.9813 8004	.9794 7131	.9774 9412	.9733 4462
5.35	.9836 4712	.9818 5426	.9799 9163	.9780 6185	.9740 1079
5.36	.9840 6672	.9823 1762	.9805 0012	.9786 1678	.9746 6217
5.37	.9844 7661	.9827 7033	.9809 9703	.9791 5915	.9752 9901
5.38	.9848 7697	.9832 1261	.9814 8256	.9796 8920	.9759 2161
5.39	.9852 6801	.9836 4466	.9819 5694	.9802 0717	.9765 3021
5.40	.9856 4991	.9840 6668	.9824 2040	.9807 1329	.9771 2509
5.41	.9860 2285	.9844 7888	.9828 7314	.9812 0779	.9777 0650
5.42	.9863 8701	.9848 8144	.9833 1537	.9816 9090	.9782 7469
5.43	.9867 4257	.9852 7456	.9837 4730	.9821 6283	.9788 2993
5.44	.9870 8972	.9856 5844	.9841 6915	.9826 2382	.9793 7245
5.45	.9874 2861	.9860 3326	.9845 8111	.9830 7407	.9799 0251
5.46	.9877 5942	.9863 9920	.9849 8337	.9835 1380	.9804 2035
5.47	.9880 8232	.9867 5645	.9853 7615	.9839 4322	.9809 2620
5.48	.9883 9748	.9871 0518	.9857 5962	.9843 6254	.9814 2030
5.49	.9887 0505	.9874 4557	.9861 3399	.9847 7196	.9819 0289

W	P(W,17)	P(W,18)	P(W,19)	P(W,20)	P(W,22)
5.50	.9890 0519	.9877 7781	.9864 9943	.9851 7168	.9823 7418
5.51	.9892 9807	.9881 0204	.9868 5613	.9855 6191	.9828 3442
5.52	.9895 8383	.9884 1845	.9872 0428	.9859 4283	.9832 8381
5.53	.9898 6263	.9887 2720	.9875 4405	.9863 1464	.9837 2259
5.54	.9901 3462	.9890 2845	.9878 7561	.9866 7753	.9841 5096
5.55	.9903 9993	.9893 2235	.9881 9915	.9870 3168	.9845 6913
5.56	.9906 5873	.9896 0908	.9885 1482	.9873 7727	.9849 7732
5.57	.9909 1114	.9898 8877	.9888 2280	.9877 1449	.9853 7573
5.58	.9911 5731	.9901 6159	.9891 2325	.9880 4351	.9857 6456
5.59	.9913 9737	.9904 2768	.9894 1633	.9883 6451	.9861 4401
5.60	.9916 3146	.9906 8718	.9897 0220	.9886 7766	.9865 1429
5.61	.9918 5970	.9909 4024	.9899 8101	.9889 8312	.9868 7557
5.62	.9920 8223	.9911 8701	.9902 5293	.9892 8106	.9872 2806
5.63	.9922 9918	.9914 2762	.9905 1809	.9895 7164	.9875 7193
5.64	.9925 1067	.9916 6220	.9907 7665	.9898 5503	.9879 0737
5.65	.9927 1682	.9918 9089	.9910 2875	.9901 3137	.9882 3457
5.66	.9929 1774	.9921 1382	.9912 7454	.9904 0083	.9885 5369
5.67	.9931 1357	.9923 3113	.9915 1415	.9906 6355	.9888 6492
5.68	.9933 0441	.9925 4292	.9917 4772	.9909 1968	.9891 6842
5.69	.9934 9038	.9927 4934	.9919 7539	.9911 6938	.9894 6436
5.70	.9936 7159	.9929 5050	.9921 9729	.9914 1277	.9897 5291
5.71	.9938 4815	.9931 4652	.9924 1355	.9916 5001	.9900 3423
5.72	.9940 2016	.9933 3753	.9926 2430	.9918 8123	.9903 0849
5.73	.9941 8773	.9935 2362	.9928 2966	.9921 0657	.9905 7583
5.74	.9943 5096	.9937 0492	.9930 2975	.9923 2616	.9908 3641
5.75	.9945 0995	.9938 8154	.9932 2470	.9925 4013	.9910 9038
5.76	.9946 6481	.9940 5358	.9934 1462	.9927 4860	.9913 3789
5.77	.9948 1563	.9942 2115	.9935 9963	.9929 5171	.9915 7909
5.78	.9949 6250	.9943 8436	.9937 7985	.9931 4958	.9918 1412
5.79	.9951 0551	.9945 4330	.9939 5538	.9933 4233	.9920 4312
5.80	.9952 4477	.9946 9809	.9941 2633	.9935 3007	.9922 6622
5.81	.9953 8035	.9948 4881	.9942 9282	.9937 1293	.9924 8357
5.82	.9955 1235	.9949 9556	.9944 5494	.9938 9101	.9926 9529
5.83	.9956 4085	.9951 3844	.9946 1280	.9940 6444	.9929 0152
5.84	.9957 6593	.9952 7753	.9947 6650	.9942 3331	.9931 0237
5.85	.9958 8768	.9954 1294	.9949 1613	.9943 9774	.9932 9799
5.86	.9960 0618	.9955 4474	.9950 6181	.9945 5783	.9934 8848
5.87	.9961 2150	.9956 7303	.9952 0361	.9947 1368	.9936 7397
5.88	.9962 3372	.9957 9789	.9953 4164	.9948 6540	.9938 5459
5.89	.9963 4293	.9959 1940	.9954 7598	.9950 1308	.9940 3043
5.90	.9964 4919	.9960 3764	.9956 0672	.9951 5683	.9942 0162
5.91	.9965 5257	.9961 5270	.9957 3396	.9952 9673	.9943 6826
5.92	.9966 5315	.9962 6464	.9958 5776	.9954 3287	.9945 3047
5.93	.9967 5099	.9963 7356	.9959 7823	.9955 6536	.9946 8836
5.94	.9968 4617	.9964 7952	.9960 9544	.9956 9428	.9948 4201
5.95	.9969 3874	.9965 8259	.9962 0947	.9958 1972	.9949 9155
5.96	.9970 2879	.9966 8285	.9963 2040	.9959 4175	.9951 3706
5.97	.9971 1635	.9967 8037	.9964 2831	.9960 6048	.9952 7865
5.98	.9972 0151	.9968 7522	.9965 3327	.9961 7597	.9954 1641
5.99	.9972 8432	.9969 6745	.9966 3535	.9962 8830	.9955 5044

W	P(W,17)	P(W,18)	P(W,19)	P(W,20)	P(W,22)
6.00	.9973 6484	.9970 5715	.9967 3463	.9963 9757	.9956 8082
6.01	.9974 4312	.9971 4436	.9968 3118	.9965 0383	.9958 0765
6.02	.9975 1923	.9972 2917	.9969 2506	.9966 0717	.9959 3101
6.03	.9975 9322	.9973 1161	.9970 1635	.9967 0767	.9960 5100
6.04	.9976 6515	.9973 9177	.9971 0510	.9968 0538	.9961 6769
6.05	.9977 3506	.9974 6968	.9971 9138	.9969 0039	.9962 8116
6.06	.9978 0301	.9975 4542	.9972 7527	.9969 9276	.9963 9151
6.07	.9978 6905	.9976 1904	.9973 5680	.9970 8255	.9964 9880
6.08	.9979 3323	.9976 9059	.9974 3606	.9971 6984	.9966 0312
6.09	.9979 9560	.9977 6012	.9975 1309	.9972 5469	.9967 0453
6.10	.9980 5620	.9978 2770	.9975 8796	.9973 3716	.9968 0312
6.11	.9981 1508	.9978 9336	.9976 6071	.9974 1731	.9968 9895
6.12	.9981 7229	.9979 5716	.9977 3140	.9974 9520	.9969 9210
6.13	.9982 2786	.9980 1914	.9978 0010	.9975 7089	.9970 8263
6.14	.9982 8185	.9980 7936	.9978 6684	.9976 4444	.9971 7061
6.15	.9983 3429	.9981 3787	.9979 3168	.9977 1590	.9972 5611
6.16	.9983 8523	.9981 9470	.9979 9468	.9977 8533	.9973 3919
6.17	.9984 3470	.9982 4989	.9980 5587	.9978 5278	.9974 1992
6.18	.9984 8275	.9983 0351	.9981 1531	.9979 1830	.9974 9835
6.19	.9985 2941	.9983 5557	.9981 7304	.9979 8194	.9975 7455
6.20	.9985 7472	.9984 0614	.9982 2911	.9980 4376	.9976 4857
6.21	.9986 1871	.9984 5524	.9982 8356	.9981 0380	.9977 2047
6.22	.9986 6143	.9985 0292	.9983 3644	.9981 6210	.9977 9031
6.23	.9987 0290	.9985 4921	.9983 8778	.9982 1873	.9978 5814
6.24	.9987 4316	.9985 9416	.9984 3764	.9982 7371	.9979 2402
6.25	.9987 8224	.9986 3779	.9984 8604	.9983 2709	.9979 8799
6.26	.9988 2017	.9986 8015	.9985 3303	.9983 7892	.9980 5012
6.27	.9988 5699	.9987 2126	.9985 7865	.9984 2924	.9981 1043
6.28	.9988 9273	.9987 6117	.9986 2293	.9984 7809	.9981 6900
6.29	.9989 2741	.9987 9990	.9986 6590	.9985 2551	.9982 2585
6.30	.9989 6106	.9988 3749	.9987 0762	.9985 7154	.9982 8105
6.31	.9989 9372	.9988 7397	.9987 4810	.9986 1621	.9983 3463
6.32	.9990 2541	.9989 0937	.9987 8739	.9986 5956	.9983 8664
6.33	.9990 5615	.9989 4371	.9988 2552	.9987 0163	.9984 3711
6.34	.9990 8598	.9989 7704	.9988 6251	.9987 4246	.9984 8610
6.35	.9991 1492	.9990 0937	.9988 9840	.9987 8208	.9985 3365
6.36	.9991 4298	.9990 4073	.9989 3322	.9988 2052	.9985 7978
6.37	.9991 7021	.9990 7116	.9989 6700	.9988 5781	.9986 2454
6.38	.9991 9662	.9991 0067	.9989 9977	.9988 9399	.9986 6798
6.39	.9992 2223	.9991 2930	.9990 3156	.9989 2908	.9987 1012
6.40	.9992 4707	.9991 5706	.9990 6239	.9989 6313	.9987 5100
6.41	.9992 7116	.9991 8399	.9990 9230	.9989 9615	.9987 9066
6.42	.9992 9452	.9992 1010	.9991 2130	.9990 2817	.9988 2913
6.43	.9993 1717	.9992 3542	.9991 4942	.9990 5923	.9988 6644
6.44	.9993 3913	.9992 5997	.9991 7669	.9990 8935	.9989 0263
6.45	.9993 6041	.9992 8377	.9992 0314	.9991 1856	.9989 3772
6.46	.9993 8105	.9993 0685	.9992 2878	.9991 4688	.9989 7176
6.47	.9994 0106	.9993 2922	.9992 5363	.9991 7433	.9990 0476
6.48	.9994 2045	.9993 5091	.9992 7773	.9992 0095	.9990 3676
6.49	.9994 3925	.9993 7193	.9993 0109	.9992 2676	.9990 6779

W	P(W,17)	P(W,18)	P(W,19)	P(W,20)	P(W,22)
6.50	.9994 5747	.9993 9231	.9993 2374	.9992 5178	.9990 9787
6.51	.9994 7513	.9994 1206	.9993 4568	.9992 7603	.9991 2703
6.52	.9994 9224	.9994 3120	.9993 6696	.9992 9953	.9991 5530
6.53	.9995 0882	.9994 4975	.9993 8757	.9993 2232	.9991 8270
6.54	.9995 2488	.9994 6772	.9994 0755	.9993 4439	.9992 0926
6.55	.9995 4045	.9994 8514	.9994 2691	.9993 6579	.9992 3500
6.56	.9995 5553	.9995 0201	.9994 4567	.9993 8652	.9992 5994
6.57	.9995 7014	.9995 1836	.9994 6384	.9994 0661	.9992 8412
6.58	.9995 8429	.9995 3420	.9994 8145	.9994 2607	.9993 0754
6.59	.9995 9800	.9995 4954	.9994 9851	.9994 4493	.9993 3024
6.60	.9996 1128	.9995 6440	.9995 1503	.9994 6320	.9993 5223
6.61	.9996 2415	.9995 7880	.9995 3104	.9994 8090	.9993 7353
6.62	.9996 3660	.9995 9274	.9995 4655	.9994 9804	.9993 9417
6.63	.9996 4867	.9996 0625	.9995 6156	.9995 1464	.9994 1417
6.64	.9996 6035	.9996 1932	.9995 7611	.9995 3072	.9994 3353
6.65	.9996 7166	.9996 3199	.9995 9019	.9995 4630	.9994 5229
6.66	.9996 8262	.9996 4425	.9996 0383	.9995 6138	.9994 7046
6.67	.9996 9322	.9996 5612	.9996 1704	.9995 7599	.9994 8805
6.68	.9997 0349	.9996 6762	.9996 2982	.9995 9013	.9995 0509
6.69	.9997 1343	.9996 7875	.9996 4220	.9996 0382	.9995 2159
6.70	.9997 2305	.9996 8952	.9996 5419	.9996 1708	.9995 3756
6.71	.9997 3236	.9996 9995	.9996 6579	.9996 2991	.9995 5303
6.72	.9997 4138	.9997 1004	.9996 7703	.9996 4234	.9995 6800
6.73	.9997 5010	.9997 1981	.9996 8790	.9996 5436	.9995 8250
6.74	.9997 5854	.9997 2927	.9996 9842	.9996 6600	.9995 9653
6.75	.9997 6672	.9997 3842	.9997 0860	.9996 7727	.9996 1011
6.76	.9997 7462	.9997 4728	.9997 1846	.9996 8818	.9996 2326
6.77	.9997 8227	.9997 5585	.9997 2800	.9996 9873	.9996 3599
6.78	.9997 8968	.9997 6414	.9997 3723	.9997 0894	.9996 4830
6.79	.9997 9684	.9997 7217	.9997 4616	.9997 1882	.9996 6022
6.80	.9998 0377	.9997 7993	.9997 5480	.9997 2839	.9996 7175
6.81	.9998 1047	.9997 8744	.9997 6316	.9997 3764	.9996 8291
6.82	.9998 1696	.9997 9471	.9997 7125	.9997 4659	.9996 9371
6.83	.9998 2323	.9998 0173	.9997 7907	.9997 5525	.9997 0415
6.84	.9998 2930	.9998 0853	.9997 8664	.9997 6362	.9997 1426
6.85	.9998 3516	.9998 1511	.9997 9396	.9997 7172	.9997 2404
6.86	.9998 4084	.9998 2147	.9998 0104	.9997 7956	.9997 3349
6.87	.9998 4632	.9998 2762	.9998 0788	.9997 8714	.9997 4264
6.88	.9998 5163	.9998 3356	.9998 1451	.9997 9447	.9997 5149
6.89	.9998 5676	.9998 3931	.9998 2091	.9998 0156	.9997 6004
6.90	.9998 6172	.9998 4487	.9998 2710	.9998 0841	.9997 6832
6.91	.9998 6652	.9998 5025	.9998 3309	.9998 1504	.9997 7632
6.92	.9998 7116	.9998 5545	.9998 3888	.9998 2145	.9997 8406
6.93	.9998 7564	.9998 6047	.9998 4447	.9998 2765	.9997 9154
6.94	.9998 7997	.9998 6533	.9998 4988	.9998 3364	.9997 9877
6.95	.9998 8416	.9998 7003	.9998 5511	.9998 3943	.9998 0577
6.96	.9998 8821	.9998 7456	.9998 6017	.9998 4503	.9998 1253
6.97	.9998 9212	.9998 7895	.9998 6505	.9998 5044	.9998 1906
6.98	.9998 9590	.9998 8319	.9998 6978	.9998 5567	.9998 2538
6.99	.9998 9956	.9998 8729	.9998 7434	.9998 6072	.9998 3149

W	P(W,17)	P(W,18)	P(W,19)	P(W,20)	P(W,22)
7.00	.9999 0309	.9998 9125	.9998 7875	.9998 6561	.9998 3739
7.01	.9999 0650	.9998 9507	.9998 8301	.9998 7033	.9998 4309
7.02	.9999 0980	.9998 9877	.9998 8713	.9998 7489	.9998 4860
7.03	.9999 1298	.9999 0234	.9998 9111	.9998 7930	.9998 5393
7.04	.9999 1606	.9999 0579	.9998 9496	.9998 8356	.9998 5908
7.05	.9999 1903	.9999 0913	.9998 9867	.9998 8767	.9998 6405
7.06	.9999 2191	.9999 1235	.9999 0226	.9998 9165	.9998 6885
7.07	.9999 2468	.9999 1546	.9999 0573	.9998 9549	.9998 7350
7.08	.9999 2736	.9999 1846	.9999 0908	.9998 9920	.9998 7798
7.09	.9999 2995	.9999 2137	.9999 1231	.9999 0278	.9998 8231
7.10	.9999 3245	.9999 2417	.9999 1543	.9999 0624	.9998 8649
7.11	.9999 3486	.9999 2688	.9999 1845	.9999 0958	.9998 9054
7.12	.9999 3719	.9999 2949	.9999 2137	.9999 1281	.9998 9444
7.13	.9999 3944	.9999 3202	.9999 2418	.9999 1593	.9998 9821
7.14	.9999 4161	.9999 3445	.9999 2690	.9999 1894	.9999 0185
7.15	.9999 4371	.9999 3681	.9999 2952	.9999 2185	.9999 0536
7.16	.9999 4574	.9999 3908	.9999 3205	.9999 2465	.9999 0876
7.17	.9999 4769	.9999 4127	.9999 3450	.9999 2736	.9999 1204
7.18	.9999 4958	.9999 4339	.9999 3686	.9999 2998	.9999 1520
7.19	.9999 5140	.9999 4544	.9999 3914	.9999 3251	.9999 1826
7.20	.9999 5316	.9999 4741	.9999 4134	.9999 3494	.9999 2120
7.21	.9999 5486	.9999 4931	.9999 4346	.9999 3730	.9999 2405
7.22	.9999 5650	.9999 5115	.9999 4551	.9999 3957	.9999 2680
7.23	.9999 5808	.9999 5293	.9999 4749	.9999 4176	.9999 2945
7.24	.9999 5960	.9999 5464	.9999 4940	.9999 4388	.9999 3201
7.25	.9999 6108	.9999 5629	.9999 5124	.9999 4592	.9999 3448
7.26	.9999 6250	.9999 5789	.9999 5302	.9999 4789	.9999 3687
7.27	.9999 6387	.9999 5942	.9999 5473	.9999 4979	.9999 3917
7.28	.9999 6519	.9999 6091	.9999 5639	.9999 5162	.9999 4139
7.29	.9999 6646	.9999 6234	.9999 5798	.9999 5339	.9999 4353
7.30	.9999 6770	.9999 6372	.9999 5952	.9999 5510	.9999 4560
7.31	.9999 6888	.9999 6505	.9999 6101	.9999 5675	.9999 4759
7.32	.9999 7003	.9999 6634	.9999 6244	.9999 5834	.9999 4951
7.33	.9999 7113	.9999 6758	.9999 6382	.9999 5987	.9999 5137
7.34	.9999 7220	.9999 6877	.9999 6516	.9999 6135	.9999 5316
7.35	.9999 7322	.9999 6993	.9999 6644	.9999 6277	.9999 5488
7.36	.9999 7422	.9999 7104	.9999 6768	.9999 6415	.9999 5655
7.37	.9999 7517	.9999 7211	.9999 6888	.9999 6548	.9999 5816
7.38	.9999 7609	.9999 7315	.9999 7003	.9999 6676	.9999 5970
7.39	.9999 7698	.9999 7414	.9999 7115	.9999 6799	.9999 6120
7.40	.9999 7784	.9999 7510	.9999 7222	.9999 6918	.9999 6264
7.41	.9999 7866	.9999 7603	.9999 7325	.9999 7032	.9999 6403
7.42	.9999 7946	.9999 7693	.9999 7425	.9999 7143	.9999 6537
7.43	.9999 8023	.9999 7779	.9999 7521	.9999 7250	.9999 6666
7.44	.9999 8097	.9999 7862	.9999 7614	.9999 7352	.9999 6790
7.45	.9999 8168	.9999 7942	.9999 7703	.9999 7451	.9999 6910
7.46	.9999 8237	.9999 8019	.9999 7789	.9999 7547	.9999 7026
7.47	.9999 8303	.9999 8093	.9999 7872	.9999 7639	.9999 7137
7.48	.9999 8367	.9999 8165	.9999 7952	.9999 7727	.9999 7244
7.49	.9999 8428	.9999 8234	.9999 8029	.9999 7813	.9999 7348

W	P(W,17)	P(W,18)	P(W,19)	P(W,20)	P(W,22)
7.50	.9999 8487	.9999 8301	.9999 8103	.9999 7895	.9999 7448
7.51	.9999 8544	.9999 8365	.9999 8175	.9999 7975	.9999 7544
7.52	.9999 8599	.9999 8426	.9999 8244	.9999 8051	.9999 7637
7.53	.9999 8652	.9999 8486	.9999 8310	.9999 8125	.9999 7726
7.54	.9999 8704	.9999 8543	.9999 8374	.9999 8196	.9999 7812
7.55	.9999 8753	.9999 8599	.9999 8436	.9999 8264	.9999 7895
7.56	.9999 8800	.9999 8652	.9999 8495	.9999 8330	.9999 7975
7.57	.9999 8846	.9999 8703	.9999 8552	.9999 8393	.9999 8052
7.58	.9999 8890	.9999 8753	.9999 8607	.9999 8455	.9999 8126
7.59	.9999 8932	.9999 8800	.9999 8661	.9999 8514	.9999 8197
7.60	.9999 8973	.9999 8846	.9999 8712	.9999 8570	.9999 8266
7.61	.9999 9012	.9999 8890	.9999 8761	.9999 8625	.9999 8332
7.62	.9999 9050	.9999 8933	.9999 8808	.9999 8677	.9999 8396
7.63	.9999 9086	.9999 8973	.9999 8854	.9999 8728	.9999 8457
7.64	.9999 9122	.9999 9013	.9999 8898	.9999 8777	.9999 8516
7.65	.9999 9155	.9999 9051	.9999 8940	.9999 8824	.9999 8573
7.66	.9999 9188	.9999 9087	.9999 8981	.9999 8869	.9999 8628
7.67	.9999 9219	.9999 9123	.9999 9020	.9999 8913	.9999 8681
7.68	.9999 9249	.9999 9156	.9999 9058	.9999 8955	.9999 8732
7.69	.9999 9278	.9999 9189	.9999 9095	.9999 8995	.9999 8781
7.70	.9999 9306	.9999 9220	.9999 9130	.9999 9034	.9999 8828
7.71	.9999 9333	.9999 9251	.9999 9163	.9999 9071	.9999 8873
7.72	.9999 9359	.9999 9280	.9999 9196	.9999 9107	.9999 8917
7.73	.9999 9384	.9999 9308	.9999 9227	.9999 9142	.9999 8959
7.74	.9999 9408	.9999 9335	.9999 9257	.9999 9175	.9999 8999
7.75	.9999 9431	.9999 9360	.9999 9286	.9999 9207	.9999 9038
7.76	.9999 9453	.9999 9385	.9999 9314	.9999 9238	.9999 9076
7.77	.9999 9474	.9999 9409	.9999 9340	.9999 9268	.9999 9112
7.78	.9999 9495	.9999 9432	.9999 9366	.9999 9296	.9999 9146
7.79	.9999 9515	.9999 9455	.9999 9391	.9999 9324	.9999 9180
7.80	.9999 9534	.9999 9476	.9999 9415	.9999 9350	.9999 9212
7.81	.9999 9552	.9999 9497	.9999 9438	.9999 9376	.9999 9243
7.82	.9999 9570	.9999 9516	.9999 9460	.9999 9400	.9999 9272
7.83	.9999 9587	.9999 9535	.9999 9481	.9999 9424	.9999 9301
7.84	.9999 9603	.9999 9554	.9999 9502	.9999 9447	.9999 9328
7.85	.9999 9619	.9999 9571	.9999 9521	.9999 9468	.9999 9355
7.86	.9999 9634	.9999 9588	.9999 9540	.9999 9489	.9999 9380
7.87	.9999 9648	.9999 9604	.9999 9558	.9999 9510	.9999 9405
7.88	.9999 9662	.9999 9620	.9999 9576	.9999 9529	.9999 9428
7.89	.9999 9675	.9999 9635	.9999 9593	.9999 9548	.9999 9451
7.90	.9999 9688	.9999 9650	.9999 9609	.9999 9566	.9999 9473
7.91	.9999 9701	.9999 9664	.9999 9624	.9999 9583	.9999 9494
7.92	.9999 9713	.9999 9677	.9999 9639	.9999 9599	.9999 9514
7.93	.9999 9724	.9999 9690	.9999 9654	.9999 9615	.9999 9533
7.94	.9999 9735	.9999 9702	.9999 9667	.9999 9631	.9999 9552
7.95	.9999 9746	.9999 9714	.9999 9681	.9999 9645	.9999 9569
7.96	.9999 9756	.9999 9725	.9999 9693	.9999 9660	.9999 9587
7.97	.9999 9766	.9999 9736	.9999 9706	.9999 9673	.9999 9603
7.98	.9999 9775	.9999 9747	.9999 9717	.9999 9686	.9999 9619
7.99	.9999 9784	.9999 9757	.9999 9729	.9999 9699	.9999 9634

W	P(W,17)	P(W,18)	P(W,19)	P(W,20)	P(W,22)
8.00	.9999 9793	.9999 9767	.9999 9740	.9999 9711	.9999 9649
8.01	.9999 9801	.9999 9776	.9999 9750	.9999 9723	.9999 9663
8.02	.9999 9809	.9999 9785	.9999 9760	.9999 9734	.9999 9677
8.03	.9999 9817	.9999 9794	.9999 9770	.9999 9744	.9999 9690
8.04	.9999 9824	.9999 9802	.9999 9779	.9999 9755	.9999 9702
8.05	.9999 9831	.9999 9810	.9999 9788	.9999 9765	.9999 9714
8.06	.9999 9838	.9999 9818	.9999 9797	.9999 9774	.9999 9726
8.07	.9999 9845	.9999 9825	.9999 9805	.9999 9783	.9999 9737
8.08	.9999 9851	.9999 9832	.9999 9813	.9999 9792	.9999 9748
8.09	.9999 9857	.9999 9839	.9999 9820	.9999 9800	.9999 9758
8.10	.9999 9863	.9999 9846	.9999 9828	.9999 9809	.9999 9768
8.11	.9999 9868	.9999 9852	.9999 9835	.9999 9816	.9999 9777
8.12	.9999 9874	.9999 9858	.9999 9841	.9999 9824	.9999 9786
8.13	.9999 9879	.9999 9864	.9999 9848	.9999 9831	.9999 9795
8.14	.9999 9884	.9999 9869	.9999 9854	.9999 9838	.9999 9803
8.15	.9999 9889	.9999 9875	.9999 9860	.9999 9845	.9999 9811
8.16	.9999 9893	.9999 9880	.9999 9866	.9999 9851	.9999 9819
8.17	.9999 9897	.9999 9885	.9999 9871	.9999 9857	.9999 9826
8.18	.9999 9902	.9999 9889	.9999 9877	.9999 9863	.9999 9833
8.19	.9999 9906	.9999 9894	.9999 9882	.9999 9868	.9999 9840
8.20	.9999 9910	.9999 9898	.9999 9886	.9999 9874	.9999 9847
8.21	.9999 9913	.9999 9903	.9999 9891	.9999 9879	.9999 9853
8.22	.9999 9917	.9999 9907	.9999 9896	.9999 9884	.9999 9859
8.23	.9999 9920	.9999 9910	.9999 9900	.9999 9889	.9999 9865
8.24	.9999 9924	.9999 9914	.9999 9904	.9999 9893	.9999 9871
8.25	.9999 9927	.9999 9918	.9999 9908	.9999 9898	.9999 9876
8.26	.9999 9930	.9999 9921	.9999 9912	.9999 9902	.9999 9881
8.27	.9999 9933	.9999 9924	.9999 9915	.9999 9906	.9999 9886
8.28	.9999 9935	.9999 9927	.9999 9919	.9999 9910	.9999 9891
8.29	.9999 9938	.9999 9930	.9999 9922	.9999 9914	.9999 9895
8.30	.9999 9941	.9999 9933	.9999 9926	.9999 9917	.9999 9900
8.31	.9999 9943	.9999 9936	.9999 9929	.9999 9921	.9999 9904
8.32	.9999 9946	.9999 9939	.9999 9932	.9999 9924	.9999 9908
8.33	.9999 9948	.9999 9941	.9999 9934	.9999 9927	.9999 9912
8.34	.9999 9950	.9999 9944	.9999 9937	.9999 9930	.9999 9915
8.35	.9999 9952	.9999 9946	.9999 9940	.9999 9933	.9999 9919
8.36	.9999 9954	.9999 9948	.9999 9942	.9999 9936	.9999 9922
8.37	.9999 9956	.9999 9951	.9999 9945	.9999 9939	.9999 9926
8.38	.9999 9958	.9999 9953	.9999 9947	.9999 9941	.9999 9929
8.39	.9999 9960	.9999 9955	.9999 9949	.9999 9944	.9999 9932
8.40	.9999 9961	.9999 9957	.9999 9951	.9999 9946	.9999 9934
8.41	.9999 9963	.9999 9958	.9999 9953	.9999 9948	.9999 9937
8.42	.9999 9965	.9999 9960	.9999 9955	.9999 9951	.9999 9940
8.43	.9999 9966	.9999 9962	.9999 9957	.9999 9953	.9999 9942
8.44	.9999 9967	.9999 9963	.9999 9959	.9999 9955	.9999 9945
8.45	.9999 9969	.9999 9965	.9999 9961	.9999 9957	.9999 9947
8.46	.9999 9970	.9999 9966	.9999 9963	.9999 9958	.9999 9949
8.47	.9999 9971	.9999 9968	.9999 9964	.9999 9960	.9999 9952
8.48	.9999 9973	.9999 9969	.9999 9966	.9999 9962	.9999 9954
8.49	.9999 9974	.9999 9971	.9999 9967	.9999 9963	.9999 9956

W	P(W,17)	P(W,18)	P(W,19)	P(W,20)	P(W,22)
8.50	.9999 9975	.9999 9972	.9999 9968	.9999 9965	.9999 9957
8.51	.9999 9976	.9999 9973	.9999 9970	.9999 9966	.9999 9959
8.52	.9999 9977	.9999 9974	.9999 9971	.9999 9968	.9999 9961
8.53	.9999 9978	.9999 9975	.9999 9972	.9999 9969	.9999 9963
8.54	.9999 9979	.9999 9976	.9999 9974	.9999 9971	.9999 9964
8.55	.9999 9980	.9999 9977	.9999 9975	.9999 9972	.9999 9966
8.56	.9999 9981	.9999 9978	.9999 9976	.9999 9973	.9999 9967
8.57	.9999 9982	.9999 9979	.9999 9977	.9999 9974	.9999 9969
8.58	.9999 9982	.9999 9980	.9999 9978	.9999 9975	.9999 9970
8.59	.9999 9983	.9999 9981	.9999 9979	.9999 9976	.9999 9971
8.60	.9999 9984	.9999 9982	.9999 9980	.9999 9977	.9999 9972
8.61	.9999 9984	.9999 9983	.9999 9980	.9999 9978	.9999 9974
8.62	.9999 9985	.9999 9983	.9999 9981	.9999 9979	.9999 9975
8.63	.9999 9986	.9999 9984	.9999 9982	.9999 9980	.9999 9976
8.64	.9999 9986	.9999 9985	.9999 9983	.9999 9981	.9999 9977
8.65	.9999 9987	.9999 9985	.9999 9984	.9999 9982	.9999 9978
8.66	.9999 9988	.9999 9986	.9999 9984	.9999 9983	.9999 9979
8.67	.9999 9988	.9999 9987	.9999 9985	.9999 9983	.9999 9980
8.68	.9999 9989	.9999 9987	.9999 9986	.9999 9984	.9999 9981
8.69	.9999 9989	.9999 9988	.9999 9986	.9999 9985	.9999 9982
8.70	.9999 9990	.9999 9988	.9999 9987	.9999 9985	.9999 9982
8.71	.9999 9990	.9999 9989	.9999 9987	.9999 9986	.9999 9983
8.72	.9999 9990	.9999 9989	.9999 9988	.9999 9987	.9999 9984
8.73	.9999 9991	.9999 9990	.9999 9989	.9999 9987	.9999 9985
8.74	.9999 9991	.9999 9990	.9999 9989	.9999 9988	.9999 9985
8.75	.9999 9992	.9999 9991	.9999 9989	.9999 9988	.9999 9986
8.76	.9999 9992	.9999 9991	.9999 9990	.9999 9989	.9999 9986
8.77	.9999 9992	.9999 9991	.9999 9990	.9999 9989	.9999 9987
8.78	.9999 9993	.9999 9992	.9999 9991	.9999 9990	.9999 9988
8.79	.9999 9993	.9999 9992	.9999 9991	.9999 9990	.9999 9988
8.80	.9999 9993	.9999 9992	.9999 9992	.9999 9991	.9999 9989
8.81	.9999 9994	.9999 9993	.9999 9992	.9999 9991	.9999 9989
8.82	.9999 9994	.9999 9993	.9999 9992	.9999 9991	.9999 9990
8.83	.9999 9994	.9999 9993	.9999 9993	.9999 9992	.9999 9990
8.84	.9999 9994	.9999 9994	.9999 9993	.9999 9992	.9999 9991
8.85	.9999 9995	.9999 9994	.9999 9993	.9999 9993	.9999 9991
8.86	.9999 9995	.9999 9994	.9999 9994	.9999 9993	.9999 9991
8.87	.9999 9995	.9999 9994	.9999 9994	.9999 9993	.9999 9992
8.88	.9999 9995	.9999 9995	.9999 9994	.9999 9993	.9999 9992
8.89	.9999 9996	.9999 9995	.9999 9994	.9999 9994	.9999 9992
8.90	.9999 9996	.9999 9995	.9999 9995	.9999 9994	.9999 9993
8.91	.9999 9996	.9999 9995	.9999 9995	.9999 9994	.9999 9993
8.92	.9999 9996	.9999 9996	.9999 9995	.9999 9995	.9999 9993
8.93	.9999 9996	.9999 9996	.9999 9995	.9999 9995	.9999 9994
8.94	.9999 9996	.9999 9996	.9999 9995	.9999 9995	.9999 9994
8.95	.9999 9997	.9999 9996	.9999 9996	.9999 9995	.9999 9994
8.96	.9999 9997	.9999 9996	.9999 9996	.9999 9995	.9999 9994
8.97	.9999 9997	.9999 9996	.9999 9996	.9999 9996	.9999 9995
8.98	.9999 9997	.9999 9997	.9999 9996	.9999 9996	.9999 9995
8.99	.9999 9997	.9999 9997	.9999 9996	.9999 9996	.9999 9995

W	P(W,17)	P(W,18)	P(W,19)	P(W,20)	P(W,22)
9.00	.9999 9997	.9999 9997	.9999 9997	.9999 9996	.9999 9995
9.01	.9999 9997	.9999 9997	.9999 9997	.9999 9996	.9999 9996
9.02	.9999 9997	.9999 9997	.9999 9997	.9999 9997	.9999 9996
9.03	.9999 9998	.9999 9997	.9999 9997	.9999 9997	.9999 9996
9.04	.9999 9998	.9999 9997	.9999 9997	.9999 9997	.9999 9996
9.05	.9999 9998	.9999 9998	.9999 9997	.9999 9997	.9999 9996
9.06	.9999 9998	.9999 9998	.9999 9997	.9999 9997	.9999 9996
9.07	.9999 9998	.9999 9998	.9999 9997	.9999 9997	.9999 9997
9.08	.9999 9998	.9999 9998	.9999 9998	.9999 9997	.9999 9997
9.09	.9999 9998	.9999 9998	.9999 9998	.9999 9997	.9999 9997
9.10	.9999 9998	.9999 9998	.9999 9998	.9999 9998	.9999 9997
9.11	.9999 9998	.9999 9998	.9999 9998	.9999 9998	.9999 9997
9.12	.9999 9998	.9999 9998	.9999 9998	.9999 9998	.9999 9997
9.13	.9999 9998	.9999 9998	.9999 9998	.9999 9998	.9999 9997
9.14	.9999 9999	.9999 9998	.9999 9998	.9999 9998	.9999 9998
9.15	.9999 9999	.9999 9998	.9999 9998	.9999 9998	.9999 9998
9.16	.9999 9999	.9999 9998	.9999 9998	.9999 9998	.9999 9998
9.17	.9999 9999	.9999 9999	.9999 9998	.9999 9998	.9999 9998
9.18	.9999 9999	.9999 9999	.9999 9998	.9999 9998	.9999 9998
9.19	.9999 9999	.9999 9999	.9999 9999	.9999 9998	.9999 9998
9.20	.9999 9999	.9999 9999	.9999 9999	.9999 9998	.9999 9998
9.21	.9999 9999	.9999 9999	.9999 9999	.9999 9999	.9999 9998
9.22	.9999 9999	.9999 9999	.9999 9999	.9999 9999	.9999 9998
9.23	.9999 9999	.9999 9999	.9999 9999	.9999 9999	.9999 9998
9.24	.9999 9999	.9999 9999	.9999 9999	.9999 9999	.9999 9998
9.25	.9999 9999	.9999 9999	.9999 9999	.9999 9999	.9999 9998
9.26	.9999 9999	.9999 9999	.9999 9999	.9999 9999	.9999 9999
9.27	.9999 9999	.9999 9999	.9999 9999	.9999 9999	.9999 9999
9.28	.9999 9999	.9999 9999	.9999 9999	.9999 9999	.9999 9999
9.29	.9999 9999	.9999 9999	.9999 9999	.9999 9999	.9999 9999
9.30	.9999 9999	.9999 9999	.9999 9999	.9999 9999	.9999 9999
9.31	.9999 9999	.9999 9999	.9999 9999	.9999 9999	.9999 9999
9.32	.9999 9999	.9999 9999	.9999 9999	.9999 9999	.9999 9999
9.33	.9999 9999	.9999 9999	.9999 9999	.9999 9999	.9999 9999
9.34	.9999 9999	.9999 9999	.9999 9999	.9999 9999	.9999 9999
9.35	.9999 9999	.9999 9999	.9999 9999	.9999 9999	.9999 9999
9.36	.9999 9999	.9999 9999	.9999 9999	.9999 9999	.9999 9999
9.37	.9999 9999	.9999 9999	.9999 9999	.9999 9999	.9999 9999
9.38	.9999 9999	.9999 9999	.9999 9999	.9999 9999	.9999 9999
9.39	1.0000 0000	.9999 9999	.9999 9999	.9999 9999	.9999 9999
9.40		.9999 9999	.9999 9999	.9999 9999	.9999 9999
9.41		.9999 9999	.9999 9999	.9999 9999	.9999 9999
9.42		1.0000 0000	.9999 9999	.9999 9999	.9999 9999
9.43			.9999 9999	.9999 9999	.9999 9999
9.44			.9999 9999	.9999 9999	.9999 9999
9.45			1.0000 0000	.9999 9999	.9999 9999
9.46				.9999 9999	.9999 9999
9.47				1.0000 0000	.9999 9999
9.48					.9999 9999
9.49					.9999 9999

W	P(W,17)	P(W,18)	P(W,19)	P(W,20)	P(W,22)
9.50					.9999 9999
9.51					1.0000 0000
9.52					
9.53					
9.54					
9.55					
9.56					
9.57					
9.58					
9.59					
9.60					
9.61					
9.62					
9.63					
9.64					
9.65					
9.66					
9.67					
9.68					
9.69					
9.70					
9.71					
9.72					
9.73					
9.74					
9.75					
9.76					
9.77					
9.78					
9.79					
9.80					
9.81					
9.82					
9.83					
9.84					
9.85					
9.86					
9.87					
9.88					
9.89					
9.90					
9.91					
9.92					
9.93					
9.94					
9.95					
9.96					
9.97					
9.98					
9.99					

W	P(W,24)	P(W,26)	P(W,28)	P(W,30)	P(W,32)
1.00					
1.01					
1.02					
1.03					
1.04					
1.05					
1.06					
1.07	.0000 0000				
1.08	.0000 0001				
1.09	.0000 0001				
1.10	.0000 0001				
1.11	.0000 0001				
1.12	.0000 0001				
1.13	.0000 0001				
1.14	.0000 0002				
1.15	.0000 0002				
1.16	.0000 0002	.0000 0000			
1.17	.0000 0003	.0000 0001			
1.18	.0000 0004	.0000 0001			
1.19	.0000 0004	.0000 0001			
1.20	.0000 0005	.0000 0001			
1.21	.0000 0006	.0000 0001			
1.22	.0000 0007	.0000 0001			
1.23	.0000 0008	.0000 0002			
1.24	.0000 0010	.0000 0002	.0000 0000		
1.25	.0000 0011	.0000 0003	.0000 0001		
1.26	.0000 0013	.0000 0003	.0000 0001		
1.27	.0000 0015	.0000 0004	.0000 0001		
1.28	.0000 0018	.0000 0004	.0000 0001		
1.29	.0000 0021	.0000 0005	.0000 0001		
1.30	.0000 0025	.0000 0006	.0000 0001		
1.31	.0000 0029	.0000 0007	.0000 0002		
1.32	.0000 0033	.0000 0008	.0000 0002	.0000 0000	
1.33	.0000 0038	.0000 0010	.0000 0002	.0000 0001	
1.34	.0000 0044	.0000 0011	.0000 0003	.0000 0001	
1.35	.0000 0051	.0000 0013	.0000 0003	.0000 0001	
1.36	.0000 0059	.0000 0016	.0000 0004	.0000 0001	
1.37	.0000 0068	.0000 0018	.0000 0005	.0000 0001	
1.38	.0000 0079	.0000 0021	.0000 0006	.0000 0002	
1.39	.0000 0090	.0000 0025	.0000 0007	.0000 0002	.0000 0000
1.40	.0000 0104	.0000 0029	.0000 0008	.0000 0002	.0000 0001
1.41	.0000 0119	.0000 0033	.0000 0009	.0000 0003	.0000 0001
1.42	.0000 0136	.0000 0039	.0000 0011	.0000 0003	.0000 0001
1.43	.0000 0155	.0000 0045	.0000 0013	.0000 0004	.0000 0001
1.44	.0000 0177	.0000 0052	.0000 0015	.0000 0004	.0000 0001
1.45	.0000 0202	.0000 0059	.0000 0017	.0000 0005	.0000 0001
1.46	.0000 0230	.0000 0068	.0000 0020	.0000 0006	.0000 0002
1.47	.0000 0262	.0000 0079	.0000 0024	.0000 0007	.0000 0002
1.48	.0000 0297	.0000 0090	.0000 0027	.0000 0008	.0000 0002
1.49	.0000 0338	.0000 0104	.0000 0032	.0000 0010	.0000 0003

W	P(W,24)	P(W,26)	P(W,28)	P(W,30)	P(W,32)
1.50	.0000 0382	.0000 0119	.0000 0037	.0000 0011	.0000 0003
1.51	.0000 0433	.0000 0136	.0000 0043	.0000 0013	.0000 0004
1.52	.0000 0489	.0000 0155	.0000 0049	.0000 0016	.0000 0005
1.53	.0000 0552	.0000 0177	.0000 0057	.0000 0018	.0000 0006
1.54	.0000 0623	.0000 0202	.0000 0065	.0000 0021	.0000 0007
1.55	.0000 0702	.0000 0230	.0000 0075	.0000 0025	.0000 0008
1.56	.0000 0790	.0000 0262	.0000 0087	.0000 0029	.0000 0009
1.57	.0000 0888	.0000 0297	.0000 0099	.0000 0033	.0000 0011
1.58	.0000 0997	.0000 0337	.0000 0114	.0000 0038	.0000 0013
1.59	.0000 1118	.0000 0382	.0000 0130	.0000 0044	.0000 0015
1.60	.0000 1253	.0000 0433	.0000 0149	.0000 0051	.0000 0018
1.61	.0000 1402	.0000 0489	.0000 0170	.0000 0059	.0000 0020
1.62	.0000 1568	.0000 0552	.0000 0194	.0000 0068	.0000 0024
1.63	.0000 1751	.0000 0623	.0000 0221	.0000 0078	.0000 0028
1.64	.0000 1954	.0000 0702	.0000 0251	.0000 0090	.0000 0032
1.65	.0000 2178	.0000 0790	.0000 0286	.0000 0103	.0000 0037
1.66	.0000 2425	.0000 0888	.0000 0324	.0000 0118	.0000 0043
1.67	.0000 2698	.0000 0997	.0000 0368	.0000 0135	.0000 0050
1.68	.0000 2998	.0000 1119	.0000 0416	.0000 0155	.0000 0057
1.69	.0000 3329	.0000 1254	.0000 0471	.0000 0176	.0000 0066
1.70	.0000 3692	.0000 1404	.0000 0532	.0000 0201	.0000 0076
1.71	.0000 4092	.0000 1570	.0000 0601	.0000 0229	.0000 0087
1.72	.0000 4530	.0000 1754	.0000 0677	.0000 0261	.0000 0100
1.73	.0000 5010	.0000 1957	.0000 0762	.0000 0296	.0000 0115
1.74	.0000 5537	.0000 2182	.0000 0858	.0000 0336	.0000 0132
1.75	.0000 6113	.0000 2431	.0000 0964	.0000 0381	.0000 0150
1.76	.0000 6743	.0000 2705	.0000 1082	.0000 0432	.0000 0172
1.77	.0000 7431	.0000 3007	.0000 1213	.0000 0488	.0000 0196
1.78	.0000 8182	.0000 3339	.0000 1359	.0000 0552	.0000 0223
1.79	.0000 9002	.0000 3705	.0000 1521	.0000 0623	.0000 0254
1.80	.0000 9895	.0000 4107	.0000 1700	.0000 0702	.0000 0289
1.81	.0001 0867	.0000 4549	.0000 1899	.0000 0791	.0000 0328
1.82	.0001 1924	.0000 5033	.0000 2118	.0000 0889	.0000 0373
1.83	.0001 3074	.0000 5564	.0000 2361	.0000 1000	.0000 0422
1.84	.0001 4322	.0000 6145	.0000 2629	.0000 1122	.0000 0478
1.85	.0001 5676	.0000 6781	.0000 2925	.0000 1258	.0000 0540
1.86	.0001 7145	.0000 7476	.0000 3250	.0000 1410	.0000 0610
1.87	.0001 8736	.0000 8234	.0000 3609	.0000 1578	.0000 0688
1.88	.0002 0459	.0000 9063	.0000 4003	.0000 1764	.0000 0776
1.89	.0002 2322	.0000 9965	.0000 4437	.0000 1970	.0000 0873
1.90	.0002 4335	.0001 0949	.0000 4912	.0000 2199	.0000 0982
1.91	.0002 6510	.0001 2019	.0000 5434	.0000 2451	.0000 1103
1.92	.0002 8856	.0001 3183	.0000 6006	.0000 2729	.0000 1238
1.93	.0003 1387	.0001 4447	.0000 6632	.0000 3037	.0000 1388
1.94	.0003 4114	.0001 5820	.0000 7316	.0000 3375	.0000 1554
1.95	.0003 7049	.0001 7309	.0000 8065	.0000 3748	.0000 1738
1.96	.0004 0208	.0001 8924	.0000 8882	.0000 4159	.0000 1943
1.97	.0004 3603	.0002 0672	.0000 9773	.0000 4609	.0000 2169
1.98	.0004 7251	.0002 2564	.0001 0745	.0000 5105	.0000 2420
1.99	.0005 1167	.0002 4609	.0001 1803	.0000 5648	.0000 2697

W	P(W,24)	P(W,26)	P(W,28)	P(W,30)	P(W,32)
2.00	.0005 5368	.0002 6820	.0001 2955	.0000 6243	.0000 3002
2.01	.0005 9872	.0002 9206	.0001 4208	.0000 6895	.0000 3339
2.02	.0006 4696	.0003 1780	.0001 5568	.0000 7608	.0000 3710
2.03	.0006 9861	.0003 4556	.0001 7045	.0000 8388	.0000 4119
2.04	.0007 5386	.0003 7545	.0001 8647	.0000 9240	.0000 4569
2.05	.0008 1292	.0004 0763	.0002 0384	.0001 0169	.0000 5062
2.06	.0008 7601	.0004 4224	.0002 2264	.0001 1182	.0000 5605
2.07	.0009 4337	.0004 7944	.0002 4299	.0001 2286	.0000 6199
2.08	.0010 1523	.0005 1939	.0002 6499	.0001 3488	.0000 6851
2.09	.0010 9185	.0005 6227	.0002 8876	.0001 4794	.0000 7564
2.10	.0011 7348	.0006 0825	.0003 1442	.0001 6215	.0000 8344
2.11	.0012 6039	.0006 5754	.0003 4210	.0001 7756	.0000 9197
2.12	.0013 5287	.0007 1032	.0003 7194	.0001 9429	.0001 0128
2.13	.0014 5121	.0007 6681	.0004 0407	.0002 1243	.0001 1144
2.14	.0015 5571	.0008 2722	.0004 3866	.0002 3207	.0001 2252
2.15	.0016 6670	.0008 9179	.0004 7586	.0002 5333	.0001 3458
2.16	.0017 8449	.0009 6074	.0005 1584	.0002 7632	.0001 4771
2.17	.0019 0944	.0010 3434	.0005 5878	.0003 0116	.0001 6198
2.18	.0020 4188	.0011 1283	.0006 0486	.0003 2799	.0001 7749
2.19	.0021 8220	.0011 9650	.0006 5427	.0003 5693	.0001 9432
2.20	.0023 3075	.0012 8562	.0007 0722	.0003 8813	.0002 1258
2.21	.0024 8794	.0013 8049	.0007 6393	.0004 2175	.0002 3236
2.22	.0026 5416	.0014 8140	.0008 2461	.0004 5794	.0002 5379
2.23	.0028 2983	.0015 8868	.0008 8950	.0004 9687	.0002 7698
2.24	.0030 1537	.0017 0266	.0009 5885	.0005 3871	.0003 0205
2.25	.0032 1123	.0018 2368	.0010 3290	.0005 8366	.0003 2913
2.26	.0034 1787	.0019 5209	.0011 1193	.0006 3190	.0003 5837
2.27	.0036 3574	.0020 8826	.0011 9622	.0006 8364	.0003 8991
2.28	.0038 6533	.0022 3256	.0012 8605	.0007 3910	.0004 2390
2.29	.0041 0713	.0023 8540	.0013 8172	.0007 9850	.0004 6051
2.30	.0043 6165	.0025 4717	.0014 8355	.0008 6207	.0004 9992
2.31	.0046 2941	.0027 1829	.0015 9187	.0009 3007	.0005 4230
2.32	.0049 1094	.0028 9920	.0017 0701	.0010 0274	.0005 8784
2.33	.0052 0678	.0030 9034	.0018 2932	.0010 8036	.0006 3675
2.34	.0055 1750	.0032 9218	.0019 5917	.0011 6321	.0006 8923
2.35	.0058 4367	.0035 0518	.0020 9693	.0012 5158	.0007 4551
2.36	.0061 8586	.0037 2983	.0022 4300	.0013 4577	.0008 0581
2.37	.0065 4468	.0039 6664	.0023 9778	.0014 4610	.0008 7038
2.38	.0069 2073	.0042 1611	.0025 6169	.0015 5290	.0009 3948
2.39	.0073 1464	.0044 7878	.0027 3516	.0016 6651	.0010 1336
2.40	.0077 2704	.0047 5519	.0029 1863	.0017 8730	.0010 9230
2.41	.0081 5857	.0050 4589	.0031 1257	.0019 1562	.0011 7660
2.42	.0086 0989	.0053 5145	.0033 1746	.0020 5187	.0012 6655
2.43	.0090 8167	.0056 7246	.0035 3378	.0021 9643	.0013 6247
2.44	.0095 7458	.0060 0951	.0037 6202	.0023 4972	.0014 6469
2.45	.0100 8931	.0063 6320	.0040 0272	.0025 1217	.0015 7354
2.46	.0106 2656	.0067 3417	.0042 5641	.0026 8421	.0016 8937
2.47	.0111 8704	.0071 2305	.0045 2362	.0028 6630	.0018 1257
2.48	.0117 7146	.0075 3048	.0048 0491	.0030 5891	.0019 4350
2.49	.0123 8055	.0079 5712	.0051 0088	.0032 6252	.0020 8257

W	P(W,24)	P(W,26)	P(W,28)	P(W,30)	P(W,32)
2.50	.0130 1505	.0084 0365	.0054 1209	.0034 7763	.0022 3018
2.51	.0136 7569	.0088 7076	.0057 3916	.0037 0475	.0023 8677
2.52	.0143 6323	.0093 5912	.0060 8270	.0039 4441	.0025 5276
2.53	.0150 7842	.0098 6946	.0064 4334	.0041 9715	.0027 2861
2.54	.0158 2202	.0104 0249	.0068 2173	.0044 6354	.0029 1480
2.55	.0165 9480	.0109 5894	.0072 1853	.0047 4414	.0031 1181
2.56	.0173 9754	.0115 3953	.0076 3439	.0050 3954	.0033 2013
2.57	.0182 3101	.0121 4503	.0080 7001	.0053 5034	.0035 4029
2.58	.0190 9599	.0127 7619	.0085 2609	.0056 7717	.0037 7281
2.59	.0199 9327	.0134 3376	.0090 0333	.0060 2065	.0040 1824
2.60	.0209 2362	.0141 1852	.0095 0245	.0063 8143	.0042 7715
2.61	.0218 8785	.0148 3126	.0100 2418	.0067 6017	.0045 5010
2.62	.0228 8674	.0155 7275	.0105 6926	.0071 5754	.0048 3770
2.63	.0239 2108	.0163 4380	.0111 3846	.0075 7423	.0051 4055
2.64	.0249 9165	.0171 4518	.0117 3252	.0080 1095	.0054 5928
2.65	.0260 9925	.0179 7772	.0123 5223	.0084 6839	.0057 9451
2.66	.0272 4465	.0188 4222	.0129 9837	.0089 4731	.0061 4692
2.67	.0284 2865	.0197 3947	.0136 7172	.0094 4842	.0065 1716
2.68	.0296 5202	.0206 7031	.0143 7309	.0099 7249	.0069 0592
2.69	.0309 1554	.0216 3554	.0151 0329	.0105 2027	.0073 1389
2.70	.0322 1997	.0226 3599	.0158 6312	.0110 9255	.0077 4180
2.71	.0335 6608	.0236 7245	.0166 5340	.0116 9010	.0081 9035
2.72	.0349 5462	.0247 4576	.0174 7497	.0123 1372	.0086 6030
2.73	.0363 8634	.0258 5673	.0183 2865	.0129 6422	.0091 5239
2.74	.0378 6199	.0270 0617	.0192 1527	.0136 4241	.0096 6739
2.75	.0393 8228	.0281 9490	.0201 3568	.0143 4911	.0102 0607
2.76	.0409 4795	.0294 2371	.0210 9070	.0150 8515	.0107 6923
2.77	.0425 5969	.0306 9341	.0220 8119	.0158 5136	.0113 5766
2.78	.0442 1821	.0320 0480	.0231 0799	.0166 4860	.0119 7218
2.79	.0459 2419	.0333 5867	.0241 7193	.0174 7771	.0126 1361
2.80	.0476 7830	.0347 5580	.0252 7387	.0183 3955	.0132 8277
2.81	.0494 8119	.0361 9697	.0264 1464	.0192 3497	.0139 8051
2.82	.0513 3351	.0376 8295	.0275 9507	.0201 6484	.0147 0768
2.83	.0532 3587	.0392 1449	.0288 1601	.0211 3001	.0154 6513
2.84	.0551 8888	.0407 9234	.0300 7829	.0221 3137	.0162 5373
2.85	.0571 9314	.0424 1723	.0313 8273	.0231 6977	.0170 7435
2.86	.0592 4921	.0440 8988	.0327 3015	.0242 4608	.0179 2785
2.87	.0613 5763	.0458 1101	.0341 2136	.0253 6118	.0188 1513
2.88	.0635 1895	.0475 8131	.0355 5717	.0265 1592	.0197 3707
2.89	.0657 3368	.0494 0146	.0370 3837	.0277 1117	.0206 9455
2.90	.0680 0229	.0512 7212	.0385 6575	.0289 4779	.0216 8847
2.91	.0703 2525	.0531 9393	.0401 4009	.0302 2663	.0227 1972
2.92	.0727 0301	.0551 6753	.0417 6214	.0315 4854	.0237 8918
2.93	.0751 3598	.0571 9352	.0434 3266	.0329 1437	.0248 9775
2.94	.0776 2456	.0592 7250	.0451 5239	.0343 2495	.0260 4632
2.95	.0801 6911	.0614 0503	.0469 2205	.0357 8112	.0272 3578
2.96	.0827 6998	.0635 9167	.0487 4234	.0372 8367	.0284 6702
2.97	.0854 2749	.0658 3293	.0506 1396	.0388 3344	.0297 4090
2.98	.0881 4191	.0681 2933	.0525 3758	.0404 3120	.0310 5832
2.99	.0909 1353	.0704 8134	.0545 1385	.0420 7775	.0324 2013

W	P(W,24)	P(W,26)	P(W,28)	P(W,30)	P(W,32)
3.00	.0937 4257	.0728 8941	.0565 4341	.0437 7385	.0338 2721
3.01	.0966 2923	.0753 5399	.0586 2688	.0455 2027	.0352 8039
3.02	.0995 7369	.0778 7548	.0607 6485	.0473 1774	.0367 8053
3.03	.1025 7611	.0804 5424	.0629 5788	.0491 6698	.0383 2846
3.04	.1056 3660	.0830 9064	.0652 0655	.0510 6871	.0399 2501
3.05	.1087 5524	.0857 8500	.0675 1136	.0530 2362	.0415 7098
3.06	.1119 3210	.0885 3762	.0698 7282	.0550 3236	.0432 6716
3.07	.1151 6720	.0913 4876	.0722 9141	.0570 9560	.0450 1435
3.08	.1184 6054	.0942 1866	.0747 6758	.0592 1395	.0468 1330
3.09	.1218 1208	.0971 4753	.0773 0175	.0613 8803	.0486 6476
3.10	.1252 2175	.1001 3554	.0798 9432	.0636 1842	.0505 6948
3.11	.1286 8947	.1031 8285	.0825 4566	.0659 0567	.0525 2815
3.12	.1322 1510	.1062 8957	.0852 5611	.0682 5033	.0545 4147
3.13	.1357 9847	.1094 5578	.0880 2598	.0706 5289	.0566 1011
3.14	.1394 3940	.1126 8153	.0908 5555	.0731 1385	.0587 3473
3.15	.1431 3766	.1159 6685	.0937 4507	.0756 3366	.0609 1595
3.16	.1468 9299	.1193 1172	.0966 9476	.0782 1273	.0631 5438
3.17	.1507 0511	.1227 1611	.0997 0481	.0808 5148	.0654 5058
3.18	.1545 7369	.1261 7992	.1027 7538	.0835 5027	.0678 0513
3.19	.1584 9838	.1297 0305	.1059 0658	.0863 0944	.0702 1854
3.20	.1624 7880	.1332 8535	.1090 9850	.0891 2930	.0726 9132
3.21	.1665 1453	.1369 2666	.1123 5122	.0920 1012	.0752 2393
3.22	.1706 0513	.1406 2675	.1156 6474	.0949 5214	.0778 1682
3.23	.1747 5012	.1443 8538	.1190 3906	.0979 5559	.0804 7040
3.24	.1789 4900	.1482 0228	.1224 7413	.1010 2063	.0831 8506
3.25	.1832 0122	.1520 7713	.1259 6987	.1041 4742	.0859 6115
3.26	.1875 0621	.1560 0959	.1295 2618	.1073 3606	.0887 9898
3.27	.1918 6338	.1599 9928	.1331 4289	.1105 8663	.0916 9884
3.28	.1962 7211	.1640 4580	.1368 1984	.1138 9917	.0946 6099
3.29	.2007 3173	.1681 4869	.1405 5680	.1172 7370	.0976 8564
3.30	.2052 4157	.1723 0749	.1443 5352	.1207 1017	.1007 7299
3.31	.2098 0090	.1765 2169	.1482 0971	.1242 0853	.1039 2318
3.32	.2144 0900	.1807 9074	.1521 2505	.1277 6868	.1071 3632
3.33	.2190 6509	.1851 1408	.1560 9919	.1313 9047	.1104 1251
3.34	.2237 6838	.1894 9109	.1601 3172	.1350 7375	.1137 5178
3.35	.2285 1805	.1939 2116	.1642 2224	.1388 1830	.1171 5414
3.36	.2333 1327	.1984 0362	.1683 7027	.1426 2387	.1206 1955
3.37	.2381 5315	.2029 3776	.1725 7532	.1464 9019	.1241 4797
3.38	.2430 3682	.2075 2287	.1768 3687	.1504 1693	.1277 3927
3.39	.2479 6335	.2121 5820	.1811 5436	.1544 0375	.1313 9332
3.40	.2529 3181	.2168 4296	.1855 2718	.1584 5026	.1351 0995
3.41	.2579 4123	.2215 7635	.1899 5472	.1625 5603	.1388 8893
3.42	.2629 9064	.2263 5753	.1944 3632	.1667 2060	.1427 3001
3.43	.2680 7903	.2311 8564	.1989 7128	.1709 4347	.1466 3291
3.44	.2732 0539	.2360 5979	.2035 5889	.1752 2411	.1505 9729
3.45	.2783 6868	.2409 7906	.2081 9840	.1795 6196	.1546 2279
3.46	.2835 6783	.2459 4252	.2128 8901	.1839 5642	.1587 0900
3.47	.2888 0178	.2509 4921	.2176 2993	.1884 0686	.1628 5548
3.48	.2940 6943	.2559 9814	.2224 2030	.1929 1260	.1670 6177
3.49	.2993 6968	.2610 8831	.2272 5927	.1974 7294	.1713 2733

W	P(W,24)	P(W,26)	P(W,28)	P(W,30)	P(W,32)
3.50	.3047 0140	.2662 1868	.2321 4593	.2020 8715	.1756 5163
3.51	.3100 6346	.2713 8820	.2370 7937	.2067 5447	.1800 3407
3.52	.3154 5471	.2765 9581	.2420 5863	.2114 7410	.1844 7404
3.53	.3208 7399	.2818 4042	.2470 8273	.2162 4521	.1889 7087
3.54	.3263 2013	.2871 2092	.2521 5069	.2210 6695	.1935 2388
3.55	.3317 9194	.2924 3618	.2572 6147	.2259 3842	.1981 3233
3.56	.3372 8824	.2977 8507	.2624 1402	.2308 5871	.2027 9548
3.57	.3428 0782	.3031 6643	.2676 0730	.2358 2687	.2075 1252
3.58	.3483 4948	.3085 7909	.2728 4019	.2408 4194	.2122 8263
3.59	.3539 1199	.3140 2185	.2781 1159	.2459 0291	.2171 0496
3.60	.3594 9414	.3194 9353	.2834 2038	.2510 0876	.2219 7861
3.61	.3650 9470	.3249 9292	.2887 6539	.2561 5845	.2269 0267
3.62	.3707 1244	.3305 1879	.2941 4548	.2613 5089	.2318 7619
3.63	.3763 4612	.3360 6991	.2995 5945	.2665 8500	.2368 9819
3.64	.3819 9450	.3416 4504	.3050 0610	.2718 5965	.2419 6766
3.65	.3876 5635	.3472 4293	.3104 8422	.2771 7371	.2470 8358
3.66	.3933 3041	.3528 6233	.3159 9259	.2825 2601	.2522 4488
3.67	.3990 1546	.3585 0197	.3215 2995	.2879 1537	.2574 5047
3.68	.4047 1026	.3641 6058	.3270 9507	.2933 4060	.2626 9926
3.69	.4104 1355	.3698 3689	.3326 8667	.2988 0048	.2679 9010
3.70	.4161 2411	.3755 2962	.3383 0347	.3042 9377	.2733 2184
3.71	.4218 4069	.3812 3749	.3439 4420	.3098 1924	.2786 9331
3.72	.4275 6208	.3869 5923	.3496 0756	.3153 7561	.2841 0329
3.73	.4332 8705	.3926 9354	.3552 9226	.3209 6160	.2895 5058
3.74	.4390 1436	.3984 3914	.3609 9698	.3265 7594	.2950 3394
3.75	.4447 4282	.4041 9475	.3667 2042	.3322 1731	.3005 5211
3.76	.4504 7121	.4099 5909	.3724 6126	.3378 8441	.3061 0382
3.77	.4561 9833	.4157 3088	.3782 1817	.3435 7592	.3116 8778
3.78	.4619 2299	.4215 0884	.3839 8985	.3492 9051	.3173 0269
3.79	.4676 4401	.4272 9171	.3897 7497	.3550 2683	.3229 4723
3.80	.4733 6021	.4330 7820	.3955 7220	.3607 8355	.3286 2007
3.81	.4790 7043	.4388 6707	.4013 8022	.3665 5931	.3343 1988
3.82	.4847 7352	.4446 5706	.4071 9770	.3723 5277	.3400 4530
3.83	.4904 6833	.4504 4691	.4130 2333	.3781 6256	.3457 9497
3.84	.4961 5375	.4562 3540	.4188 5580	.3839 8733	.3515 6752
3.85	.5018 2864	.4620 2128	.4246 9378	.3898 2571	.3573 6158
3.86	.5074 9191	.4678 0334	.4305 3597	.3956 7634	.3631 7576
3.87	.5131 4247	.4735 8036	.4363 8106	.4015 3787	.3690 0868
3.88	.5187 7924	.4793 5114	.4422 2776	.4074 0893	.3748 5894
3.89	.5244 0117	.4851 1450	.4480 7479	.4132 8816	.3807 2515
3.90	.5300 0720	.4908 6925	.4539 2085	.4191 7421	.3866 0591
3.91	.5355 9630	.4966 1424	.4597 6468	.4250 6573	.3924 9983
3.92	.5411 6747	.5023 4830	.4656 0502	.4309 6138	.3984 0551
3.93	.5467 1970	.5080 7030	.4714 4060	.4368 5981	.4043 2155
3.94	.5522 5202	.5137 7912	.4772 7019	.4427 5969	.4102 4655
3.95	.5577 6346	.5194 7365	.4830 9257	.4486 5970	.4161 7912
3.96	.5632 5308	.5251 5279	.4889 0651	.4545 5853	.4221 1788
3.97	.5687 1994	.5308 1548	.4947 1080	.4604 5486	.4280 6145
3.98	.5741 6314	.5364 6064	.5005 0427	.4663 4740	.4340 0843
3.99	.5795 8180	.5420 8724	.5062 8572	.4722 3486	.4399 5748

W	P(W,24)	P(W,26)	P(W,28)	P(W,30)	P(W,32)
4.00	.5849 7503	.5476 9425	.5120 5401	.4781 1597	.4459 0721
4.01	.5903 4198	.5532 8066	.5178 0799	.4839 8946	.4518 5629
4.02	.5956 8183	.5588 4548	.5235 4651	.4898 5410	.4578 0335
4.03	.6009 9376	.5643 8774	.5292 6849	.4957 0864	.4637 4708
4.04	.6062 7698	.5699 0649	.5349 7280	.5015 5186	.4696 8613
4.05	.6115 3070	.5754 0080	.5406 5839	.5073 8256	.4756 1921
4.06	.6167 5419	.5808 6974	.5463 2419	.5131 9955	.4815 4502
4.07	.6219 4670	.5863 1244	.5519 6915	.5190 0165	.4874 6226
4.08	.6271 0753	.5917 2801	.5575 9226	.5247 8772	.4933 6966
4.09	.6322 3597	.5971 1560	.5631 9251	.5305 5660	.4992 6598
4.10	.6373 3137	.6024 7438	.5687 6892	.5363 0718	.5051 4996
4.11	.6423 9307	.6078 0354	.5743 2053	.5420 3836	.5110 2038
4.12	.6474 2044	.6131 0229	.5798 4638	.5477 4906	.5168 7603
4.13	.6524 1287	.6183 6985	.5853 4556	.5534 3820	.5227 1573
4.14	.6573 6978	.6236 0549	.5908 1717	.5591 0475	.5285 3829
4.15	.6622 9059	.6288 0846	.5962 6033	.5647 4768	.5343 4257
4.16	.6671 7476	.6339 7808	.6016 7418	.5703 6598	.5401 2742
4.17	.6720 2177	.6391 1365	.6070 5788	.5759 5868	.5458 9173
4.18	.6768 3111	.6442 1451	.6124 1062	.5815 2482	.5516 3441
4.19	.6816 0229	.6492 8003	.6177 3160	.5870 6345	.5573 5437
4.20	.6863 3486	.6543 0958	.6230 2005	.5925 7366	.5630 5056
4.21	.6910 2837	.6593 0257	.6282 7523	.5980 5455	.5687 2196
4.22	.6956 8240	.6642 5843	.6334 9640	.6035 0525	.5743 6754
4.23	.7002 9655	.6691 7660	.6386 8288	.6089 2491	.5799 8632
4.24	.7048 7043	.6740 5654	.6438 3396	.6143 1270	.5855 7733
4.25	.7094 0368	.6788 9776	.6489 4900	.6196 6782	.5911 3962
4.26	.7138 9597	.6836 9977	.6540 2736	.6249 8948	.5966 7227
4.27	.7183 4698	.6884 6209	.6590 6843	.6302 7693	.6021 7439
4.28	.7227 5639	.6931 8428	.6640 7162	.6355 2944	.6076 4509
4.29	.7271 2392	.6978 6592	.6690 3636	.6407 4628	.6130 8353
4.30	.7314 4933	.7025 0662	.6739 6210	.6459 2678	.6184 8887
4.31	.7357 3235	.7071 0598	.6788 4833	.6510 7027	.6238 6032
4.32	.7399 7276	.7116 6364	.6836 9454	.6561 7610	.6291 9709
4.33	.7441 7037	.7161 7927	.6885 0025	.6612 4367	.6344 9842
4.34	.7483 2497	.7206 5255	.6932 6502	.6662 7237	.6397 6359
4.35	.7524 3640	.7250 8319	.6979 8840	.6712 6164	.6449 9189
4.36	.7565 0451	.7294 7089	.7026 7000	.6762 1094	.6501 8263
4.37	.7605 2917	.7338 1540	.7073 0941	.6811 1973	.6553 3515
4.38	.7645 1024	.7381 1650	.7119 0627	.6859 8751	.6604 4883
4.39	.7684 4765	.7423 7394	.7164 6025	.6908 1382	.6655 2304
4.40	.7723 4129	.7465 8755	.7209 7100	.6955 9820	.6705 5721
4.41	.7761 9111	.7507 5713	.7254 3823	.7003 4021	.6755 5078
4.42	.7799 9706	.7548 8252	.7298 6166	.7050 3945	.6805 0320
4.43	.7837 5910	.7589 6358	.7342 4102	.7096 9553	.6854 1396
4.44	.7874 7720	.7630 0019	.7385 7608	.7143 0810	.6902 8258
4.45	.7911 5138	.7669 9223	.7428 6661	.7188 7680	.6951 0859
4.46	.7947 8164	.7709 3962	.7471 1242	.7234 0132	.6998 9154
4.47	.7983 6801	.7748 4229	.7513 1332	.7278 8137	.7046 3103
4.48	.8019 1052	.7787 0018	.7554 6914	.7323 1667	.7093 2664
4.49	.8054 0924	.7825 1325	.7595 7976	.7367 0695	.7139 7803

W	P(W,24)	P(W,26)	P(W,28)	P(W,30)	P(W,32)
4.50	.8088 6423	.7862 8147	.7636 4504	.7410 5200	.7185 8482
4.51	.8122 7557	.7900 0486	.7676 6488	.7453 5160	.7231 4671
4.52	.8156 4337	.7936 8340	.7716 3919	.7496 0556	.7276 6338
4.53	.8189 6772	.7973 1713	.7755 6791	.7538 1370	.7321 3456
4.54	.8222 4876	.8009 0609	.7794 5097	.7579 7587	.7365 5998
4.55	.8254 8661	.8044 5033	.7832 8836	.7620 9194	.7409 3942
4.56	.8286 8143	.8079 4993	.7870 8005	.7661 6181	.7452 7264
4.57	.8318 3336	.8114 0496	.7908 2604	.7701 8536	.7495 5947
4.58	.8349 4257	.8148 1553	.7945 2634	.7741 6254	.7537 9972
4.59	.8380 0925	.8181 8174	.7981 8099	.7780 9328	.7579 9324
4.60	.8410 3359	.8215 0373	.8017 9004	.7819 7755	.7621 3990
4.61	.8440 1578	.8247 8162	.8053 5355	.7858 1531	.7662 3959
4.62	.8469 5603	.8280 1556	.8088 7160	.7896 0658	.7702 9221
4.63	.8498 5458	.8312 0573	.8123 4427	.7933 5136	.7742 9769
4.64	.8527 1163	.8343 5228	.8157 7168	.7970 4968	.7782 5597
4.65	.8555 2744	.8374 5541	.8191 5394	.8007 0159	.7821 6702
4.66	.8583 0225	.8405 1531	.8224 9119	.8043 0715	.7860 3082
4.67	.8610 3631	.8435 3219	.8257 8357	.8078 6643	.7898 4736
4.68	.8637 2989	.8465 0626	.8290 3125	.8113 7954	.7936 1667
4.69	.8663 8326	.8494 3775	.8322 3440	.8148 4657	.7973 3877
4.70	.8689 9670	.8523 2691	.8353 9320	.8182 6765	.8010 1372
4.71	.8715 7049	.8551 7396	.8385 0784	.8216 4291	.8046 4159
4.72	.8741 0493	.8579 7918	.8415 7853	.8249 7250	.8082 2245
4.73	.8766 0031	.8607 4281	.8446 0549	.8282 5659	.8117 5641
4.74	.8790 5695	.8634 6514	.8475 8896	.8314 9534	.8152 4357
4.75	.8814 7514	.8661 4645	.8505 2916	.8346 8896	.8186 8408
4.76	.8838 5522	.8687 8702	.8534 2634	.8378 3762	.8220 7805
4.77	.8861 9750	.8713 8715	.8562 8077	.8409 4156	.8254 2567
4.78	.8885 0231	.8739 4714	.8590 9271	.8440 0099	.8287 2709
4.79	.8907 6999	.8764 6730	.8618 6244	.8470 1614	.8319 8249
4.80	.8930 0086	.8789 4794	.8645 9024	.8499 8726	.8351 9208
4.81	.8951 9528	.8813 8940	.8672 7640	.8529 1461	.8383 5605
4.82	.8973 5358	.8837 9198	.8699 2123	.8557 9844	.8414 7464
4.83	.8994 7612	.8861 5604	.8725 2504	.8586 3904	.8445 4807
4.84	.9015 6325	.8884 8191	.8750 8813	.8614 3668	.8475 7659
4.85	.9036 1533	.8907 6993	.8776 1083	.8641 9166	.8505 6045
4.86	.9056 3271	.8930 2044	.8800 9348	.8669 0428	.8534 9991
4.87	.9076 1576	.8952 3382	.8825 3640	.8695 7484	.8563 9525
4.88	.9095 6485	.8974 1040	.8849 3993	.8722 0367	.8592 4674
4.89	.9114 8033	.8995 5055	.8873 0443	.8747 9108	.8620 5470
4.90	.9133 6258	.9016 5464	.8896 3024	.8773 3741	.8648 1941
4.91	.9152 1198	.9037 2303	.8919 1772	.8798 4300	.8675 4119
4.92	.9170 2888	.9057 5610	.8941 6723	.8823 0818	.8702 2036
4.93	.9188 1368	.9077 5421	.8963 7914	.8847 3331	.8728 5724
4.94	.9205 6673	.9097 1776	.8985 5382	.8871 1875	.8754 5217
4.95	.9222 8843	.9116 4710	.9006 9164	.8894 6486	.8780 0549
4.96	.9239 7914	.9135 4263	.9027 9298	.8917 7200	.8805 1755
4.97	.9256 3925	.9154 0474	.9048 5822	.8940 4054	.8829 8870
4.98	.9272 6914	.9172 3379	.9068 8774	.8962 7086	.8854 1931
4.99	.9288 6918	.9190 3018	.9088 8193	.8984 6334	.8878 0973

W	P(W,24)	P(W,26)	P(W,28)	P(W,30)	P(W,32)
5.00	.9304 3975	.9207 9431	.9108 4118	.9006 1836	.8901 6035
5.01	.9319 8124	.9225 2654	.9127 6588	.9027 3631	.8924 7155
5.02	.9334 9401	.9242 2729	.9146 5642	.9048 1759	.8947 4369
5.03	.9349 7846	.9258 9692	.9165 1320	.9068 6258	.8969 7717
5.04	.9364 3496	.9275 3585	.9183 3662	.9088 7168	.8991 7238
5.05	.9378 6388	.9291 4445	.9201 2707	.9108 4529	.9013 2972
5.06	.9392 6560	.9307 2312	.9218 8495	.9127 8382	.9034 4958
5.07	.9406 4051	.9322 7224	.9236 1066	.9146 8766	.9055 3237
5.08	.9419 8896	.9337 9221	.9253 0461	.9165 5723	.9075 7849
5.09	.9433 1135	.9352 8343	.9269 6719	.9183 9293	.9095 8834
5.10	.9446 0803	.9367 4627	.9285 9881	.9201 9516	.9115 6234
5.11	.9458 7938	.9381 8112	.9301 9986	.9219 6434	.9135 0090
5.12	.9471 2577	.9395 8838	.9317 7075	.9237 0088	.9154 0444
5.13	.9483 4757	.9409 6843	.9333 1188	.9254 0519	.9172 7336
5.14	.9495 4513	.9423 2166	.9348 2366	.9270 7768	.9191 0810
5.15	.9507 1883	.9436 4845	.9363 0647	.9287 1876	.9209 0906
5.16	.9518 6903	.9449 4918	.9377 6072	.9303 2884	.9226 7666
5.17	.9529 9609	.9462 2423	.9391 8682	.9319 0834	.9244 1133
5.18	.9541 0035	.9474 7399	.9405 8515	.9334 5767	.9261 1349
5.19	.9551 8218	.9486 9882	.9419 5611	.9349 7724	.9277 8356
5.20	.9562 4194	.9498 9912	.9433 0010	.9364 6745	.9294 2196
5.21	.9572 7996	.9510 7524	.9446 1750	.9379 2872	.9310 2911
5.22	.9582 9660	.9522 2756	.9459 0873	.9393 6146	.9326 0543
5.23	.9592 9220	.9533 5645	.9471 7415	.9407 6606	.9341 5135
5.24	.9602 6710	.9544 6227	.9484 1416	.9421 4295	.9356 6728
5.25	.9612 2164	.9555 4540	.9496 2915	.9434 9252	.9371 5364
5.26	.9621 5616	.9566 0618	.9508 1949	.9448 1517	.9386 1085
5.27	.9630 7100	.9576 4499	.9519 8558	.9461 1131	.9400 3933
5.28	.9639 6647	.9586 6216	.9531 2778	.9473 8134	.9414 3950
5.29	.9648 4291	.9596 5807	.9542 4648	.9486 2564	.9428 1176
5.30	.9657 0065	.9606 3306	.9553 4205	.9498 4463	.9441 5654
5.31	.9665 4000	.9615 8747	.9564 1486	.9510 3868	.9454 7423
5.32	.9673 6128	.9625 2166	.9574 6527	.9522 0818	.9467 6525
5.33	.9681 6481	.9634 3595	.9584 9367	.9533 5354	.9480 3002
5.34	.9689 5089	.9643 3069	.9595 0040	.9544 7512	.9492 6892
5.35	.9697 1984	.9652 0622	.9604 8582	.9555 7332	.9504 8236
5.36	.9704 7196	.9660 6287	.9614 5030	.9566 4851	.9516 7075
5.37	.9712 0755	.9669 0096	.9623 9418	.9577 0107	.9528 3448
5.38	.9719 2691	.9677 2082	.9633 1783	.9587 3137	.9539 7394
5.39	.9726 3033	.9685 2276	.9642 2157	.9597 3979	.9550 8953
5.40	.9733 1811	.9693 0712	.9651 0576	.9607 2668	.9561 8164
5.41	.9739 9053	.9700 7421	.9659 7075	.9616 9242	.9572 5065
5.42	.9746 4788	.9708 2432	.9668 1685	.9626 3736	.9582 9694
5.43	.9752 9043	.9715 5778	.9676 4441	.9635 6187	.9593 2089
5.44	.9759 1847	.9722 7489	.9684 5377	.9644 6629	.9603 2289
5.45	.9765 3226	.9729 7595	.9692 4523	.9653 5098	.9613 0330
5.46	.9771 3209	.9736 6124	.9700 1913	.9662 1628	.9622 6249
5.47	.9777 1821	.9743 3108	.9707 7579	.9670 6254	.9632 0084
5.48	.9782 9088	.9749 8575	.9715 1552	.9678 9010	.9641 1870
5.49	.9788 5037	.9756 2553	.9722 3863	.9686 9929	.9650 1643

W	P(W,24)	P(W,26)	P(W,28)	P(W,30)	P(W,32)
5.50	.9793 9694	.9762 5070	.9729 4544	.9694 9044	.9658 9439
5.51	.9799 3083	.9768 6155	.9736 3624	.9702 6389	.9667 5293
5.52	.9804 5230	.9774 5835	.9743 1134	.9710 1997	.9675 9239
5.53	.9809 6158	.9780 4137	.9749 7103	.9717 5898	.9684 1314
5.54	.9814 5893	.9786 1089	.9756 1560	.9724 8125	.9692 1549
5.55	.9819 4458	.9791 6715	.9762 4535	.9731 8710	.9699 9980
5.56	.9824 1876	.9797 1043	.9768 6056	.9738 7682	.9707 6639
5.57	.9828 8171	.9802 4099	.9774 6152	.9745 5074	.9715 1560
5.58	.9833 3365	.9807 5906	.9780 4850	.9752 0914	.9722 4775
5.59	.9837 7481	.9812 6491	.9786 2177	.9758 5234	.9729 6315
5.60	.9842 0541	.9817 5878	.9791 8160	.9764 8061	.9736 6214
5.61	.9846 2567	.9822 4091	.9797 2827	.9770 9426	.9743 4501
5.62	.9850 3581	.9827 1155	.9802 6203	.9776 9357	.9750 1209
5.63	.9854 3602	.9831 7092	.9807 8315	.9782 7882	.9756 6367
5.64	.9858 2652	.9836 1925	.9812 9187	.9788 5029	.9763 0006
5.65	.9862 0752	.9840 5678	.9817 8845	.9794 0826	.9769 2156
5.66	.9865 7922	.9844 8373	.9822 7315	.9799 5299	.9775 2845
5.67	.9869 4180	.9849 0032	.9827 4619	.9804 8475	.9781 2103
5.68	.9872 9548	.9853 0677	.9832 0782	.9810 0381	.9786 9958
5.69	.9876 4043	.9857 0329	.9836 5828	.9815 1042	.9792 6439
5.70	.9879 7685	.9860 9009	.9840 9781	.9820 0484	.9798 1573
5.71	.9883 0491	.9864 6738	.9845 2662	.9824 8732	.9803 5387
5.72	.9886 2481	.9868 3536	.9849 4495	.9829 5811	.9808 7908
5.73	.9889 3672	.9871 9423	.9853 5302	.9834 1744	.9813 9163
5.74	.9892 4082	.9875 4419	.9857 5104	.9838 6557	.9818 9178
5.75	.9895 3727	.9878 8544	.9861 3923	.9843 0273	.9823 7979
5.76	.9898 2625	.9882 1815	.9865 1780	.9847 2915	.9828 5590
5.77	.9901 0792	.9885 4252	.9868 8696	.9851 4505	.9833 2038
5.78	.9903 8244	.9888 5874	.9872 4692	.9855 5066	.9837 7345
5.79	.9906 4999	.9891 6697	.9875 9786	.9859 4621	.9842 1537
5.80	.9909 1070	.9894 6741	.9879 4000	.9863 3191	.9846 4638
5.81	.9911 6475	.9897 6022	.9882 7352	.9867 0797	.9850 6670
5.82	.9914 1227	.9900 4557	.9885 9862	.9870 7460	.9854 7656
5.83	.9916 5341	.9903 2364	.9889 1548	.9874 3202	.9858 7619
5.84	.9918 8834	.9905 9458	.9892 2428	.9877 8042	.9862 6582
5.85	.9921 1717	.9908 5856	.9895 2520	.9881 2000	.9866 4566
5.86	.9923 4007	.9911 1573	.9898 1843	.9884 5095	.9870 1593
5.87	.9925 5716	.9913 6626	.9901 0414	.9887 7348	.9873 7683
5.88	.9927 6857	.9916 1029	.9903 8249	.9890 8777	.9877 2857
5.89	.9929 7445	.9918 4798	.9906 5366	.9893 9400	.9880 7137
5.90	.9931 7492	.9920 7946	.9909 1780	.9896 9235	.9884 0541
5.91	.9933 7011	.9923 0490	.9911 7509	.9899 8302	.9887 3089
5.92	.9935 6014	.9925 2441	.9914 2567	.9902 6616	.9890 4802
5.93	.9937 4514	.9927 3816	.9916 6971	.9905 4196	.9893 5696
5.94	.9939 2522	.9929 4626	.9919 0735	.9908 1058	.9896 5793
5.95	.9941 0051	.9931 4886	.9921 3875	.9910 7218	.9899 5108
5.96	.9942 7111	.9933 4609	.9923 6405	.9913 2694	.9902 3661
5.97	.9944 3715	.9935 3806	.9925 8339	.9915 7500	.9905 1469
5.98	.9945 9872	.9937 2492	.9927 9692	.9918 1654	.9907 8549
5.99	.9947 5594	.9939 0677	.9930 0477	.9920 5169	.9910 4918

W	P(W,24)	P(W,26)	P(W,28)	P(W,30)	P(W,32)
6.00	.9949 0892	.9940 8375	.9932 0708	.9922 8061	.9913 0593
6.01	.9950 5776	.9942 5596	.9934 0399	.9925 0345	.9915 5590
6.02	.9952 0255	.9944 2353	.9935 9561	.9927 2036	.9917 9924
6.03	.9953 4340	.9945 8657	.9937 8209	.9929 3146	.9920 3613
6.04	.9954 8042	.9947 4519	.9939 6353	.9931 3691	.9922 6670
6.05	.9956 1368	.9948 9949	.9941 4008	.9933 3684	.9924 9111
6.06	.9957 4328	.9950 4958	.9943 1183	.9935 3138	.9927 0951
6.07	.9958 6932	.9951 9557	.9944 7892	.9937 2066	.9929 2204
6.08	.9959 9189	.9953 3756	.9946 4146	.9939 0482	.9931 2884
6.09	.9961 1107	.9954 7565	.9947 9955	.9940 8397	.9933 3005
6.10	.9962 2694	.9956 0993	.9949 5331	.9942 5824	.9935 2581
6.11	.9963 3960	.9957 4051	.9951 0285	.9944 2774	.9937 1625
6.12	.9964 4912	.9958 6746	.9952 4826	.9945 9260	.9939 0150
6.13	.9965 5558	.9959 9089	.9953 8967	.9947 5294	.9940 8169
6.14	.9966 5906	.9961 1089	.9955 2715	.9949 0885	.9942 5694
6.15	.9967 5963	.9962 2753	.9956 6082	.9950 6046	.9944 2737
6.16	.9968 5738	.9963 4091	.9957 9077	.9952 0787	.9945 9311
6.17	.9969 5237	.9964 5111	.9959 1709	.9953 5119	.9947 5427
6.18	.9970 4467	.9965 5821	.9960 3988	.9954 9052	.9949 1096
6.19	.9971 3436	.9966 6230	.9961 5922	.9956 2596	.9950 6330
6.20	.9972 2150	.9967 6344	.9962 7521	.9957 5761	.9952 1140
6.21	.9973 0616	.9968 6171	.9963 8793	.9958 8557	.9953 5537
6.22	.9973 8840	.9969 5720	.9964 9746	.9960 0993	.9954 9530
6.23	.9974 6829	.9970 4996	.9966 0389	.9961 3078	.9956 3131
6.24	.9975 4589	.9971 4008	.9967 0729	.9962 4821	.9957 6349
6.25	.9976 2126	.9972 2762	.9968 0775	.9963 6232	.9958 9194
6.26	.9976 9446	.9973 1265	.9969 0535	.9964 7318	.9960 1675
6.27	.9977 6554	.9973 9523	.9970 0015	.9965 8089	.9961 3803
6.28	.9978 3457	.9974 7544	.9970 9223	.9966 8552	.9962 5586
6.29	.9979 0159	.9975 5333	.9971 8167	.9967 8715	.9963 7033
6.30	.9979 6666	.9976 2896	.9972 6852	.9968 8587	.9964 8153
6.31	.9980 2984	.9977 0240	.9973 5287	.9969 8175	.9965 8954
6.32	.9980 9117	.9977 7371	.9974 3477	.9970 7487	.9966 9445
6.33	.9981 5070	.9978 4293	.9975 1430	.9971 6529	.9967 9635
6.34	.9982 0849	.9979 1014	.9975 9152	.9972 5309	.9968 9530
6.35	.9982 6458	.9979 7537	.9976 6648	.9973 3834	.9969 9139
6.36	.9983 1901	.9980 3869	.9977 3925	.9974 2111	.9970 8469
6.37	.9983 7184	.9981 0015	.9978 0989	.9975 0147	.9971 7528
6.38	.9984 2310	.9981 5979	.9978 7845	.9975 7947	.9972 6323
6.39	.9984 7284	.9982 1767	.9979 4499	.9976 5519	.9973 4861
6.40	.9985 2111	.9982 7384	.9980 0957	.9977 2868	.9974 3149
6.41	.9985 6793	.9983 2834	.9980 7225	.9978 0000	.9975 1194
6.42	.9986 1335	.9983 8121	.9981 3306	.9978 6923	.9975 9003
6.43	.9986 5742	.9984 3252	.9981 9207	.9979 3640	.9976 6581
6.44	.9987 0016	.9984 8228	.9982 4932	.9980 0158	.9977 3935
6.45	.9987 4162	.9985 3056	.9983 0486	.9980 6482	.9978 1071
6.46	.9987 8183	.9985 7739	.9983 5874	.9981 2617	.9978 7995
6.47	.9988 2082	.9986 2281	.9984 1101	.9981 8570	.9979 4713
6.48	.9988 5863	.9986 6686	.9984 6171	.9982 4344	.9980 1231
6.49	.9988 9530	.9987 0958	.9985 1088	.9982 9945	.9980 7554

W	P(W,24)	P(W,26)	P(W,28)	P(W,30)	P(W,32)
6.50	.9989 3086	.9987 5100	.9985 5856	.9983 5378	.9981 3687
6.51	.9989 6533	.9987 9117	.9986 0481	.9984 0647	.9981 9637
6.52	.9989 9875	.9988 3012	.9986 4965	.9984 5757	.9982 5407
6.53	.9990 3114	.9988 6788	.9986 9314	.9985 0712	.9983 1003
6.54	.9990 6255	.9989 0449	.9987 3530	.9985 5517	.9983 6430
6.55	.9990 9299	.9989 3998	.9987 7617	.9986 0175	.9984 1692
6.56	.9991 2249	.9989 7438	.9988 1579	.9986 4692	.9984 6795
6.57	.9991 5109	.9990 0772	.9988 5420	.9986 9071	.9985 1743
6.58	.9991 7880	.9990 4004	.9988 9143	.9987 3316	.9985 6539
6.59	.9992 0565	.9990 7136	.9989 2752	.9987 7431	.9986 1189
6.60	.9992 3167	.9991 0171	.9989 6249	.9988 1420	.9986 5696
6.61	.9992 5688	.9991 3112	.9989 9639	.9988 5285	.9987 0065
6.62	.9992 8131	.9991 5961	.9990 2923	.9988 9031	.9987 4300
6.63	.9993 0498	.9991 8722	.9990 6106	.9989 2662	.9987 8404
6.64	.9993 2790	.9992 1397	.9990 9190	.9989 6180	.9988 2381
6.65	.9993 5011	.9992 3989	.9991 2177	.9989 9589	.9988 6235
6.66	.9993 7162	.9992 6499	.9991 5072	.9990 2891	.9988 9970
6.67	.9993 9245	.9992 8931	.9991 7876	.9990 6091	.9989 3588
6.68	.9994 1262	.9993 1286	.9992 0592	.9990 9191	.9989 7094
6.69	.9994 3216	.9993 3567	.9992 3223	.9991 2193	.9990 0490
6.70	.9994 5108	.9993 5776	.9992 5771	.9991 5102	.9990 3780
6.71	.9994 6941	.9993 7916	.9992 8239	.9991 7919	.9990 6966
6.72	.9994 8715	.9993 9987	.9993 0628	.9992 0647	.9991 0053
6.73	.9995 0432	.9994 1993	.9993 2943	.9992 3289	.9991 3043
6.74	.9995 2095	.9994 3935	.9993 5183	.9992 5848	.9991 5938
6.75	.9995 3704	.9994 5815	.9993 7353	.9992 8326	.9991 8741
6.76	.9995 5263	.9994 7636	.9993 9454	.9993 0725	.9992 1456
6.77	.9995 6771	.9994 9398	.9994 1487	.9993 3047	.9992 4085
6.78	.9995 8230	.9995 1103	.9994 3456	.9993 5296	.9992 6630
6.79	.9995 9643	.9995 2754	.9994 5361	.9993 7472	.9992 9094
6.80	.9996 1010	.9995 4352	.9994 7206	.9993 9579	.9993 1479
6.81	.9996 2333	.9995 5898	.9994 8991	.9994 1619	.9993 3788
6.82	.9996 3614	.9995 7394	.9995 0718	.9994 3593	.9993 6023
6.83	.9996 4852	.9995 8842	.9995 2390	.9994 5503	.9993 8187
6.84	.9996 6051	.9996 0243	.9995 4008	.9994 7352	.9994 0280
6.85	.9996 7210	.9996 1598	.9995 5574	.9994 9141	.9994 2306
6.86	.9996 8332	.9996 2910	.9995 7088	.9995 0872	.9994 4267
6.87	.9996 9417	.9996 4179	.9995 8554	.9995 2547	.9994 6164
6.88	.9997 0467	.9996 5406	.9995 9971	.9995 4168	.9994 8000
6.89	.9997 1482	.9996 6593	.9996 1343	.9995 5736	.9994 9776
6.90	.9997 2464	.9996 7741	.9996 2669	.9995 7252	.9995 1494
6.91	.9997 3413	.9996 8852	.9996 3953	.9995 8719	.9995 3157
6.92	.9997 4331	.9996 9926	.9996 5194	.9996 0138	.9995 4764
6.93	.9997 5219	.9997 0964	.9996 6394	.9996 1511	.9995 6320
6.94	.9997 6078	.9997 1969	.9996 7555	.9996 2838	.9995 7824
6.95	.9997 6908	.9997 2940	.9996 8677	.9996 4122	.9995 9279
6.96	.9997 7710	.9997 3879	.9996 9762	.9996 5363	.9996 0686
6.97	.9997 8486	.9997 4787	.9997 0812	.9996 6564	.9996 2046
6.98	.9997 9236	.9997 5664	.9997 1826	.9996 7724	.9996 3362
6.99	.9997 9961	.9997 6513	.9997 2807	.9996 8846	.9996 4634

W	P(W,24)	P(W,26)	P(W,28)	P(W,30)	P(W,32)
7.00	.9998 0662	.9997 7333	.9997 3755	.9996 9931	.9996 5864
7.01	.9998 1339	.9997 8126	.9997 4672	.9997 0980	.9996 7052
7.02	.9998 1994	.9997 8892	.9997 5558	.9997 1994	.9996 8202
7.03	.9998 2626	.9997 9632	.9997 6414	.9997 2973	.9996 9313
7.04	.9998 3238	.9998 0348	.9997 7242	.9997 3920	.9997 0387
7.05	.9998 3828	.9998 1040	.9997 8041	.9997 4836	.9997 1425
7.06	.9998 4399	.9998 1708	.9997 8814	.9997 5720	.9997 2428
7.07	.9998 4950	.9998 2354	.9997 9561	.9997 6575	.9997 3398
7.08	.9998 5483	.9998 2977	.9998 0283	.9997 7401	.9997 4334
7.09	.9998 5998	.9998 3580	.9998 0980	.9997 8199	.9997 5240
7.10	.9998 6495	.9998 4162	.9998 1654	.9997 8970	.9997 6114
7.11	.9998 6975	.9998 4725	.9998 2304	.9997 9715	.9997 6960
7.12	.9998 7439	.9998 5268	.9998 2933	.9998 0435	.9997 7776
7.13	.9998 7887	.9998 5793	.9998 3540	.9998 1130	.9997 8565
7.14	.9998 8320	.9998 6300	.9998 4127	.9998 1802	.9997 9327
7.15	.9998 8737	.9998 6789	.9998 4693	.9998 2450	.9998 0063
7.16	.9998 9141	.9998 7262	.9998 5240	.9998 3077	.9998 0774
7.17	.9998 9530	.9998 7718	.9998 5768	.9998 3682	.9998 1460
7.18	.9998 9907	.9998 8159	.9998 6278	.9998 4266	.9998 2123
7.19	.9999 0270	.9998 8585	.9998 6771	.9998 4830	.9998 2764
7.20	.9999 0620	.9998 8995	.9998 7247	.9998 5375	.9998 3382
7.21	.9999 0959	.9998 9392	.9998 7706	.9998 5901	.9998 3979
7.22	.9999 1286	.9998 9775	.9998 8149	.9998 6409	.9998 4556
7.23	.9999 1601	.9999 0145	.9998 8577	.9998 6899	.9998 5112
7.24	.9999 1905	.9999 0502	.9998 8990	.9998 7373	.9998 5650
7.25	.9999 2199	.9999 0846	.9998 9389	.9998 7830	.9998 6168
7.26	.9999 2483	.9999 1178	.9998 9774	.9998 8271	.9998 6669
7.27	.9999 2757	.9999 1499	.9999 0145	.9998 8696	.9998 7152
7.28	.9999 3021	.9999 1809	.9999 0504	.9998 9107	.9998 7619
7.29	.9999 3275	.9999 2107	.9999 0850	.9998 9504	.9998 8069
7.30	.9999 3521	.9999 2396	.9999 1184	.9998 9886	.9998 8503
7.31	.9999 3758	.9999 2674	.9999 1506	.9999 0255	.9998 8923
7.32	.9999 3987	.9999 2942	.9999 1817	.9999 0612	.9998 9327
7.33	.9999 4208	.9999 3201	.9999 2117	.9999 0955	.9998 9718
7.34	.9999 4421	.9999 3451	.9999 2406	.9999 1287	.9999 0094
7.35	.9999 4626	.9999 3692	.9999 2685	.9999 1607	.9999 0458
7.36	.9999 4825	.9999 3924	.9999 2954	.9999 1915	.9999 0808
7.37	.9999 5016	.9999 4148	.9999 3214	.9999 2213	.9999 1146
7.38	.9999 5200	.9999 4364	.9999 3464	.9999 2500	.9999 1472
7.39	.9999 5378	.9999 4573	.9999 3706	.9999 2777	.9999 1787
7.40	.9999 5549	.9999 4774	.9999 3939	.9999 3044	.9999 2091
7.41	.9999 5714	.9999 4968	.9999 4163	.9999 3302	.9999 2383
7.42	.9999 5874	.9999 5155	.9999 4380	.9999 3550	.9999 2665
7.43	.9999 6027	.9999 5335	.9999 4589	.9999 3790	.9999 2938
7.44	.9999 6175	.9999 5509	.9999 4790	.9999 4021	.9999 3200
7.45	.9999 6318	.9999 5676	.9999 4985	.9999 4243	.9999 3453
7.46	.9999 6456	.9999 5838	.9999 5172	.9999 4458	.9999 3697
7.47	.9999 6589	.9999 5993	.9999 5352	.9999 4665	.9999 3932
7.48	.9999 6716	.9999 6144	.9999 5526	.9999 4865	.9999 4159
7.49	.9999 6840	.9999 6288	.9999 5694	.9999 5057	.9999 4378

W	P(W,24)	P(W,26)	P(W,28)	P(W,30)	P(W,32)
7.50	.9999 6958	.9999 6428	.9999 5855	.9999 5242	.9999 4588
7.51	.9999 7073	.9999 6562	.9999 6011	.9999 5421	.9999 4791
7.52	.9999 7183	.9999 6691	.9999 6161	.9999 5593	.9999 4987
7.53	.9999 7290	.9999 6816	.9999 6306	.9999 5759	.9999 5176
7.54	.9999 7392	.9999 6937	.9999 6445	.9999 5919	.9999 5358
7.55	.9999 7491	.9999 7052	.9999 6580	.9999 6073	.9999 5533
7.56	.9999 7586	.9999 7164	.9999 6709	.9999 6222	.9999 5702
7.57	.9999 7677	.9999 7272	.9999 6834	.9999 6365	.9999 5864
7.58	.9999 7766	.9999 7375	.9999 6954	.9999 6503	.9999 6021
7.59	.9999 7851	.9999 7475	.9999 7070	.9999 6635	.9999 6172
7.60	.9999 7933	.9999 7571	.9999 7181	.9999 6763	.9999 6317
7.61	.9999 8012	.9999 7664	.9999 7289	.9999 6887	.9999 6457
7.62	.9999 8088	.9999 7753	.9999 7392	.9999 7005	.9999 6592
7.63	.9999 8161	.9999 7839	.9999 7492	.9999 7120	.9999 6722
7.64	.9999 8231	.9999 7922	.9999 7588	.9999 7230	.9999 6848
7.65	.9999 8299	.9999 8001	.9999 7680	.9999 7336	.9999 6968
7.66	.9999 8364	.9999 8078	.9999 7769	.9999 7438	.9999 7084
7.67	.9999 8427	.9999 8152	.9999 7855	.9999 7536	.9999 7196
7.68	.9999 8488	.9999 8223	.9999 7937	.9999 7631	.9999 7304
7.69	.9999 8546	.9999 8291	.9999 8017	.9999 7722	.9999 7408
7.70	.9999 8602	.9999 8357	.9999 8093	.9999 7810	.9999 7507
7.71	.9999 8656	.9999 8421	.9999 8167	.9999 7894	.9999 7604
7.72	.9999 8708	.9999 8482	.9999 8238	.9999 7976	.9999 7696
7.73	.9999 8758	.9999 8541	.9999 8306	.9999 8054	.9999 7785
7.74	.9999 8806	.9999 8597	.9999 8372	.9999 8129	.9999 7871
7.75	.9999 8853	.9999 8652	.9999 8435	.9999 8202	.9999 7954
7.76	.9999 8897	.9999 8704	.9999 8496	.9999 8272	.9999 8033
7.77	.9999 8940	.9999 8755	.9999 8554	.9999 8339	.9999 8109
7.78	.9999 8982	.9999 8803	.9999 8610	.9999 8404	.9999 8183
7.79	.9999 9022	.9999 8850	.9999 8665	.9999 8466	.9999 8254
7.80	.9999 9060	.9999 8895	.9999 8717	.9999 8526	.9999 8322
7.81	.9999 9097	.9999 8938	.9999 8767	.9999 8583	.9999 8388
7.82	.9999 9132	.9999 8980	.9999 8815	.9999 8639	.9999 8451
7.83	.9999 9166	.9999 9020	.9999 8862	.9999 8692	.9999 8511
7.84	.9999 9199	.9999 9058	.9999 8906	.9999 8744	.9999 8570
7.85	.9999 9230	.9999 9095	.9999 8949	.9999 8793	.9999 8626
7.86	.9999 9261	.9999 9131	.9999 8991	.9999 8840	.9999 8680
7.87	.9999 9290	.9999 9165	.9999 9031	.9999 8886	.9999 8732
7.88	.9999 9318	.9999 9198	.9999 9069	.9999 8930	.9999 8782
7.89	.9999 9345	.9999 9230	.9999 9106	.9999 8972	.9999 8830
7.90	.9999 9371	.9999 9260	.9999 9141	.9999 9013	.9999 8876
7.91	.9999 9396	.9999 9290	.9999 9175	.9999 9052	.9999 8921
7.92	.9999 9420	.9999 9318	.9999 9208	.9999 9090	.9999 8963
7.93	.9999 9443	.9999 9345	.9999 9239	.9999 9126	.9999 9005
7.94	.9999 9465	.9999 9371	.9999 9269	.9999 9161	.9999 9044
7.95	.9999 9486	.9999 9396	.9999 9299	.9999 9194	.9999 9082
7.96	.9999 9507	.9999 9420	.9999 9327	.9999 9226	.9999 9119
7.97	.9999 9527	.9999 9443	.9999 9353	.9999 9257	.9999 9154
7.98	.9999 9546	.9999 9466	.9999 9379	.9999 9287	.9999 9188
7.99	.9999 9564	.9999 9487	.9999 9404	.9999 9315	.9999 9220

W	P(W,24)	P(W,26)	P(W,28)	P(W,30)	P(W,32)
8.00	.9999 9581	.9999 9507	.9999 9428	.9999 9343	.9999 9251
8.01	.9999 9598	.9999 9527	.9999 9451	.9999 9369	.9999 9281
8.02	.9999 9614	.9999 9546	.9999 9473	.9999 9394	.9999 9310
8.03	.9999 9630	.9999 9565	.9999 9494	.9999 9419	.9999 9338
8.04	.9999 9645	.9999 9582	.9999 9515	.9999 9442	.9999 9365
8.05	.9999 9659	.9999 9599	.9999 9534	.9999 9465	.9999 9390
8.06	.9999 9673	.9999 9615	.9999 9553	.9999 9486	.9999 9415
8.07	.9999 9686	.9999 9631	.9999 9571	.9999 9507	.9999 9438
8.08	.9999 9699	.9999 9646	.9999 9588	.9999 9527	.9999 9461
8.09	.9999 9711	.9999 9660	.9999 9605	.9999 9546	.9999 9483
8.10	.9999 9723	.9999 9674	.9999 9621	.9999 9564	.9999 9504
8.11	.9999 9734	.9999 9687	.9999 9636	.9999 9582	.9999 9524
8.12	.9999 9745	.9999 9700	.9999 9651	.9999 9599	.9999 9543
8.13	.9999 9755	.9999 9712	.9999 9665	.9999 9615	.9999 9562
8.14	.9999 9765	.9999 9724	.9999 9679	.9999 9631	.9999 9580
8.15	.9999 9775	.9999 9735	.9999 9692	.9999 9646	.9999 9597
8.16	.9999 9784	.9999 9746	.9999 9705	.9999 9661	.9999 9613
8.17	.9999 9793	.9999 9756	.9999 9717	.9999 9674	.9999 9629
8.18	.9999 9801	.9999 9766	.9999 9728	.9999 9688	.9999 9644
8.19	.9999 9809	.9999 9776	.9999 9740	.9999 9701	.9999 9659
8.20	.9999 9817	.9999 9785	.9999 9750	.9999 9713	.9999 9673
8.21	.9999 9825	.9999 9794	.9999 9760	.9999 9725	.9999 9686
8.22	.9999 9832	.9999 9802	.9999 9770	.9999 9736	.9999 9699
8.23	.9999 9839	.9999 9810	.9999 9780	.9999 9747	.9999 9712
8.24	.9999 9846	.9999 9818	.9999 9789	.9999 9757	.9999 9723
8.25	.9999 9852	.9999 9826	.9999 9798	.9999 9767	.9999 9735
8.26	.9999 9858	.9999 9833	.9999 9806	.9999 9777	.9999 9746
8.27	.9999 9864	.9999 9840	.9999 9814	.9999 9786	.9999 9756
8.28	.9999 9870	.9999 9847	.9999 9822	.9999 9795	.9999 9766
8.29	.9999 9875	.9999 9853	.9999 9829	.9999 9803	.9999 9776
8.30	.9999 9880	.9999 9859	.9999 9836	.9999 9812	.9999 9785
8.31	.9999 9885	.9999 9865	.9999 9843	.9999 9819	.9999 9794
8.32	.9999 9890	.9999 9870	.9999 9850	.9999 9827	.9999 9803
8.33	.9999 9894	.9999 9876	.9999 9856	.9999 9834	.9999 9811
8.34	.9999 9899	.9999 9881	.9999 9862	.9999 9841	.9999 9819
8.35	.9999 9903	.9999 9886	.9999 9868	.9999 9848	.9999 9827
8.36	.9999 9907	.9999 9891	.9999 9873	.9999 9854	.9999 9834
8.37	.9999 9911	.9999 9895	.9999 9878	.9999 9860	.9999 9841
8.38	.9999 9915	.9999 9900	.9999 9884	.9999 9866	.9999 9847
8.39	.9999 9918	.9999 9904	.9999 9888	.9999 9872	.9999 9854
8.40	.9999 9922	.9999 9908	.9999 9893	.9999 9877	.9999 9860
8.41	.9999 9925	.9999 9912	.9999 9898	.9999 9882	.9999 9866
8.42	.9999 9928	.9999 9916	.9999 9902	.9999 9887	.9999 9871
8.43	.9999 9931	.9999 9919	.9999 9906	.9999 9892	.9999 9877
8.44	.9999 9934	.9999 9923	.9999 9910	.9999 9896	.9999 9882
8.45	.9999 9937	.9999 9926	.9999 9914	.9999 9901	.9999 9887
8.46	.9999 9940	.9999 9929	.9999 9917	.9999 9905	.9999 9892
8.47	.9999 9942	.9999 9932	.9999 9921	.9999 9909	.9999 9896
8.48	.9999 9945	.9999 9935	.9999 9924	.9999 9913	.9999 9901
8.49	.9999 9947	.9999 9938	.9999 9928	.9999 9917	.9999 9905

W	P(W,24)	P(W,26)	P(W,28)	P(W,30)	P(W,32)
8.50	.9999 9949	.9999 9940	.9999 9931	.9999 9920	.9999 9909
8.51	.9999 9951	.9999 9943	.9999 9934	.9999 9924	.9999 9913
8.52	.9999 9953	.9999 9945	.9999 9936	.9999 9927	.9999 9917
8.53	.9999 9955	.9999 9948	.9999 9939	.9999 9930	.9999 9920
8.54	.9999 9957	.9999 9950	.9999 9942	.9999 9933	.9999 9924
8.55	.9999 9959	.9999 9952	.9999 9944	.9999 9936	.9999 9927
8.56	.9999 9961	.9999 9954	.9999 9947	.9999 9939	.9999 9930
8.57	.9999 9963	.9999 9956	.9999 9949	.9999 9941	.9999 9933
8.58	.9999 9964	.9999 9958	.9999 9951	.9999 9944	.9999 9936
8.59	.9999 9966	.9999 9960	.9999 9953	.9999 9946	.9999 9939
8.60	.9999 9967	.9999 9961	.9999 9955	.9999 9948	.9999 9941
8.61	.9999 9969	.9999 9963	.9999 9957	.9999 9951	.9999 9944
8.62	.9999 9970	.9999 9965	.9999 9959	.9999 9953	.9999 9946
8.63	.9999 9971	.9999 9966	.9999 9961	.9999 9955	.9999 9948
8.64	.9999 9972	.9999 9968	.9999 9962	.9999 9957	.9999 9951
8.65	.9999 9974	.9999 9969	.9999 9964	.9999 9959	.9999 9953
8.66	.9999 9975	.9999 9970	.9999 9966	.9999 9960	.9999 9955
8.67	.9999 9976	.9999 9972	.9999 9967	.9999 9962	.9999 9957
8.68	.9999 9977	.9999 9973	.9999 9968	.9999 9964	.9999 9959
8.69	.9999 9978	.9999 9974	.9999 9970	.9999 9965	.9999 9960
8.70	.9999 9979	.9999 9975	.9999 9971	.9999 9967	.9999 9962
8.71	.9999 9980	.9999 9976	.9999 9972	.9999 9968	.9999 9964
8.72	.9999 9981	.9999 9977	.9999 9974	.9999 9970	.9999 9965
8.73	.9999 9982	.9999 9978	.9999 9975	.9999 9971	.9999 9967
8.74	.9999 9982	.9999 9979	.9999 9976	.9999 9972	.9999 9968
8.75	.9999 9983	.9999 9980	.9999 9977	.9999 9973	.9999 9970
8.76	.9999 9984	.9999 9981	.9999 9978	.9999 9975	.9999 9971
8.77	.9999 9985	.9999 9982	.9999 9979	.9999 9976	.9999 9972
8.78	.9999 9985	.9999 9983	.9999 9980	.9999 9977	.9999 9973
8.79	.9999 9986	.9999 9983	.9999 9981	.9999 9978	.9999 9975
8.80	.9999 9986	.9999 9984	.9999 9981	.9999 9979	.9999 9976
8.81	.9999 9987	.9999 9985	.9999 9982	.9999 9980	.9999 9977
8.82	.9999 9988	.9999 9985	.9999 9983	.9999 9981	.9999 9978
8.83	.9999 9988	.9999 9986	.9999 9984	.9999 9981	.9999 9979
8.84	.9999 9989	.9999 9987	.9999 9985	.9999 9982	.9999 9980
8.85	.9999 9989	.9999 9987	.9999 9985	.9999 9983	.9999 9981
8.86	.9999 9990	.9999 9988	.9999 9986	.9999 9984	.9999 9981
8.87	.9999 9990	.9999 9988	.9999 9986	.9999 9984	.9999 9982
8.88	.9999 9991	.9999 9989	.9999 9987	.9999 9985	.9999 9983
8.89	.9999 9991	.9999 9989	.9999 9988	.9999 9986	.9999 9984
8.90	.9999 9991	.9999 9990	.9999 9988	.9999 9986	.9999 9985
8.91	.9999 9992	.9999 9990	.9999 9989	.9999 9987	.9999 9985
8.92	.9999 9992	.9999 9991	.9999 9989	.9999 9988	.9999 9986
8.93	.9999 9992	.9999 9991	.9999 9990	.9999 9988	.9999 9986
8.94	.9999 9993	.9999 9992	.9999 9990	.9999 9989	.9999 9987
8.95	.9999 9993	.9999 9992	.9999 9991	.9999 9989	.9999 9988
8.96	.9999 9993	.9999 9992	.9999 9991	.9999 9990	.9999 9988
8.97	.9999 9994	.9999 9993	.9999 9991	.9999 9990	.9999 9989
8.98	.9999 9994	.9999 9993	.9999 9992	.9999 9991	.9999 9989
8.99	.9999 9994	.9999 9993	.9999 9992	.9999 9991	.9999 9990

W	P(W,24)	P(W,26)	P(W,28)	P(W,30)	P(W,32)
9.00	.9999 9994	.9999 9994	.9999 9992	.9999 9991	.9999 9990
9.01	.9999 9995	.9999 9994	.9999 9993	.9999 9992	.9999 9991
9.02	.9999 9995	.9999 9994	.9999 9993	.9999 9992	.9999 9991
9.03	.9999 9995	.9999 9994	.9999 9993	.9999 9992	.9999 9991
9.04	.9999 9995	.9999 9995	.9999 9994	.9999 9993	.9999 9992
9.05	.9999 9996	.9999 9995	.9999 9994	.9999 9993	.9999 9992
9.06	.9999 9996	.9999 9995	.9999 9994	.9999 9993	.9999 9993
9.07	.9999 9996	.9999 9995	.9999 9995	.9999 9994	.9999 9993
9.08	.9999 9996	.9999 9995	.9999 9995	.9999 9994	.9999 9993
9.09	.9999 9996	.9999 9996	.9999 9995	.9999 9994	.9999 9993
9.10	.9999 9997	.9999 9996	.9999 9995	.9999 9994	.9999 9994
9.11	.9999 9997	.9999 9996	.9999 9995	.9999 9995	.9999 9994
9.12	.9999 9997	.9999 9996	.9999 9996	.9999 9995	.9999 9994
9.13	.9999 9997	.9999 9996	.9999 9996	.9999 9995	.9999 9995
9.14	.9999 9997	.9999 9997	.9999 9996	.9999 9995	.9999 9995
9.15	.9999 9997	.9999 9997	.9999 9996	.9999 9996	.9999 9995
9.16	.9999 9997	.9999 9997	.9999 9996	.9999 9996	.9999 9995
9.17	.9999 9997	.9999 9997	.9999 9997	.9999 9996	.9999 9995
9.18	.9999 9998	.9999 9997	.9999 9997	.9999 9996	.9999 9996
9.19	.9999 9998	.9999 9997	.9999 9997	.9999 9996	.9999 9996
9.20	.9999 9998	.9999 9997	.9999 9997	.9999 9997	.9999 9996
9.21	.9999 9998	.9999 9997	.9999 9997	.9999 9997	.9999 9996
9.22	.9999 9998	.9999 9998	.9999 9997	.9999 9997	.9999 9996
9.23	.9999 9998	.9999 9998	.9999 9997	.9999 9997	.9999 9997
9.24	.9999 9998	.9999 9998	.9999 9997	.9999 9997	.9999 9997
9.25	.9999 9998	.9999 9998	.9999 9998	.9999 9997	.9999 9997
9.26	.9999 9998	.9999 9998	.9999 9998	.9999 9997	.9999 9997
9.27	.9999 9998	.9999 9998	.9999 9998	.9999 9997	.9999 9997
9.28	.9999 9998	.9999 9998	.9999 9998	.9999 9998	.9999 9997
9.29	.9999 9999	.9999 9998	.9999 9998	.9999 9998	.9999 9997
9.30	.9999 9999	.9999 9998	.9999 9998	.9999 9998	.9999 9997
9.31	.9999 9999	.9999 9998	.9999 9998	.9999 9998	.9999 9998
9.32	.9999 9999	.9999 9998	.9999 9998	.9999 9998	.9999 9998
9.33	.9999 9999	.9999 9999	.9999 9998	.9999 9998	.9999 9998
9.34	.9999 9999	.9999 9999	.9999 9998	.9999 9998	.9999 9998
9.35	.9999 9999	.9999 9999	.9999 9998	.9999 9998	.9999 9998
9.36	.9999 9999	.9999 9999	.9999 9999	.9999 9998	.9999 9998
9.37	.9999 9999	.9999 9999	.9999 9999	.9999 9998	.9999 9998
9.38	.9999 9999	.9999 9999	.9999 9999	.9999 9998	.9999 9998
9.39	.9999 9999	.9999 9999	.9999 9999	.9999 9998	.9999 9998
9.40	.9999 9999	.9999 9999	.9999 9999	.9999 9999	.9999 9998
9.41	.9999 9999	.9999 9999	.9999 9999	.9999 9999	.9999 9998
9.42	.9999 9999	.9999 9999	.9999 9999	.9999 9999	.9999 9999
9.43	.9999 9999	.9999 9999	.9999 9999	.9999 9999	.9999 9999
9.44	.9999 9999	.9999 9999	.9999 9999	.9999 9999	.9999 9999
9.45	.9999 9999	.9999 9999	.9999 9999	.9999 9999	.9999 9999
9.46	.9999 9999	.9999 9999	.9999 9999	.9999 9999	.9999 9999
9.47	.9999 9999	.9999 9999	.9999 9999	.9999 9999	.9999 9999
9.48	.9999 9999	.9999 9999	.9999 9999	.9999 9999	.9999 9999
9.49	.9999 9999	.9999 9999	.9999 9999	.9999 9999	.9999 9999

W	P(W,24)	P(W,26)	P(W,28)	P(W,30)	P(W,32)
9.50	.9999 9999	.9999 9999	.9999 9999	.9999 9999	.9999 9999
9.51	.9999 9999	.9999 9999	.9999 9999	.9999 9999	.9999 9999
9.52	.9999 9999	.9999 9999	.9999 9999	.9999 9999	.9999 9999
9.53	.9999 9999	.9999 9999	.9999 9999	.9999 9999	.9999 9999
9.54	.9999 9999	.9999 9999	.9999 9999	.9999 9999	.9999 9999
9.55	.9999 9999	.9999 9999	.9999 9999	.9999 9999	.9999 9999
9.56	1.0000 0000	.9999 9999	.9999 9999	.9999 9999	.9999 9999
9.57		.9999 9999	.9999 9999	.9999 9999	.9999 9999
9.58		.9999 9999	.9999 9999	.9999 9999	.9999 9999
9.59		1.0000 0000	.9999 9999	.9999 9999	.9999 9999
9.60			.9999 9999	.9999 9999	.9999 9999
9.61			.9999 9999	.9999 9999	.9999 9999
9.62			.9999 9999	.9999 9999	.9999 9999
9.63			1.0000 0000	.9999 9999	.9999 9999
9.64				.9999 9999	.9999 9999
9.65				.9999 9999	.9999 9999
9.66				.9999 9999	.9999 9999
9.67				1.0000 0000	.9999 9999
9.68					.9999 9999
9.69					1.0000 0000
9.70					
9.71					
9.72					
9.73					
9.74					
9.75					
9.76					
9.77					
9.78					
9.79					
9.80					
9.81					
9.82					
9.83					
9.84					
9.85					
9.86					
9.87					
9.88					
9.89					
9.90					
9.91					
9.92					
9.93					
9.94					
9.95					
9.96					
9.97					
9.98					
9.99					

W	P(W,34)	P(W,36)	P(W,38)	P(W,40)	P(W,50)
1.00					
1.01					
1.02					
1.03					
1.04					
1.05					
1.06					
1.07					
1.08					
1.09					
1.10					
1.11					
1.12					
1.13					
1.14					
1.15					
1.16					
1.17					
1.18					
1.19					
1.20					
1.21					
1.22					
1.23					
1.24					
1.25					
1.26					
1.27					
1.28					
1.29					
1.30					
1.31					
1.32					
1.33					
1.34					
1.35					
1.36					
1.37					
1.38					
1.39					
1.40					
1.41					
1.42					
1.43					
1.44					
1.45					
1.46	.0000 0000				
1.47	.0000 0001				
1.48	.0000 0001				
1.49	.0000 0001				

W	P(W,34)	P(W,36)	P(W,38)	P(W,40)	P(W,50)
1.50	.0000 0001				
1.51	.0000 0001				
1.52	.0000 0002	.0000 0000			
1.53	.0000 0002	.0000 0001			
1.54	.0000 0002	.0000 0001			
1.55	.0000 0003	.0000 0001			
1.56	.0000 0003	.0000 0001			
1.57	.0000 0004	.0000 0001			
1.58	.0000 0004	.0000 0001	.0000 0000		
1.59	.0000 0005	.0000 0002	.0000 0001		
1.60	.0000 0006	.0000 0002	.0000 0001		
1.61	.0000 0007	.0000 0002	.0000 0001		
1.62	.0000 0008	.0000 0003	.0000 0001		
1.63	.0000 0010	.0000 0003	.0000 0001		
1.64	.0000 0011	.0000 0004	.0000 0001	.0000 0000	
1.65	.0000 0013	.0000 0005	.0000 0002	.0000 0001	
1.66	.0000 0016	.0000 0006	.0000 0002	.0000 0001	
1.67	.0000 0018	.0000 0007	.0000 0002	.0000 0001	
1.68	.0000 0021	.0000 0008	.0000 0003	.0000 0001	
1.69	.0000 0025	.0000 0009	.0000 0003	.0000 0001	
1.70	.0000 0029	.0000 0011	.0000 0004	.0000 0001	
1.71	.0000 0033	.0000 0013	.0000 0005	.0000 0002	
1.72	.0000 0038	.0000 0015	.0000 0006	.0000 0002	
1.73	.0000 0044	.0000 0017	.0000 0007	.0000 0003	
1.74	.0000 0051	.0000 0020	.0000 0008	.0000 0003	
1.75	.0000 0059	.0000 0023	.0000 0009	.0000 0004	
1.76	.0000 0068	.0000 0027	.0000 0011	.0000 0004	
1.77	.0000 0079	.0000 0031	.0000 0013	.0000 0005	
1.78	.0000 0090	.0000 0036	.0000 0015	.0000 0006	
1.79	.0000 0104	.0000 0042	.0000 0017	.0000 0007	
1.80	.0000 0119	.0000 0049	.0000 0020	.0000 0008	
1.81	.0000 0136	.0000 0056	.0000 0023	.0000 0010	
1.82	.0000 0156	.0000 0065	.0000 0027	.0000 0011	
1.83	.0000 0178	.0000 0075	.0000 0031	.0000 0013	
1.84	.0000 0203	.0000 0086	.0000 0036	.0000 0015	
1.85	.0000 0232	.0000 0099	.0000 0042	.0000 0018	
1.86	.0000 0264	.0000 0114	.0000 0049	.0000 0021	
1.87	.0000 0300	.0000 0130	.0000 0057	.0000 0024	
1.88	.0000 0340	.0000 0149	.0000 0065	.0000 0028	
1.89	.0000 0386	.0000 0171	.0000 0075	.0000 0033	.0000 0000
1.90	.0000 0438	.0000 0195	.0000 0087	.0000 0038	.0000 0001
1.91	.0000 0496	.0000 0222	.0000 0099	.0000 0044	.0000 0001
1.92	.0000 0560	.0000 0253	.0000 0114	.0000 0051	.0000 0001
1.93	.0000 0633	.0000 0288	.0000 0131	.0000 0059	.0000 0001
1.94	.0000 0714	.0000 0328	.0000 0150	.0000 0069	.0000 0001
1.95	.0000 0805	.0000 0372	.0000 0172	.0000 0079	.0000 0002
1.96	.0000 0906	.0000 0422	.0000 0196	.0000 0091	.0000 0002
1.97	.0000 1019	.0000 0478	.0000 0224	.0000 0105	.0000 0002
1.98	.0000 1145	.0000 0541	.0000 0255	.0000 0120	.0000 0003
1.99	.0000 1285	.0000 0611	.0000 0291	.0000 0138	.0000 0003

W	P(W,34)	P(W,36)	P(W,38)	P(W,40)	P(W,50)
2.00	.0000 1441	.0000 0691	.0000 0330	.0000 0158	.0000 0004
2.01	.0000 1614	.0000 0779	.0000 0375	.0000 0181	.0000 0005
2.02	.0000 1806	.0000 0878	.0000 0426	.0000 0206	.0000 0005
2.03	.0000 2019	.0000 0988	.0000 0483	.0000 0236	.0000 0006
2.04	.0000 2255	.0000 1111	.0000 0547	.0000 0269	.0000 0008
2.05	.0000 2516	.0000 1248	.0000 0618	.0000 0306	.0000 0009
2.06	.0000 2804	.0000 1400	.0000 0698	.0000 0348	.0000 0010
2.07	.0000 3122	.0000 1570	.0000 0788	.0000 0395	.0000 0012
2.08	.0000 3473	.0000 1758	.0000 0889	.0000 0448	.0000 0014
2.09	.0000 3860	.0000 1967	.0000 1001	.0000 0508	.0000 0017
2.10	.0000 4286	.0000 2198	.0000 1126	.0000 0576	.0000 0020
2.11	.0000 4755	.0000 2454	.0000 1265	.0000 0651	.0000 0023
2.12	.0000 5270	.0000 2738	.0000 1420	.0000 0736	.0000 0027
2.13	.0000 5836	.0000 3051	.0000 1593	.0000 0830	.0000 0031
2.14	.0000 6456	.0000 3397	.0000 1785	.0000 0936	.0000 0037
2.15	.0000 7137	.0000 3778	.0000 1997	.0000 1055	.0000 0043
2.16	.0000 7881	.0000 4199	.0000 2233	.0000 1186	.0000 0049
2.17	.0000 8696	.0000 4661	.0000 2495	.0000 1334	.0000 0057
2.18	.0000 9587	.0000 5170	.0000 2784	.0000 1497	.0000 0066
2.19	.0001 0560	.0000 5729	.0000 3104	.0000 1679	.0000 0077
2.20	.0001 1621	.0000 6343	.0000 3457	.0000 1882	.0000 0088
2.21	.0001 2779	.0000 7016	.0000 3847	.0000 2106	.0000 0102
2.22	.0001 4040	.0000 7754	.0000 4277	.0000 2355	.0000 0117
2.23	.0001 5412	.0000 8562	.0000 4750	.0000 2631	.0000 0135
2.24	.0001 6905	.0000 9446	.0000 5270	.0000 2937	.0000 0155
2.25	.0001 8526	.0001 0412	.0000 5843	.0000 3275	.0000 0178
2.26	.0002 0287	.0001 1466	.0000 6471	.0000 3648	.0000 0204
2.27	.0002 2198	.0001 2617	.0000 7161	.0000 4059	.0000 0234
2.28	.0002 4269	.0001 3872	.0000 7918	.0000 4513	.0000 0267
2.29	.0002 6511	.0001 5238	.0000 8746	.0000 5013	.0000 0305
2.30	.0002 8939	.0001 6725	.0000 9652	.0000 5563	.0000 0348
2.31	.0003 1564	.0001 8342	.0001 0643	.0000 6168	.0000 0397
2.32	.0003 4400	.0002 0098	.0001 1726	.0000 6832	.0000 0452
2.33	.0003 7462	.0002 2005	.0001 2907	.0000 7561	.0000 0513
2.34	.0004 0766	.0002 4073	.0001 4196	.0000 8360	.0000 0583
2.35	.0004 4328	.0002 6315	.0001 5600	.0000 9236	.0000 0661
2.36	.0004 8164	.0002 8743	.0001 7128	.0001 0194	.0000 0749
2.37	.0005 2294	.0003 1369	.0001 8790	.0001 1241	.0000 0848
2.38	.0005 6736	.0003 4209	.0002 0597	.0001 2386	.0000 0959
2.39	.0006 1510	.0003 7277	.0002 2559	.0001 3635	.0000 1083
2.40	.0006 6638	.0004 0589	.0002 4688	.0001 4997	.0000 1221
2.41	.0007 2141	.0004 4161	.0002 6996	.0001 6481	.0000 1376
2.42	.0007 8042	.0004 8012	.0002 9496	.0001 8097	.0000 1549
2.43	.0008 4366	.0005 2159	.0003 2201	.0001 9855	.0000 1742
2.44	.0009 1139	.0005 6622	.0003 5128	.0002 1765	.0000 1957
2.45	.0009 8387	.0006 1421	.0003 8290	.0002 3840	.0000 2196
2.46	.0010 6138	.0006 6578	.0004 1705	.0002 6091	.0000 2462
2.47	.0011 4420	.0007 2116	.0004 5389	.0002 8531	.0000 2757
2.48	.0012 3265	.0007 8058	.0004 9361	.0003 1175	.0000 3085
2.49	.0013 2704	.0008 4429	.0005 3640	.0003 4036	.0000 3448

W	P(W,34)	P(W,36)	P(W,38)	P(W,40)	P(W,50)
2.50	.0014 2770	.0009 1255	.0005 8246	.0003 7131	.0000 3849
2.51	.0015 3498	.0009 8564	.0006 3201	.0004 0475	.0000 4294
2.52	.0016 4922	.0010 6383	.0006 8526	.0004 4086	.0000 4785
2.53	.0017 7081	.0011 4743	.0007 4246	.0004 7982	.0000 5327
2.54	.0019 0012	.0012 3675	.0008 0385	.0005 2182	.0000 5924
2.55	.0020 3757	.0013 3211	.0008 6968	.0005 6707	.0000 6583
2.56	.0021 8356	.0014 3384	.0009 4023	.0006 1578	.0000 7307
2.57	.0023 3852	.0015 4232	.0010 1579	.0006 6817	.0000 8104
2.58	.0025 0291	.0016 5789	.0010 9664	.0007 2448	.0000 8980
2.59	.0026 7718	.0017 8094	.0011 8309	.0007 8496	.0000 9940
2.60	.0028 6181	.0019 1187	.0012 7548	.0008 4986	.0001 0994
2.61	.0030 5728	.0020 5108	.0013 7414	.0009 1947	.0001 2148
2.62	.0032 6412	.0021 9901	.0014 7941	.0009 9406	.0001 3411
2.63	.0034 8285	.0023 5610	.0015 9167	.0010 7393	.0001 4792
2.64	.0037 1399	.0025 2280	.0017 1130	.0011 5939	.0001 6301
2.65	.0039 5812	.0026 9958	.0018 3869	.0012 5078	.0001 7948
2.66	.0042 1580	.0028 8695	.0019 7426	.0013 4843	.0001 9744
2.67	.0044 8762	.0030 8540	.0021 1842	.0014 5270	.0002 1701
2.68	.0047 7418	.0032 9546	.0022 7163	.0015 6396	.0002 3831
2.69	.0050 7611	.0035 1766	.0024 3435	.0016 8259	.0002 6149
2.70	.0053 9404	.0037 5256	.0026 0705	.0018 0899	.0002 8667
2.71	.0057 2862	.0040 0074	.0027 9022	.0019 4359	.0003 1401
2.72	.0060 8052	.0042 6277	.0029 8437	.0020 8680	.0003 4367
2.73	.0064 5042	.0045 3927	.0031 9004	.0022 3910	.0003 7583
2.74	.0068 3903	.0048 3086	.0034 0775	.0024 0092	.0004 1065
2.75	.0072 4704	.0051 3818	.0036 3807	.0025 7278	.0004 4834
2.76	.0076 7520	.0054 6188	.0038 8158	.0027 5515	.0004 8908
2.77	.0081 2423	.0058 0262	.0041 3886	.0029 4855	.0005 3311
2.78	.0085 9491	.0061 6111	.0044 1054	.0031 5353	.0005 8063
2.79	.0090 8799	.0065 3803	.0046 9724	.0033 7063	.0006 3189
2.80	.0096 0425	.0069 3411	.0049 9960	.0036 0043	.0006 8713
2.81	.0101 4451	.0073 5008	.0053 1829	.0038 4350	.0007 4662
2.82	.0107 0955	.0077 8669	.0056 5398	.0041 0045	.0008 1064
2.83	.0113 0021	.0082 4471	.0060 0737	.0043 7190	.0008 7947
2.84	.0119 1731	.0087 2490	.0063 7917	.0046 5849	.0009 5341
2.85	.0125 6170	.0092 2807	.0067 7011	.0049 6088	.0010 3280
2.86	.0132 3422	.0097 5501	.0071 8093	.0052 7974	.0011 1795
2.87	.0139 3574	.0103 0655	.0076 1239	.0056 1576	.0012 0923
2.88	.0146 6713	.0108 8351	.0080 6527	.0059 6966	.0013 0699
2.89	.0154 2926	.0114 8675	.0085 4035	.0063 4215	.0014 1163
2.90	.0162 2302	.0121 1710	.0090 3845	.0067 3397	.0015 2353
2.91	.0170 4931	.0127 7545	.0095 6037	.0071 4589	.0016 4312
2.92	.0179 0902	.0134 6266	.0101 0695	.0075 7869	.0017 7082
2.93	.0188 0306	.0141 7963	.0106 7904	.0080 3314	.0019 0710
2.94	.0197 3232	.0149 2723	.0112 7750	.0085 1006	.0020 5241
2.95	.0206 9773	.0157 0638	.0119 0318	.0090 1026	.0022 0726
2.96	.0217 0019	.0165 1799	.0125 5699	.0095 3459	.0023 7214
2.97	.0227 4063	.0173 6297	.0132 3980	.0100 8389	.0025 4758
2.98	.0238 1995	.0182 4225	.0139 5252	.0106 5902	.0027 3412
2.99	.0249 3907	.0191 5674	.0146 9607	.0112 6087	.0029 3234

W	P(W,34)	P(W,36)	P(W,38)	P(W,40)	P(W,50)
3.00	.0260 9890	.0201 0739	.0154 7136	.0118 9032	.0031 4281
3.01	.0273 0036	.0210 9512	.0162 7932	.0125 4826	.0033 6614
3.02	.0285 4434	.0221 2087	.0171 2088	.0132 3562	.0036 0295
3.03	.0298 3176	.0231 8558	.0179 9699	.0139 5331	.0038 5388
3.04	.0311 6352	.0242 9019	.0189 0860	.0147 0227	.0041 1960
3.05	.0325 4049	.0254 3563	.0198 5666	.0154 8343	.0044 0079
3.06	.0339 6358	.0266 2283	.0208 4211	.0162 9775	.0046 9815
3.07	.0354 3364	.0278 5274	.0218 6592	.0171 4618	.0050 1241
3.08	.0369 5155	.0291 2627	.0229 2905	.0180 2968	.0053 4430
3.09	.0385 1815	.0304 4434	.0240 3245	.0189 4921	.0056 9460
3.10	.0401 3430	.0318 0788	.0251 7708	.0199 0576	.0060 6408
3.11	.0418 0082	.0332 1779	.0263 6390	.0209 0030	.0064 5353
3.12	.0435 1852	.0346 7498	.0275 9386	.0219 3380	.0068 6379
3.13	.0452 8820	.0361 8033	.0288 6791	.0230 0724	.0072 9569
3.14	.0471 1065	.0377 3472	.0301 8700	.0241 2161	.0077 5008
3.15	.0489 8664	.0393 3903	.0315 5207	.0252 7788	.0082 2784
3.16	.0509 1690	.0409 9410	.0329 6404	.0264 7702	.0087 2986
3.17	.0529 0216	.0427 0079	.0344 2383	.0277 2002	.0092 5705
3.18	.0549 4314	.0444 5991	.0359 3237	.0290 0783	.0098 1033
3.19	.0570 4051	.0462 7227	.0374 9055	.0303 4144	.0103 9064
3.20	.0591 9494	.0481 3867	.0390 9926	.0317 2178	.0109 9893
3.21	.0614 0707	.0500 5988	.0407 5938	.0331 4982	.0116 3618
3.22	.0636 7751	.0520 3665	.0424 7177	.0346 2649	.0123 0337
3.23	.0660 0684	.0540 6971	.0442 3728	.0361 5272	.0130 0149
3.24	.0683 9563	.0561 5978	.0460 5674	.0377 2944	.0137 3155
3.25	.0708 4442	.0583 0755	.0479 3095	.0393 5755	.0144 9458
3.26	.0733 5370	.0605 1367	.0498 6072	.0410 3795	.0152 9159
3.27	.0759 2395	.0627 7878	.0518 4681	.0427 7150	.0161 2362
3.28	.0785 5562	.0651 0350	.0538 8997	.0445 5908	.0169 9174
3.29	.0812 4912	.0674 8841	.0559 9094	.0464 0152	.0178 9697
3.30	.0840 0483	.0699 3406	.0581 5041	.0482 9966	.0188 4040
3.31	.0868 2311	.0724 4099	.0603 6907	.0502 5429	.0198 2307
3.32	.0897 0426	.0750 0968	.0626 4757	.0522 6621	.0208 4607
3.33	.0926 4858	.0776 4062	.0649 8653	.0543 3616	.0219 1046
3.34	.0956 5631	.0803 3422	.0673 8656	.0564 6490	.0230 1732
3.35	.0987 2766	.0830 9090	.0698 4822	.0586 5313	.0241 6771
3.36	.1018 6282	.0859 1101	.0723 7206	.0609 0154	.0253 6272
3.37	.1050 6192	.0887 9491	.0749 5857	.0632 1079	.0266 0340
3.38	.1083 2506	.0917 4287	.0776 0824	.0655 8152	.0278 9084
3.39	.1116 5232	.0947 5518	.0803 2151	.0680 1432	.0292 2608
3.40	.1150 4372	.0978 3205	.0830 9880	.0705 0977	.0306 1018
3.41	.1184 9925	.1009 7367	.0859 4047	.0730 6841	.0320 4419
3.42	.1220 1888	.1041 8021	.0888 4687	.0756 9075	.0335 2915
3.43	.1256 0251	.1074 5178	.0918 1830	.0783 7727	.0350 6609
3.44	.1292 5002	.1107 8845	.0948 5503	.0811 2840	.0366 5601
3.45	.1329 6126	.1141 9026	.0979 5728	.0839 4457	.0382 9993
3.46	.1367 3601	.1176 5722	.1011 2526	.0868 2613	.0399 9882
3.47	.1405 7405	.1211 8928	.1043 5912	.0897 7343	.0417 5366
3.48	.1444 7509	.1247 8627	.1076 5897	.0927 8675	.0435 6540
3.49	.1484 3881	.1284 4836	.1110 2489	.0958 6637	.0454 3497

W	P(W,34)	P(W,36)	P(W,38)	P(W,40)	P(W,50)
3.50	.1524 6486	.1321 7511	.1144 5690	.0990 1251	.0473 6328
3.51	.1565 5285	.1359 6641	.1179 5502	.1022 2534	.0493 5123
3.52	.1607 0234	.1398 2202	.1215 1919	.1055 0500	.0513 9968
3.53	.1649 1285	.1437 4166	.1251 4933	.1088 5161	.0535 0947
3.54	.1691 8389	.1477 2502	.1288 4532	.1122 6522	.0556 8142
3.55	.1735 1490	.1517 7173	.1326 0697	.1157 4585	.0579 1631
3.56	.1779 0530	.1558 8140	.1364 3409	.1192 9348	.0602 1491
3.57	.1823 5446	.1600 5358	.1403 2642	.1229 0804	.0625 7794
3.58	.1868 6173	.1642 8781	.1442 8368	.1265 8945	.0650 0609
3.59	.1914 2642	.1685 8355	.1483 0552	.1303 3753	.0675 0004
3.60	.1960 4778	.1729 4027	.1523 9158	.1341 5211	.0700 6040
3.61	.2007 2507	.1773 5735	.1565 4143	.1380 3295	.0726 8778
3.62	.2054 5747	.1818 3416	.1607 5463	.1419 7978	.0753 8274
3.63	.2102 4416	.1863 7004	.1650 3067	.1459 9228	.0781 4578
3.64	.2150 8426	.1909 6428	.1693 6901	.1500 7009	.0809 7740
3.65	.2199 7689	.1956 1612	.1737 6908	.1542 1281	.0838 7804
3.66	.2249 2110	.2003 2480	.1782 3026	.1584 1999	.0868 4809
3.67	.2299 1594	.2050 8948	.1827 5189	.1626 9114	.0898 8792
3.68	.2349 6041	.2099 0933	.1873 3328	.1670 2575	.0929 9785
3.69	.2400 5349	.2147 8344	.1919 7369	.1714 2323	.0961 7815
3.70	.2451 9414	.2197 1091	.1966 7235	.1758 8297	.0994 2905
3.71	.2503 8127	.2246 9078	.2014 2846	.1804 0433	.1027 5074
3.72	.2556 1378	.2297 2206	.2062 4115	.1849 8661	.1061 4336
3.73	.2608 9054	.2348 0374	.2111 0956	.1896 2908	.1096 0700
3.74	.2662 1040	.2399 3477	.2160 3277	.1943 3097	.1131 4172
3.75	.2715 7218	.2451 1407	.2210 0983	.1990 9147	.1167 4752
3.76	.2769 7467	.2503 4055	.2260 3974	.2039 0973	.1204 2435
3.77	.2824 1665	.2556 1307	.2311 2150	.2087 8488	.1241 7212
3.78	.2878 9688	.2609 3048	.2362 5406	.2137 1598	.1279 9069
3.79	.2934 1409	.2662 9158	.2414 3634	.2187 0209	.1318 7988
3.80	.2989 6700	.2716 9517	.2466 6722	.2237 4221	.1358 3945
3.81	.3045 5432	.2771 4003	.2519 4558	.2288 3532	.1398 6912
3.82	.3101 7472	.2826 2489	.2572 7023	.2339 8036	.1439 6855
3.83	.3158 2687	.2881 4847	.2626 4000	.2391 7624	.1481 3737
3.84	.3215 0942	.2937 0950	.2680 5365	.2444 2184	.1523 7514
3.85	.3272 2102	.2993 0664	.2735 0995	.2497 1600	.1566 8140
3.86	.3329 6030	.3049 3857	.2790 0763	.2550 5756	.1610 5562
3.87	.3387 2586	.3106 0393	.2845 4540	.2604 4529	.1654 9724
3.88	.3445 1632	.3163 0137	.2901 2194	.2658 7797	.1700 0562
3.89	.3503 3028	.3220 2950	.2957 3593	.2713 5433	.1745 8012
3.90	.3561 6632	.3277 8693	.3013 8601	.2768 7309	.1792 2003
3.91	.3620 2304	.3335 7225	.3070 7081	.2824 3294	.1839 2458
3.92	.3678 9900	.3393 8404	.3127 8895	.2880 3254	.1886 9299
3.93	.3737 9279	.3452 2088	.3185 3902	.2936 7055	.1935 2440
3.94	.3797 0297	.3510 8134	.3243 1961	.2993 4558	.1984 1794
3.95	.3856 2811	.3569 6396	.3301 2929	.3050 5625	.2033 7267
3.96	.3915 6678	.3628 6730	.3359 6661	.3108 0115	.2083 8763
3.97	.3975 1756	.3687 8991	.3418 3012	.3165 7884	.2134 6180
3.98	.4034 7899	.3747 3032	.3477 1837	.3223 8790	.2185 9414
3.99	.4094 4967	.3806 8706	.3536 2987	.3282 2686	.2237 8354

W	P(W,34)	P(W,36)	P(W,38)	P(W,40)	P(W,50)
4.00	.4154 2815	.3866 5869	.3595 6315	.3340 9425	.2290 2890
4.01	.4214 1303	.3926 4373	.3655 1673	.3399 8859	.2343 2903
4.02	.4274 0287	.3986 4071	.3714 8911	.3459 0840	.2396 8274
4.03	.4333 9628	.4046 4817	.3774 7881	.3518 5217	.2450 8881
4.04	.4393 9184	.4106 6465	.3834 8432	.3578 1840	.2505 4594
4.05	.4453 8815	.4166 8869	.3895 0416	.3638 0557	.2560 5286
4.06	.4513 8384	.4227 1884	.3955 3682	.3698 1217	.2616 0822
4.07	.4573 7752	.4287 5365	.4015 8080	.3758 3667	.2672 1066
4.08	.4633 6783	.4347 9167	.4076 3461	.3818 7754	.2728 5880
4.09	.4693 5341	.4408 3148	.4136 9677	.3879 3327	.2785 5121
4.10	.4753 3291	.4468 7164	.4197 6578	.3940 0231	.2842 8646
4.11	.4813 0501	.4529 1075	.4258 4016	.4000 8315	.2900 6307
4.12	.4872 6839	.4589 4739	.4319 1843	.4061 7425	.2958 7956
4.13	.4932 2174	.4649 8017	.4379 9913	.4122 7410	.3017 3442
4.14	.4991 6378	.4710 0770	.4440 8080	.4183 8118	.3076 2610
4.15	.5050 9324	.4770 2863	.4501 6198	.4244 9397	.3135 5307
4.16	.5110 0887	.4830 4158	.4562 4124	.4306 1097	.3195 1375
4.17	.5169 0942	.4890 4522	.4623 1715	.4367 3068	.3255 0656
4.18	.5227 9369	.4950 3823	.4683 8828	.4428 5160	.3315 2990
4.19	.5286 6046	.5010 1930	.4744 5324	.4489 7226	.3375 8215
4.20	.5345 0856	.5069 8712	.4805 1064	.4550 9119	.3436 6170
4.21	.5403 3683	.5129 4043	.4865 5910	.4612 0692	.3497 6690
4.22	.5461 4412	.5188 7796	.4925 9725	.4673 1800	.3558 9613
4.23	.5519 2932	.5247 9849	.4986 2377	.4734 2302	.3620 4772
4.24	.5576 9133	.5307 0079	.5046 3731	.4795 2054	.3682 2002
4.25	.5634 2907	.5365 8366	.5106 3658	.4856 0915	.3744 1138
4.26	.5691 4148	.5424 4592	.5166 2028	.4916 8749	.3806 2012
4.27	.5748 2753	.5482 8641	.5225 8713	.4977 5416	.3868 4459
4.28	.5804 8622	.5541 0401	.5285 3590	.5038 0781	.3930 8311
4.29	.5861 1655	.5598 9760	.5344 6535	.5098 4712	.3993 3403
4.30	.5917 1756	.5656 6607	.5403 7428	.5158 7076	.4055 9569
4.31	.5972 8831	.5714 0838	.5462 6148	.5218 7744	.4118 6641
4.32	.6028 2789	.5771 2347	.5521 2580	.5278 6588	.4181 4456
4.33	.6083 3540	.5828 1032	.5579 6609	.5338 3482	.4244 2848
4.34	.6138 0998	.5884 6793	.5637 8124	.5397 8303	.4307 1654
4.35	.6192 5078	.5940 9534	.5695 7015	.5457 0930	.4370 0711
4.36	.6246 5699	.5996 9159	.5753 3174	.5516 1243	.4432 9856
4.37	.6300 2782	.6052 5576	.5810 6497	.5574 9127	.4495 8929
4.38	.6353 6249	.6107 8695	.5867 6881	.5633 4467	.4558 7770
4.39	.6406 6027	.6162 8429	.5924 4227	.5691 7151	.4621 6220
4.40	.6459 2043	.6217 4693	.5980 8437	.5749 7069	.4684 4123
4.41	.6511 4229	.6271 7405	.6036 9416	.5807 4116	.4747 1324
4.42	.6563 2518	.6325 6485	.6092 7072	.5864 8186	.4809 7668
4.43	.6614 6844	.6379 1857	.6148 1316	.5921 9178	.4872 3004
4.44	.6665 7148	.6432 3445	.6203 2060	.5978 6993	.4934 7182
4.45	.6716 3369	.6485 1179	.6257 9220	.6035 1534	.4997 0054
4.46	.6766 5451	.6537 4988	.6312 2715	.6091 2707	.5059 1473
4.47	.6816 3340	.6589 4806	.6366 2465	.6147 0421	.5121 1296
4.48	.6865 6983	.6641 0569	.6419 8394	.6202 4587	.5182 9380
4.49	.6914 6333	.6692 2216	.6473 0429	.6257 5120	.5244 5587

W	P(W,34)	P(W,36)	P(W,38)	P(W,40)	P(W,50)
4.50	.6963 1341	.6742 9687	.6525 8497	.6312 1936	.5305 9779
4.51	.7011 1964	.6793 2927	.6578 2531	.6366 4956	.5367 1821
4.52	.7058 8160	.6843 1880	.6630 2465	.6420 4101	.5428 1581
4.53	.7105 9889	.6892 6498	.6681 8236	.6473 9296	.5488 8930
4.54	.7152 7114	.6941 6729	.6732 9783	.6527 0470	.5549 3739
4.55	.7198 9800	.6990 2529	.6783 7049	.6579 7552	.5609 5885
4.56	.7244 7916	.7038 3854	.6833 9979	.6632 0476	.5669 5246
4.57	.7290 1430	.7086 0662	.6883 8519	.6683 9179	.5729 1704
4.58	.7335 0315	.7133 2915	.6933 2620	.6735 3598	.5788 5140
4.59	.7379 4546	.7180 0576	.6982 2235	.6786 3675	.5847 5443
4.60	.7423 4098	.7226 3612	.7030 7319	.6836 9355	.5906 2502
4.61	.7466 8952	.7272 1991	.7078 7830	.6887 0584	.5964 6209
4.62	.7509 9088	.7317 5684	.7126 3728	.6936 7312	.6022 6460
4.63	.7552 4488	.7362 4665	.7173 4976	.6985 9491	.6080 3153
4.64	.7594 5139	.7406 8908	.7220 1539	.7034 7076	.6137 6189
4.65	.7636 1028	.7450 8391	.7266 3385	.7083 0023	.6194 5472
4.66	.7677 2144	.7494 3095	.7312 0484	.7130 8294	.6251 0911
4.67	.7717 8479	.7537 3002	.7357 2810	.7178 1851	.6307 2415
4.68	.7758 0026	.7579 8097	.7402 0336	.7225 0658	.6362 9898
4.69	.7797 6779	.7621 8365	.7446 3040	.7271 4684	.6418 3276
4.70	.7836 8737	.7663 3795	.7490 0901	.7317 3899	.6473 2469
4.71	.7875 5899	.7704 4379	.7533 3903	.7362 8274	.6527 7399
4.72	.7913 8264	.7745 0108	.7576 2028	.7407 7786	.6581 7993
4.73	.7951 5837	.7785 0978	.7618 5263	.7452 2412	.6635 4179
4.74	.7988 8620	.7824 6986	.7660 3597	.7496 2131	.6688 5888
4.75	.8025 6621	.7863 8129	.7701 7019	.7539 6926	.6741 3057
4.76	.8061 9846	.7902 4409	.7742 5524	.7582 6780	.6793 5622
4.77	.8097 8306	.7940 5828	.7782 9104	.7625 1680	.6845 3524
4.78	.8133 2011	.7978 2390	.7822 7759	.7667 1616	.6896 6708
4.79	.8168 0974	.8015 4100	.7862 1484	.7708 6578	.6947 5120
4.80	.8202 5208	.8052 0967	.7901 0283	.7749 6559	.6997 8709
4.81	.8236 4729	.8088 2999	.7939 4156	.7790 1555	.7047 7430
4.82	.8269 9553	.8124 0208	.7977 3109	.7830 1561	.7097 1237
4.83	.8302 9699	.8159 2606	.8014 7147	.7869 6580	.7146 0089
4.84	.8335 5187	.8194 0207	.8051 6278	.7908 6609	.7194 3947
4.85	.8367 6037	.8228 3026	.8088 0513	.7947 1654	.7242 2775
4.86	.8399 2271	.8262 1081	.8123 9861	.7985 1719	.7289 6541
4.87	.8430 3912	.8295 4389	.8159 4337	.8022 6811	.7336 5214
4.88	.8461 0985	.8328 2971	.8194 3954	.8059 6938	.7382 8767
4.89	.8491 3516	.8360 6848	.8228 8728	.8096 2111	.7428 7174
4.90	.8521 1530	.8392 6042	.8262 8678	.8132 2342	.7474 0413
4.91	.8550 5057	.8424 0576	.8296 3821	.8167 7644	.7518 8464
4.92	.8579 4123	.8455 0477	.8329 4179	.8202 8033	.7563 1311
4.93	.8607 8760	.8485 5768	.8361 9772	.8237 3525	.7606 8939
4.94	.8635 8998	.8515 6478	.8394 0625	.8271 4139	.7650 1335
4.95	.8663 4868	.8545 2635	.8425 6760	.8304 9894	.7692 8490
4.96	.8690 6402	.8574 4268	.8456 8205	.8338 0812	.7735 0396
4.97	.8717 3634	.8603 1408	.8487 4984	.8370 6916	.7776 7047
4.98	.8743 6598	.8631 4085	.8517 7128	.8402 8229	.7817 8442
4.99	.8769 5328	.8659 2331	.8547 4663	.8434 4776	.7858 4580

W	P(W,34)	P(W,36)	P(W,38)	P(W,40)	P(W,50)
5.00	.8794 9860	.8686 6180	.8576 7621	.8465 6585	.7898 5462
5.01	.8820 0230	.8713 5666	.8605 6031	.8496 3682	.7938 1091
5.02	.8844 6475	.8740 0823	.8633 9928	.8526 6096	.7977 1474
5.03	.8868 8632	.8766 1687	.8661 9342	.8556 3858	.8015 6618
5.04	.8892 6739	.8791 8293	.8689 4309	.8585 6999	.8053 6533
5.05	.8916 0834	.8817 0679	.8716 4862	.8614 5549	.8091 1231
5.06	.8939 0956	.8841 8882	.8743 1037	.8642 9543	.8128 0724
5.07	.8961 7145	.8866 2940	.8769 2871	.8670 9015	.8164 5029
5.08	.8983 9441	.8890 2892	.8795 0401	.8698 3998	.8200 4162
5.09	.9005 7884	.8913 8777	.8820 3664	.8725 4530	.8235 8143
5.10	.9027 2514	.8937 0635	.8845 2699	.8752 0646	.8270 6991
5.11	.9048 3372	.8959 8506	.8869 7544	.8778 2383	.8305 0728
5.12	.9069 0501	.8982 2431	.8893 8240	.8803 9780	.8338 9379
5.13	.9089 3941	.9004 2451	.8917 4826	.8829 2876	.8372 2969
5.14	.9109 3734	.9025 8608	.8940 7343	.8854 1709	.8405 1523
5.15	.9128 9922	.9047 0943	.8963 5833	.8878 6320	.8437 5070
5.16	.9148 2548	.9067 9498	.8986 0336	.8902 6750	.8469 3639
5.17	.9167 1655	.9088 4317	.9008 0896	.8926 3039	.8500 7261
5.18	.9185 7284	.9108 5441	.9029 7554	.8949 5230	.8531 5968
5.19	.9203 9478	.9128 2914	.9051 0353	.8972 3364	.8561 9792
5.20	.9221 8282	.9147 6779	.9071 9336	.8994 7484	.8591 8768
5.21	.9239 3736	.9166 7079	.9092 4547	.9016 7632	.8621 2932
5.22	.9256 5885	.9185 3858	.9112 6029	.9038 3854	.8650 2319
5.23	.9273 4771	.9203 7160	.9132 3826	.9059 6191	.8678 6967
5.24	.9290 0438	.9221 7027	.9151 7982	.9080 4688	.8706 6914
5.25	.9306 2929	.9239 3505	.9170 8542	.9100 9390	.8734 2199
5.26	.9322 2286	.9256 6637	.9189 5550	.9121 0340	.8761 2864
5.27	.9337 8553	.9273 6467	.9207 9050	.9140 7585	.8787 8948
5.28	.9353 1773	.9290 3039	.9225 9087	.9160 1168	.8814 0493
5.29	.9368 1987	.9306 6396	.9243 5706	.9179 1135	.8839 7541
5.30	.9382 9240	.9322 6583	.9260 8951	.9197 7531	.8865 0137
5.31	.9397 3574	.9338 3644	.9277 8868	.9216 0401	.8889 8323
5.32	.9411 5031	.9353 7622	.9294 5501	.9233 9792	.8914 2145
5.33	.9425 3653	.9368 8561	.9310 8894	.9251 5748	.8938 1646
5.34	.9438 9483	.9383 6504	.9326 9093	.9268 8315	.8961 6872
5.35	.9452 2563	.9398 1496	.9342 6143	.9285 7539	.8984 7870
5.36	.9465 2934	.9412 3579	.9358 0087	.9302 3465	.9007 4686
5.37	.9478 0638	.9426 2797	.9373 0970	.9318 6140	.9029 7367
5.38	.9490 5717	.9439 9192	.9387 8837	.9334 5607	.9051 5959
5.39	.9502 8211	.9453 2807	.9402 3732	.9350 1913	.9073 0511
5.40	.9514 8161	.9466 3685	.9416 5698	.9365 5103	.9094 1071
5.41	.9526 5608	.9479 1868	.9430 4781	.9380 5222	.9114 7685
5.42	.9538 0592	.9491 7399	.9444 1023	.9395 2316	.9135 0404
5.43	.9549 3153	.9504 0318	.9457 4467	.9409 6429	.9154 9275
5.44	.9560 3331	.9516 0669	.9470 5158	.9423 7605	.9174 4346
5.45	.9571 1166	.9527 8491	.9483 3138	.9437 5891	.9193 5668
5.46	.9581 6696	.9539 3827	.9495 8451	.9451 1328	.9212 3289
5.47	.9591 9959	.9550 6716	.9508 1137	.9464 3963	.9230 7258
5.48	.9602 0996	.9561 7199	.9520 1241	.9477 3839	.9248 7624
5.49	.9611 9843	.9572 5317	.9531 8803	.9490 0999	.9266 4436

W	P(W,34)	P(W,36)	P(W,38)	P(W,40)	P(W,50)
5.50	.9621 6539	.9583 1109	.9543 3866	.9502 5486	.9283 7744
5.51	.9631 1121	.9593 4615	.9554 6471	.9514 7345	.9300 7597
5.52	.9640 3626	.9603 5873	.9565 6658	.9526 6617	.9317 4043
5.53	.9649 4090	.9613 4923	.9576 4469	.9538 3346	.9333 7131
5.54	.9658 2550	.9623 1803	.9586 9944	.9549 7572	.9349 6912
5.55	.9666 9042	.9632 6551	.9597 3122	.9560 9339	.9365 3433
5.56	.9675 3602	.9641 9204	.9607 4045	.9571 8688	.9380 6742
5.57	.9683 6264	.9650 9800	.9617 2750	.9582 5660	.9395 6890
5.58	.9691 7063	.9659 8377	.9626 9277	.9593 0295	.9410 3923
5.59	.9699 6034	.9668 4969	.9636 3664	.9603 2635	.9424 7890
5.60	.9707 3211	.9676 9614	.9645 5949	.9613 2719	.9438 8839
5.61	.9714 8627	.9685 2347	.9654 6171	.9623 0586	.9452 6817
5.62	.9722 2316	.9693 3203	.9663 4367	.9632 6278	.9466 1872
5.63	.9729 4310	.9701 2218	.9672 0573	.9641 9831	.9479 4051
5.64	.9736 4641	.9708 9426	.9680 4827	.9651 1285	.9492 3400
5.65	.9743 3342	.9716 4861	.9688 7164	.9660 0679	.9504 9967
5.66	.9750 0444	.9723 8556	.9696 7619	.9668 8048	.9517 3797
5.67	.9756 5978	.9731 0545	.9704 6230	.9677 3432	.9529 4936
5.68	.9762 9974	.9738 0861	.9712 3029	.9685 6867	.9541 3430
5.69	.9769 2464	.9744 9536	.9719 8052	.9693 8389	.9552 9325
5.70	.9775 3477	.9751 6603	.9727 1334	.9701 8034	.9564 2663
5.71	.9781 3043	.9758 2092	.9734 2906	.9709 5839	.9575 3491
5.72	.9787 1190	.9764 6034	.9741 2803	.9717 1837	.9586 1852
5.73	.9792 7947	.9770 8462	.9748 1057	.9724 6064	.9596 7790
5.74	.9798 3342	.9776 9404	.9754 7701	.9731 8555	.9607 1348
5.75	.9803 7403	.9782 8891	.9761 2767	.9738 9342	.9617 2569
5.76	.9809 0159	.9788 6952	.9767 6286	.9745 8460	.9627 1494
5.77	.9814 1634	.9794 3616	.9773 8288	.9752 5941	.9636 8167
5.78	.9819 1857	.9799 8911	.9779 8805	.9759 1818	.9646 2628
5.79	.9824 0852	.9805 2867	.9785 7867	.9765 6123	.9655 4919
5.80	.9828 8647	.9810 5510	.9791 5503	.9771 8887	.9664 5080
5.81	.9833 5266	.9815 6868	.9797 1742	.9778 0142	.9673 3151
5.82	.9838 0735	.9820 6968	.9802 6614	.9783 9919	.9681 9172
5.83	.9842 5077	.9825 5836	.9808 0147	.9789 8247	.9690 3183
5.84	.9846 8316	.9830 3498	.9813 2368	.9795 5157	.9698 5221
5.85	.9851 0478	.9834 9980	.9818 3306	.9801 0678	.9706 5325
5.86	.9855 1584	.9839 5308	.9823 2987	.9806 4838	.9714 3533
5.87	.9859 1659	.9843 9505	.9828 1439	.9811 7667	.9721 9882
5.88	.9863 0724	.9848 2596	.9832 8686	.9816 9193	.9729 4410
5.89	.9866 8801	.9852 4606	.9837 4755	.9821 9442	.9736 7151
5.90	.9870 5913	.9856 5558	.9841 9672	.9826 8443	.9743 8142
5.91	.9874 2081	.9860 5475	.9846 3462	.9831 6222	.9750 7419
5.92	.9877 7326	.9864 4380	.9850 6148	.9836 2805	.9757 5016
5.93	.9881 1668	.9868 2295	.9854 7756	.9840 8218	.9764 0967
5.94	.9884 5128	.9871 9243	.9858 8308	.9845 2486	.9770 5307
5.95	.9887 7726	.9875 5244	.9862 7829	.9849 5635	.9776 8069
5.96	.9890 9481	.9879 0321	.9866 6340	.9853 7690	.9782 9285
5.97	.9894 0413	.9882 4494	.9870 3865	.9857 8674	.9788 8988
5.98	.9897 0540	.9885 7784	.9874 0426	.9861 8611	.9794 7209
5.99	.9899 9882	.9889 0210	.9877 6045	.9865 7524	.9800 3981

W	P(W,34)	P(W,36)	P(W,38)	P(W,40)	P(W,50)
6.00	.9902 8455	.9892 1792	.9881 0742	.9869 5437	.9805 9334
6.01	.9905 6278	.9895 2550	.9884 4539	.9873 2372	.9811 3299
6.02	.9908 3369	.9898 2504	.9887 7457	.9876 8352	.9816 5905
6.03	.9910 9744	.9901 1670	.9890 9515	.9880 3397	.9821 7182
6.04	.9913 5421	.9904 0069	.9894 0733	.9883 7529	.9826 7159
6.05	.9916 0415	.9906 7717	.9897 1131	.9887 0769	.9831 5864
6.06	.9918 4744	.9909 4632	.9900 0728	.9890 3138	.9836 3325
6.07	.9920 8422	.9912 0832	.9902 9543	.9893 4656	.9840 9571
6.08	.9923 1465	.9914 6334	.9905 7593	.9896 5342	.9845 4627
6.09	.9925 3890	.9917 1154	.9908 4898	.9899 5217	.9849 8521
6.10	.9927 5709	.9919 5308	.9911 1474	.9902 4299	.9854 1278
6.11	.9929 6939	.9921 8813	.9913 7339	.9905 2606	.9858 2925
6.12	.9931 7594	.9924 1684	.9916 2510	.9908 0158	.9862 3486
6.13	.9933 7686	.9926 3936	.9918 7004	.9910 6972	.9866 2987
6.14	.9935 7231	.9928 5584	.9921 0836	.9913 3065	.9870 1451
6.15	.9937 6242	.9930 6644	.9923 4023	.9915 8456	.9873 8903
6.16	.9939 4731	.9932 7129	.9925 6580	.9918 3160	.9877 5366
6.17	.9941 2712	.9934 7053	.9927 8524	.9920 7195	.9881 0863
6.18	.9943 0198	.9936 6431	.9929 9868	.9923 0576	.9884 5416
6.19	.9944 7200	.9938 5276	.9932 0627	.9925 3321	.9887 9048
6.20	.9946 3730	.9940 3601	.9934 0817	.9927 5443	.9891 1781
6.21	.9947 9802	.9942 1418	.9936 0450	.9929 6959	.9894 3635
6.22	.9949 5425	.9943 8742	.9937 9542	.9931 7883	.9897 4632
6.23	.9951 0612	.9945 5584	.9939 8104	.9933 8230	.9900 4792
6.24	.9952 5374	.9947 1956	.9941 6151	.9935 8015	.9903 4135
6.25	.9953 9721	.9948 7870	.9943 3696	.9937 7251	.9906 2682
6.26	.9955 3664	.9950 3338	.9945 0751	.9939 5953	.9909 0450
6.27	.9956 7213	.9951 8371	.9946 7328	.9941 4133	.9911 7459
6.28	.9958 0378	.9953 2980	.9948 3440	.9943 1804	.9914 3729
6.29	.9959 3170	.9954 7176	.9949 9098	.9944 8981	.9916 9276
6.30	.9960 5598	.9956 0970	.9951 4314	.9946 5674	.9919 4118
6.31	.9961 7672	.9957 4372	.9952 9100	.9948 1897	.9921 8274
6.32	.9962 9400	.9958 7393	.9954 3467	.9949 7661	.9924 1759
6.33	.9964 0792	.9960 0041	.9955 7424	.9951 2979	.9926 4592
6.34	.9965 1856	.9961 2328	.9957 0984	.9952 7862	.9928 6787
6.35	.9966 2602	.9962 4262	.9958 4156	.9954 2320	.9930 8362
6.36	.9967 3037	.9963 5852	.9959 6950	.9955 6366	.9932 9331
6.37	.9968 3170	.9964 7108	.9960 9377	.9957 0009	.9934 9710
6.38	.9969 3009	.9965 8038	.9962 1445	.9958 3261	.9936 9515
6.39	.9970 2561	.9966 8652	.9963 3165	.9959 6131	.9938 8759
6.40	.9971 1835	.9967 8957	.9964 4546	.9960 8630	.9940 7457
6.41	.9972 0838	.9968 8962	.9965 5596	.9962 0768	.9942 5623
6.42	.9972 9577	.9969 8675	.9966 6324	.9963 2553	.9944 3271
6.43	.9973 8059	.9970 8103	.9967 6740	.9964 3996	.9946 0414
6.44	.9974 6291	.9971 7255	.9968 6851	.9965 5105	.9947 7066
6.45	.9975 4280	.9972 6137	.9969 6665	.9966 5889	.9949 3239
6.46	.9976 2033	.9973 4757	.9970 6191	.9967 6358	.9950 8945
6.47	.9976 9556	.9974 3123	.9971 5436	.9968 6519	.9952 4197
6.48	.9977 6856	.9975 1241	.9972 4409	.9969 6381	.9953 9007
6.49	.9978 3937	.9975 9117	.9973 3115	.9970 5952	.9955 3387

W	P(W,34)	P(W,36)	P(W,38)	P(W,40)	P(W,50)
6.50	.9979 0808	.9976 6759	.9974 1563	.9971 5240	.9956 7348
6.51	.9979 7472	.9977 4174	.9974 9761	.9972 4252	.9958 0901
6.52	.9980 3937	.9978 1366	.9975 7713	.9973 2997	.9959 4057
6.53	.9981 0207	.9978 8343	.9976 5428	.9974 1481	.9960 6826
6.54	.9981 6288	.9979 5110	.9977 2912	.9974 9711	.9961 9220
6.55	.9982 2186	.9980 1673	.9978 0171	.9975 7696	.9963 1248
6.56	.9982 7905	.9980 8038	.9978 7212	.9976 5440	.9964 2920
6.57	.9983 3450	.9981 4211	.9979 4040	.9977 2952	.9965 4246
6.58	.9983 8827	.9982 0197	.9980 0662	.9978 0237	.9966 5235
6.59	.9984 4040	.9982 6000	.9980 7083	.9978 7302	.9967 5896
6.60	.9984 9094	.9983 1627	.9981 3309	.9979 4154	.9968 6239
6.61	.9985 3993	.9983 7082	.9981 9346	.9980 0797	.9969 6272
6.62	.9985 8742	.9984 2371	.9982 5199	.9980 7238	.9970 6004
6.63	.9986 3345	.9984 7497	.9983 0872	.9981 3483	.9971 5443
6.64	.9986 7805	.9985 2465	.9983 6372	.9981 9537	.9972 4597
6.65	.9987 2129	.9985 7281	.9984 1703	.9982 5405	.9973 3474
6.66	.9987 6318	.9986 1948	.9984 6870	.9983 1093	.9974 2082
6.67	.9988 0378	.9986 6471	.9985 1877	.9983 6607	.9975 0428
6.68	.9988 4311	.9987 0853	.9985 6729	.9984 1950	.9975 8520
6.69	.9988 8122	.9987 5099	.9986 1432	.9984 7128	.9976 6365
6.70	.9989 1814	.9987 9214	.9986 5988	.9985 2146	.9977 3970
6.71	.9989 5390	.9988 3199	.9987 0402	.9985 7008	.9978 1342
6.72	.9989 8855	.9988 7061	.9987 4679	.9986 1719	.9978 8487
6.73	.9990 2210	.9989 0801	.9987 8823	.9986 6283	.9979 5411
6.74	.9990 5460	.9989 4424	.9988 2836	.9987 0704	.9980 2122
6.75	.9990 8608	.9989 7933	.9988 6724	.9987 4987	.9980 8625
6.76	.9991 1656	.9990 1331	.9989 0489	.9987 9135	.9981 4927
6.77	.9991 4608	.9990 4622	.9989 4135	.9988 3154	.9982 1032
6.78	.9991 7466	.9990 7809	.9989 7667	.9988 7045	.9982 6947
6.79	.9992 0233	.9991 0895	.9990 1087	.9989 0814	.9983 2678
6.80	.9992 2912	.9991 3883	.9990 4398	.9989 4463	.9983 8229
6.81	.9992 5505	.9991 6775	.9990 7604	.9989 7997	.9984 3605
6.82	.9992 8016	.9991 9576	.9991 0708	.9990 1419	.9984 8813
6.83	.9993 0446	.9992 2286	.9991 3713	.9990 4731	.9985 3857
6.84	.9993 2798	.9992 4910	.9991 6622	.9990 7938	.9985 8741
6.85	.9993 5074	.9992 7450	.9991 9438	.9991 1042	.9986 3471
6.86	.9993 7277	.9992 9908	.9992 2163	.9991 4047	.9986 8051
6.87	.9993 9409	.9993 2287	.9992 4801	.9991 6956	.9987 2485
6.88	.9994 1472	.9993 4589	.9992 7354	.9991 9771	.9987 6778
6.89	.9994 3468	.9993 6816	.9992 9824	.9992 2495	.9988 0934
6.90	.9994 5399	.9993 8971	.9993 2214	.9992 5131	.9988 4956
6.91	.9994 7268	.9994 1057	.9993 4527	.9992 7682	.9988 8850
6.92	.9994 9075	.9994 3074	.9993 6765	.9993 0151	.9989 2619
6.93	.9995 0823	.9994 5026	.9993 8930	.9993 2539	.9989 6267
6.94	.9995 2515	.9994 6913	.9994 1024	.9993 4849	.9989 9797
6.95	.9995 4150	.9994 8740	.9994 3050	.9993 7084	.9990 3213
6.96	.9995 5732	.9995 0506	.9994 5009	.9993 9246	.9990 6518
6.97	.9995 7262	.9995 2214	.9994 6905	.9994 1337	.9990 9716
6.98	.9995 8741	.9995 3866	.9994 8738	.9994 3360	.9991 2810
6.99	.9996 0172	.9995 5463	.9995 0511	.9994 5316	.9991 5803

W	P(W,34)	P(W,36)	P(W,38)	P(W,40)	P(W,50)
7.00	.9996 1555	.9995 7008	.9995 2225	.9994 7208	.9991 8698
7.01	.9996 2892	.9995 8501	.9995 3882	.9994 9037	.9992 1499
7.02	.9996 4185	.9995 9945	.9995 5485	.9995 0806	.9992 4208
7.03	.9996 5435	.9996 1341	.9995 7034	.9995 2516	.9992 6827
7.04	.9996 6643	.9996 2691	.9995 8533	.9995 4170	.9992 9361
7.05	.9996 7811	.9996 3995	.9995 9981	.9995 5769	.9993 1811
7.06	.9996 8939	.9996 5256	.9996 1380	.9995 7314	.9993 4180
7.07	.9997 0030	.9996 6475	.9996 2734	.9995 8808	.9993 6471
7.08	.9997 1084	.9996 7653	.9996 4041	.9996 0252	.9993 8685
7.09	.9997 2103	.9996 8791	.9996 5305	.9996 1647	.9994 0826
7.10	.9997 3087	.9996 9891	.9996 6527	.9996 2996	.9994 2896
7.11	.9997 4039	.9997 0954	.9996 7707	.9996 4299	.9994 4897
7.12	.9997 4958	.9997 1981	.9996 8847	.9996 5559	.9994 6830
7.13	.9997 5845	.9997 2973	.9996 9949	.9996 6776	.9994 8699
7.14	.9997 6703	.9997 3932	.9997 1014	.9996 7951	.9995 0506
7.15	.9997 7532	.9997 4858	.9997 2043	.9996 9087	.9995 2251
7.16	.9997 8332	.9997 5752	.9997 3036	.9997 0185	.9995 3938
7.17	.9997 9105	.9997 6616	.9997 3996	.9997 1245	.9995 5568
7.18	.9997 9851	.9997 7451	.9997 4923	.9997 2269	.9995 7143
7.19	.9998 0572	.9997 8257	.9997 5819	.9997 3258	.9995 8664
7.20	.9998 1268	.9997 9035	.9997 6683	.9997 4214	.9996 0134
7.21	.9998 1941	.9997 9787	.9997 7519	.9997 5137	.9996 1554
7.22	.9998 2590	.9998 0513	.9997 8325	.9997 6028	.9996 2925
7.23	.9998 3217	.9998 1214	.9997 9104	.9997 6888	.9996 4250
7.24	.9998 3822	.9998 1890	.9997 9856	.9997 7719	.9996 5529
7.25	.9998 4406	.9998 2544	.9998 0582	.9997 8521	.9996 6764
7.26	.9998 4970	.9998 3174	.9998 1283	.9997 9296	.9996 7958
7.27	.9998 5514	.9998 3783	.9998 1959	.9998 0043	.9996 9110
7.28	.9998 6040	.9998 4371	.9998 2612	.9998 0765	.9997 0222
7.29	.9998 6547	.9998 4938	.9998 3243	.9998 1462	.9997 1296
7.30	.9998 7036	.9998 5485	.9998 3851	.9998 2135	.9997 2333
7.31	.9998 7509	.9998 6014	.9998 4439	.9998 2784	.9997 3334
7.32	.9998 7964	.9998 6524	.9998 5005	.9998 3410	.9997 4301
7.33	.9998 8404	.9998 7016	.9998 5552	.9998 4015	.9997 5233
7.34	.9998 8829	.9998 7490	.9998 6080	.9998 4598	.9997 6134
7.35	.9998 9238	.9998 7948	.9998 6589	.9998 5161	.9997 7003
7.36	.9998 9633	.9998 8390	.9998 7081	.9998 5705	.9997 7841
7.37	.9999 0014	.9998 8817	.9998 7555	.9998 6229	.9997 8650
7.38	.9999 0382	.9998 9228	.9998 8012	.9998 6734	.9997 9431
7.39	.9999 0736	.9998 9625	.9998 8453	.9998 7222	.9998 0185
7.40	.9999 1078	.9999 0008	.9998 8879	.9998 7693	.9998 0912
7.41	.9999 1408	.9999 0377	.9998 9289	.9998 8147	.9998 1613
7.42	.9999 1726	.9999 0733	.9998 9685	.9998 8585	.9998 2290
7.43	.9999 2033	.9999 1076	.9999 0067	.9998 9007	.9998 2942
7.44	.9999 2329	.9999 1407	.9999 0435	.9998 9414	.9998 3572
7.45	.9999 2614	.9999 1726	.9999 0790	.9998 9807	.9998 4179
7.46	.9999 2889	.9999 2034	.9999 1133	.9999 0185	.9998 4765
7.47	.9999 3154	.9999 2331	.9999 1463	.9999 0551	.9998 5330
7.48	.9999 3410	.9999 2617	.9999 1781	.9999 0903	.9998 5874
7.49	.9999 3656	.9999 2893	.9999 2088	.9999 1242	.9998 6400

W	P(W,34)	P(W,36)	P(W,38)	P(W,40)	P(W,50)
7.50	.9999 3894	.9999 3159	.9999 2384	.9999 1569	.9998 6906
7.51	.9999 4123	.9999 3415	.9999 2669	.9999 1885	.9998 7394
7.52	.9999 4343	.9999 3662	.9999 2944	.9999 2189	.9998 7865
7.53	.9999 4556	.9999 3901	.9999 3209	.9999 2482	.9998 8319
7.54	.9999 4761	.9999 4130	.9999 3464	.9999 2765	.9998 8757
7.55	.9999 4959	.9999 4351	.9999 3711	.9999 3037	.9998 9178
7.56	.9999 5149	.9999 4564	.9999 3948	.9999 3299	.9998 9585
7.57	.9999 5333	.9999 4770	.9999 4176	.9999 3552	.9998 9977
7.58	.9999 5509	.9999 4968	.9999 4397	.9999 3796	.9999 0354
7.59	.9999 5680	.9999 5158	.9999 4609	.9999 4031	.9999 0718
7.60	.9999 5844	.9999 5342	.9999 4813	.9999 4257	.9999 1069
7.61	.9999 6002	.9999 5519	.9999 5010	.9999 4475	.9999 1407
7.62	.9999 6154	.9999 5690	.9999 5200	.9999 4685	.9999 1733
7.63	.9999 6301	.9999 5854	.9999 5383	.9999 4887	.9999 2046
7.64	.9999 6442	.9999 6012	.9999 5559	.9999 5082	.9999 2349
7.65	.9999 6578	.9999 6164	.9999 5728	.9999 5270	.9999 2640
7.66	.9999 6709	.9999 6311	.9999 5892	.9999 5450	.9999 2920
7.67	.9999 6835	.9999 6453	.9999 6049	.9999 5625	.9999 3190
7.68	.9999 6956	.9999 6589	.9999 6201	.9999 5792	.9999 3451
7.69	.9999 7073	.9999 6720	.9999 6346	.9999 5954	.9999 3701
7.70	.9999 7186	.9999 6846	.9999 6487	.9999 6109	.9999 3943
7.71	.9999 7295	.9999 6967	.9999 6622	.9999 6259	.9999 4175
7.72	.9999 7399	.9999 7084	.9999 6752	.9999 6403	.9999 4399
7.73	.9999 7500	.9999 7197	.9999 6878	.9999 6542	.9999 4615
7.74	.9999 7596	.9999 7305	.9999 6998	.9999 6675	.9999 4822
7.75	.9999 7689	.9999 7410	.9999 7115	.9999 6804	.9999 5022
7.76	.9999 7779	.9999 7510	.9999 7226	.9999 6928	.9999 5214
7.77	.9999 7865	.9999 7607	.9999 7334	.9999 7047	.9999 5399
7.78	.9999 7948	.9999 7700	.9999 7438	.9999 7162	.9999 5578
7.79	.9999 8028	.9999 7789	.9999 7537	.9999 7272	.9999 5749
7.80	.9999 8105	.9999 7876	.9999 7633	.9999 7378	.9999 5914
7.81	.9999 8179	.9999 7959	.9999 7726	.9999 7481	.9999 6073
7.82	.9999 8250	.9999 8038	.9999 7815	.9999 7579	.9999 6226
7.83	.9999 8319	.9999 8115	.9999 7900	.9999 7674	.9999 6374
7.84	.9999 8385	.9999 8189	.9999 7982	.9999 7765	.9999 6515
7.85	.9999 8448	.9999 8260	.9999 8061	.9999 7852	.9999 6652
7.86	.9999 8509	.9999 8328	.9999 8138	.9999 7937	.9999 6783
7.87	.9999 8568	.9999 8394	.9999 8211	.9999 8018	.9999 6909
7.88	.9999 8624	.9999 8457	.9999 8281	.9999 8096	.9999 7030
7.89	.9999 8679	.9999 8518	.9999 8349	.9999 8171	.9999 7147
7.90	.9999 8731	.9999 8577	.9999 8414	.9999 8243	.9999 7259
7.91	.9999 8781	.9999 8633	.9999 8477	.9999 8312	.9999 7367
7.92	.9999 8829	.9999 8687	.9999 8537	.9999 8379	.9999 7471
7.93	.9999 8876	.9999 8739	.9999 8595	.9999 8443	.9999 7571
7.94	.9999 8920	.9999 8789	.9999 8651	.9999 8505	.9999 7668
7.95	.9999 8963	.9999 8837	.9999 8704	.9999 8564	.9999 7760
7.96	.9999 9005	.9999 8884	.9999 8756	.9999 8622	.9999 7849
7.97	.9999 9044	.9999 8928	.9999 8806	.9999 8676	.9999 7934
7.98	.9999 9082	.9999 8971	.9999 8853	.9999 8729	.9999 8017
7.99	.9999 9119	.9999 9012	.9999 8899	.9999 8780	.9999 8096

W	P(W,34)	P(W,36)	P(W,38)	P(W,40)	P(W,50)
8.00	.9999 9154	.9999 9052	.9999 8943	.9999 8829	.9999 8172
8.01	.9999 9188	.9999 9090	.9999 8985	.9999 8876	.9999 8245
8.02	.9999 9221	.9999 9126	.9999 9026	.9999 8921	.9999 8315
8.03	.9999 9252	.9999 9161	.9999 9065	.9999 8964	.9999 8382
8.04	.9999 9282	.9999 9195	.9999 9103	.9999 9006	.9999 8447
8.05	.9999 9311	.9999 9227	.9999 9139	.9999 9046	.9999 8510
8.06	.9999 9339	.9999 9258	.9999 9173	.9999 9084	.9999 8569
8.07	.9999 9366	.9999 9288	.9999 9207	.9999 9121	.9999 8627
8.08	.9999 9391	.9999 9317	.9999 9239	.9999 9156	.9999 8682
8.09	.9999 9416	.9999 9345	.9999 9270	.9999 9191	.9999 8736
8.10	.9999 9439	.9999 9371	.9999 9299	.9999 9223	.9999 8787
8.11	.9999 9462	.9999 9397	.9999 9328	.9999 9255	.9999 8836
8.12	.9999 9484	.9999 9421	.9999 9355	.9999 9285	.9999 8883
8.13	.9999 9505	.9999 9445	.9999 9381	.9999 9314	.9999 8928
8.14	.9999 9525	.9999 9467	.9999 9406	.9999 9342	.9999 8972
8.15	.9999 9545	.9999 9489	.9999 9430	.9999 9369	.9999 9014
8.16	.9999 9563	.9999 9510	.9999 9454	.9999 9394	.9999 9054
8.17	.9999 9581	.9999 9530	.9999 9476	.9999 9419	.9999 9092
8.18	.9999 9598	.9999 9549	.9999 9497	.9999 9443	.9999 9129
8.19	.9999 9615	.9999 9568	.9999 9518	.9999 9466	.9999 9165
8.20	.9999 9630	.9999 9585	.9999 9538	.9999 9488	.9999 9199
8.21	.9999 9646	.9999 9602	.9999 9557	.9999 9509	.9999 9232
8.22	.9999 9660	.9999 9619	.9999 9575	.9999 9529	.9999 9263
8.23	.9999 9674	.9999 9634	.9999 9592	.9999 9548	.9999 9294
8.24	.9999 9688	.9999 9649	.9999 9609	.9999 9567	.9999 9323
8.25	.9999 9700	.9999 9664	.9999 9625	.9999 9585	.9999 9351
8.26	.9999 9713	.9999 9678	.9999 9641	.9999 9602	.9999 9377
8.27	.9999 9725	.9999 9691	.9999 9656	.9999 9618	.9999 9403
8.28	.9999 9736	.9999 9704	.9999 9670	.9999 9634	.9999 9428
8.29	.9999 9747	.9999 9716	.9999 9684	.9999 9649	.9999 9451
8.30	.9999 9758	.9999 9728	.9999 9697	.9999 9664	.9999 9474
8.31	.9999 9768	.9999 9739	.9999 9709	.9999 9678	.9999 9496
8.32	.9999 9777	.9999 9750	.9999 9721	.9999 9691	.9999 9517
8.33	.9999 9787	.9999 9760	.9999 9733	.9999 9704	.9999 9537
8.34	.9999 9795	.9999 9770	.9999 9744	.9999 9716	.9999 9556
8.35	.9999 9804	.9999 9780	.9999 9755	.9999 9728	.9999 9575
8.36	.9999 9812	.9999 9789	.9999 9765	.9999 9739	.9999 9592
8.37	.9999 9820	.9999 9798	.9999 9775	.9999 9750	.9999 9609
8.38	.9999 9828	.9999 9806	.9999 9784	.9999 9761	.9999 9626
8.39	.9999 9835	.9999 9815	.9999 9793	.9999 9771	.9999 9641
8.40	.9999 9842	.9999 9822	.9999 9802	.9999 9780	.9999 9656
8.41	.9999 9848	.9999 9830	.9999 9810	.9999 9790	.9999 9671
8.42	.9999 9855	.9999 9837	.9999 9818	.9999 9799	.9999 9685
8.43	.9999 9861	.9999 9844	.9999 9826	.9999 9807	.9999 9698
8.44	.9999 9867	.9999 9850	.9999 9833	.9999 9815	.9999 9711
8.45	.9999 9872	.9999 9857	.9999 9840	.9999 9823	.9999 9723
8.46	.9999 9878	.9999 9863	.9999 9847	.9999 9830	.9999 9735
8.47	.9999 9883	.9999 9869	.9999 9853	.9999 9838	.9999 9746
8.48	.9999 9888	.9999 9874	.9999 9860	.9999 9844	.9999 9757
8.49	.9999 9893	.9999 9880	.9999 9866	.9999 9851	.9999 9767

W	P(W,34)	P(W,36)	P(W,38)	P(W,40)	P(W,50)
8.50	.9999 9897	.9999 9885	.9999 9871	.9999 9857	.9999 9777
8.51	.9999 9902	.9999 9890	.9999 9877	.9999 9863	.9999 9786
8.52	.9999 9906	.9999 9894	.9999 9882	.9999 9869	.9999 9795
8.53	.9999 9910	.9999 9899	.9999 9887	.9999 9875	.9999 9804
8.54	.9999 9914	.9999 9903	.9999 9892	.9999 9880	.9999 9812
8.55	.9999 9917	.9999 9907	.9999 9897	.9999 9885	.9999 9820
8.56	.9999 9921	.9999 9911	.9999 9901	.9999 9890	.9999 9828
8.57	.9999 9924	.9999 9915	.9999 9905	.9999 9895	.9999 9835
8.58	.9999 9927	.9999 9919	.9999 9909	.9999 9899	.9999 9842
8.59	.9999 9931	.9999 9922	.9999 9913	.9999 9904	.9999 9849
8.60	.9999 9934	.9999 9925	.9999 9917	.9999 9908	.9999 9856
8.61	.9999 9936	.9999 9929	.9999 9920	.9999 9912	.9999 9862
8.62	.9999 9939	.9999 9932	.9999 9924	.9999 9916	.9999 9868
8.63	.9999 9942	.9999 9935	.9999 9927	.9999 9919	.9999 9873
8.64	.9999 9944	.9999 9937	.9999 9930	.9999 9923	.9999 9879
8.65	.9999 9947	.9999 9940	.9999 9933	.9999 9926	.9999 9884
8.66	.9999 9949	.9999 9943	.9999 9936	.9999 9929	.9999 9889
8.67	.9999 9951	.9999 9945	.9999 9939	.9999 9932	.9999 9894
8.68	.9999 9953	.9999 9948	.9999 9942	.9999 9935	.9999 9898
8.69	.9999 9955	.9999 9950	.9999 9944	.9999 9938	.9999 9903
8.70	.9999 9957	.9999 9952	.9999 9946	.9999 9941	.9999 9907
8.71	.9999 9959	.9999 9954	.9999 9949	.9999 9943	.9999 9911
8.72	.9999 9961	.9999 9956	.9999 9951	.9999 9946	.9999 9915
8.73	.9999 9963	.9999 9958	.9999 9953	.9999 9948	.9999 9919
8.74	.9999 9964	.9999 9960	.9999 9955	.9999 9950	.9999 9922
8.75	.9999 9966	.9999 9962	.9999 9957	.9999 9952	.9999 9926
8.76	.9999 9967	.9999 9963	.9999 9959	.9999 9955	.9999 9929
8.77	.9999 9969	.9999 9965	.9999 9961	.9999 9957	.9999 9932
8.78	.9999 9970	.9999 9966	.9999 9963	.9999 9958	.9999 9935
8.79	.9999 9971	.9999 9968	.9999 9964	.9999 9960	.9999 9938
8.80	.9999 9973	.9999 9969	.9999 9966	.9999 9962	.9999 9940
8.81	.9999 9974	.9999 9971	.9999 9967	.9999 9964	.9999 9943
8.82	.9999 9975	.9999 9972	.9999 9969	.9999 9965	.9999 9946
8.83	.9999 9976	.9999 9973	.9999 9970	.9999 9967	.9999 9948
8.84	.9999 9977	.9999 9974	.9999 9971	.9999 9968	.9999 9950
8.85	.9999 9978	.9999 9975	.9999 9973	.9999 9970	.9999 9952
8.86	.9999 9979	.9999 9977	.9999 9974	.9999 9971	.9999 9954
8.87	.9999 9980	.9999 9978	.9999 9975	.9999 9972	.9999 9956
8.88	.9999 9981	.9999 9979	.9999 9976	.9999 9973	.9999 9958
8.89	.9999 9982	.9999 9979	.9999 9977	.9999 9975	.9999 9960
8.90	.9999 9983	.9999 9980	.9999 9978	.9999 9976	.9999 9962
8.91	.9999 9983	.9999 9981	.9999 9979	.9999 9977	.9999 9964
8.92	.9999 9984	.9999 9982	.9999 9980	.9999 9978	.9999 9965
8.93	.9999 9985	.9999 9983	.9999 9981	.9999 9979	.9999 9967
8.94	.9999 9985	.9999 9984	.9999 9982	.9999 9980	.9999 9968
8.95	.9999 9986	.9999 9984	.9999 9983	.9999 9981	.9999 9970
8.96	.9999 9987	.9999 9985	.9999 9983	.9999 9982	.9999 9971
8.97	.9999 9987	.9999 9986	.9999 9984	.9999 9982	.9999 9972
8.98	.9999 9988	.9999 9986	.9999 9985	.9999 9983	.9999 9974
8.99	.9999 9988	.9999 9987	.9999 9985	.9999 9984	.9999 9975

W	P(W,34)	P(W,36)	P(W,38)	P(W,40)	P(W,50)
9.00	.9999 9989	.9999 9988	.9999 9986	.9999 9985	.9999 9976
9.01	.9999 9989	.9999 9988	.9999 9987	.9999 9985	.9999 9977
9.02	.9999 9990	.9999 9989	.9999 9987	.9999 9986	.9999 9978
9.03	.9999 9990	.9999 9989	.9999 9988	.9999 9987	.9999 9979
9.04	.9999 9991	.9999 9990	.9999 9988	.9999 9987	.9999 9980
9.05	.9999 9991	.9999 9990	.9999 9989	.9999 9988	.9999 9981
9.06	.9999 9992	.9999 9991	.9999 9989	.9999 9988	.9999 9982
9.07	.9999 9992	.9999 9991	.9999 9990	.9999 9989	.9999 9982
9.08	.9999 9992	.9999 9991	.9999 9990	.9999 9989	.9999 9983
9.09	.9999 9993	.9999 9992	.9999 9991	.9999 9990	.9999 9984
9.10	.9999 9993	.9999 9992	.9999 9991	.9999 9990	.9999 9985
9.11	.9999 9993	.9999 9992	.9999 9992	.9999 9991	.9999 9985
9.12	.9999 9994	.9999 9993	.9999 9992	.9999 9991	.9999 9986
9.13	.9999 9994	.9999 9993	.9999 9992	.9999 9991	.9999 9987
9.14	.9999 9994	.9999 9993	.9999 9993	.9999 9992	.9999 9987
9.15	.9999 9994	.9999 9994	.9999 9993	.9999 9992	.9999 9988
9.16	.9999 9995	.9999 9994	.9999 9993	.9999 9993	.9999 9988
9.17	.9999 9995	.9999 9994	.9999 9994	.9999 9993	.9999 9989
9.18	.9999 9995	.9999 9995	.9999 9994	.9999 9993	.9999 9989
9.19	.9999 9995	.9999 9995	.9999 9994	.9999 9993	.9999 9990
9.20	.9999 9996	.9999 9995	.9999 9994	.9999 9994	.9999 9990
9.21	.9999 9996	.9999 9995	.9999 9995	.9999 9994	.9999 9991
9.22	.9999 9996	.9999 9995	.9999 9995	.9999 9994	.9999 9991
9.23	.9999 9996	.9999 9996	.9999 9995	.9999 9995	.9999 9992
9.24	.9999 9996	.9999 9996	.9999 9995	.9999 9995	.9999 9992
9.25	.9999 9996	.9999 9996	.9999 9996	.9999 9995	.9999 9992
9.26	.9999 9997	.9999 9996	.9999 9996	.9999 9995	.9999 9993
9.27	.9999 9997	.9999 9996	.9999 9996	.9999 9995	.9999 9993
9.28	.9999 9997	.9999 9997	.9999 9996	.9999 9996	.9999 9993
9.29	.9999 9997	.9999 9997	.9999 9996	.9999 9996	.9999 9994
9.30	.9999 9997	.9999 9997	.9999 9996	.9999 9996	.9999 9994
9.31	.9999 9997	.9999 9997	.9999 9997	.9999 9996	.9999 9994
9.32	.9999 9997	.9999 9997	.9999 9997	.9999 9996	.9999 9994
9.33	.9999 9997	.9999 9997	.9999 9997	.9999 9997	.9999 9995
9.34	.9999 9998	.9999 9997	.9999 9997	.9999 9997	.9999 9995
9.35	.9999 9998	.9999 9997	.9999 9997	.9999 9997	.9999 9995
9.36	.9999 9998	.9999 9998	.9999 9997	.9999 9997	.9999 9995
9.37	.9999 9998	.9999 9998	.9999 9997	.9999 9997	.9999 9996
9.38	.9999 9998	.9999 9998	.9999 9998	.9999 9997	.9999 9996
9.39	.9999 9998	.9999 9998	.9999 9998	.9999 9997	.9999 9996
9.40	.9999 9998	.9999 9998	.9999 9998	.9999 9997	.9999 9996
9.41	.9999 9998	.9999 9998	.9999 9998	.9999 9998	.9999 9996
9.42	.9999 9998	.9999 9998	.9999 9998	.9999 9998	.9999 9996
9.43	.9999 9998	.9999 9998	.9999 9998	.9999 9998	.9999 9997
9.44	.9999 9998	.9999 9998	.9999 9998	.9999 9998	.9999 9997
9.45	.9999 9999	.9999 9998	.9999 9998	.9999 9998	.9999 9997
9.46	.9999 9999	.9999 9998	.9999 9998	.9999 9998	.9999 9997
9.47	.9999 9999	.9999 9999	.9999 9998	.9999 9998	.9999 9997
9.48	.9999 9999	.9999 9999	.9999 9998	.9999 9998	.9999 9997
9.49	.9999 9999	.9999 9999	.9999 9998	.9999 9998	.9999 9997

W	P(W,34)	P(W,36)	P(W,38)	P(W,40)	P(W,50)
9.50	.9999 9999	.9999 9999	.9999 9999	.9999 9998	.9999 9998
9.51	.9999 9999	.9999 9999	.9999 9999	.9999 9998	.9999 9998
9.52	.9999 9999	.9999 9999	.9999 9999	.9999 9999	.9999 9998
9.53	.9999 9999	.9999 9999	.9999 9999	.9999 9999	.9999 9998
9.54	.9999 9999	.9999 9999	.9999 9999	.9999 9999	.9999 9998
9.55	.9999 9999	.9999 9999	.9999 9999	.9999 9999	.9999 9998
9.56	.9999 9999	.9999 9999	.9999 9999	.9999 9999	.9999 9998
9.57	.9999 9999	.9999 9999	.9999 9999	.9999 9999	.9999 9998
9.58	.9999 9999	.9999 9999	.9999 9999	.9999 9999	.9999 9998
9.59	.9999 9999	.9999 9999	.9999 9999	.9999 9999	.9999 9998
9.60	.9999 9999	.9999 9999	.9999 9999	.9999 9999	.9999 9998
9.61	.9999 9999	.9999 9999	.9999 9999	.9999 9999	.9999 9998
9.62	.9999 9999	.9999 9999	.9999 9999	.9999 9999	.9999 9998
9.63	.9999 9999	.9999 9999	.9999 9999	.9999 9999	.9999 9999
9.64	.9999 9999	.9999 9999	.9999 9999	.9999 9999	.9999 9999
9.65	.9999 9999	.9999 9999	.9999 9999	.9999 9999	.9999 9999
9.66	.9999 9999	.9999 9999	.9999 9999	.9999 9999	.9999 9999
9.67	.9999 9999	.9999 9999	.9999 9999	.9999 9999	.9999 9999
9.68	.9999 9999	.9999 9999	.9999 9999	.9999 9999	.9999 9999
9.69	.9999 9999	.9999 9999	.9999 9999	.9999 9999	.9999 9999
9.70	.9999 9999	.9999 9999	.9999 9999	.9999 9999	.9999 9999
9.71	.9999 9999	.9999 9999	.9999 9999	.9999 9999	.9999 9999
9.72	.9999 9999	.9999 9999	.9999 9999	.9999 9999	.9999 9999
9.73	1.0000 0000	.9999 9999	.9999 9999	.9999 9999	.9999 9999
9.74		.9999 9999	.9999 9999	.9999 9999	.9999 9999
9.75		1.0000 0000	.9999 9999	.9999 9999	.9999 9999
9.76			.9999 9999	.9999 9999	.9999 9999
9.77			.9999 9999	.9999 9999	.9999 9999
9.78			1.0000 0000	.9999 9999	.9999 9999
9.79				.9999 9999	.9999 9999
9.80				.9999 9999	.9999 9999
9.81				1.0000 0000	.9999 9999
9.82					.9999 9999
9.83					.9999 9999
9.84					.9999 9999
9.85					.9999 9999
9.86					.9999 9999
9.87					.9999 9999
9.88					.9999 9999
9.89					.9999 9999
9.90					.9999 9999
9.91					.9999 9999
9.92					.9999 9999
9.93					.9999 9999
9.94					.9999 9999
9.95					1.0000 0000
9.96					
9.97					
9.98					
9.99					

W	P(W,60)	P(W,70)	P(W,80)	P(W,90)	P(W,100)
2.00					
2.01					
2.02					
2.03					
2.04					
2.05					
2.06					
2.07					
2.08	.0000 0000				
2.09	.0000 0001				
2.10	.0000 0001				
2.11	.0000 0001				
2.12	.0000 0001				
2.13	.0000 0001				
2.14	.0000 0001				
2.15	.0000 0002				
2.16	.0000 0002				
2.17	.0000 0002				
2.18	.0000 0003				
2.19	.0000 0003				
2.20	.0000 0004				
2.21	.0000 0005				
2.22	.0000 0006				
2.23	.0000 0007				
2.24	.0000 0008				
2.25	.0000 0009	.0000 0000			
2.26	.0000 0011	.0000 0001			
2.27	.0000 0013	.0000 0001			
2.28	.0000 0015	.0000 0001			
2.29	.0000 0018	.0000 0001			
2.30	.0000 0021	.0000 0001			
2.31	.0000 0025	.0000 0001			
2.32	.0000 0029	.0000 0002			
2.33	.0000 0034	.0000 0002			
2.34	.0000 0040	.0000 0003			
2.35	.0000 0046	.0000 0003			
2.36	.0000 0054	.0000 0004			
2.37	.0000 0063	.0000 0005			
2.38	.0000 0073	.0000 0005			
2.39	.0000 0084	.0000 0006	.0000 0000		
2.40	.0000 0098	.0000 0008	.0000 0001		
2.41	.0000 0113	.0000 0009	.0000 0001		
2.42	.0000 0130	.0000 0011	.0000 0001		
2.43	.0000 0150	.0000 0013	.0000 0001		
2.44	.0000 0173	.0000 0015	.0000 0001		
2.45	.0000 0198	.0000 0018	.0000 0001		
2.46	.0000 0228	.0000 0021	.0000 0002		
2.47	.0000 0261	.0000 0024	.0000 0002		
2.48	.0000 0299	.0000 0029	.0000 0003		
2.49	.0000 0343	.0000 0034	.0000 0003		

W	P(W,60)	P(W,70)	P(W,80)	P(W,90)	P(W,100)
2.50	.0000 0391	.0000 0039	.0000 0004		
2.51	.0000 0447	.0000 0046	.0000 0005		
2.52	.0000 0509	.0000 0053	.0000 0005	.0000 0000	
2.53	.0000 0580	.0000 0062	.0000 0007	.0000 0001	
2.54	.0000 0660	.0000 0072	.0000 0008	.0000 0001	
2.55	.0000 0750	.0000 0084	.0000 0009	.0000 0001	
2.56	.0000 0851	.0000 0098	.0000 0011	.0000 0001	
2.57	.0000 0965	.0000 0113	.0000 0013	.0000 0001	
2.58	.0000 1092	.0000 0131	.0000 0015	.0000 0002	
2.59	.0000 1235	.0000 0151	.0000 0018	.0000 0002	
2.60	.0000 1396	.0000 0175	.0000 0022	.0000 0003	
2.61	.0000 1575	.0000 0201	.0000 0025	.0000 0003	
2.62	.0000 1776	.0000 0232	.0000 0030	.0000 0004	.0000 0000
2.63	.0000 2000	.0000 0267	.0000 0035	.0000 0005	.0000 0001
2.64	.0000 2249	.0000 0306	.0000 0041	.0000 0005	.0000 0001
2.65	.0000 2528	.0000 0351	.0000 0048	.0000 0007	.0000 0001
2.66	.0000 2837	.0000 0402	.0000 0056	.0000 0008	.0000 0001
2.67	.0000 3182	.0000 0460	.0000 0066	.0000 0009	.0000 0001
2.68	.0000 3564	.0000 0526	.0000 0077	.0000 0011	.0000 0002
2.69	.0000 3989	.0000 0600	.0000 0089	.0000 0013	.0000 0002
2.70	.0000 4459	.0000 0685	.0000 0104	.0000 0016	.0000 0002
2.71	.0000 4980	.0000 0779	.0000 0121	.0000 0018	.0000 0003
2.72	.0000 5556	.0000 0886	.0000 0140	.0000 0022	.0000 0003
2.73	.0000 6192	.0000 1007	.0000 0162	.0000 0026	.0000 0004
2.74	.0000 6895	.0000 1143	.0000 0187	.0000 0030	.0000 0005
2.75	.0000 7670	.0000 1295	.0000 0216	.0000 0036	.0000 0006
2.76	.0000 8523	.0000 1466	.0000 0250	.0000 0042	.0000 0007
2.77	.0000 9463	.0000 1658	.0000 0288	.0000 0049	.0000 0008
2.78	.0001 0495	.0000 1873	.0000 0331	.0000 0058	.0000 0010
2.79	.0001 1630	.0000 2113	.0000 0380	.0000 0068	.0000 0012
2.80	.0001 2875	.0000 2381	.0000 0436	.0000 0079	.0000 0014
2.81	.0001 4240	.0000 2681	.0000 0500	.0000 0092	.0000 0017
2.82	.0001 5735	.0000 3015	.0000 0572	.0000 0108	.0000 0020
2.83	.0001 7371	.0000 3387	.0000 0654	.0000 0125	.0000 0024
2.84	.0001 9159	.0000 3801	.0000 0747	.0000 0146	.0000 0028
2.85	.0002 1113	.0000 4261	.0000 0852	.0000 0169	.0000 0033
2.86	.0002 3244	.0000 4771	.0000 0970	.0000 0196	.0000 0039
2.87	.0002 5568	.0000 5337	.0000 1104	.0000 0226	.0000 0046
2.88	.0002 8100	.0000 5965	.0000 1254	.0000 0262	.0000 0054
2.89	.0003 0855	.0000 6658	.0000 1423	.0000 0302	.0000 0064
2.90	.0003 3850	.0000 7425	.0000 1613	.0000 0348	.0000 0075
2.91	.0003 7104	.0000 8272	.0000 1827	.0000 0400	.0000 0087
2.92	.0004 0636	.0000 9207	.0000 2066	.0000 0460	.0000 0102
2.93	.0004 4466	.0001 0237	.0000 2334	.0000 0528	.0000 0119
2.94	.0004 8615	.0001 1370	.0000 2634	.0000 0606	.0000 0138
2.95	.0005 3108	.0001 2617	.0000 2969	.0000 0694	.0000 0161
2.96	.0005 7966	.0001 3987	.0000 3343	.0000 0793	.0000 0187
2.97	.0006 3218	.0001 5490	.0000 3760	.0000 0906	.0000 0217
2.98	.0006 8888	.0001 7139	.0000 4224	.0000 1033	.0000 0251
2.99	.0007 5005	.0001 8945	.0000 4740	.0000 1177	.0000 0291

W	P(W,60)	P(W,70)	P(W,80)	P(W,90)	P(W,100)
3.00	.0008 1600	.0002 0921	.0000 5314	.0000 1340	.0000 0336
3.01	.0008 8703	.0002 3083	.0000 5951	.0000 1523	.0000 0387
3.02	.0009 6348	.0002 5443	.0000 6656	.0000 1729	.0000 0446
3.03	.0010 4569	.0002 8020	.0000 7438	.0000 1960	.0000 0514
3.04	.0011 3403	.0003 0828	.0000 8303	.0000 2220	.0000 0590
3.05	.0012 2887	.0003 3888	.0000 9258	.0000 2511	.0000 0677
3.06	.0013 3061	.0003 7218	.0001 0313	.0000 2837	.0000 0776
3.07	.0014 3967	.0004 0838	.0001 1477	.0000 3202	.0000 0888
3.08	.0015 5648	.0004 4770	.0001 2759	.0000 3610	.0000 1015
3.09	.0016 8151	.0004 9038	.0001 4169	.0000 4065	.0000 1159
3.10	.0018 1521	.0005 3666	.0001 5720	.0000 4572	.0000 1322
3.11	.0019 5810	.0005 8679	.0001 7423	.0000 5136	.0000 1505
3.12	.0021 1067	.0006 4106	.0001 9292	.0000 5764	.0000 1712
3.13	.0022 7346	.0006 9975	.0002 1340	.0000 6462	.0000 1945
3.14	.0024 4703	.0007 6316	.0002 3582	.0000 7235	.0000 2207
3.15	.0026 3196	.0008 3161	.0002 6036	.0000 8093	.0000 2501
3.16	.0028 2883	.0009 0545	.0002 8717	.0000 9043	.0000 2832
3.17	.0030 3828	.0009 8503	.0003 1644	.0001 0094	.0000 3201
3.18	.0032 6094	.0010 7072	.0003 4837	.0001 1254	.0000 3615
3.19	.0034 9747	.0011 6292	.0003 8316	.0001 2535	.0000 4078
3.20	.0037 4855	.0012 6203	.0004 2103	.0001 3947	.0000 4594
3.21	.0040 1490	.0013 6849	.0004 6222	.0001 5502	.0000 5170
3.22	.0042 9725	.0014 8275	.0005 0698	.0001 7213	.0000 5811
3.23	.0045 9633	.0016 0527	.0005 5557	.0001 9093	.0000 6525
3.24	.0049 1292	.0017 3656	.0006 0828	.0002 1157	.0000 7318
3.25	.0052 4783	.0018 7712	.0006 6538	.0002 3421	.0000 8198
3.26	.0056 0185	.0020 2749	.0007 2721	.0002 5901	.0000 9173
3.27	.0059 7584	.0021 8823	.0007 9409	.0002 8615	.0001 0254
3.28	.0063 7065	.0023 5992	.0008 6636	.0003 1583	.0001 1449
3.29	.0067 8715	.0025 4315	.0009 4439	.0003 4825	.0001 2770
3.30	.0072 2625	.0027 3856	.0010 2856	.0003 8363	.0001 4229
3.31	.0076 8886	.0029 4680	.0011 1929	.0004 2219	.0001 5836
3.32	.0081 7593	.0031 6853	.0012 1700	.0004 6419	.0001 7607
3.33	.0086 8842	.0034 0445	.0013 2212	.0005 0989	.0001 9556
3.34	.0092 2729	.0036 5529	.0014 3514	.0005 5957	.0002 1697
3.35	.0097 9356	.0039 2178	.0015 5653	.0006 1351	.0002 4048
3.36	.0103 8822	.0042 0470	.0016 8681	.0006 7204	.0002 6627
3.37	.0110 1230	.0045 0483	.0018 2652	.0007 3548	.0002 9452
3.38	.0116 6687	.0048 2299	.0019 7620	.0008 0418	.0003 2544
3.39	.0123 5296	.0051 6002	.0021 3645	.0008 7850	.0003 5925
3.40	.0130 7165	.0055 1679	.0023 0786	.0009 5884	.0003 9618
3.41	.0138 2404	.0058 9417	.0024 9106	.0010 4560	.0004 3648
3.42	.0146 1122	.0062 9309	.0026 8671	.0011 3921	.0004 8041
3.43	.0154 3430	.0067 1446	.0028 9550	.0012 4013	.0005 2824
3.44	.0162 9440	.0071 5924	.0031 1811	.0013 4881	.0005 8028
3.45	.0171 9265	.0076 2842	.0033 5528	.0014 6577	.0006 3684
3.46	.0181 3018	.0081 2298	.0036 0777	.0015 9151	.0006 9825
3.47	.0191 0815	.0086 4395	.0038 7636	.0017 2658	.0007 6487
3.48	.0201 2768	.0091 9236	.0041 6185	.0018 7156	.0008 3707
3.49	.0211 8994	.0097 6928	.0044 6507	.0020 2702	.0009 1523

W	P(W,60)	P(W,70)	P(W,80)	P(W,90)	P(W,100)
3.50	.0222 9608	.0103 7577	.0047 8689	.0021 9358	.0009 9978
3.51	.0234 4726	.0110 1294	.0051 2818	.0023 7190	.0010 9115
3.52	.0246 4462	.0116 8189	.0054 8985	.0025 6264	.0011 8979
3.53	.0258 8933	.0123 8375	.0058 7285	.0027 6649	.0012 9620
3.54	.0271 8252	.0131 1967	.0062 7811	.0029 8418	.0014 1087
3.55	.0285 2535	.0138 9080	.0067 0663	.0032 1646	.0015 3433
3.56	.0299 1896	.0146 9831	.0071 5942	.0034 6410	.0016 6715
3.57	.0313 6446	.0155 4339	.0076 3750	.0037 2790	.0018 0990
3.58	.0328 6299	.0164 2722	.0081 4192	.0040 0870	.0019 6318
3.59	.0344 1564	.0173 5100	.0086 7377	.0043 0735	.0021 2764
3.60	.0360 2352	.0183 1595	.0092 3413	.0046 2474	.0023 0393
3.61	.0376 8771	.0193 2329	.0098 2413	.0049 6179	.0024 9274
3.62	.0394 0927	.0203 7422	.0104 4490	.0053 1942	.0026 9478
3.63	.0411 8925	.0214 6998	.0110 9759	.0056 9861	.0029 1080
3.64	.0430 2868	.0226 1179	.0117 8339	.0061 0035	.0031 4157
3.65	.0449 2856	.0238 0089	.0125 0348	.0065 2566	.0033 8790
3.66	.0468 8988	.0250 3848	.0132 5907	.0069 7558	.0036 5060
3.67	.0489 1359	.0263 2581	.0140 5139	.0074 5118	.0039 3054
3.68	.0510 0064	.0276 6408	.0148 8166	.0079 5356	.0042 2861
3.69	.0531 5193	.0290 5451	.0157 5114	.0084 8382	.0045 4571
3.70	.0553 6833	.0304 9830	.0166 6108	.0090 4312	.0048 8280
3.71	.0576 5070	.0319 9665	.0176 1275	.0096 3262	.0052 4085
3.72	.0599 9985	.0335 5074	.0186 0743	.0102 5349	.0056 2086
3.73	.0624 1655	.0351 6174	.0196 4640	.0109 0696	.0060 2385
3.74	.0649 0156	.0368 3081	.0207 3095	.0115 9423	.0064 5088
3.75	.0674 5559	.0385 5909	.0218 6236	.0123 1655	.0069 0305
3.76	.0700 7930	.0403 4768	.0230 4193	.0130 7518	.0073 8145
3.77	.0727 7334	.0421 9771	.0242 7096	.0138 7140	.0078 8722
3.78	.0755 3828	.0441 1023	.0255 5071	.0147 0650	.0084 2152
3.79	.0783 7469	.0460 8630	.0268 8250	.0155 8178	.0089 8555
3.80	.0812 8308	.0481 2696	.0282 6758	.0164 9855	.0095 8051
3.81	.0842 6390	.0502 3319	.0297 0724	.0174 5814	.0102 0762
3.82	.0873 1757	.0524 0598	.0312 0274	.0184 6189	.0108 6815
3.83	.0904 4448	.0546 4625	.0327 5533	.0195 1113	.0115 6337
3.84	.0936 4494	.0569 5492	.0343 6624	.0206 0720	.0122 9457
3.85	.0969 1924	.0593 3285	.0360 3670	.0217 5147	.0130 6306
3.86	.1002 6760	.0617 8089	.0377 6792	.0229 4528	.0138 7017
3.87	.1036 9021	.0642 9982	.0395 6107	.0241 8997	.0147 1724
3.88	.1071 8720	.0668 9041	.0414 1732	.0254 8690	.0156 0563
3.89	.1107 5864	.0695 5337	.0433 3782	.0268 3741	.0165 3671
3.90	.1144 0456	.0722 8939	.0453 2368	.0282 4283	.0175 1186
3.91	.1181 2495	.0750 9908	.0473 7599	.0297 0451	.0185 3246
3.92	.1219 1973	.0779 8304	.0494 9580	.0312 2375	.0195 9992
3.93	.1257 8877	.0809 4181	.0516 8415	.0328 0185	.0207 1562
3.94	.1297 3189	.0839 7587	.0539 4203	.0344 4013	.0218 8097
3.95	.1337 4886	.0870 8568	.0562 7040	.0361 3984	.0230 9739
3.96	.1378 3939	.0902 7162	.0586 7019	.0379 0224	.0243 6626
3.97	.1420 0315	.0935 3405	.0611 4228	.0397 2858	.0256 8900
3.98	.1462 3974	.0968 7324	.0636 8751	.0416 2006	.0270 6700
3.99	.1505 4872	.1002 8944	.0663 0669	.0435 7787	.0285 0164

W	P(W,60)	P(W,70)	P(W,80)	P(W,90)	P(W,100)
4.00	.1549 2959	.1037 8283	.0690 0058	.0456 0317	.0299 9431
4.01	.1593 8180	.1073 5354	.0717 6990	.0476 9710	.0315 4637
4.02	.1639 0476	.1110 0165	.0746 1530	.0498 6074	.0331 5919
4.03	.1684 9781	.1147 2718	.0775 3741	.0520 9517	.0348 3409
4.04	.1731 6025	.1185 3009	.0805 3681	.0544 0142	.0365 7240
4.05	.1778 9132	.1224 1028	.0836 1400	.0567 8048	.0383 7541
4.06	.1826 9022	.1263 6762	.0867 6946	.0592 3330	.0402 4441
4.07	.1875 5610	.1304 0188	.0900 0359	.0617 6080	.0421 8065
4.08	.1924 8806	.1345 1281	.0933 1677	.0643 6384	.0441 8534
4.09	.1974 8514	.1387 0009	.0967 0928	.0670 4324	.0462 5969
4.10	.2025 4635	.1429 6333	.1001 8138	.0697 9979	.0484 0486
4.11	.2076 7065	.1473 0211	.1037 3326	.0726 3421	.0506 2197
4.12	.2128 5696	.1517 1593	.1073 6504	.0755 4717	.0529 1212
4.13	.2181 0414	.1562 0423	.1110 7681	.0785 3931	.0552 7637
4.14	.2234 1102	.1607 6642	.1148 6856	.0816 1119	.0577 1571
4.15	.2287 7638	.1654 0183	.1187 4026	.0847 6333	.0602 3114
4.16	.2341 9898	.1701 0974	.1226 9179	.0879 9620	.0628 2356
4.17	.2396 7752	.1748 8939	.1267 2299	.0913 1020	.0654 9387
4.18	.2452 1067	.1797 3994	.1308 3363	.0947 0567	.0682 4289
4.19	.2507 9706	.1846 6052	.1350 2341	.0981 8290	.0710 7140
4.20	.2564 3528	.1896 5019	.1392 9199	.1017 4212	.0739 8014
4.21	.2621 2391	.1947 0797	.1436 3894	.1053 8348	.0769 6976
4.22	.2678 6147	.1998 3282	.1480 6380	.1091 0710	.0800 4091
4.23	.2736 4646	.2050 2366	.1525 6603	.1129 1302	.0831 9412
4.24	.2794 7736	.2102 7936	.1571 4503	.1168 0120	.0864 2992
4.25	.2853 5261	.2155 9872	.1618 0015	.1207 7156	.0897 4874
4.26	.2912 7063	.2209 8054	.1665 3067	.1248 2395	.0931 5096
4.27	.2972 2980	.2264 2352	.1713 3581	.1289 5815	.0966 3691
4.28	.3032 2851	.2319 2636	.1762 1475	.1331 7388	.1002 0685
4.29	.3092 6510	.2374 8769	.1811 6658	.1374 7079	.1038 6095
4.30	.3153 3789	.2431 0611	.1861 9037	.1418 4847	.1075 9937
4.31	.3214 4521	.2487 8019	.1912 8511	.1463 0644	.1114 2213
4.32	.3275 8533	.2545 0844	.1964 4974	.1508 4417	.1153 2926
4.33	.3337 5655	.2602 8935	.2016 8315	.1554 6105	.1193 2067
4.34	.3399 5713	.2661 2138	.2069 8418	.1601 5641	.1233 9623
4.35	.3461 8533	.2720 0293	.2123 5159	.1649 2951	.1275 5572
4.36	.3524 3938	.2779 3239	.2177 8414	.1697 7956	.1317 9888
4.37	.3587 1752	.2839 0812	.2232 8050	.1747 0571	.1361 2535
4.38	.3650 1798	.2899 2844	.2288 3932	.1797 0703	.1405 3472
4.39	.3713 3899	.2959 9166	.2344 5917	.1847 8255	.1450 2651
4.40	.3776 7877	.3020 9605	.2401 3862	.1899 3123	.1496 0018
4.41	.3840 3553	.3082 3987	.2458 7615	.1951 5198	.1542 5510
4.42	.3904 0749	.3144 2133	.2516 7024	.2004 4363	.1589 9059
4.43	.3967 9287	.3206 3867	.2575 1931	.2058 0499	.1638 0590
4.44	.4031 8990	.3268 9006	.2634 2175	.2112 3478	.1687 0022
4.45	.4095 9679	.3331 7369	.2693 7589	.2167 3169	.1736 7265
4.46	.4160 1177	.3394 8772	.2753 8007	.2222 9435	.1787 2227
4.47	.4224 3309	.3458 3031	.2814 3255	.2279 2135	.1838 4804
4.48	.4288 5898	.3521 9959	.2875 3160	.2336 1121	.1890 4891
4.49	.4352 8772	.3585 9370	.2936 7543	.2393 6242	.1943 2374

W	P(W,60)	P(W,70)	P(W,80)	P(W,90)	P(W,100)
4.50	.4417 1755	.3650 1077	.2998 6224	.2451 7342	.1996 7133
4.51	.4481 4676	.3714 4890	.3060 9021	.2510 4260	.2050 9043
4.52	.4545 7364	.3779 0623	.3123 5747	.2569 6833	.2105 7974
4.53	.4609 9649	.3843 8086	.3186 6217	.2629 4892	.2161 3788
4.54	.4674 1365	.3908 7091	.3250 0240	.2689 8264	.2217 6344
4.55	.4738 2345	.3973 7449	.3313 7626	.2750 6774	.2274 5494
4.56	.4802 2425	.4038 8973	.3377 8183	.2812 0241	.2332 1085
4.57	.4866 1443	.4104 1475	.3442 1716	.2873 8484	.2390 2962
4.58	.4929 9238	.4169 4768	.3506 8031	.2936 1318	.2449 0960
4.59	.4993 5653	.4234 8667	.3571 6932	.2998 8553	.2508 4915
4.60	.5057 0532	.4300 2985	.3636 8222	.3061 9998	.2568 4654
4.61	.5120 3721	.4365 7538	.3702 1704	.3125 5461	.2629 0003
4.62	.5183 5069	.4431 2145	.3767 7182	.3189 4746	.2690 0782
4.63	.5246 4429	.4496 6624	.3833 4456	.3253 7656	.2751 6808
4.64	.5309 1653	.4562 0794	.3899 3330	.3318 3990	.2813 7896
4.65	.5371 6600	.4627 4478	.3965 3605	.3383 3548	.2876 3855
4.66	.5433 9128	.4692 7499	.4031 5086	.3448 6129	.2939 4492
4.67	.5495 9099	.4757 9683	.4097 7575	.3514 1528	.3002 9611
4.68	.5557 6380	.4823 0857	.4164 0875	.3579 9542	.3066 9015
4.69	.5619 0838	.4888 0851	.4230 4794	.3645 9965	.3131 2501
4.70	.5680 2344	.4952 9497	.4296 9135	.3712 2591	.3195 9867
4.71	.5741 0773	.5017 6630	.4363 3707	.3778 7216	.3261 0907
4.72	.5801 6001	.5082 2086	.4429 8318	.3845 3633	.3326 5415
4.73	.5861 7910	.5146 5705	.4496 2779	.3912 1636	.3392 3181
4.74	.5921 6382	.5210 7329	.4562 6900	.3979 1020	.3458 3997
4.75	.5981 1305	.5274 6802	.4629 0496	.4046 1578	.3524 7649
4.76	.6040 2569	.5338 3974	.4695 3382	.4113 3108	.3591 3928
4.77	.6099 0067	.5401 8694	.4761 5377	.4180 5404	.3658 2619
4.78	.6157 3695	.5465 0816	.4827 6298	.4247 8265	.3725 3510
4.79	.6215 3353	.5528 0197	.4893 5970	.4315 1488	.3792 6387
4.80	.6272 8945	.5590 6697	.4959 4216	.4382 4874	.3860 1036
4.81	.6330 0378	.5653 0179	.5025 0863	.4449 8224	.3927 7245
4.82	.6386 7560	.5715 0510	.5090 5742	.4517 1341	.3995 4800
4.83	.6443 0405	.5776 7559	.5155 8686	.4584 4030	.4063 3489
4.84	.6498 8830	.5838 1199	.5220 9529	.4651 6097	.4131 3099
4.85	.6554 2755	.5899 1307	.5285 8111	.4718 7351	.4199 3421
4.86	.6609 2103	.5959 7764	.5350 4273	.4785 7605	.4267 4244
4.87	.6663 6800	.6020 0451	.5414 7859	.4852 6670	.4335 5361
4.88	.6717 6777	.6079 9258	.5478 8719	.4919 4365	.4403 6564
4.89	.6771 1966	.6139 4072	.5542 6703	.4986 0507	.4471 7648
4.90	.6824 2305	.6198 4790	.5606 1666	.5052 4918	.4539 8410
4.91	.6876 7732	.6257 1309	.5669 3467	.5118 7423	.4607 8649
4.92	.6928 8191	.6315 3529	.5732 1966	.5184 7849	.4675 8166
4.93	.6980 3629	.6373 1356	.5794 7030	.5250 6027	.4743 6763
4.94	.7031 3994	.6430 4697	.5856 8526	.5316 1792	.4811 4247
4.95	.7081 9239	.6487 3466	.5918 6329	.5381 4979	.4879 0426
4.96	.7131 9320	.6543 7578	.5980 0313	.5446 5431	.4946 5110
4.97	.7181 4196	.6599 6951	.6041 0359	.5511 2990	.5013 8114
4.98	.7230 3828	.6655 1508	.6101 6351	.5575 7505	.5080 9255
4.99	.7278 8182	.6710 1177	.6161 8175	.5639 8828	.5147 8352

W	P(W,60)	P(W,70)	P(W,80)	P(W,90)	P(W,100)
5.00	.7326 7226	.6764 5886	.6221 5724	.5703 6812	.5214 5229
5.01	.7374 0930	.6818 5570	.6280 8892	.5767 1316	.5280 9712
5.02	.7420 9268	.6872 0165	.6339 7578	.5830 2204	.5347 1632
5.03	.7467 2217	.6924 9611	.6398 1685	.5892 9341	.5413 0822
5.04	.7512 9755	.6977 3853	.6456 1119	.5955 2598	.5478 7119
5.05	.7558 1867	.7029 2838	.6513 5790	.6017 1849	.5544 0365
5.06	.7602 8535	.7080 6516	.6570 5614	.6078 6972	.5609 0403
5.07	.7646 9748	.7131 4841	.6627 0508	.6139 7848	.5673 7082
5.08	.7690 5496	.7181 7772	.6683 0393	.6200 4365	.5738 0255
5.09	.7733 5771	.7231 5268	.6738 5195	.6260 6412	.5801 9778
5.10	.7776 0570	.7280 7293	.6793 4844	.6320 3883	.5865 5511
5.11	.7817 9888	.7329 3815	.6847 9273	.6379 6677	.5928 7319
5.12	.7859 3728	.7377 4804	.6901 8418	.6438 4696	.5991 5070
5.13	.7900 2090	.7425 0232	.6955 2220	.6496 7845	.6053 8638
5.14	.7940 4980	.7472 0077	.7008 0623	.6554 6036	.6115 7898
5.15	.7980 2404	.7518 4318	.7060 3574	.6611 9182	.6177 2732
5.16	.8019 4373	.7564 2936	.7112 1026	.6668 7201	.6238 3025
5.17	.8058 0896	.7609 5918	.7163 2932	.6725 0017	.6298 8666
5.18	.8096 1987	.7654 3251	.7213 9251	.6780 7555	.6358 9550
5.19	.8133 7661	.7698 4926	.7263 9945	.6835 9745	.6418 5574
5.20	.8170 7936	.7742 0937	.7313 4979	.6890 6522	.6477 6641
5.21	.8207 2831	.7785 1278	.7362 4321	.6944 7823	.6536 2656
5.22	.8243 2367	.7827 5951	.7410 7943	.6998 3591	.6594 3530
5.23	.8278 6566	.7869 4955	.7458 5821	.7051 3770	.6651 9178
5.24	.8313 5452	.7910 8294	.7505 7932	.7103 8310	.6708 9519
5.25	.8347 9052	.7951 5975	.7552 4257	.7155 7165	.6765 4476
5.26	.8381 7394	.7991 8006	.7598 4781	.7207 0291	.6821 3976
5.27	.8415 0506	.8031 4398	.7643 9492	.7257 7648	.6876 7951
5.28	.8447 8420	.8070 5164	.7688 8379	.7307 9201	.6931 6336
5.29	.8480 1166	.8109 0319	.7733 1436	.7357 4917	.6985 9070
5.30	.8511 8780	.8146 9881	.7776 8659	.7406 4766	.7039 6097
5.31	.8543 1295	.8184 3868	.7820 0046	.7454 8723	.7092 7364
5.32	.8573 8748	.8221 2303	.7862 5600	.7502 6766	.7145 2822
5.33	.8604 1175	.8257 5208	.7904 5323	.7549 8876	.7197 2427
5.34	.8633 8616	.8293 2608	.7945 9223	.7596 5036	.7248 6137
5.35	.8663 1110	.8328 4531	.7986 7309	.7642 5234	.7299 3915
5.36	.8691 8697	.8363 1005	.8026 9592	.7687 9461	.7349 5728
5.37	.8720 1418	.8397 2060	.8066 6086	.7732 7710	.7399 1544
5.38	.8747 9317	.8430 7728	.8105 6807	.7776 9977	.7448 1338
5.39	.8775 2437	.8463 8043	.8144 1775	.7820 6261	.7496 5086
5.40	.8802 0822	.8496 3039	.8182 1008	.7863 6565	.7544 2769
5.41	.8828 4517	.8528 2752	.8219 4530	.7906 0893	.7591 4371
5.42	.8854 3567	.8559 7221	.8256 2365	.7947 9253	.7637 9878
5.43	.8879 8020	.8590 6484	.8292 4541	.7989 1654	.7683 9281
5.44	.8904 7922	.8621 0582	.8328 1085	.8029 8110	.7729 2573
5.45	.8929 3321	.8650 9555	.8363 2027	.8069 8635	.7773 9751
5.46	.8953 4266	.8680 3447	.8397 7400	.8109 3247	.7818 0814
5.47	.8977 0805	.8709 2300	.8431 7237	.8148 1965	.7861 5765
5.48	.9000 2988	.8737 6160	.8465 1574	.8186 4811	.7904 4608
5.49	.9023 0864	.8765 5072	.8498 0447	.8224 1810	.7946 7352

W	P(W,60)	P(W,70)	P(W,80)	P(W,90)	P(W,100)
5.50	.9045 4484	.8792 9082	.8530 3895	.8261 2988	.7988 4008
5.51	.9067 3898	.8819 8238	.8562 1957	.8297 8373	.8029 4588
5.52	.9088 9156	.8846 2588	.8593 4674	.8333 7995	.8069 9109
5.53	.9110 0311	.8872 2181	.8624 2089	.8369 1885	.8109 7590
5.54	.9130 7414	.8897 7066	.8654 4246	.8404 0079	.8149 0050
5.55	.9151 0515	.8922 7293	.8684 1188	.8438 2611	.8187 6514
5.56	.9170 9668	.8947 2913	.8713 2962	.8471 9519	.8225 7006
5.57	.9190 4923	.8971 3978	.8741 9616	.8505 0842	.8263 1554
5.58	.9209 6333	.8995 0540	.8770 1196	.8537 6619	.8300 0187
5.59	.9228 3950	.9018 2650	.8797 7751	.8569 6893	.8336 2937
5.60	.9246 7826	.9041 0362	.8824 9331	.8601 1707	.8371 9838
5.61	.9264 8013	.9063 3728	.8851 5988	.8632 1106	.8407 0926
5.62	.9282 4564	.9085 2803	.8877 7771	.8662 5134	.8441 6236
5.63	.9299 7531	.9106 7639	.8903 4734	.8692 3840	.8475 5809
5.64	.9316 6965	.9127 8292	.8928 6928	.8721 7271	.8508 9684
5.65	.9333 2918	.9148 4815	.8953 4407	.8750 5477	.8541 7904
5.66	.9349 5444	.9168 7262	.8977 7225	.8778 8507	.8574 0513
5.67	.9365 4592	.9188 5688	.9001 5436	.8806 6413	.8605 7555
5.68	.9381 0415	.9208 0148	.9024 9095	.8833 9247	.8636 9078
5.69	.9396 2964	.9227 0697	.9047 8257	.8860 7061	.8667 5127
5.70	.9411 2291	.9245 7390	.9070 2978	.8886 9909	.8697 5754
5.71	.9425 8446	.9264 0280	.9092 3314	.8912 7846	.8727 1007
5.72	.9440 1479	.9281 9423	.9113 9321	.8938 0927	.8756 0938
5.73	.9454 1442	.9299 4875	.9135 1055	.8962 9206	.8784 5598
5.74	.9467 8384	.9316 6688	.9155 8573	.8987 2741	.8812 5042
5.75	.9481 2355	.9333 4918	.9176 1933	.9011 1588	.8839 9324
5.76	.9494 3405	.9349 9620	.9196 1190	.9034 5804	.8866 8497
5.77	.9507 1582	.9366 0847	.9215 6402	.9057 5446	.8893 2618
5.78	.9519 6936	.9381 8654	.9234 7626	.9080 0573	.8919 1743
5.79	.9531 9515	.9397 3094	.9253 4920	.9102 1243	.8944 5929
5.80	.9543 9367	.9412 4222	.9271 8340	.9123 7513	.8969 5234
5.81	.9555 6540	.9427 2089	.9289 7943	.9144 9444	.8993 9716
5.82	.9567 1080	.9441 6750	.9307 3786	.9165 7093	.9017 9434
5.83	.9578 3035	.9455 8258	.9324 5927	.9186 0519	.9041 4447
5.84	.9589 2451	.9469 6664	.9341 4422	.9205 9783	.9064 4814
5.85	.9599 9374	.9483 2021	.9357 9327	.9225 4942	.9087 0596
5.86	.9610 3850	.9496 4380	.9374 0699	.9244 6057	.9109 1852
5.87	.9620 5923	.9509 3793	.9389 8595	.9263 3186	.9130 8644
5.88	.9630 5638	.9522 0311	.9405 3069	.9281 6388	.9152 1031
5.89	.9640 3039	.9534 3985	.9420 4178	.9299 5724	.9172 9075
5.90	.9649 8169	.9546 4865	.9435 1977	.9317 1250	.9193 2836
5.91	.9659 1073	.9558 3000	.9449 6521	.9334 3028	.9213 2376
5.92	.9668 1792	.9569 8439	.9463 7864	.9351 1114	.9232 7756
5.93	.9677 0368	.9581 1233	.9477 6062	.9367 5568	.9251 9037
5.94	.9685 6844	.9592 1428	.9491 1168	.9383 6448	.9270 6280
5.95	.9694 1260	.9602 9074	.9504 3235	.9399 3811	.9288 9545
5.96	.9702 3656	.9613 4217	.9517 2318	.9414 7716	.9306 8895
5.97	.9710 4074	.9623 6904	.9529 8468	.9429 8220	.9324 4389
5.98	.9718 2551	.9633 7181	.9542 1737	.9444 5380	.9341 6088
5.99	.9725 9129	.9643 5096	.9554 2179	.9458 9253	.9358 4053

W	P(W,60)	P(W,70)	P(W,80)	P(W,90)	P(W,100)
6.00	.9733 3844	.9653 0692	.9565 9844	.9472 9894	.9374 8344
6.01	.9740 6734	.9662 4015	.9577 4783	.9486 7361	.9390 9020
6.02	.9747 7838	.9671 5109	.9588 7046	.9500 1708	.9406 6142
6.03	.9754 7193	.9680 4019	.9599 6684	.9513 2991	.9421 9769
6.04	.9761 4833	.9689 0786	.9610 3745	.9526 1265	.9436 9959
6.05	.9768 0796	.9697 5455	.9620 8279	.9538 6582	.9451 6772
6.06	.9774 5117	.9705 8066	.9631 0334	.9550 8999	.9466 0265
6.07	.9780 7829	.9713 8662	.9640 9958	.9562 8566	.9480 0497
6.08	.9786 8969	.9721 7283	.9650 7198	.9574 5339	.9493 7524
6.09	.9792 8569	.9729 3971	.9660 2101	.9585 9367	.9507 1404
6.10	.9798 6662	.9736 8765	.9669 4713	.9597 0704	.9520 2194
6.11	.9804 3281	.9744 1703	.9678 5078	.9607 9401	.9532 9949
6.12	.9809 8459	.9751 2826	.9687 3244	.9618 5507	.9545 4726
6.13	.9815 2226	.9758 2172	.9695 9253	.9628 9074	.9557 6578
6.14	.9820 4614	.9764 9777	.9704 3149	.9639 0150	.9569 5561
6.15	.9825 5654	.9771 5679	.9712 4977	.9648 8785	.9581 1728
6.16	.9830 5375	.9777 9915	.9720 4778	.9658 5026	.9592 5134
6.17	.9835 3807	.9784 2520	.9728 2594	.9667 8922	.9603 5830
6.18	.9840 0979	.9790 3529	.9735 8467	.9677 0520	.9614 3869
6.19	.9844 6920	.9796 2979	.9743 2438	.9685 9866	.9624 9304
6.20	.9849 1658	.9802 0902	.9750 4547	.9694 7005	.9635 2184
6.21	.9853 5219	.9807 7333	.9757 4834	.9703 1985	.9645 2561
6.22	.9857 7632	.9813 2304	.9764 3338	.9711 4848	.9655 0485
6.23	.9861 8922	.9818 5848	.9771 0096	.9719 5639	.9664 6004
6.24	.9865 9116	.9823 7998	.9777 5148	.9727 4402	.9673 9168
6.25	.9869 8239	.9828 8785	.9783 8530	.9735 1179	.9683 0025
6.26	.9873 6317	.9833 8239	.9790 0280	.9742 6013	.9691 8621
6.27	.9877 3374	.9838 6391	.9796 0432	.9749 8946	.9700 5004
6.28	.9880 9433	.9843 3271	.9801 9023	.9757 0017	.9708 9220
6.29	.9884 4520	.9847 8909	.9807 6087	.9763 9267	.9717 1314
6.30	.9887 8657	.9852 3332	.9813 1659	.9770 6737	.9725 1332
6.31	.9891 1867	.9856 6570	.9818 5772	.9777 2465	.9732 9317
6.32	.9894 4172	.9860 8650	.9823 8461	.9783 6490	.9740 5312
6.33	.9897 5594	.9864 9599	.9828 9756	.9789 8849	.9747 9362
6.34	.9900 6154	.9868 9444	.9833 9691	.9795 9580	.9755 1508
6.35	.9903 5874	.9872 8211	.9838 8296	.9801 8719	.9762 1792
6.36	.9906 4775	.9876 5926	.9843 5603	.9807 6302	.9769 0254
6.37	.9909 2876	.9880 2614	.9848 1642	.9813 2365	.9775 6935
6.38	.9912 0197	.9883 8300	.9852 6443	.9818 6942	.9782 1875
6.39	.9914 6757	.9887 3009	.9857 0034	.9824 0067	.9788 5112
6.40	.9917 2576	.9890 6763	.9861 2445	.9829 1775	.9794 6685
6.41	.9919 7673	.9893 9587	.9865 3703	.9834 2097	.9800 6632
6.42	.9922 2064	.9897 1502	.9869 3836	.9839 1067	.9806 4989
6.43	.9924 5769	.9900 2532	.9873 2872	.9843 8716	.9812 1794
6.44	.9926 8804	.9903 2698	.9877 0837	.9848 5075	.9817 7082
6.45	.9929 1186	.9906 2022	.9880 7756	.9853 0175	.9823 0887
6.46	.9931 2933	.9909 0525	.9884 3655	.9857 4046	.9828 3245
6.47	.9933 4060	.9911 8227	.9887 8560	.9861 6717	.9833 4190
6.48	.9935 4584	.9914 5149	.9891 2495	.9865 8217	.9838 3755
6.49	.9937 4520	.9917 1310	.9894 5483	.9869 8575	.9843 1972

W	P(W,60)	P(W,70)	P(W,80)	P(W,90)	P(W,100)
6.50	.9939 3883	.9919 6730	.9897 7548	.9873 7818	.9847 8873
6.51	.9941 2688	.9922 1427	.9900 8714	.9877 5974	.9852 4491
6.52	.9943 0950	.9924 5420	.9903 9002	.9881 3068	.9856 8855
6.53	.9944 8683	.9926 8727	.9906 8436	.9884 9129	.9861 1997
6.54	.9946 5901	.9929 1366	.9909 7036	.9888 4180	.9865 3946
6.55	.9948 2618	.9931 3354	.9912 4823	.9891 8247	.9869 4731
6.56	.9949 8846	.9933 4708	.9915 1819	.9895 1356	.9873 4380
6.57	.9951 4600	.9935 5444	.9917 8044	.9898 3529	.9877 2922
6.58	.9952 9891	.9937 5580	.9920 3517	.9901 4790	.9881 0384
6.59	.9954 4732	.9939 5129	.9922 8257	.9904 5163	.9884 6792
6.60	.9955 9134	.9941 4109	.9925 2285	.9907 4670	.9888 2174
6.61	.9957 3111	.9943 2533	.9927 5618	.9910 3333	.9891 6555
6.62	.9958 6673	.9945 0418	.9929 8275	.9913 1174	.9894 9960
6.63	.9959 9832	.9946 7777	.9932 0272	.9915 8215	.9898 2414
6.64	.9961 2599	.9948 4623	.9934 1629	.9918 4475	.9901 3942
6.65	.9962 4984	.9950 0972	.9936 2361	.9920 9975	.9904 4566
6.66	.9963 6997	.9951 6837	.9938 2485	.9923 4735	.9907 4310
6.67	.9964 8650	.9953 2230	.9940 2017	.9925 8774	.9910 3196
6.68	.9965 9952	.9954 7165	.9942 0973	.9928 2112	.9913 1248
6.69	.9967 0913	.9956 1653	.9943 9369	.9930 4767	.9915 8486
6.70	.9968 1542	.9957 5707	.9945 7220	.9932 6756	.9918 4932
6.71	.9969 1848	.9958 9340	.9947 4539	.9934 8098	.9921 0607
6.72	.9970 1841	.9960 2562	.9949 1343	.9936 8810	.9923 5531
6.73	.9971 1530	.9961 5385	.9950 7644	.9938 8908	.9925 9723
6.74	.9972 0922	.9962 7820	.9952 3457	.9940 8410	.9928 3203
6.75	.9973 0026	.9963 9878	.9953 8795	.9942 7331	.9930 5991
6.76	.9973 8851	.9965 1570	.9955 3671	.9944 5688	.9932 8104
6.77	.9974 7405	.9966 2904	.9956 8098	.9946 3495	.9934 9561
6.78	.9975 5694	.9967 3893	.9958 2087	.9948 0767	.9937 0380
6.79	.9976 3727	.9968 4545	.9959 5652	.9949 7520	.9939 0577
6.80	.9977 1511	.9969 4870	.9960 8804	.9951 3767	.9941 0170
6.81	.9977 9053	.9970 4877	.9962 1555	.9952 9522	.9942 9174
6.82	.9978 6360	.9971 4575	.9963 3916	.9954 4800	.9944 7607
6.83	.9979 3440	.9972 3973	.9964 5897	.9955 9613	.9946 5484
6.84	.9980 0297	.9973 3079	.9965 7511	.9957 3974	.9948 2820
6.85	.9980 6940	.9974 1903	.9966 8766	.9958 7896	.9949 9630
6.86	.9981 3374	.9975 0452	.9967 9673	.9960 1391	.9951 5928
6.87	.9981 9605	.9975 8734	.9969 0243	.9961 4472	.9953 1730
6.88	.9982 5640	.9976 6756	.9970 0485	.9962 7150	.9954 7048
6.89	.9983 1483	.9977 4527	.9971 0407	.9963 9436	.9956 1897
6.90	.9983 7142	.9978 2054	.9972 0021	.9965 1341	.9957 6290
6.91	.9984 2620	.9978 9343	.9972 9333	.9966 2878	.9959 0238
6.92	.9984 7924	.9979 6402	.9973 8354	.9967 4055	.9960 3756
6.93	.9985 3059	.9980 3237	.9974 7091	.9968 4883	.9961 6855
6.94	.9985 8030	.9980 9856	.9975 5553	.9969 5373	.9962 9548
6.95	.9986 2841	.9981 6264	.9976 3748	.9970 5534	.9964 1845
6.96	.9986 7497	.9982 2467	.9977 1683	.9971 5376	.9965 3759
6.97	.9987 2004	.9982 8473	.9977 9367	.9972 4908	.9966 5299
6.98	.9987 6365	.9983 4286	.9978 6806	.9973 4139	.9967 6478
6.99	.9988 0585	.9983 9913	.9979 4009	.9974 3077	.9968 7305

W	P(W,60)	P(W,70)	P(W,80)	P(W,90)	P(W,100)
7.00	.9988 4669	.9984 5359	.9980 0981	.9975 1732	.9969 7791
7.01	.9988 8620	.9985 0629	.9980 7731	.9976 0112	.9970 7946
7.02	.9989 2442	.9985 5729	.9981 4263	.9976 8225	.9971 7779
7.03	.9989 6140	.9986 0664	.9982 0586	.9977 6079	.9972 7300
7.04	.9989 9717	.9986 5438	.9982 6705	.9978 3681	.9973 6518
7.05	.9990 3177	.9987 0058	.9983 2626	.9979 1039	.9974 5442
7.06	.9990 6523	.9987 4527	.9983 8356	.9979 8161	.9975 4081
7.07	.9990 9760	.9987 8850	.9984 3899	.9980 5052	.9976 2442
7.08	.9991 2889	.9988 3032	.9984 9263	.9981 1722	.9977 0535
7.09	.9991 5916	.9988 7076	.9985 4452	.9981 8175	.9977 8368
7.10	.9991 8842	.9989 0988	.9985 9471	.9982 4419	.9978 5948
7.11	.9992 1672	.9989 4771	.9986 4326	.9983 0459	.9979 3282
7.12	.9992 4407	.9989 8429	.9986 9022	.9983 6303	.9980 0379
7.13	.9992 7052	.9990 1966	.9987 3563	.9984 1956	.9980 7245
7.14	.9992 9608	.9990 5386	.9987 7955	.9984 7423	.9981 3888
7.15	.9993 2079	.9990 8692	.9988 2202	.9985 2712	.9982 0313
7.16	.9993 4467	.9991 1889	.9988 6309	.9985 7826	.9982 6529
7.17	.9993 6775	.9991 4978	.9989 0279	.9986 2772	.9983 2541
7.18	.9993 9006	.9991 7965	.9989 4118	.9986 7554	.9983 8355
7.19	.9994 1161	.9992 0852	.9989 7829	.9987 2178	.9984 3978
7.20	.9994 3244	.9992 3642	.9990 1416	.9987 6649	.9984 9415
7.21	.9994 5256	.9992 6338	.9990 4883	.9988 0971	.9985 4672
7.22	.9994 7201	.9992 8943	.9990 8235	.9988 5149	.9985 9755
7.23	.9994 9079	.9993 1461	.9991 1473	.9988 9187	.9986 4669
7.24	.9995 0893	.9993 3893	.9991 4603	.9989 3091	.9986 9420
7.25	.9995 2646	.9993 6243	.9991 7628	.9989 6864	.9987 4012
7.26	.9995 4339	.9993 8514	.9992 0550	.9990 0510	.9987 8451
7.27	.9995 5974	.9994 0707	.9992 3373	.9990 4033	.9988 2741
7.28	.9995 7553	.9994 2825	.9992 6101	.9990 7437	.9988 6886
7.29	.9995 9078	.9994 4871	.9992 8736	.9991 0727	.9989 0893
7.30	.9996 0550	.9994 6848	.9993 1282	.9991 3905	.9989 4764
7.31	.9996 1972	.9994 8756	.9993 3740	.9991 6975	.9989 8505
7.32	.9996 3345	.9995 0599	.9993 6115	.9991 9941	.9990 2119
7.33	.9996 4670	.9995 2379	.9993 8409	.9992 2805	.9990 5610
7.34	.9996 5949	.9995 4097	.9994 0624	.9992 5572	.9990 8983
7.35	.9996 7185	.9995 5756	.9994 2762	.9992 8244	.9991 2241
7.36	.9996 8377	.9995 7358	.9994 4828	.9993 0825	.9991 5388
7.37	.9996 9527	.9995 8904	.9994 6821	.9993 3317	.9991 8427
7.38	.9997 0638	.9996 0396	.9994 8746	.9993 5724	.9992 1362
7.39	.9997 1709	.9996 1837	.9995 0605	.9993 8047	.9992 4196
7.40	.9997 2744	.9996 3228	.9995 2399	.9994 0290	.9992 6933
7.41	.9997 3742	.9996 4569	.9995 4130	.9994 2456	.9992 9575
7.42	.9997 4705	.9996 5864	.9995 5802	.9994 4546	.9993 2126
7.43	.9997 5634	.9996 7114	.9995 7415	.9994 6564	.9993 4589
7.44	.9997 6530	.9996 8320	.9995 8971	.9994 8512	.9993 6966
7.45	.9997 7394	.9996 9483	.9996 0474	.9995 0391	.9993 9261
7.46	.9997 8229	.9997 0606	.9996 1923	.9995 2206	.9994 1476
7.47	.9997 9033	.9997 1689	.9996 3322	.9995 3956	.9994 3614
7.48	.9997 9809	.9997 2733	.9996 4671	.9995 5645	.9994 5677
7.49	.9998 0557	.9997 3741	.9996 5973	.9995 7275	.9994 7668

W	P(W,60)	P(W,70)	P(W,80)	P(W,90)	P(W,100)
7.50	.9998 1279	.9997 4713	.9996 7229	.9995 8848	.9994 9589
7.51	.9998 1975	.9997 5650	.9996 8440	.9996 0365	.9995 1443
7.52	.9998 2646	.9997 6554	.9996 9608	.9996 1828	.9995 3231
7.53	.9998 3293	.9997 7426	.9997 0735	.9996 3240	.9995 4956
7.54	.9998 3917	.9997 8266	.9997 1822	.9996 4601	.9995 6621
7.55	.9998 4519	.9997 9077	.9997 2870	.9996 5915	.9995 8226
7.56	.9998 5099	.9997 9858	.9997 3881	.9996 7181	.9995 9774
7.57	.9998 5658	.9998 0612	.9997 4855	.9996 8403	.9996 1268
7.58	.9998 6196	.9998 1338	.9997 5795	.9996 9581	.9996 2708
7.59	.9998 6716	.9998 2038	.9997 6701	.9997 0716	.9996 4097
7.60	.9998 7216	.9998 2713	.9997 7574	.9997 1811	.9996 5437
7.61	.9998 7699	.9998 3364	.9997 8416	.9997 2867	.9996 6728
7.62	.9998 8164	.9998 3991	.9997 9227	.9997 3884	.9996 7973
7.63	.9998 8611	.9998 4595	.9998 0010	.9997 4866	.9996 9173
7.64	.9998 9043	.9998 5178	.9998 0763	.9997 5811	.9997 0331
7.65	.9998 9459	.9998 5739	.9998 1490	.9997 6723	.9997 1446
7.66	.9998 9860	.9998 6279	.9998 2190	.9997 7601	.9997 2521
7.67	.9999 0246	.9998 6800	.9998 2865	.9997 8448	.9997 3558
7.68	.9999 0617	.9998 7302	.9998 3515	.9997 9263	.9997 4556
7.69	.9999 0975	.9998 7786	.9998 4141	.9998 0050	.9997 5519
7.70	.9999 1320	.9998 8252	.9998 4744	.9998 0807	.9997 6447
7.71	.9999 1653	.9998 8700	.9998 5326	.9998 1537	.9997 7340
7.72	.9999 1973	.9998 9132	.9998 5886	.9998 2240	.9997 8201
7.73	.9999 2281	.9998 9549	.9998 6425	.9998 2917	.9997 9031
7.74	.9999 2578	.9998 9950	.9998 6945	.9998 3570	.9997 9831
7.75	.9999 2863	.9999 0336	.9998 7445	.9998 4198	.9998 0600
7.76	.9999 3138	.9999 0707	.9998 7927	.9998 4803	.9998 1342
7.77	.9999 3403	.9999 1065	.9998 8391	.9998 5387	.9998 2057
7.78	.9999 3658	.9999 1410	.9998 8838	.9998 5948	.9998 2745
7.79	.9999 3904	.9999 1742	.9998 9268	.9998 6489	.9998 3407
7.80	.9999 4140	.9999 2061	.9998 9683	.9998 7009	.9998 4046
7.81	.9999 4368	.9999 2369	.9999 0082	.9998 7511	.9998 4660
7.82	.9999 4587	.9999 2665	.9999 0466	.9998 7993	.9998 5252
7.83	.9999 4797	.9999 2950	.9999 0835	.9998 8458	.9998 5822
7.84	.9999 5000	.9999 3224	.9999 1191	.9998 8905	.9998 6370
7.85	.9999 5195	.9999 3488	.9999 1534	.9998 9336	.9998 6898
7.86	.9999 5383	.9999 3742	.9999 1863	.9998 9750	.9998 7407
7.87	.9999 5564	.9999 3987	.9999 2181	.9999 0149	.9998 7896
7.88	.9999 5738	.9999 4222	.9999 2486	.9999 0533	.9998 8367
7.89	.9999 5905	.9999 4448	.9999 2780	.9999 0903	.9998 8820
7.90	.9999 6066	.9999 4666	.9999 3062	.9999 1258	.9998 9257
7.91	.9999 6221	.9999 4875	.9999 3334	.9999 1601	.9998 9676
7.92	.9999 6370	.9999 5077	.9999 3596	.9999 1930	.9999 0080
7.93	.9999 6513	.9999 5271	.9999 3848	.9999 2247	.9999 0469
7.94	.9999 6651	.9999 5457	.9999 4090	.9999 2551	.9999 0843
7.95	.9999 6783	.9999 5637	.9999 4323	.9999 2845	.9999 1203
7.96	.9999 6911	.9999 5809	.9999 4547	.9999 3127	.9999 1549
7.97	.9999 7033	.9999 5975	.9999 4763	.9999 3398	.9999 1883
7.98	.9999 7151	.9999 6135	.9999 4970	.9999 3659	.9999 2203
7.99	.9999 7264	.9999 6288	.9999 5170	.9999 3910	.9999 2511

W	P(W,60)	P(W,70)	P(W,80)	P(W,90)	P(W,100)
8.00	.9999 7373	.9999 6436	.9999 5361	.9999 4151	.9999 2807
8.01	.9999 7478	.9999 6578	.9999 5546	.9999 4384	.9999 3093
8.02	.9999 7579	.9999 6714	.9999 5723	.9999 4607	.9999 3367
8.03	.9999 7676	.9999 6846	.9999 5894	.9999 4821	.9999 3630
8.04	.9999 7769	.9999 6972	.9999 6058	.9999 5028	.9999 3884
8.05	.9999 7858	.9999 7093	.9999 6215	.9999 5226	.9999 4128
8.06	.9999 7944	.9999 7209	.9999 6367	.9999 5417	.9999 4362
8.07	.9999 8027	.9999 7321	.9999 6512	.9999 5600	.9999 4587
8.08	.9999 8106	.9999 7429	.9999 6652	.9999 5777	.9999 4804
8.09	.9999 8182	.9999 7532	.9999 6787	.9999 5946	.9999 5012
8.10	.9999 8256	.9999 7632	.9999 6916	.9999 6109	.9999 5212
8.11	.9999 8326	.9999 7727	.9999 7040	.9999 6266	.9999 5405
8.12	.9999 8394	.9999 7819	.9999 7160	.9999 6416	.9999 5590
8.13	.9999 8459	.9999 7907	.9999 7274	.9999 6561	.9999 5767
8.14	.9999 8522	.9999 7992	.9999 7384	.9999 6700	.9999 5938
8.15	.9999 8582	.9999 8074	.9999 7490	.9999 6833	.9999 6102
8.16	.9999 8639	.9999 8152	.9999 7592	.9999 6961	.9999 6260
8.17	.9999 8695	.9999 8227	.9999 7690	.9999 7084	.9999 6411
8.18	.9999 8748	.9999 8299	.9999 7784	.9999 7203	.9999 6557
8.19	.9999 8799	.9999 8368	.9999 7874	.9999 7317	.9999 6697
8.20	.9999 8848	.9999 8435	.9999 7961	.9999 7426	.9999 6831
8.21	.9999 8895	.9999 8499	.9999 8044	.9999 7531	.9999 6960
8.22	.9999 8940	.9999 8560	.9999 8124	.9999 7632	.9999 7084
8.23	.9999 8984	.9999 8619	.9999 8201	.9999 7728	.9999 7203
8.24	.9999 9026	.9999 8676	.9999 8274	.9999 7821	.9999 7317
8.25	.9999 9066	.9999 8730	.9999 8345	.9999 7911	.9999 7427
8.26	.9999 9104	.9999 8783	.9999 8413	.9999 7996	.9999 7533
8.27	.9999 9141	.9999 8833	.9999 8478	.9999 8079	.9999 7634
8.28	.9999 9176	.9999 8881	.9999 8541	.9999 8158	.9999 7731
8.29	.9999 9210	.9999 8927	.9999 8601	.9999 8234	.9999 7824
8.30	.9999 9243	.9999 8971	.9999 8659	.9999 8306	.9999 7914
8.31	.9999 9274	.9999 9014	.9999 8714	.9999 8376	.9999 8000
8.32	.9999 9305	.9999 9055	.9999 8768	.9999 8443	.9999 8083
8.33	.9999 9333	.9999 9094	.9999 8819	.9999 8508	.9999 8162
8.34	.9999 9361	.9999 9132	.9999 8868	.9999 8570	.9999 8238
8.35	.9999 9388	.9999 9168	.9999 8915	.9999 8629	.9999 8311
8.36	.9999 9413	.9999 9202	.9999 8960	.9999 8686	.9999 8381
8.37	.9999 9438	.9999 9236	.9999 9003	.9999 8741	.9999 8448
8.38	.9999 9461	.9999 9267	.9999 9045	.9999 8793	.9999 8513
8.39	.9999 9484	.9999 9298	.9999 9085	.9999 8843	.9999 8575
8.40	.9999 9505	.9999 9327	.9999 9123	.9999 8892	.9999 8634
8.41	.9999 9526	.9999 9356	.9999 9159	.9999 8938	.9999 8692
8.42	.9999 9546	.9999 9383	.9999 9195	.9999 8983	.9999 8746
8.43	.9999 9565	.9999 9408	.9999 9228	.9999 9025	.9999 8799
8.44	.9999 9583	.9999 9433	.9999 9261	.9999 9066	.9999 8849
8.45	.9999 9601	.9999 9457	.9999 9292	.9999 9105	.9999 8897
8.46	.9999 9618	.9999 9480	.9999 9322	.9999 9143	.9999 8944
8.47	.9999 9634	.9999 9502	.9999 9350	.9999 9179	.9999 8988
8.48	.9999 9649	.9999 9523	.9999 9378	.9999 9214	.9999 9031
8.49	.9999 9664	.9999 9543	.9999 9404	.9999 9247	.9999 9072

W	P(W,60)	P(W,70)	P(W,80)	P(W,90)	P(W,100)
8.50	.9999 9678	.9999 9563	.9999 9429	.9999 9279	.9999 9111
8.51	.9999 9692	.9999 9581	.9999 9453	.9999 9309	.9999 9148
8.52	.9999 9705	.9999 9599	.9999 9477	.9999 9338	.9999 9184
8.53	.9999 9718	.9999 9616	.9999 9499	.9999 9366	.9999 9219
8.54	.9999 9730	.9999 9632	.9999 9520	.9999 9393	.9999 9252
8.55	.9999 9741	.9999 9648	.9999 9540	.9999 9419	.9999 9284
8.56	.9999 9752	.9999 9663	.9999 9560	.9999 9444	.9999 9314
8.57	.9999 9763	.9999 9677	.9999 9579	.9999 9468	.9999 9344
8.58	.9999 9773	.9999 9691	.9999 9597	.9999 9490	.9999 9372
8.59	.9999 9783	.9999 9704	.9999 9614	.9999 9512	.9999 9398
8.60	.9999 9792	.9999 9717	.9999 9630	.9999 9533	.9999 9424
8.61	.9999 9801	.9999 9729	.9999 9646	.9999 9553	.9999 9449
8.62	.9999 9809	.9999 9741	.9999 9661	.9999 9572	.9999 9472
8.63	.9999 9818	.9999 9752	.9999 9676	.9999 9590	.9999 9495
8.64	.9999 9825	.9999 9762	.9999 9690	.9999 9608	.9999 9517
8.65	.9999 9833	.9999 9773	.9999 9703	.9999 9625	.9999 9537
8.66	.9999 9840	.9999 9783	.9999 9716	.9999 9641	.9999 9557
8.67	.9999 9847	.9999 9792	.9999 9728	.9999 9656	.9999 9576
8.68	.9999 9854	.9999 9801	.9999 9740	.9999 9671	.9999 9595
8.69	.9999 9860	.9999 9809	.9999 9751	.9999 9686	.9999 9612
8.70	.9999 9866	.9999 9818	.9999 9762	.9999 9699	.9999 9629
8.71	.9999 9872	.9999 9826	.9999 9772	.9999 9712	.9999 9645
8.72	.9999 9877	.9999 9833	.9999 9782	.9999 9725	.9999 9660
8.73	.9999 9883	.9999 9840	.9999 9792	.9999 9737	.9999 9675
8.74	.9999 9888	.9999 9847	.9999 9801	.9999 9748	.9999 9689
8.75	.9999 9893	.9999 9854	.9999 9809	.9999 9759	.9999 9703
8.76	.9999 9897	.9999 9860	.9999 9818	.9999 9769	.9999 9716
8.77	.9999 9902	.9999 9866	.9999 9826	.9999 9779	.9999 9728
8.78	.9999 9906	.9999 9872	.9999 9833	.9999 9789	.9999 9740
8.79	.9999 9910	.9999 9878	.9999 9840	.9999 9798	.9999 9751
8.80	.9999 9914	.9999 9883	.9999 9847	.9999 9807	.9999 9762
8.81	.9999 9918	.9999 9888	.9999 9854	.9999 9816	.9999 9773
8.82	.9999 9922	.9999 9893	.9999 9861	.9999 9824	.9999 9782
8.83	.9999 9925	.9999 9898	.9999 9867	.9999 9831	.9999 9792
8.84	.9999 9928	.9999 9902	.9999 9873	.9999 9839	.9999 9801
8.85	.9999 9931	.9999 9907	.9999 9878	.9999 9846	.9999 9810
8.86	.9999 9934	.9999 9911	.9999 9883	.9999 9853	.9999 9818
8.87	.9999 9937	.9999 9915	.9999 9889	.9999 9859	.9999 9826
8.88	.9999 9940	.9999 9918	.9999 9894	.9999 9865	.9999 9834
8.89	.9999 9943	.9999 9922	.9999 9898	.9999 9871	.9999 9841
8.90	.9999 9945	.9999 9925	.9999 9903	.9999 9877	.9999 9848
8.91	.9999 9948	.9999 9929	.9999 9907	.9999 9882	.9999 9855
8.92	.9999 9950	.9999 9932	.9999 9911	.9999 9888	.9999 9861
8.93	.9999 9952	.9999 9935	.9999 9915	.9999 9893	.9999 9867
8.94	.9999 9954	.9999 9938	.9999 9919	.9999 9897	.9999 9873
8.95	.9999 9956	.9999 9941	.9999 9922	.9999 9902	.9999 9879
8.96	.9999 9958	.9999 9943	.9999 9926	.9999 9906	.9999 9884
8.97	.9999 9960	.9999 9946	.9999 9929	.9999 9910	.9999 9889
8.98	.9999 9962	.9999 9948	.9999 9932	.9999 9914	.9999 9894
8.99	.9999 9964	.9999 9951	.9999 9935	.9999 9918	.9999 9899

W	P(W,60)	P(W,70)	P(W,80)	P(W,90)	P(W,100)
9.00	.9999 9965	.9999 9953	.9999 9938	.9999 9922	.9999 9904
9.01	.9999 9967	.9999 9955	.9999 9941	.9999 9925	.9999 9908
9.02	.9999 9968	.9999 9957	.9999 9944	.9999 9929	.9999 9912
9.03	.9999 9970	.9999 9959	.9999 9946	.9999 9932	.9999 9916
9.04	.9999 9971	.9999 9961	.9999 9949	.9999 9935	.9999 9920
9.05	.9999 9972	.9999 9962	.9999 9951	.9999 9938	.9999 9923
9.06	.9999 9974	.9999 9964	.9999 9953	.9999 9941	.9999 9927
9.07	.9999 9975	.9999 9966	.9999 9955	.9999 9943	.9999 9930
9.08	.9999 9976	.9999 9967	.9999 9957	.9999 9946	.9999 9933
9.09	.9999 9977	.9999 9969	.9999 9959	.9999 9948	.9999 9936
9.10	.9999 9978	.9999 9970	.9999 9961	.9999 9951	.9999 9939
9.11	.9999 9979	.9999 9971	.9999 9963	.9999 9953	.9999 9942
9.12	.9999 9980	.9999 9973	.9999 9964	.9999 9955	.9999 9944
9.13	.9999 9981	.9999 9974	.9999 9966	.9999 9957	.9999 9947
9.14	.9999 9982	.9999 9975	.9999 9967	.9999 9959	.9999 9949
9.15	.9999 9983	.9999 9976	.9999 9969	.9999 9961	.9999 9952
9.16	.9999 9983	.9999 9977	.9999 9970	.9999 9962	.9999 9954
9.17	.9999 9984	.9999 9978	.9999 9972	.9999 9964	.9999 9956
9.18	.9999 9985	.9999 9979	.9999 9973	.9999 9966	.9999 9958
9.19	.9999 9985	.9999 9980	.9999 9974	.9999 9967	.9999 9960
9.20	.9999 9986	.9999 9981	.9999 9975	.9999 9969	.9999 9962
9.21	.9999 9987	.9999 9982	.9999 9976	.9999 9970	.9999 9963
9.22	.9999 9987	.9999 9983	.9999 9977	.9999 9972	.9999 9965
9.23	.9999 9988	.9999 9984	.9999 9978	.9999 9973	.9999 9967
9.24	.9999 9988	.9999 9984	.9999 9979	.9999 9974	.9999 9968
9.25	.9999 9989	.9999 9985	.9999 9980	.9999 9975	.9999 9969
9.26	.9999 9989	.9999 9986	.9999 9981	.9999 9976	.9999 9971
9.27	.9999 9990	.9999 9986	.9999 9982	.9999 9977	.9999 9972
9.28	.9999 9990	.9999 9987	.9999 9983	.9999 9978	.9999 9973
9.29	.9999 9991	.9999 9988	.9999 9984	.9999 9979	.9999 9975
9.30	.9999 9991	.9999 9988	.9999 9984	.9999 9980	.9999 9976
9.31	.9999 9992	.9999 9989	.9999 9985	.9999 9981	.9999 9977
9.32	.9999 9992	.9999 9989	.9999 9986	.9999 9982	.9999 9978
9.33	.9999 9992	.9999 9990	.9999 9986	.9999 9983	.9999 9979
9.34	.9999 9993	.9999 9990	.9999 9987	.9999 9984	.9999 9980
9.35	.9999 9993	.9999 9991	.9999 9988	.9999 9984	.9999 9981
9.36	.9999 9993	.9999 9991	.9999 9988	.9999 9985	.9999 9982
9.37	.9999 9994	.9999 9991	.9999 9989	.9999 9986	.9999 9983
9.38	.9999 9994	.9999 9992	.9999 9989	.9999 9986	.9999 9983
9.39	.9999 9994	.9999 9992	.9999 9990	.9999 9987	.9999 9984
9.40	.9999 9994	.9999 9992	.9999 9990	.9999 9988	.9999 9985
9.41	.9999 9995	.9999 9993	.9999 9991	.9999 9988	.9999 9985
9.42	.9999 9995	.9999 9993	.9999 9991	.9999 9989	.9999 9986
9.43	.9999 9995	.9999 9993	.9999 9991	.9999 9989	.9999 9987
9.44	.9999 9995	.9999 9994	.9999 9992	.9999 9990	.9999 9987
9.45	.9999 9996	.9999 9994	.9999 9992	.9999 9990	.9999 9988
9.46	.9999 9996	.9999 9994	.9999 9993	.9999 9991	.9999 9988
9.47	.9999 9996	.9999 9995	.9999 9993	.9999 9991	.9999 9989
9.48	.9999 9996	.9999 9995	.9999 9993	.9999 9991	.9999 9989
9.49	.9999 9996	.9999 9995	.9999 9994	.9999 9992	.9999 9990

W	P(W,60)	P(W,70)	P(W,80)	P(W,90)	P(W,100)
9.50	.9999 9996	.9999 9995	.9999 9994	.9999 9992	.9999 9990
9.51	.9999 9997	.9999 9995	.9999 9994	.9999 9993	.9999 9991
9.52	.9999 9997	.9999 9996	.9999 9994	.9999 9993	.9999 9991
9.53	.9999 9997	.9999 9996	.9999 9995	.9999 9993	.9999 9992
9.54	.9999 9997	.9999 9996	.9999 9995	.9999 9994	.9999 9992
9.55	.9999 9997	.9999 9996	.9999 9995	.9999 9994	.9999 9992
9.56	.9999 9997	.9999 9996	.9999 9995	.9999 9994	.9999 9993
9.57	.9999 9997	.9999 9997	.9999 9995	.9999 9994	.9999 9993
9.58	.9999 9997	.9999 9997	.9999 9996	.9999 9995	.9999 9993
9.59	.9999 9998	.9999 9997	.9999 9996	.9999 9995	.9999 9994
9.60	.9999 9998	.9999 9997	.9999 9996	.9999 9995	.9999 9994
9.61	.9999 9998	.9999 9997	.9999 9996	.9999 9995	.9999 9994
9.62	.9999 9998	.9999 9997	.9999 9996	.9999 9995	.9999 9994
9.63	.9999 9998	.9999 9997	.9999 9996	.9999 9996	.9999 9995
9.64	.9999 9998	.9999 9997	.9999 9997	.9999 9996	.9999 9995
9.65	.9999 9998	.9999 9998	.9999 9997	.9999 9996	.9999 9995
9.66	.9999 9998	.9999 9998	.9999 9997	.9999 9996	.9999 9995
9.67	.9999 9998	.9999 9998	.9999 9997	.9999 9996	.9999 9996
9.68	.9999 9998	.9999 9998	.9999 9997	.9999 9997	.9999 9996
9.69	.9999 9998	.9999 9998	.9999 9997	.9999 9997	.9999 9996
9.70	.9999 9998	.9999 9998	.9999 9997	.9999 9997	.9999 9996
9.71	.9999 9999	.9999 9998	.9999 9998	.9999 9997	.9999 9996
9.72	.9999 9999	.9999 9998	.9999 9998	.9999 9997	.9999 9996
9.73	.9999 9999	.9999 9998	.9999 9998	.9999 9997	.9999 9997
9.74	.9999 9999	.9999 9998	.9999 9998	.9999 9997	.9999 9997
9.75	.9999 9999	.9999 9998	.9999 9998	.9999 9997	.9999 9997
9.76	.9999 9999	.9999 9998	.9999 9998	.9999 9998	.9999 9997
9.77	.9999 9999	.9999 9998	.9999 9998	.9999 9998	.9999 9997
9.78	.9999 9999	.9999 9999	.9999 9998	.9999 9998	.9999 9997
9.79	.9999 9999	.9999 9999	.9999 9998	.9999 9998	.9999 9997
9.80	.9999 9999	.9999 9999	.9999 9998	.9999 9998	.9999 9997
9.81	.9999 9999	.9999 9999	.9999 9998	.9999 9998	.9999 9998
9.82	.9999 9999	.9999 9999	.9999 9998	.9999 9998	.9999 9998
9.83	.9999 9999	.9999 9999	.9999 9998	.9999 9998	.9999 9998
9.84	.9999 9999	.9999 9999	.9999 9999	.9999 9998	.9999 9998
9.85	.9999 9999	.9999 9999	.9999 9999	.9999 9998	.9999 9998
9.86	.9999 9999	.9999 9999	.9999 9999	.9999 9998	.9999 9998
9.87	.9999 9999	.9999 9999	.9999 9999	.9999 9998	.9999 9998
9.88	.9999 9999	.9999 9999	.9999 9999	.9999 9998	.9999 9998
9.89	.9999 9999	.9999 9999	.9999 9999	.9999 9998	.9999 9998
9.90	.9999 9999	.9999 9999	.9999 9999	.9999 9999	.9999 9998
9.91	.9999 9999	.9999 9999	.9999 9999	.9999 9999	.9999 9998
9.92	.9999 9999	.9999 9999	.9999 9999	.9999 9999	.9999 9998
9.93	.9999 9999	.9999 9999	.9999 9999	.9999 9999	.9999 9998
9.94	.9999 9999	.9999 9999	.9999 9999	.9999 9999	.9999 9998
9.95	.9999 9999	.9999 9999	.9999 9999	.9999 9999	.9999 9999
9.96	.9999 9999	.9999 9999	.9999 9999	.9999 9999	.9999 9999
9.97	.9999 9999	.9999 9999	.9999 9999	.9999 9999	.9999 9999
9.98	.9999 9999	.9999 9999	.9999 9999	.9999 9999	.9999 9999
9.99	.9999 9999	.9999 9999	.9999 9999	.9999 9999	.9999 9999

W	P(W,60)	P(W,70)	P(W,80)	P(W,90)	P(W,100)
10.00	.9999 9999	.9999 9999	.9999 9999	.9999 9999	.9999 9999
10.01	.9999 9999	.9999 9999	.9999 9999	.9999 9999	.9999 9999
10.02	.9999 9999	.9999 9999	.9999 9999	.9999 9999	.9999 9999
10.03	.9999 9999	.9999 9999	.9999 9999	.9999 9999	.9999 9999
10.04	.9999 9999	.9999 9999	.9999 9999	.9999 9999	.9999 9999
10.05	1.0000 0000	.9999 9999	.9999 9999	.9999 9999	.9999 9999
10.06		.9999 9999	.9999 9999	.9999 9999	.9999 9999
10.07		.9999 9999	.9999 9999	.9999 9999	.9999 9999
10.08		.9999 9999	.9999 9999	.9999 9999	.9999 9999
10.09		.9999 9999	.9999 9999	.9999 9999	.9999 9999
10.10		.9999 9999	.9999 9999	.9999 9999	.9999 9999
10.11		.9999 9999	.9999 9999	.9999 9999	.9999 9999
10.12		.9999 9999	.9999 9999	.9999 9999	.9999 9999
10.13		1.0000 0000	.9999 9999	.9999 9999	.9999 9999
10.14			.9999 9999	.9999 9999	.9999 9999
10.15			.9999 9999	.9999 9999	.9999 9999
10.16			.9999 9999	.9999 9999	.9999 9999
10.17			.9999 9999	.9999 9999	.9999 9999
10.18			.9999 9999	.9999 9999	.9999 9999
10.19			.9999 9999	.9999 9999	.9999 9999
10.20			.9999 9999	.9999 9999	.9999 9999
10.21			.9999 9999	.9999 9999	.9999 9999
10.22			1.0000 0000	.9999 9999	.9999 9999
10.23				.9999 9999	.9999 9999
10.24				.9999 9999	.9999 9999
10.25				.9999 9999	.9999 9999
10.26				.9999 9999	.9999 9999
10.27				.9999 9999	.9999 9999
10.28				.9999 9999	.9999 9999
10.29				.9999 9999	.9999 9999
10.30				.9999 9999	.9999 9999
10.31				.9999 9999	.9999 9999
10.32				1.0000 0000	.9999 9999
10.33					.9999 9999
10.34					.9999 9999
10.35					.9999 9999
10.36					.9999 9999
10.37					.9999 9999
10.38					.9999 9999
10.39					.9999 9999
10.40					.9999 9999
10.41					.9999 9999
10.42					.9999 9999
10.43					.9999 9999
10.44					.9999 9999
10.45					.9999 9999
10.46					1.0000 0000
10.47					
10.48					
10.49					

Table A5

PERCENTAGE POINTS OF THE RANGE

[Values of the Range W Corresponding to Cumulative Probability P for Samples of Size n From $N(\mu, 1)$]

PERCENTAGE POINTS OF THE RANGE

P \ n	2	3	4	5	6	7
.0001	0.000177	0.019047	0.092394	0.205489	0.334167	0.464516
.0005	0.000886	0.042594	0.158155	0.308222	0.463700	0.612589
.0010	0.001772	0.060245	0.199446	0.367392	0.534736	0.691347
.0050	0.008862	0.134847	0.342702	0.554904	0.748983	0.921826
.0100	0.017725	0.190945	0.433676	0.665015	0.869515	1.048144
.0250	0.044319	0.303071	0.594643	0.849672	1.065952	1.250500
.0500	0.088681	0.431402	0.759533	1.029940	1.252886	1.440141
.1000	0.177712	0.618352	0.979366	1.261398	1.488195	1.676051
.2000	0.358287	0.900092	1.285672	1.573441	1.799995	1.985445
.3000	0.544926	1.138259	1.531485	1.818447	2.042028	2.223993
.4000	0.741614	1.362597	1.756529	2.040097	2.259641	2.437704
.5000	0.953873	1.587788	1.978321	2.256883	2.471652	2.645453
.6000	1.190232	1.826320	2.210281	2.482427	2.691658	2.860733
.7000	1.465738	2.094590	2.468799	2.732888	2.935559	3.099199
.8000	1.812388	2.423529	2.783758	3.037317	3.231739	3.388684
.9000	2.326174	2.902380	3.240446	3.478281	3.660721	3.808098
.9500	2.771808	3.314493	3.633160	3.857656	4.030092	4.169554
.9750	3.169822	3.682268	3.984015	4.197026	4.360906	4.493624
.9900	3.642773	4.120303	4.402801	4.602821	4.757047	4.882166
.9950	3.969745	4.424235	4.694087	4.885585	5.033479	5.153613
.9990	4.653508	5.063453	5.308804	5.483754	5.619332	5.729754
.9995	4.922533	5.316400	5.552855	5.721773	5.852849	5.959710
.9999	5.502128	5.864157	6.082863	6.239691	6.361709	6.461391

P \ n	8	9	10	11	12	13
.0001	0.590186	0.708709	0.819433	0.922513	1.018443	1.107819
.0005	0.751013	0.878357	0.995219	1.102585	1.201493	1.292919
.0010	0.834826	0.965507	1.084583	1.193404	1.293251	1.385253
.0050	1.075282	1.212115	1.334928	1.445920	1.546898	1.639328
.0100	1.204819	1.343386	1.467033	1.578304	1.679205	1.771332
.0250	1.410019	1.549720	1.673518	1.784355	1.884475	1.975612
.0500	1.600413	1.739852	1.862844	1.972583	2.071455	2.161277
.1000	1.835449	1.973327	2.094446	2.202195	2.299057	2.386902
.2000	2.141656	2.276121	2.393843	2.498316	2.592064	2.676969
.3000	2.376728	2.507898	2.622556	2.724195	2.815328	2.897817
.4000	2.586852	2.714772	2.826491	2.925467	3.014177	3.094450
.5000	2.790841	2.915438	3.024202	3.120531	3.206854	3.284960
.6000	3.002059	3.123122	3.228778	3.322347	3.406194	3.482065
.7000	3.235931	3.353046	3.455258	3.545785	3.626919	3.700346
.8000	3.519834	3.632192	3.730280	3.817183	3.895093	3.965627
.9000	3.931349	4.037023	4.129346	4.211200	4.284635	4.351158
.9500	4.286309	4.386509	4.474124	4.551864	4.621655	4.684920
.9750	4.604857	4.700411	4.784033	4.858286	4.924993	4.985497
.9900	4.987183	5.077506	5.156635	5.226963	5.290196	5.347592
.9950	5.254550	5.341439	5.417616	5.485364	5.546312	5.601663
.9990	5.822728	5.902906	5.973307	6.036000	6.092467	6.143802
.9995	6.049760	6.127468	6.195739	6.256567	6.311378	6.361227
.9999	6.545529	6.618235	6.682187	6.739225	6.790667	6.837489

PERCENTAGE POINTS OF THE RANGE

P \ n	14	15	16	17	18	19
.0001	1.191258	1.269336	1.342579	1.411460	1.476395	1.537756
.0005	1.377729	1.456683	1.530433	1.599544	1.664502	1.725726
.0010	1.470384	1.549474	1.623228	1.692245	1.757038	1.818046
.0050	1.724404	1.803104	1.876237	1.944472	2.008372	2.068413
.0100	1.855958	1.934115	2.006645	2.074243	2.137488	2.196867
.0250	2.059129	2.136114	2.207443	2.273835	2.335885	2.394088
.0500	2.243459	2.319117	2.389145	2.454273	2.515097	2.572117
.1000	2.467168	2.540983	2.609247	2.672690	2.731908	2.787396
.2000	2.754467	2.825680	2.891495	2.952631	3.009675	3.063109
.3000	2.973079	3.042214	3.106097	3.165428	3.220781	3.272627
.4000	3.167678	3.234938	3.297083	3.354799	3.408646	3.459083
.5000	3.356208	3.421651	3.482119	3.538281	3.590681	3.639766
.6000	3.551278	3.614858	3.673612	3.728188	3.779115	3.826829
.7000	3.767343	3.828898	3.885792	3.938651	3.987986	4.034216
.8000	4.030005	4.089172	4.143877	4.194716	4.242179	4.286668
.9000	4.411913	4.467782	4.519464	4.567519	4.612403	4.654494
.9500	4.742732	4.795924	4.845154	4.890951	4.933745	4.973892
.9750	5.040817	5.091743	5.138897	5.182782	5.223806	5.262307
.9900	5.400105	5.448476	5.493291	5.535020	5.574047	5.610690
.9950	5.652328	5.699017	5.742289	5.782597	5.820307	5.855724
.9990	6.190836	6.234215	6.274452	6.311958	6.347071	6.380070
.9995	6.406915	6.449067	6.488177	6.524643	6.558790	6.590889
.9999	6.880434	6.920082	6.956890	6.991229	7.023401	7.053657

P \ n	20	22	24	26	28	30
.0001	1.595868	1.703468	1.801126	1.890368	1.972413	2.048246
.0005	1.783582	1.890416	1.987093	2.075236	2.156123	2.230775
.0010	1.875647	1.981896	2.077934	2.165415	2.245638	2.319635
.0050	2.125000	2.229148	2.323063	2.408455	2.486648	2.558691
.0100	2.252791	2.355636	2.448296	2.532490	2.609547	2.680513
.0250	2.448862	2.549498	2.640076	2.722319	2.797547	2.866800
.0500	2.625753	2.724238	2.812829	2.893230	2.966750	3.034415
.1000	2.839570	2.935330	3.021432	3.099550	3.170969	3.236693
.2000	3.113340	3.205511	3.288366	3.363534	3.432252	3.495491
.3000	3.321364	3.410792	3.491185	3.564123	3.630811	3.692188
.4000	3.506497	3.593503	3.671730	3.742714	3.807625	3.867378
.5000	3.685915	3.770611	3.846776	3.915903	3.979129	4.037343
.6000	3.871692	3.954046	4.028125	4.095376	4.156902	4.213563
.7000	4.077692	4.157522	4.229355	4.294588	4.354286	4.409280
.8000	4.328517	4.405388	4.474592	4.537464	4.595024	4.648069
.9000	4.694105	4.766907	4.832495	4.892122	4.946746	4.997113
.9500	5.011689	5.081193	5.143852	5.200850	5.253094	5.301290
.9750	5.298566	5.365277	5.425452	5.480220	5.530445	5.576798
.9900	5.645215	5.708769	5.766138	5.818385	5.866325	5.910592
.9950	5.889103	5.950573	6.006087	6.056666	6.103092	6.145978
.9990	6.411187	6.468538	6.520381	6.567656	6.611084	6.651228
.9995	6.621165	6.676980	6.727453	6.773495	6.815801	6.854919
.9999	7.082207	7.134873	7.182535	7.226039	7.266039	7.303044

PERCENTAGE POINTS OF THE RANGE

P \ n	32	34	36	38	40	50
.0001	2.118671	2.184353	2.245845	2.303612	2.358048	2.590591
.0005	2.300019	2.364536	2.424887	2.481541	2.534899	2.762552
.0010	2.388241	2.452137	2.511889	2.567966	2.620769	2.845954
.0050	2.625423	2.687528	2.745569	2.800012	2.851256	3.069616
.0100	2.746228	2.807370	2.864498	2.918079	2.968503	3.183321
.0250	2.930905	2.990535	3.046240	3.098477	3.147630	3.357005
.0500	3.097040	3.155286	3.209692	3.260710	3.308716	3.513200
.1000	3.297516	3.354083	3.406923	3.456472	3.503096	3.701734
.2000	3.554019	3.608457	3.659314	3.707009	3.751894	3.943206
.3000	3.749002	3.801853	3.851234	3.897552	3.941149	4.127044
.4000	3.922697	3.974166	4.022264	4.067386	4.109863	4.291064
.5000	4.091247	4.141409	4.188295	4.232287	4.273708	4.450482
.6000	4.266041	4.314888	4.360553	4.403408	4.443766	4.616090
.7000	4.460228	4.507662	4.552018	4.593654	4.632872	4.800425
.8000	4.697229	4.743013	4.785838	4.826050	4.863937	5.025917
.9000	5.043816	5.087334	5.128057	5.166312	5.202370	5.356687
.9500	5.346000	5.387678	5.426697	5.463363	5.497935	5.646026
.9750	5.619817	5.659933	5.697502	5.732818	5.766127	5.908917
.9900	5.951695	5.990041	6.025967	6.059751	6.091626	6.228393
.9950	6.185810	6.222982	6.257818	6.290585	6.321508	6.454269
.9990	6.688538	6.723377	6.756044	6.786787	6.815814	6.940585
.9995	6.891284	6.925248	6.957102	6.987085	7.015400	7.137164
.9999	7.337461	7.369622	7.399796	7.428210	7.455053	7.570596

P \ n	60	70	80	90	100	
.0001	2.775319	2.927786	3.057128	3.169148	3.267737	
.0005	2.943168	3.092146	3.218493	3.327905	3.424199	
.0010	3.024532	3.171801	3.296691	3.404839	3.500024	
.0050	3.242655	3.385324	3.506313	3.611097	3.703340	
.0100	3.353527	3.493863	3.612885	3.715980	3.806747	
.0250	3.522895	3.659695	3.775746	3.876294	3.964843	
.0500	3.675244	3.808909	3.922333	4.020632	4.107228	
.1000	3.859209	3.989161	4.099483	4.195135	4.279426	
.2000	4.094984	4.220324	4.326797	4.419166	4.500610	
.3000	4.274625	4.396573	4.500222	4.590182	4.669535	
.4000	4.435016	4.554032	4.655239	4.743118	4.820666	
.5000	4.591013	4.707269	4.806177	4.892098	4.967946	
.6000	4.753185	4.866667	4.963266	5.047218	5.121358	
.7000	4.933836	5.044345	5.138468	5.220308	5.292614	
.8000	5.155024	5.262057	5.353283	5.432652	5.502811	
.9000	5.479870	5.582115	5.669346	5.745304	5.812497	
.9500	5.764388	5.862730	5.946701	6.019871	6.084638	
.9750	6.023168	6.118178	6.199362	6.270146	6.332834	
.9900	6.337964	6.429173	6.507175	6.575233	6.635542	
.9950	6.560722	6.649396	6.725272	6.791507	6.850223	
.9990	7.040804	7.124400	7.196010	7.258580	7.314094	
.9995	7.235032	7.316708	7.386704	7.447885	7.502183	
.9999	7.663588	7.741276	7.807913	7.866200	7.917964	

Table A6

MOMENTS OF THE RANGE W FOR SAMPLES OF SIZE n FROM $N(\mu, 1)$

MOMENTS OF THE RANGE FOR SAMPLES OF n FROM $N(\mu,1)$

n	E(W)	σ^2_W	$\alpha_{3:W}$	$\alpha_{4:W}$
2	1.12837 91671	.72676 04553	.9952 7175	3.869 1773
3	1.69256 87506	.78919 77107	.6460 7471	3.286 4021
4	2.05875 07460	.77406 24738	.5229 5734	3.188 3555
5	2.32592 89473	.74663 76009	.4655 1383	3.169 1478
6	2.53441 27212	.71917 13092	.4349 7555	3.169 6424
7	2.70435 67512	.69423 11313	.4175 5240	3.175 9064
8	2.84720 06121	.67212 36717	.4072 5611	3.183 7977
9	2.97002 63244	.65259 62151	.4011 3245	3.191 9210
10	3.07750 54617	.63528 97762	.3975 8678	3.199 7848
11	3.17287 27038	.61986 43117	.3956 9856	3.207 2265
12	3.25845 52798	.60602 85277	.3949 0804	3.214 2105
13	3.33598 03541	.59354 11244	.3948 6050	3.220 7503
14	3.40676 31082	.58220 42445	.3953 2354	3.226 8773
15	3.47182 68899	.57185 57265	.3961 4066	3.232 6279
16	3.53198 27861	.56236 21426	.3972 0409	3.238 0376
17	3.58788 39618	.55361 30572	.3984 3819	3.243 1394
18	3.64006 37579	.54551 64487	.3997 8908	3.247 9628
19	3.68896 30232	.53799 51043	.4012 1787	3.252 5340
20	3.73495 01196	.53098 37904	.4026 9623	3.256 8763
21	3.77833 58298	.52442 70274	.4042 0335	3.261 0099
22	3.81938 46434	.51827 73314	.4057 2387	3.264 9529
23	3.85832 34233	.51249 38181	.4072 4641	3.268 7211
24	3.89534 81485	.50704 10861	.4087 6255	3.272 3285
25	3.93062 92195	.50188 83188	.4102 6606	3.275 7877
26	3.96431 56795	.49700 85564	.4117 5237	3.279 1097
27	3.99653 86040	.49237 81028	.4132 1818	3.282 3044
28	4.02741 38482	.48797 60384	.4146 6112	3.285 3810
29	4.05704 42921	.48378 38184	.4160 7955	3.288 3472
30	4.08552 16883	.47978 49392	.4174 7239	3.291 2106
31	4.11292 81953	.47596 46599	.4188 3901	3.293 9775
32	4.13933 76559	.47230 97683	.4201 7907	3.296 6540
33	4.16481 66719	.46880 83838	.4214 9251	3.299 2456
34	4.18942 55115	.46544 97900	.4227 7944	3.301 7572
35	4.21321 88792	.46222 42928	.4240 4013	3.304 1933
36	4.23624 65735	.45912 30982	.4252 7496	3.306 5582
37	4.25855 40507	.45613 82080	.4264 8438	3.308 8557
38	4.28018 29105	.45326 23296	.4276 6890	3.311 0893
39	4.30117 13155	.45048 87982	.4288 2909	3.313 2624
40	4.32155 43564	.44781 15084	.4299 6552	3.315 3779
41	4.34136 43695	.44522 48562	.4310 7881	3.317 4387
42	4.36063 12150	.44272 36864	.4321 6955	3.319 4474
43	4.37938 25208	.44030 32479	.4332 3836	3.321 4065
44	4.39764 38975	.43795 91537	.4342 8586	3.323 3181
45	4.41543 91280	.43568 73457	.4353 1265	3.325 1845
46	4.43279 03360	.43348 40636	.4363 1932	3.327 0076
47	4.44971 81351	.43134 58177	.4373 0645	3.328 7892
48	4.46624 17617	.42926 93638	.4382 7462	3.330 5311
49	4.48237 91942	.42725 16817	.4392 2438	3.332 2350
50	4.49814 72588	.42528 99556	.4401 5628	3.333 9024

MOMENTS OF THE RANGE FOR SAMPLES OF n FROM $N(\mu,1)$

n	E(W)	σ^2_W	$\alpha_{3:W}$	$\alpha_{4:W}$
51	4.51356 17253	.42338 15568	.4410 7083	3.335 5347
52	4.52863 73928	.42152 40275	.4419 6854	3.337 1333
53	4.54338 81668	.41971 50671	.4428 4992	3.338 6994
54	4.55782 71291	.41795 25197	.4437 1543	3.340 2344
55	4.57196 66012	.41623 43619	.4445 6553	3.341 7393
56	4.58581 82013	.41455 86931	.4454 0068	3.343 2152
57	4.59939 28961	.41292 37256	.4462 2129	3.344 6632
58	4.61270 10487	.41132 77766	.4470 2779	3.346 0843
59	4.62575 24613	.40976 92598	.4478 2058	3.347 4793
60	4.63855 64145	.40824 66789	.4486 0004	3.348 8491
61	4.65112 17036	.40675 86207	.4493 6654	3.350 1947
62	4.66345 66714	.40530 37495	.4501 2045	3.351 5168
63	4.67556 92383	.40388 08018	.4508 6211	3.352 8161
64	4.68746 69302	.40248 85808	.4515 9186	3.354 0933
65	4.69915 69040	.40112 59526	.4523 1001	3.355 3493
66	4.71064 59712	.39979 18416	.4530 1689	3.356 5846
67	4.72194 06193	.39848 52266	.4537 1278	3.357 7998
68	4.73304 70321	.39720 51377	.4543 9799	3.358 9955
69	4.74397 11082	.39595 06527	.4550 7278	3.360 1724
70	4.75471 84777	.39472 08940	.4557 3743	3.361 3310
71	4.76529 45186	.39351 50265	.4563 9220	3.362 4718
72	4.77570 43714	.39233 22541	.4570 3735	3.363 5953
73	4.78595 29522	.39117 18179	.4576 7310	3.364 7021
74	4.79604 49664	.39003 29940	.4582 9971	3.365 7924
75	4.80598 49196	.38891 50914	.4589 1739	3.366 8669
76	4.81577 71291	.38781 74497	.4595 2637	3.367 9259
77	4.82542 57340	.38673 94380	.4601 2686	3.368 9699
78	4.83493 47049	.38568 04527	.4607 1905	3.369 9992
79	4.84430 78526	.38463 99165	.4613 0316	3.371 0143
80	4.85354 88369	.38361 72763	.4618 7936	3.372 0154
81	4.86266 11740	.38261 20024	.4624 4786	3.373 0030
82	4.87164 82439	.38162 35871	.4630 0882	3.373 9773
83	4.88051 32976	.38065 15435	.4635 6241	3.374 9388
84	4.88925 94630	.37969 54044	.4641 0882	3.375 8877
85	4.89788 97515	.37875 47214	.4646 4820	3.376 8244
86	4.90640 70634	.37782 90636	.4651 8070	3.377 7490
87	4.91481 41933	.37691 80172	.4657 0649	3.378 6620
88	4.92311 38348	.37602 11844	.4662 2570	3.379 5635
89	4.93130 85861	.37513 81825	.4667 3849	3.380 4538
90	4.93940 09535	.37426 86432	.4672 4499	3.381 3334
91	4.94739 33562	.37341 22122	.4677 4534	3.382 2022
92	4.95528 81299	.37256 85481	.4682 3966	3.383 0607
93	4.96308 75311	.37173 73222	.4687 2809	3.383 9089
94	4.97079 37398	.37091 82175	.4692 1075	3.384 7472
95	4.97840 88637	.37011 09284	.4696 8776	3.385 5757
96	4.98593 49408	.36931 51602	.4701 5923	3.386 3948
97	4.99337 39426	.36853 06286	.4706 2527	3.387 2044
98	5.00072 77771	.36775 70590	.4710 8601	3.388 0050
99	5.00799 82910	.36699 41863	.4715 4154	3.388 7966
100	5.01518 72729	.36624 17546	.4719 9196	3.389 5794

Table A7

CONSTANTS FOR CONSTRUCTING $\bar{X}$ AND R CHARTS

	$\bar{X}$ chart	R chart	
n	A_2	D_3	D_4
2	1.880	0	3.267
3	1.023	0	2.575
4	0.729	0	2.282
5	0.577	0	2.115
6	0.483	0	2.004
7	0.419	0.076	1.924
8	0.373	0.136	1.864
9	0.337	0.184	1.816
10	0.308	0.223	1.777
11	0.285	0.256	1.744
12	0.266	0.284	1.716
13	0.249	0.308	1.692
14	0.235	0.329	1.671
15	0.223	0.348	1.652
16	0.212	0.364	1.636
17	0.203	0.379	1.621
18	0.194	0.392	1.608
19	0.187	0.404	1.596
20	0.180	0.414	1.586
21	0.173	0.425	1.575
22	0.167	0.434	1.566
23	0.162	0.443	1.557
24	0.157	0.452	1.548
25	0.153	0.459	1.541

Table A8

APPROXIMATE UPPER 5% CRITICAL VALUES OF THE DISTRIBUTION OF V

n	k	kN		kN		kN		kN		kN	
25	2	34	.204	50	.277	100	.342	500	.384	∞	.389
			(.017)		(.089)		(.063)		–		–
			(.118)		(.023)		(.020)		–		–
50		66	.136	100	.197	200	.246	1000	.274		.276
			(.042)		(.071)		–		–		–
			(.150)		(.027)		–		–		–
75		100	.112	150	.159	300	.192	1500	.215		.226
			(.063)		–		–		–		–
			(.020)		–		–		–		–
100		134	.099	200	.139	400	.169	2000	.193		.193
25	3	33	.190	51	.282	99	.336	501	.370		.381
			(.058)		(.026)		(.042)		–		–
			(.013)		(.026)		(.083)		–		–
50		66	.134	99	.190	201	.235	999	.265		.276
			(.055)		(.051)		–		–		–
			(.020)		(.026)		–		–		–
75		99	.110	150	.157	300	.193	1500	.218		.220
			(.037)		–		–		–		–
			(.037)		–		–		–		–
100		132	.096	201	.136	399	.166	2001	.187		.191
25	4	32	.174	52	.263	100	.316	500	.349		.363
			(.019)		(.050)		(.065)		–		–
			(.145)		(.015)		(.065)		–		–
50		68	.132	100	.183	200	.226	1000	.253		.256
			(.052)		(.035)		–		–		–
			(.015)		(.035)		–		–		–
75		100	.107	152	.150	300	.182	1500	.203		.212
			(.065)		–		–		–		–
			(.025)		–		–		–		–
100		132	.089	200	.130	400	.158	2000	.179		.182
25	5	35	.186	50	.245	100	.302	500	.336		.343
			(.044)		(.025)		(.043)		–		–
			(.234)		(.094)		(.043)		–		–
50		65	.119	100	.174	200	.211	1000	.238		.245
			(.067)		(.053)		–		–		–
			(.067)		(.020)		–		–		–
75		100	.101	150	.141	300	.174	1500	.194		.200
			(.043)		–		–		–		–
			(.043)		–		–		–		–
100		135	.088	200	.123	400	.150	2000	.167		.174
25	6	36	.184	48	.230	102	.291	498	.322		.330
			(.031)		(.054)		(.027)		–		–
			(.237)		(.054)		(.027)		–		–
50		66	.115	102	.168	198	.202	1002	.226		.231
			(.053)		(.037)		–		–		–
			(.053)		(.099)		–		–		–
75		102	.098	150	.135	300	.165	1500	.185		.190
			(.035)		–		–		–		–
			(.035)		–		–		–		–
100		132	.082	198	.116	402	.142	1998	.161		.165

Table A9

APPROXIMATE UPPER 1% CRITICAL VALUES OF THE DISTRIBUTION OF V

n	k	kN		kN		kN		kN		kN	
25	2	34	.269	50	.368	100	.454	500	.500	∞	.507
			(.017)		(.004)		(.005)		–		–
			(.001)		(.023)		(.020)		–		–
50		66	.181	100	.260	200	.319	1000	.359		.366
			(.008)		(.009)		–		–		–
			(.042)		(.027)		–		–		–
75		100	.148	150	.209	300	.255	1500	.283		.297
			(.005)		–		–		–		–
			(.020)		–		–		–		–
100		134	.132	200	.182	400	.227	2000	.251		.258
25	3	33	.239	51	.345	99	.418	501	.460		.470
			(.013)		(.009)		(.007)		–		–
			(.002)		(.026)		(.007)		–		–
50		66	.167	99	.238	201	.293	999	.328		.336
			(.007)		(.013)		–		–		–
			(.020)		(.013)		–		–		–
75		99	.137	150	.195	300	.237	1500	.272		.270
			(.006)		–		–		–		–
			(.006)		–		–		–		–
100		132	.119	201	.169	399	.205	2001	.233		.238
25	4	32	.211	52	.323	100	.383	500	.426		.447
			(.001)		(.003)		(.009)		–		–
			(.001)		(.015)		(.009)		–		–
50		68	.158	100	.224	200	.267	1000	.305		.306
			(.015)		(.006)		–		–		–
			(.015)		(.015)		–		–		–
75		100	.130	152	.183	300	.218	1500	.246		.255
			(.009)		–		–		–		–
			(.025)		–		–		–		–
100		132	.108	200	.156	400	.190	2000	.218		.217
25	5	35	.222	50	.291	100	.358	500	.398		.412
			(.004)		(.004)		(.013)		–		–
			(.004)		(.004)		(.003)		–		–
50		65	.140	100	.206	200	.251	1000	.283		.293
			(.002)		(.007)		–		–		–
			(.002)		(.007)		–		–		–
75		100	.121	150	.170	300	.210	1500	.229		.238
			(.003)		–		–		–		–
			(.013)		–		–		–		–
100		135	.103	200	.145	400	.178	2000	.201		.205
25	6	36	.218	48	.272	102	.340	498	.376		.385
			(.001)		(.008)		(.006)		–		–
			(.001)		(.054)		(.027)		–		–
50		66	.137	102	.198	198	.238	1002	.267		.273
			(.009)		(.011)		–		–		–
			(.053)		(.003)		–		–		–
75		102	.115	150	.159	300	.195	1500	.218		.221
			(.009)		–		–		–		–
			(.009)		–		–		–		–
100		132	.096	198	.138	402	.167	1998	.190		.193

Appendix B

Tables Based on the Studentized Range

SOURCES OF TABLES

Tables B1–B3	WADC TR 58–484, Vol. II (Harter, Clemm and Guthrie)
Tables B4–B6	Freshly recomputed (Harter and Clemm) [for an earlier version, see *Biometrics* **13** (1957), 511-536 (Harter)]
Table B7	*Biometrika Tables for Statisticians*, Vol. I (3rd ed.), Table 30, p. 201 (Pearson and Hartley) [reprinted from *Biometrics* **38**, 393-409 (David)]
Table B8	Abridged from Pearson and Hartley's Table 29c

Table B1

PROBABILITY INTEGRAL $P(Q, \nu, n)$ OF THE STUDENTIZED RANGE $Q = w/s$ FOR SAMPLES OF SIZE n FROM A NORMAL POPULATION WITH ν DEGREES OF FREEDOM FOR THE INDEPENDENT ESTIMATE s^2 OF THE POPULATION VARIANCE

$\nu = 1$

Q \ n	2	3	4	5	6	7	8
0.0	.000000	.000000	.000000	.000000	.000000	.000000	.000000
0.1	.044941	.002745	.000201	.000017	.000002	.000000	.000000
0.2	.089439	.010846	.001574	.000260	.000047	.000009	.000002
0.3	.133075	.023917	.005123	.001243	.000332	.000096	.000030
0.4	.175480	.041369	.011566	.003645	.001259	.000469	.000185
0.5	.216347	.062483	.021275	.008121	.003380	.001508	.000712
0.6	.255442	.086478	.034292	.015153	.007262	.003710	.001997
0.7	.292603	.112582	.050390	.024980	.013356	.007576	.004507
0.8	.327736	.140078	.069163	.037594	.021923	.013498	.008680
0.9	.360806	.168339	.090104	.052785	.033008	.021698	.014841
1.0	.391827	.196839	.112679	.070206	.046475	.032212	.023150
1.2	.447950	.252970	.160743	.110059	.079409	.059578	.046080
1.4	.496785	.306202	.209976	.153828	.117951	.093529	.076105
1.6	.539190	.355415	.258083	.198766	.159334	.131502	.110972
1.8	.576047	.400233	.303719	.242966	.201381	.171238	.148454
2.0	.608173	.440712	.346222	.285262	.242601	.211053	.186766
2.2	.636290	.477126	.385373	.325037	.282085	.249828	.224644
2.4	.661012	.509845	.421209	.362037	.319344	.286889	.261273
2.6	.682855	.539261	.453906	.396231	.354168	.321883	.296176
2.8	.702253	.565753	.483705	.427717	.386527	.354664	.329113
3.0	.719562	.589667	.510868	.456661	.416493	.385222	.360001
3.2	.735082	.611315	.535656	.483257	.444198	.413628	.388853
3.4	.749060	.630969	.558313	.507708	.469798	.439995	.415744
3.6	.761703	.648868	.579064	.530212	.493460	.464458	.440780
3.8	.773185	.665218	.598111	.550954	.515349	.487161	.464082
4.0	.783653	.680198	.615635	.570105	.535621	.508246	.485776
4.2	.793230	.693962	.631794	.587819	.554423	.527848	.505987
4.4	.802022	.706644	.646730	.604235	.571889	.546094	.524836
4.6	.810118	.718361	.660567	.619480	.588140	.563103	.542435
4.8	.817595	.729215	.673414	.633663	.603286	.578980	.558887
5.0	.824520	.739292	.685368	.646884	.617428	.593825	.574288
5.2	.830951	.748671	.696515	.659232	.630654	.607726	.588726
5.4	.836937	.757419	.706930	.670785	.643045	.620763	.602280
5.6	.842522	.765596	.716679	.681614	.654672	.633009	.615023
5.8	.847744	.773255	.725822	.691781	.665599	.644528	.627019
6.0	.852637	.780441	.734412	.701343	.675885	.655380	.638329
6.4	.861550	.793557	.750115	.718848	.694738	.675290	.659097
6.8	.869461	.805224	.764109	.734471	.711587	.693106	.677702
7.2	.876528	.815665	.776652	.748493	.726725	.709130	.694450
7.6	.882877	.825060	.787953	.761140	.740394	.723609	.709595
8.0	.888611	.833557	.798186	.772602	.752791	.736752	.723351
8.4	.893815	.841278	.807491	.783035	.764083	.748729	.735894
8.8	.898559	.848322	.815988	.792567	.774407	.759686	.747375
9.2	.902900	.854774	.823777	.801310	.783881	.769746	.757919
9.6	.906887	.860704	.830941	.809356	.792603	.779011	.767635
10.0	.910561	.866174	.837551	.816784	.800659	.787572	.776614
11.0	.918600	.878149	.852036	.833072	.818334	.806363	.796334
12.0	.925318	.888170	.864168	.846725	.833159	.822135	.812894
13.0	.931016	.896676	.874474	.858329	.845767	.835554	.826989
14.0	.935909	.903986	.883335	.868311	.856617	.847105	.839127

$\nu = 1$

Q\n	2	3	4	5	6	7	8
15.0	.940156	.910333	.891033	.876986	.866049	.857151	.849685
16.0	.943876	.915896	.897782	.884595	.874324	.865966	.858952
17.0	.947162	.920811	.903747	.891321	.881641	.873763	.867149
18.0	.950085	.925185	.909057	.897309	.888156	.880706	.874451
19.0	.952702	.929102	.913813	.902674	.893995	.886928	.880995
20.0	.955059	.932630	.918097	.907508	.899256	.892536	.886894
22.0	.959133	.938731	.925507	.915870	.908357	.902239	.897100
24.0	.962530	.943820	.931689	.922848	.915954	.910339	.905623
26.0	.965407	.948129	.936926	.928759	.922390	.917203	.912845
28.0	.967873	.951825	.941418	.933830	.927913	.923092	.919042
30.0	.970012	.955030	.945313	.938228	.932703	.928201	.924418
32.0	.971883	.957835	.948724	.942079	.936896	.932674	.929126
34.0	.973535	.960312	.951734	.945478	.940599	.936623	.933282
36.0	.975004	.962513	.954410	.948501	.943891	.940135	.936979
38.0	.976318	.964484	.956806	.951206	.946838	.943279	.940288
40.0	.977501	.966257	.958963	.953642	.949491	.946109	.943267
45.0	.980000	.970003	.963517	.958786	.955095	.952087	.949559
50.0	.981998	.973000	.967162	.962903	.959580	.956872	.954596
55.0	.983634	.975453	.970145	.966272	.963251	.960788	.958719
60.0	.984998	.977498	.972631	.969081	.966311	.964053	.962156
65.0	.986151	.979228	.974735	.971458	.968900	.966816	.965064
70.0	.987140	.980711	.976539	.973495	.971120	.969185	.967558
75.0	.987997	.981997	.978102	.975261	.973045	.971238	.969719
80.0	.988747	.983121	.979471	.976807	.974729	.973035	.971611
85.0	.989409	.984114	.980678	.978171	.976215	.974620	.973280
90.0	.989997	.984996	.981751	.979383	.977535	.976030	.974764
95.0	.990524	.985786	.982711	.980468	.978717	.977291	.976091
100.0	.990997	.986496	.983575	.981444	.979781	.978426	.977286
105.0	.991426	.987139	.984357	.982328	.980744	.979453	.978368
110.0	.991816	.987724	.985068	.983131	.981619	.980387	.979351
115.0	.992172	.988258	.985717	.983864	.982418	.981239	.980248
120.0	.992498	.988747	.986312	.984536	.983150	.982021	.981071
125.0	.992798	.989197	.986860	.985155	.983824	.982740	.981828
130.0	.993075	.989612	.987365	.985726	.984446	.983403	.982527
135.0	.993331	.989997	.987833	.986254	.985022	.984018	.983174
140.0	.993569	.990354	.988267	.986745	.985557	.984589	.983775
145.0	.993791	.990687	.988672	.987202	.986055	.985120	.984334
150.0	.993998	.990997	.989050	.987629	.986520	.985616	.984856
155.0	.994192	.991288	.989403	.988028	.986955	.986080	.985345
160.0	.994373	.991560	.989734	.988402	.987362	.986515	.985803
165.0	.994544	.991816	.990045	.988753	.987745	.986923	.986233
170.0	.994704	.992056	.990338	.989084	.988105	.987308	.986638
175.0	.994855	.992283	.990614	.989396	.988445	.987671	.987019
180.0	.994998	.992498	.990875	.989690	.988766	.988013	.987380
190.0	.995262	.992892	.991355	.990233	.989357	.988644	.988044
200.0	.995498	.993248	.991787	.990721	.989890	.989212	.988642
210.0	.995713	.993569	.992178	.991163	.990371	.989725	.989183
220.0	.995908	.993862	.992534	.991565	.990809	.990192	.989674
230.0	.996086	.994128	.992858	.991931	.991208	.990619	.990123
240.0	.996249	.994373	.993156	.992268	.991575	.991010	.990535

$\nu = 1$

Q\n	2	3	4	5	6	7	8
250.0	.996399	.994598	.993430	.992577	.991912	.991369	.990913
260.0	.996537	.994806	.993682	.992862	.992223	.991701	.991263
270.0	.996666	.994998	.993916	.993127	.992511	.992008	.991586
280.0	.996785	.995177	.994133	.993372	.992778	.992294	.991887
290.0	.996895	.995343	.994336	.993601	.993027	.992560	.992167
300.0	.996999	.995498	.994525	.993814	.993260	.992808	.992428
310.0	.997096	.995644	.994701	.994014	.993477	.993040	.992672
320.0	.997187	.995780	.994867	.994201	.993681	.993257	.992901
330.0	.997272	.995908	.995022	.994376	.993872	.993461	.993116
340.0	.997352	.996028	.995169	.994542	.994053	.993654	.993319
350.0	.997428	.996142	.995307	.994698	.994222	.993835	.993509
360.0	.997499	.996249	.995437	.994845	.994383	.994006	.993690
370.0	.997567	.996350	.995560	.994984	.994535	.994168	.993860
380.0	.997631	.996446	.995677	.995116	.994679	.994322	.994022
390.0	.997692	.996537	.995788	.995242	.994815	.994467	.994175
400.0	.997749	.996624	.995893	.995360	.994945	.994606	.994321
420.0	.997856	.996785	.996089	.995581	.995185	.994863	.994591
440.0	.997954	.996931	.996267	.995782	.995404	.995096	.994837
460.0	.998043	.997064	.996429	.995966	.995604	.995309	.995061
480.0	.998124	.997187	.996578	.996134	.995787	.995505	.995267
500.0	.998199	.997299	.996715	.996288	.995956	.995684	.995457
520.0	.998269	.997403	.996841	.996431	.996111	.995850	.995631
540.0	.998333	.997499	.996958	.996563	.996255	.996004	.995793
560.0	.998392	.997588	.997067	.996686	.996389	.996147	.995943
580.0	.998448	.997672	.997168	.996800	.996514	.996280	.996083
600.0	.998499	.997749	.997262	.996907	.996630	.996404	.996214
620.0	.998548	.997822	.997351	.997007	.996738	.996520	.996336
640.0	.998593	.997890	.997433	.997100	.996840	.996629	.996450
660.0	.998636	.997954	.997511	.997188	.996936	.996731	.996558
680.0	.998676	.998014	.997584	.997271	.997026	.996827	.996659
700.0	.998714	.998071	.997653	.997349	.997111	.996917	.996755
720.0	.998750	.998124	.997719	.997422	.997191	.997003	.996845
740.0	.998783	.998175	.997780	.997492	.997267	.997084	.996930
760.0	.998815	.998223	.997839	.997558	.997339	.997161	.997011
780.0	.998846	.998269	.997894	.997621	.997407	.997234	.997088
800.0	.998875	.998312	.997947	.997680	.997472	.997303	.997160
820.0	.998902	.998353	.997997	.997737	.997534	.997369	.997230
840.0	.998928	.998392	.998044	.997791	.997593	.997431	.997296
860.0	.998953	.998430	.998090	.997842	.997649	.997491	.997358
880.0	.998977	.998465	.998133	.997891	.997702	.997548	.997418
900.0	.999000	.998499	.998175	.997938	.997753	.997602	.997476
920.0	.999021	.998532	.998215	.997983	.997802	.997655	.997531
940.0	.999042	.998563	.998253	.998026	.997849	.997705	.997583
960.0	.999062	.998593	.998289	.998067	.997894	.997752	.997634
980.0	.999081	.998622	.998324	.998106	.997937	.997798	.997682
1000.0	.999100	.998650	.998357	.998144	.997978	.997842	.997728
1100.0	.999182	.998772	.998507	.998313	.998162	.998038	.997935
1200.0	.999250	.998875	.998631	.998453	.998315	.998202	.998107
1300.0	.999307	.998961	.998736	.998572	.998444	.998340	.998253
1400.0	.999357	.999035	.998827	.998674	.998556	.998459	.998377

$\nu = 1$

Q \ n	2	3	4	5	6	7	8
1500.0	.999400	.999100	.998905	.998763	.998652	.998561	.998486
1600.0	.999437	.999156	.998973	.998840	.998736	.998651	.998580
1700.0	.999470	.999206	.999034	.998908	.998810	.998731	.998664
1800.0	.999500	.999250	.999087	.998969	.998877	.998801	.998738
1900.0	.999526	.999289	.999135	.999023	.998936	.998864	.998804
2000.0	.999550	.999325	.999179	.999072	.998989	.998921	.998864

$\nu = 1$

Q \ n	9	10	11	12	13	14	15
0.0	.000000	.000000	.000000	.000000	.000000	.000000	.000000
0.1	.000000	.000000	.000000	.000000	.000000	.000000	.000000
0.2	.000000	.000000	.000000	.000000	.000000	.000000	.000000
0.3	.000010	.000003	.000001	.000000	.000000	.000000	.000000
0.4	.000077	.000034	.000015	.000007	.000004	.000002	.000001
0.5	.000353	.000182	.000097	.000054	.000031	.000018	.000011
0.6	.001123	.000656	.000395	.000245	.000156	.000101	.000067
0.7	.002790	.001786	.001176	.000795	.000549	.000386	.000277
0.8	.005786	.003974	.002801	.002019	.001483	.001109	.000842
0.9	.010485	.007611	.005653	.004283	.003301	.002583	.002049
1.0	.017134	.012995	.010061	.007928	.006344	.005144	.004221
1.2	.036521	.029531	.024284	.020255	.017105	.014599	.012579
1.4	.063212	.053391	.045728	.039628	.034691	.030635	.027261
1.6	.095304	.083020	.073175	.065139	.058477	.052880	.048124
1.8	.130671	.116436	.104803	.095133	.086978	.080016	.074009
2.0	.167490	.151817	.138823	.127875	.118524	.110446	.103396
2.2	.204398	.187739	.173775	.161888	.151637	.142701	.134836
2.4	.240470	.223195	.208589	.196056	.185168	.175609	.167139
2.6	.275132	.257529	.242543	.229604	.218295	.208311	.199420
2.8	.308062	.290348	.275186	.262026	.250471	.240224	.231060
3.0	.339111	.321447	.306261	.293026	.281359	.270975	.261656
3.2	.368244	.350748	.335650	.322446	.310770	.300346	.290965
3.4	.395498	.378251	.363323	.350230	.338621	.328231	.318859
3.6	.420950	.404010	.389309	.376385	.364899	.354599	.345288
3.8	.444702	.428107	.413673	.400958	.389636	.379464	.370254
4.0	.466865	.450639	.436498	.424019	.412890	.402875	.393795
4.2	.487554	.471709	.457878	.445654	.434736	.424898	.415967
4.4	.506880	.491422	.477910	.465950	.455256	.445609	.436842
4.6	.524951	.509879	.496688	.485000	.474536	.465088	.456492
4.8	.541867	.527177	.514306	.502889	.492660	.483414	.474997
5.0	.557720	.543405	.530850	.519705	.509709	.500668	.492430
5.2	.572597	.558648	.546403	.535524	.525761	.516923	.508866
5.4	.586576	.572982	.561041	.550423	.540888	.532252	.524373
5.6	.599728	.586479	.574832	.564470	.555158	.546720	.539018
5.8	.612119	.599203	.587842	.577728	.568634	.560390	.552861
6.0	.623808	.611213	.600129	.590256	.581374	.573319	.565959
6.4	.645292	.633305	.622745	.613331	.604855	.597161	.590127
6.8	.664556	.653132	.643059	.634073	.625977	.618623	.611895
7.2	.681912	.671008	.661387	.652799	.645057	.638021	.631580
7.6	.697618	.687195	.677994	.669775	.662363	.655623	.649451
8.0	.711891	.701913	.693101	.685225	.678120	.671656	.665735
8.4	.724913	.715348	.706895	.699339	.692519	.686313	.680626
8.8	.736837	.727653	.719536	.712277	.705722	.699756	.694288
9.2	.747792	.738964	.731158	.724175	.717868	.712127	.706862
9.6	.757890	.749392	.741876	.735151	.729076	.723543	.718470
10.0	.767225	.759035	.751790	.745306	.739447	.734110	.729215
11.0	.787735	.780230	.773588	.767640	.762264	.757364	.752869
12.0	.804967	.798046	.791917	.786428	.781464	.776940	.772787
13.0	.819639	.813221	.807535	.802441	.797834	.793633	.789776
14.0	.832278	.826296	.820995	.816245	.811948	.808029	.804431

$\nu = 1$

Q\n	9	10	11	12	13	14	15
15.0	.843276	.837675	.832712	.828263	.824238	.820567	.817195
16.0	.852929	.847665	.843000	.838818	.835033	.831581	.828410
17.0	.861470	.856505	.852105	.848160	.844589	.841332	.838340
18.0	.869078	.864381	.860218	.856484	.853105	.850022	.847190
19.0	.875898	.871442	.867492	.863949	.860742	.857816	.855128
20.0	.882046	.877808	.874049	.870679	.867628	.864844	.862287
22.0	.892685	.888824	.885401	.882330	.879550	.877013	.874682
24.0	.901570	.898025	.894882	.892062	.889509	.887179	.885038
26.0	.909099	.905824	.902918	.900312	.897952	.895798	.893819
28.0	.915561	.912517	.909816	.907393	.905200	.903197	.901357
30.0	.921167	.918323	.915801	.913538	.911488	.909618	.907898
32.0	.926076	.923408	.921042	.918919	.916996	.915241	.913628
34.0	.930411	.927899	.925670	.923671	.921860	.920207	.918688
36.0	.934266	.931892	.929786	.927897	.926186	.924624	.923189
38.0	.937716	.935467	.933471	.931681	.930059	.928579	.927218
40.0	.940823	.938686	.936789	.935088	.933547	.932140	.930847
45.0	.947386	.945485	.943798	.942284	.940914	.939662	.938512
50.0	.952639	.950928	.949409	.948046	.946811	.945684	.944649
55.0	.956940	.955383	.954002	.952762	.951639	.950615	.949673
60.0	.960524	.959097	.957830	.956694	.955664	.954725	.953861
65.0	.963558	.962240	.961071	.960022	.959071	.958204	.957406
70.0	.966159	.964935	.963849	.962875	.961992	.961186	.960445
75.0	.968414	.967271	.966258	.965348	.964524	.963772	.963080
80.0	.970387	.969315	.968365	.967512	.966740	.966034	.965386
85.0	.972128	.971119	.970225	.969422	.968695	.968031	.967421
90.0	.973675	.972723	.971878	.971120	.970433	.969806	.969230
95.0	.975060	.974158	.973358	.972639	.971989	.971394	.970848
100.0	.976307	.975450	.974689	.974007	.973388	.972824	.972305
105.0	.977435	.976618	.975894	.975244	.974655	.974118	.973623
110.0	.978460	.977681	.976989	.976369	.975807	.975294	.974822
115.0	.979396	.978651	.977990	.977396	.976858	.976367	.975916
120.0	.980255	.979540	.978906	.978338	.977822	.977352	.976919
125.0	.981044	.980358	.979750	.979204	.978709	.978257	.977842
130.0	.981773	.981114	.980529	.980003	.979528	.979094	.978694
135.0	.982448	.981813	.981250	.980744	.980286	.979868	.979483
140.0	.983075	.982462	.981919	.981431	.980990	.980586	.980216
145.0	.983658	.983067	.982542	.982072	.981645	.981256	.980898
150.0	.984203	.983631	.983124	.982669	.982257	.981880	.981534
155.0	.984713	.984159	.983669	.983228	.982829	.982465	.982130
160.0	.985190	.984654	.984179	.983752	.983366	.983013	.982688
165.0	.985639	.985119	.984658	.984244	.983870	.983527	.983213
170.0	.986061	.985557	.985109	.984708	.984344	.984012	.983706
175.0	.986459	.985969	.985535	.985145	.984791	.984469	.984172
180.0	.986836	.986359	.985936	.985557	.985214	.984900	.984612
190.0	.987528	.987077	.986677	.986317	.985992	.985695	.985421
200.0	.988152	.987723	.987343	.987001	.986692	.986410	.986150
210.0	.988716	.988308	.987945	.987620	.987326	.987057	.986810
220.0	.989229	.988839	.988493	.988183	.987902	.987645	.987409
230.0	.989697	.989324	.988994	.988697	.988428	.988182	.987957
240.0	.990126	.989769	.989452	.989168	.988910	.988675	.988458

$\nu = 1$

Q \ n	9	10	11	12	13	14	15
250.0	.990521	.990178	.989874	.989601	.989353	.989128	.988920
260.0	.990886	.990556	.990263	.990001	.989763	.989546	.989346
270.0	.991223	.990906	.990624	.990371	.990142	.989933	.989741
280.0	.991537	.991231	.990959	.990715	.990494	.990292	.990107
290.0	.991829	.991533	.991271	.991035	.990822	.990627	.990448
300.0	.992101	.991815	.991562	.991334	.991128	.990940	.990767
310.0	.992356	.992079	.991834	.991613	.991414	.991232	.991064
320.0	.992595	.992327	.992089	.991876	.991682	.991506	.991344
330.0	.992819	.992559	.992329	.992122	.991934	.991763	.991606
340.0	.993030	.992778	.992554	.992353	.992172	.992005	.991853
350.0	.993229	.992984	.992767	.992572	.992395	.992234	.992086
360.0	.993417	.993179	.992968	.992778	.992606	.992450	.992305
370.0	.993595	.993364	.993158	.992973	.992806	.992654	.992513
380.0	.993764	.993538	.993338	.993158	.992996	.992847	.992710
390.0	.993924	.993704	.993509	.993334	.993175	.993030	.992897
400.0	.994076	.993861	.993671	.993500	.993346	.993205	.993075
420.0	.994358	.994154	.993972	.993810	.993663	.993528	.993405
440.0	.994614	.994419	.994246	.994091	.993951	.993822	.993704
460.0	.994848	.994662	.994497	.994348	.994214	.994091	.993978
480.0	.995063	.994884	.994726	.994584	.994455	.994337	.994229
500.0	.995261	.995089	.994937	.994800	.994677	.994564	.994460
520.0	.995443	.995278	.995132	.995000	.994881	.994773	.994673
540.0	.995612	.995453	.995312	.995185	.995071	.994966	.994870
560.0	.995768	.995615	.995479	.995357	.995247	.995146	.995053
580.0	.995914	.995766	.995635	.995517	.995411	.995313	.995224
600.0	.996050	.995908	.995781	.995667	.995564	.995470	.995383
620.0	.996178	.996040	.995917	.995807	.995707	.995616	.995532
640.0	.996297	.996163	.996044	.995938	.995841	.995753	.995672
660.0	.996410	.996280	.996164	.996061	.995967	.995882	.995803
680.0	.996515	.996389	.996277	.996177	.996086	.996003	.995926
700.0	.996615	.996492	.996383	.996286	.996198	.996117	.996043
720.0	.996709	.996590	.996484	.996389	.996303	.996225	.996153
740.0	.996798	.996682	.996579	.996487	.996403	.996327	.996257
760.0	.996882	.996769	.996669	.996579	.996498	.996423	.996355
780.0	.996962	.996852	.996754	.996667	.996588	.996515	.996449
800.0	.997038	.996931	.996836	.996750	.996673	.996602	.996537
820.0	.997110	.997006	.996913	.996829	.996754	.996685	.996622
840.0	.997179	.997077	.996986	.996905	.996831	.996764	.996702
860.0	.997244	.997145	.997056	.996977	.996905	.996839	.996779
880.0	.997307	.997210	.997123	.997046	.996975	.996911	.996852
900.0	.997367	.997272	.997187	.997111	.997043	.996980	.996922
920.0	.997424	.997331	.997248	.997174	.997107	.997045	.996989
940.0	.997479	.997388	.997307	.997234	.997168	.997108	.997053
960.0	.997532	.997442	.997363	.997292	.997227	.997169	.997114
980.0	.997582	.997494	.997417	.997347	.997284	.997226	.997173
1000.0	.997630	.997545	.997468	.997400	.997338	.997282	.997230
1100.0	.997846	.997768	.997699	.997636	.997580	.997529	.997482
1200.0	.998025	.997954	.997890	.997833	.997782	.997735	.997692
1300.0	.998177	.998111	.998053	.998000	.997953	.997909	.997869
1400.0	.998307	.998246	.998192	.998143	.998099	.998058	.998021

$\nu = 1$

Q\n	9	10	11	12	13	14	15
1500.0	.998420	.998363	.998312	.998267	.998226	.998188	.998153
1600.0	.998519	.998465	.998418	.998375	.998336	.998301	.998269
1700.0	.998606	.998556	.998511	.998471	.998434	.998401	.998371
1800.0	.998683	.998636	.998594	.998556	.998521	.998490	.998461
1900.0	.998753	.998708	.998668	.998632	.998599	.998569	.998542
2000.0	.998815	.998772	.998734	.998700	.998669	.998641	.998615

$\nu = 1$

Q \ n	16	17	18	19	20	22	24
0.0	.000000	.000000	.000000	.000000	.000000	.000000	.000000
0.1	.000000	.000000	.000000	.000000	.000000	.000000	.000000
0.2	.000000	.000000	.000000	.000000	.000000	.000000	.000000
0.3	.000000	.000000	.000000	.000000	.000000	.000000	.000000
0.4	.000000	.000000	.000000	.000000	.000000	.000000	.000000
0.5	.000007	.000004	.000003	.000002	.000001	.000000	.000000
0.6	.000045	.000031	.000022	.000015	.000011	.000006	.000003
0.7	.000202	.000149	.000111	.000084	.000065	.000039	.000024
0.8	.000648	.000505	.000398	.000316	.000254	.000168	.000115
0.9	.001644	.001334	.001093	.000903	.000753	.000534	.000389
1.0	.003501	.002931	.002475	.002106	.001804	.001350	.001033
1.2	.010928	.009566	.008429	.007472	.006660	.005369	.004402
1.4	.024423	.022013	.019947	.018163	.016611	.014056	.012055
1.6	.044041	.040506	.037420	.034707	.032307	.028262	.024995
1.8	.068777	.064184	.060121	.056505	.053266	.047715	.043136
2.0	.097191	.091687	.086772	.082355	.078366	.071442	.065640
2.2	.127856	.121618	.116005	.110928	.106310	.098221	.091362
2.4	.159576	.152776	.146624	.141027	.135911	.126885	.119160
2.6	.191440	.184232	.177681	.171697	.166204	.156457	.148056
2.8	.222803	.215315	.208486	.202227	.196463	.186188	.177281
3.0	.253233	.245571	.238563	.232121	.226174	.215533	.206265
3.2	.282463	.274710	.267602	.261054	.254994	.244119	.234611
3.4	.310346	.302567	.295420	.288823	.282708	.271705	.262054
3.6	.336815	.329058	.321920	.315321	.309195	.298147	.288431
3.8	.361859	.354163	.347070	.340504	.334400	.323373	.313653
4.0	.385507	.377898	.370878	.364371	.358315	.347359	.337682
4.2	.407806	.400306	.393378	.386950	.380963	.370115	.360517
4.4	.428822	.421444	.414623	.408289	.402383	.391672	.382181
4.6	.448623	.441377	.434673	.428443	.422630	.412076	.402713
4.8	.467284	.460177	.453597	.447477	.441764	.431382	.422160
5.0	.484877	.477912	.471460	.465456	.459847	.449647	.440578
5.2	.501473	.494653	.488330	.482444	.476943	.466930	.458021
5.4	.517140	.510465	.504273	.498506	.493113	.483292	.474546
5.6	.531944	.525411	.519350	.513701	.508418	.498790	.490210
5.8	.545943	.539551	.533619	.528088	.522913	.513478	.505064
6.0	.559194	.552941	.547135	.541721	.536653	.527409	.519161
6.4	.583656	.577672	.572112	.566923	.562064	.553194	.545272
6.8	.605703	.599973	.594646	.589673	.585014	.576503	.568895
7.2	.625649	.620159	.615053	.610284	.605814	.597644	.590336
7.6	.643765	.638500	.633601	.629024	.624733	.616885	.609862
8.0	.660279	.655224	.650519	.646123	.641999	.634456	.627701
8.4	.675384	.670526	.666003	.661776	.657810	.650552	.644050
8.8	.689246	.684572	.680220	.676151	.672333	.665344	.659081
9.2	.702007	.697506	.693314	.689394	.685714	.678977	.672938
9.6	.713790	.709450	.705408	.701627	.698077	.691578	.685749
10.0	.724699	.720511	.716609	.712958	.709531	.703254	.697623
11.0	.748720	.744871	.741284	.737927	.734774	.728998	.723813
12.0	.768953	.765396	.762079	.758975	.756059	.750714	.745915
13.0	.786215	.782910	.779828	.776943	.774233	.769263	.764800
14.0	.801108	.798023	.795146	.792452	.789921	.785280	.781111

$\nu = 1$

Q \ n	16	17	18	19	20	22	24
15.0	.814081	.811190	.808494	.805969	.803596	.799244	.795334
16.0	.825481	.822762	.820225	.817849	.815616	.811521	.807840
17.0	.835575	.833008	.830614	.828371	.826263	.822397	.818921
18.0	.844574	.842144	.839877	.837753	.835757	.832096	.828804
19.0	.852645	.850338	.848186	.846170	.844275	.840798	.837673
20.0	.859923	.857728	.855680	.853762	.851958	.848649	.845674
22.0	.872527	.870526	.868659	.866910	.865266	.862248	.859535
24.0	.883059	.881221	.879506	.877899	.876388	.873616	.871122
26.0	.891989	.890290	.888704	.887218	.885821	.883257	.880951
28.0	.899656	.898076	.896601	.895220	.893921	.891536	.889392
30.0	.906309	.904833	.903455	.902164	.900951	.898723	.896719
32.0	.912137	.910752	.909459	.908248	.907109	.905018	.903138
34.0	.917284	.915979	.914761	.913620	.912548	.910578	.908807
36.0	.921862	.920629	.919478	.918400	.917386	.915525	.913851
38.0	.925961	.924792	.923701	.922679	.921718	.919954	.918367
40.0	.929651	.928541	.927504	.926533	.925619	.923942	.922434
45.0	.937448	.936460	.935538	.934674	.933861	.932369	.931027
50.0	.943691	.942801	.941971	.941193	.940461	.939117	.937908
55.0	.948802	.947992	.947237	.946529	.945864	.944642	.943542
60.0	.953062	.952320	.951628	.950979	.950368	.949248	.948239
65.0	.956669	.955984	.955344	.954745	.954181	.953146	.952216
70.0	.959761	.959124	.958530	.957974	.957450	.956489	.955625
75.0	.962441	.961847	.961292	.960773	.960284	.959387	.958580
80.0	.964787	.964230	.963710	.963223	.962764	.961923	.961166
85.0	.966857	.966332	.965843	.965384	.964953	.964161	.963449
90.0	.968697	.968202	.967739	.967306	.966899	.966151	.965478
95.0	.970343	.969874	.969436	.969026	.968640	.967931	.967294
100.0	.971826	.971380	.970964	.970574	.970207	.969534	.968928
105.0	.973167	.972742	.972346	.971974	.971625	.970984	.970407
110.0	.974386	.973981	.973602	.973248	.972914	.972302	.971752
115.0	.975499	.975111	.974750	.974410	.974092	.973506	.972979
120.0	.976520	.976148	.975801	.975476	.975171	.974610	.974105
125.0	.977458	.977102	.976769	.976457	.976163	.975625	.975140
130.0	.978325	.977982	.977662	.977362	.977080	.976562	.976096
135.0	.979128	.978798	.978489	.978200	.977929	.977430	.976981
140.0	.979873	.979555	.979257	.978979	.978717	.978236	.977803
145.0	.980567	.980259	.979972	.979703	.979450	.978986	.978568
150.0	.981215	.980917	.980640	.980380	.980135	.979686	.979282
155.0	.981820	.981533	.981264	.981013	.980776	.980341	.979950
160.0	.982388	.982110	.981850	.981606	.981377	.980956	.980577
165.0	.982922	.982652	.982399	.982163	.981941	.981533	.981165
170.0	.983424	.983162	.982917	.982688	.982472	.982076	.981719
175.0	.983898	.983643	.983405	.983182	.982973	.982588	.982241
180.0	.984345	.984097	.983866	.983649	.983445	.983071	.982735
190.0	.985169	.984934	.984715	.984510	.984317	.983962	.983643
200.0	.985910	.985687	.985479	.985284	.985101	.984764	.984461
210.0	.986581	.986369	.986171	.985985	.985810	.985489	.985201
220.0	.987191	.986988	.986799	.986622	.986455	.986149	.985873
230.0	.987748	.987554	.987373	.987203	.987044	.986751	.986488
240.0	.988258	.988073	.987899	.987737	.987584	.987303	.987050

$\nu = 1$

Q \ n	16	17	18	19	20	22	24
250.0	.988728	.988550	.988383	.988227	.988080	.987811	.987568
260.0	.989161	.988990	.988830	.988680	.988539	.988280	.988046
270.0	.989563	.989398	.989244	.989099	.988963	.988714	.988489
280.0	.989936	.989776	.989628	.989488	.989357	.989117	.988900
290.0	.990283	.990129	.989985	.989851	.989724	.989492	.989283
300.0	.990607	.990458	.990319	.990189	.990067	.989842	.989640
310.0	.990910	.990766	.990631	.990506	.990387	.990170	.989974
320.0	.991194	.991054	.990924	.990802	.990688	.990477	.990288
330.0	.991460	.991325	.991199	.991081	.990970	.990766	.990582
340.0	.991712	.991580	.991458	.991343	.991235	.991037	.990859
350.0	.991948	.991821	.991702	.991591	.991486	.991293	.991120
360.0	.992172	.992048	.991933	.991824	.991722	.991535	.991367
370.0	.992384	.992263	.992151	.992045	.991946	.991764	.991600
380.0	.992584	.992467	.992357	.992254	.992158	.991981	.991821
390.0	.992774	.992660	.992553	.992453	.992359	.992186	.992031
400.0	.992955	.992843	.992739	.992642	.992550	.992382	.992230
420.0	.993290	.993184	.993085	.992992	.992905	.992744	.992600
440.0	.993595	.993494	.993399	.993311	.993227	.993074	.992936
460.0	.993874	.993777	.993686	.993601	.993522	.993375	.993243
480.0	.994129	.994036	.993949	.993868	.993792	.993651	.993525
500.0	.994364	.994275	.994191	.994113	.994040	.993905	.993784
520.0	.994581	.994495	.994415	.994340	.994269	.994140	.994023
540.0	.994781	.994699	.994622	.994549	.994481	.994357	.994244
560.0	.994968	.994888	.994814	.994744	.994679	.994558	.994450
580.0	.995141	.995064	.994993	.994925	.994862	.994746	.994641
600.0	.995303	.995229	.995159	.995094	.995033	.994921	.994820
620.0	.995455	.995383	.995316	.995253	.995193	.995085	.994987
640.0	.995597	.995527	.995462	.995401	.995344	.995238	.995144
660.0	.995730	.995663	.995599	.995540	.995485	.995383	.995291
680.0	.995856	.995790	.995729	.995672	.995618	.995519	.995429
700.0	.995974	.995910	.995851	.995795	.995743	.995647	.995560
720.0	.996086	.996024	.995966	.995912	.995861	.995767	.995683
740.0	.996192	.996131	.996075	.996022	.995973	.995882	.995800
760.0	.996292	.996233	.996179	.996127	.996079	.995990	.995910
780.0	.996387	.996330	.996276	.996226	.996179	.996093	.996015
800.0	.996477	.996422	.996370	.996321	.996275	.996191	.996115
820.0	.996563	.996509	.996458	.996411	.996366	.996284	.996210
840.0	.996645	.996592	.996542	.996496	.996452	.996372	.996300
860.0	.996723	.996671	.996623	.996577	.996535	.996456	.996386
880.0	.996798	.996747	.996700	.996655	.996614	.996537	.996468
900.0	.996869	.996819	.996773	.996730	.996689	.996614	.996547
920.0	.996937	.996888	.996843	.996801	.996761	.996688	.996622
940.0	.997002	.996955	.996910	.996869	.996830	.996758	.996694
960.0	.997064	.997018	.996975	.996934	.996896	.996826	.996762
980.0	.997124	.997079	.997036	.996997	.996959	.996890	.996829
1000.0	.997182	.997137	.997096	.997057	.997020	.996953	.996892
1100.0	.997438	.997398	.997360	.997324	.997291	.997230	.997175
1200.0	.997652	.997614	.997580	.997547	.997517	.997460	.997410
1300.0	.997832	.997798	.997766	.997736	.997708	.997656	.997609
1400.0	.997987	.997955	.997925	.997898	.997871	.997823	.997780

$\nu = 1$

Q \ n	16	17	18	19	20	22	24
1500.0	.998121	.998092	.998064	.998038	.998013	.997968	.997928
1600.0	.998239	.998211	.998185	.998160	.998137	.998095	.998057
1700.0	.998342	.998316	.998292	.998269	.998247	.998207	.998172
1800.0	.998434	.998410	.998386	.998365	.998344	.998307	.998273
1900.0	.998517	.998493	.998471	.998451	.998432	.998396	.998364
2000.0	.998591	.998569	.998548	.998528	.998510	.998476	.998446

$\nu = 1$

Q \ n	26	28	30	32	34	36	38
0.0	.000000	.000000	.000000	.000000	.000000	.000000	.000000
0.2	.000000	.000000	.000000	.000000	.000000	.000000	.000000
0.4	.000000	.000000	.000000	.000000	.000000	.000000	.000000
0.6	.000002	.000001	.000001	.000000	.000000	.000000	.000000
0.8	.000080	.000057	.000042	.000031	.000023	.000018	.000014
1.0	.000805	.000637	.000512	.000417	.000343	.000285	.000239
1.2	.003661	.003083	.002625	.002256	.001955	.001708	.001502
1.4	.010457	.009161	.008094	.007205	.006457	.005820	.005274
1.6	.022313	.020077	.018192	.016584	.015199	.013997	.012945
1.8	.039300	.036043	.033247	.030823	.028703	.026834	.025176
2.0	.060708	.056463	.052773	.049534	.046669	.044116	.041828
2.2	.085466	.080341	.075841	.071856	.068301	.065108	.062223
2.4	.112465	.106598	.101408	.096781	.092625	.088869	.085456
2.6	.140726	.134263	.128512	.123357	.118703	.114476	.110617
2.8	.169467	.162543	.156355	.150782	.145730	.141125	.136904
3.0	.198100	.190835	.184317	.178427	.173070	.168170	.163667
3.2	.226204	.218699	.211945	.205824	.200241	.195122	.190405
3.4	.253495	.245834	.238922	.232641	.226900	.221625	.216754
3.6	.279793	.272043	.265035	.258655	.252812	.247433	.242457
3.8	.304993	.297208	.290156	.283723	.277823	.272383	.267344
4.0	.329045	.321268	.314210	.307765	.301844	.296377	.291307
4.2	.351938	.344200	.337170	.330741	.324828	.319363	.314288
4.4	.373685	.366014	.359036	.352647	.346765	.341322	.336265
4.6	.394321	.386735	.379827	.373497	.367663	.362261	.357236
4.8	.413887	.406401	.399578	.393320	.387548	.382200	.377221
5.0	.432434	.425058	.418331	.412155	.406456	.401171	.396248
5.2	.450013	.442756	.436132	.430047	.424428	.419213	.414354
5.4	.466680	.459546	.453030	.447041	.441508	.436370	.431580
5.6	.482488	.475480	.469076	.463187	.457742	.452685	.447968
5.8	.497488	.490608	.484318	.478530	.473178	.468203	.463562
6.0	.511730	.504979	.498803	.493119	.487859	.482970	.478406
6.4	.538128	.531632	.525684	.520206	.515134	.510416	.506008
6.8	.562028	.555781	.550057	.544782	.539894	.535345	.531094
7.2	.583736	.577727	.572219	.567140	.562433	.558049	.553950
7.6	.603515	.597734	.592433	.587542	.583006	.578781	.574830
8.0	.621594	.616030	.610924	.606213	.601842	.597769	.593958
8.4	.638170	.632810	.627891	.623349	.619135	.615207	.611530
8.8	.653414	.648247	.643503	.639122	.635056	.631265	.627716
9.2	.667472	.662487	.657909	.653680	.649755	.646093	.642665
9.6	.680472	.675659	.671237	.667152	.663359	.659820	.656507
10.0	.692525	.687873	.683599	.679650	.675982	.672560	.669354
11.0	.719117	.714830	.710889	.707246	.703862	.700704	.697744
12.0	.741567	.737596	.733945	.730569	.727431	.724502	.721757
13.0	.760754	.757059	.753660	.750517	.747595	.744867	.742310
14.0	.777331	.773877	.770700	.767762	.765030	.762478	.760086
15.0	.791788	.788548	.785567	.782809	.780244	.777849	.775604
16.0	.804503	.801452	.798645	.796048	.793633	.791377	.789261
17.0	.815769	.812888	.810236	.807783	.805501	.803369	.801370
18.0	.825819	.823089	.820578	.818253	.816091	.814071	.812177
19.0	.834838	.832245	.829860	.827652	.825598	.823679	.821879

ν = 1

Q\n	26	28	30	32	34	36	38
20.0	.842975	.840507	.838236	.836133	.834177	.832350	.830636
22.0	.857073	.854822	.852749	.850831	.849047	.847379	.845815
24.0	.868860	.866791	.864886	.863123	.861482	.859950	.858511
26.0	.878859	.876945	.875183	.873552	.872034	.870616	.869286
28.0	.887446	.885666	.884027	.882510	.881098	.879779	.878541
30.0	.894900	.893237	.891705	.890287	.888968	.887735	.886578
32.0	.901431	.899870	.898432	.897101	.895863	.894706	.893620
34.0	.907199	.905729	.904375	.903121	.901954	.900864	.899841
36.0	.912331	.910942	.909662	.908477	.907374	.906343	.905376
38.0	.916927	.915609	.914396	.913273	.912227	.911250	.910333
40.0	.921065	.919813	.918660	.917592	.916598	.915669	.914798
45.0	.929809	.928695	.927669	.926718	.925834	.925008	.924232
50.0	.936811	.935808	.934883	.934027	.933231	.932486	.931788
55.0	.942544	.941631	.940791	.940012	.939288	.938610	.937975
60.0	.947324	.946487	.945716	.945002	.944338	.943717	.943134
65.0	.951371	.950597	.949886	.949226	.948613	.948039	.947501
70.0	.954840	.954122	.953461	.952848	.952278	.951746	.951246
75.0	.957847	.957177	.956560	.955988	.955456	.954959	.954492
80.0	.960479	.959851	.959272	.958736	.958237	.957771	.957333
85.0	.962802	.962211	.961666	.961161	.960692	.960253	.959841
90.0	.964867	.964308	.963794	.963317	.962874	.962459	.962070
95.0	.966715	.966186	.965698	.965247	.964826	.964433	.964065
100.0	.968378	.967875	.967412	.966983	.966584	.966211	.965860
105.0	.969883	.969404	.968963	.968554	.968174	.967819	.967485
110.0	.971252	.970794	.970373	.969983	.969620	.969281	.968962
115.0	.972501	.972064	.971661	.971287	.970940	.970616	.970311
120.0	.973646	.973227	.972841	.972483	.972150	.971839	.971547
125.0	.974700	.974298	.973927	.973584	.973264	.972965	.972685
130.0	.975673	.975286	.974929	.974599	.974292	.974005	.973735
135.0	.976574	.976201	.975858	.975540	.975244	.974967	.974708
140.0	.977410	.977051	.976719	.976413	.976128	.975861	.975611
145.0	.978189	.977842	.977522	.977226	.976951	.976693	.976451
150.0	.978916	.978580	.978271	.977985	.977719	.977470	.977236
155.0	.979596	.979271	.978972	.978695	.978437	.978196	.977970
160.0	.980233	.979918	.979629	.979361	.979111	.978877	.978658
165.0	.980832	.980527	.980246	.979986	.979744	.979517	.979305
170.0	.981396	.981100	.980827	.980574	.980339	.980120	.979914
175.0	.981927	.981639	.981375	.981129	.980901	.980688	.980487
180.0	.982429	.982149	.981892	.981653	.981431	.981224	.981029
190.0	.983354	.983089	.982845	.982619	.982408	.982212	.982027
200.0	.984186	.983934	.983702	.983488	.983288	.983101	.982926
210.0	.984939	.984699	.984478	.984274	.984084	.983906	.983739
220.0	.985623	.985394	.985184	.984989	.984807	.984637	.984478
230.0	.986248	.986029	.985828	.985641	.985467	.985305	.985153
240.0	.986821	.986611	.986418	.986239	.986073	.985917	.985771
250.0	.987348	.987147	.986962	.986790	.986630	.986481	.986340
260.0	.987835	.987641	.987463	.987298	.987144	.987000	.986866
270.0	.988285	.988099	.987927	.987768	.987620	.987482	.987352
280.0	.988704	.988524	.988358	.988205	.988062	.987929	.987804
290.0	.989093	.988920	.988760	.988612	.988474	.988345	.988224

$\nu = 1$

Q\n	26	28	30	32	34	36	38
300.0	.989457	.989289	.989134	.988991	.988858	.988734	.988617
310.0	.989797	.989634	.989485	.989346	.989218	.989097	.988984
320.0	.990116	.989958	.989814	.989679	.989554	.989438	.989328
330.0	.990415	.990263	.990122	.989992	.989871	.989758	.989652
340.0	.990697	.990549	.990413	.990286	.990169	.990059	.989956
350.0	.990963	.990819	.990687	.990564	.990450	.990343	.990243
360.0	.991214	.991074	.990945	.990826	.990715	.990611	.990514
370.0	.991451	.991315	.991190	.991074	.990966	.990865	.990770
380.0	.991676	.991544	.991422	.991309	.991204	.991105	.991013
390.0	.991890	.991761	.991642	.991532	.991429	.991333	.991244
400.0	.992092	.991967	.991851	.991743	.991643	.991550	.991462
420.0	.992469	.992349	.992239	.992137	.992041	.991952	.991869
440.0	.992811	.992697	.992592	.992494	.992403	.992318	.992239
460.0	.993124	.993014	.992914	.992820	.992733	.992652	.992576
480.0	.993410	.993305	.993209	.993119	.993036	.992958	.992885
500.0	.993674	.993573	.993481	.993395	.993315	.993240	.993170
520.0	.993917	.993820	.993731	.993649	.993572	.993500	.993433
540.0	.994143	.994049	.993963	.993884	.993810	.993741	.993676
560.0	.994352	.994262	.994179	.994102	.994031	.993964	.993902
580.0	.994546	.994460	.994380	.994306	.994237	.994172	.994112
600.0	.994728	.994644	.994567	.994496	.994429	.994367	.994308
620.0	.994898	.994817	.994742	.994673	.994609	.994548	.994492
640.0	.995058	.994979	.994907	.994840	.994777	.994719	.994664
660.0	.995208	.995131	.995061	.994996	.994935	.994879	.994826
680.0	.995348	.995274	.995206	.995143	.995084	.995029	.994978
700.0	.995481	.995409	.995343	.995282	.995225	.995171	.995121
720.0	.995607	.995537	.995473	.995413	.995357	.995306	.995257
740.0	.995726	.995658	.995595	.995537	.995483	.995432	.995385
760.0	.995838	.995772	.995711	.995654	.995602	.995553	.995506
780.0	.995945	.995880	.995821	.995766	.995715	.995667	.995622
800.0	.996046	.995983	.995925	.995872	.995822	.995775	.995731
820.0	.996143	.996081	.996025	.995972	.995924	.995878	.995835
840.0	.996234	.996175	.996119	.996068	.996021	.995976	.995934
860.0	.996322	.996263	.996210	.996160	.996113	.996070	.996029
880.0	.996406	.996348	.996296	.996247	.996202	.996159	.996119
900.0	.996485	.996430	.996378	.996330	.996286	.996244	.996205
920.0	.996562	.996507	.996457	.996410	.996367	.996326	.996288
940.0	.996635	.996581	.996532	.996486	.996444	.996404	.996367
960.0	.996705	.996653	.996604	.996560	.996518	.996479	.996443
980.0	.996772	.996721	.996674	.996630	.996589	.996551	.996515
1000.0	.996837	.996787	.996740	.996697	.996657	.996620	.996585
1100.0	.997124	.997079	.997037	.996998	.996961	.996927	.996895
1200.0	.997364	.997322	.997284	.997248	.997214	.997183	.997154
1300.0	.997567	.997528	.997492	.997459	.997429	.997400	.997373
1400.0	.997741	.997705	.997672	.997641	.997612	.997586	.997561
1500.0	.997891	.997858	.997827	.997798	.997772	.997747	.997723
1600.0	.998023	.997992	.997963	.997936	.997911	.997887	.997866
1700.0	.998139	.998110	.998082	.998057	.998034	.998012	.997991
1800.0	.998243	.998215	.998189	.998165	.998143	.998122	.998103
1900.0	.998335	.998309	.998284	.998262	.998241	.998221	.998203

$\nu = 1$

Q \ n	26	28	30	32	34	36	38
2000.0	.998418	.998393	.998370	.998349	.998329	.998310	.998292

$\nu = 1$

Q\n	40	50	60	70	80	90	100
0.0	.000000	.000000	.000000	.000000	.000000	.000000	.000000
0.1	.000000	.000000	.000000	.000000	.000000	.000000	.000000
0.2	.000000	.000000	.000000	.000000	.000000	.000000	.000000
0.3	.000000	.000000	.000000	.000000	.000000	.000000	.000000
0.4	.000000	.000000	.000000	.000000	.000000	.000000	.000000
0.5	.000000	.000000	.000000	.000000	.000000	.000000	.000000
0.6	.000000	.000000	.000000	.000000	.000000	.000000	.000000
0.7	.000001	.000000	.000000	.000000	.000000	.000000	.000000
0.8	.000011	.000004	.000001	.000001	.000000	.000000	.000000
0.9	.000055	.000023	.000011	.000006	.000003	.000002	.000001
1.0	.000202	.000096	.000052	.000031	.000019	.000013	.000009
1.1	.000570	.000305	.000181	.000116	.000079	.000056	.000041
1.2	.001329	.000776	.000497	.000340	.000244	.000182	.000140
1.3	.002675	.001676	.001140	.000820	.000616	.000478	.000381
1.4	.004803	.003186	.002272	.001703	.001326	.001062	.000870
1.5	.007878	.005477	.004060	.003147	.002522	.002073	.001739
1.6	.012018	.008685	.006649	.005299	.004351	.003654	.003125
1.7	.017287	.012907	.010152	.008280	.006937	.005932	.005155
1.8	.023696	.018187	.014637	.012175	.010375	.009007	.007936
1.9	.031211	.024529	.020131	.017026	.014723	.012948	.011542
2.0	.039765	.031895	.026621	.022842	.020001	.017787	.016014
2.1	.049265	.040220	.034064	.029595	.026197	.023524	.021363
2.2	.059603	.049419	.042394	.037236	.033275	.030132	.027572
2.3	.070666	.059395	.051528	.045693	.041175	.037561	.034599
2.4	.082339	.070045	.061374	.054886	.049824	.045749	.042388
2.5	.094511	.081265	.071837	.064727	.059143	.054621	.050872
2.6	.107077	.092956	.082822	.075127	.069047	.064098	.059975
2.7	.119942	.105023	.094237	.085997	.079452	.074099	.069621
2.8	.133019	.117379	.105997	.097253	.090275	.084544	.079733
2.9	.146231	.129944	.118021	.108817	.101440	.095358	.090235
3.0	.159509	.142648	.130238	.120616	.112873	.106468	.101056
3.1	.172796	.155428	.142584	.132584	.124508	.117809	.112132
3.2	.186040	.168230	.155000	.144662	.136287	.129319	.123400
3.3	.199199	.181006	.167437	.156798	.148155	.140945	.134807
3.4	.212238	.193716	.179852	.168947	.160065	.152638	.146302
3.5	.225125	.206325	.192206	.181069	.171975	.164356	.157843
3.6	.237836	.218805	.204467	.193129	.183850	.176060	.169390
3.7	.250352	.231132	.216610	.205098	.195658	.187719	.180910
3.8	.262657	.243285	.228610	.216952	.207374	.199304	.192373
3.9	.274738	.255249	.240450	.228669	.218973	.210792	.203755
4.0	.286586	.267011	.252114	.240232	.230437	.222161	.215033
4.1	.298194	.278563	.263590	.251628	.241751	.233395	.226190
4.2	.309558	.289895	.274869	.262844	.252902	.244480	.237210
4.3	.320676	.301003	.285943	.273872	.263879	.255404	.248081
4.4	.331546	.311884	.296806	.284705	.274674	.266158	.258792
4.5	.342169	.322536	.307456	.295338	.285281	.276735	.269336
4.6	.352545	.332957	.317890	.305767	.295695	.287128	.279705
4.7	.362678	.343149	.328107	.315990	.305913	.297334	.289895
4.8	.372570	.353113	.338108	.326006	.315933	.307350	.299902
4.9	.382224	.362852	.347892	.335815	.325754	.317174	.309724

$\nu = 1$

Q\n	40	50	60	70	80	90	100
5.0	.391646	.372367	.357462	.345417	.335375	.326805	.319359
5.1	.400840	.381662	.366820	.354815	.344798	.336244	.328807
5.2	.409809	.390741	.375969	.364010	.354024	.345491	.338068
5.3	.418560	.399608	.384912	.373005	.363055	.354548	.347143
5.4	.427097	.408267	.393652	.381802	.371893	.363416	.356034
5.5	.435426	.416723	.402193	.390404	.380541	.372097	.364741
5.6	.443551	.424980	.410540	.398816	.389001	.380595	.373268
5.7	.451479	.433042	.418696	.407041	.397278	.388912	.381616
5.8	.459215	.440915	.426666	.415082	.405373	.397050	.389789
5.9	.466763	.448604	.434454	.422943	.413292	.405014	.397790
6.0	.474129	.456112	.442064	.430630	.421037	.412807	.405621
6.4	.501877	.484441	.470813	.459700	.450361	.442336	.435320
6.8	.527107	.510257	.497063	.486285	.477216	.469412	.462583
7.2	.550103	.533834	.521072	.510634	.501839	.494265	.487630
7.6	.571120	.555415	.543079	.532976	.524456	.517112	.510673
8.0	.590380	.575218	.563295	.553521	.545271	.538154	.531910
8.4	.608077	.593436	.581910	.572454	.564467	.557572	.551520
8.8	.624382	.610238	.599093	.589943	.582209	.575529	.569663
9.2	.639445	.625772	.614992	.606134	.598644	.592171	.586484
9.6	.653393	.640169	.629735	.621158	.613900	.607626	.602111
10.0	.666342	.653543	.643438	.635128	.628093	.622009	.616660
11.0	.694962	.683132	.673780	.666081	.659558	.653913	.648946
12.0	.719176	.708194	.699504	.692344	.686274	.681018	.676391
13.0	.739905	.729667	.721560	.714877	.709208	.704297	.699971
14.0	.757836	.748255	.740664	.734402	.729089	.724484	.720427
15.0	.773491	.764491	.757358	.751472	.746476	.742144	.738327
16.0	.787271	.778790	.772065	.766515	.761802	.757715	.754112
17.0	.799489	.791473	.785115	.779865	.775407	.771540	.768131
18.0	.810394	.802796	.796768	.791790	.787561	.783893	.780658
19.0	.820186	.812965	.807235	.802503	.798482	.794994	.791918
20.0	.829023	.822146	.816688	.812179	.808347	.805022	.802090
22.0	.844343	.838065	.833080	.828961	.825461	.822423	.819743
24.0	.857158	.851384	.846800	.843011	.839790	.836994	.834527
26.0	.868033	.862691	.858447	.854940	.851958	.849369	.847085
28.0	.877376	.872406	.868457	.865193	.862417	.860008	.857882
30.0	.885488	.880842	.877150	.874098	.871503	.869250	.867261
32.0	.892597	.888235	.884770	.881904	.879467	.877351	.875484
34.0	.898878	.894768	.891502	.888802	.886506	.884511	.882752
36.0	.904466	.900581	.897494	.894941	.892770	.890884	.889220
38.0	.909470	.905787	.902860	.900439	.898380	.896592	.895015
40.0	.913977	.910476	.907693	.905392	.903434	.901735	.900235
45.0	.923502	.920386	.917909	.915860	.914118	.912604	.911269
50.0	.931130	.928323	.926092	.924246	.922676	.921313	.920109
55.0	.937376	.934823	.932793	.931114	.929685	.928445	.927350
60.0	.942585	.940243	.938381	.936841	.935531	.934393	.933389
65.0	.946994	.944831	.943112	.941690	.940480	.939429	.938502
70.0	.950775	.948766	.947169	.945848	.944724	.943748	.942886
75.0	.954053	.952177	.950686	.949453	.948404	.947492	.946688
80.0	.956921	.955163	.953765	.952608	.951624	.950769	.950015
85.0	.959453	.957797	.956481	.955393	.954466	.953662	.952952

$\nu = 1$

Q \ n	40	50	60	70	80	90	100
90.0	.961704	.960140	.958897	.957868	.956993	.956233	.955562
95.0	.963718	.962236	.961058	.960084	.959255	.958535	.957899
100.0	.965531	.964123	.963004	.962078	.961290	.960606	.960002
105.0	.967171	.965830	.964764	.963882	.963132	.962480	.961905
110.0	.968662	.967382	.966365	.965523	.964807	.964185	.963636
115.0	.970024	.968800	.967826	.967021	.966336	.965741	.965216
120.0	.971272	.970099	.969166	.968394	.967738	.967167	.966664
125.0	.972421	.971295	.970399	.969658	.969028	.968480	.967997
130.0	.973481	.972398	.971537	.970824	.970218	.969692	.969227
135.0	.974463	.973420	.972591	.971905	.971321	.970814	.970366
140.0	.975375	.974369	.973569	.972908	.972345	.971856	.971424
145.0	.976224	.975252	.974480	.973841	.973298	.972826	.972409
150.0	.977016	.976077	.975331	.974713	.974188	.973731	.973328
155.0	.977757	.976849	.976126	.975528	.975020	.974578	.974188
160.0	.978452	.977572	.976872	.976293	.975800	.975372	.974995
165.0	.979105	.978251	.977573	.977011	.976533	.976118	.975752
170.0	.979719	.978891	.978232	.977687	.977223	.976821	.976465
175.0	.980299	.979494	.978854	.978324	.977874	.977483	.977137
180.0	.980846	.980063	.979441	.978926	.978488	.978108	.977772
190.0	.981854	.981112	.980523	.980035	.979620	.979260	.978942
200.0	.982761	.982057	.981497	.981033	.980639	.980297	.979994
210.0	.983582	.982911	.982378	.981936	.981561	.981235	.980947
220.0	.984328	.983688	.983178	.982757	.982399	.982088	.981813
230.0	.985009	.984397	.983910	.983507	.983164	.982866	.982603
240.0	.985634	.985047	.984580	.984194	.983865	.983580	.983328
250.0	.986208	.985645	.985197	.984826	.984511	.984237	.983995
260.0	.986739	.986197	.985766	.985410	.985106	.984843	.984610
270.0	.987230	.986708	.986293	.985950	.985658	.985404	.985180
280.0	.987686	.987183	.986783	.986452	.986170	.985926	.985710
290.0	.988110	.987625	.987238	.986919	.986647	.986411	.986202
300.0	.988507	.988037	.987664	.987355	.987092	.986864	.986662
310.0	.988877	.988423	.988062	.987763	.987508	.987287	.987092
320.0	.989225	.988785	.988435	.988145	.987899	.987685	.987496
330.0	.989552	.989125	.988785	.988504	.988265	.988058	.987875
340.0	.989859	.989444	.989115	.988842	.988610	.988409	.988231
350.0	.990149	.989746	.989426	.989161	.988936	.988740	.988567
360.0	.990422	.990031	.989720	.989462	.989243	.989053	.988885
370.0	.990681	.990300	.989997	.989747	.989534	.989349	.989185
380.0	.990926	.990555	.990261	.990017	.989809	.989629	.989470
390.0	.991159	.990798	.990510	.990273	.990071	.989895	.989740
400.0	.991380	.991028	.990748	.990516	.990319	.990148	.989996
420.0	.991790	.991455	.991188	.990968	.990780	.990617	.990473
440.0	.992164	.991843	.991589	.991378	.991199	.991043	.990906
460.0	.992504	.992198	.991954	.991753	.991582	.991433	.991301
480.0	.992817	.992523	.992290	.992097	.991932	.991790	.991664
500.0	.993104	.992822	.992598	.992413	.992255	.992118	.991997
520.0	.993369	.993098	.992883	.992704	.992553	.992421	.992305
540.0	.993615	.993354	.993146	.992975	.992829	.992702	.992590
560.0	.993843	.993591	.993391	.993226	.993085	.992962	.992854
580.0	.994055	.993812	.993619	.993459	.993323	.993205	.993101

$\nu = 1$

Q \ n	40	50	60	70	80	90	100
600.0	.994253	.994018	.993832	.993677	.993546	.993432	.993331
620.0	.994439	.994211	.994031	.993881	.993754	.993644	.993546
640.0	.994612	.994392	.994217	.994072	.993949	.993842	.993748
660.0	.994776	.994562	.994392	.994252	.994133	.994029	.993937
680.0	.994929	.994722	.994557	.994421	.994305	.994204	.994115
700.0	.995074	.994873	.994713	.994580	.994468	.994370	.994284
720.0	.995211	.995015	.994860	.994731	.994621	.994526	.994442
740.0	.995340	.995150	.994999	.994873	.994767	.994674	.994593
760.0	.995463	.995278	.995130	.995008	.994905	.994814	.994735
780.0	.995579	.995399	.995255	.995136	.995035	.994947	.994870
800.0	.995690	.995514	.995374	.995258	.995159	.995074	.994998
820.0	.995795	.995623	.995487	.995374	.995277	.995194	.995120
840.0	.995895	.995727	.995594	.995484	.995390	.995308	.995236
860.0	.995991	.995827	.995696	.995589	.995497	.995417	.995347
880.0	.996082	.995922	.995794	.995689	.995599	.995522	.995453
900.0	.996169	.996012	.995888	.995785	.995697	.995621	.995554
920.0	.996252	.996099	.995977	.995876	.995791	.995716	.995651
940.0	.996332	.996182	.996063	.995964	.995880	.995807	.995743
960.0	.996408	.996261	.996145	.996048	.995966	.995895	.995832
980.0	.996482	.996338	.996223	.996129	.996048	.995979	.995917
1000.0	.996552	.996411	.996299	.996206	.996127	.996059	.995998
1100.0	.996865	.996737	.996635	.996551	.996479	.996417	.996362
1200.0	.997127	.997009	.996916	.996839	.996773	.996716	.996665
1300.0	.997348	.997239	.997153	.997082	.997021	.996968	.996922
1400.0	.997537	.997436	.997356	.997290	.997234	.997185	.997142
1500.0	.997701	.997607	.997533	.997471	.997418	.997373	.997332
1600.0	.997845	.997757	.997687	.997629	.997580	.997537	.997499
1700.0	.997972	.997889	.997823	.997768	.997722	.997682	.997646
1800.0	.998084	.998006	.997944	.997892	.997849	.997811	.997777
1900.0	.998185	.998111	.998052	.998003	.997962	.997926	.997894
2000.0	.998276	.998205	.998149	.998103	.998064	.998029	.997999

$\nu = 2$

Q \ n	2	3	4	5	6	7	8
0.0	.000000	.000000	.000000	.000000	.000000	.000000	.000000
0.1	.049938	.002749	.000168	.000011	.000001	.000000	.000000
0.2	.099504	.010905	.001326	.000176	.000025	.000004	.000001
0.3	.148340	.024205	.004372	.000862	.000183	.000042	.000010
0.4	.196116	.042230	.010042	.002601	.000725	.000215	.000067
0.5	.242536	.064443	.018853	.005990	.002041	.000738	.000281
0.6	.287348	.090223	.031086	.011592	.004620	.001949	.000863
0.7	.330350	.118906	.046791	.019854	.008972	.004277	.002134
0.8	.371391	.149822	.065818	.031057	.015552	.008186	.004496
0.9	.410365	.182325	.087860	.045299	.024695	.014104	.008379
1.0	.447214	.215818	.112501	.062502	.036585	.022362	.014177
1.2	.514496	.283723	.167655	.104803	.068561	.046556	.032612
1.4	.573462	.350178	.227406	.155162	.110134	.080719	.060749
1.6	.624695	.412981	.288359	.210270	.158679	.123097	.097679
1.8	.668965	.470904	.347967	.267111	.211259	.171118	.141325
2.0	.707107	.523439	.404553	.323336	.265258	.222165	.189224
2.2	.739940	.570553	.457163	.377327	.318650	.274009	.239086
2.4	.768221	.612499	.505377	.428095	.370033	.324967	.289058
2.6	.792624	.649684	.549131	.475134	.418538	.373892	.337786
2.8	.813733	.682575	.588585	.518275	.463704	.420079	.384369
3.0	.832050	.711650	.624022	.557569	.505360	.463161	.428269
3.2	.847998	.737363	.655781	.593200	.543526	.503006	.469220
3.4	.861934	.760131	.684222	.625422	.578345	.539642	.507142
3.6	.874157	.780327	.709693	.654522	.610023	.573196	.542085
3.8	.884918	.798280	.732523	.680791	.638800	.603851	.574174
4.0	.894427	.814278	.753011	.704511	.664927	.631819	.603580
4.2	.902861	.828571	.771428	.725948	.688650	.657321	.630496
4.4	.910366	.841374	.788014	.745343	.710202	.680574	.655121
4.6	.917070	.852872	.802981	.762916	.729801	.701788	.677651
4.8	.923077	.863227	.816515	.778865	.747644	.721157	.698274
5.0	.928477	.872577	.828781	.793365	.763912	.738860	.717167
5.2	.933346	.881040	.839921	.806573	.778766	.755061	.734491
5.4	.937749	.888721	.850061	.818624	.792351	.769907	.750395
5.6	.941742	.895709	.859311	.829643	.804797	.783532	.765014
5.8	.945373	.902082	.867766	.839735	.816217	.796054	.778470
6.0	.948683	.907906	.875511	.848997	.826714	.807581	.790873
6.4	.954480	.918140	.889157	.865356	.845293	.828022	.812904
6.8	.959366	.926799	.900740	.879281	.861148	.845504	.831783
7.2	.963518	.934183	.910645	.891216	.874765	.860545	.848053
7.6	.967075	.940525	.919173	.901512	.886531	.873562	.862153
8.0	.970142	.946009	.926560	.910446	.896757	.884891	.874439
8.4	.972806	.950780	.932999	.918244	.905693	.894802	.885198
8.8	.975133	.954955	.938641	.925086	.913543	.903516	.894666
9.2	.977176	.958627	.943610	.931119	.920471	.911213	.903036
9.6	.978980	.961873	.948008	.936463	.926613	.918043	.910468
10.0	.980581	.964756	.951917	.941218	.932083	.924128	.917093
11.0	.983870	.970693	.959979	.951034	.943385	.936715	.930809
12.0	.986394	.975257	.966188	.958606	.952114	.946447	.941425
13.0	.988372	.978839	.971067	.964562	.958987	.954117	.949797
14.0	.989949	.981701	.974968	.969328	.964492	.960264	.956511

$\nu = 2$

Q\n	2	3	4	5	6	7	8
15.0	.991228	.984021	.978134	.973200	.968966	.965262	.961973
16.0	.992278	.985929	.980739	.976387	.972650	.969380	.966475
17.0	.993151	.987515	.982907	.979039	.975718	.972810	.970227
18.0	.993884	.988849	.984729	.981271	.978300	.975698	.973386
19.0	.994505	.989980	.986276	.983166	.980493	.978151	.976070
20.0	.995037	.990948	.987600	.984788	.982370	.980253	.978369
22.0	.995893	.992507	.989734	.987403	.985398	.983641	.982079
24.0	.996546	.993697	.991361	.989398	.987710	.986229	.984912
26.0	.997054	.994624	.992631	.990956	.989514	.988250	.987125
28.0	.997459	.995361	.993641	.992194	.990949	.989857	.988885
30.0	.997785	.995957	.994457	.993195	.992109	.991157	.990309
32.0	.998053	.996444	.995125	.994015	.993060	.992222	.991476
34.0	.998274	.996849	.995680	.994696	.993849	.993106	.992444
36.0	.998460	.997189	.996145	.995267	.994511	.993847	.993257
38.0	.998618	.997476	.996539	.995750	.995071	.994476	.993945
40.0	.998752	.997721	.996875	.996163	.995550	.995012	.994533
45.0	.999014	.998199	.997530	.996967	.996482	.996056	.995677
50.0	.999201	.998541	.997998	.997542	.997149	.996804	.996497
55.0	.999339	.998794	.998345	.997968	.997643	.997358	.997104
60.0	.999445	.998986	.998609	.998292	.998019	.997779	.997565
65.0	.999527	.999136	.998815	.998544	.998312	.998107	.997925
70.0	.999592	.999255	.998978	.998745	.998544	.998368	.998211
75.0	.999645	.999351	.999110	.998906	.998731	.998578	.998441
80.0	.999688	.999429	.999217	.999039	.998885	.998750	.998630
85.0	.999723	.999495	.999307	.999148	.999012	.998892	.998786
90.0	.999753	.999549	.999381	.999240	.999119	.999012	.998917
95.0	.999778	.999595	.999445	.999318	.999209	.999113	.999028
100.0	.999800	.999635	.999499	.999385	.999286	.999200	.999123
105.0	.999819	.999669	.999546	.999442	.999352	.999274	.999204
110.0	.999835	.999698	.999586	.999491	.999410	.999338	.999275
115.0	.999849	.999724	.999621	.999535	.999460	.999395	.999336
120.0	.999861	.999746	.999652	.999573	.999504	.999444	.999391
125.0	.999872	.999766	.999679	.999606	.999543	.999488	.999438
130.0	.999882	.999784	.999703	.999636	.999577	.999526	.999481
135.0	.999890	.999800	.999725	.999662	.999608	.999561	.999518
140.0	.999898	.999814	.999744	.999686	.999636	.999592	.999552
145.0	.999905	.999826	.999762	.999707	.999660	.999619	.999583
150.0	.999911	.999838	.999777	.999726	.999683	.999644	.999610
155.0	.999917	.999848	.999791	.999744	.999703	.999667	.999635
160.0	.999922	.999857	.999804	.999760	.999721	.999687	.999657
165.0	.999927	.999866	.999816	.999774	.999738	.999706	.999678
170.0	.999931	.999874	.999827	.999787	.999753	.999723	.999696
175.0	.999935	.999881	.999836	.999799	.999767	.999739	.999713
180.0	.999938	.999887	.999845	.999810	.999780	.999753	.999729
190.0	.999945	.999899	.999861	.999829	.999802	.999778	.999757
200.0	.999950	.999909	.999875	.999846	.999821	.999800	.999781
210.0	.999955	.999917	.999886	.999860	.999838	.999818	.999801
220.0	.999959	.999925	.999896	.999873	.999852	.999835	.999819
230.0	.999962	.999931	.999905	.999884	.999865	.999849	.999834
240.0	.999965	.999937	.999913	.999893	.999876	.999861	.999848

$\nu = 2$

Q \ n	2	3	4	5	6	7	8
250.0	.999968	.999942	.999920	.999902	.999886	.999872	.999860
260.0	.999970	.999946	.999926	.999909	.999894	.999882	.999870
270.0	.999973	.999950	.999931	.999916	.999902	.999890	.999880
280.0	.999974	.999953	.999936	.999921	.999909	.999898	.999888
290.0	.999976	.999957	.999940	.999927	.999915	.999905	.999896
300.0	.999978	.999959	.999944	.999932	.999921	.999911	.999902
310.0	.999979	.999962	.999948	.999936	.999926	.999917	.999909
320.0	.999980	.999964	.999951	.999940	.999930	.999922	.999914
330.0	.999982	.999966	.999954	.999943	.999934	.999926	.999919
340.0	.999983	.999968	.999957	.999947	.999938	.999931	.999924
350.0	.999984	.999970	.999959	.999950	.999942	.999935	.999928
360.0	.999985	.999972	.999961	.999952	.999945	.999938	.999932
370.0	.999985	.999973	.999963	.999955	.999948	.999942	.999936
380.0	.999986	.999975	.999965	.999957	.999951	.999945	.999939
390.0	.999987	.999976	.999967	.999960	.999953	.999947	.999942
400.0	.999987	.999977	.999969	.999962	.999955	.999950	.999945
420.0	.999989	.999979	.999972	.999965	.999960	.999955	.999950
440.0	.999990	.999981	.999974	.999968	.999963	.999959	.999955
460.0	.999991	.999983	.999976	.999971	.999966	.999962	.999959
480.0	.999991	.999984	.999978	.999973	.999969	.999965	.999962
500.0	.999992	.999985	.999980	.999975	.999971	.999968	.999965
520.0	.999993	.999986	.999981	.999977	.999974	.999970	.999968
540.0	.999993	.999987	.999983	.999979	.999976	.999973	.999970
560.0	.999994	.999988	.999984	.999980	.999977	.999974	.999972
580.0	.999994	.999989	.999985	.999982	.999979	.999976	.999974
600.0	.999994	.999990	.999986	.999983	.999980	.999978	.999976
620.0	.999995	.999990	.999987	.999984	.999981	.999979	.999977
640.0	1.00000	.999991	.999988	.999985	.999983	.999980	.999979
660.0		.999992	.999988	.999986	.999984	.999982	.999980
680.0		.999992	.999989	.999987	.999985	.999983	.999981
700.0		.999993	.999990	.999987	.999985	.999984	.999982
720.0		.999993	.999990	.999988	.999986	.999985	.999983
740.0		.999993	.999991	.999989	.999987	.999985	.999984
760.0		.999994	.999991	.999989	.999988	.999986	.999985
780.0		.999994	.999992	.999990	.999988	.999987	.999986
800.0		.999994	.999992	.999990	.999989	.999987	.999986
820.0		.999995	.999993	.999991	.999989	.999988	.999987
840.0		.999995	.999993	.999991	.999990	.999989	.999988
860.0		1.00000	.999993	.999992	.999990	.999989	.999988
880.0			.999994	.999992	.999991	.999990	.999989
900.0			.999994	.999992	.999991	.999990	.999989
920.0			.999994	.999993	.999992	.999991	.999990
940.0			.999994	.999993	.999992	.999991	.999990
960.0			.999995	.999993	.999992	.999991	.999990
980.0			.999995	.999994	.999993	.999992	.999991
1000.0			.999995	.999994	.999993	.999992	.999991
1100.0			1.00000	.999995	.999994	.999993	.999993
1200.0				1.00000	1.00000	.999994	.999994
1300.0						1.00000	.999995
1400.0							1.00000

ν = 2

Q\n	9	10	11	12	13	14	15
0.0	.000000	.000000	.000000	.000000	.000000	.000000	.000000
0.1	.000000	.000000	.000000	.000000	.000000	.000000	.000000
0.2	.000000	.000000	.000000	.000000	.000000	.000000	.000000
0.3	.000003	.000001	.000000	.000000	.000000	.000000	.000000
0.4	.000022	.000008	.000003	.000001	.000000	.000000	.000000
0.5	.000112	.000047	.000020	.000009	.000004	.000002	.000001
0.6	.000399	.000192	.000095	.000049	.000026	.000014	.000008
0.7	.001108	.000596	.000331	.000189	.000110	.000066	.000040
0.8	.002562	.001508	.000913	.000567	.000360	.000233	.000154
0.9	.005150	.003260	.002118	.001408	.000955	.000660	.000464
1.0	.009272	.006230	.004286	.003011	.002154	.001567	.001158
1.2	.023454	.017252	.012942	.009876	.007652	.006009	.004776
1.4	.046747	.036660	.029223	.023628	.019345	.016015	.013390
1.6	.078987	.064901	.054062	.045573	.038818	.033370	.028921
1.8	.118615	.100917	.086861	.075517	.066231	.058536	.052090
2.0	.163417	.142783	.125996	.112136	.100545	.090743	.082371
2.2	.211136	.188336	.169439	.153560	.140059	.128461	.118407
2.4	.259826	.235602	.215225	.197864	.182910	.169904	.158498
2.6	.307989	.282981	.261695	.243358	.227397	.213378	.200968
2.8	.354567	.329296	.307578	.288700	.272128	.257457	.244371
3.0	.398881	.373748	.351977	.332912	.316060	.301042	.287564
3.2	.440543	.415844	.394307	.375331	.358461	.343345	.329708
3.4	.479379	.455323	.434231	.415550	.398861	.383839	.370230
3.6	.515362	.492089	.471588	.453350	.436991	.422209	.408768
3.8	.548562	.526161	.506347	.488655	.472729	.458292	.445123
4.0	.579110	.557627	.538560	.521480	.506058	.492038	.479216
4.2	.607169	.586623	.568332	.551902	.537029	.523474	.511048
4.4	.632917	.613306	.595801	.580039	.565738	.552676	.540679
4.6	.656539	.637844	.621121	.606029	.592308	.579754	.568202
4.8	.678212	.660408	.644448	.630018	.616877	.604833	.593732
5.0	.698107	.681160	.665940	.652158	.639586	.628046	.617396
5.2	.716384	.700256	.685749	.672592	.660574	.649529	.639323
5.4	.733190	.717842	.704018	.691462	.679980	.669414	.659640
5.6	.748662	.734054	.720878	.708899	.697930	.687827	.678472
5.8	.762921	.749013	.736454	.725023	.714546	.704887	.695935
6.0	.776080	.762833	.750859	.739949	.729941	.720706	.712141
6.4	.799490	.787454	.776555	.766609	.757470	.749024	.741180
6.8	.819586	.808625	.798685	.789600	.781242	.773508	.766318
7.2	.836932	.826924	.817836	.809520	.801862	.794769	.788166
7.6	.851983	.842821	.834492	.826863	.819830	.813310	.807237
8.0	.865112	.856701	.849047	.842031	.835558	.829553	.823955
8.4	.876620	.868877	.861827	.855359	.849387	.843844	.838673
8.8	.886755	.879609	.873098	.867120	.861599	.856470	.851683
9.2	.895722	.889110	.883081	.877544	.872426	.867671	.863230
9.6	.903687	.897555	.891960	.886819	.882066	.877646	.873518
10.0	.910793	.905091	.899888	.895104	.890679	.886563	.882718
11.0	.925514	.920717	.916335	.912303	.908570	.905095	.901846
12.0	.936917	.932831	.929096	.925656	.922470	.919502	.916726
13.0	.945918	.942399	.939180	.936215	.933466	.930905	.928508
14.0	.953139	.950080	.947279	.944698	.942305	.940075	.937986

$\nu = 2$

Q \ n	9	10	11	12	13	14	15
15.0	.959017	.956334	.953876	.951611	.949510	.947551	.945716
16.0	.963863	.961491	.959319	.957315	.955456	.953723	.952099
17.0	.967903	.965792	.963858	.962074	.960419	.958875	.957429
18.0	.971305	.969415	.967683	.966085	.964602	.963218	.961922
19.0	.974197	.972495	.970935	.969495	.968159	.966912	.965744
20.0	.976675	.975134	.973722	.972419	.971209	.970080	.969022
22.0	.980672	.979393	.978220	.977138	.976133	.975195	.974315
24.0	.983726	.982648	.981659	.980746	.979898	.979107	.978364
26.0	.986112	.985190	.984346	.983565	.982841	.982164	.981529
28.0	.988010	.987214	.986484	.985809	.985183	.984598	.984050
30.0	.989545	.988850	.988213	.987624	.987078	.986567	.986088
32.0	.990804	.990192	.989631	.989113	.988632	.988182	.987761
34.0	.991848	.991306	.990808	.990349	.989922	.989523	.989149
36.0	.992725	.992240	.991796	.991386	.991005	.990648	.990314
38.0	.993467	.993032	.992633	.992264	.991922	.991602	.991302
40.0	.994102	.993709	.993348	.993015	.992706	.992417	.992146
45.0	.995336	.995025	.994740	.994476	.994232	.994003	.993788
50.0	.996220	.995968	.995737	.995523	.995324	.995139	.994965
55.0	.996875	.996666	.996475	.996298	.996134	.995981	.995837
60.0	.997373	.997198	.997037	.996888	.996750	.996621	.996500
65.0	.997761	.997612	.997475	.997348	.997230	.997120	.997017
70.0	.998069	.997940	.997822	.997713	.997611	.997516	.997427
75.0	.998318	.998205	.998102	.998007	.997919	.997836	.997758
80.0	.998521	.998422	.998332	.998248	.998170	.998098	.998030
85.0	.998690	.998602	.998522	.998448	.998379	.998315	.998254
90.0	.998831	.998753	.998682	.998616	.998554	.998497	.998443
95.0	.998951	.998881	.998817	.998757	.998702	.998651	.998602
100.0	.999053	.998990	.998932	.998878	.998829	.998782	.998738
105.0	.999141	.999084	.999031	.998983	.998937	.998895	.998856
110.0	.999217	.999165	.999117	.999073	.999032	.998993	.998957
115.0	.999284	.999236	.999192	.999152	.999114	.999079	.999046
120.0	.999342	.999298	.999258	.999221	.999186	.999154	.999124
125.0	.999394	.999353	.999316	.999282	.999250	.999220	.999192
130.0	.999440	.999402	.999368	.999336	.999307	.999279	.999253
135.0	.999480	.999446	.999414	.999384	.999357	.999332	.999308
140.0	.999517	.999485	.999455	.999428	.999402	.999378	.999356
145.0	.999550	.999519	.999492	.999466	.999443	.999420	.999400
150.0	.999579	.999551	.999525	.999501	.999479	.999458	.999439
155.0	.999606	.999579	.999555	.999533	.999512	.999493	.999475
160.0	.999630	.999605	.999583	.999562	.999542	.999524	.999507
165.0	.999652	.999629	.999608	.999588	.999570	.999552	.999536
170.0	.999672	.999650	.999630	.999612	.999594	.999578	.999563
175.0	.999691	.999670	.999651	.999634	.999617	.999602	.999588
180.0	.999708	.999688	.999670	.999654	.999638	.999624	.999610
190.0	.999738	.999720	.999704	.999689	.999675	.999662	.999650
200.0	.999763	.999747	.999733	.999719	.999707	.999695	.999684
210.0	.999785	.999771	.999758	.999746	.999734	.999724	.999714
220.0	.999804	.999791	.999779	.999768	.999758	.999748	.999739
230.0	.999821	.999809	.999798	.999788	.999778	.999770	.999761
240.0	.999836	.999825	.999814	.999805	.999797	.999788	.999781

$\nu = 2$

Q\n	9	10	11	12	13	14	15
250.0	.999848	.999838	.999829	.999820	.999812	.999805	.999798
260.0	.999860	.999851	.999842	.999834	.999827	.999820	.999813
270.0	.999870	.999861	.999853	.999846	.999839	.999833	.999827
280.0	.999879	.999871	.999864	.999857	.999850	.999845	.999839
290.0	.999887	.999880	.999873	.999867	.999861	.999855	.999850
300.0	.999895	.999888	.999881	.999875	.999870	.999865	.999860
310.0	.999901	.999895	.999889	.999883	.999878	.999873	.999869
320.0	.999907	.999901	.999896	.999890	.999886	.999881	.999877
330.0	.999913	.999907	.999902	.999897	.999892	.999888	.999884
340.0	.999918	.999913	.999908	.999903	.999899	.999895	.999891
350.0	.999923	.999918	.999913	.999908	.999904	.999901	.999897
360.0	.999927	.999922	.999918	.999913	.999910	.999906	.999903
370.0	.999931	.999926	.999922	.999918	.999914	.999911	.999908
380.0	.999934	.999930	.999926	.999922	.999919	.999916	.999913
390.0	.999938	.999934	.999930	.999926	.999923	.999920	.999917
400.0	.999941	.999937	.999933	.999930	.999927	.999924	.999921
420.0	.999946	.999943	.999939	.999936	.999934	.999931	.999928
440.0	.999951	.999948	.999945	.999942	.999939	.999937	.999935
460.0	.999955	.999952	.999949	.999947	.999945	.999942	.999940
480.0	.999959	.999956	.999954	.999951	.999949	.999947	.999945
500.0	.999962	.999960	.999957	.999955	.999953	.999951	.999949
520.0	.999965	.999963	.999960	.999958	.999957	.999955	.999953
540.0	.999968	.999965	.999963	.999962	.999960	.999958	.999957
560.0	.999970	.999968	.999966	.999964	.999963	.999961	.999960
580.0	.999972	.999970	.999968	.999967	.999965	.999964	.999962
600.0	.999974	.999972	.999970	.999969	.999967	.999966	.999965
620.0	.999975	.999974	.999972	.999971	.999970	.999968	.999967
640.0	.999977	.999975	.999974	.999973	.999971	.999970	.999969
660.0	.999978	.999977	.999975	.999974	.999973	.999972	.999971
680.0	.999980	.999978	.999977	.999976	.999975	.999974	.999973
700.0	.999981	.999979	.999978	.999977	.999976	.999975	.999974
720.0	.999982	.999981	.999979	.999978	.999977	.999976	.999976
740.0	.999983	.999982	.999980	.999980	.999979	.999978	.999977
760.0	.999984	.999983	.999981	.999981	.999980	.999979	.999978
780.0	.999984	.999983	.999982	.999982	.999981	.999980	.999979
800.0	.999985	.999984	.999983	.999982	.999982	.999981	.999980
820.0	.999986	.999985	.999984	.999983	.999983	.999982	.999981
840.0	.999987	.999986	.999985	.999984	.999983	.999983	.999982
860.0	.999987	.999986	.999986	.999985	.999984	.999984	.999983
880.0	.999988	.999987	.999986	.999986	.999985	.999984	.999984
900.0	.999988	.999988	.999987	.999986	.999986	.999985	.999984
920.0	.999989	.999988	.999987	.999987	.999986	.999986	.999985
940.0	.999989	.999989	.999988	.999987	.999987	.999986	.999986
960.0	.999990	.999989	.999988	.999988	.999987	.999987	.999986
980.0	.999990	.999989	.999989	.999988	.999988	.999987	.999987
1000.0	.999991	.999990	.999989	.999989	.999988	.999988	.999987
1100.0	.999992	.999992	.999991	.999991	.999990	.999990	.999990
1200.0	.999993	.999993	.999993	.999992	.999992	.999992	.999991
1300.0	.999994	.999994	.999994	.999993	.999993	.999993	.999993
1400.0	1.00000	.999995	.999995	.999994	.999994	.999994	.999994

$\nu = 2$

Q\n	9	10	11	12	13	14	15
1500.0		1.00000	1.00000	1.00000	.999995	.999995	.999994
1600.0					1.00000	1.00000	1.00000

$\nu = 2$

Q\n	16	17	18	19	20	22	24
0.0	.000000	.000000	.000000	.000000	.000000	.000000	.000000
0.2	.000000	.000000	.000000	.000000	.000000	.000000	.000000
0.4	.000000	.000000	.000000	.000000	.000000	.000000	.000000
0.6	.000004	.000002	.000001	.000001	.000001	.000000	.000000
0.8	.000104	.000071	.000049	.000034	.000024	.000013	.000007
1.0	.000867	.000657	.000503	.000390	.000305	.000191	.000124
1.2	.003838	.003115	.002551	.002107	.001753	.001238	.000896
1.4	.011295	.009604	.008226	.007093	.006154	.004708	.003671
1.6	.025250	.022191	.019620	.017440	.015581	.012601	.010352
1.8	.046638	.041987	.037987	.034524	.031506	.026528	.022626
2.0	.075159	.068895	.063418	.058598	.054332	.047141	.041343
2.2	.109621	.101888	.095038	.088934	.083466	.074097	.066379
2.4	.148418	.139452	.131429	.124211	.117685	.106355	.096868
2.6	.189905	.179980	.171028	.162911	.155519	.142551	.131549
2.8	.232621	.222009	.212373	.203583	.195530	.181285	.169070
3.0	.275391	.264335	.254243	.244990	.236471	.221300	.208177
3.2	.317332	.306040	.295688	.286155	.277344	.261562	.247814
3.4	.357828	.346469	.336016	.326357	.317398	.301277	.287150
3.6	.396477	.385182	.374756	.365094	.356106	.339869	.325568
3.8	.433046	.421917	.411616	.402045	.393122	.376945	.362635
4.0	.467427	.456536	.446434	.437027	.428238	.412259	.398072
4.2	.499599	.489000	.479149	.469959	.461357	.445677	.431713
4.4	.529602	.519331	.509767	.500831	.492453	.477149	.463480
4.6	.557519	.547596	.538344	.529686	.521557	.506681	.493362
4.8	.583452	.573891	.564963	.556598	.548735	.534320	.521387
5.0	.607521	.598324	.589727	.581662	.574074	.560142	.547618
5.2	.629848	.621014	.612748	.604986	.597675	.584235	.572133
5.4	.650557	.642081	.634141	.626680	.619646	.606699	.595024
5.6	.669770	.661642	.654022	.646856	.640095	.627637	.616388
5.8	.687601	.679811	.672502	.665623	.659129	.647151	.636322
6.0	.704160	.696695	.689687	.683086	.676851	.665341	.654924
6.4	.733862	.727008	.720566	.714492	.708748	.698128	.688499
6.8	.759602	.753305	.747381	.741790	.736499	.726703	.717807
7.2	.781994	.776203	.770750	.765599	.760721	.751680	.743459
7.6	.801556	.796220	.791193	.786442	.781939	.773586	.765982
8.0	.818715	.813791	.809148	.804758	.800595	.792867	.785825
8.4	.833830	.829276	.824981	.820917	.817062	.809900	.803369
8.8	.847198	.842979	.838997	.835228	.831651	.825003	.818935
9.2	.859067	.855150	.851451	.847949	.844625	.838442	.832796
9.6	.869646	.866002	.862560	.859299	.856203	.850443	.845180
10.0	.879110	.875712	.872502	.869461	.866573	.861196	.856281
11.0	.898796	.895921	.893204	.890628	.888180	.883620	.879447
12.0	.914118	.911659	.909334	.907128	.905031	.901123	.897544
13.0	.926256	.924132	.922122	.920215	.918401	.915019	.911920
14.0	.936023	.934171	.932418	.930754	.929172	.926220	.923513
15.0	.943991	.942363	.940822	.939359	.937967	.935370	.932988
16.0	.950572	.949131	.947766	.946471	.945238	.942936	.940825
17.0	.956068	.954783	.953567	.952412	.951312	.949260	.947377
18.0	.960702	.959550	.958460	.957424	.956438	.954597	.952907
19.0	.964645	.963607	.962623	.961689	.960800	.959140	.957616

$\nu = 2$

Q\n	16	17	18	19	20	22	24
20.0	.968026	.967086	.966195	.965349	.964543	.963039	.961657
22.0	.973487	.972706	.971965	.971261	.970591	.969340	.968190
24.0	.977666	.977006	.976381	.975787	.975221	.974164	.973193
26.0	.980932	.980368	.979833	.979325	.978841	.977937	.977106
28.0	.983533	.983045	.982583	.982144	.981725	.980943	.980224
30.0	.985637	.985212	.984808	.984424	.984059	.983376	.982748
32.0	.987364	.986989	.986633	.986295	.985973	.985372	.984819
34.0	.988797	.988464	.988149	.987849	.987563	.987030	.986539
36.0	.990000	.989703	.989421	.989153	.988898	.988422	.987983
38.0	.991019	.990752	.990499	.990259	.990030	.989601	.989207
40.0	.991891	.991650	.991421	.991204	.990997	.990610	.990254
45.0	.993586	.993395	.993214	.993042	.992878	.992572	.992290
50.0	.994801	.994646	.994500	.994360	.994227	.993978	.993750
55.0	.995701	.995573	.995452	.995336	.995226	.995021	.994832
60.0	.996386	.996279	.996176	.996079	.995987	.995814	.995655
65.0	.996920	.996828	.996741	.996658	.996579	.996432	.996296
70.0	.997344	.997264	.997189	.997118	.997050	.996923	.996806
75.0	.997685	.997616	.997551	.997489	.997429	.997319	.997217
80.0	.997965	.997905	.997847	.997792	.997740	.997643	.997553
85.0	.998197	.998144	.998093	.998044	.997998	.997912	.997832
90.0	.998392	.998344	.998299	.998255	.998214	.998137	.998066
95.0	.998557	.998514	.998473	.998434	.998397	.998328	.998264
100.0	.998697	.998658	.998622	.998587	.998553	.998491	.998433
105.0	.998818	.998783	.998750	.998718	.998688	.998631	.998579
110.0	.998923	.998891	.998861	.998832	.998804	.998752	.998705
115.0	.999015	.998985	.998957	.998931	.998906	.998859	.998815
120.0	.999095	.999068	.999043	.999018	.998995	.998952	.998912
125.0	.999166	.999141	.999118	.999095	.999074	.999034	.998997
130.0	.999229	.999206	.999184	.999163	.999144	.999107	.999073
135.0	.999285	.999264	.999243	.999224	.999206	.999172	.999140
140.0	.999335	.999315	.999296	.999279	.999261	.999230	.999200
145.0	.999380	.999362	.999344	.999327	.999312	.999282	.999254
150.0	.999421	.999403	.999387	.999371	.999357	.999329	.999303
155.0	.999458	.999441	.999426	.999411	.999397	.999371	.999348
160.0	.999491	.999476	.999461	.999448	.999435	.999410	.999388
165.0	.999521	.999507	.999493	.999481	.999468	.999445	.999424
170.0	.999549	.999536	.999523	.999511	.999499	.999477	.999458
175.0	.999574	.999562	.999550	.999538	.999527	.999507	.999488
180.0	.999598	.999586	.999574	.999563	.999553	.999534	.999516
190.0	.999639	.999628	.999618	.999608	.999599	.999582	.999566
200.0	.999674	.999664	.999655	.999646	.999638	.999622	.999608
210.0	.999704	.999696	.999687	.999679	.999672	.999658	.999644
220.0	.999731	.999723	.999715	.999708	.999701	.999688	.999676
230.0	.999754	.999746	.999739	.999733	.999726	.999714	.999704
240.0	.999774	.999767	.999761	.999754	.999749	.999738	.999728
250.0	.999791	.999785	.999779	.999774	.999768	.999758	.999749
260.0	.999807	.999801	.999796	.999791	.999786	.999777	.999768
270.0	.999821	.999816	.999811	.999806	.999801	.999793	.999785
280.0	.999834	.999829	.999824	.999820	.999815	.999807	.999800
290.0	.999845	.999840	.999836	.999832	.999828	.999820	.999814

$\nu = 2$

Q\n	16	17	18	19	20	22	24
300.0	.999855	.999851	.999847	.999843	.999839	.999832	.999826
310.0	.999864	.999860	.999856	.999853	.999849	.999843	.999837
320.0	.999873	.999869	.999865	.999862	.999859	.999852	.999847
330.0	.999880	.999877	.999873	.999870	.999867	.999861	.999856
340.0	.999887	.999884	.999881	.999878	.999875	.999869	.999864
350.0	.999894	.999890	.999887	.999885	.999882	.999877	.999872
360.0	.999899	.999896	.999894	.999891	.999888	.999883	.999879
370.0	.999905	.999902	.999899	.999897	.999894	.999890	.999885
380.0	.999910	.999907	.999904	.999902	.999900	.999895	.999891
390.0	.999914	.999912	.999909	.999907	.999905	.999901	.999897
400.0	.999919	.999916	.999914	.999912	.999909	.999906	.999902
420.0	.999926	.999924	.999922	.999920	.999918	.999914	.999911
440.0	.999933	.999931	.999929	.999927	.999925	.999922	.999919
460.0	.999938	.999937	.999935	.999933	.999932	.999929	.999926
480.0	.999943	.999942	.999940	.999939	.999937	.999934	.999932
500.0	.999948	.999946	.999945	.999943	.999942	.999940	.999937
520.0	.999952	.999950	.999949	.999948	.999946	.999944	.999942
540.0	.999955	.999954	.999953	.999951	.999950	.999948	.999946
560.0	.999958	.999957	.999956	.999955	.999954	.999952	.999950
580.0	.999961	.999960	.999959	.999958	.999957	.999955	.999953
600.0	.999964	.999963	.999962	.999961	.999960	.999958	.999956
620.0	.999966	.999965	.999964	.999963	.999962	.999961	.999959
640.0	.999968	.999967	.999966	.999965	.999965	.999963	.999962
660.0	.999970	.999969	.999968	.999968	.999967	.999965	.999964
680.0	.999972	.999971	.999970	.999969	.999969	.999967	.999966
700.0	.999973	.999973	.999972	.999971	.999970	.999969	.999968
720.0	.999975	.999974	.999973	.999973	.999972	.999971	.999970
740.0	.999976	.999975	.999975	.999974	.999974	.999972	.999971
760.0	.999977	.999977	.999976	.999976	.999975	.999974	.999973
780.0	.999979	.999978	.999977	.999977	.999976	.999975	.999974
800.0	.999980	.999979	.999978	.999978	.999977	.999976	.999975
820.0	.999981	.999980	.999979	.999979	.999978	.999978	.999977
840.0	.999982	.999981	.999980	.999980	.999979	.999979	.999978
860.0	.999982	.999982	.999981	.999981	.999980	.999980	.999979
880.0	.999983	.999983	.999982	.999982	.999981	.999980	.999980
900.0	.999984	.999983	.999983	.999983	.999982	.999981	.999981
920.0	.999985	.999984	.999984	.999983	.999983	.999982	.999981
940.0	.999985	.999985	.999984	.999984	.999984	.999983	.999982
960.0	.999986	.999985	.999985	.999985	.999984	.999984	.999983
980.0	.999986	.999986	.999986	.999985	.999985	.999984	.999984
1000.0	.999987	.999987	.999986	.999986	.999986	.999985	.999984
1100.0	.999989	.999989	.999989	.999988	.999988	.999988	.999987
1200.0	.999991	.999991	.999990	.999990	.999990	.999990	.999989
1300.0	.999992	.999992	.999992	.999992	.999991	.999991	.999991
1400.0	.999993	.999993	.999993	.999993	.999993	.999992	.999992
1500.0	.999994	.999994	.999994	.999994	.999994	.999993	.999993
1600.0	.999995	.999995	.999995	.999994	.999994	.999994	.999994
1700.0	1.00000	1.00000	1.00000	1.00000	.999995	.999995	.999995
1800.0					1.00000	1.00000	1.00000

$\nu = 2$

Q\n	26	28	30	32	34	36	38
0.0	.000000	.000000	.000000	.000000	.000000	.000000	.000000
0.2	.000000	.000000	.000000	.000000	.000000	.000000	.000000
0.4	.000000	.000000	.000000	.000000	.000000	.000000	.000000
0.6	.000000	.000000	.000000	.000000	.000000	.000000	.000000
0.8	.000004	.000002	.000001	.000001	.000001	.000000	.000000
1.0	.000082	.000056	.000039	.000028	.000020	.000014	.000011
1.2	.000662	.000498	.000381	.000296	.000232	.000185	.000149
1.4	.002911	.002341	.001907	.001572	.001308	.001099	.000930
1.6	.008618	.007259	.006177	.005305	.004592	.004004	.003515
1.8	.019511	.016986	.014913	.013191	.011745	.010519	.009472
2.0	.036593	.032648	.029333	.026518	.024105	.022019	.020203
2.2	.059930	.054474	.049807	.045778	.042269	.039192	.036474
2.4	.088816	.081904	.075912	.070672	.066053	.061954	.058295
2.6	.122097	.113890	.106698	.100344	.094690	.089627	.085067
2.8	.158472	.149186	.140977	.133666	.127109	.121195	.115831
3.0	.196701	.186568	.177548	.169461	.162163	.155541	.149501
3.2	.235711	.224959	.215331	.206651	.198779	.191599	.185021
3.4	.274644	.263475	.253427	.244326	.236036	.228444	.221461
3.6	.312848	.301439	.291132	.281761	.273194	.265322	.258057
3.8	.349857	.338354	.327925	.318413	.309689	.301649	.294209
4.0	.385360	.373879	.363440	.353891	.345111	.336999	.329473
4.2	.419163	.407797	.397436	.387935	.379179	.371072	.363536
4.4	.451165	.439985	.429771	.420385	.411717	.403676	.396188
4.6	.481334	.470393	.460376	.451155	.442625	.434699	.427306
4.8	.509685	.499020	.489240	.480221	.471865	.464090	.456828
5.0	.536266	.525903	.516385	.507596	.499442	.491845	.484741
5.2	.561146	.551103	.541865	.533325	.525391	.517991	.511063
5.4	.584410	.574695	.565749	.557468	.549767	.542577	.535839
5.6	.606149	.596765	.588115	.580099	.572639	.565667	.559127
5.8	.626454	.617402	.609048	.601301	.594084	.587333	.580997
6.0	.645421	.636696	.628637	.621157	.614182	.607655	.601523
6.4	.679700	.671607	.664121	.657162	.650666	.644577	.638851
6.8	.709666	.702168	.695224	.688761	.682721	.677053	.671719
7.2	.735926	.728981	.722541	.716542	.710930	.705660	.700694
7.6	.759007	.752570	.746597	.741027	.735813	.730912	.726292
8.0	.779360	.773389	.767843	.762668	.757820	.753261	.748960
8.4	.797368	.791822	.786668	.781855	.777344	.773099	.769092
8.8	.813357	.808198	.803401	.798920	.794717	.790760	.787023
9.2	.827602	.822796	.818325	.814146	.810225	.806532	.803043
9.6	.840336	.835851	.831677	.827775	.824111	.820660	.817398
10.0	.851756	.847565	.843662	.840012	.836584	.833354	.830300
11.0	.875602	.872037	.868715	.865606	.862684	.859928	.857321
12.0	.894243	.891181	.888326	.885653	.883139	.880767	.878522
13.0	.909061	.906407	.903931	.901611	.899430	.897370	.895420
14.0	.921015	.918695	.916531	.914502	.912593	.910790	.909083
15.0	.930789	.928746	.926839	.925051	.923368	.921779	.920273
16.0	.938875	.937063	.935371	.933785	.932292	.930881	.929544
17.0	.945637	.944020	.942510	.941093	.939760	.938500	.937306
18.0	.951345	.949894	.948539	.947267	.946069	.944938	.943865
19.0	.956207	.954898	.953674	.952527	.951446	.950424	.949456

ν = 2

Q\n	26	28	30	32	34	36	38
20.0	.960380	.959193	.958084	.957043	.956063	.955136	.954258
22.0	.967127	.966139	.965216	.964349	.963532	.962760	.962028
24.0	.972295	.971460	.970680	.969947	.969257	.968604	.967985
26.0	.976338	.975624	.974956	.974329	.973738	.973179	.972649
28.0	.979560	.978942	.978364	.977821	.977310	.976826	.976367
30.0	.982168	.981628	.981123	.980649	.980202	.979779	.979379
32.0	.984308	.983832	.983387	.982970	.982576	.982204	.981851
34.0	.986086	.985663	.985269	.984898	.984548	.984218	.983905
36.0	.987578	.987201	.986848	.986517	.986205	.985910	.985629
38.0	.988843	.988504	.988187	.987890	.987609	.987344	.987092
40.0	.989925	.989618	.989332	.989063	.988810	.988570	.988342
45.0	.992030	.991787	.991560	.991347	.991147	.990957	.990776
50.0	.993539	.993342	.993158	.992985	.992822	.992668	.992522
55.0	.994657	.994494	.994342	.994199	.994064	.993936	.993815
60.0	.995508	.995371	.995243	.995123	.995009	.994902	.994800
65.0	.996171	.996054	.995945	.995842	.995746	.995654	.995567
70.0	.996697	.996597	.996503	.996414	.996331	.996252	.996177
75.0	.997122	.997035	.996953	.996875	.996803	.996734	.996669
80.0	.997470	.997393	.997321	.997253	.997189	.997129	.997071
85.0	.997759	.997690	.997627	.997566	.997510	.997456	.997405
90.0	.998001	.997940	.997883	.997829	.997778	.997731	.997685
95.0	.998205	.998151	.998099	.998051	.998006	.997963	.997922
100.0	.998380	.998331	.998285	.998241	.998200	.998161	.998125
105.0	.998531	.998486	.998444	.998404	.998367	.998332	.998299
110.0	.998661	.998620	.998582	.998546	.998512	.998480	.998450
115.0	.998775	.998738	.998703	.998670	.998639	.998609	.998582
120.0	.998875	.998840	.998808	.998778	.998750	.998723	.998697
125.0	.998963	.998931	.998902	.998874	.998848	.998823	.998799
130.0	.999041	.999012	.998985	.998959	.998935	.998912	.998890
135.0	.999111	.999084	.999058	.999034	.999012	.998991	.998971
140.0	.999173	.999148	.999124	.999102	.999081	.999061	.999043
145.0	.999229	.999206	.999184	.999163	.999143	.999125	.999108
150.0	.999280	.999258	.999237	.999218	.999200	.999182	.999166
155.0	.999325	.999305	.999286	.999267	.999250	.999234	.999219
160.0	.999367	.999348	.999329	.999313	.999296	.999281	.999267
165.0	.999405	.999387	.999370	.999354	.999338	.999324	.999311
170.0	.999439	.999422	.999406	.999391	.999377	.999363	.999351
175.0	.999471	.999455	.999439	.999425	.999412	.999399	.999387
180.0	.999500	.999484	.999470	.999457	.999444	.999432	.999421
190.0	.999551	.999537	.999524	.999512	.999501	.999490	.999480
200.0	.999595	.999582	.999571	.999560	.999550	.999540	.999531
210.0	.999632	.999621	.999611	.999601	.999592	.999583	.999574
220.0	.999665	.999655	.999645	.999636	.999628	.999620	.999612
230.0	.999694	.999684	.999675	.999667	.999659	.999652	.999645
240.0	.999719	.999710	.999702	.999694	.999687	.999681	.999674
250.0	.999741	.999733	.999725	.999718	.999712	.999706	.999700
260.0	.999760	.999753	.999746	.999740	.999734	.999728	.999722
270.0	.999778	.999771	.999764	.999759	.999753	.999748	.999743
280.0	.999793	.999787	.999781	.999775	.999770	.999765	.999761
290.0	.999807	.999801	.999796	.999791	.999786	.999781	.999777

ν = 2

Q\n	26	28	30	32	34	36	38
300.0	.999820	.999814	.999809	.999804	.999800	.999796	.999791
310.0	.999831	.999826	.999821	.999817	.999813	.999808	.999805
320.0	.999842	.999837	.999832	.999828	.999824	.999820	.999817
330.0	.999851	.999847	.999842	.999838	.999835	.999831	.999828
340.0	.999860	.999855	.999851	.999848	.999844	.999841	.999838
350.0	.999868	.999864	.999860	.999856	.999853	.999850	.999847
360.0	.999875	.999871	.999868	.999864	.999861	.999858	.999855
370.0	.999882	.999878	.999875	.999871	.999868	.999866	.999863
380.0	.999888	.999884	.999881	.999878	.999875	.999873	.999870
390.0	.999893	.999890	.999887	.999884	.999882	.999879	.999877
400.0	.999899	.999896	.999893	.999890	.999887	.999885	.999883
420.0	.999908	.999905	.999903	.999900	.999898	.999896	.999894
440.0	.999916	.999914	.999911	.999909	.999907	.999905	.999903
460.0	.999923	.999921	.999919	.999917	.999915	.999913	.999911
480.0	.999930	.999927	.999925	.999924	.999922	.999920	.999919
500.0	.999935	.999933	.999931	.999930	.999928	.999926	.999925
520.0	.999940	.999938	.999936	.999935	.999933	.999932	.999931
540.0	.999944	.999943	.999941	.999940	.999938	.999937	.999936
560.0	.999948	.999947	.999945	.999944	.999943	.999941	.999940
580.0	.999952	.999950	.999949	.999948	.999946	.999945	.999944
600.0	.999955	.999954	.999952	.999951	.999950	.999949	.999948
620.0	.999958	.999957	.999955	.999954	.999953	.999952	.999951
640.0	.999960	.999959	.999958	.999957	.999956	.999955	.999954
660.0	.999963	.999962	.999961	.999960	.999959	.999958	.999957
680.0	.999965	.999964	.999963	.999962	.999961	.999960	.999959
700.0	.999967	.999966	.999965	.999964	.999963	.999962	.999962
720.0	.999969	.999968	.999967	.999966	.999965	.999964	.999964
740.0	.999970	.999969	.999969	.999968	.999967	.999966	.999966
760.0	.999972	.999971	.999970	.999970	.999969	.999968	.999967
780.0	.999973	.999973	.999972	.999971	.999970	.999970	.999969
800.0	.999975	.999974	.999973	.999972	.999972	.999971	.999971
820.0	.999976	.999975	.999974	.999974	.999973	.999973	.999972
840.0	.999977	.999976	.999976	.999975	.999974	.999974	.999973
860.0	.999978	.999977	.999977	.999976	.999976	.999975	.999975
880.0	.999979	.999978	.999978	.999977	.999977	.999976	.999976
900.0	.999980	.999979	.999979	.999978	.999978	.999977	.999977
920.0	.999981	.999980	.999980	.999979	.999979	.999978	.999978
940.0	.999982	.999981	.999981	.999980	.999980	.999979	.999979
960.0	.999982	.999982	.999981	.999981	.999980	.999980	.999980
980.0	.999983	.999983	.999982	.999982	.999981	.999981	.999980
1000.0	.999984	.999983	.999983	.999982	.999982	.999982	.999981
1100.0	.999987	.999986	.999986	.999985	.999985	.999985	.999984
1200.0	.999989	.999988	.999988	.999988	.999987	.999987	.999987
1300.0	.999990	.999990	.999990	.999990	.999989	.999989	.999989
1400.0	.999992	.999991	.999991	.999991	.999991	.999991	.999990
1500.0	.999993	.999993	.999992	.999992	.999992	.999992	.999992
1600.0	.999994	.999993	.999993	.999993	.999993	.999993	.999993
1700.0	.999994	.999994	.999994	.999994	.999994	.999994	.999994
1800.0	.999995	.999995	.999995	.999995	.999994	.999994	.999994
1900.0	1.00000	1.00000	1.00000	1.00000	1.00000	.999995	.999995

$\nu = 2$

Q\n	26	28	30	32	34	36	38
2000.0						1.00000	1.00000

$\nu = 2$

Q\n	40	50	60	70	80	90	100
0.0	.000000	.000000	.000000	.000000	.000000	.000000	.000000
0.1	.000000	.000000	.000000	.000000	.000000	.000000	.000000
0.2	.000000	.000000	.000000	.000000	.000000	.000000	.000000
0.3	.000000	.000000	.000000	.000000	.000000	.000000	.000000
0.4	.000000	.000000	.000000	.000000	.000000	.000000	.000000
0.5	.000000	.000000	.000000	.000000	.000000	.000000	.000000
0.6	.000000	.000000	.000000	.000000	.000000	.000000	.000000
0.7	.000000	.000000	.000000	.000000	.000000	.000000	.000000
0.8	.000000	.000000	.000000	.000000	.000000	.000000	.000000
0.9	.000001	.000000	.000000	.000000	.000000	.000000	.000000
1.0	.000008	.000002	.000001	.000000	.000000	.000000	.000000
1.1	.000035	.000012	.000005	.000002	.000001	.000001	.000000
1.2	.000120	.000048	.000022	.000011	.000006	.000004	.000002
1.3	.000335	.000150	.000077	.000043	.000026	.000016	.000011
1.4	.000794	.000393	.000219	.000132	.000085	.000057	.000040
1.5	.001654	.000891	.000532	.000341	.000232	.000164	.000120
1.6	.003104	.001792	.001134	.000766	.000543	.000400	.000304
1.7	.005345	.003272	.002175	.001533	.001129	.000860	.000673
1.8	.008571	.005515	.003823	.002793	.002122	.001663	.001335
1.9	.012950	.008697	.006247	.004707	.003675	.002949	.002419
2.0	.018611	.012968	.009607	.007432	.005939	.004865	.004066
2.1	.025637	.018443	.014033	.011109	.009057	.007554	.006417
2.2	.034059	.025197	.019625	.015850	.013151	.011142	.009598
2.3	.043867	.033261	.026441	.021733	.018313	.015729	.013718
2.4	.055009	.042625	.034504	.028803	.024601	.021388	.018858
2.5	.067402	.053244	.043797	.037067	.032043	.028157	.025067
2.6	.080938	.065045	.054274	.046501	.040631	.036045	.032366
2.7	.095496	.077935	.065866	.057054	.050332	.045033	.040747
2.8	.110943	.091802	.078483	.068654	.061088	.055076	.050179
2.9	.127145	.106528	.092021	.081213	.072826	.066112	.060607
3.0	.143967	.121992	.106371	.094633	.085456	.078062	.071964
3.1	.161281	.138071	.121419	.108809	.098883	.090839	.084170
3.2	.178966	.154648	.137053	.123635	.113008	.104349	.097135
3.3	.196910	.171609	.153163	.139004	.127728	.118495	.110768
3.4	.215011	.188851	.169644	.154815	.142944	.133180	.124977
3.5	.233176	.206277	.186401	.170971	.158561	.148312	.139669
3.6	.251325	.223801	.203342	.187380	.174488	.163800	.154756
3.7	.269386	.241344	.220387	.203961	.190642	.179560	.170154
3.8	.287296	.258838	.237462	.220637	.206943	.195514	.185785
3.9	.305005	.276223	.254502	.237339	.223323	.211589	.201575
4.0	.322466	.293446	.271450	.254007	.239717	.227721	.217458
4.1	.339642	.310462	.288257	.270587	.256070	.243852	.233374
4.2	.356504	.327235	.304879	.287033	.272331	.259928	.249269
4.3	.373026	.343733	.321279	.303304	.288458	.275905	.265096
4.4	.389190	.359929	.337428	.319365	.304412	.291742	.280812
4.5	.404980	.375804	.353300	.335189	.320161	.307405	.296380
4.6	.420386	.391341	.368874	.350749	.335680	.322864	.311770
4.7	.435402	.406528	.384134	.366027	.350943	.338093	.326953
4.8	.450022	.421355	.399066	.381006	.365934	.353073	.341908
4.9	.464246	.435818	.413661	.395674	.380637	.367786	.356615

$\nu = 2$

Q\n	40	50	60	70	80	90	100
5.0	.478074	.449912	.427914	.410021	.395039	.382219	.371059
5.1	.491510	.463636	.441818	.424041	.409133	.396359	.385226
5.2	.504556	.476991	.455373	.437729	.422912	.410199	.399108
5.3	.517219	.489980	.468578	.451083	.436371	.423734	.412696
5.4	.529504	.502606	.481434	.464102	.449508	.436958	.425986
5.5	.541420	.514875	.493945	.476787	.462323	.449871	.438974
5.6	.552974	.526790	.506114	.489140	.474816	.462471	.451658
5.7	.564175	.538360	.517945	.501165	.486988	.474759	.464039
5.8	.575031	.549592	.529444	.512865	.498843	.486737	.476116
5.9	.585551	.560492	.540618	.524246	.510386	.498408	.487892
6.0	.595746	.571069	.551473	.535313	.521619	.509776	.499370
6.4	.633449	.610308	.591849	.576566	.563574	.552305	.542378
6.8	.666681	.645045	.627720	.613332	.601066	.590402	.580987
7.2	.696002	.675806	.659583	.646073	.634530	.624474	.615580
7.6	.721922	.703082	.687908	.675243	.664401	.654939	.646558
8.0	.744890	.727315	.713128	.701264	.691090	.682199	.674313
8.4	.765299	.748896	.735629	.724516	.714973	.706622	.699207
8.8	.783484	.768164	.755750	.745338	.736385	.728542	.721571
9.2	.799737	.785413	.773789	.764027	.755624	.748255	.741701
9.6	.814306	.800897	.790002	.780842	.772950	.766023	.759857
10.0	.827404	.814837	.804613	.796010	.788590	.782074	.776270
11.0	.854849	.844098	.835332	.827940	.821555	.815939	.810930
12.0	.876391	.867118	.859542	.853144	.847611	.842738	.838387
13.0	.893569	.885503	.878906	.873327	.868497	.864240	.860436
14.0	.907462	.900393	.894605	.889706	.885460	.881716	.878368
15.0	.918843	.912604	.907490	.903159	.899403	.896089	.893124
16.0	.928274	.922731	.918185	.914331	.910988	.908037	.905395
17.0	.936171	.931217	.927151	.923703	.920711	.918068	.915701
18.0	.942846	.938394	.934738	.931636	.928943	.926564	.924433
19.0	.948535	.944514	.941210	.938407	.935972	.933820	.931892
20.0	.953423	.949774	.946775	.944229	.942018	.940063	.938311
22.0	.961333	.958290	.955789	.953664	.951818	.950185	.948721
24.0	.967397	.964824	.962707	.960908	.959344	.957961	.956721
26.0	.972145	.969941	.968127	.966586	.965245	.964059	.962996
28.0	.975931	.974023	.972452	.971117	.969956	.968928	.968006
30.0	.978997	.977330	.975956	.974789	.973773	.972874	.972068
32.0	.981515	.980045	.978835	.977805	.976910	.976117	.975406
34.0	.983606	.982302	.981227	.980313	.979517	.978813	.978182
36.0	.985363	.984197	.983236	.982419	.981708	.981079	.980514
38.0	.986852	.985804	.984940	.984206	.983566	.983000	.982492
40.0	.988126	.987178	.986398	.985734	.985156	.984644	.984185
45.0	.990605	.989855	.989236	.988710	.988252	.987846	.987482
50.0	.992383	.991774	.991272	.990844	.990473	.990143	.989848
55.0	.993700	.993196	.992780	.992427	.992119	.991846	.991602
60.0	.994703	.994279	.993930	.993632	.993373	.993144	.992938
65.0	.995485	.995123	.994825	.994572	.994351	.994155	.993979
70.0	.996106	.995794	.995536	.995317	.995127	.994958	.994807
75.0	.996607	.996335	.996110	.995920	.995754	.995606	.995474
80.0	.997017	.996778	.996581	.996413	.996267	.996137	.996021
85.0	.997357	.997145	.996970	.996822	.996692	.996578	.996475

$\nu = 2$

Q\n	40	50	60	70	80	90	100
90.0	.997642	.997453	.997297	.997165	.997049	.996947	.996855
95.0	.997883	.997714	.997574	.997455	.997351	.997259	.997177
100.0	.998090	.997936	.997810	.997703	.997609	.997526	.997452
105.0	.998267	.998128	.998014	.997916	.997831	.997756	.997688
110.0	.998421	.998294	.998190	.998101	.998024	.997955	.997893
115.0	.998555	.998439	.998344	.998262	.998191	.998129	.998072
120.0	.998673	.998566	.998479	.998404	.998339	.998281	.998230
125.0	.998777	.998679	.998598	.998529	.998469	.998416	.998368
130.0	.998869	.998778	.998704	.998640	.998584	.998535	.998491
135.0	.998951	.998867	.998798	.998739	.998687	.998642	.998601
140.0	.999025	.998947	.998882	.998827	.998779	.998737	.998699
145.0	.999091	.999018	.998958	.998907	.998862	.998823	.998787
150.0	.999150	.999082	.999026	.998978	.998937	.998900	.998867
155.0	.999204	.999141	.999088	.999043	.999004	.998969	.998938
160.0	.999253	.999193	.999144	.999102	.999065	.999033	.999004
165.0	.999298	.999242	.999195	.999155	.999121	.999091	.999063
170.0	.999339	.999285	.999242	.999204	.999172	.999143	.999117
175.0	.999376	.999326	.999284	.999249	.999219	.999191	.999167
180.0	.999410	.999363	.999324	.999290	.999261	.999236	.999213
190.0	.999470	.999428	.999393	.999363	.999337	.999314	.999293
200.0	.999522	.999484	.999452	.999425	.999402	.999381	.999362
210.0	.999566	.999532	.999503	.999479	.999457	.999438	.999422
220.0	.999605	.999573	.999547	.999525	.999505	.999488	.999473
230.0	.999639	.999610	.999586	.999565	.999548	.999532	.999518
240.0	.999668	.999641	.999619	.999601	.999584	.999570	.999557
250.0	.999694	.999670	.999649	.999632	.999617	.999604	.999592
260.0	.999717	.999694	.999676	.999660	.999646	.999634	.999623
270.0	.999738	.999717	.999699	.999685	.999672	.999660	.999650
280.0	.999756	.999737	.999720	.999707	.999695	.999684	.999675
290.0	.999773	.999754	.999739	.999727	.999715	.999705	.999697
300.0	.999788	.999770	.999756	.999744	.999734	.999725	.999716
310.0	.999801	.999785	.999772	.999761	.999751	.999742	.999734
320.0	.999813	.999798	.999786	.999775	.999766	.999758	.999751
330.0	.999824	.999810	.999799	.999789	.999780	.999773	.999766
340.0	.999835	.999821	.999810	.999801	.999793	.999786	.999779
350.0	.999844	.999831	.999821	.999812	.999805	.999798	.999792
360.0	.999852	.999841	.999831	.999823	.999815	.999809	.999803
370.0	.999860	.999849	.999840	.999832	.999825	.999819	.999814
380.0	.999868	.999857	.999848	.999841	.999834	.999828	.999823
390.0	.999874	.999864	.999856	.999849	.999843	.999837	.999832
400.0	.999880	.999871	.999863	.999856	.999850	.999845	.999841
420.0	.999892	.999883	.999876	.999870	.999864	.999860	.999855
440.0	.999901	.999893	.999887	.999881	.999876	.999872	.999868
460.0	.999910	.999902	.999896	.999891	.999887	.999883	.999879
480.0	.999917	.999910	.999905	.999900	.999896	.999892	.999889
500.0	.999924	.999917	.999912	.999908	.999904	.999901	.999898
520.0	.999929	.999924	.999919	.999915	.999911	.999908	.999906
540.0	.999934	.999929	.999925	.999921	.999918	.999915	.999912
560.0	.999939	.999934	.999930	.999927	.999924	.999921	.999919
580.0	.999943	.999939	.999935	.999932	.999929	.999926	.999924

$\nu = 2$

Q\n	40	50	60	70	80	90	100
600.0	.999947	.999943	.999939	.999936	.999933	.999931	.999929
620.0	.999950	.999946	.999943	.999940	.999938	.999936	.999934
640.0	.999953	.999950	.999946	.999944	.999942	.999940	.999938
660.0	.999956	.999953	.999950	.999947	.999945	.999943	.999941
680.0	.999959	.999955	.999953	.999950	.999948	.999946	.999945
700.0	.999961	.999958	.999955	.999953	.999951	.999949	.999948
720.0	.999963	.999960	.999958	.999956	.999954	.999952	.999951
740.0	.999965	.999962	.999960	.999958	.999956	.999955	.999953
760.0	.999967	.999964	.999962	.999960	.999959	.999957	.999956
780.0	.999969	.999966	.999964	.999962	.999961	.999959	.999958
800.0	.999970	.999968	.999966	.999964	.999963	.999961	.999960
820.0	.999972	.999969	.999967	.999966	.999964	.999963	.999962
840.0	.999973	.999971	.999969	.999967	.999966	.999965	.999964
860.0	.999974	.999972	.999970	.999969	.999968	.999967	.999965
880.0	.999975	.999973	.999972	.999970	.999969	.999968	.999967
900.0	.999976	.999974	.999973	.999972	.999970	.999969	.999968
920.0	.999977	.999976	.999974	.999973	.999972	.999971	.999970
940.0	.999978	.999977	.999975	.999974	.999973	.999972	.999971
960.0	.999979	.999978	.999976	.999975	.999974	.999973	.999972
980.0	.999980	.999978	.999977	.999976	.999975	.999974	.999973
1000.0	.999981	.999979	.999978	.999977	.999976	.999975	.999974
1100.0	.999984	.999983	.999982	.999981	.999980	.999980	.999979
1200.0	.999987	.999986	.999985	.999984	.999983	.999983	.999982
1300.0	.999989	.999988	.999987	.999986	.999986	.999985	.999985
1400.0	.999990	.999989	.999989	.999988	.999988	.999987	.999987
1500.0	.999992	.999991	.999990	.999990	.999989	.999989	.999989
1600.0	.999993	.999992	.999991	.999991	.999991	.999990	.999990
1700.0	.999993	.999993	.999992	.999992	.999992	.999991	.999991
1800.0	.999994	.999994	.999993	.999993	.999993	.999992	.999992
1900.0	.999995	.999994	.999994	.999994	.999993	.999993	.999993
2000.0	1.00000	.999995	.999995	.999994	.999994	.999994	.999994

$\nu = 3$

Q\n	2	3	4	5	6	7	8
0.0	.000000	.000000	.000000	.000000	.000000	.000000	.000000
0.1	.051925	.002750	.000155	.000009	.000001	.000000	.000000
0.2	.103500	.010925	.001229	.000148	.000019	.000003	.000000
0.3	.154401	.024303	.004073	.000728	.000138	.000028	.000006
0.4	.204309	.042528	.009412	.002219	.000555	.000146	.000040
0.5	.252940	.065134	.017801	.005171	.001590	.000514	.000174
0.6	.300041	.091572	.029597	.010145	.003671	.001394	.000553
0.7	.345400	.121236	.044959	.017637	.007284	.003150	.001420
0.8	.388845	.153496	.063855	.028022	.012912	.006215	.003109
0.9	.430249	.187724	.086088	.041529	.020977	.011038	.006022
1.0	.469522	.223316	.111334	.058219	.031790	.018034	.010582
1.2	.541517	.296410	.169141	.100664	.062217	.039752	.026146
1.4	.604821	.369007	.233481	.153248	.103937	.072535	.051891
1.6	.659836	.438382	.300595	.212771	.154922	.115596	.088096
1.8	.707225	.502804	.367342	.275839	.212222	.166734	.133380
2.0	.747785	.561371	.431416	.339474	.272761	.223127	.185357
2.2	.782354	.613789	.491328	.401386	.333850	.281986	.241339
2.4	.811747	.660181	.546268	.460012	.393415	.340947	.298838
2.6	.836715	.700916	.595938	.514420	.450025	.398218	.355830
2.8	.857929	.736497	.640385	.564167	.502808	.452582	.410827
3.0	.875973	.767474	.679870	.609164	.551331	.503302	.462841
3.2	.891350	.794396	.714778	.649549	.595476	.550019	.511296
3.4	.904484	.817782	.745542	.685599	.635336	.592644	.555931
3.6	.915733	.838103	.772608	.717662	.671137	.631269	.596706
3.8	.925396	.855779	.796404	.746117	.703176	.666098	.633729
4.0	.933724	.871179	.817327	.771341	.731783	.697399	.667202
4.2	.940925	.884620	.835737	.793692	.757292	.725470	.697376
4.4	.947171	.896377	.851955	.813504	.780027	.750613	.724524
4.6	.952607	.906685	.866264	.831079	.800293	.773122	.748925
4.8	.957354	.915746	.878911	.846686	.818367	.793273	.770847
5.0	.961514	.923731	.890109	.860566	.834501	.811324	.790544
5.2	.965169	.930785	.900047	.872929	.848920	.827505	.808249
5.4	.968392	.937033	.908883	.883961	.861825	.842025	.824177
5.6	.971242	.942582	.916759	.893822	.873393	.855072	.838520
5.8	.973770	.947522	.923793	.902654	.883778	.866812	.851451
6.0	.976019	.951932	.930089	.910580	.893118	.877391	.863125
6.4	.979818	.959416	.940815	.924126	.909127	.895570	.883232
6.8	.982873	.965464	.949521	.935162	.922213	.910474	.899761
7.2	.985353	.970396	.956646	.944222	.932987	.922775	.913435
7.6	.987384	.974451	.962523	.951715	.941918	.932994	.924816
8.0	.989062	.977812	.967407	.957957	.949373	.941539	.934348
8.4	.990460	.980618	.971495	.963191	.955635	.948729	.942380
8.8	.991633	.982978	.974939	.967609	.960929	.954814	.949186
9.2	.992623	.984976	.977859	.971360	.965429	.959993	.954985
9.6	.993465	.986677	.980350	.974564	.969277	.964426	.959953
10.0	.994184	.988134	.982485	.977314	.972584	.968240	.964230
11.0	.995578	.990961	.986639	.982672	.979035	.975689	.972594
12.0	.996563	.992964	.989588	.986483	.983632	.981004	.978572
13.0	.997277	.994421	.991735	.989262	.986989	.984891	.982947
14.0	.997808	.995503	.993335	.991335	.989494	.987794	.986218

$\nu = 3$

Ω\n	2	3	4	5	6	7	8
15.0	.998209	.996325	.994549	.992909	.991400	.990004	.988709
16.0	.998519	.996958	.995486	.994127	.992874	.991715	.990638
17.0	.998761	.997455	.996222	.995082	.994031	.993058	.992155
18.0	.998954	.997849	.996806	.995842	.994952	.994128	.993362
19.0	.999108	.998167	.997277	.996453	.995693	.994990	.994335
20.0	.999234	.998425	.997659	.996951	.996297	.995691	.995128
22.0	.999423	.998812	.998235	.997699	.997205	.996747	.996321
24.0	.999554	.999083	.998636	.998222	.997840	.997485	.997155
26.0	.999649	.999277	.998925	.998598	.998296	.998016	.997756
28.0	.999718	.999420	.999137	.998875	.998633	.998408	.998199
30.0	.999771	.999528	.999298	.999084	.998887	.998703	.998533
32.0	.999811	.999611	.999421	.999244	.999081	.998930	.998789
34.0	.999842	.999675	.999516	.999369	.999233	.999107	.998989
36.0	.999867	.999726	.999592	.999468	.999353	.999247	.999147
38.0	.999887	.999767	.999653	.999547	.999450	.999359	.999274
40.0	.999903	.999800	.999702	.999612	.999528	.999450	.999377
45.0	.999932	.999859	.999791	.999727	.999668	.999613	.999562
50.0	.999950	.999897	.999847	.999801	.999758	.999718	.999680
55.0	.999963	.999923	.999885	.999850	.999818	.999788	.999760
60.0	.999971	.999941	.999912	.999885	.999860	.999836	.999815
65.0	.999977	.999953	.999930	.999909	.999890	.999871	.999854
70.0	.999982	.999963	.999944	.999927	.999912	.999897	.999883
75.0	.999985	.999970	.999955	.999941	.999928	.999916	.999905
80.0	.999988	.999975	.999963	.999951	.999941	.999931	.999922
85.0	.999990	.999979	.999969	.999959	.999951	.999942	.999935
90.0	.999991	.999982	.999974	.999966	.999958	.999951	.999945
95.0	.999993	.999985	.999978	.999971	.999965	.999959	.999953
100.0	.999994	.999987	.999981	.999975	.999970	.999965	.999960
105.0	.999995	.999989	.999983	.999978	.999974	.999969	.999965
110.0	1.00000	.999990	.999986	.999981	.999977	.999973	.999970
115.0		.999992	.999987	.999984	.999980	.999977	.999974
120.0		.999993	.999989	.999986	.999982	.999979	.999977
125.0		.999993	.999990	.999987	.999984	.999982	.999979
130.0		.999994	.999991	.999989	.999986	.999984	.999982
135.0		.999995	.999992	.999990	.999988	.999986	.999984
140.0		1.00000	.999993	.999991	.999989	.999987	.999985
145.0			.999994	.999992	.999990	.999988	.999987
150.0			.999994	.999993	.999991	.999989	.999988
155.0			.999995	.999993	.999992	.999990	.999989
160.0			1.00000	.999994	.999993	.999991	.999990
165.0				.999994	.999993	.999992	.999991
170.0				.999995	.999994	.999993	.999992
175.0				1.00000	.999994	.999993	.999993
180.0					.999995	.999994	.999993
190.0					1.00000	.999995	.999994
200.0						1.00000	.999995
210.0							1.00000

$\nu = 3$

Q\n	9	10	11	12	13	14	15
0.0	.000000	.000000	.000000	.000000	.000000	.000000	.000000
0.1	.000000	.000000	.000000	.000000	.000000	.000000	.000000
0.2	.000000	.000000	.000000	.000000	.000000	.000000	.000000
0.3	.000001	.000000	.000000	.000000	.000000	.000000	.000000
0.4	.000012	.000004	.000001	.000000	.000000	.000000	.000000
0.5	.000061	.000023	.000009	.000003	.000001	.000001	.000000
0.6	.000228	.000098	.000043	.000020	.000009	.000004	.000002
0.7	.000664	.000321	.000160	.000082	.000043	.000023	.000013
0.8	.001610	.000860	.000472	.000266	.000154	.000090	.000054
0.9	.003393	.001967	.001171	.000713	.000444	.000281	.000182
1.0	.006397	.003971	.002525	.001640	.001086	.000732	.000501
1.2	.017640	.012173	.008570	.006143	.004474	.003307	.002477
1.4	.037936	.028266	.021418	.016474	.012842	.010132	.008083
1.6	.068384	.053941	.043154	.034960	.028640	.023699	.019789
1.8	.108375	.089262	.074401	.062670	.053285	.045687	.039470
2.0	.156038	.132878	.114303	.099202	.086778	.076447	.067774
2.2	.208905	.182615	.161007	.143031	.127915	.115080	.104089
2.4	.264488	.236062	.212241	.192056	.174785	.159877	.146908
2.6	.320625	.290999	.265779	.244090	.225270	.208808	.194305
2.8	.375632	.345604	.319711	.297172	.277390	.259898	.244328
3.0	.428315	.398521	.372554	.349723	.329494	.311447	.295247
3.2	.477912	.448826	.423249	.400573	.380322	.362120	.345666
3.4	.524003	.495960	.471114	.448929	.428986	.410948	.394545
3.6	.566423	.539643	.515762	.494311	.474919	.457285	.441168
3.8	.605188	.579797	.557032	.536477	.517804	.500748	.485092
4.0	.640428	.616488	.594920	.575360	.557517	.541155	.526079
4.2	.672346	.649866	.629530	.611016	.594066	.578469	.564052
4.4	.701184	.680139	.661032	.643579	.627549	.612755	.599042
4.6	.727197	.707539	.689634	.673231	.658123	.644143	.631153
4.8	.750642	.732307	.715561	.700178	.685976	.672804	.660537
5.0	.771768	.754683	.739040	.724637	.711311	.698926	.687370
5.2	.790805	.774895	.760295	.746824	.734336	.722709	.711841
5.4	.807970	.793156	.779535	.766945	.755252	.744348	.734141
5.6	.823459	.809665	.796959	.785195	.774254	.764034	.754455
5.8	.837448	.824601	.812748	.801757	.791520	.781946	.772960
6.0	.850097	.838126	.827066	.816796	.807218	.798250	.789823
6.4	.871931	.861519	.851874	.842898	.834508	.826635	.819224
6.8	.889925	.880842	.872410	.864547	.857184	.850264	.843738
7.2	.904841	.896889	.889495	.882588	.876111	.870014	.864257
7.6	.917278	.910292	.903786	.897700	.891985	.886599	.881508
8.0	.927710	.921550	.915805	.910424	.905366	.900595	.896079
8.4	.936511	.931058	.925967	.921195	.916703	.912463	.908446
8.8	.943977	.939133	.934606	.930358	.926357	.922576	.918993
9.2	.950345	.946026	.941986	.938193	.934617	.931236	.928029
9.6	.955805	.951941	.948324	.944925	.941719	.938686	.935807
10.0	.960509	.957040	.953791	.950736	.947853	.945124	.942532
11.0	.969719	.967034	.964515	.962144	.959904	.957782	.955764
12.0	.976308	.974192	.972206	.970334	.968564	.966884	.965287
13.0	.981136	.979442	.977850	.976349	.974928	.973580	.972297
14.0	.984748	.983372	.982079	.980858	.979703	.978605	.977560

$\nu = 3$

Q\n	9	10	11	12	13	14	15
15.0	.987501	.986370	.985305	.984301	.983349	.982444	.981583
16.0	.989634	.988693	.987807	.986971	.986178	.985425	.984707
17.0	.991311	.990520	.989776	.989073	.988406	.987772	.987168
18.0	.992647	.991976	.991345	.990748	.990183	.989645	.989132
19.0	.993724	.993151	.992611	.992100	.991616	.991156	.990717
20.0	.994601	.994107	.993642	.993202	.992785	.992388	.992009
22.0	.995922	.995548	.995196	.994863	.994547	.994246	.993959
24.0	.996847	.996557	.996284	.996025	.995780	.995547	.995324
26.0	.997512	.997283	.997067	.996863	.996669	.996485	.996309
28.0	.998003	.997819	.997645	.997481	.997326	.997177	.997036
30.0	.998373	.998223	.998082	.997948	.997821	.997700	.997584
32.0	.998657	.998533	.998416	.998306	.998201	.998101	.998005
34.0	.998879	.998775	.998678	.998585	.998498	.998414	.998334
36.0	.999055	.998967	.998885	.998807	.998733	.998662	.998595
38.0	.999195	.999121	.999051	.998984	.998921	.998861	.998804
40.0	.999309	.999246	.999185	.999128	.999074	.999023	.998974
45.0	.999514	.999469	.999427	.999387	.999349	.999312	.999278
50.0	.999645	.999613	.999582	.999552	.999525	.999498	.999473
55.0	.999733	.999709	.999685	.999663	.999642	.999622	.999603
60.0	.999795	.999775	.999758	.999741	.999724	.999709	.999694
65.0	.999838	.999823	.999809	.999796	.999783	.999771	.999759
70.0	.999870	.999858	.999847	.999836	.999826	.999817	.999807
75.0	.999895	.999885	.999876	.999867	.999859	.999851	.999843
80.0	.999913	.999905	.999898	.999890	.999884	.999877	.999871
85.0	.999928	.999921	.999915	.999909	.999903	.999897	.999892
90.0	.999939	.999933	.999928	.999923	.999918	.999914	.999909
95.0	.999948	.999943	.999939	.999934	.999930	.999927	.999923
100.0	.999956	.999951	.999948	.999944	.999940	.999937	.999934
105.0	.999962	.999958	.999955	.999951	.999948	.999946	.999943
110.0	.999967	.999963	.999961	.999958	.999955	.999953	.999950
115.0	.999971	.999968	.999965	.999963	.999961	.999959	.999956
120.0	.999974	.999972	.999970	.999967	.999965	.999964	.999962
125.0	.999977	.999975	.999973	.999971	.999969	.999968	.999966
130.0	.999980	.999978	.999976	.999974	.999973	.999971	.999970
135.0	.999982	.999980	.999979	.999977	.999976	.999974	.999973
140.0	.999984	.999982	.999981	.999980	.999978	.999977	.999976
145.0	.999985	.999984	.999983	.999982	.999980	.999979	.999978
150.0	.999987	.999986	.999984	.999983	.999982	.999981	.999980
155.0	.999988	.999987	.999986	.999985	.999984	.999983	.999982
160.0	.999989	.999988	.999987	.999986	.999985	.999985	.999984
165.0	.999990	.999989	.999988	.999987	.999987	.999986	.999985
170.0	.999991	.999990	.999989	.999989	.999988	.999987	.999987
175.0	.999992	.999991	.999990	.999990	.999989	.999988	.999988
180.0	.999992	.999992	.999991	.999990	.999990	.999989	.999989
190.0	.999994	.999993	.999992	.999992	.999991	.999991	.999990
200.0	.999994	.999994	.999993	.999993	.999993	.999992	.999992
210.0	1.00000	.999995	.999994	.999994	.999994	.999993	.999993
220.0		1.00000	1.00000	.999995	.999994	.999994	.999994
230.0				1.00000	1.00000	.999995	.999995
240.0						1.00000	1.00000

$\nu = 3$

Q\n	16	17	18	19	20	22	24
0.0	.000000	.000000	.000000	.000000	.000000	.000000	.000000
0.2	.000000	.000000	.000000	.000000	.000000	.000000	.000000
0.4	.000000	.000000	.000000	.000000	.000000	.000000	.000000
0.6	.000001	.000001	.000000	.000000	.000000	.000000	.000000
0.8	.000033	.000021	.000013	.000008	.000005	.000002	.000001
1.0	.000348	.000245	.000175	.000126	.000092	.000051	.000029
1.2	.001878	.001439	.001115	.000871	.000687	.000438	.000287
1.4	.006512	.005294	.004340	.003585	.002983	.002105	.001520
1.6	.016660	.014131	.012069	.010372	.008966	.006805	.005262
1.8	.034332	.030049	.026449	.023403	.020806	.016659	.013543
2.0	.060429	.054161	.048774	.044113	.040057	.033386	.028181
2.2	.094603	.086359	.079149	.072805	.067195	.057757	.050175
2.4	.135546	.125529	.116647	.108729	.101636	.089491	.079508
2.6	.181446	.169978	.159696	.150434	.142052	.127494	.115308
2.8	.230388	.217839	.206487	.196172	.186762	.170228	.156181
3.0	.280625	.267361	.255273	.244213	.234054	.216034	.200540
3.2	.330714	.317064	.304548	.293030	.282390	.263368	.246848
3.4	.379555	.365796	.353117	.341389	.330506	.310919	.293766
3.6	.426370	.412725	.400096	.388366	.377437	.357658	.340213
3.8	.470657	.457295	.444882	.433312	.422496	.402826	.385372
4.0	.512131	.499176	.487103	.475815	.465231	.445905	.428667
4.2	.550673	.538210	.526563	.515645	.505383	.486576	.469724
4.4	.586282	.574366	.563202	.552714	.542832	.524668	.508330
4.6	.619037	.607698	.597052	.587029	.577569	.560131	.544391
4.8	.649072	.638321	.628209	.618671	.609653	.592991	.577906
5.0	.676550	.666385	.656809	.647762	.639196	.623334	.608934
5.2	.701649	.692059	.683011	.674452	.666336	.651279	.637578
5.4	.724553	.715521	.706987	.698904	.691230	.676970	.663965
5.6	.745446	.736947	.728908	.721285	.714040	.700557	.688238
5.8	.764500	.756509	.748943	.741762	.734930	.722197	.710543
6.0	.781881	.774372	.767255	.760493	.754055	.742042	.731029
6.4	.812225	.805598	.799305	.793317	.787607	.776929	.767114
6.8	.837566	.831713	.826148	.820845	.815782	.806297	.797559
7.2	.858805	.853628	.848700	.843999	.839506	.831076	.823296
7.6	.876681	.872092	.867720	.863546	.859552	.852050	.845115
8.0	.891794	.887717	.883830	.880115	.876558	.869869	.863677
8.4	.904631	.900999	.897533	.894219	.891044	.885066	.879526
8.8	.915587	.912342	.909243	.906278	.903436	.898082	.893115
9.2	.924979	.922072	.919294	.916635	.914084	.909276	.904811
9.6	.933068	.930456	.927958	.925567	.923271	.918942	.914919
10.0	.940065	.937711	.935460	.933302	.931232	.927323	.923689
11.0	.953841	.952005	.950247	.948561	.946942	.943882	.941032
12.0	.963764	.962308	.960914	.959576	.958290	.955857	.953590
13.0	.971072	.969901	.968779	.967702	.966666	.964705	.962875
14.0	.976562	.975608	.974693	.973814	.972968	.971367	.969872
15.0	.980760	.979973	.979218	.978492	.977794	.976472	.975236
16.0	.984021	.983365	.982735	.982130	.981547	.980443	.979412
17.0	.986591	.986038	.985508	.984998	.984507	.983577	.982707
18.0	.988641	.988172	.987721	.987288	.986871	.986080	.985340
19.0	.990297	.989895	.989509	.989138	.988781	.988103	.987469

$\nu = 3$

Q\n	16	17	18	19	20	22	24
20.0	.991648	.991301	.990968	.990648	.990339	.989755	.989207
22.0	.993684	.993421	.993169	.992926	.992692	.992248	.991832
24.0	.995111	.994907	.994711	.994523	.994341	.993996	.993673
26.0	.996140	.995979	.995824	.995674	.995531	.995258	.995002
28.0	.996900	.996770	.996646	.996526	.996410	.996190	.995985
30.0	.997474	.997368	.997266	.997168	.997073	.996894	.996726
32.0	.997914	.997827	.997742	.997661	.997583	.997435	.997296
34.0	.998258	.998185	.998115	.998047	.997982	.997858	.997742
36.0	.998531	.998469	.998409	.998352	.998297	.998193	.998095
38.0	.998749	.998696	.998646	.998597	.998550	.998461	.998378
40.0	.998926	.998881	.998838	.998796	.998756	.998679	.998607
45.0	.999244	.999213	.999182	.999153	.999124	.999070	.999020
50.0	.999448	.999425	.999403	.999381	.999361	.999321	.999284
55.0	.999585	.999568	.999551	.999535	.999519	.999489	.999462
60.0	.999680	.999667	.999654	.999641	.999629	.999606	.999585
65.0	.999748	.999738	.999728	.999718	.999708	.999690	.999673
70.0	.999798	.999790	.999782	.999774	.999766	.999752	.999738
75.0	.999836	.999829	.999822	.999816	.999810	.999798	.999787
80.0	.999865	.999859	.999854	.999848	.999843	.999834	.999825
85.0	.999887	.999883	.999878	.999874	.999869	.999861	.999854
90.0	.999905	.999901	.999897	.999893	.999890	.999883	.999877
95.0	.999919	.999916	.999913	.999909	.999906	.999901	.999895
100.0	.999931	.999928	.999925	.999922	.999920	.999915	.999910
105.0	.999940	.999938	.999935	.999933	.999931	.999926	.999922
110.0	.999948	.999946	.999944	.999942	.999940	.999936	.999932
115.0	.999954	.999953	.999951	.999949	.999947	.999944	.999941
120.0	.999960	.999958	.999957	.999955	.999953	.999951	.999948
125.0	.999965	.999963	.999962	.999960	.999959	.999956	.999954
130.0	.999968	.999967	.999966	.999965	.999963	.999961	.999959
135.0	.999972	.999971	.999969	.999968	.999967	.999965	.999963
140.0	.999975	.999974	.999973	.999972	.999971	.999969	.999967
145.0	.999977	.999976	.999975	.999974	.999974	.999972	.999970
150.0	.999979	.999979	.999978	.999977	.999976	.999975	.999973
155.0	.999981	.999981	.999980	.999979	.999978	.999977	.999976
160.0	.999983	.999982	.999982	.999981	.999980	.999979	.999978
165.0	.999985	.999984	.999983	.999983	.999982	.999981	.999980
170.0	.999986	.999985	.999985	.999984	.999984	.999983	.999982
175.0	.999987	.999987	.999986	.999985	.999985	.999984	.999983
180.0	.999988	.999988	.999987	.999987	.999986	.999985	.999985
190.0	.999990	.999989	.999989	.999989	.999988	.999988	.999987
200.0	.999991	.999991	.999991	.999990	.999990	.999989	.999989
210.0	.999993	.999992	.999992	.999992	.999991	.999991	.999990
220.0	.999993	.999993	.999993	.999993	.999992	.999992	.999992
230.0	.999994	.999994	.999994	.999994	.999993	.999993	.999993
240.0	.999995	.999995	.999995	.999994	.999994	.999994	.999993
250.0	1.00000	1.00000	1.00000	1.00000	.999995	.999995	.999994
260.0					1.00000	1.00000	.999995
270.0							1.00000

$\nu = 3$

Q\n	26	28	30	32	34	36	38
0.0	.000000	.000000	.000000	.000000	.000000	.000000	.000000
0.2	.000000	.000000	.000000	.000000	.000000	.000000	.000000
0.4	.000000	.000000	.000000	.000000	.000000	.000000	.000000
0.6	.000000	.000000	.000000	.000000	.000000	.000000	.000000
0.8	.000001	.000000	.000000	.000000	.000000	.000000	.000000
1.0	.000017	.000010	.000006	.000004	.000003	.000002	.000001
1.2	.000193	.000132	.000093	.000066	.000048	.000035	.000026
1.4	.001119	.000839	.000639	.000493	.000385	.000305	.000243
1.6	.004135	.003296	.002660	.002171	.001790	.001490	.001250
1.8	.011157	.009299	.007830	.006654	.005701	.004921	.004276
2.0	.024049	.020722	.018007	.015767	.013899	.012328	.010994
2.2	.043990	.038879	.034607	.030999	.027925	.025284	.022999
2.4	.071189	.064175	.058201	.053064	.048612	.044725	.041308
2.6	.104980	.096132	.088480	.081807	.075945	.070761	.066149
2.8	.144112	.133639	.124471	.116384	.109202	.102784	.097018
3.0	.187076	.175269	.164830	.155536	.147208	.139703	.132906
3.2	.232359	.219540	.208114	.197862	.188607	.180210	.172553
3.4	.278603	.265090	.252963	.242009	.232062	.222982	.214658
3.6	.324690	.310770	.298205	.286794	.276377	.266822	.258021
3.8	.369753	.355674	.342902	.331249	.320563	.310722	.301620
4.0	.413167	.399131	.386344	.374630	.363849	.353882	.344634
4.2	.454508	.440676	.428028	.416401	.405665	.395709	.386443
4.4	.493522	.480015	.467625	.456201	.445622	.435785	.426607
4.6	.530080	.516988	.504944	.493810	.483473	.473840	.464830
4.8	.564152	.551535	.539900	.529119	.519089	.509721	.500942
5.0	.595773	.583672	.572487	.562103	.552423	.543365	.534862
5.2	.625027	.613464	.602755	.592795	.583493	.574776	.566580
5.4	.652029	.641012	.630791	.621269	.612363	.604004	.596134
5.6	.676910	.666437	.656706	.647627	.639124	.631132	.623599
5.8	.699811	.689872	.680626	.671987	.663886	.656264	.649070
6.0	.720873	.711455	.702682	.694476	.686771	.679514	.672659
6.4	.758040	.749606	.741731	.734351	.727408	.720857	.714657
6.8	.789464	.781925	.774874	.768253	.762016	.756120	.750533
7.2	.816075	.809339	.803030	.797097	.791500	.786203	.781177
7.6	.838669	.832648	.827000	.821683	.816661	.811904	.807385
8.0	.857914	.852524	.847464	.842695	.838186	.833910	.829846
8.4	.874365	.869533	.864992	.860708	.856655	.852808	.849148
8.8	.888482	.884141	.880058	.876204	.872554	.869088	.865788
9.2	.900643	.896735	.893057	.889582	.886289	.883160	.880179
9.6	.911160	.907634	.904313	.901173	.898197	.895367	.892669
10.0	.920292	.917103	.914097	.911254	.908557	.905992	.903547
11.0	.938365	.935858	.933493	.931253	.929127	.927102	.925169
12.0	.951465	.949466	.947579	.945790	.944090	.942471	.940924
13.0	.961160	.959544	.958018	.956571	.955195	.953883	.952629
14.0	.968470	.967149	.965899	.964714	.963587	.962512	.961484
15.0	.974077	.972984	.971950	.970968	.970035	.969143	.968291
16.0	.978443	.977529	.976665	.975844	.975063	.974317	.973604
17.0	.981890	.981119	.980390	.979697	.979037	.978407	.977805
18.0	.984645	.983990	.983369	.982779	.982218	.981681	.981168
19.0	.986873	.986311	.985779	.985273	.984791	.984331	.983890

$\nu = 3$

Q\n	26	28	30	32	34	36	38
20.0	.988693	.988207	.987748	.987311	.986894	.986497	.986116
22.0	.991441	.991072	.990722	.990390	.990073	.989771	.989481
24.0	.993370	.993083	.992811	.992553	.992307	.992071	.991846
26.0	.994762	.994535	.994320	.994115	.993920	.993733	.993555
28.0	.995791	.995608	.995435	.995270	.995113	.994963	.994819
30.0	.996568	.996419	.996277	.996143	.996015	.995892	.995774
32.0	.997166	.997042	.996925	.996814	.996708	.996606	.996509
34.0	.997632	.997529	.997431	.997338	.997249	.997165	.997083
36.0	.998002	.997915	.997832	.997754	.997679	.997607	.997538
38.0	.998299	.998225	.998154	.998087	.998023	.997962	.997904
40.0	.998540	.998476	.998416	.998358	.998303	.998251	.998200
45.0	.998972	.998927	.998885	.998844	.998805	.998768	.998733
50.0	.999250	.999217	.999185	.999156	.999128	.999100	.999075
55.0	.999435	.999411	.999387	.999365	.999344	.999323	.999304
60.0	.999565	.999546	.999528	.999510	.999494	.999478	.999463
65.0	.999657	.999642	.999628	.999615	.999602	.999589	.999577
70.0	.999726	.999714	.999702	.999691	.999681	.999671	.999661
75.0	.999777	.999767	.999758	.999749	.999740	.999732	.999725
80.0	.999816	.999808	.999800	.999793	.999786	.999779	.999773
85.0	.999847	.999840	.999833	.999827	.999822	.999816	.999811
90.0	.999871	.999865	.999860	.999855	.999850	.999845	.999840
95.0	.999890	.999885	.999881	.999876	.999872	.999868	.999864
100.0	.999906	.999902	.999898	.999894	.999890	.999887	.999884
105.0	.999919	.999915	.999912	.999908	.999905	.999902	.999899
110.0	.999929	.999926	.999923	.999920	.999918	.999915	.999913
115.0	.999938	.999935	.999933	.999930	.999928	.999926	.999923
120.0	.999945	.999943	.999941	.999939	.999936	.999935	.999933
125.0	.999952	.999950	.999948	.999946	.999944	.999942	.999940
130.0	.999957	.999955	.999953	.999952	.999950	.999948	.999947
135.0	.999962	.999960	.999958	.999957	.999955	.999954	.999953
140.0	.999966	.999964	.999963	.999961	.999960	.999959	.999958
145.0	.999969	.999968	.999966	.999965	.999964	.999963	.999962
150.0	.999972	.999971	.999970	.999969	.999967	.999966	.999965
155.0	.999975	.999974	.999972	.999971	.999971	.999970	.999969
160.0	.999977	.999976	.999975	.999974	.999973	.999972	.999972
165.0	.999979	.999978	.999977	.999976	.999976	.999975	.999974
170.0	.999981	.999980	.999979	.999978	.999978	.999977	.999976
175.0	.999982	.999982	.999981	.999980	.999980	.999979	.999978
180.0	.999984	.999983	.999982	.999982	.999981	.999981	.999980
190.0	.999986	.999986	.999985	.999985	.999984	.999983	.999983
200.0	.999988	.999988	.999987	.999987	.999986	.999986	.999985
210.0	.999990	.999989	.999989	.999989	.999988	.999988	.999987
220.0	.999991	.999991	.999990	.999990	.999990	.999989	.999989
230.0	.999992	.999992	.999992	.999991	.999991	.999991	.999990
240.0	.999993	.999993	.999993	.999992	.999992	.999992	.999992
250.0	.999994	.999994	.999993	.999993	.999993	.999993	.999993
260.0	.999995	.999994	.999994	.999994	.999994	.999994	.999993
270.0	1.00000	.999995	.999995	.999995	.999994	.999994	.999994
280.0		1.00000	1.00000	1.00000	.999995	.999995	.999995
290.0					1.00000	1.00000	1.00000

$\nu = 3$

Q\n	40	50	60	70	80	90	100
0.0	.000000	.000000	.000000	.000000	.000000	.000000	.000000
0.1	.000000	.000000	.000000	.000000	.000000	.000000	.000000
0.2	.000000	.000000	.000000	.000000	.000000	.000000	.000000
0.3	.000000	.000000	.000000	.000000	.000000	.000000	.000000
0.4	.000000	.000000	.000000	.000000	.000000	.000000	.000000
0.5	.000000	.000000	.000000	.000000	.000000	.000000	.000000
0.6	.000000	.000000	.000000	.000000	.000000	.000000	.000000
0.7	.000000	.000000	.000000	.000000	.000000	.000000	.000000
0.8	.000000	.000000	.000000	.000000	.000000	.000000	.000000
0.9	.000000	.000000	.000000	.000000	.000000	.000000	.000000
1.0	.000001	.000000	.000000	.000000	.000000	.000000	.000000
1.1	.000005	.000001	.000000	.000000	.000000	.000000	.000000
1.2	.000020	.000006	.000002	.000001	.000000	.000000	.000000
1.3	.000068	.000023	.000009	.000004	.000002	.000001	.000001
1.4	.000196	.000075	.000034	.000017	.000009	.000005	.000003
1.5	.000485	.000209	.000103	.000056	.000032	.000020	.000013
1.6	.001057	.000501	.000267	.000156	.000097	.000063	.000043
1.7	.002075	.001067	.000610	.000377	.000247	.000169	.000120
1.8	.003738	.002060	.001250	.000812	.000556	.000396	.000292
1.9	.006260	.003661	.002335	.001585	.001128	.000832	.000632
2.0	.009855	.006067	.004042	.002848	.002094	.001592	.001242
2.1	.014717	.009476	.006554	.004772	.003611	.002816	.002249
2.2	.021008	.014066	.010055	.007532	.005843	.004660	.003798
2.3	.028843	.019990	.014708	.011296	.008958	.007285	.006045
2.4	.038288	.027356	.020649	.016211	.013108	.010846	.009141
2.5	.049358	.036232	.027976	.022396	.018423	.015478	.013227
2.6	.062023	.046639	.036746	.029933	.025001	.021293	.018421
2.7	.076209	.058556	.046976	.038865	.032908	.028370	.024814
2.8	.091811	.071923	.058642	.049199	.042170	.036755	.032466
2.9	.108698	.086651	.071689	.060905	.052782	.046458	.041403
3.0	.126721	.102625	.086032	.073924	.064706	.057461	.051620
3.1	.145723	.119714	.101565	.088172	.077876	.069714	.063084
3.2	.165542	.137775	.118165	.103545	.092207	.083148	.075737
3.3	.186017	.156662	.135701	.119927	.107595	.097671	.089501
3.4	.206995	.176228	.154036	.137193	.123927	.113182	.104284
3.5	.228329	.196328	.173032	.155212	.141082	.129568	.119981
3.6	.249883	.216827	.192556	.173857	.158937	.146712	.136483
3.7	.271534	.237595	.212480	.193001	.177369	.164496	.153675
3.8	.293171	.258515	.232682	.212523	.196260	.182804	.171446
3.9	.314696	.279478	.253051	.232310	.215496	.201523	.189683
4.0	.336021	.300390	.273484	.252258	.234971	.220547	.208281
4.1	.357074	.321164	.293891	.272270	.254586	.239776	.227140
4.2	.377790	.341727	.314190	.292259	.274251	.259118	.246165
4.3	.398118	.362015	.334308	.312148	.293886	.278489	.265272
4.4	.418014	.381973	.354183	.331870	.313417	.297812	.284381
4.5	.437443	.401555	.373763	.351364	.332781	.317022	.303424
4.6	.456378	.420725	.393001	.370579	.351922	.336058	.322336
4.7	.474799	.439453	.411860	.389473	.370792	.354868	.341064
4.8	.492691	.457714	.430311	.408009	.389350	.373408	.359559
4.9	.510045	.475492	.448328	.426158	.407562	.391640	.377781

$\nu = 3$

Q\n	40	50	60	70	80	90	100
5.0	.526857	.492773	.465893	.443895	.425400	.409531	.395694
5.1	.543125	.509551	.482992	.461201	.442842	.427057	.413270
5.2	.558852	.525820	.499616	.478064	.459868	.444196	.430483
5.3	.574042	.541580	.515758	.494473	.476466	.460930	.447316
5.4	.588703	.556833	.531417	.510422	.492627	.477249	.463753
5.5	.602845	.571584	.546593	.525907	.508344	.493142	.479783
5.6	.616477	.585838	.561289	.540929	.523614	.508605	.495397
5.7	.629613	.599605	.575509	.555489	.538436	.523633	.510592
5.8	.642263	.612893	.589261	.569591	.552812	.538228	.525363
5.9	.654443	.625713	.602551	.583242	.566746	.552390	.539712
6.0	.666165	.638077	.615390	.596447	.580242	.566122	.553640
6.4	.708774	.683217	.662438	.644991	.629995	.616872	.605228
6.8	.745225	.722077	.703155	.687193	.673417	.661322	.650554
7.2	.776396	.755485	.738312	.723769	.711177	.700087	.690190
7.6	.803082	.784212	.768655	.755437	.743960	.733827	.724764
8.0	.825972	.808946	.794863	.782864	.772420	.763180	.754898
8.4	.845658	.830287	.817537	.806647	.797149	.788730	.781172
8.8	.862639	.848748	.837196	.827309	.818670	.811000	.804105
9.2	.877333	.864762	.854284	.845301	.837438	.830448	.824156
9.6	.890093	.878696	.869180	.861007	.853845	.847469	.841724
10.0	.901209	.890859	.882202	.874757	.868225	.862403	.857152
11.0	.923321	.915118	.908232	.902294	.897070	.892405	.888189
12.0	.939443	.932861	.927322	.922534	.918314	.914539	.911123
13.0	.951429	.946084	.941577	.937674	.934229	.931144	.928348
14.0	.960499	.956109	.952402	.949187	.946347	.943799	.941489
15.0	.967475	.963832	.960751	.958077	.955712	.953589	.951662
16.0	.972920	.969867	.967283	.965038	.963050	.961265	.959644
17.0	.977227	.974646	.972460	.970558	.968874	.967361	.965986
18.0	.980676	.978476	.976611	.974988	.973550	.972257	.971082
19.0	.983468	.981579	.979976	.978581	.977344	.976231	.975220
20.0	.985751	.984117	.982731	.981523	.980452	.979488	.978612
22.0	.989203	.987959	.986902	.985981	.985163	.984427	.983758
24.0	.991630	.990662	.989838	.989121	.988483	.987909	.987387
26.0	.993383	.992616	.991963	.991393	.990887	.990431	.990016
28.0	.994681	.994062	.993536	.993077	.992668	.992300	.991965
30.0	.995661	.995156	.994725	.994350	.994016	.993715	.993441
32.0	.996416	.995997	.995641	.995330	.995054	.994804	.994577
34.0	.997005	.996655	.996357	.996097	.995865	.995657	.995466
36.0	.997472	.997177	.996925	.996705	.996509	.996333	.996172
38.0	.997848	.997595	.997381	.997193	.997026	.996876	.996739
40.0	.998152	.997935	.997751	.997590	.997446	.997317	.997199
45.0	.998699	.998546	.998416	.998302	.998201	.998110	.998026
50.0	.999050	.998938	.998843	.998760	.998686	.998619	.998558
55.0	.999285	.999201	.999129	.999067	.999011	.998960	.998915
60.0	.999449	.999384	.999328	.999280	.999237	.999198	.999163
65.0	.999566	.999515	.999471	.999433	.999399	.999369	.999341
70.0	.999652	.999611	.999576	.999546	.999519	.999494	.999472
75.0	.999717	.999684	.999655	.999631	.999608	.999589	.999570
80.0	.999767	.999739	.999716	.999695	.999677	.999661	.999646
85.0	.999806	.999783	.999763	.999746	.999731	.999717	.999705

$\nu = 3$

Q\n	40	50	60	70	80	90	100
90.0	.999836	.999817	.999800	.999786	.999773	.999762	.999751
95.0	.999861	.999844	.999830	.999818	.999807	.999797	.999788
100.0	.999880	.999866	.999854	.999844	.999835	.999826	.999818
105.0	.999897	.999885	.999874	.999865	.999857	.999850	.999843
110.0	.999910	.999900	.999891	.999883	.999876	.999869	.999863
115.0	.999921	.999912	.999904	.999897	.999891	.999886	.999881
120.0	.999931	.999923	.999916	.999910	.999904	.999899	.999895
125.0	.999939	.999932	.999925	.999920	.999915	.999911	.999907
130.0	.999946	.999939	.999934	.999929	.999925	.999921	.999917
135.0	.999951	.999946	.999941	.999936	.999933	.999929	.999926
140.0	.999956	.999951	.999947	.999943	.999940	.999937	.999934
145.0	.999961	.999956	.999952	.999949	.999946	.999943	.999940
150.0	.999965	.999960	.999957	.999954	.999951	.999948	.999946
155.0	.999968	.999964	.999961	.999958	.999955	.999953	.999951
160.0	.999971	.999967	.999964	.999962	.999960	.999957	.999956
165.0	.999973	.999970	.999968	.999965	.999963	.999961	.999960
170.0	.999976	.999973	.999970	.999968	.999966	.999965	.999963
175.0	.999978	.999975	.999973	.999971	.999969	.999967	.999966
180.0	.999979	.999977	.999975	.999973	.999972	.999970	.999969
190.0	.999983	.999980	.999979	.999977	.999976	.999975	.999973
200.0	.999985	.999983	.999982	.999980	.999979	.999978	.999977
210.0	.999987	.999986	.999984	.999983	.999982	.999981	.999980
220.0	.999989	.999987	.999986	.999985	.999984	.999984	.999983
230.0	.999990	.999989	.999988	.999987	.999986	.999986	.999985
240.0	.999991	.999990	.999989	.999989	.999988	.999987	.999987
250.0	.999992	.999991	.999991	.999990	.999989	.999989	.999988
260.0	.999993	.999992	.999992	.999991	.999991	.999990	.999990
270.0	.999994	.999993	.999993	.999992	.999992	.999991	.999991
280.0	.999995	.999994	.999993	.999993	.999992	.999992	.999992
290.0	1.00000	.999995	.999994	.999994	.999993	.999993	.999993
300.0		1.00000	.999995	.999994	.999994	.999994	.999993
310.0			1.00000	.999995	.999994	.999994	.999994
320.0				1.00000	.999995	.999995	.999994
330.0					1.00000	1.00000	.999995
340.0							1.00000

$\nu = 4$

Q\n	2	3	4	5	6	7	8
0.0	.000000	.000000	.000000	.000000	.000000	.000000	.000000
0.1	.052977	.002750	.000149	.000008	.000001	.000000	.000000
0.2	.105626	.010935	.001178	.000133	.000016	.000002	.000000
0.3	.157625	.024352	.003912	.000660	.000117	.000022	.000004
0.4	.208669	.042679	.009068	.002021	.000472	.000116	.000029
0.5	.258479	.065487	.017214	.004739	.001366	.000412	.000129
0.6	.306803	.092266	.028746	.009364	.003189	.001132	.000418
0.7	.353426	.122447	.043877	.016407	.006401	.002599	.001094
0.8	.398168	.155426	.062640	.026290	.011487	.005212	.002448
0.9	.440887	.190590	.084906	.039304	.018900	.009417	.004848
1.0	.481481	.227340	.110410	.055595	.029014	.015655	.008709
1.2	.556061	.303358	.169575	.097838	.058243	.035694	.022461
1.4	.621762	.379513	.236481	.151436	.099633	.067210	.046377
1.6	.678868	.452776	.307234	.213395	.151686	.110149	.081543
1.8	.727961	.521100	.378357	.280193	.211617	.162751	.127230
2.0	.769800	.583307	.447133	.348490	.276164	.222234	.181325
2.2	.805225	.638907	.511688	.415540	.342226	.285527	.241021
2.4	.835077	.687908	.570911	.479345	.407246	.349805	.303446
2.6	.860155	.730640	.624301	.538623	.469346	.412782	.366081
2.8	.881185	.767618	.671800	.592695	.527299	.472806	.426956
3.0	.898808	.799442	.713644	.641337	.580434	.528810	.484683
3.2	.913582	.826730	.750240	.684636	.628498	.580219	.538397
3.4	.925979	.850077	.782083	.722883	.671534	.626825	.587654
3.6	.936397	.870031	.809695	.756477	.709776	.668681	.632325
3.8	.945172	.887081	.833588	.785871	.743572	.706008	.672496
4.0	.952579	.901659	.854239	.811522	.773321	.739125	.708395
4.2	.958850	.914137	.872084	.833874	.799439	.768400	.740328
4.4	.964172	.924833	.887510	.853338	.822334	.794215	.768642
4.6	.968704	.934019	.900856	.870287	.842386	.816944	.793692
4.8	.972574	.941925	.912417	.885055	.859947	.836942	.815824
5.0	.975890	.948744	.922448	.897933	.875330	.854533	.835367
5.2	.978739	.954641	.931167	.909177	.888817	.870011	.852620
5.4	.981196	.959752	.938759	.919009	.900653	.883640	.867857
5.6	.983320	.964193	.945385	.927621	.911054	.895651	.881322
5.8	.985162	.968063	.951180	.935178	.920208	.906250	.893233
6.0	.986764	.971444	.956259	.941822	.928276	.915615	.903780
6.4	.989386	.977003	.964650	.952839	.941703	.931248	.921437
6.8	.991404	.981308	.971183	.961456	.952247	.943570	.935399
7.2	.992974	.984676	.976315	.968251	.960590	.953349	.946511
7.6	.994208	.987334	.980381	.973653	.967241	.961165	.955414
8.0	.995187	.989452	.983630	.977981	.972584	.967457	.962595
8.4	.995971	.991152	.986247	.981475	.976906	.972557	.968425
8.8	.996604	.992529	.988371	.984316	.980427	.976719	.973190
9.2	.997119	.993652	.990107	.986643	.983315	.980138	.977110
9.6	.997541	.994575	.991536	.988561	.985700	.982963	.980353
10.0	.997889	.995338	.992719	.990153	.987680	.985313	.983052
11.0	.998527	.996739	.994896	.993085	.991335	.989656	.988049
12.0	.998942	.997654	.996323	.995012	.993742	.992522	.991352
13.0	.999222	.998272	.997288	.996317	.995376	.994469	.993599
14.0	.999416	.998700	.997958	.997225	.996513	.995827	.995168

$\nu = 4$

Q\n	2	3	4	5	6	7	8
15.0	.999553	.999004	.998435	.997871	.997324	.996795	.996287
16.0	.999652	.999225	.998781	.998341	.997913	.997500	.997102
17.0	.999725	.999388	.999037	.998688	.998349	.998022	.997707
18.0	.999780	.999510	.999229	.998950	.998678	.998415	.998162
19.0	.999822	.999604	.999376	.999150	.998929	.998716	.998511
20.0	.999855	.999676	.999490	.999304	.999124	.998949	.998781
22.0	.999900	.999777	.999649	.999521	.999397	.999276	.999160
24.0	.999929	.999842	.999751	.999660	.999572	.999486	.999403
26.0	.999948	.999885	.999818	.999752	.999688	.999625	.999565
28.0	.999962	.999914	.999865	.999815	.999767	.999720	.999675
30.0	.999971	.999935	.999897	.999859	.999823	.999787	.999753
32.0	.999977	.999949	.999920	.999891	.999863	.999835	.999808
34.0	.999982	.999960	.999937	.999914	.999892	.999870	.999849
36.0	.999986	.999968	.999950	.999932	.999914	.999897	.999880
38.0	.999989	.999974	.999960	.999945	.999931	.999917	.999903
40.0	.999991	.999979	.999967	.999955	.999943	.999932	.999921
45.0	.999994	.999987	.999979	.999972	.999965	.999957	.999951
50.0	1.00000	.999991	.999986	.999982	.999977	.999972	.999967
55.0		.999994	.999991	.999987	.999984	.999981	.999978
60.0		1.00000	.999993	.999991	.999989	.999986	.999984
65.0			1.00000	.999994	.999992	.999990	.999989
70.0				1.00000	.999994	.999993	.999992
75.0					1.00000	.999994	.999994
80.0						1.00000	1.00000

$\nu = 4$

Q\n	9	10	11	12	13	14	15
0.0	.000000	.000000	.000000	.000000	.000000	.000000	.000000
0.1	.000000	.000000	.000000	.000000	.000000	.000000	.000000
0.2	.000000	.000000	.000000	.000000	.000000	.000000	.000000
0.3	.000001	.000000	.000000	.000000	.000000	.000000	.000000
0.4	.000008	.000002	.000001	.000000	.000000	.000000	.000000
0.5	.000042	.000014	.000005	.000002	.000001	.000000	.000000
0.6	.000160	.000063	.000026	.000011	.000005	.000002	.000001
0.7	.000477	.000214	.000099	.000047	.000023	.000011	.000006
0.8	.001187	.000593	.000304	.000160	.000086	.000047	.000026
0.9	.002571	.001401	.000782	.000447	.000261	.000155	.000094
1.0	.004981	.002921	.001753	.001075	.000672	.000427	.000276
1.2	.014475	.009532	.006402	.004376	.003041	.002144	.001533
1.4	.032660	.023426	.017083	.012646	.009489	.007210	.005540
1.6	.061419	.046983	.036445	.028629	.022746	.018260	.014798
1.8	.100926	.081114	.065960	.054205	.044972	.037635	.031745
2.0	.149784	.125100	.105520	.089796	.077028	.066555	.057886
2.2	.205584	.176995	.153654	.134389	.118331	.104828	.093379
2.4	.265561	.234240	.208068	.185987	.167195	.151074	.137143
2.6	.327096	.294213	.266215	.242169	.221354	.203208	.187285
2.8	.388002	.354600	.325715	.300541	.278445	.258927	.241584
3.0	.446637	.413564	.384591	.359032	.336339	.316073	.297877
3.2	.501890	.469785	.441355	.416017	.393304	.372833	.354293
3.4	.553100	.522414	.494989	.470337	.448056	.427820	.409358
3.6	.599964	.570983	.544880	.521242	.499730	.480063	.462008
3.8	.642435	.615319	.590731	.568324	.547810	.528950	.511543
4.0	.680643	.655454	.632479	.611427	.592055	.574158	.557563
4.2	.714828	.691556	.670223	.650582	.632426	.615582	.599902
4.4	.745292	.723881	.704166	.685938	.669024	.653274	.638559
4.6	.772364	.752725	.734570	.717725	.702038	.687384	.673651
4.8	.796377	.778403	.761730	.746209	.731712	.718129	.705366
5.0	.817653	.801228	.785944	.771676	.758312	.745760	.733937
5.2	.836496	.821500	.807508	.794411	.782116	.770541	.759615
5.4	.853182	.839498	.826699	.814691	.803393	.792736	.782656
5.6	.867965	.855480	.843776	.832773	.822401	.812598	.803311
5.8	.881070	.869677	.858975	.848896	.839378	.830367	.821817
6.0	.892699	.882298	.872511	.863277	.854544	.846264	.838397
6.4	.912216	.903532	.895335	.887579	.880223	.873231	.866570
6.8	.927697	.920422	.913538	.907008	.900800	.894887	.889243
7.2	.940049	.933931	.928128	.922613	.917360	.912347	.907554
7.6	.949966	.944799	.939888	.935213	.930752	.926489	.922406
8.0	.957980	.953596	.949422	.945443	.941641	.938002	.934513
8.4	.964498	.960760	.957198	.953796	.950543	.947425	.944434
8.8	.969832	.966631	.963577	.960657	.957862	.955181	.952605
9.2	.974224	.971471	.968841	.966324	.963912	.961597	.959372
9.6	.977862	.975483	.973209	.971031	.968942	.966935	.965004
10.0	.980893	.978829	.976854	.974962	.973145	.971399	.969717
11.0	.986511	.985038	.983627	.982272	.980970	.979716	.978508
12.0	.990231	.989156	.988124	.987132	.986178	.985258	.984371
13.0	.992765	.991963	.991193	.990453	.989740	.989052	.988387
14.0	.994534	.993926	.993341	.992778	.992235	.991712	.991206

ν = 4

Q\n	9	10	11	12	13	14	15
15.0	.995799	.995329	.994877	.994442	.994023	.993617	.993226
16.0	.996720	.996352	.995998	.995657	.995328	.995010	.994702
17.0	.997403	.997112	.996830	.996559	.996298	.996045	.995800
18.0	.997919	.997684	.997458	.997240	.997030	.996827	.996630
19.0	.998313	.998122	.997939	.997762	.997591	.997425	.997265
20.0	.998618	.998462	.998312	.998166	.998026	.997890	.997759
22.0	.999048	.998940	.998836	.998736	.998639	.998545	.998454
24.0	.999324	.999247	.999172	.999101	.999032	.998965	.998900
26.0	.999506	.999450	.999396	.999344	.999293	.999244	.999196
28.0	.999631	.999589	.999549	.999510	.999472	.999435	.999400
30.0	.999719	.999687	.999656	.999627	.999598	.999570	.999543
32.0	.999783	.999758	.999734	.999711	.999688	.999667	.999646
34.0	.999829	.999810	.999791	.999772	.999755	.999738	.999721
36.0	.999864	.999848	.999833	.999819	.999805	.999791	.999778
38.0	.999890	.999878	.999865	.999854	.999842	.999831	.999821
40.0	.999910	.999900	.999890	.999881	.999871	.999862	.999854
45.0	.999944	.999937	.999931	.999925	.999919	.999914	.999908
50.0	.999963	.999959	.999955	.999951	.999947	.999943	.999940
55.0	.999975	.999972	.999969	.999966	.999964	.999961	.999959
60.0	.999982	.999980	.999978	.999976	.999974	.999973	.999971
65.0	.999987	.999986	.999984	.999983	.999981	.999980	.999979
70.0	.999990	.999989	.999988	.999987	.999986	.999985	.999984
75.0	.999993	.999992	.999991	.999990	.999989	.999989	.999988
80.0	.999994	.999994	.999993	.999992	.999992	.999991	.999991
85.0	1.00000	1.00000	.999995	.999994	.999994	.999993	.999993
90.0			1.00000	1.00000	.999995	.999995	.999994
95.0					1.00000	1.00000	1.00000

$\nu = 4$

Q\n	16	17	18	19	20	22	24
0.0	.000000	.000000	.000000	.000000	.000000	.000000	.000000
0.2	.000000	.000000	.000000	.000000	.000000	.000000	.000000
0.4	.000000	.000000	.000000	.000000	.000000	.000000	.000000
0.6	.000000	.000000	.000000	.000000	.000000	.000000	.000000
0.8	.000015	.000009	.000005	.000003	.000002	.000001	.000000
1.0	.000181	.000121	.000081	.000056	.000038	.000019	.000010
1.2	.001110	.000813	.000602	.000450	.000340	.000199	.000120
1.4	.004302	.003373	.002668	.002128	.001711	.001129	.000764
1.6	.012097	.009968	.008274	.006915	.005815	.004185	.003074
1.8	.026969	.023064	.019845	.017171	.014935	.011460	.008943
2.0	.050650	.044563	.039406	.035009	.031238	.025164	.020557
2.2	.083601	.075193	.067918	.061586	.056047	.046877	.039666
2.4	.125027	.114424	.105094	.096842	.089510	.077102	.067066
2.6	.173230	.160758	.149633	.139666	.130697	.115251	.102473
2.8	.226091	.212183	.199641	.188284	.177961	.159925	.144728
3.0	.281460	.266583	.253044	.240677	.229341	.209302	.192160
3.2	.337427	.322020	.307894	.294896	.282899	.261480	.242928
3.4	.392446	.376894	.362543	.349257	.336922	.314718	.295282
3.6	.445370	.429984	.415708	.402424	.390029	.367559	.347715
3.8	.495420	.480438	.466473	.453420	.441189	.418882	.399032
4.0	.542125	.527719	.514238	.501589	.489692	.467883	.448348
4.2	.585259	.571544	.558666	.546542	.535103	.514039	.495065
4.4	.624773	.611820	.599619	.588100	.577202	.557054	.538815
4.6	.660746	.648588	.637106	.626238	.615929	.596808	.579422
4.8	.693342	.681986	.671235	.661037	.651343	.633307	.616845
5.0	.722772	.712205	.702180	.692652	.683578	.666648	.651144
5.2	.749276	.739471	.730153	.721280	.712816	.696987	.682446
5.4	.773101	.764024	.755383	.747141	.739268	.724511	.710920
5.6	.794493	.786103	.778103	.770463	.763154	.749430	.736758
5.8	.813687	.805940	.798545	.791473	.784698	.771956	.760165
6.0	.830905	.823758	.816926	.810386	.804114	.792298	.781343
6.4	.860214	.854136	.848314	.842729	.837363	.827226	.817796
6.8	.883846	.878676	.873715	.868948	.864361	.855675	.847572
7.2	.902963	.898558	.894326	.890253	.886328	.878883	.871921
7.6	.918491	.914730	.911111	.907624	.904260	.897869	.891880
8.0	.931164	.927942	.924839	.921846	.918956	.913458	.908296
8.4	.941558	.938789	.936120	.933544	.931053	.926310	.921851
8.8	.950127	.947739	.945436	.943210	.941058	.936954	.933090
9.2	.957228	.955162	.953167	.951238	.949372	.945809	.942452
9.6	.963144	.961349	.959615	.957938	.956313	.953211	.950284
10.0	.968096	.966532	.965019	.963555	.962137	.959426	.956867
11.0	.977341	.976214	.975123	.974066	.973040	.971078	.969222
12.0	.983514	.982684	.981881	.981102	.980346	.978898	.977526
13.0	.987745	.987123	.986521	.985936	.985368	.984279	.983247
14.0	.990716	.990242	.989782	.989335	.988902	.988069	.987279
15.0	.992847	.992479	.992123	.991777	.991440	.990794	.990181
16.0	.994404	.994116	.993836	.993564	.993299	.992791	.992308
17.0	.995563	.995334	.995111	.994894	.994683	.994278	.993893
18.0	.996439	.996254	.996075	.995900	.995730	.995404	.995093
19.0	.997110	.996960	.996814	.996672	.996533	.996268	.996015

$\nu = 4$

Q\n	16	17	18	19	20	22	24
20.0	.997631	.997508	.997388	.997271	.997157	.996939	.996731
22.0	.998365	.998280	.998197	.998116	.998037	.997886	.997741
24.0	.998837	.998776	.998716	.998659	.998602	.998494	.998391
26.0	.999150	.999106	.999062	.999020	.998979	.998899	.998824
28.0	.999365	.999332	.999299	.999268	.999237	.999177	.999121
30.0	.999516	.999491	.999466	.999442	.999418	.999373	.999330
32.0	.999625	.999605	.999586	.999567	.999549	.999514	.999481
34.0	.999705	.999690	.999674	.999660	.999645	.999618	.999591
36.0	.999765	.999752	.999740	.999729	.999717	.999695	.999674
38.0	.999810	.999800	.999790	.999781	.999772	.999754	.999737
40.0	.999845	.999837	.999829	.999821	.999814	.999799	.999785
45.0	.999903	.999898	.999893	.999888	.999883	.999874	.999865
50.0	.999936	.999933	.999930	.999926	.999923	.999917	.999911
55.0	.999956	.999954	.999952	.999950	.999947	.999943	.999939
60.0	.999969	.999968	.999966	.999964	.999963	.999960	.999957
65.0	.999978	.999976	.999975	.999974	.999973	.999971	.999969
70.0	.999983	.999982	.999982	.999981	.999980	.999978	.999977
75.0	.999987	.999987	.999986	.999985	.999985	.999984	.999982
80.0	.999990	.999990	.999989	.999989	.999988	.999987	.999986
85.0	.999992	.999992	.999992	.999991	.999991	.999990	.999989
90.0	.999994	.999994	.999993	.999993	.999993	.999992	.999992
95.0	1.00000	.999995	.999995	.999994	.999994	.999994	.999993
100.0		1.00000	1.00000	1.00000	1.00000	.999995	.999994
105.0						1.00000	1.00000

$\nu = 4$

Q\n	26	28	30	32	34	36	38
0.0	.000000	.000000	.000000	.000000	.000000	.000000	.000000
0.2	.000000	.000000	.000000	.000000	.000000	.000000	.000000
0.4	.000000	.000000	.000000	.000000	.000000	.000000	.000000
0.6	.000000	.000000	.000000	.000000	.000000	.000000	.000000
0.8	.000000	.000000	.000000	.000000	.000000	.000000	.000000
1.0	.000005	.000003	.000002	.000001	.000001	.000000	.000000
1.2	.000074	.000047	.000031	.000020	.000014	.000009	.000007
1.4	.000528	.000373	.000268	.000195	.000145	.000108	.000082
1.6	.002299	.001747	.001347	.001052	.000831	.000663	.000535
1.8	.007083	.005684	.004615	.003786	.003136	.002619	.002205
2.0	.016999	.014210	.011994	.010211	.008760	.007569	.006582
2.2	.033908	.029248	.025430	.022270	.019629	.017402	.015509
2.4	.058837	.052009	.046282	.041433	.037292	.033730	.030644
2.6	.091771	.082711	.074969	.068295	.062499	.057432	.052972
2.8	.131781	.120642	.110976	.102524	.095082	.088489	.082616
3.0	.177349	.164437	.153091	.143052	.134114	.126110	.118906
3.2	.226710	.212414	.199723	.188382	.178190	.168983	.160626
3.4	.278123	.262859	.249189	.236874	.225720	.215568	.206289
3.6	.330050	.314212	.299923	.286962	.275144	.264322	.254370
3.8	.381235	.365172	.350590	.337284	.325084	.313851	.303470
4.0	.430727	.414731	.400132	.386742	.374405	.362995	.352404
4.2	.477857	.462160	.447766	.434506	.422239	.410847	.400233
4.4	.522199	.506975	.492958	.479995	.467960	.456745	.446261
4.6	.563519	.548893	.535379	.522839	.511159	.500242	.490008
4.8	.601733	.587789	.574864	.562835	.551599	.541070	.531174
5.0	.636866	.623652	.611370	.599910	.589179	.579099	.569603
5.2	.669017	.656557	.644947	.634088	.623898	.614306	.605252
5.4	.698336	.686632	.675702	.665459	.655827	.646743	.638154
5.6	.724999	.714040	.703785	.694156	.685085	.676517	.668402
5.8	.749201	.738963	.729366	.720340	.711823	.703767	.696125
6.0	.771137	.761591	.752628	.744185	.736208	.728651	.721474
6.4	.808983	.800714	.792930	.785577	.778613	.772000	.765706
6.8	.839979	.832838	.826099	.819720	.813665	.807905	.802411
7.2	.865382	.859220	.853393	.847868	.842614	.837607	.832825
7.6	.886245	.880925	.875886	.871101	.866544	.862195	.858036
8.0	.903432	.898833	.894470	.890321	.886366	.882587	.878968
8.4	.917642	.913658	.909874	.906272	.902834	.899545	.896393
8.8	.929440	.925980	.922691	.919556	.916561	.913694	.910943
9.2	.939276	.936263	.933396	.930662	.928047	.925542	.923137
9.6	.947513	.944882	.942376	.939984	.937696	.935501	.933394
10.0	.954442	.952137	.949941	.947843	.945834	.943907	.942055
11.0	.967460	.965784	.964183	.962653	.961185	.959775	.958419
12.0	.976222	.974979	.973792	.972655	.971564	.970515	.969505
13.0	.982265	.981328	.980432	.979573	.978749	.977955	.977191
14.0	.986527	.985810	.985123	.984464	.983831	.983221	.982634
15.0	.989596	.989038	.988504	.987991	.987498	.987023	.986565
16.0	.991847	.991408	.990986	.990582	.990193	.989818	.989456
17.0	.993526	.993175	.992839	.992516	.992205	.991906	.991617
18.0	.994797	.994514	.994243	.993982	.993731	.993489	.993256
19.0	.995773	.995543	.995321	.995109	.994904	.994707	.994516

$\nu = 4$

Q\n	26	28	30	32	34	36	38
20.0	.996532	.996342	.996160	.995985	.995817	.995654	.995497
22.0	.997604	.997472	.997345	.997224	.997107	.996994	.996884
24.0	.998293	.998199	.998108	.998021	.997937	.997856	.997778
26.0	.998752	.998683	.998616	.998553	.998491	.998432	.998375
28.0	.999067	.999015	.998965	.998918	.998872	.998827	.998784
30.0	.999289	.999249	.999211	.999175	.999140	.999106	.999073
32.0	.999449	.999418	.999388	.999360	.999333	.999306	.999281
34.0	.999566	.999542	.999519	.999496	.999475	.999454	.999434
36.0	.999654	.999634	.999616	.999598	.999581	.999564	.999548
38.0	.999721	.999705	.999690	.999676	.999662	.999648	.999635
40.0	.999772	.999759	.999747	.999735	.999724	.999713	.999702
45.0	.999857	.999849	.999841	.999834	.999827	.999820	.999813
50.0	.999906	.999901	.999896	.999891	.999886	.999882	.999877
55.0	.999936	.999932	.999929	.999925	.999922	.999919	.999916
60.0	.999955	.999952	.999950	.999947	.999945	.999943	.999941
65.0	.999967	.999965	.999963	.999962	.999960	.999958	.999957
70.0	.999975	.999974	.999973	.999971	.999970	.999969	.999968
75.0	.999981	.999980	.999979	.999978	.999977	.999976	.999976
80.0	.999986	.999985	.999984	.999983	.999982	.999982	.999981
85.0	.999989	.999988	.999987	.999987	.999986	.999986	.999985
90.0	.999991	.999990	.999990	.999990	.999989	.999989	.999988
95.0	.999993	.999992	.999992	.999992	.999991	.999991	.999990
100.0	.999994	.999994	.999993	.999993	.999993	.999993	.999992
105.0	1.00000	.999995	.999995	.999994	.999994	.999994	.999994
110.0		1.00000	1.00000	1.00000	1.00000	.999995	.999995
115.0						1.00000	1.00000

$\nu = 4$

Q\n	40	50	60	70	80	90	100
0.0	.000000	.000000	.000000	.000000	.000000	.000000	.000000
0.1	.000000	.000000	.000000	.000000	.000000	.000000	.000000
0.2	.000000	.000000	.000000	.000000	.000000	.000000	.000000
0.3	.000000	.000000	.000000	.000000	.000000	.000000	.000000
0.4	.000000	.000000	.000000	.000000	.000000	.000000	.000000
0.5	.000000	.000000	.000000	.000000	.000000	.000000	.000000
0.6	.000000	.000000	.000000	.000000	.000000	.000000	.000000
0.7	.000000	.000000	.000000	.000000	.000000	.000000	.000000
0.8	.000000	.000000	.000000	.000000	.000000	.000000	.000000
0.9	.000000	.000000	.000000	.000000	.000000	.000000	.000000
1.0	.000000	.000000	.000000	.000000	.000000	.000000	.000000
1.1	.000001	.000000	.000000	.000000	.000000	.000000	.000000
1.2	.000005	.000001	.000000	.000000	.000000	.000000	.000000
1.3	.000019	.000005	.000002	.000001	.000000	.000000	.000000
1.4	.000063	.000019	.000007	.000003	.000001	.000001	.000000
1.5	.000178	.000063	.000026	.000012	.000006	.000003	.000002
1.6	.000435	.000173	.000079	.000040	.000022	.000013	.000008
1.7	.000947	.000416	.000207	.000113	.000067	.000041	.000027
1.8	.001870	.000896	.000481	.000281	.000174	.000114	.000077
1.9	.003399	.001754	.001004	.000619	.000404	.000275	.000195
2.0	.005757	.003170	.001916	.001239	.000843	.000598	.000437
2.1	.009178	.005346	.003389	.002284	.001613	.001181	.000891
2.2	.013890	.008500	.005618	.003926	.002862	.002157	.001670
2.3	.020094	.012843	.008806	.006353	.004764	.003682	.002916
2.4	.027953	.018566	.013150	.009758	.007500	.005926	.004789
2.5	.037578	.025825	.018826	.014322	.011253	.009069	.007459
2.6	.049027	.034735	.025980	.020208	.016191	.013279	.011096
2.7	.062302	.045360	.034715	.027543	.022457	.018708	.015856
2.8	.077356	.057716	.045090	.036417	.030163	.025482	.021873
2.9	.094096	.071771	.057120	.046878	.039379	.033690	.029251
3.0	.112392	.087452	.070775	.058932	.050139	.043387	.038060
3.1	.132088	.104649	.085989	.072544	.062437	.054588	.048334
3.2	.153009	.123228	.102660	.087645	.076228	.067272	.060071
3.3	.174967	.143033	.120665	.104138	.091440	.081388	.073237
3.4	.197773	.163896	.139857	.121901	.107973	.096852	.087768
3.5	.221240	.185643	.160083	.140797	.125706	.113563	.103574
3.6	.245185	.208101	.181179	.160678	.144506	.131400	.120550
3.7	.269438	.231098	.202984	.181389	.164229	.150230	.138573
3.8	.293842	.254474	.225336	.202778	.184729	.169916	.157513
3.9	.318252	.278077	.248084	.224694	.205859	.190315	.177234
4.0	.342540	.301767	.271082	.246991	.227477	.211288	.197601
4.1	.366593	.325417	.294199	.269534	.249446	.232700	.218480
4.2	.390312	.348917	.317313	.292197	.271637	.254420	.239741
4.3	.413615	.372165	.340315	.314864	.293931	.276328	.261264
4.4	.436431	.395077	.363108	.337432	.316220	.298312	.282933
4.5	.458704	.417579	.385609	.359808	.338405	.320270	.304644
4.6	.480386	.439611	.407745	.381913	.360401	.342111	.326303
4.7	.501442	.461122	.429455	.403676	.382130	.363752	.347822
4.8	.521847	.482072	.450688	.425039	.403527	.385123	.369128
4.9	.541581	.502431	.471403	.445951	.424536	.406163	.390154

$\nu = 4$

Q\n	40	50	60	70	80	90	100
5.0	.560635	.522174	.491567	.466372	.445110	.426818	.410842
5.1	.579002	.541286	.511154	.486270	.465209	.447046	.431145
5.2	.596684	.559757	.530148	.505619	.484803	.466808	.451022
5.3	.613685	.577583	.548536	.524401	.503868	.486077	.470439
5.4	.630012	.594764	.566310	.542603	.522385	.504831	.489370
5.5	.645679	.611305	.583470	.560218	.540342	.523051	.507795
5.6	.660698	.627212	.600016	.577241	.557732	.540727	.525697
5.7	.675087	.642496	.615954	.593674	.574550	.557850	.543067
5.8	.688861	.657170	.631292	.609521	.590798	.574419	.559898
5.9	.702040	.671247	.646040	.624788	.606477	.590433	.576189
6.0	.714643	.684744	.660210	.639484	.621594	.605896	.591938
6.4	.759702	.733274	.711403	.692793	.676631	.662370	.649628
6.8	.797162	.773948	.754600	.738040	.723583	.710768	.699271
7.2	.828249	.807931	.790896	.776242	.763394	.751962	.741670
7.6	.854051	.836296	.821337	.808414	.797041	.786890	.777724
8.0	.875497	.859989	.846866	.835489	.825445	.816454	.808316
8.4	.893367	.879812	.868301	.858288	.849426	.841474	.834261
8.8	.908301	.896439	.886332	.877519	.869699	.862667	.856278
9.2	.920825	.910426	.901541	.893774	.886869	.880650	.874989
9.6	.931366	.922231	.914406	.907552	.901448	.895941	.890921
10.0	.940272	.932228	.925324	.919265	.913860	.908977	.904521
11.0	.957112	.951197	.946098	.941606	.937586	.933943	.930611
12.0	.968531	.964112	.960289	.956913	.953883	.951132	.948610
13.0	.976452	.973100	.970191	.967617	.965302	.963197	.961264
14.0	.982066	.979484	.977240	.975250	.973458	.971826	.970326
15.0	.986123	.984107	.982352	.980793	.979388	.978107	.976928
16.0	.989106	.987512	.986123	.984887	.983772	.982755	.981818
17.0	.991337	.990062	.988949	.987958	.987064	.986247	.985494
18.0	.993030	.991999	.991098	.990295	.989570	.988907	.988296
19.0	.994332	.993490	.992753	.992097	.991503	.990961	.990460
20.0	.995345	.994651	.994044	.993502	.993012	.992564	.992151
22.0	.996779	.996296	.995872	.995495	.995153	.994839	.994550
24.0	.997703	.997357	.997053	.996782	.996537	.996312	.996104
26.0	.998319	.998065	.997842	.997643	.997462	.997297	.997144
28.0	.998742	.998552	.998385	.998235	.998099	.997975	.997860
30.0	.999041	.998895	.998767	.998653	.998549	.998454	.998366
32.0	.999256	.999143	.999043	.998954	.998874	.998800	.998731
34.0	.999414	.999325	.999247	.999176	.999113	.999054	.999000
36.0	.999533	.999461	.999399	.999343	.999292	.999245	.999202
38.0	.999623	.999565	.999514	.999469	.999428	.999390	.999355
40.0	.999692	.999645	.999604	.999566	.999533	.999502	.999473
45.0	.999807	.999777	.999751	.999728	.999707	.999688	.999670
50.0	.999873	.999853	.999836	.999821	.999807	.999794	.999782
55.0	.999913	.999900	.999888	.999877	.999868	.999859	.999851
60.0	.999939	.999929	.999921	.999913	.999907	.999900	.999895
65.0	.999955	.999948	.999942	.999937	.999932	.999928	.999923
70.0	.999967	.999962	.999957	.999953	.999949	.999946	.999943
75.0	.999975	.999971	.999967	.999964	.999962	.999959	.999957
80.0	.999980	.999977	.999975	.999972	.999970	.999968	.999966
85.0	.999985	.999982	.999980	.999978	.999977	.999975	.999974

$\nu = 4$

Q\n	40	50	60	70	80	90	100
90.0	.999988	.999986	.999984	.999983	.999981	.999980	.999979
95.0	.999990	.999989	.999987	.999986	.999985	.999984	.999983
100.0	.999992	.999991	.999990	.999989	.999988	.999987	.999986
105.0	.999993	.999992	.999991	.999991	.999990	.999989	.999989
110.0	.999995	.999994	.999993	.999992	.999992	.999991	.999991
115.0	1.00000	.999995	.999994	.999994	.999993	.999993	.999992
120.0		1.00000	1.00000	.999995	.999994	.999994	.999993
125.0				1.00000	.999995	.999995	.999994
130.0					1.00000	1.00000	1.00000

$\nu = 5$

Q\n	2	3	4	5	6	7	8
0.0	.000000	.000000	.000000	.000000	.000000	.000000	.000000
0.1	.053614	.002750	.000145	.000008	.000000	.000000	.000000
0.2	.106941	.010941	.001146	.000125	.000014	.000002	.000000
0.3	.159619	.024382	.003811	.000619	.000105	.000018	.000003
0.4	.211367	.042770	.008850	.001900	.000424	.000099	.000024
0.5	.261907	.065701	.016839	.004472	.001234	.000354	.000105
0.6	.310991	.092690	.028196	.008875	.002898	.000981	.000344
0.7	.358401	.123190	.043166	.015627	.005860	.002275	.000912
0.8	.403951	.156616	.061823	.025172	.010598	.004611	.002069
0.9	.447493	.192369	.084083	.037843	.017579	.008423	.004156
1.0	.488916	.229851	.109722	.053834	.027212	.014161	.007574
1.2	.565125	.307747	.169702	.095834	.055544	.033020	.020103
1.4	.632345	.386224	.238248	.149976	.096541	.063515	.042652
1.6	.690775	.462061	.311408	.213470	.149131	.106134	.076860
1.8	.740938	.532991	.385498	.282759	.210723	.159513	.122533
2.0	.783563	.597638	.457516	.354277	.277985	.220994	.177863
2.2	.819482	.655361	.525300	.424953	.347549	.287358	.240046
2.4	.849553	.706075	.587502	.492454	.416501	.355459	.305972
2.6	.874607	.750071	.643454	.555215	.482600	.422627	.372752
2.8	.895408	.787870	.693008	.612355	.544327	.486847	.438018
3.0	.912641	.820108	.736371	.663530	.600797	.546764	.500038
3.2	.926900	.847455	.773968	.708782	.651636	.601607	.557685
3.4	.938695	.870567	.806342	.748407	.696839	.651059	.610347
3.6	.948458	.890052	.834080	.782849	.736647	.695135	.657808
3.8	.956546	.906458	.857763	.812624	.771450	.734070	.700134
4.0	.963257	.920264	.877937	.838264	.801714	.768230	.737578
4.2	.968837	.931886	.895100	.860285	.827929	.798050	.770499
4.4	.973487	.941676	.909695	.879166	.850574	.823987	.799314
4.6	.977372	.949935	.922109	.895343	.870104	.846490	.824451
4.8	.980625	.956912	.932674	.909200	.886931	.865981	.846330
5.0	.983359	.962817	.941675	.921075	.901426	.882850	.865348
5.2	.985661	.967827	.949355	.931259	.913914	.897445	.881866
5.4	.987606	.972085	.955919	.940002	.924681	.910075	.896209
5.6	.989255	.975715	.961539	.947520	.933973	.921012	.908668
5.8	.990656	.978815	.966361	.953995	.942002	.930492	.919497
6.0	.991851	.981471	.970506	.959580	.948950	.938717	.928916
6.4	.993749	.985714	.977164	.968589	.960199	.952083	.944273
6.8	.995152	.988873	.982151	.975373	.968710	.962236	.955983
7.2	.996202	.991251	.985922	.980525	.975197	.970003	.964970
7.6	.996995	.993057	.988799	.984469	.980182	.975989	.971914
8.0	.997601	.994442	.991013	.987516	.984042	.980635	.977317
8.4	.998069	.995515	.992733	.989888	.987055	.984270	.981552
8.8	.998432	.996352	.994080	.991750	.989425	.987135	.984895
9.2	.998718	.997012	.995143	.993223	.991302	.989408	.987553
9.6	.998944	.997535	.995989	.994396	.992801	.991225	.989679
10.0	.999125	.997954	.996666	.995338	.994005	.992687	.991392
11.0	.999438	.998681	.997846	.996982	.996112	.995249	.994400
12.0	.999626	.999122	.998563	.997983	.997398	.996816	.996243
13.0	.999744	.999398	.999014	.998614	.998210	.997807	.997410
14.0	.999821	.999577	.999306	.999024	.998738	.998453	.998171

$\nu = 5$

Q\n	2	3	4	5	6	7	8
15.0	.999871	.999696	.999501	.999297	.999091	.998885	.998681
16.0	.999906	.999777	.999634	.999484	.999332	.999180	.999030
17.0	.999930	.999834	.999727	.999615	.999501	.999387	.999275
18.0	.999947	.999874	.999793	.999708	.999621	.999535	.999449
19.0	.999959	.999903	.999841	.999775	.999709	.999642	.999576
20.0	.999968	.999925	.999876	.999825	.999773	.999721	.999669
22.0	.999980	.999953	.999922	.999890	.999857	.999825	.999792
24.0	.999987	.999969	.999949	.999928	.999907	.999885	.999864
26.0	.999991	.999979	.999966	.999952	.999937	.999923	.999908
28.0	.999994	.999986	.999976	.999966	.999956	.999946	.999936
30.0	1.00000	.999990	.999983	.999976	.999969	.999962	.999955
32.0		.999993	.999988	.999983	.999977	.999972	.999967
34.0		.999994	.999991	.999987	.999983	.999979	.999976
36.0		1.00000	.999993	.999990	.999987	.999985	.999982
38.0			.999995	.999993	.999990	.999988	.999986
40.0			1.00000	.999994	.999993	.999991	.999989
45.0				1.00000	1.00000	.999995	.999994
50.0						1.00000	1.00000

$\nu = 5$

Q\n	9	10	11	12	13	14	15
0.0	.000000	.000000	.000000	.000000	.000000	.000000	.000000
0.1	.000000	.000000	.000000	.000000	.000000	.000000	.000000
0.2	.000000	.000000	.000000	.000000	.000000	.000000	.000000
0.3	.000001	.000000	.000000	.000000	.000000	.000000	.000000
0.4	.000006	.000002	.000000	.000000	.000000	.000000	.000000
0.5	.000032	.000010	.000003	.000001	.000000	.000000	.000000
0.6	.000124	.000046	.000018	.000007	.000003	.000001	.000000
0.7	.000377	.000161	.000070	.000031	.000014	.000007	.000003
0.8	.000956	.000454	.000221	.000110	.000056	.000029	.000015
0.9	.002107	.001096	.000583	.000317	.000176	.000100	.000057
1.0	.004156	.002335	.001341	.000786	.000469	.000285	.000176
1.2	.012513	.007949	.005146	.003389	.002268	.001540	.001061
1.4	.029188	.020325	.014381	.010325	.007514	.005536	.004126
1.6	.056560	.042238	.031971	.024499	.018986	.014868	.011755
1.8	.095408	.075212	.059965	.048305	.039282	.032223	.026644
2.0	.144783	.119084	.098879	.082814	.069910	.059445	.050884
2.2	.202436	.172206	.147656	.127525	.110867	.096970	.085288
2.4	.265470	.232006	.204109	.180655	.160782	.143821	.129248
2.6	.330941	.295608	.265514	.239695	.217390	.197999	.181040
2.8	.396264	.360311	.329144	.301952	.278084	.257016	.238322
3.0	.459410	.423876	.392614	.364956	.340355	.318365	.298616
3.2	.518954	.484629	.454054	.426683	.402066	.379828	.359654
3.4	.574013	.541450	.512136	.485633	.461571	.439638	.419571
3.6	.624151	.593695	.566031	.540806	.517718	.496513	.476971
3.8	.669262	.641095	.615310	.591626	.569799	.549619	.530905
4.0	.709477	.683653	.659854	.637855	.617459	.598495	.580814
4.2	.745071	.721557	.699758	.679496	.660613	.642969	.626442
4.4	.776406	.755106	.735258	.716720	.699364	.683078	.667759
4.6	.803882	.784664	.766674	.749800	.733939	.718998	.704894
4.8	.827906	.810616	.794367	.779068	.764636	.750996	.738079
5.0	.848870	.833348	.818709	.804879	.791791	.779385	.767603
5.2	.867144	.853229	.840062	.827587	.815748	.804496	.793782
5.4	.883063	.870599	.858772	.847535	.836845	.826660	.816941
5.6	.896930	.885770	.875153	.865042	.855401	.846195	.837393
5.8	.909013	.899021	.889493	.880400	.871711	.863398	.855436
6.0	.919549	.910600	.902049	.893872	.886044	.878543	.871345
6.4	.936776	.929587	.922692	.916076	.909722	.903614	.897736
6.8	.949960	.944164	.938589	.933223	.928057	.923078	.918276
7.2	.960107	.955414	.950889	.946524	.942310	.938241	.934309
7.6	.967967	.964149	.960460	.956893	.953444	.950108	.946877
8.0	.974096	.970975	.967952	.965025	.962190	.959442	.956779
8.4	.978909	.976343	.973854	.971440	.969099	.966827	.964621
8.8	.982714	.980593	.978533	.976533	.974590	.972703	.970869
9.2	.985743	.983981	.982267	.980601	.978982	.977407	.975874
9.6	.988169	.986698	.985265	.983871	.982514	.981194	.979908
10.0	.990126	.988891	.987688	.986515	.985373	.984261	.983177
11.0	.993567	.992753	.991959	.991183	.990426	.989688	.988968
12.0	.995680	.995128	.994589	.994062	.993547	.993044	.992553
13.0	.997019	.996636	.996261	.995894	.995535	.995184	.994841
14.0	.997894	.997621	.997355	.997094	.996838	.996588	.996343

ν = 5

Q\n	9	10	11	12	13	14	15
15.0	.998480	.998282	.998089	.997899	.997714	.997532	.997354
16.0	.998882	.998736	.998593	.998453	.998316	.998181	.998049
17.0	.999163	.999054	.998947	.998842	.998738	.998637	.998538
18.0	.999365	.999281	.999200	.999119	.999041	.998964	.998888
19.0	.999511	.999446	.999383	.999321	.999260	.999201	.999142
20.0	.999618	.999568	.999519	.999470	.999423	.999376	.999330
22.0	.999760	.999728	.999697	.999667	.999637	.999607	.999578
24.0	.999843	.999822	.999802	.999782	.999762	.999743	.999724
26.0	.999894	.999880	.999866	.999853	.999839	.999826	.999813
28.0	.999926	.999917	.999907	.999898	.999888	.999879	.999870
30.0	.999948	.999941	.999934	.999927	.999921	.999914	.999908
32.0	.999962	.999957	.999952	.999947	.999942	.999937	.999933
34.0	.999972	.999968	.999964	.999961	.999957	.999954	.999950
36.0	.999979	.999976	.999973	.999970	.999968	.999965	.999962
38.0	.999984	.999982	.999979	.999977	.999975	.999973	.999971
40.0	.999987	.999986	.999984	.999982	.999981	.999979	.999978
45.0	.999993	.999992	.999991	.999990	.999989	.999988	.999988
50.0	1.00000	1.00000	.999995	.999994	.999994	.999993	.999993
55.0			1.00000	1.00000	1.00000	1.00000	1.00000

$\nu = 5$

Q\n	16	17	18	19	20	22	24
0.0	.000000	.000000	.000000	.000000	.000000	.000000	.000000
0.2	.000000	.000000	.000000	.000000	.000000	.000000	.000000
0.4	.000000	.000000	.000000	.000000	.000000	.000000	.000000
0.6	.000000	.000000	.000000	.000000	.000000	.000000	.000000
0.8	.000008	.000005	.000003	.000001	.000001	.000000	.000000
1.0	.000110	.000070	.000045	.000030	.000020	.000009	.000004
1.2	.000740	.000522	.000373	.000269	.000196	.000107	.000060
1.4	.003108	.002365	.001816	.001406	.001098	.000684	.000438
1.6	.009376	.007541	.006111	.004987	.004097	.002816	.001978
1.8	.022193	.018613	.015709	.013336	.011383	.008420	.006341
2.0	.043824	.037957	.033049	.028916	.025415	.019879	.015781
2.2	.075397	.066969	.059744	.053514	.048116	.039302	.032501
2.4	.116650	.105696	.096120	.087710	.080287	.067857	.057945
2.6	.166129	.152951	.141250	.130815	.121472	.105500	.092423
2.8	.221655	.206727	.193302	.181182	.170199	.151108	.135137
3.0	.280805	.264675	.250015	.236644	.224408	.202842	.184479
3.2	.341283	.324492	.309096	.294933	.281866	.258569	.238436
3.4	.401148	.384179	.368501	.353977	.340484	.316190	.294935
3.6	.458904	.442153	.426579	.412061	.398496	.373869	.352095
3.8	.513502	.497274	.482104	.467889	.454540	.430133	.408358
4.0	.564287	.548800	.534254	.520563	.507650	.483896	.462538
4.2	.610923	.596320	.582548	.569534	.557214	.534430	.513806
4.4	.653319	.639680	.626771	.614532	.602906	.581307	.561641
4.6	.691554	.678912	.666910	.655496	.644623	.624340	.605777
4.8	.725824	.714177	.703089	.692516	.682419	.663515	.646135
5.0	.756395	.745715	.735523	.725781	.716457	.698945	.682779
5.2	.783566	.773810	.764478	.755540	.746968	.730823	.715865
5.4	.807653	.798765	.790247	.782073	.774222	.759391	.745609
5.6	.828965	.820885	.813128	.805672	.798497	.784916	.772259
5.8	.847799	.840464	.833412	.826623	.820080	.807672	.796076
6.0	.864430	.857779	.851376	.845202	.839245	.827926	.817324
6.4	.892075	.886615	.881345	.876253	.871327	.861939	.853109
6.8	.913639	.909158	.904824	.900627	.896561	.888788	.881453
7.2	.930505	.926822	.923253	.919792	.916432	.909997	.903907
7.6	.943747	.940712	.937767	.934906	.932126	.926790	.921728
8.0	.954194	.951685	.949246	.946875	.944569	.940133	.935917
8.4	.962479	.960396	.958370	.956398	.954478	.950780	.947259
8.8	.969085	.967350	.965660	.964014	.962409	.959315	.956365
9.2	.974383	.972931	.971515	.970136	.968789	.966191	.963710
9.6	.978656	.977435	.976245	.975083	.973950	.971760	.969665
10.0	.982121	.981091	.980085	.979104	.978145	.976292	.974517
11.0	.988264	.987577	.986906	.986250	.985609	.984366	.983174
12.0	.992072	.991603	.991144	.990694	.990254	.989402	.988582
13.0	.994505	.994177	.993856	.993541	.993232	.992634	.992058
14.0	.996103	.995869	.995639	.995414	.995193	.994765	.994352
15.0	.997179	.997009	.996841	.996677	.996516	.996203	.995902
16.0	.997920	.997794	.997670	.997548	.997429	.997197	.996973
17.0	.998441	.998346	.998252	.998161	.998071	.997896	.997727
18.0	.998814	.998741	.998670	.998600	.998531	.998397	.998268
19.0	.999085	.999029	.998974	.998919	.998866	.998763	.998663

$\nu = 5$

Q\n	16	17	18	19	20	22	24
20.0	.999286	.999242	.999198	.999156	.999114	.999033	.998955
22.0	.999550	.999522	.999495	.999468	.999441	.999390	.999340
24.0	.999705	.999687	.999669	.999651	.999634	.999600	.999568
26.0	.999801	.999788	.999776	.999764	.999753	.999730	.999708
28.0	.999862	.999853	.999844	.999836	.999828	.999812	.999797
30.0	.999901	.999895	.999889	.999883	.999877	.999866	.999855
32.0	.999928	.999924	.999919	.999915	.999911	.999902	.999894
34.0	.999947	.999943	.999940	.999937	.999934	.999928	.999922
36.0	.999960	.999957	.999955	.999952	.999950	.999945	.999941
38.0	.999969	.999967	.999966	.999964	.999962	.999958	.999955
40.0	.999976	.999975	.999973	.999972	.999970	.999968	.999965
45.0	.999987	.999986	.999985	.999984	.999983	.999982	.999980
50.0	.999992	.999992	.999991	.999991	.999990	.999989	.999988
55.0	1.00000	.999995	.999994	.999994	.999994	.999993	.999993
60.0		1.00000	1.00000	1.00000	1.00000	1.00000	1.00000

$\nu = 5$

Q\n	26	28	30	32	34	36	38
0.0	.000000	.000000	.000000	.000000	.000000	.000000	.000000
0.2	.000000	.000000	.000000	.000000	.000000	.000000	.000000
0.4	.000000	.000000	.000000	.000000	.000000	.000000	.000000
0.6	.000000	.000000	.000000	.000000	.000000	.000000	.000000
0.8	.000000	.000000	.000000	.000000	.000000	.000000	.000000
1.0	.000002	.000001	.000001	.000000	.000000	.000000	.000000
1.2	.000035	.000021	.000013	.000008	.000005	.000003	.000002
1.4	.000287	.000192	.000131	.000091	.000064	.000046	.000033
1.6	.001417	.001033	.000764	.000574	.000436	.000336	.000261
1.8	.004851	.003765	.002959	.002353	.001890	.001533	.001254
2.0	.012694	.010331	.008496	.007053	.005906	.004984	.004236
2.2	.027172	.022937	.019532	.016762	.014487	.012602	.011026
2.4	.049933	.043378	.037957	.033430	.029617	.026379	.023611
2.6	.081587	.072511	.064836	.058290	.052664	.047795	.043554
2.8	.121632	.110103	.100177	.091565	.084042	.077429	.071583
3.0	.168692	.155001	.143038	.132512	.123193	.114897	.107473
3.2	.220886	.205468	.191828	.179686	.168818	.159039	.150200
3.4	.276190	.259541	.244660	.231283	.219197	.208226	.198226
3.6	.332701	.315316	.299640	.285433	.272495	.260663	.249800
3.8	.388800	.371128	.355074	.340421	.326988	.314625	.303204
4.0	.443215	.425637	.409565	.394807	.381199	.368605	.356911
4.2	.495029	.477847	.462050	.447467	.433953	.421388	.409668
4.4	.543638	.527079	.511781	.497593	.484389	.472061	.460516
4.6	.588701	.572924	.558286	.544657	.531924	.519992	.508780
4.8	.630080	.615187	.601318	.588358	.576210	.564789	.554026
5.0	.667790	.653836	.640799	.628578	.617088	.606256	.596020
5.2	.701950	.688955	.676778	.665331	.654541	.644343	.634682
5.4	.732749	.720705	.709390	.698727	.688651	.679108	.670047
5.6	.760416	.749297	.738826	.728936	.719572	.710684	.702230
5.8	.785201	.774967	.765309	.756169	.747497	.739252	.731396
6.0	.807358	.797961	.789076	.780651	.772646	.765021	.757744
6.4	.844777	.836894	.829414	.822300	.815519	.809043	.802846
6.8	.874511	.867922	.861653	.855676	.849964	.844496	.839252
7.2	.898127	.892628	.887385	.882373	.877575	.872972	.868549
7.6	.916914	.912323	.907937	.903738	.899709	.895839	.892114
8.0	.931900	.928062	.924389	.920867	.917483	.914227	.911089
8.4	.943898	.940682	.937600	.934640	.931793	.929050	.926404
8.8	.953544	.950842	.948249	.945756	.943355	.941040	.938803
9.2	.961336	.959058	.956870	.954764	.952734	.950774	.948879
9.6	.967659	.965733	.963880	.962095	.960373	.958710	.957100
10.0	.972816	.971181	.969607	.968089	.966624	.965207	.963836
11.0	.982029	.980926	.979863	.978836	.977843	.976881	.975949
12.0	.987793	.987033	.986299	.985589	.984902	.984235	.983589
13.0	.991503	.990968	.990450	.989949	.989464	.988993	.988535
14.0	.993954	.993569	.993197	.992837	.992487	.992148	.991818
15.0	.995611	.995330	.995058	.994794	.994538	.994289	.994047
16.0	.996757	.996547	.996345	.996148	.995958	.995772	.995592
17.0	.997564	.997406	.997253	.997105	.996961	.996821	.996684
18.0	.998143	.998023	.997906	.997792	.997681	.997574	.997469
19.0	.998566	.998472	.998382	.998294	.998208	.998124	.998043

$\nu = 5$

Q\n	26	28	30	32	34	36	38
20.0	.998879	.998806	.998734	.998665	.998598	.998533	.998469
22.0	.999292	.999246	.999201	.999157	.999114	.999072	.999032
24.0	.999536	.999506	.999476	.999447	.999419	.999391	.999365
26.0	.999686	.999665	.999645	.999625	.999606	.999588	.999570
28.0	.999782	.999767	.999753	.999739	.999726	.999713	.999700
30.0	.999844	.999834	.999824	.999814	.999805	.999795	.999786
32.0	.999887	.999879	.999872	.999865	.999858	.999851	.999844
34.0	.999916	.999910	.999905	.999900	.999894	.999889	.999884
36.0	.999937	.999932	.999928	.999924	.999920	.999917	.999913
38.0	.999951	.999948	.999945	.999942	.999939	.999936	.999933
40.0	.999962	.999960	.999957	.999955	.999953	.999950	.999948
45.0	.999979	.999978	.999976	.999975	.999974	.999972	.999971
50.0	.999988	.999987	.999986	.999985	.999984	.999984	.999983
55.0	.999992	.999992	.999991	.999991	.999990	.999990	.999989
60.0	.999995	.999995	.999994	.999994	.999994	.999993	.999993
65.0	1.00000	1.00000	1.00000	1.00000	1.00000	1.00000	1.00000

$\nu = 5$

Q\n	40	50	60	70	80	90	100
0.0	.000000	.000000	.000000	.000000	.000000	.000000	.000000
0.1	.000000	.000000	.000000	.000000	.000000	.000000	.000000
0.2	.000000	.000000	.000000	.000000	.000000	.000000	.000000
0.3	.000000	.000000	.000000	.000000	.000000	.000000	.000000
0.4	.000000	.000000	.000000	.000000	.000000	.000000	.000000
0.5	.000000	.000000	.000000	.000000	.000000	.000000	.000000
0.6	.000000	.000000	.000000	.000000	.000000	.000000	.000000
0.7	.000000	.000000	.000000	.000000	.000000	.000000	.000000
0.8	.000000	.000000	.000000	.000000	.000000	.000000	.000000
0.9	.000000	.000000	.000000	.000000	.000000	.000000	.000000
1.0	.000000	.000000	.000000	.000000	.000000	.000000	.000000
1.1	.000000	.000000	.000000	.000000	.000000	.000000	.000000
1.2	.000001	.000000	.000000	.000000	.000000	.000000	.000000
1.3	.000007	.000001	.000000	.000000	.000000	.000000	.000000
1.4	.000024	.000006	.000002	.000001	.000000	.000000	.000000
1.5	.000076	.000022	.000008	.000003	.000001	.000001	.000000
1.6	.000205	.000069	.000027	.000012	.000006	.000003	.000002
1.7	.000486	.000185	.000081	.000040	.000021	.000012	.000007
1.8	.001034	.000436	.000209	.000110	.000063	.000038	.000024
1.9	.002013	.000927	.000479	.000270	.000163	.000103	.000068
2.0	.003623	.001801	.000995	.000594	.000376	.000249	.000172
2.1	.006102	.003243	.001896	.001189	.000787	.000543	.000388
2.2	.009700	.005467	.003361	.002202	.001514	.001082	.000798
2.3	.014666	.008704	.005591	.003806	.002708	.001995	.001512
2.4	.021228	.013189	.008808	.006202	.004546	.003440	.002671
2.5	.029573	.019137	.013230	.009598	.007225	.005599	.004443
2.6	.039839	.026734	.019060	.014202	.010946	.008665	.007008
2.7	.052104	.036121	.026471	.020202	.015903	.012829	.010556
2.8	.066388	.047388	.035597	.027755	.022267	.018270	.015266
2.9	.082650	.060570	.046523	.036982	.030179	.025143	.021302
3.0	.100799	.075648	.059284	.047954	.039740	.033568	.028797
3.1	.120697	.092554	.073866	.060699	.051007	.043627	.037852
3.2	.142176	.111178	.090208	.075198	.063995	.055358	.048526
3.3	.165038	.131375	.108210	.091388	.078673	.068760	.060839
3.4	.189074	.152972	.127740	.109171	.094972	.083789	.074771
3.5	.214064	.175780	.148637	.128418	.112793	.100369	.090266
3.6	.239791	.199600	.170728	.148978	.132005	.118393	.107236
3.7	.266043	.224231	.193826	.170684	.152461	.137730	.125569
3.8	.292620	.249472	.217742	.193359	.174000	.158233	.145131
3.9	.319336	.275133	.242288	.216824	.196450	.179744	.165776
4.0	.346020	.301033	.267282	.240901	.219641	.202098	.187346
4.1	.372521	.327007	.292553	.265417	.243403	.225130	.209684
4.2	.398704	.352903	.317941	.290209	.267572	.248679	.232630
4.3	.424455	.378588	.343301	.315125	.291993	.272589	.256030
4.4	.449676	.403941	.368500	.340025	.316522	.296713	.279735
4.5	.474285	.428863	.393423	.364785	.341028	.320915	.303608
4.6	.498217	.453266	.417970	.389292	.365390	.345070	.327520
4.7	.521420	.477079	.442052	.413449	.389504	.369068	.351355
4.8	.543856	.500243	.465599	.437173	.413277	.392807	.375007
4.9	.565496	.522714	.488550	.460391	.436628	.416202	.398384

ν = 5

Ω\n	40	50	60	70	80	90	100
5.0	.586323	.544457	.510857	.483047	.459491	.439177	.421406
5.1	.606328	.565447	.532483	.505091	.481809	.461670	.444002
5.2	.625510	.585669	.553402	.526488	.503537	.483627	.466115
5.3	.643873	.605115	.573594	.547208	.524638	.505005	.487695
5.4	.661428	.623784	.593047	.567232	.545086	.525772	.508703
5.5	.678188	.641680	.611759	.586548	.564862	.545902	.529109
5.6	.694172	.658812	.629728	.605150	.583952	.565376	.548889
5.7	.709401	.675193	.646962	.623037	.602350	.584183	.568027
5.8	.723896	.690838	.663470	.640212	.620056	.602317	.586513
5.9	.737683	.705768	.679265	.656685	.637072	.619777	.604341
6.0	.750787	.720002	.694364	.672466	.653406	.636566	.621512
6.4	.796906	.770440	.748172	.728987	.712161	.697197	.683738
6.8	.834214	.811641	.792487	.775865	.761196	.748077	.736219
7.2	.864293	.845131	.828754	.814456	.801771	.790374	.780030
7.6	.888524	.872294	.858339	.846094	.835181	.825338	.816372
8.0	.908061	.894324	.882451	.871987	.862626	.854154	.846414
8.4	.923847	.912213	.902114	.893179	.885159	.877880	.871213
8.8	.936641	.926774	.918176	.910544	.903675	.897424	.891686
9.2	.947046	.938661	.931330	.924804	.918916	.913546	.908606
9.6	.955541	.948399	.942135	.936546	.931491	.926873	.922617
10.0	.962507	.956406	.951042	.946244	.941897	.937919	.934247
11.0	.975044	.970877	.967193	.963883	.960873	.958108	.955548
12.0	.982960	.980059	.977483	.975161	.973042	.971092	.969282
13.0	.988090	.986031	.984197	.982540	.981024	.979626	.978325
14.0	.991497	.990009	.988681	.987477	.986375	.985356	.984408
15.0	.993811	.992718	.991740	.990852	.990038	.989284	.988582
16.0	.995416	.994600	.993869	.993204	.992594	.992028	.991500
17.0	.996551	.995933	.995378	.994874	.994410	.993979	.993578
18.0	.997368	.996893	.996467	.996079	.995722	.995390	.995080
19.0	.997964	.997596	.997264	.996962	.996684	.996425	.996184
20.0	.998407	.998117	.997856	.997619	.997400	.997196	.997006
22.0	.998992	.998808	.998642	.998490	.998350	.998220	.998098
24.0	.999339	.999217	.999107	.999007	.998915	.998829	.998748
26.0	.999552	.999469	.999395	.999326	.999263	.999205	.999150
28.0	.999688	.999630	.999578	.999530	.999486	.999445	.999407
30.0	.999777	.999736	.999699	.999665	.999633	.999604	.999576
32.0	.999838	.999808	.999781	.999756	.999732	.999711	.999691
34.0	.999880	.999857	.999837	.999818	.999801	.999785	.999770
36.0	.999909	.999892	.999877	.999863	.999850	.999838	.999827
38.0	.999931	.999918	.999906	.999895	.999885	.999876	.999867
40.0	.999946	.999936	.999927	.999919	.999911	.999904	.999897
45.0	.999970	.999964	.999959	.999954	.999950	.999946	.999942
50.0	.999982	.999979	.999976	.999973	.999970	.999968	.999966
55.0	.999989	.999987	.999985	.999983	.999982	.999980	.999979
60.0	.999993	.999991	.999990	.999989	.999988	.999987	.999986
65.0	1.00000	.999994	.999993	.999993	.999992	.999991	.999991
70.0		1.00000	1.00000	.999995	.999994	.999994	.999994
75.0				1.00000	1.00000	1.00000	1.00000

ν = 6

Q\n	2	3	4	5	6	7	8
0.0	.000000	.000000	.000000	.000000	.000000	.000000	.000000
0.1	.054039	.002751	.000142	.000008	.000000	.000000	.000000
0.2	.107834	.010945	.001124	.000119	.000013	.000001	.000000
0.3	.160973	.024402	.003742	.000591	.000096	.000016	.000003
0.4	.213198	.042831	.008700	.001818	.000393	.000088	.000020
0.5	.264235	.065845	.016580	.004290	.001146	.000317	.000090
0.6	.313836	.092976	.027811	.008540	.002705	.000884	.000298
0.7	.361781	.123692	.042663	.015088	.005495	.002063	.000797
0.8	.407883	.157424	.061238	.024392	.009991	.004212	.001825
0.9	.451988	.193580	.083482	.036811	.016667	.007753	.003703
1.0	.493979	.231568	.109200	.052574	.025949	.013138	.006818
1.2	.571308	.310772	.169723	.094350	.053596	.031129	.018473
1.4	.639574	.390884	.239406	.148818	.094230	.060812	.039977
1.6	.698918	.468550	.314279	.213364	.147113	.103079	.073366
1.8	.749815	.541346	.390517	.284435	.209841	.156906	.118875
2.0	.792969	.607744	.464909	.358318	.279066	.219775	.174982
2.2	.829204	.666985	.535073	.431698	.351240	.288397	.238943
2.4	.859390	.718908	.599471	.501978	.423170	.359392	.307495
2.6	.884378	.763770	.657298	.567363	.492329	.429785	.377464
2.8	.904963	.802093	.708326	.626798	.556942	.497257	.446157
3.0	.921859	.834540	.752736	.679835	.615944	.560204	.511542
3.2	.935694	.861825	.790967	.726474	.668852	.617678	.572257
3.4	.947007	.884651	.823603	.767017	.715615	.669265	.627539
3.6	.956250	.903677	.851283	.801945	.756482	.714944	.677093
3.8	.963803	.919497	.874649	.831832	.791883	.754964	.720966
4.0	.969980	.932632	.894306	.857272	.822341	.789737	.759435
4.2	.975038	.943530	.910806	.878846	.848413	.819757	.792911
4.4	.979185	.952573	.924637	.897095	.870647	.845553	.821875
4.6	.982592	.960081	.936223	.912507	.889560	.867639	.846826
4.8	.985399	.966322	.945931	.925510	.905620	.886504	.868254
5.0	.987715	.971516	.954069	.936480	.919246	.902593	.886614
5.2	.989632	.975847	.960898	.945736	.930802	.916301	.902326
5.4	.991223	.979465	.966636	.953553	.940605	.927978	.915761
5.6	.992547	.982494	.971464	.960162	.948926	.937927	.927246
5.8	.993651	.985036	.975534	.965756	.955997	.946408	.937068
6.0	.994576	.987174	.978973	.970498	.962011	.953645	.945471
6.4	.996006	.990501	.984352	.977954	.971506	.965115	.958839
6.8	.997025	.992890	.988240	.983373	.978443	.973534	.968691
7.2	.997759	.994623	.991076	.987345	.983549	.979754	.975997
7.6	.998295	.995894	.993165	.990282	.987338	.984384	.981451
8.0	.998689	.996834	.994717	.992472	.990171	.987857	.985553
8.4	.998983	.997537	.995881	.994119	.992309	.990483	.988661
8.8	.999204	.998068	.996762	.995369	.993934	.992484	.991034
9.2	.999372	.998471	.997434	.996325	.995180	.994021	.992860
9.6	.999500	.998782	.997952	.997062	.996143	.995210	.994274
10.0	.999599	.999022	.998353	.997635	.996892	.996136	.995377
11.0	.999762	.999418	.999017	.998586	.998137	.997680	.997219
12.0	.999853	.999640	.999391	.999122	.998842	.998556	.998267
13.0	.999907	.999770	.999611	.999438	.999257	.999072	.998886
14.0	.999939	.999849	.999744	.999629	.999510	.999387	.999263

$\nu = 6$

Q\n	2	3	4	5	6	7	8
15.0	.999959	.999898	.999827	.999749	.999668	.999585	.999500
16.0	.999971	.999930	.999880	.999827	.999770	.999712	.999654
17.0	.999980	.999950	.999915	.999877	.999838	.999797	.999755
18.0	.999986	.999964	.999939	.999912	.999883	.999854	.999824
19.0	.999989	.999974	.999956	.999936	.999915	.999893	.999871
20.0	.999992	.999981	.999967	.999952	.999937	.999920	.999904
22.0	1.00000	.999989	.999981	.999973	.999964	.999954	.999945
24.0		.999993	.999989	.999984	.999978	.999973	.999967
26.0		1.00000	.999993	.999990	.999986	.999983	.999979
28.0			1.00000	.999993	.999991	.999989	.999987
30.0				1.00000	.999994	.999993	.999991
32.0					1.00000	.999995	.999994
34.0						1.00000	1.00000

$\nu = 6$

Q\n	9	10	11	12	13	14	15
0.0	.000000	.000000	.000000	.000000	.000000	.000000	.000000
0.1	.000000	.000000	.000000	.000000	.000000	.000000	.000000
0.2	.000000	.000000	.000000	.000000	.000000	.000000	.000000
0.3	.000001	.000000	.000000	.000000	.000000	.000000	.000000
0.4	.000005	.000001	.000000	.000000	.000000	.000000	.000000
0.5	.000027	.000008	.000002	.000001	.000000	.000000	.000000
0.6	.000103	.000037	.000014	.000005	.000002	.000001	.000000
0.7	.000317	.000129	.000054	.000023	.000010	.000005	.000002
0.8	.000812	.000371	.000173	.000083	.000040	.000020	.000010
0.9	.001813	.000909	.000466	.000244	.000130	.000071	.000039
1.0	.003622	.001967	.001091	.000617	.000355	.000208	.000124
1.2	.011188	.006907	.004341	.002774	.001800	.001185	.000791
1.4	.026743	.018185	.012555	.008792	.006238	.004481	.003255
1.6	.052996	.038815	.028796	.021620	.016412	.012587	.009746
1.8	.091189	.070769	.055516	.043988	.035177	.028374	.023068
2.0	.140771	.114351	.093729	.077469	.064525	.054129	.045709
2.2	.199678	.168215	.142773	.122022	.104958	.090818	.079016
2.4	.264964	.229843	.200617	.176118	.155436	.137862	.122835
2.6	.333450	.296193	.264452	.237241	.213772	.193417	.175667
2.8	.402226	.364264	.331287	.302488	.277206	.254904	.235139
3.0	.468933	.431475	.398400	.369064	.342929	.319548	.298546
3.2	.531866	.495836	.463581	.434597	.408454	.384787	.363287
3.4	.589940	.555982	.525225	.497278	.471805	.448512	.427148
3.6	.642595	.611106	.582296	.555871	.531566	.509151	.488424
3.8	.689675	.660848	.634246	.609645	.586843	.565659	.545932
4.0	.731306	.705186	.680900	.658282	.637176	.617443	.598955
4.2	.767803	.744325	.722353	.701762	.682436	.664266	.647153
4.4	.799585	.778614	.758875	.740277	.722731	.706155	.690472
4.6	.827120	.808479	.790843	.774148	.758327	.743316	.729055
4.8	.850884	.834375	.818686	.803770	.789579	.776064	.763178
5.0	.871338	.856756	.842843	.829567	.816890	.804776	.793189
5.2	.888910	.876055	.863746	.851960	.840671	.829851	.819473
5.4	.903988	.892670	.881797	.871356	.861326	.851687	.842418
5.6	.916920	.906961	.897368	.888130	.879233	.870662	.862401
5.8	.928010	.919251	.910790	.902623	.894740	.887129	.879778
6.0	.937524	.929818	.922358	.915141	.908160	.901407	.894872
6.4	.952707	.946736	.940932	.935295	.929822	.924511	.919354
6.8	.963942	.959300	.954772	.950360	.946065	.941883	.937813
7.2	.972299	.968675	.965129	.961665	.958283	.954984	.951764
7.6	.978557	.975712	.972922	.970190	.967518	.964904	.962350
8.0	.983274	.981028	.978822	.976657	.974535	.972456	.970421
8.4	.986855	.985072	.983317	.981592	.979899	.978238	.976609
8.8	.989594	.988171	.986767	.985385	.984026	.982692	.981382
9.2	.991704	.990561	.989431	.988318	.987222	.986145	.985086
9.6	.993342	.992417	.991503	.990602	.989713	.988839	.987979
10.0	.994621	.993869	.993126	.992392	.991667	.990954	.990251
11.0	.996759	.996300	.995846	.995396	.994952	.994513	.994080
12.0	.997978	.997689	.997402	.997118	.996837	.996559	.996284
13.0	.998698	.998511	.998325	.998140	.997957	.997776	.997597
14.0	.999139	.999014	.998890	.998767	.998645	.998524	.998404

$\nu = 6$

Q\n	9	10	11	12	13	14	15
15.0	.999416	.999331	.999246	.999162	.999079	.998996	.998914
16.0	.999595	.999536	.999477	.999418	.999360	.999302	.999245
17.0	.999713	.999671	.999630	.999588	.999546	.999505	.999465
18.0	.999793	.999763	.999733	.999703	.999673	.999643	.999614
19.0	.999849	.999827	.999804	.999782	.999760	.999738	.999717
20.0	.999888	.999871	.999855	.999838	.999822	.999805	.999789
22.0	.999935	.999926	.999916	.999907	.999897	.999888	.999879
24.0	.999961	.999955	.999950	.999944	.999938	.999933	.999927
26.0	.999976	.999972	.999969	.999965	.999961	.999958	.999954
28.0	.999984	.999982	.999980	.999977	.999975	.999973	.999970
30.0	.999990	.999988	.999986	.999985	.999983	.999982	.999980
32.0	.999993	.999992	.999991	.999990	.999989	.999988	.999987
34.0	1.00000	.999994	.999994	.999993	.999992	.999991	.999991
36.0		1.00000	1.00000	.999995	.999994	.999994	.999993
38.0				1.00000	1.00000	1.00000	1.00000

$\nu = 6$

Q\n	16	17	18	19	20	22	24
0.0	.000000	.000000	.000000	.000000	.000000	.000000	.000000
0.2	.000000	.000000	.000000	.000000	.000000	.000000	.000000
0.4	.000000	.000000	.000000	.000000	.000000	.000000	.000000
0.6	.000000	.000000	.000000	.000000	.000000	.000000	.000000
0.8	.000005	.000003	.000001	.000001	.000000	.000000	.000000
1.0	.000075	.000046	.000028	.000018	.000011	.000005	.000002
1.2	.000535	.000366	.000253	.000177	.000125	.000064	.000034
1.4	.002390	.001772	.001327	.001002	.000763	.000452	.000276
1.6	.007614	.005998	.004761	.003807	.003065	.002024	.001367
1.8	.018894	.015583	.012934	.010800	.009069	.006496	.004740
2.0	.038837	.033188	.028511	.024616	.021353	.016274	.012597
2.2	.069100	.060717	.053587	.047490	.042250	.033799	.027388
2.4	.109912	.098738	.089027	.080547	.073110	.060768	.051051
2.6	.160110	.146411	.134296	.123536	.113943	.097651	.084436
2.8	.217545	.201820	.187710	.175004	.163523	.143654	.127139
3.0	.279608	.262470	.246909	.232734	.219783	.197016	.177708
3.2	.343689	.325770	.309335	.294220	.280282	.255456	.234047
3.4	.407496	.389368	.372602	.357057	.342609	.316591	.293835
3.6	.469208	.451351	.434715	.419185	.404655	.378242	.354861
3.8	.527521	.510301	.494161	.479003	.464741	.438606	.415232
4.0	.581601	.565279	.549899	.535382	.521655	.496324	.473470
4.2	.631008	.615750	.601307	.587613	.574609	.550467	.528518
4.4	.675609	.661504	.648098	.635338	.623177	.600479	.579704
4.6	.715488	.702566	.690239	.678467	.667210	.646103	.626671
4.8	.750877	.739122	.727874	.717099	.706766	.687312	.669308
5.0	.782096	.771462	.761260	.751461	.742039	.724237	.707685
5.2	.809509	.799934	.790724	.781857	.773312	.757113	.741992
5.4	.833497	.824904	.816621	.808629	.800912	.786240	.772493
5.6	.854433	.846743	.839314	.832134	.825187	.811945	.799498
5.8	.872674	.865804	.859156	.852719	.846481	.834564	.823327
6.0	.888546	.882417	.876478	.870717	.865127	.854423	.844304
6.4	.914346	.909480	.904751	.900152	.895678	.887079	.878912
6.8	.933850	.929990	.926230	.922565	.918991	.912102	.905534
7.2	.948623	.945557	.942565	.939642	.936787	.931270	.925993
7.6	.959853	.957411	.955024	.952689	.950405	.945981	.941737
8.0	.968428	.966477	.964567	.962696	.960863	.957305	.953886
8.4	.975012	.973447	.971912	.970406	.968930	.966061	.963297
8.8	.980096	.978834	.977595	.976380	.975186	.972862	.970620
9.2	.984046	.983023	.982019	.981033	.980063	.978174	.976348
9.6	.987132	.986300	.985482	.984678	.983887	.982344	.980851
10.0	.989560	.988879	.988210	.987551	.986903	.985637	.984410
11.0	.993654	.993233	.992819	.992410	.992008	.991221	.990456
12.0	.996013	.995746	.995482	.995222	.994965	.994462	.993972
13.0	.997420	.997245	.997073	.996903	.996734	.996404	.996083
14.0	.998286	.998169	.998053	.997939	.997826	.997604	.997388
15.0	.998833	.998753	.998674	.998595	.998518	.998366	.998217
16.0	.999188	.999132	.999077	.999022	.998968	.998861	.998757
17.0	.999424	.999385	.999345	.999306	.999267	.999191	.999117
18.0	.999585	.999556	.999527	.999499	.999471	.999416	.999362
19.0	.999695	.999674	.999653	.999632	.999612	.999571	.999531

$\nu = 6$

Q\n	16	17	18	19	20	22	24
20.0	.999773	.999757	.999742	.999726	.999711	.999680	.999651
22.0	.999869	.999860	.999851	.999842	.999833	.999816	.999799
24.0	.999921	.999916	.999910	.999905	.999900	.999889	.999879
26.0	.999951	.999947	.999944	.999940	.999937	.999930	.999924
28.0	.999968	.999966	.999964	.999961	.999959	.999955	.999951
30.0	.999979	.999977	.999976	.999974	.999973	.999970	.999967
32.0	.999986	.999984	.999983	.999982	.999981	.999979	.999978
34.0	.999990	.999989	.999988	.999988	.999987	.999986	.999984
36.0	.999993	.999992	.999992	.999991	.999991	.999990	.999989
38.0	.999995	.999994	.999994	.999994	.999993	.999993	.999992
40.0	1.00000	1.00000	1.00000	1.00000	1.00000	.999995	.999994
45.0						1.00000	1.00000

$\nu = 6$

Q\n	26	28	30	32	34	36	38
0.0	.000000	.000000	.000000	.000000	.000000	.000000	.000000
0.2	.000000	.000000	.000000	.000000	.000000	.000000	.000000
0.4	.000000	.000000	.000000	.000000	.000000	.000000	.000000
0.6	.000000	.000000	.000000	.000000	.000000	.000000	.000000
0.8	.000000	.000000	.000000	.000000	.000000	.000000	.000000
1.0	.000001	.000000	.000000	.000000	.000000	.000000	.000000
1.2	.000019	.000010	.000006	.000004	.000002	.000001	.000001
1.4	.000172	.000110	.000072	.000048	.000032	.000022	.000015
1.6	.000943	.000662	.000473	.000342	.000252	.000187	.000141
1.8	.003518	.002650	.002023	.001564	.001222	.000965	.000769
2.0	.009886	.007855	.006311	.005121	.004195	.003464	.002883
2.2	.022447	.018587	.015532	.013088	.011112	.009500	.008173
2.4	.043296	.037032	.031916	.027698	.024189	.021245	.018758
2.6	.073588	.064588	.057051	.050684	.045264	.040617	.036607
2.8	.113267	.101508	.091454	.082794	.075283	.068728	.062974
3.0	.161182	.146919	.134518	.123662	.114102	.105636	.098099
3.2	.215431	.199125	.184746	.171991	.160614	.150415	.141231
3.4	.273784	.256000	.240133	.225898	.213065	.201444	.190877
3.6	.334027	.315353	.298523	.283280	.269415	.256751	.245140
3.8	.394205	.375184	.357895	.342111	.327641	.314327	.302035
4.0	.452738	.433839	.416534	.400624	.385942	.372348	.359721
4.2	.508464	.490059	.473099	.457411	.442851	.429296	.416639
4.4	.560603	.542970	.526629	.511436	.497264	.484007	.471573
4.6	.608706	.592035	.576511	.562010	.548424	.535663	.523646
4.8	.652583	.636992	.622411	.608736	.595874	.583748	.572290
5.0	.692243	.677790	.664222	.651450	.639397	.627997	.617190
5.2	.727829	.714526	.701996	.690162	.678961	.668336	.658236
5.4	.759575	.747401	.735899	.725006	.714667	.704834	.695465
5.6	.787764	.776675	.766169	.756194	.746704	.737656	.729016
5.8	.812706	.802642	.793084	.783988	.775315	.767030	.759101
6.0	.834715	.825607	.816939	.808673	.800774	.793215	.785969
6.4	.871140	.863727	.856645	.849867	.843369	.837129	.831129
6.8	.899261	.893258	.887504	.881981	.876670	.871557	.866627
7.2	.920938	.916086	.911424	.906936	.902612	.898438	.894406
7.6	.937661	.933740	.929963	.926321	.922803	.919402	.916110
8.0	.950594	.947421	.944358	.941399	.938536	.935764	.933076
8.4	.960631	.958057	.955568	.953160	.950826	.948563	.946366
8.8	.968454	.966359	.964331	.962366	.960459	.958608	.956808
9.2	.974581	.972870	.971212	.969603	.968040	.966521	.965043
9.6	.979404	.978001	.976640	.975318	.974033	.972782	.971565
10.0	.983220	.982066	.980944	.979854	.978793	.977760	.976753
11.0	.989713	.988990	.988287	.987601	.986933	.986282	.985646
12.0	.993496	.993031	.992579	.992137	.991706	.991285	.990873
13.0	.995770	.995464	.995165	.994874	.994589	.994311	.994038
14.0	.997177	.996971	.996770	.996573	.996381	.996192	.996008
15.0	.998072	.997930	.997792	.997656	.997523	.997394	.997266
16.0	.998656	.998556	.998459	.998363	.998270	.998179	.998089
17.0	.999044	.998973	.998904	.998836	.998769	.998703	.998639
18.0	.999309	.999257	.999207	.999157	.999109	.999061	.999014
19.0	.999492	.999454	.999417	.999380	.999345	.999309	.999275

$\nu = 6$

Q\n	26	28	30	32	34	36	38
20.0	.999622	.999593	.999565	.999538	.999511	.999485	.999459
22.0	.999782	.999765	.999749	.999733	.999718	.999702	.999687
24.0	.999868	.999858	.999849	.999839	.999829	.999820	.999811
26.0	.999917	.999911	.999905	.999899	.999893	.999887	.999881
28.0	.999947	.999942	.999938	.999935	.999931	.999927	.999923
30.0	.999964	.999962	.999959	.999956	.999954	.999951	.999949
32.0	.999976	.999974	.999972	.999970	.999968	.999967	.999965
34.0	.999983	.999982	.999980	.999979	.999978	.999977	.999975
36.0	.999988	.999987	.999986	.999985	.999984	.999983	.999982
38.0	.999991	.999991	.999990	.999989	.999989	.999988	.999987
40.0	.999993	.999993	.999993	.999992	.999992	.999991	.999991
45.0	1.00000	1.00000	1.00000	1.00000	1.00000	1.00000	1.00000

$\nu = 6$

Q\n	40	50	60	70	80	90	100
0.0	.000000	.000000	.000000	.000000	.000000	.000000	.000000
0.1	.000000	.000000	.000000	.000000	.000000	.000000	.000000
0.2	.000000	.000000	.000000	.000000	.000000	.000000	.000000
0.3	.000000	.000000	.000000	.000000	.000000	.000000	.000000
0.4	.000000	.000000	.000000	.000000	.000000	.000000	.000000
0.5	.000000	.000000	.000000	.000000	.000000	.000000	.000000
0.6	.000000	.000000	.000000	.000000	.000000	.000000	.000000
0.7	.000000	.000000	.000000	.000000	.000000	.000000	.000000
0.8	.000000	.000000	.000000	.000000	.000000	.000000	.000000
0.9	.000000	.000000	.000000	.000000	.000000	.000000	.000000
1.0	.000000	.000000	.000000	.000000	.000000	.000000	.000000
1.1	.000000	.000000	.000000	.000000	.000000	.000000	.000000
1.2	.000001	.000000	.000000	.000000	.000000	.000000	.000000
1.3	.000003	.000000	.000000	.000000	.000000	.000000	.000000
1.4	.000011	.000002	.000001	.000000	.000000	.000000	.000000
1.5	.000037	.000009	.000003	.000001	.000000	.000000	.000000
1.6	.000107	.000031	.000011	.000004	.000002	.000001	.000000
1.7	.000272	.000091	.000035	.000016	.000008	.000004	.000002
1.8	.000618	.000232	.000100	.000048	.000025	.000014	.000008
1.9	.001274	.000528	.000249	.000129	.000072	.000042	.000026
2.0	.002417	.001093	.000555	.000307	.000182	.000113	.000074
2.1	.004265	.002083	.001130	.000662	.000412	.000269	.000182
2.2	.007073	.003694	.002123	.001309	.000852	.000579	.000407
2.3	.011110	.006158	.003722	.002399	.001624	.001143	.000831
2.4	.016643	.009723	.006147	.004120	.002888	.002098	.001568
2.5	.023914	.014640	.009633	.006685	.004833	.003609	.002767
2.6	.033126	.021145	.014418	.010320	.007669	.005870	.004603
2.7	.044426	.029440	.020723	.015251	.011615	.009089	.007272
2.8	.057897	.039680	.028742	.021686	.016883	.013477	.010978
2.9	.073557	.051965	.038622	.029801	.023667	.019231	.015920
3.0	.091360	.066335	.050462	.039732	.032124	.026526	.022283
3.1	.111201	.082769	.064304	.051567	.042375	.035503	.030221
3.2	.132927	.101194	.080136	.065340	.054488	.046260	.039851
3.3	.156344	.121485	.097893	.081034	.068486	.058847	.051250
3.4	.181232	.143480	.117464	.098584	.084342	.073268	.064447
3.5	.207353	.166985	.138701	.117883	.101983	.089483	.079427
3.6	.234459	.191785	.161425	.138787	.121298	.107410	.096135
3.7	.262305	.217655	.185439	.161126	.142146	.126932	.114477
3.8	.290651	.244365	.210531	.184712	.164359	.147905	.134328
3.9	.319272	.271689	.236485	.209343	.187754	.170161	.155540
4.0	.347959	.299409	.263087	.234813	.212137	.193521	.177947
4.1	.376522	.327322	.290129	.260920	.237312	.217796	.201369
4.2	.404791	.355239	.317416	.287466	.263083	.242799	.225626
4.3	.432620	.382991	.344765	.314262	.289263	.268340	.250533
4.4	.459882	.410426	.372011	.341136	.315672	.294243	.275912
4.5	.486472	.437414	.399005	.367927	.342146	.320336	.301592
4.6	.512304	.463841	.425617	.394494	.368532	.346463	.327412
4.7	.537310	.489615	.451735	.420709	.394696	.372480	.353226
4.8	.561439	.514659	.477264	.446464	.420516	.398261	.378897
4.9	.584652	.538912	.502124	.471666	.445888	.423691	.404307

ν = 6

Q\n	40	50	60	70	80	90	100
5.0	.606927	.562329	.526253	.496237	.470725	.448672	.429349
5.1	.628250	.584877	.549600	.520114	.494950	.473120	.453931
5.2	.648619	.606535	.572130	.543246	.518503	.496966	.477977
5.3	.668038	.627290	.593816	.565598	.541337	.520153	.501421
5.4	.686521	.647142	.614643	.587140	.563415	.542635	.524211
5.5	.704085	.666094	.634605	.607858	.584709	.564378	.546305
5.6	.720752	.684158	.653701	.627741	.605205	.585357	.567671
5.7	.736548	.701349	.671940	.646788	.624891	.605557	.588289
5.8	.751503	.717689	.689332	.665004	.643766	.624968	.608142
5.9	.765647	.733202	.705896	.682400	.661834	.643590	.627225
6.0	.779013	.747912	.721651	.698989	.679105	.661425	.645536
6.4	.825351	.799317	.777071	.757680	.740516	.725135	.711215
6.8	.861869	.840286	.821661	.805289	.790692	.777526	.765542
7.2	.890506	.872716	.857237	.843535	.831243	.820096	.809900
7.6	.912920	.898301	.885492	.874085	.863799	.854429	.845822
8.0	.930468	.918467	.907888	.898420	.889844	.882001	.874771
8.4	.944232	.934375	.925642	.917792	.910653	.904103	.898047
8.8	.955058	.946951	.939736	.933225	.927285	.921819	.916752
9.2	.963604	.956921	.950950	.945544	.940598	.936035	.931795
9.6	.970378	.964854	.959902	.955405	.951280	.947466	.943915
10.0	.975771	.971191	.967072	.963323	.959876	.956682	.953704
11.0	.985024	.982114	.979481	.977071	.974846	.972776	.970838
12.0	.990471	.988580	.986862	.985282	.983819	.982453	.981171
13.0	.993772	.992516	.991370	.990314	.989332	.988414	.987551
14.0	.995828	.994975	.994196	.993475	.992804	.992175	.991583
15.0	.997141	.996552	.996011	.995510	.995043	.994604	.994190
16.0	.998001	.997585	.997203	.996849	.996518	.996207	.995913
17.0	.998576	.998278	.998003	.997748	.997510	.997286	.997074
18.0	.998969	.998751	.998551	.998365	.998190	.998026	.997871
19.0	.999241	.999080	.998932	.998794	.998665	.998543	.998428
20.0	.999434	.999313	.999202	.999099	.999001	.998910	.998823
22.0	.999673	.999602	.999538	.999477	.999420	.999367	.999316
24.0	.999802	.999760	.999720	.999683	.999649	.999616	.999585
26.0	.999876	.999849	.999824	.999801	.999779	.999758	.999739
28.0	.999919	.999902	.999886	.999871	.999856	.999843	.999830
30.0	.999946	.999935	.999924	.999914	.999904	.999895	.999887
32.0	.999963	.999955	.999948	.999941	.999934	.999928	.999922
34.0	.999974	.999969	.999963	.999959	.999954	.999950	.999946
36.0	.999982	.999978	.999974	.999970	.999967	.999964	.999961
38.0	.999987	.999984	.999981	.999979	.999976	.999974	.999972
40.0	.999990	.999988	.999986	.999984	.999982	.999981	.999979
45.0	1.00000	.999994	.999993	.999992	.999991	.999990	.999990
50.0		1.00000	1.00000	1.00000	1.00000	.999995	.999994
55.0						1.00000	1.00000

$\nu = 7$

Q\n	2	3	4	5	6	7	8
0.0	.000000	.000000	.000000	.000000	.000000	.000000	.000000
0.1	.054350	.002751	.000140	.000007	.000000	.000000	.000000
0.2	.108479	.010948	.001109	.000115	.000012	.000001	.000000
0.3	.161951	.024416	.003692	.000571	.000091	.000015	.000003
0.4	.214521	.042875	.008591	.001759	.000370	.000080	.000018
0.5	.265918	.065949	.016389	.004159	.001084	.000291	.000080
0.6	.315892	.093181	.027528	.008297	.002566	.000816	.000267
0.7	.364226	.124054	.042290	.014693	.005233	.001914	.000718
0.8	.410728	.158008	.060800	.023816	.009552	.003928	.001656
0.9	.455242	.194457	.083025	.036044	.015999	.007272	.003385
1.0	.497646	.232816	.108793	.051629	.025017	.012396	.006280
1.2	.575793	.312983	.169702	.093210	.052127	.029724	.017281
1.4	.644824	.394309	.240221	.147888	.092441	.058751	.037967
1.6	.704835	.473344	.316376	.213198	.145493	.100686	.070665
1.8	.756267	.547542	.394241	.285610	.209043	.154783	.115960
2.0	.799800	.615258	.470449	.361304	.279756	.218670	.172585
2.2	.836253	.675638	.542443	.436782	.353953	.289023	.237876
2.4	.866501	.728459	.608528	.509233	.428225	.362291	.308475
2.6	.891413	.773947	.667786	.576668	.499803	.435251	.380983
2.8	.911805	.812626	.719922	.637886	.566701	.505325	.452435
3.0	.928418	.845178	.765091	.692348	.627694	.570692	.520535
3.2	.941904	.872351	.803744	.740017	.682202	.630251	.583719
3.4	.952823	.894892	.836498	.781198	.730135	.683496	.641082
3.6	.961650	.913499	.864040	.816408	.771747	.730377	.692259
3.8	.968779	.928806	.887062	.846267	.807504	.771155	.737281
4.0	.974536	.941367	.906221	.871429	.837983	.806284	.776449
4.2	.979188	.951659	.922113	.892531	.863802	.836316	.810222
4.4	.982949	.960086	.935268	.910168	.885571	.861842	.839143
4.6	.985995	.966986	.946141	.924872	.903860	.883442	.863777
4.8	.988465	.972638	.955124	.937111	.919189	.901659	.884675
5.0	.990473	.977273	.962546	.947291	.932017	.916989	.902351
5.2	.992109	.981077	.968680	.955756	.942741	.929870	.917273
5.4	.993444	.984206	.973755	.962798	.951706	.940685	.929852
5.6	.994537	.986783	.977959	.968659	.959200	.949763	.940450
5.8	.995434	.988911	.981446	.973542	.965470	.957384	.949377
6.0	.996172	.990671	.984344	.977617	.970719	.963787	.956900
6.4	.997286	.993343	.988771	.983871	.978815	.973702	.968594
6.8	.998053	.995199	.991865	.988270	.984539	.980748	.976942
7.2	.998587	.996500	.994047	.991389	.988616	.985786	.982935
7.6	.998963	.997422	.995601	.993618	.991542	.989416	.987266
8.0	.999231	.998082	.996718	.995227	.993661	.992051	.990419
8.4	.999424	.998559	.997529	.996398	.995207	.993980	.992732
8.8	.999564	.998908	.998122	.997258	.996346	.995403	.994443
9.2	.999668	.999164	.998561	.997896	.997191	.996461	.995717
9.6	.999744	.999356	.998888	.998372	.997824	.997255	.996674
10.0	.999801	.999499	.999134	.998730	.998301	.997855	.997399
11.0	.999891	.999724	.999522	.999297	.999057	.998807	.998550
12.0	.999938	.999841	.999725	.999594	.999455	.999309	.999159
13.0	.999963	.999905	.999835	.999757	.999673	.999585	.999495
14.0	.999977	.999942	.999898	.999850	.999796	.999743	.999687

$\nu = 7$

Q\n	2	3	4	5	6	7	8
15.0	.999986	.999963	.999935	.999905	.999871	.999836	.999800
16.0	.999991	.999976	.999958	.999938	.999916	.999893	.999869
17.0	.999994	.999984	.999972	.999958	.999944	.999928	.999913
18.0	1.00000	.999989	.999981	.999972	.999962	.999951	.999940
19.0		.999992	.999987	.999980	.999973	.999966	.999958
20.0		.999995	.999991	.999986	.999981	.999976	.999971
22.0		1.00000	1.00000	.999993	.999990	.999987	.999985
24.0				1.00000	.999995	.999993	.999991
26.0					1.00000	1.00000	1.00000

$\nu = 7$

Q\n	9	10	11	12	13	14	15
0.0	.000000	.000000	.000000	.000000	.000000	.000000	.000000
0.1	.000000	.000000	.000000	.000000	.000000	.000000	.000000
0.2	.000000	.000000	.000000	.000000	.000000	.000000	.000000
0.3	.000000	.000000	.000000	.000000	.000000	.000000	.000000
0.4	.000004	.000001	.000000	.000000	.000000	.000000	.000000
0.5	.000023	.000007	.000002	.000001	.000000	.000000	.000000
0.6	.000090	.000031	.000011	.000004	.000001	.000001	.000000
0.7	.000277	.000109	.000044	.000018	.000008	.000003	.000001
0.8	.000716	.000316	.000143	.000066	.000031	.000015	.000007
0.9	.001612	.000785	.000390	.000198	.000102	.000054	.000029
1.0	.003251	.001718	.000926	.000508	.000284	.000161	.000093
1.2	.010238	.006174	.003787	.002360	.001493	.000958	.000623
1.4	.024933	.016626	.011248	.007714	.005358	.003766	.002677
1.6	.050276	.036236	.026438	.019511	.014554	.010966	.008341
1.8	.087871	.067312	.052094	.040704	.032091	.025514	.020444
2.0	.137505	.110548	.089635	.073261	.060326	.050022	.041749
2.2	.197307	.164879	.138752	.117539	.100187	.085891	.074034
2.4	.264322	.227873	.197590	.172267	.150957	.132916	.117555
2.6	.335197	.296383	.263307	.234969	.210564	.189438	.171061
2.8	.406756	.367167	.332712	.302596	.276156	.252843	.232203
3.0	.476357	.437349	.402797	.372083	.344683	.320151	.298109
3.2	.542045	.504664	.471056	.440755	.413356	.388505	.365900
3.4	.602551	.567523	.535627	.506521	.479899	.455488	.433049
3.6	.657203	.624965	.595289	.567928	.542654	.519262	.497567
3.8	.705797	.676553	.649379	.624101	.600554	.578583	.558049
4.0	.748461	.722239	.697673	.674645	.653036	.632733	.613630
4.2	.785545	.762249	.740269	.719525	.699934	.681416	.663891
4.4	.817523	.796978	.777471	.758952	.741365	.724652	.708755
4.6	.844929	.826913	.809712	.793298	.777632	.762675	.748385
4.8	.868305	.852576	.837485	.823018	.809150	.795855	.783102
5.0	.888173	.874486	.861298	.848602	.836386	.824630	.813314
5.2	.905016	.893135	.881643	.870539	.859817	.849466	.839470
5.4	.919270	.908975	.898981	.889293	.879910	.870823	.862025
5.6	.931321	.922408	.913730	.905293	.897097	.889140	.881417
5.8	.941503	.933792	.926263	.918923	.911775	.904819	.898052
6.0	.950107	.943436	.936906	.930525	.924297	.918223	.912301
6.4	.963530	.958535	.953622	.948801	.944077	.939452	.934927
6.8	.973154	.969401	.965696	.962049	.958462	.954941	.951484
7.2	.980086	.977255	.974451	.971682	.968952	.966264	.963620
7.6	.985111	.982964	.980832	.978720	.976634	.974576	.972546
8.0	.988779	.987141	.985510	.983892	.982290	.980706	.979142
8.4	.991476	.990218	.988963	.987717	.986480	.985255	.984043
8.8	.993474	.992501	.991530	.990564	.989603	.988651	.987707
9.2	.994965	.994209	.993452	.992698	.991948	.991203	.990465
9.6	.996086	.995494	.994902	.994310	.993721	.993135	.992553
10.0	.996936	.996470	.996003	.995535	.995070	.994606	.994146
11.0	.998289	.998025	.997760	.997495	.997229	.996965	.996702
12.0	.999006	.998852	.998696	.998540	.998384	.998227	.998072
13.0	.999402	.999309	.999214	.999119	.999024	.998929	.998834
14.0	.999629	.999571	.999512	.999452	.999393	.999333	.999274

$\nu = 7$

Q\n	9	10	11	12	13	14	15
15.0	.999763	.999726	.999688	.999650	.999612	.999573	.999535
16.0	.999845	.999821	.999796	.999771	.999745	.999720	.999695
17.0	.999896	.999880	.999863	.999846	.999829	.999812	.999795
18.0	.999929	.999918	.999906	.999895	.999883	.999871	.999860
19.0	.999951	.999943	.999935	.999927	.999919	.999910	.999902
20.0	.999965	.999959	.999954	.999948	.999942	.999936	.999931
22.0	.999982	.999979	.999976	.999973	.999970	.999967	.999963
24.0	.999990	.999988	.999987	.999985	.999983	.999981	.999980
26.0	.999994	.999993	.999992	.999991	.999990	.999989	.999988
28.0	1.00000	1.00000	1.00000	.999995	.999994	.999994	.999993
30.0				1.00000	1.00000	1.00000	1.00000

$\nu = 7$

Q\n	16	17	18	19	20	22	24
0.0	.000000	.000000	.000000	.000000	.000000	.000000	.000000
0.2	.000000	.000000	.000000	.000000	.000000	.000000	.000000
0.4	.000000	.000000	.000000	.000000	.000000	.000000	.000000
0.6	.000000	.000000	.000000	.000000	.000000	.000000	.000000
0.8	.000004	.000002	.000001	.000000	.000000	.000000	.000000
1.0	.000054	.000032	.000019	.000012	.000007	.000003	.000001
1.2	.000410	.000273	.000184	.000125	.000086	.000042	.000021
1.4	.001923	.001395	.001022	.000755	.000562	.000319	.000186
1.6	.006400	.004951	.003861	.003032	.002398	.001529	.000998
1.8	.016503	.013413	.010972	.009030	.007475	.005203	.003692
2.0	.035058	.029608	.025139	.021452	.018393	.013699	.010367
2.2	.064136	.055826	.048808	.042850	.037768	.029659	.023599
2.4	.104405	.093089	.083306	.074807	.067394	.055192	.045694
2.6	.155001	.140904	.128479	.117484	.107719	.091233	.077970
2.8	.213856	.197487	.182830	.169660	.157790	.137328	.120417
3.0	.278238	.260266	.243961	.229126	.215589	.191848	.171786
3.2	.345279	.326414	.309110	.293198	.278530	.252430	.229962
3.4	.412372	.393274	.375592	.359187	.343934	.316459	.292434
3.6	.477403	.458625	.441103	.424721	.409377	.381450	.356703
3.8	.538824	.520793	.503853	.487912	.472887	.445295	.420566
4.0	.595631	.578646	.562596	.547407	.533013	.506374	.482264
4.2	.647287	.631535	.616575	.602347	.588800	.563561	.540522
4.4	.693620	.679195	.665433	.652290	.639723	.616174	.594518
4.6	.734722	.721646	.709123	.697117	.685597	.663896	.643810
4.8	.770862	.759107	.747809	.736942	.726481	.706686	.688258
5.0	.802417	.791918	.781797	.772032	.762606	.744697	.727940
5.2	.829817	.820489	.811471	.802749	.794308	.778213	.763083
5.4	.853505	.845252	.837253	.829498	.821976	.807587	.794007
5.6	.873919	.866639	.859568	.852699	.846022	.833213	.821079
5.8	.891468	.885062	.878828	.872760	.866851	.855486	.844684
6.0	.906529	.900902	.895416	.890067	.884849	.874791	.865203
6.4	.930501	.926173	.921941	.917801	.913752	.905913	.898403
6.8	.948095	.944770	.941511	.938316	.935182	.929096	.923240
7.2	.961020	.958465	.955954	.953487	.951064	.946342	.941783
7.6	.970546	.968577	.966639	.964731	.962853	.959186	.955635
8.0	.977598	.976075	.974573	.973093	.971634	.968779	.966007
8.4	.982845	.981662	.980494	.979341	.978203	.975973	.973802
8.8	.986774	.985850	.984937	.984035	.983144	.981394	.979688
9.2	.989733	.989008	.988291	.987582	.986880	.985501	.984154
9.6	.991976	.991405	.990838	.990278	.989723	.988631	.987562
10.0	.993688	.993235	.992785	.992340	.991899	.991030	.990178
11.0	.996440	.996180	.995921	.995665	.995411	.994909	.994415
12.0	.997917	.997763	.997609	.997457	.997306	.997007	.996712
13.0	.998740	.998646	.998552	.998459	.998366	.998183	.998002
14.0	.999214	.999155	.999096	.999038	.998979	.998864	.998749
15.0	.999497	.999459	.999421	.999383	.999345	.999270	.999196
16.0	.999670	.999644	.999619	.999594	.999569	.999520	.999471
17.0	.999778	.999761	.999744	.999727	.999711	.999677	.999644
18.0	.999848	.999836	.999825	.999813	.999802	.999779	.999756
19.0	.999894	.999886	.999878	.999870	.999861	.999845	.999829

$\nu = 7$

Q\n	16	17	18	19	20	22	24
20.0	.999925	.999919	.999913	.999907	.999902	.999890	.999879
22.0	.999960	.999957	.999954	.999951	.999948	.999942	.999936
24.0	.999978	.999976	.999975	.999973	.999971	.999968	.999964
26.0	.999987	.999986	.999985	.999984	.999983	.999981	.999979
28.0	.999992	.999992	.999991	.999991	.999990	.999989	.999988
30.0	1.00000	.999995	.999994	.999994	.999994	.999993	.999992
32.0		1.00000	1.00000	1.00000	1.00000	1.00000	1.00000

$\nu = 7$

Q\n	26	28	30	32	34	36	38
0.0	.000000	.000000	.000000	.000000	.000000	.000000	.000000
0.2	.000000	.000000	.000000	.000000	.000000	.000000	.000000
0.4	.000000	.000000	.000000	.000000	.000000	.000000	.000000
0.6	.000000	.000000	.000000	.000000	.000000	.000000	.000000
0.8	.000000	.000000	.000000	.000000	.000000	.000000	.000000
1.0	.000000	.000000	.000000	.000000	.000000	.000000	.000000
1.2	.000011	.000006	.000003	.000002	.000001	.000001	.000000
1.4	.000112	.000068	.000043	.000027	.000018	.000012	.000008
1.6	.000665	.000452	.000312	.000219	.000156	.000112	.000082
1.8	.002665	.001954	.001453	.001095	.000835	.000643	.000500
2.0	.007957	.006187	.004866	.003868	.003105	.002514	.002053
2.2	.019000	.015460	.012700	.010525	.008792	.007398	.006267
2.4	.038201	.032217	.027388	.023450	.020212	.017526	.015281
2.6	.067175	.058298	.050928	.044757	.039549	.035123	.031336
2.8	.106300	.094407	.084305	.075661	.068212	.061754	.056122
3.0	.154684	.139987	.127267	.116184	.106471	.097910	.090327
3.2	.210471	.193442	.178471	.165231	.153461	.142945	.133509
3.4	.271283	.252546	.235854	.220908	.207460	.195309	.184286
3.6	.334642	.314868	.297054	.280933	.266282	.252914	.240676
3.8	.398284	.378109	.359760	.343004	.327643	.313513	.300474
4.0	.460339	.440315	.421952	.405052	.389445	.374986	.361553
4.2	.519404	.499970	.482023	.465392	.449935	.435527	.422063
4.4	.574527	.556011	.538803	.522765	.507774	.493727	.480531
4.6	.625155	.607775	.591536	.576322	.562032	.548578	.535885
4.8	.671050	.654937	.639809	.625572	.612141	.599445	.587418
5.0	.712217	.697428	.683485	.670308	.657831	.645993	.634740
5.2	.748828	.735365	.722624	.710541	.699060	.688131	.677711
5.4	.781162	.768989	.757428	.746430	.735947	.725941	.716373
5.6	.809563	.798614	.788185	.778235	.768725	.759623	.750899
5.8	.834401	.824596	.815231	.806272	.797690	.789456	.781546
6.0	.856049	.847298	.838920	.830886	.823172	.815756	.808618
6.4	.891199	.884280	.877627	.871222	.865049	.859092	.853338
6.8	.917600	.912163	.906916	.901848	.896948	.892205	.887611
7.2	.937377	.933117	.928993	.924998	.921125	.917368	.913718
7.6	.952193	.948855	.945617	.942473	.939417	.936446	.933554
8.0	.963313	.960696	.958150	.955674	.953263	.950914	.948624
8.4	.971689	.969631	.967626	.965671	.963765	.961906	.960090
8.8	.978023	.976400	.974816	.973269	.971759	.970283	.968840
9.2	.982838	.981552	.980296	.979068	.977867	.976692	.975543
9.6	.986517	.985495	.984495	.983516	.982557	.981619	.980699
10.0	.989344	.988528	.987728	.986944	.986176	.985423	.984685
11.0	.993931	.993456	.992989	.992531	.992081	.991639	.991205
12.0	.996423	.996138	.995858	.995582	.995311	.995045	.994783
13.0	.997823	.997648	.997475	.997305	.997137	.996972	.996810
14.0	.998637	.998526	.998416	.998308	.998202	.998097	.997994
15.0	.999123	.999051	.998980	.998910	.998841	.998773	.998706
16.0	.999423	.999375	.999328	.999281	.999235	.999190	.999145
17.0	.999611	.999579	.999547	.999516	.999485	.999454	.999424
18.0	.999733	.999711	.999689	.999667	.999646	.999625	.999604
19.0	.999814	.999798	.999783	.999767	.999752	.999737	.999723

$\nu = 7$

Q\n	26	28	30	32	34	36	38
20.0	.999868	.999856	.999845	.999834	.999824	.999813	.999803
22.0	.999930	.999924	.999918	.999913	.999907	.999901	.999896
24.0	.999961	.999958	.999955	.999951	.999948	.999945	.999942
26.0	.999977	.999976	.999974	.999972	.999970	.999968	.999966
28.0	.999986	.999985	.999984	.999983	.999982	.999981	.999980
30.0	.999992	.999991	.999990	.999989	.999989	.999988	.999987
32.0	.999995	.999994	.999994	.999993	.999993	.999992	.999992
34.0	1.00000	1.00000	1.00000	1.00000	1.00000	.999995	.999995
36.0						1.00000	1.00000

$\nu = 7$

Q\n	40	50	60	70	80	90	100
0.0	.000000	.000000	.000000	.000000	.000000	.000000	.000000
0.1	.000000	.000000	.000000	.000000	.000000	.000000	.000000
0.2	.000000	.000000	.000000	.000000	.000000	.000000	.000000
0.3	.000000	.000000	.000000	.000000	.000000	.000000	.000000
0.4	.000000	.000000	.000000	.000000	.000000	.000000	.000000
0.5	.000000	.000000	.000000	.000000	.000000	.000000	.000000
0.6	.000000	.000000	.000000	.000000	.000000	.000000	.000000
0.7	.000000	.000000	.000000	.000000	.000000	.000000	.000000
0.8	.000000	.000000	.000000	.000000	.000000	.000000	.000000
0.9	.000000	.000000	.000000	.000000	.000000	.000000	.000000
1.0	.000000	.000000	.000000	.000000	.000000	.000000	.000000
1.1	.000000	.000000	.000000	.000000	.000000	.000000	.000000
1.2	.000000	.000000	.000000	.000000	.000000	.000000	.000000
1.3	.000001	.000000	.000000	.000000	.000000	.000000	.000000
1.4	.000005	.000001	.000000	.000000	.000000	.000000	.000000
1.5	.000020	.000004	.000001	.000000	.000000	.000000	.000000
1.6	.000061	.000015	.000005	.000002	.000001	.000000	.000000
1.7	.000164	.000048	.000017	.000007	.000003	.000001	.000001
1.8	.000393	.000132	.000052	.000023	.000011	.000006	.000003
1.9	.000851	.000320	.000138	.000066	.000034	.000019	.000011
2.0	.001689	.000700	.000329	.000169	.000094	.000055	.000034
2.1	.003104	.001401	.000708	.000390	.000229	.000142	.000091
2.2	.005341	.002599	.001402	.000816	.000504	.000327	.000220
2.3	.008675	.004512	.002576	.001577	.001019	.000687	.000479
2.4	.013393	.007389	.004438	.002839	.001908	.001333	.000961
2.5	.019776	.011499	.007224	.004808	.003345	.002412	.001790
2.6	.028076	.017110	.011189	.007712	.005536	.004105	.003125
2.7	.038498	.024468	.016587	.011797	.008707	.006620	.005157
2.8	.051185	.033785	.023653	.017303	.013095	.010183	.008096
2.9	.066212	.045217	.032591	.024454	.018928	.015021	.012164
3.0	.083579	.058861	.043554	.033436	.026413	.021347	.017578
3.1	.103220	.074749	.056640	.044394	.035720	.029351	.024534
3.2	.125007	.092847	.071887	.057414	.046975	.039182	.033202
3.3	.148757	.113059	.089271	.072529	.060249	.050945	.043709
3.4	.174248	.135241	.108712	.089712	.075561	.064692	.056135
3.5	.201230	.159202	.130079	.108884	.092875	.080424	.070510
3.6	.229433	.184722	.153201	.129920	.112106	.098092	.086817
3.7	.258582	.211557	.177873	.152654	.133126	.117599	.104988
3.8	.288405	.239453	.203871	.176892	.155771	.138813	.124916
3.9	.318639	.268154	.230955	.202420	.179852	.161566	.146459
4.0	.349038	.297409	.258883	.229010	.205158	.185670	.169447
4.1	.379376	.326978	.287416	.256431	.231473	.210921	.193691
4.2	.409449	.356636	.316324	.284453	.258572	.237105	.218989
4.3	.439078	.386180	.345389	.312858	.286238	.264008	.245135
4.4	.468109	.415426	.374412	.341436	.314260	.291421	.271920
4.5	.496413	.444214	.403213	.369996	.342439	.319142	.299144
4.6	.523883	.472405	.431633	.398365	.370592	.346983	.326616
4.7	.550435	.499884	.459532	.426386	.398553	.374770	.354156
4.8	.576004	.526556	.486792	.453924	.426174	.402345	.381601
4.9	.600544	.552344	.513316	.480865	.453325	.429568	.408801

$\nu = 7$

Q\n	40	50	60	70	80	90	100
5.0	.624026	.577193	.539024	.507111	.479895	.456317	.435627
5.1	.646432	.601059	.563854	.532582	.505792	.482488	.461963
5.2	.667759	.623918	.587759	.557218	.530939	.507993	.487713
5.3	.688014	.645754	.610708	.580969	.555276	.532760	.512795
5.4	.707211	.666564	.632682	.603802	.578756	.556731	.537142
5.5	.725372	.686355	.653671	.625696	.601347	.579865	.560703
5.6	.742525	.705139	.673676	.646640	.623026	.602129	.583437
5.7	.758702	.722937	.692707	.666632	.643782	.623503	.605317
5.8	.773938	.739775	.710778	.685677	.663614	.643978	.626324
5.9	.788270	.755681	.727910	.703789	.682524	.663549	.646449
6.0	.801739	.770688	.744129	.720986	.700526	.682223	.665693
6.4	.847774	.822438	.800474	.781117	.763832	.748233	.734031
6.8	.883156	.862717	.844801	.828861	.814510	.801463	.789507
7.2	.910172	.893798	.879312	.866321	.854543	.843770	.833842
7.6	.930739	.917671	.906019	.895498	.885904	.877083	.868916
8.0	.946390	.935976	.926627	.918137	.910357	.903171	.896491
8.4	.958316	.950015	.942519	.935679	.929382	.923545	.918100
8.8	.967429	.960802	.954788	.949276	.944183	.939446	.935015
9.2	.974417	.969114	.964280	.959833	.955712	.951867	.948260
9.6	.979798	.975542	.971647	.968053	.964712	.961587	.958649
10.0	.983961	.980533	.977386	.974473	.971758	.969214	.966817
11.0	.990778	.988750	.986875	.985129	.983493	.981953	.980496
12.0	.994525	.993294	.992150	.991080	.990073	.989122	.988220
13.0	.996650	.995883	.995169	.994498	.993865	.993265	.992694
14.0	.997892	.997404	.996946	.996516	.996109	.995722	.995354
15.0	.998640	.998321	.998022	.997740	.997472	.997218	.996975
16.0	.999101	.998889	.998689	.998501	.998321	.998151	.997988
17.0	.999394	.999249	.999113	.998985	.998862	.998746	.998634
18.0	.999583	.999483	.999389	.999299	.999215	.999133	.999056
19.0	.999708	.999638	.999571	.999508	.999448	.999391	.999336
20.0	.999792	.999742	.999694	.999649	.999606	.999565	.999526
22.0	.999890	.999863	.999838	.999814	.999791	.999769	.999748
24.0	.999939	.999924	.999910	.999896	.999883	.999871	.999859
26.0	.999964	.999956	.999947	.999939	.999932	.999925	.999918
28.0	.999978	.999973	.999968	.999963	.999959	.999954	.999950
30.0	.999987	.999983	.999980	.999977	.999974	.999971	.999969
32.0	.999991	.999989	.999987	.999985	.999983	.999982	.999980
34.0	.999994	.999993	.999992	.999990	.999989	.999988	.999987
36.0	1.00000	1.00000	.999994	.999993	.999993	.999992	.999991
38.0			1.00000	1.00000	.999995	.999994	.999994
40.0					1.00000	1.00000	1.00000

ν = 8

Q\n	2	3	4	5	6	7	8
0.0	.000000	.000000	.000000	.000000	.000000	.000000	.000000
0.1	.054595	.002752	.000138	.000007	.000000	.000000	.000000
0.2	.108967	.010950	.001096	.000112	.000012	.000001	.000000
0.3	.162691	.024427	.003654	.000556	.000087	.000014	.000002
0.4	.215522	.042908	.008507	.001715	.000354	.000075	.000016
0.5	.267190	.066027	.016244	.004060	.001038	.000272	.000073
0.6	.317448	.093336	.027310	.008111	.002463	.000766	.000244
0.7	.366075	.124328	.042002	.014391	.005035	.001803	.000661
0.8	.412881	.158449	.060459	.023375	.009218	.003716	.001533
0.9	.457706	.195123	.082666	.035451	.015489	.006911	.003150
1.0	.500424	.233764	.108469	.050894	.024300	.011833	.005879
1.2	.579194	.314671	.169666	.092309	.050979	.028639	.016373
1.4	.648808	.396934	.240825	.147129	.091019	.057131	.036403
1.6	.709329	.477030	.317975	.213019	.144170	.098764	.068519
1.8	.761167	.552320	.397117	.286476	.208342	.153030	.113588
2.0	.804984	.621064	.474759	.363604	.280220	.217692	.170572
2.2	.841595	.682332	.548204	.440758	.356033	.289416	.236896
2.4	.871878	.735845	.615628	.514953	.432196	.364520	.309137
2.6	.896714	.781806	.676015	.584036	.505740	.439574	.383718
2.8	.916938	.820737	.729012	.646680	.574494	.511781	.457442
3.0	.933312	.853336	.774752	.702267	.637095	.579131	.527786
3.2	.946507	.880383	.813696	.750726	.692875	.640382	.593001
3.4	.957103	.902655	.846489	.792367	.741713	.694950	.652058
3.6	.965590	.920889	.873859	.827734	.783865	.742759	.704528
3.8	.972376	.935750	.896543	.857494	.819831	.784080	.750427
4.0	.977796	.947821	.915241	.882352	.850236	.819406	.790079
4.2	.982125	.957604	.930591	.902995	.875755	.849345	.823990
4.4	.985582	.965521	.943155	.920063	.897052	.874545	.852762
4.6	.988346	.971922	.953416	.934130	.914747	.895642	.877018
4.8	.990558	.977098	.961787	.945697	.929404	.913233	.897369
5.0	.992330	.981285	.968613	.955195	.941517	.927857	.914380
5.2	.993753	.984674	.974177	.962988	.951512	.939989	.928562
5.4	.994899	.987421	.978717	.969381	.959755	.950040	.940362
5.6	.995822	.989651	.982423	.974627	.966550	.958362	.950171
5.8	.996568	.991465	.985452	.978936	.972153	.965250	.958319
6.0	.997173	.992942	.987931	.982477	.976776	.970953	.965087
6.4	.998064	.995135	.991635	.987795	.983753	.979597	.975386
6.8	.998659	.996611	.994145	.991421	.988537	.985556	.982521
7.2	.999060	.997613	.995860	.993912	.991840	.989688	.987488
7.6	.999334	.998301	.997043	.995638	.994138	.992574	.990969
8.0	.999522	.998778	.997867	.996845	.995750	.994605	.993425
8.4	.999654	.999112	.998446	.997697	.996891	.996045	.995173
8.8	.999747	.999349	.998857	.998303	.997705	.997076	.996426
9.2	.999813	.999518	.999152	.998738	.998291	.997820	.997331
9.6	.999861	.999639	.999365	.999054	.998717	.998361	.997991
10.0	.999895	.999728	.999521	.999285	.999029	.998758	.998476
11.0	.999947	.999861	.999754	.999632	.999499	.999358	.999211
12.0	.999971	.999926	.999868	.999802	.999730	.999654	.999574
13.0	.999984	.999959	.999926	.999889	.999849	.999806	.999760
14.0	.999991	.999976	.999957	.999936	.999912	.999887	.999861

$\nu = 8$

Q\n	2	3	4	5	6	7	8
15.0	.999995	.999986	.999974	.999962	.999947	.999932	.999916
16.0	1.00000	.999991	.999984	.999976	.999968	.999958	.999948
17.0		.999994	.999990	.999985	.999979	.999974	.999967
18.0		1.00000	.999994	.999990	.999987	.999983	.999979
19.0			1.00000	.999994	.999991	.999989	.999986
20.0				1.00000	.999994	.999992	.999990
22.0					1.00000	1.00000	1.00000

$\nu = 8$

Q\n	9	10	11	12	13	14	15
0.0	.000000	.000000	.000000	.000000	.000000	.000000	.000000
0.1	.000000	.000000	.000000	.000000	.000000	.000000	.000000
0.2	.000000	.000000	.000000	.000000	.000000	.000000	.000000
0.3	.000000	.000000	.000000	.000000	.000000	.000000	.000000
0.4	.000004	.000001	.000000	.000000	.000000	.000000	.000000
0.5	.000020	.000006	.000002	.000000	.000000	.000000	.000000
0.6	.000080	.000027	.000009	.000003	.000001	.000000	.000000
0.7	.000248	.000095	.000037	.000015	.000006	.000003	.000001
0.8	.000646	.000278	.000122	.000055	.000025	.000012	.000006
0.9	.001466	.000697	.000337	.000167	.000084	.000043	.000022
1.0	.002979	.001539	.000810	.000434	.000236	.000131	.000073
1.2	.009524	.005633	.003385	.002066	.001279	.000802	.000510
1.4	.023541	.015444	.010271	.006920	.004719	.003256	.002271
1.6	.048135	.034227	.024621	.017906	.013157	.009763	.007311
1.8	.085197	.064552	.049385	.038129	.029694	.023315	.018447
2.0	.134805	.107434	.086309	.069867	.056965	.046762	.038631
2.2	.195270	.162065	.135396	.113827	.096262	.081865	.069989
2.4	.263653	.226117	.194970	.168978	.147166	.128760	.113146
2.6	.336472	.296370	.262187	.232918	.207739	.185981	.167095
2.8	.410329	.369390	.333704	.302486	.275076	.250918	.229548
3.0	.482334	.442049	.406267	.374399	.345934	.320430	.297510
3.2	.550309	.511832	.477109	.445711	.417256	.391407	.367865
3.4	.612821	.576950	.544135	.514078	.486502	.461154	.437807
3.6	.669096	.636303	.605953	.577846	.551785	.527588	.505085
3.8	.718884	.689379	.661797	.636007	.611878	.589279	.568088
4.0	.762319	.736111	.711397	.688098	.666125	.645392	.625810
4.2	.799784	.776745	.754853	.734065	.714326	.695578	.677760
4.4	.831807	.811722	.792508	.774147	.756607	.739852	.723841
4.6	.858983	.841586	.824847	.808760	.793312	.778480	.764239
4.8	.881915	.866925	.852425	.838423	.824912	.811883	.799319
5.0	.901182	.888317	.875815	.863687	.851938	.840561	.829550
5.2	.917318	.906309	.895566	.885104	.874931	.865045	.855444
5.4	.930799	.921399	.912192	.903194	.894414	.885857	.877520
5.6	.942046	.934031	.926154	.918432	.910875	.903487	.896271
5.8	.951419	.944592	.937861	.931244	.924750	.918386	.912154
6.0	.959229	.953414	.947667	.942002	.936429	.930954	.925582
6.4	.971158	.966940	.962751	.958603	.954506	.950464	.946482
6.8	.979459	.976392	.973333	.970294	.967280	.964298	.961350
7.2	.985260	.983021	.980780	.978546	.976324	.974119	.971934
7.6	.989338	.987694	.986044	.984395	.982751	.981115	.979491
8.0	.992224	.991010	.989789	.988565	.987342	.986123	.984910
8.4	.994282	.993379	.992469	.991556	.990641	.989728	.988817
8.8	.995760	.995084	.994402	.993716	.993028	.992340	.991652
9.2	.996831	.996321	.995806	.995287	.994766	.994245	.993723
9.6	.997612	.997225	.996834	.996439	.996042	.995644	.995246
10.0	.998187	.997891	.997592	.997289	.996985	.996679	.996373
11.0	.999059	.998904	.998746	.998587	.998425	.998263	.998101
12.0	.999491	.999406	.999320	.999232	.999143	.999054	.998964
13.0	.999714	.999665	.999616	.999567	.999516	.999465	.999414
14.0	.999833	.999805	.999776	.999747	.999717	.999687	.999657

$\nu = 8$

Q\n	9	10	11	12	13	14	15
15.0	.999900	.999883	.999865	.999848	.999830	.999812	.999793
16.0	.999938	.999927	.999917	.999906	.999895	.999883	.999872
17.0	.999961	.999954	.999947	.999940	.999933	.999926	.999919
18.0	.999975	.999970	.999966	.999961	.999956	.999952	.999947
19.0	.999983	.999980	.999977	.999974	.999971	.999968	.999965
20.0	.999989	.999987	.999985	.999983	.999980	.999978	.999976
22.0	.999995	.999994	.999993	.999992	.999991	.999990	.999989
24.0	1.00000	1.00000	1.00000	1.00000	1.00000	.999995	.999994
26.0						1.00000	1.00000

$\nu = 8$

Q\n	16	17	18	19	20	22	24
0.0	.000000	.000000	.000000	.000000	.000000	.000000	.000000
0.2	.000000	.000000	.000000	.000000	.000000	.000000	.000000
0.4	.000000	.000000	.000000	.000000	.000000	.000000	.000000
0.6	.000000	.000000	.000000	.000000	.000000	.000000	.000000
0.8	.000003	.000001	.000001	.000000	.000000	.000000	.000000
1.0	.000042	.000024	.000014	.000008	.000005	.000002	.000001
1.2	.000328	.000214	.000141	.000093	.000063	.000029	.000014
1.4	.001601	.001139	.000818	.000593	.000433	.000237	.000133
1.6	.005523	.004206	.003228	.002496	.001943	.001201	.000760
1.8	.014702	.011797	.009527	.007741	.006326	.004292	.002970
2.0	.032107	.026835	.022549	.019043	.016159	.011790	.008742
2.2	.060133	.051907	.045005	.039182	.034247	.026452	.020704
2.4	.099832	.088425	.078606	.070118	.062749	.050709	.041432
2.6	.150632	.136222	.123559	.112390	.102504	.085902	.072645
2.8	.210576	.193674	.178568	.165022	.152840	.131914	.114710
3.0	.276850	.258173	.241242	.225852	.211826	.187277	.166600
3.2	.346372	.326701	.308656	.292064	.276775	.249591	.226228
3.4	.416259	.396333	.377869	.360726	.344781	.316052	.290937
3.6	.484124	.464567	.446289	.429179	.413137	.383904	.357976
3.8	.548191	.529485	.511873	.495270	.479596	.450756	.424857
4.0	.607298	.589778	.573178	.557432	.542480	.514737	.489554
4.2	.660814	.644684	.629317	.614663	.600676	.574534	.550583
4.4	.708534	.693891	.679872	.666442	.653566	.629346	.606976
4.6	.750561	.737417	.724782	.712627	.700927	.678796	.658211
4.8	.787202	.775514	.764235	.753346	.742829	.722836	.704121
5.0	.818892	.808575	.798586	.788912	.779539	.761643	.744799
5.2	.846122	.837070	.828280	.819742	.811448	.795549	.780510
5.4	.869402	.861497	.853801	.846306	.839007	.824968	.811629
5.6	.889225	.882348	.875636	.869086	.862692	.850354	.838586
5.8	.906055	.900089	.894254	.888547	.882966	.872166	.861827
6.0	.920313	.915148	.910087	.905127	.900268	.890842	.881789
6.4	.942563	.938708	.934917	.931191	.927528	.920392	.913500
6.8	.958440	.955569	.952738	.949947	.947198	.941820	.936602
7.2	.969771	.967632	.965518	.963430	.961367	.957321	.953380
7.6	.977879	.976282	.974700	.973134	.971585	.968538	.965561
8.0	.983704	.982507	.981320	.980142	.978976	.976676	.974422
8.4	.987911	.987010	.986115	.985226	.984344	.982601	.980890
8.8	.990968	.990286	.989607	.988933	.988263	.986938	.985632
9.2	.993203	.992684	.992167	.991653	.991141	.990128	.989128
9.6	.994848	.994451	.994055	.993660	.993268	.992489	.991720
10.0	.996067	.995762	.995456	.995152	.994849	.994248	.993652
11.0	.997938	.997774	.997611	.997449	.997286	.996963	.996642
12.0	.998874	.998784	.998694	.998603	.998513	.998333	.998154
13.0	.999363	.999311	.999259	.999208	.999156	.999052	.998949
14.0	.999627	.999596	.999566	.999535	.999505	.999443	.999382
15.0	.999775	.999756	.999738	.999719	.999701	.999663	.999626
16.0	.999860	.999849	.999837	.999826	.999814	.999791	.999767
17.0	.999911	.999904	.999896	.999889	.999882	.999867	.999852
18.0	.999942	.999937	.999933	.999928	.999923	.999913	.999903
19.0	.999962	.999958	.999955	.999952	.999949	.999942	.999936

$\nu = 8$

Q\n	16	17	18	19	20	22	24
20.0	.999974	.999972	.999970	.999968	.999965	.999961	.999956
22.0	.999988	.999986	.999985	.999984	.999983	.999981	.999979
24.0	.999994	.999993	.999993	.999992	.999991	.999990	.999989
26.0	1.00000	1.00000	1.00000	1.00000	1.00000	.999995	.999994
28.0						1.00000	1.00000

ν = 8

Q\n	26	28	30	32	34	36	38
0.0	.000000	.000000	.000000	.000000	.000000	.000000	.000000
0.2	.000000	.000000	.000000	.000000	.000000	.000000	.000000
0.4	.000000	.000000	.000000	.000000	.000000	.000000	.000000
0.6	.000000	.000000	.000000	.000000	.000000	.000000	.000000
0.8	.000000	.000000	.000000	.000000	.000000	.000000	.000000
1.0	.000000	.000000	.000000	.000000	.000000	.000000	.000000
1.2	.000007	.000004	.000002	.000001	.000001	.000000	.000000
1.4	.000077	.000045	.000027	.000017	.000011	.000007	.000004
1.6	.000491	.000323	.000217	.000148	.000102	.000072	.000051
1.8	.002092	.001497	.001087	.000800	.000596	.000449	.000342
2.0	.006577	.005014	.003868	.003017	.002377	.001890	.001516
2.2	.016401	.013135	.010623	.008670	.007134	.005916	.004940
2.4	.034190	.028468	.023898	.020211	.017211	.014748	.012711
2.6	.061940	.053205	.046011	.040036	.035035	.030817	.027238
2.8	.100426	.088463	.078361	.069768	.062408	.056066	.050570
3.0	.149037	.134004	.121047	.109806	.099997	.091391	.083803
3.2	.206001	.188373	.172915	.159285	.147204	.136445	.126821
3.4	.268841	.249289	.231896	.216347	.202384	.189792	.178393
3.6	.334852	.314125	.295459	.278577	.263248	.249277	.236501
3.8	.401488	.380309	.361035	.343430	.327292	.312450	.298759
4.0	.466603	.445604	.426322	.408557	.392139	.376923	.362781
4.2	.528564	.508250	.489452	.472004	.455766	.440613	.426440
4.4	.586252	.566996	.549056	.532296	.516601	.501870	.488014
4.6	.639012	.621061	.604236	.588429	.573547	.559506	.546234
4.8	.686565	.670058	.654504	.639819	.625928	.612762	.600263
5.0	.728913	.713904	.699696	.686222	.673422	.661242	.649635
5.2	.766261	.752739	.739886	.727649	.715981	.704838	.694183
5.4	.798939	.786848	.775313	.764293	.753749	.743648	.733960
5.6	.827348	.816604	.806319	.796461	.787003	.777916	.769176
5.8	.851920	.842419	.833297	.824530	.816094	.807969	.800135
6.0	.873088	.864720	.856664	.848901	.841413	.834185	.827200
6.4	.906841	.900405	.894180	.888154	.882319	.876662	.871175
6.8	.931539	.926625	.921854	.917219	.912714	.908333	.904070
7.2	.949541	.945803	.942161	.938613	.935153	.931780	.928489
7.6	.962651	.959810	.957034	.954323	.951673	.949082	.946549
8.0	.972214	.970052	.967935	.965862	.963832	.961843	.959895
8.4	.979209	.977560	.975942	.974355	.972797	.971269	.969770
8.8	.984349	.983086	.981846	.980627	.979429	.978252	.977095
9.2	.988143	.987173	.986218	.985279	.984354	.983444	.982549
9.6	.990960	.990212	.989473	.988746	.988029	.987323	.986628
10.0	.993064	.992483	.991910	.991344	.990786	.990236	.989694
11.0	.996324	.996009	.995697	.995389	.995085	.994784	.994486
12.0	.997977	.997801	.997626	.997453	.997282	.997112	.996944
13.0	.998847	.998745	.998644	.998544	.998445	.998346	.998249
14.0	.999322	.999261	.999201	.999141	.999082	.999023	.998965
15.0	.999589	.999552	.999515	.999479	.999442	.999406	.999371
16.0	.999744	.999721	.999698	.999675	.999652	.999630	.999607
17.0	.999837	.999822	.999807	.999793	.999778	.999763	.999749
18.0	.999894	.999884	.999874	.999865	.999855	.999845	.999836
19.0	.999929	.999923	.999916	.999910	.999903	.999897	.999891

$\nu = 8$

Q\n	26	28	30	32	34	36	38
20.0	.999952	.999948	.999943	.999939	.999934	.999930	.999926
22.0	.999977	.999975	.999973	.999970	.999968	.999966	.999964
24.0	.999988	.999987	.999986	.999985	.999984	.999983	.999982
26.0	.999994	.999993	.999992	.999992	.999991	.999991	.999990
28.0	1.00000	1.00000	1.00000	1.00000	1.00000	.999995	.999994
30.0						1.00000	1.00000

$\nu = 8$

Q\n	40	50	60	70	80	90	100
0.0	.000000	.000000	.000000	.000000	.000000	.000000	.000000
0.1	.000000	.000000	.000000	.000000	.000000	.000000	.000000
0.2	.000000	.000000	.000000	.000000	.000000	.000000	.000000
0.3	.000000	.000000	.000000	.000000	.000000	.000000	.000000
0.4	.000000	.000000	.000000	.000000	.000000	.000000	.000000
0.5	.000000	.000000	.000000	.000000	.000000	.000000	.000000
0.6	.000000	.000000	.000000	.000000	.000000	.000000	.000000
0.7	.000000	.000000	.000000	.000000	.000000	.000000	.000000
0.8	.000000	.000000	.000000	.000000	.000000	.000000	.000000
0.9	.000000	.000000	.000000	.000000	.000000	.000000	.000000
1.0	.000000	.000000	.000000	.000000	.000000	.000000	.000000
1.1	.000000	.000000	.000000	.000000	.000000	.000000	.000000
1.2	.000000	.000000	.000000	.000000	.000000	.000000	.000000
1.3	.000001	.000000	.000000	.000000	.000000	.000000	.000000
1.4	.000003	.000000	.000000	.000000	.000000	.000000	.000000
1.5	.000011	.000002	.000000	.000000	.000000	.000000	.000000
1.6	.000037	.000008	.000002	.000001	.000000	.000000	.000000
1.7	.000104	.000027	.000009	.000003	.000001	.000001	.000000
1.8	.000263	.000080	.000028	.000011	.000005	.000002	.000001
1.9	.000594	.000204	.000081	.000036	.000017	.000009	.000005
2.0	.001225	.000468	.000204	.000098	.000051	.000028	.000017
2.1	.002335	.000979	.000463	.000240	.000133	.000078	.000048
2.2	.004152	.001891	.000961	.000530	.000311	.000193	.000124
2.3	.006945	.003404	.001842	.001074	.000663	.000429	.000288
2.4	.011014	.005760	.003297	.002018	.001302	.000877	.000611
2.5	.016663	.009234	.005554	.003552	.002383	.001661	.001195
2.6	.024182	.014112	.008874	.005901	.004099	.002948	.002182
2.7	.033822	.020675	.013528	.009315	.006674	.004937	.003749
2.8	.045780	.029176	.019785	.014057	.010356	.007855	.006103
2.9	.060183	.039824	.027889	.020361	.015397	.011946	.009474
3.0	.077080	.052768	.038045	.028519	.022038	.017451	.014099
3.1	.096445	.068088	.050400	.038662	.030495	.024598	.020209
3.2	.118178	.085794	.065042	.050948	.040940	.033580	.028013
3.3	.142115	.105825	.081991	.065456	.053495	.044552	.037685
3.4	.168036	.128057	.101201	.082204	.068225	.057614	.049353
3.5	.195686	.152311	.122564	.101143	.085133	.072809	.063092
3.6	.224779	.178366	.145921	.122172	.104165	.090124	.078925
3.7	.255016	.205967	.171070	.145138	.125212	.109490	.096816
3.8	.286094	.234840	.197777	.169847	.148121	.130791	.116683
3.9	.317717	.264703	.225785	.196075	.172702	.153868	.138394
4.0	.349605	.295274	.254828	.223579	.198735	.178527	.161784
4.1	.381496	.326280	.284638	.252104	.225984	.204553	.186656
4.2	.413152	.357463	.314952	.281393	.254204	.231715	.212796
4.3	.444366	.388585	.345521	.311195	.283148	.259774	.239976
4.4	.474953	.419430	.376112	.341270	.312575	.288491	.267963
4.5	.504762	.449811	.406513	.371394	.342255	.317637	.296528
4.6	.533666	.479561	.436537	.401361	.371973	.346991	.325451
4.7	.561563	.508544	.466017	.430989	.401534	.376350	.354521
4.8	.588377	.536646	.494813	.460116	.430761	.405525	.383545
4.9	.614054	.563776	.522807	.488603	.459499	.434351	.412347

$\nu = 8$

Q\n	40	50	60	70	80	90	100
5.0	.638557	.589866	.549903	.516334	.487616	.462682	.440769
5.1	.661867	.614867	.576029	.543215	.514999	.490390	.468676
5.2	.683980	.638745	.601127	.569168	.541557	.517372	.495949
5.3	.704904	.661486	.625160	.594139	.567216	.543539	.522490
5.4	.724657	.683085	.648104	.618086	.591921	.568824	.548219
5.5	.743264	.703549	.669949	.640983	.615632	.593173	.573072
5.6	.760761	.722896	.690697	.662817	.638323	.616549	.597001
5.7	.777183	.741150	.710359	.683587	.659981	.638928	.619973
5.8	.792575	.758341	.728954	.703301	.680604	.660299	.641966
5.9	.806980	.774506	.746507	.721974	.700196	.680657	.662970
6.0	.820445	.789682	.763048	.739628	.718774	.700011	.682984
6.4	.865849	.841355	.819834	.800669	.783414	.767737	.753383
6.8	.899919	.880672	.863552	.848147	.834150	.821328	.809503
7.2	.925276	.910275	.896795	.884558	.873354	.863021	.853431
7.6	.944071	.932433	.921884	.912236	.903345	.895097	.887404
8.0	.957986	.948974	.940745	.933171	.926152	.919609	.913478
8.4	.968297	.961320	.954906	.948972	.943445	.938272	.933406
8.8	.975957	.970546	.965546	.960896	.956549	.952464	.948609
9.2	.981668	.977461	.973555	.969909	.966486	.963261	.960208
9.6	.985943	.982663	.979604	.976738	.974039	.971489	.969069
10.0	.989159	.986591	.984188	.981929	.979797	.977776	.975854
11.0	.994193	.992776	.991439	.990175	.988974	.987831	.986738
12.0	.996778	.995974	.995211	.994486	.993794	.993133	.992499
13.0	.998152	.997683	.997236	.996809	.996401	.996009	.995633
14.0	.998907	.998626	.998357	.998099	.997852	.997614	.997386
15.0	.999335	.999162	.998996	.998837	.998684	.998536	.998394
16.0	.999585	.999476	.999371	.999270	.999173	.999079	.998989
17.0	.999735	.999664	.999597	.999531	.999469	.999408	.999349
18.0	.999827	.999780	.999736	.999693	.999651	.999611	.999572
19.0	.999884	.999853	.999823	.999795	.999767	.999740	.999713
20.0	.999921	.999900	.999880	.999860	.999841	.999823	.999805
22.0	.999962	.999952	.999942	.999932	.999923	.999914	.999905
24.0	.999980	.999975	.999970	.999965	.999960	.999955	.999951
26.0	.999989	.999987	.999984	.999981	.999978	.999976	.999973
28.0	.999994	.999992	.999991	.999989	.999988	.999986	.999985
30.0	1.00000	1.00000	.999995	.999994	.999993	.999992	.999991
32.0			1.00000	1.00000	1.00000	1.00000	.999995
34.0							1.00000

$\nu = 9$

Q\n	2	3	4	5	6	7	8
0.0	.000000	.000000	.000000	.000000	.000000	.000000	.000000
0.1	.054799	.002753	.000137	.000007	.000000	.000000	.000000
0.2	.109348	.010952	.001087	.000109	.000011	.000001	.000000
0.3	.163270	.024435	.003623	.000544	.000083	.000013	.000002
0.4	.216305	.042934	.008442	.001680	.000341	.000071	.000015
0.5	.268186	.066087	.016128	.003982	.001002	.000258	.000068
0.6	.318666	.093457	.027137	.007966	.002382	.000728	.000227
0.7	.367523	.124542	.041773	.014153	.004881	.001718	.000618
0.8	.414567	.158795	.060186	.023025	.008957	.003553	.001438
0.9	.459636	.195645	.082377	.034979	.015088	.006629	.002969
1.0	.502601	.234509	.108205	.050307	.023732	.011391	.005568
1.2	.581860	.316001	.169624	.091578	.050059	.027776	.015659
1.4	.651935	.399009	.241290	.146500	.089861	.055823	.035152
1.6	.712856	.479953	.319235	.212845	.143072	.097187	.066773
1.8	.765014	.556118	.399405	.287139	.207728	.151562	.111623
2.0	.809053	.625687	.478211	.365431	.280546	.216833	.168864
2.2	.845782	.687665	.552835	.443956	.357680	.289671	.236012
2.4	.876083	.741728	.621347	.519584	.435404	.366289	.309601
2.6	.900849	.788058	.682647	.590022	.510577	.443086	.385909
2.8	.920928	.827173	.736331	.653832	.580871	.517076	.461539
3.0	.937097	.859789	.782515	.710329	.644797	.586080	.533771
3.2	.950048	.886705	.821665	.759411	.701614	.648733	.600688
3.4	.960374	.908733	.854452	.801391	.751167	.704381	.661151
3.6	.968578	.926636	.881639	.836840	.793720	.752921	.714671
3.8	.975082	.941110	.904004	.866466	.829801	.794639	.761254
4.0	.980227	.952761	.922285	.891016	.860082	.830062	.801245
4.2	.984294	.962113	.937153	.911226	.885286	.859850	.835196
4.4	.987507	.969601	.949201	.927777	.906127	.884702	.863759
4.6	.990046	.975589	.958937	.941276	.923271	.905308	.887617
4.8	.992053	.980375	.966789	.952254	.937319	.922312	.907432
5.0	.993642	.984198	.973114	.961164	.948798	.936291	.923817
5.2	.994900	.987254	.978208	.968385	.958157	.947753	.937320
5.4	.995900	.989699	.982309	.974235	.965779	.957133	.948422
5.6	.996695	.991656	.985613	.978972	.971982	.964801	.957534
5.8	.997328	.993226	.988277	.982810	.977029	.971065	.965007
6.0	.997834	.994487	.990428	.985922	.981138	.976183	.971131
6.4	.998565	.996321	.993574	.990500	.987212	.983784	.980267
6.8	.999038	.997519	.995645	.993533	.991260	.988877	.986420
7.2	.999347	.998309	.997018	.995556	.993974	.992307	.990581
7.6	.999552	.998834	.997938	.996917	.995807	.994633	.993413
8.0	.999689	.999188	.998559	.997840	.997055	.996222	.995354
8.4	.999782	.999429	.998983	.998472	.997912	.997316	.996693
8.8	.999845	.999594	.999275	.998909	.998506	.998076	.997626
9.2	.999889	.999708	.999479	.999213	.998921	.998609	.998281
9.6	.999920	.999789	.999621	.999428	.999214	.998985	.998745
10.0	.999942	.999845	.999723	.999580	.999423	.999254	.999075
11.0	.999972	.999926	.999868	.999799	.999723	.999641	.999555
12.0	.999986	.999963	.999934	.999899	.999861	.999819	.999775
13.0	.999993	.999981	.999965	.999947	.999927	.999905	.999882
14.0	1.00000	.999990	.999981	.999971	.999960	.999948	.999935

$\nu = 9$

Q\n	2	3	4	5	6	7	8
15.0		.999994	.999989	.999984	.999977	.999971	.999963
16.0		1.00000	.999994	.999991	.999987	.999983	.999979
17.0			1.00000	.999994	.999992	.999990	.999987
18.0				1.00000	1.00000	.999994	.999992
19.0						1.00000	1.00000

$\nu = 9$

Q\n	9	10	11	12	13	14	15
0.0	.000000	.000000	.000000	.000000	.000000	.000000	.000000
0.1	.000000	.000000	.000000	.000000	.000000	.000000	.000000
0.2	.000000	.000000	.000000	.000000	.000000	.000000	.000000
0.3	.000000	.000000	.000000	.000000	.000000	.000000	.000000
0.4	.000003	.000001	.000000	.000000	.000000	.000000	.000000
0.5	.000018	.000005	.000001	.000000	.000000	.000000	.000000
0.6	.000073	.000024	.000008	.000003	.000001	.000000	.000000
0.7	.000227	.000085	.000033	.000013	.000005	.000002	.000001
0.8	.000594	.000251	.000108	.000047	.000021	.000010	.000004
0.9	.001356	.000631	.000299	.000144	.000071	.000035	.000018
1.0	.002772	.001405	.000724	.000380	.000202	.000109	.000060
1.2	.008970	.005219	.003082	.001847	.001122	.000691	.000430
1.4	.022440	.014517	.009514	.006313	.004238	.002877	.001974
1.6	.046408	.032620	.023181	.016646	.012073	.008839	.006530
1.8	.082998	.062298	.047189	.036058	.027783	.021577	.016883
2.0	.132540	.104840	.083556	.067076	.054220	.044115	.036118
2.2	.193511	.159668	.132558	.110706	.092982	.078519	.066645
2.4	.263005	.224559	.192693	.166148	.143925	.125226	.109414
2.6	.337439	.296251	.261134	.231079	.205251	.182965	.163657
2.8	.413227	.371149	.334419	.302265	.274029	.249151	.227161
3.0	.487263	.445907	.409084	.376234	.346857	.320520	.296846
3.2	.557171	.517787	.482128	.449801	.420447	.393740	.369392
3.4	.621368	.584818	.551247	.520396	.492014	.465867	.441742
3.6	.678986	.645773	.614891	.586177	.559464	.534591	.511405
3.8	.729736	.700072	.672196	.646013	.621421	.598310	.576575
4.0	.773757	.747632	.722855	.699378	.677142	.656079	.636118
4.2	.811465	.788719	.766971	.746207	.726396	.707500	.689473
4.4	.843439	.823816	.804922	.786760	.769322	.752587	.736529
4.6	.870331	.853528	.837246	.821504	.806304	.791638	.777493
4.8	.892802	.878497	.864560	.851014	.837868	.825125	.812778
5.0	.911484	.899361	.887492	.875903	.864606	.853609	.842911
5.2	.926954	.916717	.906651	.896780	.887121	.877682	.868467
5.4	.939728	.931106	.922594	.914216	.905989	.897923	.890023
5.6	.950253	.943005	.935823	.928732	.921745	.914875	.908126
5.8	.958913	.952827	.946778	.940786	.934867	.929029	.923280
6.0	.966034	.960927	.955837	.950781	.945772	.940821	.935934
6.4	.976699	.973104	.969503	.965909	.962333	.958783	.955265
6.8	.983914	.981380	.978829	.976274	.973723	.971180	.968652
7.2	.988815	.987020	.985209	.983387	.981563	.979739	.977921
7.6	.992160	.990883	.989590	.988287	.986977	.985665	.984354
8.0	.994459	.993545	.992616	.991679	.990734	.989786	.988836
8.4	.996050	.995391	.994721	.994042	.993357	.992668	.991976
8.8	.997160	.996682	.996194	.995700	.995200	.994696	.994190
9.2	.997941	.997591	.997234	.996871	.996504	.996133	.995760
9.6	.998494	.998237	.997973	.997705	.997434	.997159	.996883
10.0	.998890	.998699	.998503	.998304	.998102	.997897	.997691
11.0	.999464	.999371	.999275	.999177	.999077	.998976	.998874
12.0	.999729	.999681	.999632	.999582	.999531	.999479	.999426
13.0	.999857	.999832	.999806	.999779	.999752	.999724	.999696
14.0	.999922	.999908	.999894	.999879	.999864	.999848	.999833

$\nu = 9$

Q\n	9	10	11	12	13	14	15
15.0	.999956	.999948	.999940	.999931	.999923	.999914	.999905
16.0	.999974	.999970	.999965	.999960	.999955	.999950	.999944
17.0	.999984	.999982	.999979	.999976	.999973	.999970	.999966
18.0	.999990	.999989	.999987	.999985	.999983	.999981	.999979
19.0	.999994	.999993	.999992	.999991	.999989	.999988	.999987
20.0	1.00000	1.00000	.999995	.999994	.999993	.999992	.999992
22.0			1.00000	1.00000	1.00000	1.00000	1.00000

$\nu = 9$

Q\n	16	17	18	19	20	22	24
0.0	.000000	.000000	.000000	.000000	.000000	.000000	.000000
0.2	.000000	.000000	.000000	.000000	.000000	.000000	.000000
0.4	.000000	.000000	.000000	.000000	.000000	.000000	.000000
0.6	.000000	.000000	.000000	.000000	.000000	.000000	.000000
0.8	.000002	.000001	.000000	.000000	.000000	.000000	.000000
1.0	.000033	.000019	.000011	.000006	.000004	.000001	.000000
1.2	.000272	.000173	.000112	.000073	.000048	.000021	.000010
1.4	.001369	.000958	.000676	.000482	.000346	.000183	.000099
1.6	.004865	.003654	.002766	.002108	.001618	.000972	.000598
1.8	.013304	.010555	.008427	.006769	.005468	.003626	.002453
2.0	.029744	.024633	.020507	.017158	.014424	.010330	.007519
2.2	.056842	.048704	.041913	.036218	.031420	.023906	.018435
2.4	.095980	.084514	.074684	.066222	.058908	.047036	.037974
2.6	.146864	.132201	.119352	.108051	.098079	.081412	.068194
2.8	.207660	.190311	.174830	.160973	.148535	.127239	.109812
3.0	.275509	.256228	.238761	.222897	.208455	.183225	.162036
3.2	.347147	.326780	.308093	.290913	.275086	.246967	.222834
3.4	.419445	.398803	.379659	.361876	.345328	.315506	.289440
3.6	.489763	.469537	.450607	.432866	.416216	.385844	.358880
3.8	.556116	.536839	.518655	.501483	.485249	.455326	.428404
4.0	.617190	.599230	.582173	.565959	.550534	.521845	.495735
4.2	.672270	.655846	.640155	.625156	.610807	.583910	.559186
4.4	.721119	.706328	.692124	.678478	.665361	.640605	.617650
4.6	.763853	.750697	.738007	.725762	.713943	.691500	.670531
4.8	.800820	.789239	.778023	.767159	.756632	.736539	.717639
5.0	.832510	.822399	.812573	.803021	.793737	.775931	.759081
5.2	.859477	.850710	.842161	.833827	.825702	.810053	.795167
5.4	.882292	.874730	.867335	.860107	.853041	.839382	.826326
5.6	.901504	.895009	.888643	.882403	.876290	.864433	.853051
5.8	.917625	.912065	.906603	.901238	.895970	.885722	.875846
6.0	.931116	.926369	.921695	.917095	.912570	.903743	.895207
6.4	.951782	.948337	.944934	.941574	.938257	.931755	.925430
6.8	.966141	.963650	.961181	.958737	.956317	.951556	.946901
7.2	.976110	.974309	.972520	.970743	.968981	.965502	.962086
7.6	.983045	.981740	.980441	.979148	.977864	.975320	.972814
8.0	.987886	.986938	.985991	.985048	.984109	.982246	.980404
8.4	.991284	.990591	.989898	.989208	.988519	.987149	.985791
8.8	.993682	.993173	.992664	.992155	.991647	.990636	.989631
9.2	.995386	.995010	.994633	.994257	.993880	.993129	.992382
9.6	.996605	.996325	.996045	.995765	.995484	.994924	.994365
10.0	.997483	.997274	.997064	.996854	.996644	.996223	.995803
11.0	.998770	.998667	.998562	.998457	.998352	.998141	.997930
12.0	.999373	.999319	.999265	.999211	.999156	.999047	.998937
13.0	.999667	.999639	.999610	.999580	.999551	.999492	.999433
14.0	.999817	.999801	.999785	.999769	.999752	.999719	.999686
15.0	.999896	.999887	.999877	.999868	.999859	.999840	.999821
16.0	.999939	.999934	.999928	.999923	.999917	.999906	.999895
17.0	.999963	.999960	.999957	.999953	.999950	.999943	.999936
18.0	.999977	.999975	.999973	.999971	.999969	.999965	.999961
19.0	.999986	.999984	.999983	.999982	.999980	.999978	.999975

$\nu = 9$

Q\n	16	17	18	19	20	22	24
20.0	.999991	.999990	.999989	.999988	.999987	.999986	.999984
22.0	1.00000	1.00000	1.00000	.999995	.999994	.999994	.999993
24.0				1.00000	1.00000	1.00000	1.00000

$\nu = 9$

Q\n	26	28	30	32	34	36	38
0.0	.000000	.000000	.000000	.000000	.000000	.000000	.000000
0.2	.000000	.000000	.000000	.000000	.000000	.000000	.000000
0.4	.000000	.000000	.000000	.000000	.000000	.000000	.000000
0.6	.000000	.000000	.000000	.000000	.000000	.000000	.000000
0.8	.000000	.000000	.000000	.000000	.000000	.000000	.000000
1.0	.000000	.000000	.000000	.000000	.000000	.000000	.000000
1.2	.000005	.000002	.000001	.000001	.000000	.000000	.000000
1.4	.000055	.000032	.000018	.000011	.000007	.000004	.000003
1.6	.000376	.000241	.000157	.000104	.000070	.000048	.000033
1.8	.001689	.001182	.000839	.000604	.000441	.000325	.000243
2.0	.005554	.004159	.003152	.002416	.001871	.001463	.001154
2.2	.014390	.011357	.009055	.007286	.005913	.004837	.003985
2.4	.030966	.025483	.021146	.017681	.014889	.012619	.010759
2.6	.057595	.049010	.041992	.036206	.031398	.027375	.023986
2.8	.095417	.083423	.073351	.064830	.057574	.051356	.045997
3.0	.144098	.128800	.115664	.104313	.094448	.085830	.078262
3.2	.201981	.183846	.167983	.154032	.141701	.130751	.120987
3.4	.266522	.246263	.228264	.212198	.197794	.184830	.173116
3.6	.334823	.313259	.293846	.276298	.260376	.245879	.232635
3.8	.404080	.382017	.361928	.343573	.326748	.311277	.297010
4.0	.471888	.450034	.429942	.411414	.394279	.378389	.363618
4.2	.536392	.515316	.495776	.477611	.460684	.444872	.430070
4.4	.596313	.576431	.557862	.540479	.524172	.508842	.494404
4.6	.650899	.632482	.615169	.598863	.583477	.568932	.555160
4.8	.699831	.683025	.667137	.652092	.637822	.624266	.611371
5.0	.743116	.727969	.713577	.699884	.686837	.674390	.662499
5.2	.780991	.767478	.754581	.742259	.730470	.719180	.708354
5.4	.813838	.801884	.790429	.779443	.768895	.758758	.749005
5.6	.842120	.831616	.821516	.811796	.802433	.793407	.784699
5.8	.866328	.857151	.848298	.839751	.831495	.823514	.815793
6.0	.886953	.878970	.871247	.863771	.856530	.849513	.842708
6.4	.919279	.913300	.907485	.901829	.896327	.890971	.885755
6.8	.942353	.937911	.933575	.929340	.925204	.921165	.917217
7.2	.958735	.955451	.952234	.949081	.945992	.942966	.940001
7.6	.970348	.967923	.965540	.963199	.960899	.958640	.956421
8.0	.978587	.976795	.975030	.973291	.971579	.969894	.968235
8.4	.984448	.983121	.981811	.980517	.979242	.977983	.976742
8.8	.988635	.987648	.986672	.985708	.984754	.983812	.982882
9.2	.991640	.990904	.990174	.989452	.988737	.988029	.987330
9.6	.993809	.993257	.992709	.992166	.991627	.991094	.990566
10.0	.995385	.994968	.994555	.994144	.993736	.993332	.992932
11.0	.997719	.997509	.997299	.997091	.996883	.996677	.996472
12.0	.998827	.998716	.998606	.998497	.998388	.998279	.998171
13.0	.999373	.999313	.999254	.999194	.999135	.999076	.999017
14.0	.999653	.999620	.999586	.999553	.999520	.999486	.999453
15.0	.999802	.999783	.999763	.999744	.999725	.999706	.999686
16.0	.999883	.999872	.999861	.999849	.999838	.999826	.999815
17.0	.999929	.999923	.999916	.999909	.999902	.999895	.999888
18.0	.999956	.999952	.999948	.999943	.999939	.999935	.999930
19.0	.999972	.999970	.999967	.999964	.999961	.999959	.999956

$\nu = 9$

Q\n	26	28	30	32	34	36	38
20.0	.999982	.999980	.999979	.999977	.999975	.999973	.999971
22.0	.999992	.999991	.999990	.999990	.999989	.999988	.999987
24.0	1.00000	1.00000	1.00000	1.00000	.999995	.999994	.999994
26.0					1.00000	1.00000	1.00000

$\nu = 9$

Q\n	40	50	60	70	80	90	100
0.0	.000000	.000000	.000000	.000000	.000000	.000000	.000000
0.1	.000000	.000000	.000000	.000000	.000000	.000000	.000000
0.2	.000000	.000000	.000000	.000000	.000000	.000000	.000000
0.3	.000000	.000000	.000000	.000000	.000000	.000000	.000000
0.4	.000000	.000000	.000000	.000000	.000000	.000000	.000000
0.5	.000000	.000000	.000000	.000000	.000000	.000000	.000000
0.6	.000000	.000000	.000000	.000000	.000000	.000000	.000000
0.7	.000000	.000000	.000000	.000000	.000000	.000000	.000000
0.8	.000000	.000000	.000000	.000000	.000000	.000000	.000000
0.9	.000000	.000000	.000000	.000000	.000000	.000000	.000000
1.0	.000000	.000000	.000000	.000000	.000000	.000000	.000000
1.1	.000000	.000000	.000000	.000000	.000000	.000000	.000000
1.2	.000000	.000000	.000000	.000000	.000000	.000000	.000000
1.3	.000000	.000000	.000000	.000000	.000000	.000000	.000000
1.4	.000002	.000000	.000000	.000000	.000000	.000000	.000000
1.5	.000007	.000001	.000000	.000000	.000000	.000000	.000000
1.6	.000023	.000005	.000001	.000000	.000000	.000000	.000000
1.7	.000070	.000017	.000005	.000002	.000001	.000000	.000000
1.8	.000183	.000050	.000017	.000006	.000003	.000001	.000001
1.9	.000429	.000135	.000050	.000021	.000009	.000005	.000002
2.0	.000918	.000325	.000132	.000060	.000029	.000015	.000009
2.1	.001806	.000707	.000314	.000154	.000081	.000045	.000027
2.2	.003306	.001415	.000680	.000356	.000200	.000118	.000073
2.3	.005678	.002632	.001354	.000754	.000446	.000277	.000180
2.4	.009224	.004589	.002509	.001473	.000915	.000594	.000400
2.5	.014263	.007556	.004362	.002687	.001741	.001175	.000820
2.6	.021112	.011831	.007169	.004608	.003102	.002167	.001561
2.7	.030062	.017718	.011213	.007488	.005215	.003758	.002784
2.8	.041354	.025505	.016783	.011598	.008329	.006169	.004688
2.9	.055163	.035443	.024157	.017218	.012710	.009651	.007501
3.0	.071586	.047727	.033580	.024611	.018625	.014464	.011474
3.1	.090636	.062486	.045249	.034011	.026324	.020862	.016859
3.2	.112244	.079773	.059295	.045601	.036023	.029080	.023898
3.3	.136267	.099561	.075782	.059508	.047889	.039312	.032804
3.4	.162497	.121754	.094701	.075788	.062031	.051704	.043750
3.5	.190673	.146187	.115972	.094433	.078494	.066344	.056855
3.6	.220500	.172642	.139452	.115364	.097255	.083255	.072181
3.7	.251659	.200860	.164946	.138447	.118233	.102401	.089729
3.8	.283819	.230550	.192215	.163492	.141287	.123684	.109442
3.9	.316656	.261407	.220989	.190274	.166231	.146958	.131207
4.0	.349854	.293123	.250983	.218535	.192841	.172032	.154867
4.1	.383120	.325393	.281901	.248001	.220868	.198683	.180223
4.2	.416184	.357927	.313452	.278391	.250046	.226663	.207051
4.3	.448807	.390454	.345355	.309423	.280104	.255715	.235105
4.4	.480780	.422729	.377345	.340827	.310771	.285575	.264133
4.5	.511926	.454534	.409180	.372349	.341787	.315982	.293878
4.6	.542098	.485679	.440643	.403753	.372908	.346688	.324090
4.7	.571180	.516004	.471542	.434826	.403908	.377458	.354531
4.8	.599084	.545377	.501714	.465382	.434583	.408077	.384977
4.9	.625746	.573693	.531022	.495260	.464753	.438351	.415226

$\nu = 9$

Q\n	40	50	60	70	80	90	100
5.0	.651125	.600872	.559354	.524323	.494263	.468110	.445095
5.1	.675198	.626858	.586624	.552460	.522981	.497207	.474422
5.2	.697963	.651614	.612767	.579585	.550801	.525517	.503071
5.3	.719428	.675120	.637740	.605629	.577637	.552939	.530926
5.4	.739615	.697374	.661515	.630546	.603423	.579392	.557892
5.5	.758556	.718385	.684082	.654307	.628114	.604815	.583896
5.6	.776289	.738173	.705443	.676897	.651680	.629165	.608881
5.7	.792860	.756768	.725612	.698316	.674106	.652413	.632809
5.8	.808318	.774206	.744612	.718572	.695389	.674547	.655653
5.9	.822715	.790530	.762473	.737685	.715538	.695564	.677404
6.0	.836104	.805783	.779232	.755683	.734571	.715472	.698062
6.4	.880675	.857093	.836110	.817242	.800122	.784466	.770056
6.8	.913359	.895292	.879000	.864183	.850603	.838075	.826449
7.2	.937094	.923382	.910879	.899398	.888788	.878925	.869712
7.6	.954240	.943889	.934362	.925543	.917334	.909655	.902441
8.0	.966602	.958808	.951575	.944834	.938522	.932585	.926981
8.4	.975519	.969651	.964168	.959028	.954189	.949618	.945284
8.8	.981964	.977540	.973383	.969465	.965760	.962245	.958901
9.2	.986638	.983295	.980137	.977147	.974309	.971608	.969029
9.6	.990043	.987508	.985103	.982817	.980639	.978560	.976570
10.0	.992535	.990606	.988768	.987014	.985339	.983735	.982197
11.0	.996269	.995274	.994319	.993401	.992519	.991670	.990851
12.0	.998063	.997535	.997024	.996531	.996055	.995594	.995149
13.0	.998958	.998669	.998387	.998115	.997851	.997594	.997346
14.0	.999420	.999257	.999098	.998943	.998792	.998646	.998503
15.0	.999667	.999572	.999480	.999389	.999301	.999215	.999131
16.0	.999803	.999747	.999692	.999637	.999584	.999533	.999482
17.0	.999881	.999846	.999812	.999779	.999747	.999715	.999684
18.0	.999926	.999904	.999883	.999862	.999842	.999822	.999802
19.0	.999953	.999939	.999926	.999912	.999899	.999886	.999874
20.0	.999970	.999961	.999952	.999943	.999934	.999926	.999918
22.0	.999986	.999982	.999979	.999975	.999971	.999967	.999963
24.0	.999994	.999992	.999990	.999988	.999986	.999984	.999983
26.0	1.00000	1.00000	.999995	.999994	.999993	.999992	.999991
28.0			1.00000	1.00000	1.00000	1.00000	1.00000

$\nu = 10$

Q\n	2	3	4	5	6	7	8
0.0	.000000	.000000	.000000	.000000	.000000	.000000	.000000
0.1	.054973	.002754	.000136	.000007	.000000	.000000	.000000
0.2	.109654	.010953	.001079	.000107	.000011	.000001	.000000
0.3	.163735	.024442	.003599	.000535	.000081	.000012	.000002
0.4	.216934	.042954	.008389	.001652	.000331	.000068	.000014
0.5	.268986	.066136	.016035	.003919	.000974	.000247	.000064
0.6	.319644	.093554	.026997	.007848	.002318	.000698	.000214
0.7	.368688	.124713	.041586	.013961	.004757	.001651	.000584
0.8	.415923	.159074	.059963	.022741	.008746	.003422	.001364
0.9	.461189	.196065	.082139	.034596	.014763	.006403	.002827
1.0	.504352	.235109	.107986	.049826	.023271	.011036	.005321
1.2	.584007	.317076	.169583	.090975	.049304	.027075	.015083
1.4	.654453	.400691	.241658	.145972	.088901	.054746	.034129
1.6	.715699	.482328	.320253	.212682	.142147	.095871	.065325
1.8	.768114	.559210	.401271	.287662	.207191	.150317	.109969
2.0	.812330	.629455	.481037	.366918	.280782	.216077	.167399
2.2	.849151	.692014	.556640	.446586	.359018	.289838	.235219
2.4	.879462	.746525	.626053	.523412	.438052	.367728	.309935
2.6	.904163	.793150	.688107	.594983	.514599	.446000	.387705
2.8	.924115	.832404	.742353	.659766	.586190	.521503	.464960
3.0	.940110	.865017	.788889	.717013	.651228	.591909	.538802
3.2	.952852	.891808	.828188	.766597	.708904	.655743	.607169
3.4	.962949	.913614	.860943	.808834	.759036	.712287	.668817
3.6	.970917	.931225	.887949	.844317	.801892	.761416	.723205
3.8	.977183	.945361	.910018	.873791	.838029	.803427	.770331
4.0	.982100	.956651	.927922	.898045	.868158	.838884	.810561
4.2	.985951	.965633	.942365	.917854	.893048	.868488	.844486
4.4	.988963	.972758	.953962	.933936	.913459	.892992	.872812
4.6	.991319	.978400	.963243	.946931	.930098	.913131	.896271
4.8	.993162	.982860	.970651	.957393	.943599	.929592	.915576
5.0	.994603	.986384	.976554	.965793	.954516	.942987	.931380
5.2	.995732	.989169	.981253	.972526	.963320	.953853	.944267
5.4	.996617	.991369	.984993	.977916	.970408	.962645	.954745
5.6	.997313	.993109	.987968	.982229	.976108	.969747	.963246
5.8	.997860	.994487	.990337	.985680	.980688	.975479	.970133
6.0	.998291	.995580	.992225	.988442	.984370	.980103	.975708
6.4	.998901	.997137	.994934	.992429	.989711	.986843	.983871
6.8	.999285	.998127	.996669	.994998	.993175	.991240	.989224
7.2	.999530	.998762	.997788	.996666	.995434	.994121	.992747
7.6	.999687	.999173	.998516	.997756	.996918	.996021	.995078
8.0	.999790	.999441	.998994	.998475	.997900	.997282	.996631
8.4	.999857	.999618	.999312	.998953	.998555	.998127	.997673
8.8	.999901	.999737	.999524	.999275	.998997	.998697	.998378
9.2	.999932	.999817	.999667	.999492	.999297	.999085	.998860
9.6	.999952	.999871	.999765	.999641	.999502	.999352	.999191
10.0	.999966	.999908	.999833	.999744	.999645	.999537	.999421
11.0	.999985	.999959	.999926	.999886	.999841	.999792	.999740
12.0	.999993	.999981	.999965	.999947	.999925	.999902	.999877
13.0	1.00000	.999991	.999983	.999974	.999963	.999952	.999939
14.0		1.00000	.999991	.999987	.999981	.999975	.999969

$\nu = 10$

Q\n	2	3	4	5	6	7	8
15.0			1.00000	.999993	.999990	.999987	.999983
16.0				1.00000	.999994	.999993	.999991
17.0					1.00000	1.00000	.999995
18.0							1.00000

$\nu = 10$

Q\n	9	10	11	12	13	14	15
0.0	.000000	.000000	.000000	.000000	.000000	.000000	.000000
0.1	.000000	.000000	.000000	.000000	.000000	.000000	.000000
0.2	.000000	.000000	.000000	.000000	.000000	.000000	.000000
0.3	.000000	.000000	.000000	.000000	.000000	.000000	.000000
0.4	.000003	.000001	.000000	.000000	.000000	.000000	.000000
0.5	.000017	.000005	.000001	.000000	.000000	.000000	.000000
0.6	.000067	.000022	.000007	.000002	.000001	.000000	.000000
0.7	.000211	.000078	.000029	.000011	.000004	.000002	.000001
0.8	.000554	.000229	.000097	.000041	.000018	.000008	.000004
0.9	.001270	.000581	.000270	.000128	.000062	.000030	.000015
1.0	.002609	.001301	.000659	.000339	.000177	.000094	.000051
1.2	.008527	.004892	.002846	.001679	.001004	.000607	.000372
1.4	.021546	.013773	.008912	.005835	.003864	.002587	.001749
1.6	.044985	.031307	.022013	.015634	.011209	.008111	.005920
1.8	.081159	.060424	.045375	.034359	.026226	.020171	.015628
2.0	.130614	.102647	.081241	.064742	.051936	.041927	.034052
2.2	.191981	.157604	.130130	.108049	.090202	.075695	.063837
2.4	.262395	.223177	.190701	.163691	.141126	.122187	.106218
2.6	.338193	.296077	.260161	.229433	.203050	.180316	.160654
2.8	.415629	.372577	.334949	.301988	.273039	.247542	.225018
3.0	.491406	.449138	.411423	.377724	.347558	.320498	.296168
3.2	.562971	.522825	.486369	.453245	.423113	.395662	.370611
3.4	.628603	.591497	.557294	.525770	.496698	.469863	.445062
3.6	.687349	.653815	.622504	.593289	.566029	.540582	.516809
3.8	.738888	.709135	.681045	.654557	.629590	.606056	.583866
4.0	.783361	.757361	.732575	.708988	.686559	.665240	.644975
4.2	.821218	.798777	.777204	.756508	.736678	.717690	.699515
4.4	.853086	.833912	.815343	.797403	.780098	.763422	.747362
4.6	.879670	.863421	.847582	.832184	.817244	.802765	.788745
4.8	.901684	.888005	.874592	.861483	.848696	.836242	.824125
5.0	.919809	.908352	.897061	.885971	.875104	.864473	.854085
5.2	.934663	.925106	.915645	.906312	.897128	.888108	.879262
5.4	.946793	.938847	.930947	.923124	.915397	.907781	.900287
5.6	.956675	.950082	.943503	.936966	.930487	.924081	.917759
5.8	.964709	.959248	.953780	.948329	.942911	.937539	.932222
6.0	.971234	.966714	.962176	.957638	.953116	.948620	.944159
6.4	.980827	.977735	.974613	.971477	.968337	.965201	.962076
6.8	.987148	.985030	.982883	.980717	.978539	.976356	.974173
7.2	.991326	.989870	.988389	.986889	.985377	.983856	.982330
7.6	.994100	.993094	.992068	.991026	.989972	.988909	.987841
8.0	.995953	.995254	.994539	.993811	.993073	.992328	.991576
8.4	.997200	.996711	.996210	.995698	.995179	.994652	.994121
8.8	.998046	.997701	.997347	.996985	.996617	.996243	.995866
9.2	.998624	.998380	.998128	.997870	.997607	.997340	.997070
9.6	.999023	.998848	.998667	.998482	.998293	.998101	.997907
10.0	.999300	.999174	.999044	.998910	.998773	.998634	.998493
11.0	.999685	.999627	.999568	.999506	.999443	.999379	.999314
12.0	.999851	.999824	.999795	.999766	.999735	.999704	.999673
13.0	.999926	.999913	.999898	.999884	.999869	.999853	.999837
14.0	.999962	.999955	.999948	.999940	.999932	.999924	.999916

$\nu = 10$

Q\n	9	10	11	12	13	14	15
15.0	.999980	.999976	.999972	.999968	.999964	.999959	.999955
16.0	.999989	.999987	.999984	.999982	.999980	.999977	.999975
17.0	.999994	.999992	.999991	.999990	.999988	.999987	.999986
18.0	1.00000	1.00000	.999995	.999994	.999993	.999992	.999992
19.0			1.00000	1.00000	1.00000	1.00000	.999995
20.0							1.00000

$\nu = 10$

Q\n	16	17	18	19	20	22	24
0.0	.000000	.000000	.000000	.000000	.000000	.000000	.000000
0.2	.000000	.000000	.000000	.000000	.000000	.000000	.000000
0.4	.000000	.000000	.000000	.000000	.000000	.000000	.000000
0.6	.000000	.000000	.000000	.000000	.000000	.000000	.000000
0.8	.000002	.000001	.000000	.000000	.000000	.000000	.000000
1.0	.000028	.000015	.000008	.000005	.000003	.000001	.000000
1.2	.000231	.000145	.000092	.000059	.000038	.000016	.000007
1.4	.001195	.000824	.000573	.000402	.000284	.000146	.000077
1.6	.004357	.003232	.002416	.001819	.001379	.000807	.000484
1.8	.012192	.009574	.007566	.006015	.004809	.003124	.002069
2.0	.027815	.022845	.018861	.015649	.013045	.009186	.006575
2.2	.054091	.046040	.039355	.033779	.029105	.021845	.016618
2.4	.092693	.081190	.071364	.062937	.055682	.043977	.035118
2.6	.143585	.128715	.115716	.104314	.094281	.077583	.064423
2.8	.205063	.187332	.171532	.157414	.144764	.123166	.105569
3.0	.274243	.254437	.236505	.220232	.205431	.179618	.157998
3.2	.347709	.326733	.307485	.289790	.273492	.244556	.219754
3.4	.422112	.400843	.381104	.362757	.345678	.314894	.287989
3.6	.494580	.473772	.454273	.435978	.418794	.387416	.359536
3.8	.562930	.543163	.524485	.506820	.490097	.459223	.431399
4.0	.625708	.607380	.589938	.573326	.557495	.527986	.501065
4.2	.682118	.665462	.649510	.634227	.619577	.592042	.566654
4.4	.731898	.717008	.702671	.688862	.675557	.650369	.626929
4.6	.775176	.762046	.749342	.737049	.725153	.702486	.681220
4.8	.812344	.800894	.789768	.778959	.768456	.748333	.729319
5.0	.843945	.834051	.824401	.814991	.805817	.788151	.771351
5.2	.870594	.862108	.853804	.845680	.837734	.822367	.807670
5.4	.892920	.885685	.878584	.871617	.864784	.851516	.838763
5.6	.911525	.905387	.899345	.893403	.887560	.876173	.865180
5.8	.926966	.921777	.916658	.911611	.906637	.896914	.887488
6.0	.939740	.935366	.931042	.926770	.922552	.914281	.906233
6.4	.958967	.955878	.952813	.949774	.946762	.940827	.935016
6.8	.971993	.969821	.967659	.965508	.963371	.959141	.954978
7.2	.980803	.979277	.977753	.976234	.974721	.971716	.968745
7.6	.986768	.985694	.984619	.983545	.982473	.980338	.978219
8.0	.990820	.990062	.989301	.988540	.987779	.986259	.984746
8.4	.993586	.993048	.992507	.991966	.991423	.990337	.989253
8.8	.995485	.995101	.994715	.994327	.993939	.993160	.992380
9.2	.996797	.996521	.996244	.995965	.995685	.995123	.994560
9.6	.997710	.997511	.997310	.997108	.996906	.996498	.996088
10.0	.998349	.998205	.998059	.997912	.997764	.997467	.997167
11.0	.999248	.999181	.999113	.999044	.998975	.998836	.998696
12.0	.999641	.999609	.999576	.999543	.999509	.999441	.999373
13.0	.999821	.999805	.999788	.999772	.999755	.999721	.999686
14.0	.999907	.999899	.999890	.999882	.999873	.999855	.999837
15.0	.999950	.999946	.999941	.999936	.999932	.999922	.999912
16.0	.999972	.999970	.999967	.999965	.999962	.999957	.999951
17.0	.999984	.999983	.999981	.999980	.999978	.999975	.999972
18.0	.999991	.999990	.999989	.999988	.999987	.999985	.999983
19.0	.999994	.999994	.999993	.999993	.999992	.999991	.999990

$\nu = 10$

Q\n	16	17	18	19	20	22	24
20.0	1.00000	1.00000	1.00000	1.00000	1.00000	.999995	.999994
22.0						1.00000	1.00000

$\nu = 10$

Q\n	26	28	30	32	34	36	38
0.0	.000000	.000000	.000000	.000000	.000000	.000000	.000000
0.2	.000000	.000000	.000000	.000000	.000000	.000000	.000000
0.4	.000000	.000000	.000000	.000000	.000000	.000000	.000000
0.6	.000000	.000000	.000000	.000000	.000000	.000000	.000000
0.8	.000000	.000000	.000000	.000000	.000000	.000000	.000000
1.0	.000000	.000000	.000000	.000000	.000000	.000000	.000000
1.2	.000003	.000002	.000001	.000000	.000000	.000000	.000000
1.4	.000041	.000023	.000013	.000008	.000004	.000003	.000002
1.6	.000297	.000186	.000118	.000077	.000050	.000034	.000023
1.8	.001396	.000957	.000666	.000470	.000336	.000243	.000178
2.0	.004776	.003517	.002622	.001978	.001508	.001160	.000901
2.2	.012797	.009965	.007840	.006227	.004989	.004029	.003279
2.4	.028328	.023061	.018933	.015665	.013054	.010951	.009243
2.6	.053939	.045504	.038655	.033047	.028420	.024575	.021358
2.8	.091100	.079103	.069078	.060641	.053494	.047402	.042179
3.0	.139750	.124238	.110965	.099539	.089646	.081036	.073506
3.2	.198358	.179789	.163583	.149365	.136831	.125731	.115859
3.4	.264348	.243468	.224939	.208423	.193640	.180356	.168376
3.6	.334651	.312345	.292268	.274130	.257684	.242723	.229070
3.8	.406229	.383378	.362563	.343539	.326100	.310067	.295288
4.0	.476430	.453819	.433006	.413797	.396020	.379528	.364192
4.2	.543188	.521446	.501251	.482452	.464911	.448511	.433146
4.4	.605073	.584655	.565541	.547614	.530768	.514910	.499955
4.6	.661240	.642438	.624716	.607986	.592166	.577184	.562975
4.8	.711332	.694299	.678146	.662809	.648226	.634344	.621111
5.0	.755365	.740140	.725625	.711772	.698537	.685879	.673759
5.2	.793611	.780153	.767262	.754904	.743045	.731656	.720708
5.4	.826505	.814719	.803381	.792467	.781955	.771821	.762046
5.6	.854568	.844324	.834432	.824875	.815638	.806704	.798059
5.8	.878354	.869505	.860930	.852619	.844561	.836745	.829160
6.0	.898408	.890802	.883409	.876222	.869235	.862439	.855827
6.4	.929331	.923775	.918345	.913040	.907857	.902793	.897844
6.8	.950886	.946867	.942922	.939051	.935254	.931530	.927877
7.2	.965812	.962920	.960071	.957266	.954505	.951788	.949116
7.6	.976120	.974044	.971992	.969965	.967965	.965992	.964045
8.0	.983242	.981751	.980273	.978809	.977361	.975929	.974514
8.4	.988174	.987100	.986033	.984975	.983926	.982886	.981856
8.8	.991602	.990826	.990054	.989286	.988524	.987767	.987017
9.2	.993996	.993433	.992872	.992313	.991757	.991205	.990656
9.6	.995678	.995268	.994858	.994449	.994042	.993637	.993233
10.0	.996867	.996566	.996265	.995965	.995665	.995366	.995069
11.0	.998554	.998412	.998270	.998127	.997984	.997842	.997700
12.0	.999304	.999234	.999164	.999094	.999024	.998953	.998883
13.0	.999651	.999615	.999580	.999544	.999508	.999472	.999436
14.0	.999818	.999799	.999781	.999762	.999743	.999724	.999705
15.0	.999902	.999892	.999882	.999871	.999861	.999850	.999840
16.0	.999945	.999940	.999934	.999928	.999922	.999917	.999911
17.0	.999969	.999965	.999962	.999959	.999955	.999952	.999949
18.0	.999982	.999980	.999978	.999976	.999974	.999972	.999970
19.0	.999989	.999988	.999986	.999985	.999984	.999983	.999982

ν = 10

Q\n	26	28	30	32	34	36	38
20.0	.999993	.999992	.999992	.999991	.999990	.999989	.999989
22.0	1.00000	1.00000	1.00000	1.00000	1.00000	1.00000	1.00000

ν = 10

Q\n	40	50	60	70	80	90	100
0.0	.000000	.000000	.000000	.000000	.000000	.000000	.000000
0.1	.000000	.000000	.000000	.000000	.000000	.000000	.000000
0.2	.000000	.000000	.000000	.000000	.000000	.000000	.000000
0.3	.000000	.000000	.000000	.000000	.000000	.000000	.000000
0.4	.000000	.000000	.000000	.000000	.000000	.000000	.000000
0.5	.000000	.000000	.000000	.000000	.000000	.000000	.000000
0.6	.000000	.000000	.000000	.000000	.000000	.000000	.000000
0.7	.000000	.000000	.000000	.000000	.000000	.000000	.000000
0.8	.000000	.000000	.000000	.000000	.000000	.000000	.000000
0.9	.000000	.000000	.000000	.000000	.000000	.000000	.000000
1.0	.000000	.000000	.000000	.000000	.000000	.000000	.000000
1.1	.000000	.000000	.000000	.000000	.000000	.000000	.000000
1.2	.000000	.000000	.000000	.000000	.000000	.000000	.000000
1.3	.000000	.000000	.000000	.000000	.000000	.000000	.000000
1.4	.000001	.000000	.000000	.000000	.000000	.000000	.000000
1.5	.000004	.000001	.000000	.000000	.000000	.000000	.000000
1.6	.000016	.000003	.000001	.000000	.000000	.000000	.000000
1.7	.000048	.000010	.000003	.000001	.000000	.000000	.000000
1.8	.000132	.000033	.000010	.000003	.000001	.000001	.000000
1.9	.000320	.000093	.000032	.000012	.000005	.000002	.000001
2.0	.000706	.000232	.000088	.000038	.000017	.000009	.000005
2.1	.001430	.000525	.000220	.000102	.000051	.000027	.000015
2.2	.002687	.001085	.000494	.000246	.000132	.000075	.000045
2.3	.004727	.002079	.001020	.000543	.000308	.000185	.000115
2.4	.007847	.003724	.001950	.001100	.000659	.000413	.000270
2.5	.012375	.006284	.003489	.002073	.001300	.000851	.000577
2.6	.018649	.010060	.005886	.003663	.002393	.001626	.001141
2.7	.026990	.015372	.009425	.006113	.004144	.002912	.002107
2.8	.037678	.022533	.014411	.009700	.006798	.004922	.003661
2.9	.050931	.031831	.021147	.014719	.010628	.007906	.006027
3.0	.066889	.043504	.029911	.021458	.015918	.012133	.009459
3.1	.085606	.057723	.040942	.030186	.022947	.017882	.014224
3.2	.107046	.074582	.054415	.041127	.031965	.025414	.020589
3.3	.131088	.094094	.070435	.054451	.043183	.034964	.028800
3.4	.157536	.116188	.089031	.070257	.056750	.046718	.039069
3.5	.186133	.140718	.110153	.088571	.072751	.060804	.051558
3.6	.216574	.167474	.133677	.109344	.091201	.077287	.066368
3.7	.248523	.196194	.159418	.132462	.112043	.096161	.083537
3.8	.281629	.226575	.187136	.157746	.135156	.117354	.103037
3.9	.315536	.258294	.216554	.184968	.160360	.140734	.124775
4.0	.349901	.291017	.247367	.213863	.187433	.166116	.148606
4.1	.384396	.324411	.279258	.244141	.216114	.193273	.174335
4.2	.418723	.358154	.311908	.275496	.246121	.221948	.201729
4.3	.452612	.391945	.345005	.307623	.277158	.251863	.230532
4.4	.485829	.425508	.378256	.340220	.308931	.282731	.260470
4.5	.518173	.458599	.411387	.373003	.341149	.314267	.291262
4.6	.549479	.491001	.444153	.405707	.373539	.346191	.322632
4.7	.579615	.522533	.476337	.438093	.405845	.378241	.354313
4.8	.608481	.553046	.507753	.469946	.437837	.410173	.386053
4.9	.636006	.582420	.538244	.501084	.469309	.441767	.417620

$\nu = 10$

Q\n	40	50	60	70	80	90	100
5.0	.662142	.610565	.567684	.531352	.500085	.472828	.448808
5.1	.686866	.637416	.595975	.560622	.530014	.503187	.479431
5.2	.710175	.662932	.623043	.588794	.558972	.532703	.509334
5.3	.732081	.687093	.648839	.615792	.586863	.561258	.538381
5.4	.752609	.709895	.673332	.641563	.613613	.588761	.566466
5.5	.771796	.731352	.696512	.666075	.639168	.615141	.593504
5.6	.789688	.751487	.718382	.689312	.663496	.640350	.619429
5.7	.806335	.770335	.738959	.711273	.686580	.664356	.644199
5.8	.821795	.787938	.758272	.731972	.708419	.687145	.667786
5.9	.836127	.804345	.776355	.751431	.729025	.708716	.690177
6.0	.849391	.819609	.793251	.769683	.748418	.729080	.711374
6.4	.893006	.870361	.849972	.831468	.814555	.798994	.784596
6.8	.924294	.907361	.891897	.877689	.864562	.852368	.840987
7.2	.946486	.933959	.922381	.911635	.901615	.892233	.883413
7.6	.962125	.952915	.944318	.936268	.928705	.921575	.914830
8.0	.973115	.966365	.960009	.954014	.948344	.942968	.937857
8.4	.980836	.975892	.971202	.966750	.962516	.958481	.954628
8.8	.986272	.982646	.979185	.975881	.972724	.969702	.966804
9.2	.990110	.987445	.984886	.982432	.980077	.977814	.975637
9.6	.992833	.990867	.988970	.987143	.985383	.983687	.982050
10.0	.994773	.993317	.991906	.990542	.989224	.987949	.986717
11.0	.997558	.996856	.996170	.995502	.994852	.994219	.993604
12.0	.998813	.998463	.998119	.997782	.997453	.997131	.996817
13.0	.999400	.999220	.999042	.998867	.998695	.998527	.998362
14.0	.999686	.999590	.999495	.999401	.999309	.999218	.999129
15.0	.999830	.999777	.999725	.999673	.999622	.999572	.999523
16.0	.999905	.999875	.999846	.999816	.999787	.999759	.999731
17.0	.999945	.999928	.999911	.999894	.999877	.999860	.999844
18.0	.999968	.999957	.999947	.999937	.999927	.999917	.999907
19.0	.999980	.999974	.999968	.999962	.999956	.999950	.999943
20.0	.999988	.999984	.999980	.999976	.999972	.999969	.999965
22.0	1.00000	.999993	.999992	.999990	.999989	.999987	.999986
24.0		1.00000	1.00000	1.00000	1.00000	.999994	.999994
26.0						1.00000	1.00000

$\nu = 11$

Q\n	2	3	4	5	6	7	8
0.0	.000000	.000000	.000000	.000000	.000000	.000000	.000000
0.1	.055126	.002755	.000135	.000007	.000000	.000000	.000000
0.2	.109906	.010955	.001073	.000106	.000011	.000001	.000000
0.3	.164116	.024447	.003579	.000527	.000079	.000012	.000002
0.4	.217451	.042971	.008345	.001629	.000323	.000065	.000013
0.5	.269643	.066176	.015958	.003868	.000950	.000238	.000061
0.6	.320448	.093634	.026881	.007752	.002265	.000673	.000204
0.7	.369644	.124855	.041431	.013802	.004656	.001596	.000557
0.8	.417037	.159302	.059778	.022506	.008573	.003316	.001305
0.9	.462465	.196411	.081941	.034277	.014495	.006219	.002711
1.0	.505792	.235604	.107802	.049426	.022889	.010744	.005120
1.2	.585772	.317963	.169543	.090468	.048674	.026493	.014609
1.4	.656525	.402083	.241958	.145521	.088092	.053844	.033278
1.6	.718039	.484296	.321094	.212533	.141358	.094757	.064105
1.8	.770665	.561775	.402821	.288085	.206720	.149247	.108559
2.0	.815026	.632586	.483396	.368152	.280957	.215411	.166132
2.2	.851921	.695629	.559822	.448788	.360125	.289948	.234509
2.4	.882236	.750511	.629995	.526631	.440277	.368921	.310182
2.6	.906877	.797376	.692682	.599165	.517998	.448458	.389206
2.8	.926718	.836739	.747395	.664771	.590697	.525262	.467863
3.0	.942562	.869337	.794217	.722648	.656682	.596872	.543097
3.2	.955124	.896011	.833625	.772644	.715082	.661715	.612711
3.4	.965026	.917616	.866334	.815077	.765690	.719014	.675372
3.6	.972792	.934969	.893165	.850564	.808779	.768625	.730489
3.8	.978858	.948808	.914962	.879880	.844930	.810856	.778053
4.0	.983582	.959783	.932528	.903853	.874895	.846302	.818449
4.2	.987251	.968447	.946592	.923295	.899483	.875709	.852309
4.4	.990097	.975262	.957793	.938954	.919493	.899873	.880384
4.6	.992302	.980609	.966679	.951499	.935671	.919575	.903456
4.8	.994009	.984796	.973705	.961507	.948682	.935537	.922280
5.0	.995331	.988070	.979248	.969465	.959101	.948406	.937551
5.2	.996355	.990630	.983614	.975777	.967419	.958741	.949882
5.4	.997149	.992630	.987051	.980776	.974044	.967016	.959804
5.6	.997765	.994194	.989755	.984732	.979313	.973628	.967767
5.8	.998244	.995418	.991882	.987860	.983500	.978904	.974146
6.0	.998617	.996376	.993557	.990334	.986824	.983110	.979250
6.4	.999136	.997718	.995918	.993841	.991563	.989134	.986594
6.8	.999454	.998550	.997391	.996046	.994559	.992966	.991290
7.2	.999651	.999068	.998317	.997439	.996463	.995412	.994301
7.6	.999775	.999395	.998903	.998325	.997680	.996982	.996242
8.0	.999853	.999603	.999278	.998894	.998465	.997998	.997501
8.4	.999903	.999737	.999520	.999263	.998974	.998659	.998323
8.8	.999935	.999824	.999677	.999504	.999308	.999093	.998864
9.2	.999956	.999881	.999781	.999662	.999528	.999381	.999224
9.6	.999970	.999918	.999850	.999768	.999676	.999574	.999465
10.0	.999979	.999944	.999896	.999839	.999775	.999704	.999627
11.0	.999991	.999977	.999957	.999933	.999906	.999876	.999844
12.0	1.00000	.999990	.999981	.999971	.999959	.999945	.999931
13.0		1.00000	.999991	.999986	.999981	.999975	.999968
14.0			1.00000	.999993	.999991	.999988	.999984

$\nu = 11$

Q\n	2	3	4	5	6	7	8
15.0				1.00000	1.00000	.999994	.999992
16.0						1.00000	1.00000

$\nu = 11$

Q\n	9	10	11	12	13	14	15
0.0	.000000	.000000	.000000	.000000	.000000	.000000	.000000
0.1	.000000	.000000	.000000	.000000	.000000	.000000	.000000
0.2	.000000	.000000	.000000	.000000	.000000	.000000	.000000
0.3	.000000	.000000	.000000	.000000	.000000	.000000	.000000
0.4	.000003	.000001	.000000	.000000	.000000	.000000	.000000
0.5	.000016	.000004	.000001	.000000	.000000	.000000	.000000
0.6	.000063	.000020	.000006	.000002	.000001	.000000	.000000
0.7	.000198	.000072	.000026	.000010	.000004	.000001	.000001
0.8	.000522	.000213	.000088	.000037	.000016	.000007	.000003
0.9	.001202	.000541	.000248	.000115	.000055	.000026	.000013
1.0	.002478	.001218	.000608	.000308	.000158	.000083	.000044
1.2	.008166	.004627	.002658	.001546	.000911	.000543	.000328
1.4	.020807	.013163	.008423	.005451	.003566	.002357	.001574
1.6	.043793	.030213	.021048	.014803	.010507	.007523	.005433
1.8	.079599	.058842	.043852	.032940	.024934	.019013	.014601
2.0	.128957	.100770	.079268	.062762	.050008	.040089	.032326
2.2	.190642	.155811	.128029	.105761	.087817	.073282	.061446
2.4	.261829	.221947	.188947	.161541	.138686	.119547	.103451
2.6	.338795	.295877	.259268	.227957	.201096	.177976	.158010
2.8	.417655	.373760	.335352	.301687	.272116	.246078	.223090
3.0	.494942	.451888	.413398	.378959	.348103	.320408	.295503
3.2	.567943	.527148	.490006	.456190	.425379	.397275	.371606
3.4	.634813	.597246	.562508	.530406	.500737	.473302	.447909
3.6	.694521	.660737	.629076	.599442	.571717	.545776	.521495
3.8	.746715	.716921	.688676	.661946	.636673	.612786	.590209
4.0	.791542	.765689	.740933	.717280	.694711	.673192	.652681
4.2	.829482	.807346	.785963	.765362	.745548	.726510	.708231
4.4	.861208	.842461	.824213	.806503	.789349	.772758	.756726
4.6	.887476	.871741	.856321	.841258	.826579	.812298	.798419
4.8	.909049	.895938	.883011	.870313	.857870	.845701	.833816
5.0	.926651	.915790	.905024	.894394	.883928	.873645	.863558
5.2	.940939	.931982	.923062	.914215	.905466	.896835	.888335
5.4	.952489	.945129	.937768	.930438	.923161	.915956	.908835
5.6	.961797	.955766	.949711	.943658	.937630	.931641	.925703
5.8	.969281	.964348	.959378	.954395	.949415	.944454	.939520
6.0	.975289	.971260	.967188	.963092	.958988	.954888	.950800
6.4	.983971	.981287	.978560	.975803	.973027	.970241	.967451
6.8	.989550	.987762	.985937	.984084	.982210	.980323	.978425
7.2	.993144	.991949	.990725	.989477	.988212	.986932	.985643
7.6	.995468	.994666	.993841	.992998	.992141	.991272	.990393
8.0	.996979	.996438	.995879	.995307	.994724	.994131	.993530
8.4	.997969	.997601	.997220	.996830	.996430	.996024	.995611
8.8	.998623	.998370	.998109	.997840	.997565	.997285	.996999
9.2	.999057	.998883	.998703	.998517	.998326	.998131	.997932
9.6	.999349	.999228	.999102	.998972	.998839	.998702	.998563
10.0	.999546	.999462	.999373	.999282	.999188	.999092	.998994
11.0	.999809	.999773	.999735	.999696	.999656	.999614	.999572
12.0	.999916	.999899	.999882	.999865	.999847	.999828	.999809
13.0	.999961	.999953	.999945	.999937	.999928	.999920	.999911
14.0	.999981	.999977	.999973	.999969	.999965	.999961	.999956

$\nu = 11$

Q\n	9	10	11	12	13	14	15
15.0	.999990	.999989	.999987	.999985	.999982	.999980	.999978
16.0	.999995	.999994	.999993	.999992	.999991	.999990	.999988
17.0	1.00000	1.00000	1.00000	1.00000	.999995	.999994	.999994
18.0					1.00000	1.00000	1.00000

ν =11

Q\n	16	17	18	19	20	22	24
0.0	.000000	.000000	.000000	.000000	.000000	.000000	.000000
0.2	.000000	.000000	.000000	.000000	.000000	.000000	.000000
0.4	.000000	.000000	.000000	.000000	.000000	.000000	.000000
0.6	.000000	.000000	.000000	.000000	.000000	.000000	.000000
0.8	.000001	.000001	.000000	.000000	.000000	.000000	.000000
1.0	.000023	.000013	.000007	.000004	.000002	.000001	.000000
1.2	.000200	.000123	.000077	.000048	.000031	.000013	.000005
1.4	.001061	.000722	.000495	.000343	.000239	.000119	.000061
1.6	.003955	.002901	.002144	.001596	.001196	.000684	.000401
1.8	.011288	.008784	.006878	.005417	.004290	.002734	.001777
2.0	.026212	.021369	.017510	.014417	.011927	.008270	.005828
2.2	.051760	.043792	.037207	.031739	.027179	.020147	.015135
2.4	.089858	.078332	.068519	.060133	.052938	.041395	.032726
2.6	.140709	.125667	.112546	.101065	.090987	.074282	.061191
2.8	.202740	.184679	.168605	.154264	.141435	.119590	.101860
3.0	.273061	.252795	.234455	.217823	.202710	.176392	.154403
3.2	.348125	.326611	.306867	.288716	.272002	.242345	.216955
3.4	.424384	.402562	.382295	.363448	.345898	.314257	.286606
3.6	.498752	.477434	.457433	.438649	.420990	.388717	.360019
3.8	.568864	.548674	.529565	.511467	.494314	.462598	.433970
4.0	.633131	.614495	.596724	.579770	.563587	.533361	.505724
4.2	.690686	.673847	.657683	.642165	.627262	.599182	.573219
4.4	.741242	.726292	.711860	.697927	.684475	.658935	.635088
4.6	.784943	.771863	.759173	.746862	.734920	.712095	.690599
4.8	.822221	.810915	.799896	.789162	.778705	.758601	.739525
5.0	.853674	.843997	.834530	.825272	.816220	.798725	.782014
5.2	.879975	.871760	.863695	.855781	.848019	.832945	.818462
5.4	.901808	.894880	.888058	.881342	.874737	.861856	.849413
5.6	.919825	.914014	.908275	.902611	.897024	.886090	.875478
5.8	.934623	.929770	.924963	.920209	.915508	.906277	.897279
6.0	.946733	.942692	.938682	.934706	.930767	.923007	.915414
6.4	.964663	.961881	.959110	.956352	.953609	.948178	.942828
6.8	.976523	.974618	.972714	.970813	.968917	.965146	.961411
7.2	.984345	.983043	.981738	.980431	.979124	.976516	.973920
7.6	.989507	.988616	.987720	.986822	.985921	.984118	.982317
8.0	.992923	.992311	.991695	.991075	.990453	.989205	.987953
8.4	.995193	.994771	.994345	.993916	.993485	.992618	.991746
8.8	.996710	.996417	.996121	.995823	.995523	.994918	.994308
9.2	.997730	.997526	.997320	.997111	.996901	.996476	.996047
9.6	.998422	.998278	.998133	.997986	.997838	.997538	.997235
10.0	.998894	.998792	.998689	.998585	.998480	.998267	.998052
11.0	.999529	.999485	.999440	.999395	.999349	.999256	.999161
12.0	.999789	.999769	.999749	.999728	.999708	.999665	.999622
13.0	.999901	.999892	.999882	.999873	.999863	.999843	.999822
14.0	.999952	.999947	.999943	.999938	.999933	.999923	.999913
15.0	.999976	.999973	.999971	.999968	.999966	.999961	.999956
16.0	.999987	.999986	.999985	.999983	.999982	.999979	.999977
17.0	.999993	.999992	.999992	.999991	.999990	.999989	.999987
18.0	1.00000	1.00000	1.00000	.999995	.999995	.999994	.999993
19.0				1.00000	1.00000	1.00000	1.00000

ν = 11

Q\n	26	28	30	32	34	36	38
0.0	.000000	.000000	.000000	.000000	.000000	.000000	.000000
0.2	.000000	.000000	.000000	.000000	.000000	.000000	.000000
0.4	.000000	.000000	.000000	.000000	.000000	.000000	.000000
0.6	.000000	.000000	.000000	.000000	.000000	.000000	.000000
0.8	.000000	.000000	.000000	.000000	.000000	.000000	.000000
1.0	.000000	.000000	.000000	.000000	.000000	.000000	.000000
1.2	.000002	.000001	.000001	.000000	.000000	.000000	.000000
1.4	.000032	.000017	.000010	.000005	.000003	.000002	.000001
1.6	.000240	.000147	.000091	.000058	.000037	.000024	.000016
1.8	.001176	.000792	.000541	.000375	.000263	.000187	.000134
2.0	.004169	.003023	.002220	.001650	.001239	.000940	.000720
2.2	.011511	.008854	.006881	.005399	.004274	.003411	.002743
2.4	.026135	.021065	.017123	.014029	.011578	.009620	.008044
2.6	.050824	.042535	.035847	.030406	.025945	.022262	.019201
2.8	.087344	.075362	.065396	.057049	.050011	.044043	.038951
3.0	.135895	.120210	.106833	.095355	.085454	.076867	.069384
3.2	.195085	.176140	.159640	.145197	.132495	.121274	.111322
3.4	.262322	.240892	.221896	.204984	.189870	.176309	.164101
3.6	.334394	.311423	.290753	.272087	.255174	.239801	.225785
3.8	.408043	.384487	.363018	.343393	.325402	.308864	.293623
4.0	.480389	.457102	.435644	.415821	.397465	.380430	.364584
4.2	.549164	.526832	.506057	.486690	.468600	.451670	.435797
4.4	.612790	.591908	.572319	.553913	.536590	.520260	.504843
4.6	.670337	.651216	.633148	.616053	.599857	.584493	.569899
4.8	.721415	.704209	.687847	.672271	.657428	.643269	.629748
5.0	.766049	.750790	.736196	.722230	.708852	.696026	.683721
5.2	.804547	.791177	.778326	.765968	.754076	.742626	.731593
5.4	.837399	.825801	.814603	.803788	.793339	.783238	.773470
5.6	.865186	.855207	.845534	.836156	.827063	.818242	.809682
5.8	.888518	.879991	.871695	.863625	.855773	.848133	.840697
6.0	.907994	.900748	.893675	.886773	.880038	.873466	.867052
6.4	.937567	.932399	.927326	.922349	.917467	.912680	.907987
6.8	.957719	.954074	.950479	.946937	.943448	.940013	.936632
7.2	.971343	.968789	.966259	.963758	.961285	.958843	.956430
7.6	.980522	.978736	.976962	.975202	.973458	.971729	.970017
8.0	.986702	.985454	.984211	.982974	.981744	.980523	.979311
8.4	.990872	.989998	.989125	.988254	.987387	.986525	.985666
8.8	.993695	.993081	.992466	.991852	.991239	.990628	.990019
9.2	.995616	.995182	.994747	.994312	.993877	.993443	.993009
9.6	.996929	.996622	.996313	.996003	.995693	.995383	.995073
10.0	.997834	.997614	.997394	.997172	.996950	.996728	.996505
11.0	.999065	.998968	.998870	.998772	.998673	.998574	.998474
12.0	.999578	.999533	.999488	.999443	.999397	.999351	.999305
13.0	.999801	.999780	.999758	.999736	.999714	.999692	.999670
14.0	.999902	.999892	.999881	.999870	.999859	.999848	.999837
15.0	.999950	.999945	.999939	.999934	.999928	.999922	.999917
16.0	.999974	.999971	.999968	.999965	.999962	.999959	.999956
17.0	.999986	.999984	.999983	.999981	.999979	.999978	.999976
18.0	.999992	.999991	.999990	.999989	.999988	.999987	.999986
19.0	1.00000	.999995	.999994	.999994	.999993	.999993	.999992

$\nu = 11$

Q\n	26	28	30	32	34	36	38
20.0		1.00000	1.00000	1.00000	1.00000	1.00000	1.00000

$\nu = 11$

Q\n	40	50	60	70	80	90	100
0.0	.000000	.000000	.000000	.000000	.000000	.000000	.000000
0.1	.000000	.000000	.000000	.000000	.000000	.000000	.000000
0.2	.000000	.000000	.000000	.000000	.000000	.000000	.000000
0.3	.000000	.000000	.000000	.000000	.000000	.000000	.000000
0.4	.000000	.000000	.000000	.000000	.000000	.000000	.000000
0.5	.000000	.000000	.000000	.000000	.000000	.000000	.000000
0.6	.000000	.000000	.000000	.000000	.000000	.000000	.000000
0.7	.000000	.000000	.000000	.000000	.000000	.000000	.000000
0.8	.000000	.000000	.000000	.000000	.000000	.000000	.000000
0.9	.000000	.000000	.000000	.000000	.000000	.000000	.000000
1.0	.000000	.000000	.000000	.000000	.000000	.000000	.000000
1.1	.000000	.000000	.000000	.000000	.000000	.000000	.000000
1.2	.000000	.000000	.000000	.000000	.000000	.000000	.000000
1.3	.000000	.000000	.000000	.000000	.000000	.000000	.000000
1.4	.000001	.000000	.000000	.000000	.000000	.000000	.000000
1.5	.000003	.000000	.000000	.000000	.000000	.000000	.000000
1.6	.000011	.000002	.000000	.000000	.000000	.000000	.000000
1.7	.000035	.000007	.000002	.000000	.000000	.000000	.000000
1.8	.000098	.000023	.000006	.000002	.000001	.000000	.000000
1.9	.000245	.000066	.000021	.000008	.000003	.000001	.000001
2.0	.000556	.000171	.000061	.000025	.000011	.000005	.000003
2.1	.001155	.000399	.000158	.000069	.000033	.000017	.000009
2.2	.002222	.000850	.000368	.000175	.000090	.000049	.000028
2.3	.003995	.001673	.000784	.000400	.000219	.000126	.000076
2.4	.006765	.003071	.001543	.000838	.000484	.000294	.000186
2.5	.010863	.005300	.002836	.001628	.000989	.000628	.000415
2.6	.016641	.008660	.004900	.002957	.001877	.001242	.000850
2.7	.024444	.013479	.008020	.005059	.003342	.002292	.001621
2.8	.034585	.020092	.012508	.008211	.005621	.003982	.002901
2.9	.047322	.028816	.018684	.012714	.008989	.006555	.004906
3.0	.062835	.039925	.026858	.018879	.013740	.010288	.007887
3.1	.081215	.053631	.037301	.027002	.020176	.015471	.012121
3.2	.102460	.070069	.050231	.037344	.028578	.022392	.017893
3.3	.126473	.089286	.065792	.050113	.039191	.031317	.025478
3.4	.153074	.111242	.084050	.065449	.052206	.042470	.035120
3.5	.182009	.135810	.104984	.083413	.067746	.056019	.047021
3.6	.212969	.162792	.128495	.103990	.085861	.072065	.061320
3.7	.245605	.191923	.154408	.127084	.106522	.090636	.078092
3.8	.279543	.222896	.182489	.152531	.129631	.111688	.097338
3.9	.314405	.255370	.212452	.180105	.155019	.135106	.118992
4.0	.349816	.288987	.243979	.209537	.182464	.160714	.142920
4.1	.385420	.323387	.276732	.240521	.211700	.188285	.168935
4.2	.420888	.358221	.310366	.272732	.242429	.217553	.196800
4.3	.455924	.393157	.344543	.305840	.274337	.248224	.226249
4.4	.490266	.427892	.378937	.339516	.307103	.279992	.256989
4.5	.523692	.462150	.413248	.373446	.340410	.312544	.288720
4.6	.556019	.495695	.447203	.407337	.373956	.345575	.321137
4.7	.587099	.528322	.480558	.440921	.407456	.378794	.353947
4.8	.616822	.559864	.513106	.473961	.440654	.411929	.386870
4.9	.645107	.590189	.544672	.506250	.473320	.444733	.419648

$\nu = 11$

Q\n	40	50	60	70	80	90	100
5.0	.671904	.619195	.575114	.537614	.505253	.476988	.452048
5.1	.697188	.646811	.604321	.567910	.536286	.508504	.483862
5.2	.720956	.672992	.632213	.597027	.566279	.539121	.514913
5.3	.743222	.697716	.658734	.624878	.595124	.568707	.545051
5.4	.764017	.720981	.683852	.651407	.622736	.597159	.574153
5.5	.783384	.742803	.707556	.676575	.649059	.624399	.602125
5.6	.801372	.763210	.729851	.700369	.674056	.650371	.628895
5.7	.818042	.782242	.750758	.722788	.697709	.675042	.654413
5.8	.833457	.799948	.770310	.743848	.720019	.698397	.678649
5.9	.847684	.816383	.788547	.763578	.740999	.720437	.701593
6.0	.860791	.831607	.805520	.782014	.760676	.741174	.723245
6.4	.903385	.881670	.861901	.843805	.827147	.811733	.797402
6.8	.933304	.917442	.902782	.889186	.876526	.864690	.853583
7.2	.954049	.942601	.931885	.921838	.912392	.903485	.895061
7.6	.968323	.960119	.952358	.945014	.938053	.931441	.925147
8.0	.978109	.972252	.966660	.961326	.956236	.951372	.946714
8.4	.984813	.980636	.976616	.972756	.969050	.965489	.962064
8.8	.989413	.986430	.983540	.980750	.978057	.975457	.972946
9.2	.992577	.990443	.988363	.986343	.984386	.982489	.980650
9.6	.994764	.993231	.991730	.990266	.988841	.987455	.986107
10.0	.996283	.995177	.994090	.993025	.991985	.990970	.989981
11.0	.998374	.997875	.997380	.996891	.996410	.995938	.995475
12.0	.999259	.999026	.998792	.998561	.998332	.998106	.997884
13.0	.999648	.999535	.999422	.999308	.999196	.999085	.998975
14.0	.999826	.999770	.999712	.999655	.999598	.999542	.999486
15.0	.999911	.999882	.999852	.999822	.999792	.999763	.999733
16.0	.999953	.999937	.999921	.999905	.999889	.999873	.999857
17.0	.999974	.999966	.999957	.999948	.999939	.999930	.999921
18.0	.999986	.999981	.999976	.999971	.999966	.999961	.999956
19.0	.999992	.999989	.999986	.999983	.999980	.999977	.999974
20.0	1.00000	.999993	.999992	.999990	.999988	.999986	.999985
22.0		1.00000	1.00000	1.00000	1.00000	.999995	.999994
24.0						1.00000	1.00000

$\nu = 12$

Q\n	2	3	4	5	6	7	8
0.0	.000000	.000000	.000000	.000000	.000000	.000000	.000000
0.1	.055260	.002756	.000135	.000007	.000000	.000000	.000000
0.2	.110116	.010955	.001068	.000104	.000010	.000001	.000000
0.3	.164436	.024452	.003562	.000521	.000077	.000012	.000002
0.4	.217883	.042985	.008308	.001610	.000316	.000063	.000013
0.5	.270193	.066209	.015894	.003824	.000931	.000230	.000058
0.6	.321120	.093700	.026784	.007671	.002221	.000653	.000195
0.7	.370444	.124972	.041301	.013669	.004571	.001551	.000535
0.8	.417969	.159493	.059621	.022308	.008428	.003228	.001255
0.9	.463531	.196701	.081772	.034008	.014271	.006065	.002616
1.0	.506996	.236018	.107644	.049087	.022568	.010500	.004953
1.2	.587249	.318708	.169506	.090037	.048140	.026002	.014212
1.4	.658259	.403252	.242205	.145133	.087401	.053078	.032558
1.6	.719997	.485954	.321800	.212396	.140677	.093802	.063065
1.8	.772801	.563939	.404130	.288434	.206303	.148320	.107343
2.0	.817283	.635228	.485393	.369193	.281090	.214820	.165025
2.2	.854238	.698681	.562523	.450659	.361058	.290021	.233872
2.4	.884553	.753876	.633346	.529377	.442173	.369928	.310367
2.6	.909141	.800941	.696572	.602738	.520909	.450562	.390480
2.8	.928884	.840390	.751678	.669051	.594567	.528497	.470359
3.0	.944595	.872967	.798736	.727463	.661368	.601153	.546808
3.2	.957002	.899530	.838226	.777801	.720386	.666867	.617509
3.4	.966735	.920955	.870880	.820388	.771390	.724810	.681044
3.6	.974327	.938077	.897546	.855859	.814660	.774820	.736782
3.8	.980221	.951656	.919094	.885018	.850801	.817217	.784702
4.0	.984780	.962355	.936355	.908728	.880597	.852626	.825213
4.2	.988296	.970742	.950082	.927832	.904896	.881830	.858982
4.4	.991000	.977289	.960934	.943110	.924536	.905669	.886803
4.6	.993078	.982383	.969473	.955255	.940295	.924963	.909505
4.8	.994673	.986337	.976168	.964862	.952864	.940470	.927882
5.0	.995896	.989400	.981401	.972432	.962841	.952864	.942663
5.2	.996834	.991772	.985484	.978380	.970732	.962725	.954492
5.4	.997553	.993606	.988664	.983044	.976955	.970545	.963918
5.6	.998106	.995025	.991141	.986696	.981854	.976730	.971408
5.8	.998531	.996123	.993068	.989553	.985704	.981612	.977344
6.0	.998858	.996973	.994568	.991787	.988728	.985462	.982042
6.4	.999305	.998144	.996648	.994902	.992967	.990886	.988692
6.8	.999573	.998851	.997914	.996813	.995584	.994255	.992845
7.2	.999734	.999282	.998691	.997991	.997206	.996353	.995444
7.6	.999833	.999547	.999170	.998722	.998217	.997666	.997076
8.0	.999894	.999711	.999469	.999180	.998852	.998493	.998108
8.4	.999932	.999814	.999656	.999468	.999254	.999018	.998765
8.8	.999956	.999878	.999775	.999651	.999510	.999354	.999186
9.2	.999971	.999920	.999852	.999769	.999675	.999571	.999459
9.6	.999981	.999947	.999901	.999846	.999783	.999713	.999637
10.0	.999987	.999964	.999933	.999896	.999853	.999806	.999754
11.0	.999995	.999986	.999974	.999959	.999943	.999924	.999903
12.0	1.00000	.999994	.999989	.999983	.999976	.999968	.999960
13.0		1.00000	1.00000	.999993	.999990	.999986	.999983
14.0				1.00000	1.00000	.999994	.999992

$\nu = 12$

Q\n	2	3	4	5	6	7	8
15.0						1.00000	1.00000

ν = 12

Q\n	9	10	11	12	13	14	15
0.0	.000000	.000000	.000000	.000000	.000000	.000000	.000000
0.1	.000000	.000000	.000000	.000000	.000000	.000000	.000000
0.2	.000000	.000000	.000000	.000000	.000000	.000000	.000000
0.3	.000000	.000000	.000000	.000000	.000000	.000000	.000000
0.4	.000003	.000001	.000000	.000000	.000000	.000000	.000000
0.5	.000015	.000004	.000001	.000000	.000000	.000000	.000000
0.6	.000059	.000018	.000006	.000002	.000001	.000000	.000000
0.7	.000187	.000067	.000024	.000009	.000003	.000001	.000000
0.8	.000496	.000199	.000081	.000034	.000014	.000006	.000003
0.9	.001145	.000509	.000230	.000105	.000049	.000023	.000011
1.0	.002370	.001151	.000567	.000283	.000143	.000074	.000038
1.2	.007866	.004410	.002504	.001439	.000837	.000493	.000293
1.4	.020187	.012654	.008018	.005136	.003324	.002173	.001434
1.6	.042781	.029289	.020238	.014110	.009925	.007040	.005035
1.8	.078258	.057490	.042556	.031739	.023846	.018043	.013746
2.0	.127518	.099145	.077568	.061062	.048360	.038525	.030864
2.2	.189461	.154239	.126196	.103769	.085748	.071197	.059389
2.4	.261308	.220848	.187394	.159644	.136542	.117234	.101034
2.6	.339285	.295666	.258450	.226630	.199351	.175895	.155667
2.8	.419389	.374756	.335663	.301379	.271261	.244746	.221349
3.0	.497999	.454260	.415091	.380001	.348535	.320279	.294864
3.2	.572258	.530902	.493164	.458741	.427332	.398651	.372433
3.4	.640206	.602251	.567055	.534453	.504262	.476298	.450382
3.6	.700743	.666762	.634813	.604824	.576699	.550330	.525603
3.8	.753488	.723685	.695329	.668407	.642881	.618695	.595786
4.0	.798594	.772900	.748199	.724514	.701843	.680167	.659454
4.2	.836571	.814733	.793547	.773057	.753282	.734224	.715875
4.4	.868135	.849791	.831853	.814372	.797379	.780889	.764905
4.6	.894088	.878828	.863800	.849058	.834636	.820554	.806825
4.8	.915241	.902646	.890166	.877851	.865735	.853841	.842185
5.0	.932357	.922028	.911737	.901529	.891436	.881480	.871679
5.2	.946126	.937699	.929262	.920854	.912503	.904230	.896053
5.4	.957152	.950305	.943419	.936527	.929656	.922823	.916044
5.6	.965950	.960403	.954803	.949177	.943548	.937931	.932340
5.8	.972950	.968467	.963925	.959347	.954750	.950150	.945558
6.0	.978509	.974891	.971215	.967497	.963755	.959998	.956238
6.4	.986411	.984062	.981661	.979221	.976751	.974261	.971757
6.8	.991372	.989847	.988281	.986683	.985059	.983415	.981755
7.2	.994489	.993497	.992475	.991427	.990359	.989274	.988175
7.6	.996455	.995807	.995137	.994448	.993743	.993026	.992297
8.0	.997701	.997275	.996834	.996379	.995912	.995436	.994951
8.4	.998497	.998215	.997922	.997620	.997309	.996991	.996667
8.8	.999008	.998820	.998625	.998422	.998214	.998001	.997782
9.2	.999339	.999213	.999082	.998945	.998805	.998660	.998513
9.6	.999556	.999471	.999382	.999289	.999193	.999095	.998994
10.0	.999699	.999641	.999580	.999516	.999451	.999383	.999314
11.0	.999881	.999858	.999834	.999808	.999782	.999755	.999727
12.0	.999951	.999941	.999931	.999920	.999909	.999897	.999886
13.0	.999978	.999974	.999970	.999965	.999960	.999955	.999950
14.0	.999990	.999988	.999986	.999984	.999982	.999979	.999977

$\nu = 12$

Q\n	9	10	11	12	13	14	15
15.0	1.00000	.999994	.999993	.999992	.999991	.999990	.999989
16.0		1.00000	1.00000	1.00000	1.00000	1.00000	.999994
17.0							1.00000

$\nu = 12$

Q\n	16	17	18	19	20	22	24
0.0	.000000	.000000	.000000	.000000	.000000	.000000	.000000
0.2	.000000	.000000	.000000	.000000	.000000	.000000	.000000
0.4	.000000	.000000	.000000	.000000	.000000	.000000	.000000
0.6	.000000	.000000	.000000	.000000	.000000	.000000	.000000
0.8	.000001	.000001	.000000	.000000	.000000	.000000	.000000
1.0	.000020	.000011	.000006	.000003	.000002	.000001	.000000
1.2	.000177	.000107	.000066	.000041	.000026	.000010	.000004
1.4	.000955	.000642	.000435	.000298	.000205	.000100	.000050
1.6	.003629	.002636	.001928	.001421	.001053	.000590	.000339
1.8	.010542	.008135	.006316	.004932	.003873	.002426	.001550
2.0	.024861	.020131	.016383	.013396	.011005	.007523	.005227
2.2	.049760	.041872	.035379	.030011	.025554	.018727	.013908
2.4	.087389	.075850	.066056	.057712	.050578	.039189	.030697
2.6	.138166	.122979	.109758	.098214	.088105	.071409	.058393
2.8	.200654	.182304	.165993	.151459	.138477	.116424	.098591
3.0	.271963	.251289	.232589	.215641	.200252	.173493	.151184
3.2	.348437	.326444	.306257	.287700	.270615	.240316	.214404
3.4	.426346	.404032	.383294	.364000	.346028	.313619	.285300
3.6	.502409	.480638	.460191	.440971	.422888	.389813	.360378
3.8	.574086	.553526	.534039	.515559	.498025	.465558	.436208
4.0	.639669	.620770	.602716	.585464	.568973	.538117	.509843
4.2	.698217	.681231	.664894	.649179	.634061	.605512	.579046
4.4	.749425	.734442	.719945	.705919	.692351	.666523	.642333
4.6	.793455	.780442	.767785	.755478	.743514	.720580	.698907
4.8	.830777	.819621	.808720	.798073	.787677	.767627	.748529
5.0	.862043	.852581	.843297	.834193	.825270	.807966	.791368
5.2	.887982	.880027	.872192	.864483	.856902	.842127	.827868
5.4	.909330	.902690	.896129	.889653	.883265	.870761	.858627
5.6	.926785	.921275	.915815	.910410	.905064	.894559	.884314
5.8	.940983	.936431	.931910	.927423	.922974	.914200	.905606
6.0	.952483	.948737	.945008	.941298	.937612	.930320	.923148
6.4	.969245	.966729	.964213	.961701	.959195	.954210	.949274
6.8	.980083	.978404	.976718	.975030	.973340	.969965	.966602
7.2	.987064	.985946	.984820	.983689	.982554	.980278	.978001
7.6	.991559	.990813	.990061	.989304	.988542	.987010	.985470
8.0	.994458	.993960	.993456	.992948	.992436	.991403	.990361
8.4	.996337	.996002	.995664	.995321	.994976	.994277	.993571
8.8	.997560	.997334	.997105	.996874	.996640	.996165	.995684
9.2	.998362	.998209	.998053	.997895	.997736	.997412	.997082
9.6	.998891	.998787	.998680	.998572	.998462	.998240	.998013
10.0	.999243	.999171	.999098	.999023	.998948	.998794	.998637
11.0	.999698	.999669	.999639	.999609	.999578	.999515	.999450
12.0	.999873	.999861	.999848	.999835	.999822	.999795	.999767
13.0	.999944	.999939	.999933	.999927	.999921	.999909	.999897
14.0	.999974	.999972	.999969	.999966	.999964	.999958	.999952
15.0	.999988	.999986	.999985	.999984	.999983	.999980	.999977
16.0	.999994	.999993	.999993	.999992	.999991	.999990	.999989
17.0	1.00000	1.00000	1.00000	1.00000	1.00000	.999995	.999994
18.0						1.00000	1.00000

$\nu = 12$

Q\n	26	28	30	32	34	36	38
0.0	.000000	.000000	.000000	.000000	.000000	.000000	.000000
0.2	.000000	.000000	.000000	.000000	.000000	.000000	.000000
0.4	.000000	.000000	.000000	.000000	.000000	.000000	.000000
0.6	.000000	.000000	.000000	.000000	.000000	.000000	.000000
0.8	.000000	.000000	.000000	.000000	.000000	.000000	.000000
1.0	.000000	.000000	.000000	.000000	.000000	.000000	.000000
1.2	.000002	.000001	.000000	.000000	.000000	.000000	.000000
1.4	.000025	.000013	.000007	.000004	.000002	.000001	.000001
1.6	.000199	.000119	.000072	.000045	.000028	.000018	.000012
1.8	.001008	.000667	.000448	.000305	.000210	.000147	.000104
2.0	.003687	.002636	.001909	.001398	.001036	.000775	.000585
2.2	.010456	.007950	.006108	.004739	.003709	.002928	.002329
2.4	.024287	.019395	.015622	.012682	.010372	.008541	.007078
2.6	.048142	.039992	.033456	.028170	.023863	.020328	.017408
2.8	.084048	.072093	.062192	.053937	.047008	.041159	.036193
3.0	.132456	.116629	.103171	.091661	.081764	.073211	.065783
3.2	.192117	.172844	.156089	.141454	.128612	.117295	.107281
3.4	.260440	.238518	.219105	.201844	.186437	.172635	.160229
3.6	.334086	.310516	.289311	.270171	.252838	.237095	.222754
3.8	.409599	.385406	.363346	.343176	.324684	.307689	.292030
4.0	.483880	.459986	.437944	.417567	.398687	.381157	.364848
4.2	.554472	.531615	.510320	.490443	.471856	.454447	.438113
4.4	.619654	.598367	.578360	.559529	.541780	.525028	.509194
4.6	.678416	.659027	.640663	.623253	.606729	.591028	.576093
4.8	.730337	.713002	.696473	.680702	.665641	.651246	.637476
5.0	.775454	.760194	.745557	.731512	.718026	.705070	.692614
5.2	.814115	.800855	.788068	.775737	.763839	.752357	.741268
5.4	.846862	.835462	.824418	.813719	.803353	.793307	.783567
5.6	.874334	.864621	.855172	.845981	.837041	.828345	.819886
5.8	.897199	.888984	.880961	.873130	.865487	.858028	.850748
6.0	.916106	.909199	.902432	.895804	.889316	.882965	.876749
6.4	.944395	.939581	.934836	.930162	.925562	.921037	.916586
6.8	.963261	.959947	.956664	.953417	.950206	.947033	.943900
7.2	.975727	.973462	.971210	.968972	.966752	.964551	.962370
7.6	.983927	.982384	.980844	.979310	.977783	.976265	.974755
8.0	.989314	.988264	.987212	.986162	.985114	.984068	.983027
8.4	.992858	.992142	.991423	.990703	.989983	.989264	.988545
8.8	.995198	.994707	.994215	.993720	.993224	.992728	.992231
9.2	.996749	.996412	.996073	.995731	.995389	.995045	.994701
9.6	.997783	.997550	.997316	.997079	.996841	.996602	.996363
10.0	.998477	.998315	.998152	.997987	.997821	.997654	.997487
11.0	.999384	.999317	.999249	.999181	.999112	.999042	.998971
12.0	.999739	.999710	.999681	.999651	.999621	.999591	.999560
13.0	.999884	.999871	.999858	.999845	.999831	.999817	.999803
14.0	.999946	.999940	.999934	.999928	.999921	.999915	.999908
15.0	.999974	.999971	.999968	.999965	.999962	.999959	.999956
16.0	.999987	.999986	.999984	.999983	.999981	.999979	.999978
17.0	.999993	.999993	.999992	.999991	.999990	.999989	.999988
18.0	1.00000	1.00000	1.00000	1.00000	.999995	.999994	.999994
19.0					1.00000	1.00000	1.00000

$\nu = 12$

Q\n	40	50	60	70	80	90	100
0.0	.000000	.000000	.000000	.000000	.000000	.000000	.000000
0.1	.000000	.000000	.000000	.000000	.000000	.000000	.000000
0.2	.000000	.000000	.000000	.000000	.000000	.000000	.000000
0.3	.000000	.000000	.000000	.000000	.000000	.000000	.000000
0.4	.000000	.000000	.000000	.000000	.000000	.000000	.000000
0.5	.000000	.000000	.000000	.000000	.000000	.000000	.000000
0.6	.000000	.000000	.000000	.000000	.000000	.000000	.000000
0.7	.000000	.000000	.000000	.000000	.000000	.000000	.000000
0.8	.000000	.000000	.000000	.000000	.000000	.000000	.000000
0.9	.000000	.000000	.000000	.000000	.000000	.000000	.000000
1.0	.000000	.000000	.000000	.000000	.000000	.000000	.000000
1.1	.000000	.000000	.000000	.000000	.000000	.000000	.000000
1.2	.000000	.000000	.000000	.000000	.000000	.000000	.000000
1.3	.000000	.000000	.000000	.000000	.000000	.000000	.000000
1.4	.000000	.000000	.000000	.000000	.000000	.000000	.000000
1.5	.000002	.000000	.000000	.000000	.000000	.000000	.000000
1.6	.000008	.000001	.000000	.000000	.000000	.000000	.000000
1.7	.000026	.000005	.000001	.000000	.000000	.000000	.000000
1.8	.000074	.000016	.000004	.000001	.000000	.000000	.000000
1.9	.000192	.000048	.000014	.000005	.000002	.000001	.000000
2.0	.000446	.000129	.000043	.000016	.000007	.000003	.000002
2.1	.000949	.000309	.000116	.000049	.000022	.000011	.000006
2.2	.001866	.000678	.000279	.000127	.000063	.000033	.000018
2.3	.003423	.001368	.000614	.000301	.000158	.000088	.000052
2.4	.005901	.002569	.001241	.000650	.000363	.000214	.000131
2.5	.009634	.004526	.002338	.001299	.000765	.000473	.000304
2.6	.014981	.007535	.004131	.002420	.001495	.000964	.000644
2.7	.022307	.011931	.006900	.004238	.002731	.001830	.001266
2.8	.031954	.018062	.010959	.007024	.004702	.003261	.002330
2.9	.044214	.026270	.016645	.011084	.007680	.005495	.004040
3.0	.059303	.036861	.024289	.016744	.011967	.008808	.006643
3.1	.077351	.050085	.034194	.024323	.017878	.013498	.010422
3.2	.098386	.066114	.046613	.034113	.025722	.019874	.015672
3.3	.122338	.085029	.061729	.046359	.035775	.028229	.022693
3.4	.149042	.106821	.079642	.061237	.048264	.038820	.031758
3.5	.178251	.131385	.100366	.078846	.063351	.051852	.043102
3.6	.209655	.158533	.123822	.099201	.081120	.067463	.056904
3.7	.242891	.188006	.149852	.122229	.101573	.085715	.073273
3.8	.277570	.219490	.178225	.147781	.124631	.106591	.092242
3.9	.313288	.252629	.208654	.175638	.150142	.129996	.113768
4.0	.349645	.287045	.240808	.205527	.177888	.155766	.137738
4.1	.386256	.322355	.274331	.237130	.207598	.183676	.163970
4.2	.422763	.358180	.308854	.270106	.238962	.213454	.192229
4.3	.458842	.394161	.344012	.304100	.271649	.244794	.222238
4.4	.494209	.429965	.379451	.338757	.305314	.277370	.253692
4.5	.528619	.465293	.414843	.373737	.339614	.310845	.286268
4.6	.561870	.499881	.449888	.408718	.374220	.344888	.319639
4.7	.593802	.533506	.484317	.443405	.408819	.379180	.353485
4.8	.624292	.565985	.517902	.477535	.443128	.413423	.387498
4.9	.653253	.597169	.550449	.510881	.476892	.447345	.421393

$\nu = 12$

Q\n	40	50	60	70	80	90	100
5.0	.680631	.626948	.581802	.543249	.509891	.480701	.454912
5.1	.706399	.655245	.611838	.574481	.541936	.513283	.487826
5.2	.730555	.682011	.640468	.604454	.572875	.544911	.519936
5.3	.753118	.707223	.667633	.633074	.602586	.575440	.551076
5.4	.774122	.730880	.693298	.660277	.630978	.604755	.581109
5.5	.793614	.753002	.717452	.686024	.657986	.632770	.609931
5.6	.811654	.773620	.740104	.710299	.683573	.659425	.637462
5.7	.828306	.792782	.761277	.733106	.707720	.684683	.663648
5.8	.843643	.810543	.781009	.754462	.730429	.708530	.688457
5.9	.857737	.826964	.799347	.774401	.751718	.730967	.711879
6.0	.870665	.842112	.816349	.792966	.771616	.752011	.733917
6.4	.912209	.891400	.872259	.854595	.838227	.822997	.808771
6.8	.940807	.925946	.912057	.899061	.886871	.875405	.864588
7.2	.960209	.949736	.939816	.930426	.921529	.913084	.905051
7.6	.973256	.965935	.958922	.952219	.945813	.939685	.933816
8.0	.981990	.976894	.971965	.967215	.962643	.958240	.953998
8.4	.987829	.984286	.980832	.977479	.974232	.971087	.968042
8.8	.991735	.989271	.986851	.984489	.982187	.979948	.977769
9.2	.994357	.992639	.990941	.989275	.987644	.986051	.984495
9.6	.996123	.994921	.993727	.992549	.991392	.990257	.989145
10.0	.997319	.996474	.995631	.994796	.993973	.993163	.992367
11.0	.998901	.998543	.998183	.997823	.997466	.997112	.996762
12.0	.999529	.999372	.999213	.999053	.998893	.998734	.998576
13.0	.999789	.999718	.999645	.999571	.999497	.999424	.999350
14.0	.999902	.999868	.999834	.999798	.999763	.999728	.999692
15.0	.999953	.999936	.999919	.999902	.999884	.999867	.999849
16.0	.999976	.999968	.999959	.999950	.999941	.999932	.999923
17.0	.999988	.999983	.999979	.999974	.999969	.999965	.999960
18.0	.999993	.999991	.999989	.999986	.999984	.999981	.999978
19.0	1.00000	1.00000	.999994	.999992	.999991	.999989	.999988
20.0			1.00000	1.00000	.999995	.999994	.999993
22.0					1.00000	1.00000	1.00000

$\nu = 13$

Q\n	2	3	4	5	6	7	8
0.0	.000000	.000000	.000000	.000000	.000000	.000000	.000000
0.1	.055378	.002757	.000134	.000007	.000000	.000000	.000000
0.2	.110295	.010956	.001063	.000103	.000010	.000001	.000000
0.3	.164706	.024456	.003548	.000515	.000076	.000011	.000002
0.4	.218249	.042997	.008277	.001594	.000310	.000061	.000012
0.5	.270659	.066237	.015839	.003788	.000915	.000224	.000056
0.6	.321690	.093756	.026700	.007602	.002184	.000636	.000188
0.7	.371122	.125072	.041189	.013556	.004499	.001513	.000516
0.8	.418759	.159656	.059487	.022140	.008305	.003153	.001214
0.9	.464437	.196946	.081627	.033778	.014079	.005935	.002536
1.0	.508018	.236370	.107508	.048797	.022294	.010293	.004812
1.2	.588504	.319342	.169472	.089665	.047682	.025583	.013875
1.4	.659733	.404250	.242414	.144796	.086804	.052418	.031942
1.6	.721661	.487368	.322401	.212272	.140084	.092974	.062166
1.8	.774616	.565788	.405249	.288726	.205934	.147509	.106284
2.0	.819200	.637488	.487107	.370083	.281193	.214293	.164050
2.2	.856204	.701293	.564846	.452269	.361855	.290067	.233299
2.4	.886518	.756755	.636229	.531747	.443809	.370789	.310509
2.6	.911058	.803989	.699919	.605828	.523432	.452384	.391575
2.8	.930714	.843506	.755363	.672753	.597928	.531311	.472530
3.0	.946309	.876059	.802618	.731625	.665439	.604884	.550049
3.2	.958579	.902520	.842170	.782254	.724989	.671359	.621706
3.4	.968164	.923782	.874766	.824962	.776329	.729857	.686004
3.6	.975604	.940698	.901276	.860403	.819742	.780202	.742273
3.8	.981350	.954045	.922596	.889410	.855854	.822725	.790489
4.0	.985767	.964501	.939581	.912874	.885481	.858077	.831077
4.2	.989150	.972645	.953007	.931669	.909509	.887080	.864738
4.4	.991734	.978959	.963549	.946603	.928808	.910610	.892310
4.6	.993704	.983834	.971784	.958389	.944184	.929526	.914660
4.8	.995204	.987587	.978188	.967640	.956356	.944617	.932622
5.0	.996344	.990470	.983153	.974869	.965939	.956582	.946956
5.2	.997210	.992682	.986991	.980500	.973452	.966021	.958330
5.4	.997868	.994377	.989954	.984874	.979324	.973438	.967314
5.6	.998369	.995675	.992238	.988265	.983901	.979249	.974384
5.8	.998750	.996669	.993997	.990892	.987463	.983790	.979933
6.0	.999040	.997430	.995352	.992925	.990231	.987334	.984280
6.4	.999430	.998463	.997201	.995715	.994052	.992250	.990338
6.8	.999658	.999073	.998303	.997388	.996359	.995236	.994038
7.2	.999793	.999435	.998962	.998396	.997755	.997053	.996299
7.6	.999873	.999653	.999359	.999006	.998605	.998163	.997687
8.0	.999922	.999784	.999600	.999378	.999125	.998845	.998542
8.4	.999951	.999865	.999748	.999607	.999446	.999267	.999073
8.8	.999969	.999914	.999840	.999750	.999646	.999531	.999405
9.2	.999980	.999945	.999897	.999839	.999771	.999697	.999615
9.6	.999987	.999964	.999933	.999895	.999851	.999802	.999748
10.0	.999992	.999977	.999956	.999931	.999902	.999869	.999834
11.0	1.00000	.999991	.999984	.999975	.999964	.999952	.999939
12.0		1.00000	.999994	.999990	.999986	.999981	.999976
13.0			1.00000	1.00000	.999994	.999992	.999990
14.0					1.00000	1.00000	1.00000

ν =13

Q\n	9	10	11	12	13	14	15
0.0	.000000	.000000	.000000	.000000	.000000	.000000	.000000
0.1	.000000	.000000	.000000	.000000	.000000	.000000	.000000
0.2	.000000	.000000	.000000	.000000	.000000	.000000	.000000
0.3	.000000	.000000	.000000	.000000	.000000	.000000	.000000
0.4	.000003	.000001	.000000	.000000	.000000	.000000	.000000
0.5	.000014	.000004	.000001	.000000	.000000	.000000	.000000
0.6	.000057	.000017	.000005	.000002	.000001	.000000	.000000
0.7	.000179	.000063	.000023	.000008	.000003	.000001	.000000
0.8	.000475	.000188	.000076	.000031	.000013	.000005	.000002
0.9	.001099	.000483	.000215	.000097	.000045	.000021	.000010
1.0	.002280	.001095	.000533	.000263	.000132	.000067	.000034
1.2	.007613	.004227	.002376	.001351	.000777	.000452	.000266
1.4	.019658	.012222	.007678	.004872	.003123	.002021	.001320
1.6	.041910	.028499	.019548	.013524	.009435	.006637	.004705
1.8	.077095	.056320	.041440	.030710	.022918	.017221	.013025
2.0	.126257	.097726	.076087	.059587	.046935	.037178	.029610
2.2	.188413	.152850	.124582	.102021	.083938	.069377	.057599
2.4	.260829	.219861	.186010	.157960	.134643	.115191	.098905
2.6	.339692	.295454	.257703	.225432	.197784	.174035	.153577
2.8	.420890	.375607	.335907	.301074	.270470	.243532	.219773
3.0	.500670	.456329	.416559	.380891	.348882	.320126	.294256
3.2	.576039	.534197	.495935	.460975	.429034	.399839	.373131
3.4	.644936	.606652	.571059	.538019	.507367	.478935	.452553
3.6	.706194	.672058	.639868	.609576	.581105	.554359	.529240
3.8	.759408	.729620	.701183	.674108	.648370	.623930	.600734
4.0	.804736	.779207	.754576	.730882	.708139	.686338	.665460
4.2	.842717	.821166	.800177	.779808	.760089	.741031	.722636
4.4	.874108	.856140	.838499	.821244	.804415	.788034	.772113
4.6	.899755	.884930	.870269	.855832	.841657	.827773	.814197
4.8	.920510	.908382	.896313	.884355	.872546	.860915	.849481
5.0	.937175	.927324	.917463	.907641	.897892	.888242	.878711
5.2	.950471	.942513	.934508	.926496	.918506	.910564	.902686
5.4	.961024	.954625	.948158	.941658	.935151	.928656	.922189
5.6	.969365	.964238	.959035	.953785	.948510	.943227	.937948
5.8	.975938	.971840	.967667	.963442	.959182	.954902	.950613
6.0	.981104	.977836	.974497	.971105	.967675	.964219	.960747
6.4	.988337	.986265	.984136	.981961	.979751	.977513	.975254
6.8	.992777	.991465	.990111	.988721	.987303	.985861	.984400
7.2	.995503	.994671	.993809	.992921	.992012	.991084	.990140
7.6	.997182	.996652	.996101	.995533	.994948	.994350	.993740
8.0	.998220	.997881	.997528	.997161	.996784	.996397	.996002
8.4	.998866	.998648	.998420	.998183	.997938	.997687	.997429
8.8	.999271	.999130	.998981	.998827	.998667	.998503	.998334
9.2	.999527	.999435	.999338	.999236	.999131	.999023	.998912
9.6	.999691	.999630	.999565	.999498	.999429	.999357	.999283
10.0	.999796	.999755	.999712	.999668	.999621	.999573	.999524
11.0	.999925	.999909	.999893	.999876	.999859	.999841	.999822
12.0	.999971	.999965	.999958	.999952	.999945	.999937	.999930
13.0	.999988	.999985	.999983	.999980	.999977	.999974	.999971
14.0	.999995	.999994	.999993	.999991	.999990	.999989	.999987

$\nu = 13$

Q\n	9	10	11	12	13	14	15
15.0	1.00000	1.00000	1.00000	1.00000	1.00000	.999995	.999994
16.0						1.00000	1.00000

$\nu = 13$

Q\n	16	17	18	19	20	22	24
0.0	.000000	.000000	.000000	.000000	.000000	.000000	.000000
0.2	.000000	.000000	.000000	.000000	.000000	.000000	.000000
0.4	.000000	.000000	.000000	.000000	.000000	.000000	.000000
0.6	.000000	.000000	.000000	.000000	.000000	.000000	.000000
0.8	.000001	.000000	.000000	.000000	.000000	.000000	.000000
1.0	.000018	.000009	.000005	.000003	.000001	.000000	.000000
1.2	.000158	.000095	.000058	.000035	.000022	.000009	.000003
1.4	.000870	.000579	.000388	.000262	.000179	.000085	.000041
1.6	.003362	.002419	.001754	.001280	.000940	.000517	.000291
1.8	.009915	.007594	.005851	.004534	.003532	.002178	.001369
2.0	.023708	.019079	.015430	.012537	.010233	.006906	.004735
2.2	.048027	.040213	.033806	.028530	.024167	.017525	.012877
2.4	.085219	.073675	.063904	.055603	.048528	.037284	.028956
2.6	.135904	.120592	.107288	.095694	.085563	.068886	.055948
2.8	.198772	.180168	.163648	.148946	.135832	.113605	.095691
3.0	.270946	.249907	.230886	.213657	.198024	.170874	.148287
3.2	.348673	.326250	.305666	.286745	.269327	.238453	.212075
3.4	.428061	.405305	.384144	.364447	.346095	.312993	.284071
3.6	.505644	.483471	.462624	.443012	.424548	.390748	.360647
3.8	.578724	.557839	.538016	.519196	.501320	.468178	.438177
4.0	.645475	.626351	.608052	.590540	.573778	.542360	.513517
4.2	.704894	.687791	.671309	.655429	.640127	.611171	.584262
4.4	.756655	.741659	.727118	.713023	.699363	.673298	.648816
4.6	.800940	.788005	.775395	.763108	.751139	.728134	.706324
4.8	.838258	.827255	.816475	.805923	.795598	.775626	.756535
5.0	.869313	.860058	.850954	.842004	.833213	.816110	.799643
5.2	.894886	.887176	.879561	.872050	.864645	.850166	.836136
5.4	.915764	.909389	.903074	.896823	.890642	.878501	.866668
5.6	.932687	.927451	.922247	.917082	.911960	.901859	.891964
5.8	.946326	.942047	.937783	.933540	.929321	.920971	.912754
6.0	.957266	.953784	.950305	.946835	.943378	.936512	.929726
6.4	.972979	.970693	.968400	.966103	.963806	.959217	.954650
6.8	.982923	.981433	.979934	.978427	.976914	.973879	.970841
7.2	.989183	.988216	.987239	.986254	.985263	.983267	.981259
7.6	.993120	.992491	.991855	.991212	.990564	.989253	.987929
8.0	.995599	.995190	.994775	.994354	.993929	.993068	.992195
8.4	.997166	.996898	.996626	.996350	.996071	.995504	.994927
8.8	.998161	.997985	.997806	.997624	.997440	.997065	.996682
9.2	.998798	.998681	.998563	.998442	.998320	.998070	.997815
9.6	.999207	.999130	.999051	.998970	.998888	.998721	.998550
10.0	.999473	.999421	.999368	.999314	.999259	.999146	.999030
11.0	.999803	.999783	.999763	.999742	.999721	.999678	.999633
12.0	.999922	.999914	.999906	.999898	.999889	.999872	.999854
13.0	.999968	.999964	.999961	.999958	.999954	.999947	.999939
14.0	.999986	.999985	.999983	.999982	.999980	.999977	.999973
15.0	.999994	.999993	.999992	.999992	.999991	.999989	.999988
16.0	1.00000	1.00000	1.00000	1.00000	1.00000	.999995	.999994
17.0						1.00000	1.00000

$\nu = 13$

Q\n	26	28	30	32	34	36	38
0.0	.000000	.000000	.000000	.000000	.000000	.000000	.000000
0.2	.000000	.000000	.000000	.000000	.000000	.000000	.000000
0.4	.000000	.000000	.000000	.000000	.000000	.000000	.000000
0.6	.000000	.000000	.000000	.000000	.000000	.000000	.000000
0.8	.000000	.000000	.000000	.000000	.000000	.000000	.000000
1.0	.000000	.000000	.000000	.000000	.000000	.000000	.000000
1.2	.000001	.000001	.000000	.000000	.000000	.000000	.000000
1.4	.000021	.000011	.000006	.000003	.000002	.000001	.000001
1.6	.000167	.000098	.000059	.000036	.000022	.000014	.000009
1.8	.000876	.000570	.000377	.000253	.000172	.000118	.000082
2.0	.003296	.002326	.001662	.001202	.000879	.000649	.000484
2.2	.009578	.007205	.005477	.004204	.003257	.002544	.002003
2.4	.022714	.017983	.014360	.011558	.009373	.007653	.006290
2.6	.045810	.037794	.031399	.026257	.022091	.018691	.015899
2.8	.081134	.069214	.059382	.051218	.044396	.038661	.033813
3.0	.129370	.113425	.099905	.088377	.078494	.069980	.062611
3.2	.189416	.169852	.152876	.138076	.125116	.113720	.103660
3.4	.258691	.236327	.216541	.198967	.183300	.169285	.156707
3.6	.333750	.309637	.287947	.268376	.250664	.234587	.219954
3.8	.410951	.386179	.363581	.342915	.323967	.306554	.290515
4.0	.486990	.462545	.439975	.419092	.399733	.381752	.365018
4.2	.559226	.535901	.514137	.493798	.474761	.456915	.440160
4.4	.625808	.604166	.583788	.564577	.546446	.529312	.513102
4.6	.685646	.666032	.647415	.629730	.612917	.596918	.581678
4.8	.738294	.720864	.704203	.688271	.673026	.658429	.644444
5.0	.783801	.768565	.753910	.739813	.726248	.713189	.700611
5.2	.822556	.809419	.796714	.784429	.772547	.761053	.749932
5.4	.855153	.843955	.833074	.822502	.812231	.802254	.792559
5.6	.882287	.872835	.863608	.854606	.845826	.837264	.828914
5.8	.904682	.896765	.889007	.881410	.873973	.866695	.859575
6.0	.923035	.916448	.909970	.903604	.897353	.891217	.885195
6.4	.950116	.945623	.941178	.936784	.932446	.928164	.923941
6.8	.967808	.964786	.961781	.958796	.955836	.952901	.949994
7.2	.979244	.977228	.975215	.973208	.971209	.969220	.967243
7.6	.986596	.985257	.983915	.982572	.981230	.979891	.978556
8.0	.991313	.990424	.989531	.988634	.987736	.986837	.985939
8.4	.994342	.993751	.993156	.992557	.991956	.991352	.990748
8.8	.996293	.995899	.995501	.995100	.994697	.994291	.993884
9.2	.997555	.997291	.997024	.996754	.996483	.996209	.995934
9.6	.998375	.998198	.998018	.997836	.997652	.997466	.997280
10.0	.998912	.998792	.998670	.998546	.998421	.998295	.998168
11.0	.999587	.999541	.999493	.999445	.999396	.999346	.999296
12.0	.999836	.999817	.999797	.999778	.999758	.999737	.999717
13.0	.999931	.999923	.999915	.999907	.999898	.999890	.999881
14.0	.999970	.999966	.999963	.999959	.999955	.999952	.999948
15.0	.999986	.999985	.999983	.999981	.999980	.999978	.999976
16.0	.999994	.999993	.999992	.999991	.999990	.999989	.999989
17.0	1.00000	1.00000	1.00000	1.00000	1.00000	.999995	.999994
18.0						1.00000	1.00000

$\nu = 13$

Q\n	40	50	60	70	80	90	100
0.0	.000000	.000000	.000000	.000000	.000000	.000000	.000000
0.1	.000000	.000000	.000000	.000000	.000000	.000000	.000000
0.2	.000000	.000000	.000000	.000000	.000000	.000000	.000000
0.3	.000000	.000000	.000000	.000000	.000000	.000000	.000000
0.4	.000000	.000000	.000000	.000000	.000000	.000000	.000000
0.5	.000000	.000000	.000000	.000000	.000000	.000000	.000000
0.6	.000000	.000000	.000000	.000000	.000000	.000000	.000000
0.7	.000000	.000000	.000000	.000000	.000000	.000000	.000000
0.8	.000000	.000000	.000000	.000000	.000000	.000000	.000000
0.9	.000000	.000000	.000000	.000000	.000000	.000000	.000000
1.0	.000000	.000000	.000000	.000000	.000000	.000000	.000000
1.1	.000000	.000000	.000000	.000000	.000000	.000000	.000000
1.2	.000000	.000000	.000000	.000000	.000000	.000000	.000000
1.3	.000000	.000000	.000000	.000000	.000000	.000000	.000000
1.4	.000000	.000000	.000000	.000000	.000000	.000000	.000000
1.5	.000001	.000000	.000000	.000000	.000000	.000000	.000000
1.6	.000006	.000001	.000000	.000000	.000000	.000000	.000000
1.7	.000019	.000003	.000001	.000000	.000000	.000000	.000000
1.8	.000058	.000011	.000003	.000001	.000000	.000000	.000000
1.9	.000153	.000036	.000010	.000003	.000001	.000000	.000000
2.0	.000364	.000099	.000031	.000011	.000005	.000002	.000001
2.1	.000792	.000244	.000087	.000035	.000015	.000007	.000004
2.2	.001589	.000549	.000216	.000094	.000045	.000023	.000012
2.3	.002967	.001134	.000488	.000230	.000117	.000063	.000036
2.4	.005201	.002175	.001013	.000513	.000277	.000158	.000094
2.5	.008620	.003907	.001952	.001051	.000601	.000361	.000226
2.6	.013591	.006619	.003521	.002005	.001206	.000759	.000495
2.7	.020494	.010648	.005993	.003589	.002258	.001479	.001002
2.8	.029694	.016354	.009684	.006066	.003974	.002701	.001893
2.9	.041513	.024098	.014938	.009744	.006621	.004652	.003361
3.0	.056203	.034215	.022105	.014958	.010505	.007605	.005648
3.1	.073927	.046988	.031517	.022047	.015952	.011866	.009033
3.2	.094746	.062622	.043458	.031331	.023291	.017756	.013825
3.3	.118613	.081236	.058147	.043085	.032827	.025591	.020337
3.4	.145382	.102847	.075719	.057523	.044820	.035659	.028872
3.5	.174815	.127375	.096217	.074778	.059468	.048199	.039694
3.6	.206600	.154645	.119589	.094894	.076888	.063384	.053016
3.7	.240367	.184403	.145692	.117825	.097112	.081308	.068983
3.8	.275709	.216331	.174303	.143439	.120087	.101984	.087660
3.9	.312201	.250061	.205134	.171523	.145675	.125338	.109030
4.0	.349418	.285198	.237843	.201803	.173663	.151219	.132998
4.1	.386948	.321334	.272057	.233954	.203780	.179408	.159392
4.2	.424406	.358065	.307387	.267617	.235708	.209629	.187981
4.3	.461441	.395004	.343441	.302416	.269096	.241564	.218481
4.4	.497746	.431791	.379841	.337973	.303579	.274869	.250574
4.5	.533055	.468101	.416229	.373919	.338791	.309186	.283917
4.6	.567149	.503649	.452278	.409905	.374373	.344160	.318162
4.7	.599852	.538189	.487698	.445610	.409988	.379444	.352961
4.8	.631033	.571522	.522237	.480748	.445325	.414713	.387982
4.9	.660599	.603488	.555684	.515068	.480106	.449670	.422914

ν = 13

Q\n	40	50	60	70	80	90	100
5.0	.688490	.633966	.587869	.548360	.514089	.484047	.457473
5.1	.714679	.662873	.618658	.580451	.547069	.517615	.491406
5.2	.739167	.690156	.647954	.611205	.578876	.550177	.524497
5.3	.761973	.715792	.675693	.640520	.609378	.581573	.556562
5.4	.783138	.739783	.701839	.668328	.638476	.611677	.587452
5.5	.802715	.762151	.726382	.694587	.666100	.640395	.617050
5.6	.820770	.782933	.749333	.719281	.692210	.667663	.645271
5.7	.837375	.802182	.770719	.742415	.716788	.693442	.672056
5.8	.852608	.819958	.790584	.764013	.739837	.717717	.697373
5.9	.866551	.836333	.808982	.784112	.761379	.740492	.721211
6.0	.879287	.851379	.825976	.802761	.781448	.761788	.743575
6.4	.919776	.899841	.881323	.864102	.848044	.833025	.818934
6.8	.947116	.933183	.920025	.907609	.895883	.884789	.874271
7.2	.965279	.955683	.946493	.937717	.929339	.921336	.913683
7.6	.977226	.970676	.964330	.958207	.952309	.946630	.941158
8.0	.985041	.980593	.976239	.972002	.967890	.963903	.960038
8.4	.990143	.987128	.984151	.981233	.978382	.975601	.972891
8.8	.993476	.991431	.989397	.987390	.985419	.983486	.981594
9.2	.995658	.994268	.992877	.991497	.990134	.988792	.987473
9.6	.997092	.996144	.995190	.994239	.993296	.992364	.991444
10.0	.998040	.997391	.996734	.996076	.995422	.994772	.994130
11.0	.999246	.998988	.998724	.998458	.998190	.997924	.997658
12.0	.999696	.999590	.999480	.999369	.999256	.999143	.999030
13.0	.999872	.999826	.999779	.999731	.999682	.999632	.999583
14.0	.999944	.999923	.999902	.999880	.999858	.999836	.999813
15.0	.999974	.999965	.999955	.999945	.999934	.999924	.999913
16.0	.999988	.999983	.999978	.999974	.999969	.999963	.999958
17.0	.999994	.999992	.999989	.999987	.999984	.999982	.999979
18.0	1.00000	1.00000	.999995	.999993	.999992	.999991	.999989
19.0			1.00000	1.00000	1.00000	1.00000	.999994
20.0							1.00000

$\nu = 14$

Q\n	2	3	4	5	6	7	8
0.0	.000000	.000000	.000000	.000000	.000000	.000000	.000000
0.1	.055482	.002758	.000134	.000006	.000000	.000000	.000000
0.2	.110448	.010957	.001060	.000102	.000010	.000001	.000000
0.3	.164939	.024459	.003536	.000510	.000074	.000011	.000002
0.4	.218564	.043007	.008250	.001580	.000305	.000060	.000012
0.5	.271059	.066261	.015791	.003756	.000901	.000219	.000054
0.6	.322180	.093805	.026628	.007543	.002152	.000622	.000182
0.7	.371704	.125158	.041093	.013458	.004438	.001480	.000500
0.8	.419438	.159795	.059370	.021994	.008200	.003090	.001179
0.9	.465215	.197158	.081502	.033580	.013915	.005824	.002467
1.0	.508897	.236673	.107390	.048546	.022057	.010115	.004692
1.2	.589582	.319888	.169440	.089341	.047285	.025221	.013585
1.4	.660999	.405110	.242591	.144500	.086284	.051845	.031408
1.6	.723093	.488590	.322919	.212159	.139562	.092249	.061382
1.8	.776177	.567387	.406218	.288975	.205603	.146793	.105353
2.0	.820848	.639443	.488595	.370854	.281274	.213822	.163185
2.2	.857894	.703553	.566864	.453669	.362543	.290096	.232781
2.4	.888204	.759245	.638737	.533814	.445236	.371534	.310618
2.6	.912701	.806623	.702831	.608527	.525641	.453978	.392527
2.8	.932279	.846196	.758566	.675987	.600874	.533783	.474436
3.0	.947771	.878724	.805988	.735260	.669009	.608167	.552906
3.2	.959921	.905091	.845587	.786136	.729023	.675310	.625408
3.4	.969376	.926204	.878123	.828941	.780650	.734292	.690378
3.6	.976684	.942936	.904488	.864345	.824175	.784922	.747109
3.8	.982299	.956075	.925600	.893205	.860247	.827540	.795571
4.0	.986592	.966316	.942336	.916440	.889711	.862824	.836207
4.2	.989860	.974246	.955490	.934953	.913483	.891629	.869753
4.4	.992341	.980354	.965756	.949574	.932466	.914869	.897081
4.6	.994218	.985038	.973721	.961038	.947495	.933435	.919100
4.8	.995636	.988618	.979870	.969971	.959307	.948146	.936677
5.0	.996706	.991346	.984600	.976899	.968538	.959722	.950602
5.2	.997512	.993421	.988226	.982251	.975717	.968782	.961565
5.4	.998119	.994997	.991001	.986373	.981279	.975842	.970151
5.6	.998576	.996193	.993121	.989540	.985576	.981323	.976849
5.8	.998920	.997100	.994738	.991969	.988889	.985567	.982058
6.0	.999180	.997788	.995972	.993831	.991438	.988847	.986099
6.4	.999525	.998707	.997630	.996349	.994906	.993331	.991649
6.8	.999722	.999239	.998597	.997828	.996955	.995997	.994968
7.2	.999836	.999548	.999163	.998698	.998168	.997583	.996952
7.6	.999902	.999729	.999496	.999213	.998889	.998530	.998141
8.0	.999941	.999836	.999694	.999520	.999321	.999099	.998858
8.4	.999964	.999899	.999812	.999705	.999581	.999443	.999292
8.8	.999978	.999938	.999883	.999816	.999739	.999652	.999557
9.2	.999986	.999961	.999927	.999885	.999836	.999781	.999721
9.6	.999991	.999975	.999954	.999927	.999896	.999861	.999822
10.0	.999994	.999984	.999970	.999953	.999933	.999910	.999885
11.0	1.00000	.999995	.999990	.999984	.999977	.999969	.999960
12.0		1.00000	1.00000	.999994	.999992	.999989	.999985
13.0				1.00000	1.00000	1.00000	.999994
14.0							1.00000

$\nu = 14$

Q\n	9	10	11	12	13	14	15
0.0	.000000	.000000	.000000	.000000	.000000	.000000	.000000
0.1	.000000	.000000	.000000	.000000	.000000	.000000	.000000
0.2	.000000	.000000	.000000	.000000	.000000	.000000	.000000
0.3	.000000	.000000	.000000	.000000	.000000	.000000	.000000
0.4	.000002	.000000	.000000	.000000	.000000	.000000	.000000
0.5	.000013	.000003	.000001	.000000	.000000	.000000	.000000
0.6	.000054	.000016	.000005	.000002	.000000	.000000	.000000
0.7	.000172	.000060	.000021	.000008	.000003	.000001	.000000
0.8	.000456	.000179	.000071	.000029	.000012	.000005	.000002
0.9	.001059	.000461	.000203	.000091	.000041	.000019	.000009
1.0	.002203	.001048	.000505	.000246	.000122	.000061	.000031
1.2	.007397	.004073	.002268	.001277	.000727	.000419	.000244
1.4	.019202	.011853	.007388	.004650	.002954	.001895	.001226
1.6	.041154	.027815	.018954	.013022	.009018	.006295	.004428
1.8	.076076	.055298	.040468	.029817	.022117	.016514	.012410
2.0	.125142	.096476	.074786	.058294	.045691	.036006	.028524
2.2	.187477	.151616	.123150	.100475	.082341	.067776	.056028
2.4	.260390	.218972	.184768	.156455	.132950	.113374	.097015
2.6	.340034	.295245	.257018	.224347	.196372	.172361	.151702
2.8	.422205	.376343	.336102	.300778	.269739	.242423	.218340
3.0	.503025	.458151	.417847	.381662	.349166	.319960	.293681
3.2	.579383	.537114	.498388	.462950	.430534	.400876	.373727
3.4	.649120	.610553	.574615	.541188	.510128	.481277	.454477
3.6	.711011	.676751	.644358	.613805	.585030	.557954	.532485
3.8	.764627	.734869	.706377	.679178	.653263	.628603	.605157
4.0	.810133	.784770	.760218	.736534	.713741	.691842	.670825
4.2	.848095	.826817	.806023	.785779	.766126	.747084	.728662
4.4	.879308	.861692	.844332	.827296	.810630	.794364	.778514
4.6	.904659	.890235	.875916	.861765	.847828	.834137	.820714
4.8	.925041	.913338	.901645	.890017	.878497	.867115	.855895
5.0	.941289	.931866	.922396	.912927	.903496	.894131	.884854
5.2	.954152	.946611	.938993	.931339	.923679	.916039	.908439
5.4	.964277	.958272	.952178	.946028	.939848	.933659	.927477
5.6	.972210	.967447	.962594	.957676	.952716	.947731	.942735
5.8	.978404	.974638	.970786	.966869	.962905	.958908	.954890
6.0	.983226	.980255	.977206	.974095	.970938	.967745	.964526
6.4	.989880	.988038	.986138	.984188	.982198	.980176	.978128
6.8	.993879	.992741	.991560	.990343	.989096	.987823	.986528
7.2	.996281	.995576	.994843	.994084	.993303	.992503	.991687
7.6	.997726	.997289	.996832	.996357	.995868	.995365	.994851
8.0	.998600	.998327	.998041	.997743	.997435	.997118	.996793
8.4	.999131	.998959	.998779	.998591	.998396	.998195	.997989
8.8	.999455	.999347	.999233	.999113	.998989	.998861	.998729
9.2	.999656	.999587	.999514	.999437	.999358	.999276	.999191
9.6	.999780	.999736	.999689	.999640	.999588	.999535	.999480
10.0	.999858	.999830	.999799	.999767	.999734	.999699	.999663
11.0	.999951	.999941	.999930	.999919	.999907	.999895	.999882
12.0	.999982	.999978	.999974	.999970	.999966	.999961	.999956
13.0	.999993	.999992	.999990	.999988	.999987	.999985	.999983
14.0	1.00000	1.00000	1.00000	1.00000	.999995	.999994	.999993

ν = 14

Q\n	9	10	11	12	13	14	15
15.0					1.00000	1.00000	1.00000

$\nu = 14$

Q\n	16	17	18	19	20	22	24
0.0	.000000	.000000	.000000	.000000	.000000	.000000	.000000
0.2	.000000	.000000	.000000	.000000	.000000	.000000	.000000
0.4	.000000	.000000	.000000	.000000	.000000	.000000	.000000
0.6	.000000	.000000	.000000	.000000	.000000	.000000	.000000
0.8	.000001	.000000	.000000	.000000	.000000	.000000	.000000
1.0	.000016	.000008	.000004	.000002	.000001	.000000	.000000
1.2	.000143	.000085	.000051	.000031	.000019	.000007	.000003
1.4	.000800	.000527	.000350	.000234	.000158	.000073	.000035
1.6	.003138	.002240	.001610	.001165	.000848	.000458	.000253
1.8	.009383	.007137	.005461	.004201	.003250	.001974	.001223
2.0	.022713	.018176	.014615	.011806	.009579	.006387	.004327
2.2	.046511	.038767	.032439	.027247	.022970	.016496	.012002
2.4	.083297	.071754	.062007	.053750	.046730	.035623	.027447
2.6	.133878	.118460	.105085	.093451	.083305	.066654	.053794
2.8	.197067	.178236	.161532	.146682	.133454	.111078	.093099
3.0	.270004	.248638	.229328	.211847	.195996	.168499	.145667
3.2	.348854	.326043	.305100	.285849	.268131	.236737	.209940
3.4	.429574	.406420	.384876	.364816	.346118	.312388	.282918
3.6	.508531	.485996	.464790	.444824	.426014	.391557	.360849
3.8	.582875	.561701	.541579	.522455	.504271	.470520	.439928
4.0	.650671	.631352	.612838	.595097	.578096	.546177	.516820
4.2	.710856	.693659	.677058	.661037	.645578	.616266	.588965
4.4	.763091	.748097	.733529	.719383	.705651	.679389	.654659
4.6	.807573	.794723	.782169	.769912	.757952	.734905	.712991
4.8	.844852	.834000	.823344	.812891	.802643	.782765	.763704
5.0	.875681	.866625	.857695	.848898	.840237	.823341	.807016
5.2	.900892	.893411	.886006	.878683	.871448	.857259	.843458
5.4	.921317	.915189	.909102	.903063	.897076	.885281	.873741
5.6	.937739	.932754	.927786	.922843	.917929	.908206	.898642
5.8	.950860	.946826	.942796	.938775	.934768	.926808	.918942
6.0	.961289	.958040	.954787	.951532	.948281	.941802	.935372
6.4	.976059	.973973	.971874	.969766	.967652	.963415	.959178
6.8	.985215	.983887	.982546	.981195	.979834	.977095	.974339
7.2	.990857	.990015	.989162	.988299	.987429	.985669	.983890
7.6	.994326	.993792	.993249	.992700	.992144	.991017	.989872
8.0	.996460	.996121	.995775	.995425	.995070	.994347	.993611
8.4	.997777	.997561	.997340	.997116	.996888	.996424	.995949
8.8	.998594	.998455	.998314	.998170	.998023	.997723	.997416
9.2	.999104	.999014	.998923	.998830	.998735	.998540	.998341
9.6	.999424	.999366	.999306	.999246	.999184	.999057	.998926
10.0	.999626	.999588	.999550	.999510	.999469	.999386	.999300
11.0	.999869	.999855	.999841	.999827	.999812	.999782	.999751
12.0	.999951	.999946	.999941	.999936	.999930	.999919	.999907
13.0	.999981	.999979	.999977	.999975	.999973	.999968	.999963
14.0	.999992	.999991	.999990	.999990	.999989	.999987	.999985
15.0	1.00000	1.00000	1.00000	1.00000	1.00000	.999994	.999993
16.0						1.00000	1.00000

$\nu = 14$

Q\n	26	28	30	32	34	36	38
0.0	.000000	.000000	.000000	.000000	.000000	.000000	.000000
0.2	.000000	.000000	.000000	.000000	.000000	.000000	.000000
0.4	.000000	.000000	.000000	.000000	.000000	.000000	.000000
0.6	.000000	.000000	.000000	.000000	.000000	.000000	.000000
0.8	.000000	.000000	.000000	.000000	.000000	.000000	.000000
1.0	.000000	.000000	.000000	.000000	.000000	.000000	.000000
1.2	.000001	.000000	.000000	.000000	.000000	.000000	.000000
1.4	.000017	.000009	.000004	.000002	.000001	.000001	.000000
1.6	.000143	.000082	.000048	.000029	.000017	.000011	.000007
1.8	.000771	.000494	.000322	.000212	.000142	.000096	.000066
2.0	.002975	.002073	.001464	.001046	.000755	.000551	.000406
2.2	.008839	.006583	.004954	.003765	.002888	.002234	.001742
2.4	.021359	.016774	.013287	.010609	.008535	.006914	.005638
2.6	.043766	.035875	.029614	.024605	.020568	.017292	.014615
2.8	.078539	.066660	.056898	.048824	.042104	.036478	.031742
3.0	.126586	.110543	.096976	.085439	.075578	.067107	.059798
3.2	.186949	.167127	.149955	.135012	.121953	.110493	.100399
3.4	.257068	.234303	.214179	.196324	.180425	.166221	.153491
3.6	.333402	.308792	.286660	.266698	.248640	.232260	.217362
3.8	.412139	.386838	.363749	.342627	.323262	.305467	.289079
4.0	.489781	.464837	.441783	.420438	.400641	.382245	.365121
4.2	.563516	.539768	.517580	.496821	.477373	.459127	.441986
4.4	.631363	.609408	.588699	.569148	.550672	.533192	.516638
4.6	.692160	.672356	.653520	.635596	.618527	.602262	.586749
4.8	.745438	.727939	.711175	.695110	.679710	.664940	.650766
5.0	.791261	.776065	.761413	.747286	.733664	.720525	.707848
5.2	.830056	.817051	.804440	.792215	.780364	.768877	.757740
5.4	.862470	.851476	.840760	.830321	.820155	.810257	.800619
5.6	.889255	.880055	.871047	.862233	.853615	.845189	.836955
5.8	.911187	.903552	.896047	.888676	.881440	.874342	.867380
6.0	.929007	.922717	.916510	.910393	.904368	.898439	.892605
6.4	.954954	.950753	.946582	.942445	.938348	.934293	.930282
6.8	.971576	.968812	.966054	.963305	.960569	.957849	.955147
7.2	.982097	.980296	.978490	.976684	.974878	.973076	.971280
7.6	.988713	.987545	.986370	.985190	.984006	.982821	.981637
8.0	.992863	.992106	.991343	.990574	.989800	.989024	.988246
8.4	.995466	.994975	.994479	.993978	.993473	.992964	.992454
8.8	.997103	.996784	.996460	.996133	.995803	.995469	.995134
9.2	.998136	.997928	.997717	.997502	.997285	.997066	.996844
9.6	.998793	.998656	.998517	.998375	.998232	.998087	.997941
10.0	.999212	.999121	.999029	.998936	.998841	.998745	.998647
11.0	.999719	.999686	.999652	.999618	.999583	.999547	.999511
12.0	.999895	.999882	.999869	.999856	.999843	.999829	.999815
13.0	.999958	.999953	.999948	.999943	.999938	.999932	.999927
14.0	.999983	.999981	.999979	.999976	.999974	.999972	.999969
15.0	.999993	.999992	.999991	.999990	.999989	.999988	.999987
16.0	1.00000	1.00000	1.00000	1.00000	.999995	.999994	.999994
17.0					1.00000	1.00000	1.00000

$\nu = 14$

Q\n	40	50	60	70	80	90	100
0.0	.000000	.000000	.000000	.000000	.000000	.000000	.000000
0.1	.000000	.000000	.000000	.000000	.000000	.000000	.000000
0.2	.000000	.000000	.000000	.000000	.000000	.000000	.000000
0.3	.000000	.000000	.000000	.000000	.000000	.000000	.000000
0.4	.000000	.000000	.000000	.000000	.000000	.000000	.000000
0.5	.000000	.000000	.000000	.000000	.000000	.000000	.000000
0.6	.000000	.000000	.000000	.000000	.000000	.000000	.000000
0.7	.000000	.000000	.000000	.000000	.000000	.000000	.000000
0.8	.000000	.000000	.000000	.000000	.000000	.000000	.000000
0.9	.000000	.000000	.000000	.000000	.000000	.000000	.000000
1.0	.000000	.000000	.000000	.000000	.000000	.000000	.000000
1.1	.000000	.000000	.000000	.000000	.000000	.000000	.000000
1.2	.000000	.000000	.000000	.000000	.000000	.000000	.000000
1.3	.000000	.000000	.000000	.000000	.000000	.000000	.000000
1.4	.000000	.000000	.000000	.000000	.000000	.000000	.000000
1.5	.000001	.000000	.000000	.000000	.000000	.000000	.000000
1.6	.000004	.000001	.000000	.000000	.000000	.000000	.000000
1.7	.000015	.000002	.000000	.000000	.000000	.000000	.000000
1.8	.000046	.000008	.000002	.000001	.000000	.000000	.000000
1.9	.000124	.000027	.000007	.000002	.000001	.000000	.000000
2.0	.000302	.000077	.000023	.000008	.000003	.000001	.000001
2.1	.000670	.000196	.000067	.000025	.000011	.000005	.000002
2.2	.001368	.000451	.000170	.000071	.000032	.000016	.000008
2.3	.002598	.000952	.000394	.000179	.000088	.000046	.000025
2.4	.004625	.001863	.000837	.000410	.000215	.000119	.000069
2.5	.007774	.003406	.001648	.000861	.000479	.000280	.000171
2.6	.012415	.005865	.003031	.001680	.000985	.000605	.000386
2.7	.018940	.009575	.005251	.003068	.001887	.001210	.000803
2.8	.027735	.014904	.008621	.005283	.003390	.002260	.001555
2.9	.039148	.022230	.013494	.008630	.005756	.003974	.002823
3.0	.053463	.031912	.020233	.013450	.009288	.006618	.004841
3.1	.070875	.044262	.029193	.020098	.014323	.010503	.007887
3.2	.091474	.059521	.040688	.028916	.021205	.015959	.012274
3.3	.115241	.077837	.054970	.040211	.030265	.023321	.018329
3.4	.142046	.099258	.072206	.054228	.041792	.032903	.026376
3.5	.171663	.123726	.092471	.071133	.056016	.044977	.036709
3.6	.203779	.151083	.115738	.091003	.073090	.059747	.049573
3.7	.238017	.181080	.141880	.113815	.093075	.077342	.065145
3.8	.273956	.213397	.170685	.139455	.115941	.097802	.083522
3.9	.311152	.247656	.201863	.167722	.141568	.121077	.104715
4.0	.349155	.283446	.235066	.198340	.169752	.147029	.128647
4.1	.387528	.320336	.269906	.230978	.200222	.175447	.155160
4.2	.425860	.357899	.305973	.265262	.232651	.206053	.184026
4.3	.463776	.395721	.342851	.300797	.266674	.238520	.214958
4.4	.500944	.433416	.380137	.337181	.301907	.272488	.247625
4.5	.537078	.470633	.417446	.374019	.337958	.307579	.281668
4.6	.571943	.507066	.454425	.410936	.374444	.343411	.316717
4.7	.605350	.542449	.490762	.447587	.411002	.379615	.352399
4.8	.637157	.576567	.526183	.483659	.447295	.415839	.388358
4.9	.667265	.609246	.560460	.518884	.483021	.451759	.424255

$\nu = 14$

Q\n	40	50	60	70	80	90	100
5.0	.695612	.640358	.593408	.553030	.517918	.487087	.459782
5.1	.722170	.669813	.624884	.585911	.551762	.521571	.494666
5.2	.746940	.697556	.654783	.617379	.584370	.554998	.528669
5.3	.769947	.723564	.683037	.647326	.615598	.587194	.561592
5.4	.791235	.747840	.709609	.675678	.645339	.618022	.593271
5.5	.810865	.770409	.734489	.702392	.673519	.647381	.623582
5.6	.828907	.791315	.757691	.727452	.700094	.675202	.652431
5.7	.845441	.810616	.779248	.750865	.725049	.701445	.679757
5.8	.860554	.828380	.799208	.772659	.748388	.726095	.705525
5.9	.874333	.844684	.817631	.792877	.770137	.749158	.729725
6.0	.886869	.859609	.834588	.811574	.790335	.770660	.752366
6.4	.926318	.907214	.889307	.872532	.856797	.842007	.828072
6.8	.952465	.939390	.926919	.915060	.903786	.893061	.882845
7.2	.969491	.960682	.952159	.943951	.936061	.928479	.921191
7.6	.980453	.974578	.968824	.963223	.957789	.952523	.947422
8.0	.987466	.983570	.979714	.975928	.972224	.968609	.965085
8.4	.991941	.989363	.986789	.984242	.981734	.979271	.976856
8.8	.994796	.993090	.991374	.989665	.987971	.986299	.984652
9.2	.996622	.995491	.994346	.993198	.992055	.990922	.989801
9.6	.997793	.997041	.996275	.995503	.994731	.993963	.993200
10.0	.998549	.998046	.997532	.997011	.996489	.995966	.995446
11.0	.999475	.999287	.999093	.998894	.998694	.998492	.998289
12.0	.999801	.999728	.999652	.999574	.999494	.999414	.999332
13.0	.999921	.999891	.999860	.999828	.999796	.999762	.999729
14.0	.999967	.999955	.999942	.999928	.999914	.999900	.999885
15.0	.999986	.999980	.999974	.999968	.999962	.999956	.999949
16.0	.999994	.999991	.999988	.999986	.999983	.999980	.999977
17.0	1.00000	1.00000	.999995	.999993	.999992	.999990	.999989
18.0			1.00000	1.00000	1.00000	1.00000	.999995
19.0							1.00000

$\nu = 15$

Q\n	2	3	4	5	6	7	8
0.0	.000000	.000000	.000000	.000000	.000000	.000000	.000000
0.1	.055574	.002759	.000133	.000006	.000000	.000000	.000000
0.2	.110581	.010957	.001056	.000102	.000010	.000001	.000000
0.3	.165140	.024462	.003525	.000506	.000073	.000011	.000002
0.4	.218837	.043016	.008226	.001568	.000301	.000058	.000011
0.5	.271406	.066282	.015750	.003729	.000889	.000214	.000052
0.6	.322605	.093847	.026566	.007491	.002125	.000609	.000177
0.7	.372210	.125233	.041009	.013373	.004385	.001452	.000487
0.8	.420028	.159916	.059269	.021867	.008108	.003035	.001149
0.9	.465890	.197341	.081392	.033406	.013771	.005727	.002408
1.0	.509660	.236937	.107286	.048326	.021851	.009961	.004588
1.2	.590519	.320364	.169411	.089057	.046937	.024906	.013333
1.4	.662100	.405860	.242745	.144238	.085826	.051342	.030942
1.6	.724337	.489657	.323370	.212056	.139101	.091609	.060692
1.8	.777533	.568783	.407065	.289188	.205307	.146157	.104528
2.0	.822281	.641151	.489897	.371526	.281339	.213398	.162414
2.2	.859362	.705528	.568634	.454898	.363144	.290112	.232312
2.4	.889668	.761422	.640938	.535634	.446491	.372185	.310704
2.6	.914125	.808924	.705388	.610905	.527590	.455384	.393363
2.8	.933634	.848543	.761377	.678838	.603479	.535972	.476125
3.0	.949034	.881045	.808942	.738461	.672165	.611077	.555443
3.2	.961077	.907324	.848577	.789551	.732588	.678814	.628701
3.4	.970417	.928303	.881053	.832434	.784461	.738220	.694266
3.6	.977607	.944867	.907283	.867796	.828077	.789094	.751400
3.8	.983107	.957822	.928203	.896515	.864102	.831784	.800069
4.0	.987291	.967870	.944713	.919539	.893407	.866993	.840733
4.2	.990459	.975609	.957623	.937793	.916940	.895607	.874158
4.4	.992849	.981536	.967641	.952130	.935633	.918575	.901252
4.6	.994646	.986052	.975365	.963302	.950343	.936817	.922960
4.8	.995994	.989479	.981288	.971952	.961831	.951179	.940181
5.0	.997003	.992072	.985811	.978612	.970744	.962403	.953731
5.2	.997758	.994029	.989253	.983717	.977625	.971122	.964320
5.4	.998321	.995503	.991864	.987617	.982913	.977862	.972550
5.6	.998742	.996612	.993842	.990589	.986964	.983052	.978916
5.8	.999056	.997446	.995338	.992848	.990060	.987035	.983824
6.0	.999291	.998073	.996469	.994564	.992421	.990086	.987597
6.4	.999598	.998898	.997968	.996853	.995588	.994199	.992709
6.8	.999770	.999366	.998824	.998169	.997421	.996596	.995704
7.2	.999867	.999632	.999314	.998928	.998485	.997992	.997458
7.6	.999923	.999785	.999597	.999368	.999103	.998808	.998486
8.0	.999954	.999873	.999761	.999624	.999465	.999287	.999092
8.4	.999973	.999924	.999857	.999774	.999678	.999570	.999451
8.8	.999984	.999954	.999913	.999863	.999804	.999738	.999665
9.2	.999990	.999972	.999947	.999916	.999880	.999839	.999794
9.6	.999994	.999983	.999967	.999948	.999925	.999900	.999872
10.0	1.00000	.999989	.999980	.999967	.999953	.999937	.999919
11.0		1.00000	.999993	.999989	.999985	.999980	.999974
12.0			1.00000	1.00000	.999995	.999993	.999991
13.0					1.00000	1.00000	1.00000

$\nu = 15$

Q\n	9	10	11	12	13	14	15
0.0	.000000	.000000	.000000	.000000	.000000	.000000	.000000
0.1	.000000	.000000	.000000	.000000	.000000	.000000	.000000
0.2	.000000	.000000	.000000	.000000	.000000	.000000	.000000
0.3	.000000	.000000	.000000	.000000	.000000	.000000	.000000
0.4	.000002	.000000	.000000	.000000	.000000	.000000	.000000
0.5	.000013	.000003	.000001	.000000	.000000	.000000	.000000
0.6	.000052	.000016	.000005	.000001	.000000	.000000	.000000
0.7	.000166	.000057	.000020	.000007	.000003	.000001	.000000
0.8	.000441	.000171	.000068	.000027	.000011	.000004	.000002
0.9	.001025	.000442	.000193	.000085	.000038	.000017	.000008
1.0	.002138	.001008	.000481	.000233	.000114	.000056	.000028
1.2	.007210	.003940	.002176	.001215	.000685	.000391	.000225
1.4	.018805	.011533	.007138	.004459	.002811	.001788	.001147
1.6	.040490	.027217	.018437	.012587	.008659	.006003	.004192
1.8	.075176	.054398	.039615	.029037	.021420	.015901	.011878
2.0	.124150	.095366	.073634	.057153	.044595	.034978	.027575
2.2	.186637	.150511	.121872	.099098	.080921	.066357	.054640
2.4	.259986	.218167	.183650	.155102	.131432	.111747	.095327
2.6	.340324	.295044	.256389	.223360	.195092	.170849	.150010
2.8	.423365	.376986	.336259	.300494	.269063	.241407	.217033
3.0	.505118	.459769	.418985	.382336	.349401	.319789	.293141
3.2	.582362	.539715	.500575	.464710	.431866	.401791	.374242
3.4	.652848	.614036	.577794	.544025	.512599	.483372	.456196
3.6	.715299	.680940	.648375	.617595	.588553	.561182	.535402
3.8	.769263	.739547	.711018	.683718	.657652	.632803	.609138
4.0	.814913	.789713	.765248	.741585	.718759	.696781	.675649
4.2	.852839	.831821	.811215	.791099	.771519	.752504	.734068
4.4	.883873	.866584	.849490	.832665	.816160	.800010	.784238
4.6	.908941	.894886	.880884	.867003	.853292	.839787	.826515
4.8	.928973	.917657	.906309	.894988	.883737	.872591	.861574
5.0	.944835	.935798	.926682	.917537	.908399	.899299	.890260
5.2	.957302	.950133	.942863	.935533	.928175	.920813	.913468
5.4	.967039	.961383	.955620	.949783	.943899	.937988	.932067
5.6	.974606	.970163	.965617	.960994	.956315	.951598	.946857
5.8	.980463	.976984	.973412	.969766	.966063	.962318	.958541
6.0	.984982	.982266	.979467	.976601	.973681	.970719	.967724
6.4	.991132	.989485	.987777	.986019	.984218	.982381	.980515
6.8	.994756	.993760	.992723	.991649	.990545	.989415	.988261
7.2	.996887	.996285	.995655	.995001	.994326	.993632	.992921
7.6	.998142	.997776	.997393	.996994	.996581	.996154	.995717
8.0	.998883	.998660	.998426	.998182	.997928	.997665	.997395
8.4	.999323	.999187	.999043	.998892	.998736	.998573	.998406
8.8	.999586	.999502	.999413	.999320	.999223	.999122	.999017
9.2	.999745	.999693	.999637	.999579	.999518	.999455	.999389
9.6	.999841	.999808	.999774	.999737	.999699	.999659	.999617
10.0	.999900	.999879	.999857	.999834	.999810	.999784	.999758
11.0	.999967	.999961	.999953	.999946	.999937	.999929	.999920
12.0	.999989	.999986	.999984	.999981	.999978	.999975	.999972
13.0	1.00000	.999995	.999994	.999993	.999992	.999991	.999990
14.0		1.00000	1.00000	1.00000	1.00000	1.00000	1.00000

$\nu = 15$

Q\n	16	17	18	19	20	22	24
0.0	.000000	.000000	.000000	.000000	.000000	.000000	.000000
0.2	.000000	.000000	.000000	.000000	.000000	.000000	.000000
0.4	.000000	.000000	.000000	.000000	.000000	.000000	.000000
0.6	.000000	.000000	.000000	.000000	.000000	.000000	.000000
0.8	.000001	.000000	.000000	.000000	.000000	.000000	.000000
1.0	.000014	.000007	.000004	.000002	.000001	.000000	.000000
1.2	.000131	.000077	.000046	.000027	.000016	.000006	.000002
1.4	.000742	.000484	.000318	.000211	.000141	.000064	.000030
1.6	.002949	.002089	.001489	.001069	.000772	.000410	.000223
1.8	.008926	.006747	.005129	.003920	.003012	.001805	.001103
2.0	.021847	.017392	.013911	.011177	.009019	.005947	.003984
2.2	.045174	.037495	.031241	.026127	.021928	.015606	.011250
2.4	.081584	.070045	.060324	.052108	.045143	.034165	.026130
2.6	.132054	.116542	.103108	.091441	.081285	.064666	.051884
2.8	.195515	.176482	.159613	.144634	.131304	.108801	.090771
3.0	.269130	.247469	.227898	.210190	.194142	.166335	.143286
3.2	.348992	.325829	.304561	.285011	.267020	.235155	.207978
3.4	.430921	.407405	.385514	.365122	.346111	.311807	.281837
3.6	.511125	.488264	.466732	.446445	.427321	.392263	.361001
3.8	.586613	.565182	.544792	.525393	.506932	.472627	.441496
4.0	.655350	.635862	.617160	.599216	.582000	.549630	.519809
4.2	.716216	.698943	.682243	.666102	.650505	.620881	.593231
4.4	.768858	.753876	.739295	.725112	.711324	.684900	.659955
4.6	.813491	.800730	.788239	.776021	.764078	.741012	.719020
4.8	.850706	.840001	.829469	.819117	.808949	.789178	.770162
5.0	.881301	.872434	.863672	.855022	.846491	.829802	.813625
5.2	.906156	.898891	.891683	.884540	.877468	.863559	.849985
5.4	.926151	.920250	.914375	.908534	.902731	.891264	.880004
5.6	.942103	.937346	.932595	.927856	.923134	.913764	.904513
5.8	.954743	.950931	.947113	.943294	.939480	.931880	.924341
6.0	.964703	.961664	.958612	.955551	.952487	.946361	.940256
6.4	.978624	.976713	.974785	.972844	.970892	.966966	.963025
6.8	.987088	.985897	.984692	.983474	.982245	.979762	.977253
7.2	.992196	.991458	.990708	.989949	.989180	.987621	.986037
7.6	.995269	.994812	.994347	.993874	.993395	.992419	.991423
8.0	.997118	.996835	.996546	.996252	.995952	.995342	.994716
8.4	.998234	.998058	.997877	.997694	.997507	.997123	.996730
8.8	.998910	.998800	.998687	.998572	.998454	.998213	.997964
9.2	.999322	.999253	.999181	.999109	.999034	.998882	.998724
9.6	.999575	.999531	.999486	.999439	.999392	.999295	.999195
10.0	.999731	.999703	.999674	.999645	.999614	.999552	.999487
11.0	.999911	.999902	.999892	.999882	.999872	.999850	.999828
12.0	.999969	.999966	.999962	.999959	.999955	.999947	.999939
13.0	.999989	.999987	.999986	.999985	.999983	.999980	.999978
14.0	1.00000	1.00000	.999995	.999994	.999993	.999992	.999991
15.0			1.00000	1.00000	1.00000	1.00000	1.00000

$\nu = 15$

Q\n	26	28	30	32	34	36	38
0.0	.000000	.000000	.000000	.000000	.000000	.000000	.000000
0.2	.000000	.000000	.000000	.000000	.000000	.000000	.000000
0.4	.000000	.000000	.000000	.000000	.000000	.000000	.000000
0.6	.000000	.000000	.000000	.000000	.000000	.000000	.000000
0.8	.000000	.000000	.000000	.000000	.000000	.000000	.000000
1.0	.000000	.000000	.000000	.000000	.000000	.000000	.000000
1.2	.000001	.000000	.000000	.000000	.000000	.000000	.000000
1.4	.000014	.000007	.000004	.000002	.000001	.000001	.000000
1.6	.000124	.000070	.000040	.000024	.000014	.000009	.000005
1.8	.000686	.000433	.000278	.000181	.000120	.000080	.000054
2.0	.002708	.001866	.001302	.000919	.000656	.000474	.000345
2.2	.008209	.006057	.004516	.003400	.002584	.001980	.001530
2.4	.020181	.015731	.012367	.009800	.007824	.006291	.005092
2.6	.041961	.034189	.028051	.023165	.019247	.016084	.013513
2.8	.076216	.064380	.054689	.046702	.040080	.034558	.029927
3.0	.124063	.107938	.094334	.082796	.072961	.064537	.057288
3.2	.184687	.164634	.147290	.132222	.119078	.107566	.097446
3.4	.255557	.232428	.211998	.193888	.177781	.163409	.150544
3.6	.333049	.307985	.285448	.265127	.246753	.230096	.214958
3.8	.413192	.387406	.363865	.342325	.322576	.304429	.287721
4.0	.492305	.466903	.443407	.421638	.401436	.382658	.365174
4.2	.567411	.543280	.520706	.499564	.479739	.461126	.443629
4.4	.636408	.614174	.593169	.573311	.554521	.536727	.519859
4.6	.698064	.678098	.659073	.640937	.623642	.607139	.591380
4.8	.751891	.734344	.717499	.701325	.685793	.670873	.656535
5.0	.797967	.782826	.768192	.754052	.740391	.727191	.714434
5.2	.836761	.823894	.811385	.799230	.787422	.775954	.764816
5.4	.868971	.858177	.847628	.837325	.827270	.817458	.807886
5.6	.895402	.886445	.877649	.869021	.860563	.852276	.844159
5.8	.916880	.909513	.902249	.895095	.888054	.881131	.874326
6.0	.934191	.928178	.922226	.916343	.910533	.904802	.899150
6.4	.959081	.955144	.951222	.947321	.943446	.939601	.935788
6.8	.974728	.972192	.969653	.967115	.964581	.962055	.959539
7.2	.984435	.982819	.981194	.979562	.977926	.976289	.974652
7.6	.990412	.989388	.988354	.987312	.986264	.985212	.984156
8.0	.994079	.993431	.992775	.992112	.991443	.990769	.990092
8.4	.996328	.995918	.995501	.995079	.994653	.994222	.993788
8.8	.997710	.997450	.997185	.996916	.996643	.996368	.996089
9.2	.998562	.998397	.998228	.998056	.997881	.997704	.997525
9.6	.999091	.998985	.998876	.998766	.998653	.998539	.998424
10.0	.999421	.999352	.999282	.999211	.999138	.999064	.998989
11.0	.999806	.999782	.999758	.999733	.999708	.999682	.999656
12.0	.999931	.999923	.999914	.999905	.999896	.999887	.999877
13.0	.999974	.999971	.999968	.999965	.999961	.999958	.999954
14.0	.999990	.999989	.999987	.999986	.999985	.999983	.999982
15.0	1.00000	1.00000	.999995	.999994	.999994	.999993	.999993
16.0			1.00000	1.00000	1.00000	1.00000	1.00000

$\nu = 15$

Q\n	40	50	60	70	80	90	100
0.0	.000000	.000000	.000000	.000000	.000000	.000000	.000000
0.1	.000000	.000000	.000000	.000000	.000000	.000000	.000000
0.2	.000000	.000000	.000000	.000000	.000000	.000000	.000000
0.3	.000000	.000000	.000000	.000000	.000000	.000000	.000000
0.4	.000000	.000000	.000000	.000000	.000000	.000000	.000000
0.5	.000000	.000000	.000000	.000000	.000000	.000000	.000000
0.6	.000000	.000000	.000000	.000000	.000000	.000000	.000000
0.7	.000000	.000000	.000000	.000000	.000000	.000000	.000000
0.8	.000000	.000000	.000000	.000000	.000000	.000000	.000000
0.9	.000000	.000000	.000000	.000000	.000000	.000000	.000000
1.0	.000000	.000000	.000000	.000000	.000000	.000000	.000000
1.1	.000000	.000000	.000000	.000000	.000000	.000000	.000000
1.2	.000000	.000000	.000000	.000000	.000000	.000000	.000000
1.3	.000000	.000000	.000000	.000000	.000000	.000000	.000000
1.4	.000000	.000000	.000000	.000000	.000000	.000000	.000000
1.5	.000001	.000000	.000000	.000000	.000000	.000000	.000000
1.6	.000003	.000000	.000000	.000000	.000000	.000000	.000000
1.7	.000012	.000002	.000000	.000000	.000000	.000000	.000000
1.8	.000037	.000006	.000001	.000000	.000000	.000000	.000000
1.9	.000102	.000021	.000005	.000002	.000000	.000000	.000000
2.0	.000254	.000062	.000018	.000006	.000002	.000001	.000000
2.1	.000573	.000160	.000052	.000019	.000008	.000003	.000002
2.2	.001191	.000376	.000136	.000055	.000024	.000011	.000006
2.3	.002296	.000809	.000322	.000141	.000067	.000034	.000018
2.4	.004146	.001611	.000700	.000332	.000169	.000091	.000051
2.5	.007061	.002995	.001405	.000713	.000386	.000220	.000131
2.6	.011411	.005236	.002632	.001422	.000813	.000488	.000305
2.7	.017597	.008667	.004636	.002647	.001592	.000999	.000651
2.8	.026023	.013661	.007728	.004637	.002917	.001908	.001290
2.9	.037062	.020609	.012262	.007695	.005041	.003421	.002392
3.0	.051024	.029892	.018616	.012166	.008266	.005801	.004182
3.1	.068137	.041848	.027161	.018415	.012934	.009354	.006933
3.2	.088518	.056749	.038240	.026806	.019402	.014421	.010961
3.3	.112174	.074774	.052135	.037671	.028022	.021352	.016603
3.4	.138995	.096001	.069045	.051287	.039111	.030485	.024203
3.5	.168762	.120392	.089075	.067852	.052931	.042118	.034079
3.6	.201167	.147808	.112220	.087471	.069665	.056489	.046507
3.7	.235826	.178006	.138376	.110149	.089404	.073757	.061694
3.8	.272307	.210666	.167338	.135789	.112144	.093991	.079769
3.9	.310145	.245401	.198818	.164201	.137781	.117164	.100770
4.0	.348871	.281785	.232463	.195112	.166124	.143157	.124641
4.1	.388021	.319368	.267872	.228185	.196900	.171763	.151238
4.2	.427161	.357698	.304615	.263033	.229777	.202706	.180337
4.3	.465889	.396337	.342255	.299244	.264379	.235652	.211650
4.4	.503854	.434873	.380361	.336392	.300300	.270224	.244836
4.5	.540749	.472932	.418525	.374059	.337128	.306027	.279521
4.6	.576322	.510185	.456370	.411843	.374455	.342657	.315312
4.7	.610373	.546347	.493558	.449374	.411891	.379717	.351816
4.8	.642751	.581188	.529798	.486317	.449075	.416831	.388648
4.9	.673349	.614522	.564843	.522381	.485684	.453652	.425448

$\nu = 15$

Q\n	40	50	60	70	80	90	100
5.0	.702102	.646212	.598494	.557320	.521432	.489868	.461882
5.1	.728984	.676162	.630599	.590930	.556079	.525206	.497654
5.2	.753996	.704316	.661047	.623056	.589428	.559438	.532508
5.3	.777168	.730650	.689764	.653580	.621325	.592375	.566229
5.4	.798548	.755169	.716713	.682424	.651653	.623870	.598640
5.5	.818203	.777903	.741886	.709543	.680336	.653815	.629607
5.6	.836211	.798901	.765300	.734923	.707328	.682137	.659030
5.7	.852659	.818227	.786991	.758574	.732614	.708794	.686845
5.8	.867639	.835955	.807015	.780527	.756200	.733772	.713015
5.9	.881247	.852170	.825437	.800831	.778117	.757081	.737532
6.0	.893579	.866960	.842335	.819546	.798410	.778750	.760407
6.4	.932011	.913697	.896381	.880049	.864643	.850094	.836330
6.8	.957035	.944750	.932924	.921594	.910757	.900393	.890477
7.2	.973018	.964916	.957001	.949318	.941883	.934699	.927759
7.6	.983099	.977815	.972587	.967457	.962444	.957558	.952799
8.0	.989412	.985988	.982563	.979171	.975830	.972548	.969331
8.4	.993351	.991139	.988905	.986676	.984464	.982278	.980122
8.8	.995809	.994379	.992925	.991463	.990004	.988554	.987117
9.2	.997344	.996419	.995471	.994513	.993552	.992592	.991636
9.6	.998307	.997706	.997087	.996458	.995824	.995188	.994553
10.0	.998913	.998522	.998116	.997702	.997282	.996860	.996437
11.0	.999630	.999492	.999348	.999199	.999047	.998893	.998738
12.0	.999868	.999817	.999764	.999709	.999652	.999594	.999535
13.0	.999950	.999931	.999911	.999889	.999867	.999845	.999822
14.0	.999980	.999973	.999965	.999956	.999947	.999938	.999929
15.0	.999992	.999989	.999985	.999982	.999978	.999974	.999970
16.0	1.00000	1.00000	.999994	.999992	.999990	.999989	.999987
17.0			1.00000	1.00000	1.00000	.999995	.999994
18.0						1.00000	1.00000

$\nu = 16$

Q\n	2	3	4	5	6	7	8
0.0	.000000	.000000	.000000	.000000	.000000	.000000	.000000
0.1	.055653	.002759	.000133	.000006	.000000	.000000	.000000
0.2	.110698	.010958	.001053	.000101	.000010	.000001	.000000
0.3	.165317	.024465	.003516	.000503	.000072	.000011	.000002
0.4	.219076	.043024	.008206	.001557	.000297	.000057	.000011
0.5	.271711	.066301	.015713	.003705	.000878	.000210	.000051
0.6	.322977	.093884	.026511	.007446	.002101	.000598	.000172
0.7	.372654	.125298	.040935	.013298	.004338	.001428	.000475
0.8	.420545	.160022	.059179	.021756	.008027	.002987	.001123
0.9	.466483	.197503	.081294	.033254	.013646	.005643	.002357
1.0	.510328	.237168	.107193	.048133	.021670	.009825	.004497
1.2	.591340	.320781	.169384	.088805	.046630	.024628	.013112
1.4	.663066	.406519	.242878	.144005	.085420	.050898	.030530
1.6	.725428	.490595	.323766	.211962	.138689	.091041	.060080
1.8	.778724	.570012	.407811	.289374	.205040	.145589	.103793
2.0	.823537	.642656	.491047	.372119	.281390	.213014	.161721
2.2	.860649	.707269	.570199	.455985	.363673	.290119	.231886
2.4	.890951	.763339	.642885	.537247	.447604	.372759	.310771
2.6	.915371	.810950	.707650	.613015	.529324	.456634	.394103
2.8	.934818	.850608	.763863	.681369	.605798	.537924	.477630
3.0	.950135	.883084	.811552	.741303	.674977	.613677	.557713
3.2	.962083	.909282	.851214	.792578	.735761	.681943	.631648
3.4	.971319	.930138	.883632	.835525	.787849	.741725	.697745
3.6	.978405	.946552	.909735	.870841	.831537	.792809	.755234
3.8	.983803	.959338	.930480	.899428	.867510	.835553	.804078
4.0	.987891	.969214	.946783	.922254	.896664	.870683	.844755
4.2	.990970	.976783	.959472	.940270	.919973	.899114	.878057
4.4	.993281	.982548	.969267	.954349	.938397	.921826	.904928
4.6	.995007	.986915	.976775	.965258	.952816	.939768	.926343
4.8	.996294	.990208	.982497	.973651	.964008	.953810	.943234
5.0	.997251	.992682	.986837	.980071	.972636	.964714	.956440
5.2	.997961	.994536	.990116	.984958	.979249	.973125	.966690
5.4	.998487	.995922	.992585	.988663	.984294	.979579	.974597
5.6	.998877	.996957	.994440	.991464	.988128	.984510	.980667
5.8	.999166	.997728	.995831	.993575	.991034	.988263	.985307
6.0	.999379	.998303	.996873	.995165	.993231	.991113	.988844
6.4	.999655	.999049	.998237	.997258	.996140	.994906	.993575
6.8	.999807	.999465	.999002	.998439	.997792	.997074	.996295
7.2	.999891	.999696	.999431	.999106	.998731	.998312	.997855
7.6	.999938	.999826	.999673	.999485	.999266	.999020	.998752
8.0	.999964	.999900	.999810	.999700	.999572	.999427	.999269
8.4	.999979	.999941	.999889	.999824	.999748	.999662	.999568
8.8	.999988	.999965	.999934	.999896	.999851	.999799	.999743
9.2	.999993	.999979	.999961	.999938	.999910	.999879	.999845
9.6	1.00000	.999988	.999976	.999962	.999946	.999927	.999906
10.0		.999992	.999986	.999977	.999967	.999955	.999942
11.0		1.00000	1.00000	.999993	.999990	.999986	.999982
12.0				1.00000	1.00000	1.00000	.999994
13.0							1.00000

$\nu = 16$

Q\n	9	10	11	12	13	14	15
0.0	.000000	.000000	.000000	.000000	.000000	.000000	.000000
0.1	.000000	.000000	.000000	.000000	.000000	.000000	.000000
0.2	.000000	.000000	.000000	.000000	.000000	.000000	.000000
0.3	.000000	.000000	.000000	.000000	.000000	.000000	.000000
0.4	.000002	.000000	.000000	.000000	.000000	.000000	.000000
0.5	.000013	.000003	.000001	.000000	.000000	.000000	.000000
0.6	.000050	.000015	.000004	.000001	.000000	.000000	.000000
0.7	.000160	.000055	.000019	.000007	.000002	.000001	.000000
0.8	.000428	.000165	.000064	.000025	.000010	.000004	.000002
0.9	.000996	.000426	.000184	.000081	.000036	.000016	.000007
1.0	.002081	.000974	.000461	.000221	.000107	.000052	.000026
1.2	.007047	.003824	.002097	.001161	.000650	.000367	.000210
1.4	.018457	.011253	.006920	.004294	.002687	.001696	.001080
1.6	.039904	.026690	.017983	.012207	.008347	.005750	.003989
1.8	.074375	.053600	.038861	.028348	.020807	.015365	.011414
2.0	.123262	.094374	.072607	.056139	.043624	.034069	.026738
2.2	.185878	.149516	.120724	.097863	.079651	.065090	.053403
2.4	.259614	.217435	.182637	.153880	.130063	.110283	.093809
2.6	.340574	.294851	.255812	.222459	.193927	.169476	.148477
2.8	.424398	.377552	.336386	.300223	.268438	.240473	.215837
3.0	.506992	.461216	.420000	.382930	.349598	.319617	.292633
3.2	.585033	.542050	.502540	.466288	.433057	.402604	.374692
3.4	.656193	.617167	.580656	.546580	.514826	.485260	.457741
3.6	.719142	.684704	.651991	.621012	.591733	.564099	.538038
3.8	.773409	.743742	.715190	.687809	.661614	.636600	.612741
4.0	.819175	.794134	.769759	.746127	.723280	.701241	.680013
4.2	.857054	.836281	.815858	.795867	.776365	.757385	.738947
4.4	.887911	.870927	.854084	.837460	.821111	.805078	.789386
4.6	.912710	.898994	.885287	.871659	.858163	.844837	.831710
4.8	.932414	.921450	.910420	.899382	.888383	.877459	.866636
5.0	.947919	.939231	.930437	.921588	.912721	.903867	.895051
5.2	.960023	.953187	.946231	.939195	.932111	.925005	.917897
5.4	.969408	.964060	.958594	.953039	.947422	.941763	.936081
5.6	.976645	.972482	.968208	.963848	.959421	.954945	.950434
5.8	.982201	.978972	.975645	.972238	.968767	.965246	.961686
6.0	.986451	.983955	.981373	.978721	.976010	.973252	.970455
6.4	.992161	.990678	.989135	.987540	.985902	.984226	.982518
6.8	.995463	.994585	.993667	.992714	.991731	.990721	.989688
7.2	.997365	.996846	.996301	.995734	.995145	.994539	.993916
7.6	.998463	.998155	.997831	.997492	.997140	.996776	.996401
8.0	.999097	.998914	.998721	.998518	.998307	.998087	.997861
8.4	.999466	.999356	.999240	.999118	.998991	.998858	.998722
8.8	.999681	.999615	.999545	.999471	.999394	.999314	.999230
9.2	.999808	.999768	.999725	.999680	.999633	.999584	.999533
9.6	.999883	.999859	.999833	.999805	.999776	.999746	.999714
10.0	.999928	.999913	.999897	.999880	.999862	.999843	.999824
11.0	.999978	.999973	.999968	.999963	.999957	.999951	.999945
12.0	.999993	.999991	.999990	.999988	.999986	.999984	.999982
13.0	1.00000	1.00000	1.00000	1.00000	1.00000	.999994	.999994
						1.00000	1.00000

$\nu = 16$

Q\n	16	17	18	19	20	22	24
0.0	.000000	.000000	.000000	.000000	.000000	.000000	.000000
0.2	.000000	.000000	.000000	.000000	.000000	.000000	.000000
0.4	.000000	.000000	.000000	.000000	.000000	.000000	.000000
0.6	.000000	.000000	.000000	.000000	.000000	.000000	.000000
0.8	.000001	.000000	.000000	.000000	.000000	.000000	.000000
1.0	.000013	.000007	.000003	.000002	.000001	.000000	.000000
1.2	.000121	.000070	.000041	.000024	.000015	.000005	.000002
1.4	.000693	.000449	.000292	.000192	.000127	.000057	.000026
1.6	.002787	.001960	.001388	.000989	.000709	.000371	.000199
1.8	.008529	.006410	.004843	.003679	.002810	.001663	.001003
2.0	.021085	.016706	.013297	.010630	.008535	.005570	.003692
2.2	.043986	.036369	.030183	.025140	.021013	.014829	.010599
2.4	.080047	.068515	.058820	.050645	.043731	.032874	.024969
2.6	.130403	.114810	.101324	.089631	.079469	.062884	.050178
2.8	.194098	.174882	.157867	.142770	.129352	.106738	.088668
3.0	.268320	.246390	.226583	.208668	.192443	.164356	.141113
3.2	.349099	.325615	.304049	.284226	.265986	.233691	.206169
3.4	.432128	.408283	.386075	.365380	.346081	.311252	.280824
3.6	.513470	.490313	.468485	.447905	.428494	.392886	.361115
3.8	.590001	.568338	.547707	.528059	.509346	.474536	.442910
4.0	.659588	.639952	.621083	.602958	.585550	.552774	.522530
4.2	.721061	.703728	.686944	.670700	.654984	.625084	.597121
4.4	.774055	.759095	.744510	.730302	.716470	.689911	.664781
4.6	.818804	.806134	.793708	.781535	.769616	.746550	.724500
4.8	.855935	.845374	.834963	.824712	.814626	.794970	.776011
5.0	.886293	.877607	.869005	.860498	.852093	.835608	.819583
5.2	.910804	.903741	.896717	.889744	.882828	.869189	.855836
5.4	.930389	.924699	.919021	.913363	.907733	.896575	.885584
5.6	.945900	.941352	.936799	.932249	.927706	.918665	.909708
5.8	.958096	.954485	.950859	.947225	.943587	.936318	.929082
6.0	.967627	.964775	.961904	.959018	.956123	.950318	.944512
6.4	.980783	.979024	.977246	.975452	.973644	.969996	.966319
6.8	.988633	.987561	.986472	.985370	.984255	.981995	.979702
7.2	.993279	.992628	.991966	.991293	.990611	.989222	.987806
7.6	.996016	.995623	.995221	.994812	.994396	.993546	.992675
8.0	.997629	.997390	.997146	.996897	.996644	.996124	.995589
8.4	.998580	.998435	.998287	.998135	.997980	.997662	.997333
8.8	.999144	.999056	.998965	.998872	.998777	.998581	.998378
9.2	.999480	.999426	.999370	.999313	.999254	.999133	.999008
9.6	.999682	.999648	.999613	.999578	.999541	.999466	.999388
10.0	.999803	.999782	.999761	.999739	.999716	.999669	.999620
11.0	.999939	.999932	.999925	.999918	.999911	.999896	.999880
12.0	.999980	.999978	.999975	.999973	.999970	.999965	.999960
13.0	.999993	.999992	.999991	.999991	.999990	.999988	.999986
14.0	1.00000	1.00000	1.00000	1.00000	1.00000	1.00000	.999995
15.0							1.00000

$\nu = 16$

Q\n	26	28	30	32	34	36	38
0.0	.000000	.000000	.000000	.000000	.000000	.000000	.000000
0.2	.000000	.000000	.000000	.000000	.000000	.000000	.000000
0.4	.000000	.000000	.000000	.000000	.000000	.000000	.000000
0.6	.000000	.000000	.000000	.000000	.000000	.000000	.000000
0.8	.000000	.000000	.000000	.000000	.000000	.000000	.000000
1.0	.000000	.000000	.000000	.000000	.000000	.000000	.000000
1.2	.000001	.000000	.000000	.000000	.000000	.000000	.000000
1.4	.000012	.000006	.000003	.000001	.000001	.000000	.000000
1.6	.000108	.000060	.000034	.000020	.000012	.000007	.000004
1.8	.000615	.000384	.000243	.000156	.000102	.000067	.000045
2.0	.002483	.001692	.001168	.000816	.000576	.000411	.000297
2.2	.007667	.005607	.004144	.003093	.002330	.001770	.001355
2.4	.019151	.014822	.011570	.009103	.007217	.005761	.004630
2.6	.040355	.032695	.026673	.021902	.018094	.015034	.012559
2.8	.074123	.062333	.052711	.044810	.038281	.032856	.028324
3.0	.121766	.105570	.091939	.080406	.070601	.062224	.055036
3.2	.182607	.162346	.144847	.129670	.116453	.104899	.094762
3.4	.254151	.230688	.209978	.191638	.175342	.160818	.147833
3.6	.332699	.307217	.284307	.263655	.244991	.228081	.212723
3.8	.414133	.387901	.363943	.342017	.321913	.303441	.286437
4.0	.494601	.468780	.444876	.422715	.402139	.383007	.365191
4.2	.570966	.546488	.523561	.502067	.481895	.462943	.445117
4.4	.641012	.618530	.597259	.577122	.558047	.539964	.522808
4.6	.703442	.683338	.664148	.645826	.628329	.611611	.595630
4.8	.757749	.740173	.723264	.707000	.691356	.676307	.661825
5.0	.804029	.788952	.774348	.760209	.746523	.733277	.720456
5.2	.842790	.830063	.817661	.805583	.793827	.782388	.771259
5.4	.874781	.864182	.853798	.843634	.833691	.823971	.814470
5.6	.900859	.892133	.883543	.875095	.866795	.858646	.850649
5.8	.921898	.914782	.907746	.900799	.893946	.887193	.880540
6.0	.938723	.932967	.927253	.921590	.915985	.910441	.904962
6.4	.962627	.958929	.955235	.951550	.947880	.944229	.940600
6.8	.977386	.975053	.972710	.970360	.968007	.965656	.963309
7.2	.986368	.984913	.983444	.981965	.980479	.978987	.977492
7.6	.991787	.990885	.989972	.989048	.988116	.987178	.986235
8.0	.995042	.994485	.993918	.993344	.992762	.992175	.991583
8.4	.996996	.996651	.996300	.995943	.995580	.995214	.994843
8.8	.998170	.997956	.997738	.997516	.997290	.997060	.996828
9.2	.998878	.998745	.998609	.998470	.998329	.998185	.998039
9.6	.999307	.999224	.999139	.999052	.998963	.998872	.998780
10.0	.999569	.999517	.999463	.999408	.999352	.999294	.999236
11.0	.999864	.999847	.999829	.999811	.999793	.999774	.999755
12.0	.999955	.999949	.999943	.999937	.999930	.999924	.999917
13.0	.999984	.999982	.999980	.999978	.999975	.999973	.999971
14.0	.999994	.999993	.999993	.999992	.999991	.999990	.999989
15.0	1.00000	1.00000	1.00000	1.00000	1.00000	1.00000	1.00000

$\nu = 16$

Q\n	40	50	60	70	80	90	100
0.0	.000000	.000000	.000000	.000000	.000000	.000000	.000000
0.1	.000000	.000000	.000000	.000000	.000000	.000000	.000000
0.2	.000000	.000000	.000000	.000000	.000000	.000000	.000000
0.3	.000000	.000000	.000000	.000000	.000000	.000000	.000000
0.4	.000000	.000000	.000000	.000000	.000000	.000000	.000000
0.5	.000000	.000000	.000000	.000000	.000000	.000000	.000000
0.6	.000000	.000000	.000000	.000000	.000000	.000000	.000000
0.7	.000000	.000000	.000000	.000000	.000000	.000000	.000000
0.8	.000000	.000000	.000000	.000000	.000000	.000000	.000000
0.9	.000000	.000000	.000000	.000000	.000000	.000000	.000000
1.0	.000000	.000000	.000000	.000000	.000000	.000000	.000000
1.1	.000000	.000000	.000000	.000000	.000000	.000000	.000000
1.2	.000000	.000000	.000000	.000000	.000000	.000000	.000000
1.3	.000000	.000000	.000000	.000000	.000000	.000000	.000000
1.4	.000000	.000000	.000000	.000000	.000000	.000000	.000000
1.5	.000001	.000000	.000000	.000000	.000000	.000000	.000000
1.6	.000003	.000000	.000000	.000000	.000000	.000000	.000000
1.7	.000009	.000001	.000000	.000000	.000000	.000000	.000000
1.8	.000030	.000005	.000001	.000000	.000000	.000000	.000000
1.9	.000085	.000017	.000004	.000001	.000000	.000000	.000000
2.0	.000216	.000050	.000014	.000004	.000001	.000001	.000000
2.1	.000496	.000132	.000041	.000014	.000006	.000002	.000001
2.2	.001046	.000316	.000110	.000043	.000018	.000008	.000004
2.3	.002046	.000694	.000267	.000113	.000052	.000025	.000013
2.4	.003744	.001406	.000591	.000272	.000134	.000070	.000039
2.5	.006453	.002654	.001209	.000597	.000315	.000175	.000102
2.6	.010545	.004707	.002305	.001214	.000678	.000398	.000243
2.7	.016428	.007892	.004123	.002301	.001355	.000834	.000532
2.8	.024518	.012587	.006971	.004098	.002529	.001624	.001079
2.9	.035210	.019193	.011203	.006903	.004445	.002967	.002043
3.0	.048842	.028109	.017207	.011063	.007401	.005117	.003637
3.1	.065668	.039698	.025373	.016952	.011741	.008378	.006131
3.2	.085836	.054259	.036065	.024950	.017833	.013096	.009840
3.3	.109374	.072003	.049593	.035415	.026048	.019635	.015111
3.4	.136192	.093032	.066187	.048650	.036727	.028350	.022300
3.5	.166083	.117336	.085981	.064885	.050161	.039568	.031750
3.6	.198741	.144787	.108995	.084253	.066563	.053555	.043763
3.7	.233780	.175155	.135143	.106785	.086054	.070502	.058577
3.8	.270754	.208119	.164232	.132404	.108654	.090505	.076352
3.9	.309182	.243285	.195978	.160931	.134280	.113561	.097151
4.0	.348574	.280213	.230021	.192098	.162748	.139567	.120941
4.1	.388444	.318434	.265948	.225561	.193791	.168328	.147592
4.2	.428331	.357475	.303314	.260925	.227072	.199568	.176889
4.3	.467814	.396873	.341659	.297758	.262202	.232945	.208540
4.4	.506517	.436191	.380529	.335616	.298759	.268072	.242197
4.5	.544116	.475033	.419491	.374054	.336309	.304534	.277472
4.6	.580344	.513047	.458142	.412647	.374420	.341906	.313953
4.7	.614986	.549933	.496125	.451000	.412678	.379766	.351222
4.8	.647884	.585442	.533126	.488757	.450697	.417715	.388873
4.9	.678926	.619379	.568884	.525605	.488130	.455379	.426518

$\nu = 16$

Q\n	40	50	60	70	80	90	100
5.0	.708045	.651598	.603186	.561281	.524674	.492427	.463803
5.1	.735212	.681998	.635870	.595568	.560070	.528565	.500408
5.2	.760432	.710519	.666818	.628300	.594107	.563547	.536059
5.3	.783739	.737140	.695954	.659352	.626621	.597172	.570525
5.4	.805186	.761868	.723239	.688642	.657489	.629284	.603616
5.5	.824846	.784736	.748667	.716124	.686629	.659767	.635189
5.6	.842803	.805800	.772258	.741785	.713995	.688544	.665139
5.7	.859152	.825128	.794055	.765638	.739571	.715572	.693397
5.8	.873991	.842803	.814116	.787718	.763369	.740839	.719927
5.9	.887424	.858915	.832516	.808080	.785421	.764358	.744721
6.0	.899552	.873560	.849338	.826791	.805780	.786160	.767795
6.4	.936998	.919429	.902684	.886787	.871711	.857409	.843827
6.8	.960967	.949408	.938184	.927356	.916938	.906925	.897304
7.2	.975995	.968527	.961165	.953966	.946956	.940146	.933537
7.6	.985288	.980522	.975761	.971054	.966423	.961884	.957443
8.0	.990987	.987967	.984917	.981871	.978851	.975866	.972926
8.4	.994469	.992561	.990617	.988659	.986704	.984759	.982831
8.8	.996593	.995389	.994152	.992898	.991636	.990375	.989119
9.2	.997891	.997130	.996343	.995539	.994727	.993911	.993094
9.6	.998687	.998204	.997702	.997187	.996663	.996135	.995604
10.0	.999177	.998870	.998548	.998216	.997878	.997536	.997191
11.0	.999736	.999634	.999526	.999414	.999298	.999180	.999061
12.0	.999911	.999876	.999838	.999799	.999758	.999716	.999673
13.0	.999968	.999956	.999942	.999928	.999913	.999897	.999881
14.0	.999988	.999983	.999978	.999973	.999967	.999961	.999955
15.0	1.00000	.999994	.999991	.999989	.999987	.999985	.999982
16.0		1.00000	1.00000	1.00000	.999995	.999994	.999993
17.0					1.00000	1.00000	1.00000

$\nu = 17$

Q\n	2	3	4	5	6	7	8
0.0	.000000	.000000	.000000	.000000	.000000	.000000	.000000
0.1	.055722	.002760	.000132	.000006	.000000	.000000	.000000
0.2	.110801	.010958	.001051	.000100	.000010	.000001	.000000
0.3	.165473	.024467	.003507	.000500	.000071	.000010	.000002
0.4	.219287	.043031	.008187	.001548	.000294	.000056	.000011
0.5	.271980	.066317	.015681	.003684	.000869	.000207	.000050
0.6	.323306	.093916	.026462	.007406	.002080	.000589	.000169
0.7	.373046	.125356	.040869	.013232	.004297	.001406	.000465
0.8	.421002	.160116	.059099	.021657	.007956	.002944	.001100
0.9	.467006	.197645	.081208	.033118	.013534	.005568	.002312
1.0	.510919	.237373	.107111	.047960	.021509	.009706	.004418
1.2	.592066	.321151	.169360	.088581	.046357	.024381	.012917
1.4	.663919	.407103	.242996	.143796	.085058	.050502	.030165
1.6	.726393	.491427	.324117	.211876	.138320	.090533	.059534
1.8	.779776	.571103	.408474	.289537	.204798	.145077	.103133
2.0	.824647	.643993	.492071	.372646	.281433	.212666	.161095
2.2	.861786	.708815	.571593	.456955	.364142	.290120	.231496
2.4	.892083	.765042	.644621	.538687	.448597	.373269	.310825
2.6	.916471	.812748	.709665	.614902	.530876	.457754	.394763
2.8	.935861	.852438	.766077	.683632	.607877	.539677	.478982
3.0	.951104	.884888	.813875	.743842	.677497	.616012	.559756
3.2	.962965	.911012	.853557	.795280	.738603	.684754	.634302
3.4	.972109	.931756	.885919	.838279	.790880	.744871	.700876
3.6	.979101	.948032	.911904	.873549	.834627	.796138	.758681
3.8	.984408	.960667	.932488	.902009	.870544	.838923	.807675
4.0	.988410	.970386	.948602	.924653	.899553	.873971	.848352
4.2	.991411	.977802	.961089	.942449	.922654	.902227	.881532
4.4	.993651	.983423	.970682	.956291	.940829	.924699	.908189
4.6	.995315	.987657	.977996	.966961	.954981	.942363	.929331
4.8	.996549	.990831	.983538	.975123	.965904	.956111	.945915
5.0	.997459	.993201	.987715	.981328	.974273	.966722	.958805
5.2	.998131	.994965	.990849	.986019	.980646	.974855	.968745
5.4	.998625	.996274	.993193	.989551	.985473	.981052	.976360
5.6	.998988	.997244	.994941	.992201	.989115	.985751	.982163
5.8	.999255	.997961	.996241	.994183	.991853	.989300	.986566
6.0	.999451	.998491	.997207	.995663	.993906	.991973	.989894
6.4	.999701	.999171	.998456	.997588	.996592	.995488	.994291
6.8	.999836	.999543	.999143	.998655	.998090	.997461	.996774
7.2	.999909	.999746	.999522	.999246	.998925	.998566	.998172
7.6	.999949	.999858	.999731	.999575	.999392	.999186	.998959
8.0	.999972	.999920	.999848	.999758	.999653	.999534	.999403
8.4	.999984	.999954	.999913	.999861	.999801	.999732	.999656
8.8	.999991	.999974	.999950	.999920	.999884	.999844	.999799
9.2	.999995	.999985	.999971	.999953	.999932	.999909	.999882
9.6	1.00000	.999991	.999983	.999972	.999960	.999946	.999930
10.0		.999995	.999990	.999983	.999976	.999968	.999958
11.0		1.00000	1.00000	1.00000	.999993	.999991	.999988
12.0					1.00000	1.00000	1.00000

$\nu = 17$

Q\n	9	10	11	12	13	14	15
0.0	.000000	.000000	.000000	.000000	.000000	.000000	.000000
0.1	.000000	.000000	.000000	.000000	.000000	.000000	.000000
0.2	.000000	.000000	.000000	.000000	.000000	.000000	.000000
0.3	.000000	.000000	.000000	.000000	.000000	.000000	.000000
0.4	.000002	.000000	.000000	.000000	.000000	.000000	.000000
0.5	.000012	.000003	.000001	.000000	.000000	.000000	.000000
0.6	.000049	.000014	.000004	.000001	.000000	.000000	.000000
0.7	.000156	.000053	.000018	.000006	.000002	.000001	.000000
0.8	.000416	.000159	.000062	.000024	.000010	.000004	.000002
0.9	.000970	.000412	.000177	.000077	.000034	.000015	.000007
1.0	.002031	.000944	.000443	.000211	.000101	.000049	.000024
1.2	.006903	.003723	.002028	.001115	.000619	.000347	.000196
1.4	.018149	.011006	.006729	.004149	.002580	.001618	.001022
1.6	.039382	.026223	.017582	.011872	.008073	.005529	.003812
1.8	.073658	.052887	.038189	.027737	.020265	.014892	.011007
2.0	.122462	.093483	.071685	.055230	.042757	.033260	.025995
2.2	.185190	.148616	.119687	.096750	.078508	.063952	.052295
2.4	.259271	.216767	.181715	.152771	.128821	.108958	.092438
2.6	.340792	.294667	.255279	.221634	.192864	.168224	.147081
2.8	.425323	.378055	.336491	.299965	.267858	.239613	.214738
3.0	.508679	.462517	.420910	.383458	.349764	.319447	.292156
3.2	.587442	.544158	.504314	.467713	.434130	.403331	.375088
3.4	.659210	.619997	.583245	.548895	.516843	.486969	.459139
3.6	.722605	.688103	.655264	.624109	.594620	.566750	.540434
3.8	.777139	.747527	.718962	.691514	.665210	.640050	.616018
4.0	.822999	.798113	.773829	.750233	.727377	.705289	.683979
4.2	.860823	.840281	.820033	.800167	.780744	.761804	.743373
4.4	.891507	.874807	.858199	.841766	.825569	.809651	.794042
4.6	.916050	.902646	.889213	.875823	.862530	.849375	.836391
4.8	.935447	.924805	.914067	.903293	.892529	.881813	.871174
5.0	.950622	.942249	.933750	.925172	.916556	.907931	.899323
5.2	.962392	.955855	.949183	.942415	.935582	.928711	.921822
5.4	.971456	.966384	.961183	.955882	.950507	.945079	.939615
5.6	.978395	.974480	.970448	.966322	.962122	.957864	.953562
5.8	.983681	.980672	.977561	.974365	.971101	.967780	.964414
6.0	.987692	.985387	.982995	.980530	.978004	.975427	.972807
6.4	.993016	.991672	.990270	.988817	.987319	.985782	.984213
6.8	.996039	.995260	.994443	.993592	.992711	.991804	.990873
7.2	.997748	.997297	.996822	.996326	.995810	.995276	.994727
7.6	.998714	.998453	.998176	.997887	.997584	.997271	.996948
8.0	.999261	.999109	.998948	.998778	.998601	.998417	.998226
8.4	.999573	.999484	.999389	.999289	.999185	.999076	.998963
8.8	.999751	.999698	.999642	.999584	.999522	.999457	.999390
9.2	.999853	.999822	.999789	.999754	.999717	.999678	.999638
9.6	.999913	.999894	.999874	.999853	.999831	.999808	.999784
10.0	.999948	.999937	.999925	.999912	.999898	.999884	.999870
11.0	.999985	.999982	.999978	.999974	.999970	.999966	.999962
12.0	1.00000	.999994	.999993	.999992	.999991	.999989	.999988
13.0		1.00000	1.00000	1.00000	1.00000	1.00000	1.00000

$\nu = 17$

Q\n	16	17	18	19	20	22	24
0.0	.000000	.000000	.000000	.000000	.000000	.000000	.000000
0.2	.000000	.000000	.000000	.000000	.000000	.000000	.000000
0.4	.000000	.000000	.000000	.000000	.000000	.000000	.000000
0.6	.000000	.000000	.000000	.000000	.000000	.000000	.000000
0.8	.000001	.000000	.000000	.000000	.000000	.000000	.000000
1.0	.000012	.000006	.000003	.000002	.000001	.000000	.000000
1.2	.000112	.000065	.000038	.000022	.000013	.000005	.000002
1.4	.000651	.000418	.000271	.000176	.000116	.000051	.000023
1.6	.002647	.001850	.001301	.000921	.000656	.000338	.000178
1.8	.008182	.006116	.004596	.003472	.002636	.001542	.000919
2.0	.020412	.016101	.012757	.010152	.008112	.005243	.003441
2.2	.042925	.035365	.029242	.024265	.020204	.014147	.010031
2.4	.078661	.067137	.057469	.049334	.042468	.031724	.023941
2.6	.128902	.113237	.099706	.087992	.077828	.061279	.048647
2.8	.192798	.173418	.156270	.141069	.127571	.104861	.086759
3.0	.267567	.245392	.225369	.207267	.190879	.162540	.139123
3.2	.349181	.325403	.303565	.283492	.265023	.232335	.204497
3.4	.433218	.409071	.386572	.365598	.346035	.310723	.279874
3.6	.515602	.492176	.470077	.449228	.429553	.393440	.361200
3.8	.593086	.571215	.550365	.530490	.511547	.476274	.444194
4.0	.663446	.643679	.624663	.606375	.588794	.555649	.525020
4.2	.725464	.708082	.691228	.674895	.659076	.628930	.600686
4.4	.778764	.763831	.749251	.735027	.721160	.694489	.669198
4.6	.823600	.811020	.798663	.786537	.774649	.751596	.729505
4.8	.860634	.850210	.839918	.829767	.819764	.800227	.781334
5.0	.890754	.882238	.873790	.865420	.857137	.840854	.824980
5.2	.914933	.908058	.901209	.894396	.887627	.874247	.861109
5.4	.934129	.928633	.923138	.917653	.912184	.901319	.890582
5.6	.949228	.944871	.940501	.936124	.931747	.923013	.914332
5.8	.961012	.957583	.954132	.950666	.947190	.940227	.933271
6.0	.970151	.967466	.964758	.962030	.959289	.953776	.948243
6.4	.982614	.980990	.979344	.977680	.975999	.972599	.969161
6.8	.989921	.988950	.987963	.986960	.985945	.983880	.981777
7.2	.994163	.993587	.992999	.992400	.991791	.990549	.989277
7.6	.996615	.996273	.995924	.995568	.995204	.994460	.993695
8.0	.998029	.997827	.997619	.997407	.997191	.996746	.996286
8.4	.998846	.998726	.998603	.998476	.998347	.998080	.997804
8.8	.999320	.999249	.999175	.999099	.999022	.998861	.998695
9.2	.999597	.999554	.999509	.999464	.999417	.999320	.999219
9.6	.999759	.999733	.999706	.999678	.999650	.999591	.999530
10.0	.999854	.999838	.999822	.999805	.999788	.999752	.999714
11.0	.999957	.999952	.999947	.999942	.999937	.999926	.999915
12.0	.999987	.999985	.999984	.999982	.999980	.999977	.999973
13.0	1.00000	1.00000	.999995	.999994	.999993	.999992	.999991
14.0			1.00000	1.00000	1.00000	1.00000	1.00000

$\nu = 17$

Q\n	26	28	30	32	34	36	38
0.0	.000000	.000000	.000000	.000000	.000000	.000000	.000000
0.2	.000000	.000000	.000000	.000000	.000000	.000000	.000000
0.4	.000000	.000000	.000000	.000000	.000000	.000000	.000000
0.6	.000000	.000000	.000000	.000000	.000000	.000000	.000000
0.8	.000000	.000000	.000000	.000000	.000000	.000000	.000000
1.0	.000000	.000000	.000000	.000000	.000000	.000000	.000000
1.2	.000001	.000000	.000000	.000000	.000000	.000000	.000000
1.4	.000011	.000005	.000002	.000001	.000001	.000000	.000000
1.6	.000096	.000053	.000029	.000017	.000010	.000006	.000003
1.8	.000557	.000343	.000215	.000136	.000088	.000057	.000038
2.0	.002291	.001546	.001056	.000730	.000511	.000361	.000257
2.2	.007196	.005220	.003826	.002832	.002115	.001594	.001210
2.4	.018241	.014024	.010874	.008499	.006692	.005307	.004236
2.6	.038919	.031364	.025450	.020785	.017079	.014114	.011727
2.8	.072229	.060485	.050932	.043111	.036672	.031339	.026900
3.0	.119666	.103411	.089759	.078236	.068462	.060133	.053005
3.2	.180688	.160239	.142602	.127328	.114048	.102460	.092310
3.4	.252839	.229070	.208104	.189552	.173085	.158424	.145332
3.6	.332354	.306487	.283232	.262276	.243344	.226201	.210640
3.8	.414981	.388336	.363991	.341708	.321274	.302501	.285222
4.0	.496700	.470492	.446212	.423688	.402767	.383306	.365179
4.2	.574226	.549431	.526180	.504362	.483870	.464605	.446474
4.4	.645234	.622530	.601018	.580628	.561292	.542944	.525522
4.6	.708364	.688143	.668808	.650321	.632642	.615730	.599547
4.8	.763093	.745500	.728543	.712206	.696467	.681305	.666695
5.0	.809535	.794530	.779965	.765836	.752137	.738858	.725986
5.2	.848239	.835652	.823360	.811364	.799667	.788264	.777153
5.4	.880001	.869592	.859371	.849343	.839515	.829888	.820463
5.6	.905730	.897225	.888832	.880559	.872414	.864400	.856522
5.8	.926345	.919465	.912646	.905896	.899223	.892632	.886129
6.0	.942711	.937193	.931701	.926245	.920831	.915466	.910153
6.4	.965696	.962216	.958728	.955241	.951759	.948288	.944831
6.8	.979646	.977493	.975324	.973143	.970954	.968761	.966566
7.2	.987981	.986665	.985333	.983988	.982633	.981269	.979899
7.6	.992912	.992114	.991303	.990480	.989649	.988809	.987963
8.0	.995814	.995332	.994840	.994339	.993832	.993318	.992798
8.4	.997520	.997228	.996930	.996626	.996316	.996002	.995684
8.8	.998523	.998346	.998165	.997980	.997792	.997600	.997405
9.2	.999115	.999008	.998897	.998784	.998669	.998551	.998432
9.6	.999466	.999401	.999333	.999264	.999193	.999120	.999047
10.0	.999675	.999635	.999594	.999551	.999507	.999462	.999417
11.0	.999903	.999891	.999878	.999865	.999851	.999838	.999823
12.0	.999969	.999965	.999961	.999957	.999953	.999948	.999944
13.0	.999990	.999989	.999987	.999986	.999984	.999983	.999981
14.0	1.00000	1.00000	1.00000	.999995	.999994	.999994	.999993
15.0				1.00000	1.00000	1.00000	1.00000

$\nu = 17$

Q\n	40	50	60	70	80	90	100
0.0	.000000	.000000	.000000	.000000	.000000	.000000	.000000
0.1	.000000	.000000	.000000	.000000	.000000	.000000	.000000
0.2	.000000	.000000	.000000	.000000	.000000	.000000	.000000
0.3	.000000	.000000	.000000	.000000	.000000	.000000	.000000
0.4	.000000	.000000	.000000	.000000	.000000	.000000	.000000
0.5	.000000	.000000	.000000	.000000	.000000	.000000	.000000
0.6	.000000	.000000	.000000	.000000	.000000	.000000	.000000
0.7	.000000	.000000	.000000	.000000	.000000	.000000	.000000
0.8	.000000	.000000	.000000	.000000	.000000	.000000	.000000
0.9	.000000	.000000	.000000	.000000	.000000	.000000	.000000
1.0	.000000	.000000	.000000	.000000	.000000	.000000	.000000
1.1	.000000	.000000	.000000	.000000	.000000	.000000	.000000
1.2	.000000	.000000	.000000	.000000	.000000	.000000	.000000
1.3	.000000	.000000	.000000	.000000	.000000	.000000	.000000
1.4	.000000	.000000	.000000	.000000	.000000	.000000	.000000
1.5	.000000	.000000	.000000	.000000	.000000	.000000	.000000
1.6	.000002	.000000	.000000	.000000	.000000	.000000	.000000
1.7	.000008	.000001	.000000	.000000	.000000	.000000	.000000
1.8	.000025	.000004	.000001	.000000	.000000	.000000	.000000
1.9	.000072	.000013	.000003	.000001	.000000	.000000	.000000
2.0	.000185	.000041	.000011	.000003	.000001	.000000	.000000
2.1	.000433	.000110	.000033	.000011	.000004	.000002	.000001
2.2	.000926	.000269	.000090	.000034	.000014	.000006	.000003
2.3	.001837	.000601	.000223	.000091	.000041	.000019	.000010
2.4	.003403	.001236	.000504	.000225	.000108	.000055	.000030
2.5	.005932	.002369	.001049	.000505	.000259	.000141	.000080
2.6	.009794	.004257	.002032	.001045	.000571	.000328	.000196
2.7	.015402	.007226	.003690	.002015	.001162	.000701	.000440
2.8	.023185	.011653	.006322	.003645	.002208	.001394	.000910
2.9	.033557	.017948	.010286	.006228	.003943	.002591	.001757
3.0	.046879	.026526	.015974	.010109	.006662	.004541	.003184
3.1	.063432	.037771	.023790	.015671	.010708	.007544	.005453
3.2	.083391	.052011	.034120	.023308	.016459	.011948	.008878
3.3	.106808	.069483	.047302	.033399	.024299	.018127	.013812
3.4	.133610	.090316	.063592	.046273	.034594	.026455	.020624
3.5	.163603	.114522	.083152	.062189	.047661	.037282	.029676
3.6	.196485	.141992	.106028	.081309	.063741	.050902	.041295
3.7	.231866	.172504	.132152	.103689	.082985	.067535	.055751
3.8	.269291	.205738	.161344	.129270	.105437	.087304	.073229
3.9	.308263	.241296	.193322	.157887	.131032	.110231	.093820
4.0	.348272	.278724	.227725	.189276	.159599	.136231	.117513
4.1	.388809	.317536	.264129	.223092	.190877	.165118	.144195
4.2	.429393	.357237	.302071	.258929	.224523	.196619	.173658
4.3	.469578	.397342	.341072	.296338	.260138	.230388	.205611
4.4	.508967	.437391	.380654	.334856	.297284	.266026	.239698
4.5	.547219	.476963	.420361	.374014	.335507	.303100	.275517
4.6	.584052	.515688	.459767	.413365	.374352	.341164	.312640
4.7	.619241	.553247	.498493	.452489	.413379	.379775	.350626
4.8	.652616	.589376	.536205	.491008	.452182	.418507	.389045
4.9	.684062	.623870	.572627	.528590	.490390	.456965	.427486

$\nu = 17$

Q\n	40	50	60	70	80	90	100
5.0	.713508	.656574	.607533	.564954	.527679	.494793	.465571
5.1	.740928	.687382	.640751	.599871	.563775	.531681	.502960
5.2	.766328	.716235	.672157	.633163	.598454	.567366	.539359
5.3	.789744	.743109	.701672	.664701	.631539	.601633	.574521
5.4	.811237	.768016	.729258	.694397	.662903	.634316	.608247
5.5	.830885	.790993	.754908	.722205	.692460	.665294	.640382
5.6	.848779	.812100	.778648	.748113	.720161	.694486	.670815
5.7	.865020	.831412	.800524	.772137	.745994	.721848	.699477
5.8	.879714	.849020	.820603	.794318	.769972	.747369	.726329
5.9	.892969	.865020	.838963	.814715	.792133	.771065	.751366
6.0	.904896	.879514	.855696	.833402	.812534	.792974	.774607
6.4	.941391	.924524	.908325	.892853	.878105	.864054	.850661
6.8	.964372	.953480	.942818	.932463	.922445	.912772	.903438
7.2	.978525	.971627	.964768	.958014	.951399	.944940	.938644
7.6	.987112	.982800	.978455	.974127	.969844	.965623	.961473
8.0	.992274	.989600	.986875	.984134	.981397	.978679	.975987
8.4	.995362	.993711	.992011	.990287	.988553	.986819	.985092
8.8	.997207	.996188	.995131	.994050	.992957	.991857	.990755
9.2	.998310	.997680	.997023	.996346	.995658	.994961	.994261
9.6	.998972	.998581	.998171	.997747	.997313	.996873	.996428
10.0	.999370	.999127	.998871	.998604	.998330	.998051	.997768
11.0	.999809	.999733	.999652	.999566	.999478	.999387	.999295
12.0	.999939	.999914	.999888	.999859	.999830	.999799	.999768
13.0	.999980	.999971	.999962	.999952	.999942	.999931	.999920
14.0	.999993	.999990	.999986	.999983	.999979	.999975	.999971
15.0	1.00000	1.00000	.999995	.999994	.999992	.999991	.999989
16.0			1.00000	1.00000	1.00000	1.00000	1.00000

$\nu = 18$

Q\n	2	3	4	5	6	7	8
0.0	.000000	.000000	.000000	.000000	.000000	.000000	.000000
0.1	.055782	.002760	.000132	.000006	.000000	.000000	.000000
0.2	.110892	.010959	.001048	.000100	.000009	.000001	.000000
0.3	.165613	.024469	.003500	.000497	.000071	.000010	.000001
0.4	.219476	.043037	.008171	.001540	.000291	.000055	.000011
0.5	.272219	.066331	.015653	.003665	.000860	.000204	.000049
0.6	.323599	.093945	.026418	.007370	.002061	.000581	.000165
0.7	.373394	.125407	.040810	.013173	.004260	.001387	.000456
0.8	.421408	.160200	.059028	.021569	.007893	.002907	.001080
0.9	.467472	.197772	.081130	.032997	.013435	.005502	.002273
1.0	.511446	.237555	.107037	.047806	.021365	.009599	.004347
1.2	.592713	.321481	.169337	.088380	.046113	.024161	.012743
1.4	.664679	.407624	.243100	.143608	.084732	.050147	.029838
1.6	.727252	.492170	.324430	.211797	.137987	.090075	.059044
1.8	.780713	.572078	.409066	.289681	.204578	.144615	.102537
2.0	.825637	.645187	.492987	.373116	.281467	.212348	.160527
2.2	.862798	.710196	.572842	.457824	.364561	.290115	.231139
2.4	.893091	.766564	.646177	.539982	.449490	.373725	.310867
2.6	.917448	.814355	.711473	.616599	.532274	.458761	.395355
2.8	.936787	.854073	.768062	.685667	.609751	.541259	.480203
3.0	.951962	.886498	.815955	.746125	.679770	.618123	.561604
3.2	.963746	.912552	.855653	.797707	.741164	.687294	.636705
3.4	.972807	.933193	.887961	.840748	.793608	.747710	.703710
3.6	.979714	.949344	.913837	.875971	.837402	.799138	.761796
3.8	.984939	.961841	.934271	.904313	.873263	.841952	.810919
4.0	.988864	.971418	.950212	.926786	.902134	.876919	.851588
4.2	.991794	.978696	.962515	.944380	.925040	.905008	.884647
4.4	.993971	.984186	.971924	.958005	.942984	.927255	.911100
4.6	.995581	.988301	.979063	.968456	.956890	.944661	.931986
4.8	.996767	.991369	.984442	.976408	.967567	.958138	.948287
5.0	.997637	.993647	.988473	.982419	.975701	.968482	.960885
5.2	.998275	.995331	.991479	.986935	.981856	.976361	.970541
5.4	.998741	.996572	.993711	.990312	.986488	.982325	.977891
5.6	.999081	.997485	.995364	.992828	.989958	.986817	.983454
5.8	.999330	.998155	.996585	.994697	.992548	.990185	.987643
6.0	.999510	.998647	.997485	.996081	.994475	.992702	.990786
6.4	.999738	.999271	.998635	.997860	.996967	.995972	.994890
6.8	.999859	.999605	.999257	.998830	.998333	.997777	.997168
7.2	.999924	.999785	.999594	.999357	.999081	.998770	.998427
7.6	.999958	.999882	.999776	.999645	.999490	.999316	.999123
8.0	.999977	.999935	.999876	.999802	.999716	.999617	.999508
8.4	.999987	.999964	.999931	.999889	.999840	.999784	.999722
8.8	.999993	.999979	.999961	.999937	.999909	.999877	.999842
9.2	1.00000	.999988	.999978	.999964	.999948	.999930	.999909
9.6		.999993	.999987	.999979	.999970	.999959	.999947
10.0		1.00000	.999992	.999988	.999982	.999976	.999969
11.0			1.00000	1.00000	1.00000	.999993	.999992
12.0						1.00000	1.00000

ν = 18

Q\n	9	10	11	12	13	14	15
0.0	.000000	.000000	.000000	.000000	.000000	.000000	.000000
0.1	.000000	.000000	.000000	.000000	.000000	.000000	.000000
0.2	.000000	.000000	.000000	.000000	.000000	.000000	.000000
0.3	.000000	.000000	.000000	.000000	.000000	.000000	.000000
0.4	.000002	.000000	.000000	.000000	.000000	.000000	.000000
0.5	.000012	.000003	.000001	.000000	.000000	.000000	.000000
0.6	.000048	.000014	.000004	.000001	.000000	.000000	.000000
0.7	.000152	.000051	.000017	.000006	.000002	.000001	.000000
0.8	.000406	.000154	.000059	.000023	.000009	.000004	.000001
0.9	.000948	.000400	.000170	.000073	.000032	.000014	.000006
1.0	.001987	.000917	.000428	.000202	.000096	.000046	.000023
1.2	.006775	.003634	.001967	.001075	.000593	.000330	.000185
1.4	.017874	.010786	.006561	.004022	.002486	.001549	.000972
1.6	.038914	.025805	.017225	.011575	.007831	.005334	.003658
1.8	.073012	.052246	.037586	.027191	.019781	.014472	.010647
2.0	.121737	.092677	.070854	.054413	.041978	.032535	.025331
2.2	.184563	.147798	.118747	.095742	.077475	.062925	.051297
2.4	.258954	.216156	.180874	.151759	.127691	.107753	.091194
2.6	.340982	.294492	.254787	.220876	.191888	.167077	.145805
2.8	.426156	.378504	.336578	.299721	.267320	.238819	.213725
3.0	.510206	.463695	.421731	.383930	.349905	.319281	.291708
3.2	.589628	.546072	.505925	.469005	.435101	.403987	.375440
3.4	.661947	.622568	.585601	.551002	.518681	.488526	.460411
3.6	.725744	.691191	.658241	.626931	.597253	.569169	.542623
3.8	.780513	.750958	.722390	.694887	.668488	.643200	.619015
4.0	.826449	.801712	.777519	.753964	.731106	.708980	.687601
4.2	.864212	.843888	.823807	.804063	.784720	.765825	.747406
4.4	.894728	.878292	.861906	.845656	.829605	.813799	.798273
4.6	.919029	.905914	.892736	.879568	.866466	.853475	.840627
4.8	.938138	.927792	.917323	.906793	.896249	.885729	.875263
5.0	.953006	.944921	.936691	.928364	.919978	.911566	.903154
5.2	.964469	.958203	.951789	.945265	.938663	.932008	.925321
5.4	.973240	.968416	.963453	.958383	.953228	.948010	.942746
5.6	.979909	.976215	.972399	.968484	.964488	.960427	.956315
5.8	.984952	.982137	.979217	.976210	.973130	.969989	.966798
6.0	.988750	.986612	.984387	.982087	.979725	.977308	.974846
6.4	.993733	.992509	.991228	.989897	.988522	.987107	.985659
6.8	.996514	.995818	.995086	.994322	.993528	.992709	.991866
7.2	.998058	.997663	.997246	.996809	.996354	.995882	.995394
7.6	.998914	.998690	.998452	.998202	.997941	.997670	.997389
8.0	.999389	.999262	.999126	.998983	.998833	.998677	.998514
8.4	.999654	.999581	.999503	.999421	.999335	.999244	.999150
8.8	.999803	.999761	.999716	.999668	.999618	.999566	.999511
9.2	.999886	.999862	.999836	.999808	.999779	.999748	.999716
9.6	.999934	.999920	.999905	.999888	.999871	.999853	.999834
10.0	.999961	.999953	.999944	.999934	.999924	.999913	.999902
11.0	.999989	.999987	.999985	.999982	.999979	.999976	.999973
12.0	1.00000	1.00000	1.00000	.999995	.999994	.999993	.999992
13.0				1.00000	1.00000	1.00000	1.00000

ν = 18

Q\n	16	17	18	19	20	22	24
0.0	.000000	.000000	.000000	.000000	.000000	.000000	.000000
0.2	.000000	.000000	.000000	.000000	.000000	.000000	.000000
0.4	.000000	.000000	.000000	.000000	.000000	.000000	.000000
0.6	.000000	.000000	.000000	.000000	.000000	.000000	.000000
0.8	.000001	.000000	.000000	.000000	.000000	.000000	.000000
1.0	.000011	.000005	.000003	.000001	.000001	.000000	.000000
1.2	.000105	.000060	.000035	.000020	.000012	.000004	.000002
1.4	.000615	.000392	.000252	.000163	.000106	.000046	.000020
1.6	.002525	.001754	.001226	.000862	.000610	.000311	.000162
1.8	.007876	.005858	.004379	.003291	.002485	.001438	.000847
2.0	.019812	.015564	.012279	.009729	.007741	.004958	.003224
2.2	.041970	.034464	.028399	.023483	.019483	.013543	.009530
2.4	.077405	.065890	.056248	.048151	.041331	.030693	.023023
2.6	.127532	.111802	.098233	.086501	.076336	.059825	.047265
2.8	.191603	.172073	.154804	.139509	.125940	.103146	.085019
3.0	.266866	.244466	.224245	.205971	.189436	.160866	.137292
3.2	.349244	.325196	.303107	.282803	.264125	.231074	.202947
3.4	.434206	.409783	.387016	.365786	.345979	.310221	.278982
3.6	.517550	.493877	.471530	.450434	.430516	.393936	.361261
3.8	.595908	.573849	.552799	.532718	.513564	.477865	.445366
4.0	.666974	.647092	.627943	.609509	.591771	.558290	.527307
4.2	.729483	.712063	.695149	.678740	.662828	.632464	.603966
4.4	.783051	.768149	.753579	.739347	.725455	.698690	.673260
4.6	.827949	.815459	.803171	.791097	.779243	.756212	.734095
4.8	.864876	.854586	.844409	.834355	.824435	.805020	.786199
5.0	.894762	.886408	.878106	.869867	.861701	.845616	.829892
5.2	.918621	.911923	.905238	.898576	.891947	.878815	.865884
5.4	.937450	.932134	.926809	.921484	.916166	.905577	.895083
5.6	.952163	.947982	.943779	.939563	.935339	.926890	.918468
5.8	.963567	.960302	.957010	.953698	.950371	.943689	.936994
6.0	.972344	.969810	.967249	.964665	.962062	.956816	.951535
6.4	.984180	.982675	.981146	.979597	.978030	.974852	.971628
6.8	.991003	.990120	.989220	.988305	.987376	.985483	.983548
7.2	.994893	.994380	.993854	.993319	.992773	.991656	.990509
7.6	.997099	.996801	.996496	.996183	.995864	.995209	.994533
8.0	.998347	.998174	.997996	.997814	.997628	.997245	.996847
8.4	.999053	.998953	.998849	.998743	.998634	.998410	.998176
8.8	.999454	.999396	.999335	.999273	.999209	.999077	.998940
9.2	.999683	.999649	.999613	.999577	.999539	.999461	.999380
9.6	.999815	.999794	.999773	.999752	.999729	.999683	.999635
10.0	.999891	.999879	.999866	.999853	.999840	.999812	.999783
11.0	.999970	.999966	.999963	.999959	.999955	.999947	.999939
12.0	.999991	.999990	.999989	.999988	.999987	.999984	.999982
13.0	1.00000	1.00000	1.00000	1.00000	1.00000	1.00000	.999994
14.0							1.00000

$\nu = 18$

Q\n	26	28	30	32	34	36	38
0.0	.000000	.000000	.000000	.000000	.000000	.000000	.000000
0.2	.000000	.000000	.000000	.000000	.000000	.000000	.000000
0.4	.000000	.000000	.000000	.000000	.000000	.000000	.000000
0.6	.000000	.000000	.000000	.000000	.000000	.000000	.000000
0.8	.000000	.000000	.000000	.000000	.000000	.000000	.000000
1.0	.000000	.000000	.000000	.000000	.000000	.000000	.000000
1.2	.000001	.000000	.000000	.000000	.000000	.000000	.000000
1.4	.000009	.000004	.000002	.000001	.000000	.000000	.000000
1.6	.000086	.000046	.000026	.000014	.000008	.000005	.000003
1.8	.000508	.000309	.000191	.000120	.000076	.000049	.000032
2.0	.002126	.001421	.000962	.000659	.000456	.000319	.000226
2.2	.006785	.004884	.003552	.002608	.001933	.001445	.001089
2.4	.017434	.013320	.010263	.007970	.006236	.004913	.003897
2.6	.037627	.030172	.024359	.019792	.016180	.013302	.010996
2.8	.070507	.058810	.049322	.041580	.035225	.029979	.025627
3.0	.117738	.101432	.087766	.076256	.066515	.058234	.051165
3.2	.178912	.158292	.140530	.125170	.111837	.100220	.090063
3.4	.251613	.227561	.206360	.187615	.170991	.156205	.143017
3.6	.332019	.305793	.282220	.260981	.241802	.224442	.208696
3.8	.415749	.388721	.364018	.341402	.320662	.301608	.284074
4.0	.498628	.472064	.447434	.424574	.403330	.383563	.365148
4.2	.577229	.552143	.528595	.506478	.485689	.466131	.447717
4.4	.649121	.626217	.604486	.583865	.564290	.545698	.528030
4.6	.712886	.692564	.673103	.654469	.636627	.619540	.603172
4.8	.767988	.750389	.733397	.717000	.701180	.685919	.671197
5.0	.814559	.799629	.785109	.771000	.757298	.743995	.731083
5.2	.853185	.840738	.828556	.816646	.805011	.793652	.782566
5.4	.884713	.874488	.864425	.854533	.844819	.835287	.825940
5.6	.910100	.901806	.893601	.885496	.877501	.869621	.861860
5.8	.930308	.923650	.917035	.910472	.903971	.897537	.891176
6.0	.946238	.940942	.935657	.930395	.925162	.919965	.914809
6.4	.968369	.965086	.961788	.958482	.955174	.951868	.948569
6.8	.981581	.979588	.977575	.975545	.973503	.971453	.969397
7.2	.989336	.988142	.986930	.985703	.984464	.983214	.981955
7.6	.993839	.993130	.992407	.991672	.990927	.990173	.989411
8.0	.996438	.996018	.995589	.995151	.994706	.994254	.993796
8.4	.997935	.997686	.997432	.997171	.996906	.996635	.996361
8.8	.998797	.998650	.998499	.998343	.998185	.998024	.997859
9.2	.999295	.999208	.999117	.999025	.998930	.998833	.998735
9.6	.999584	.999532	.999478	.999422	.999366	.999307	.999248
10.0	.999753	.999721	.999689	.999655	.999621	.999586	.999550
11.0	.999930	.999921	.999912	.999902	.999892	.999882	.999871
12.0	.999979	.999976	.999974	.999971	.999968	.999964	.999961
13.0	.999993	.999993	.999992	.999991	.999990	.999989	.999988
14.0	1.00000	1.00000	1.00000	1.00000	1.00000	1.00000	1.00000

ν = 18

Q\n	40	50	60	70	80	90	100
0.0	.000000	.000000	.000000	.000000	.000000	.000000	.000000
0.1	.000000	.000000	.000000	.000000	.000000	.000000	.000000
0.2	.000000	.000000	.000000	.000000	.000000	.000000	.000000
0.3	.000000	.000000	.000000	.000000	.000000	.000000	.000000
0.4	.000000	.000000	.000000	.000000	.000000	.000000	.000000
0.5	.000000	.000000	.000000	.000000	.000000	.000000	.000000
0.6	.000000	.000000	.000000	.000000	.000000	.000000	.000000
0.7	.000000	.000000	.000000	.000000	.000000	.000000	.000000
0.8	.000000	.000000	.000000	.000000	.000000	.000000	.000000
0.9	.000000	.000000	.000000	.000000	.000000	.000000	.000000
1.0	.000000	.000000	.000000	.000000	.000000	.000000	.000000
1.1	.000000	.000000	.000000	.000000	.000000	.000000	.000000
1.2	.000000	.000000	.000000	.000000	.000000	.000000	.000000
1.3	.000000	.000000	.000000	.000000	.000000	.000000	.000000
1.4	.000000	.000000	.000000	.000000	.000000	.000000	.000000
1.5	.000000	.000000	.000000	.000000	.000000	.000000	.000000
1.6	.000002	.000000	.000000	.000000	.000000	.000000	.000000
1.7	.000006	.000001	.000000	.000000	.000000	.000000	.000000
1.8	.000021	.000003	.000001	.000000	.000000	.000000	.000000
1.9	.000062	.000011	.000002	.000001	.000000	.000000	.000000
2.0	.000161	.000034	.000008	.000002	.000001	.000000	.000000
2.1	.000381	.000093	.000026	.000009	.000003	.000001	.000000
2.2	.000827	.000231	.000074	.000027	.000011	.000005	.000002
2.3	.001660	.000524	.000188	.000075	.000032	.000015	.000007
2.4	.003111	.001095	.000433	.000188	.000088	.000044	.000023
2.5	.005480	.002128	.000917	.000430	.000216	.000114	.000064
2.6	.009136	.003872	.001804	.000906	.000484	.000272	.000160
2.7	.014496	.006648	.003322	.001777	.001004	.000595	.000366
2.8	.021998	.010834	.005764	.003262	.001941	.001204	.000774
2.9	.032073	.016846	.009486	.005647	.003519	.002277	.001521
3.0	.045105	.025112	.014886	.009279	.006027	.004051	.002803
3.1	.061398	.036038	.022380	.014544	.009809	.006825	.004875
3.2	.081154	.049973	.032374	.021848	.015249	.010946	.008047
3.3	.104447	.067183	.045227	.031589	.022743	.016796	.012675
3.4	.131223	.087822	.061226	.044122	.032679	.024766	.019140
3.5	.161299	.111925	.080556	.059731	.045396	.035225	.027820
3.6	.194380	.139400	.103290	.078607	.061166	.048494	.039068
3.7	.230072	.170034	.129377	.100829	.080165	.064821	.053178
3.8	.267911	.203509	.158651	.126359	.102462	.084357	.070364
3.9	.307387	.239424	.190835	.155046	.128011	.107147	.090745
4.0	.347968	.277313	.225564	.186631	.156657	.133123	.114330
4.1	.389128	.316674	.262406	.220766	.188140	.162112	.141024
4.2	.430361	.356991	.300883	.257037	.222117	.193844	.170626
4.3	.471200	.397756	.340496	.294982	.258179	.227970	.202848
4.4	.511230	.438488	.380745	.334115	.295873	.264079	.237328
4.5	.550091	.478745	.421151	.373949	.334725	.301724	.273653
4.6	.587487	.518134	.461265	.414012	.374258	.340437	.311375
4.7	.623180	.556321	.500687	.453861	.414010	.379752	.350034
4.8	.656994	.593028	.539065	.493095	.453550	.419222	.389176
4.9	.688808	.628037	.576107	.531365	.492486	.458427	.428367

ν = 18

Q\n	40	50	60	70	80	90	100
5.0	.718551	.661188	.611574	.568373	.530476	.496991	.467206
5.1	.746195	.692370	.645286	.603878	.567228	.534585	.505334
5.2	.771749	.721521	.677113	.637690	.602505	.570928	.542436
5.3	.795255	.748620	.706974	.669675	.636122	.605795	.578253
5.4	.816777	.773680	.734828	.699741	.667944	.639010	.612571
5.5	.836399	.796744	.760673	.727843	.697881	.670444	.645228
5.6	.854220	.817876	.784537	.753968	.725886	.700015	.676108
5.7	.870347	.837159	.806473	.778138	.751945	.727678	.705137
5.8	.884892	.854688	.826550	.800396	.776076	.753423	.732279
5.9	.897971	.870569	.844858	.820810	.798322	.777270	.757529
6.0	.909699	.884909	.861491	.839458	.818745	.799262	.780911
6.4	.945281	.929074	.913398	.898337	.883912	.870113	.856914
6.8	.967338	.957058	.946918	.937009	.927373	.918026	.908972
7.2	.980689	.974303	.967903	.961558	.955309	.949178	.943177
7.6	.988643	.984731	.980756	.976770	.972802	.968871	.964989
8.0	.993333	.990957	.988515	.986042	.983557	.981076	.978608
8.4	.996083	.994646	.993156	.991633	.990091	.988542	.986990
8.8	.997692	.996825	.995918	.994984	.994032	.993070	.992101
9.2	.998634	.998110	.997558	.996986	.996400	.995804	.995201
9.6	.999187	.998870	.998533	.998182	.997821	.997452	.997078
10.0	.999513	.999320	.999114	.998898	.998675	.998447	.998214
11.0	.999860	.999803	.999742	.999676	.999608	.999538	.999466
12.0	.999958	.999940	.999921	.999901	.999879	.999857	.999834
13.0	.999987	.999981	.999975	.999968	.999961	.999954	.999946
14.0	1.00000	.999994	.999991	.999989	.999987	.999984	.999982
15.0		1.00000	1.00000	1.00000	1.00000	.999994	.999993
16.0						1.00000	1.00000

ν = 19

Q\n	2	3	4	5	6	7	8
0.0	.000000	.000000	.000000	.000000	.000000	.000000	.000000
0.1	.055833	.002760	.000132	.000006	.000000	.000000	.000000
0.2	.110974	.010959	.001046	.000099	.000009	.000001	.000000
0.3	.165737	.024471	.003493	.000494	.000070	.000010	.000001
0.4	.219644	.043042	.008157	.001532	.000288	.000055	.000010
0.5	.272434	.066344	.015627	.003648	.000853	.000201	.000048
0.6	.323862	.093971	.026379	.007338	.002044	.000573	.000162
0.7	.373707	.125453	.040757	.013120	.004227	.001370	.000448
0.8	.421772	.160275	.058964	.021490	.007836	.002873	.001062
0.9	.467889	.197886	.081060	.032888	.013346	.005443	.002237
1.0	.511917	.237718	.106971	.047668	.021236	.009504	.004284
1.2	.593292	.321777	.169316	.088198	.045893	.023963	.012588
1.4	.665361	.408092	.243192	.143437	.084438	.049827	.029545
1.6	.728023	.492837	.324711	.211725	.137685	.089661	.058602
1.8	.781553	.572954	.409599	.289809	.204377	.144194	.101998
2.0	.826523	.646261	.493812	.373540	.281496	.212058	.160010
2.2	.863705	.711439	.573969	.458609	.364938	.290108	.230811
2.4	.893993	.767932	.647581	.541151	.450297	.374135	.310901
2.6	.918322	.815799	.713104	.618133	.533539	.459674	.395889
2.8	.937614	.855540	.769852	.687508	.611449	.542694	.481311
3.0	.952728	.887941	.817829	.748188	.681829	.620039	.563285
3.2	.964441	.913931	.857539	.799899	.743484	.689600	.638892
3.4	.973426	.934478	.889795	.842975	.796075	.750287	.706287
3.6	.980257	.950513	.915568	.878151	.839908	.801856	.764625
3.8	.985408	.962885	.935864	.906381	.875713	.844691	.813860
4.0	.989263	.972333	.951646	.928695	.904453	.879576	.854513
4.2	.992131	.979485	.963781	.946102	.927176	.907507	.887454
4.4	.994251	.984857	.973022	.959527	.944906	.929543	.913715
4.6	.995812	.988865	.980001	.969778	.958585	.946709	.934360
4.8	.996955	.991838	.985234	.977539	.969037	.959936	.950396
5.0	.997790	.994032	.989133	.983373	.976956	.970034	.962726
5.2	.998398	.995645	.992024	.987731	.982914	.977682	.972122
5.4	.998840	.996827	.994157	.990970	.987370	.983435	.979231
5.6	.999160	.997690	.995727	.993367	.990686	.987740	.984575
5.8	.999392	.998320	.996878	.995135	.993144	.990945	.988572
6.0	.999560	.998778	.997720	.996435	.994959	.993323	.991550
6.4	.999769	.999353	.998784	.998087	.997281	.996379	.995395
6.8	.999878	.999656	.999351	.998973	.998533	.998038	.997495
7.2	.999935	.999816	.999652	.999447	.999207	.998935	.998636
7.6	.999965	.999901	.999812	.999700	.999569	.999420	.999254
8.0	.999981	.999947	.999898	.999837	.999764	.999682	.999590
8.4	.999990	.999971	.999944	.999910	.999870	.999824	.999773
8.8	.999994	.999984	.999969	.999950	.999928	.999902	.999874
9.2	1.00000	.999991	.999983	.999972	.999960	.999945	.999929
9.6		.999995	.999990	.999984	.999977	.999969	.999960
10.0		1.00000	.999994	.999991	.999987	.999982	.999977
11.0			1.00000	1.00000	1.00000	1.00000	.999994
12.0							1.00000

ν = 19

Q\n	9	10	11	12	13	14	15
0.0	.000000	.000000	.000000	.000000	.000000	.000000	.000000
0.1	.000000	.000000	.000000	.000000	.000000	.000000	.000000
0.2	.000000	.000000	.000000	.000000	.000000	.000000	.000000
0.3	.000000	.000000	.000000	.000000	.000000	.000000	.000000
0.4	.000002	.000000	.000000	.000000	.000000	.000000	.000000
0.5	.000011	.000003	.000001	.000000	.000000	.000000	.000000
0.6	.000046	.000013	.000004	.000001	.000000	.000000	.000000
0.7	.000148	.000049	.000017	.000006	.000002	.000001	.000000
0.8	.000397	.000150	.000057	.000022	.000009	.000003	.000001
0.9	.000928	.000389	.000165	.000070	.000030	.000013	.000006
1.0	.001948	.000894	.000414	.000194	.000092	.000044	.000021
1.2	.006662	.003555	.001913	.001039	.000569	.000315	.000176
1.4	.017627	.010590	.006410	.003910	.002403	.001488	.000929
1.6	.038493	.025430	.016904	.011309	.007616	.005162	.003521
1.8	.072427	.051667	.037043	.026699	.019348	.014096	.010326
2.0	.121079	.091945	.070101	.053673	.041275	.031881	.024734
2.2	.183989	.147051	.117889	.094824	.076536	.061993	.050393
2.4	.258660	.215593	.180102	.150833	.126658	.106653	.090059
2.6	.341150	.294326	.254331	.220176	.190991	.166024	.144633
2.8	.426911	.378909	.336651	.299490	.266819	.238083	.212789
3.0	.511596	.464767	.422476	.384356	.350026	.319119	.291287
3.2	.591619	.547818	.507395	.470184	.435985	.404581	.375754
3.4	.664441	.624914	.587754	.552929	.520362	.489950	.461573
3.6	.728601	.694007	.660961	.629513	.599665	.571386	.544631
3.8	.783580	.754083	.725518	.697971	.671489	.646088	.621764
4.0	.829577	.804983	.780880	.757369	.734516	.712360	.690923
4.2	.867275	.847158	.827236	.807610	.788347	.769499	.751098
4.4	.897629	.881440	.865263	.849185	.833274	.817578	.802134
4.6	.921700	.908852	.895912	.882953	.870032	.857197	.844480
4.8	.940541	.930465	.920245	.909942	.899603	.889268	.878966
5.0	.955123	.947301	.939318	.931221	.923049	.914836	.906606
5.2	.966304	.960282	.954102	.947802	.941411	.934956	.928458
5.4	.974806	.970204	.965457	.960595	.955642	.950616	.945536
5.6	.981229	.977732	.974110	.970384	.966572	.962691	.958752
5.8	.986053	.983409	.980659	.977821	.974906	.971927	.968895
6.0	.989659	.987668	.985590	.983437	.981220	.978947	.976625
6.4	.994339	.993220	.992044	.990819	.989551	.988243	.986901
6.8	.996909	.996284	.995625	.994934	.994216	.993473	.992706
7.2	.998311	.997963	.997595	.997208	.996803	.996383	.995949
7.6	.999074	.998881	.998675	.998458	.998231	.997994	.997748
8.0	.999490	.999382	.999267	.999145	.999018	.998884	.998745
8.4	.999717	.999657	.999592	.999524	.999452	.999376	.999297
8.8	.999842	.999808	.999772	.999733	.999692	.999649	.999604
9.2	.999911	.999892	.999871	.999849	.999826	.999801	.999775
9.6	.999949	.999938	.999926	.999914	.999900	.999886	.999871
10.0	.999971	.999965	.999958	.999950	.999943	.999934	.999926
11.0	.999992	.999991	.999989	.999987	.999985	.999983	.999980
12.0	1.00000	1.00000	1.00000	1.00000	1.00000	1.00000	.999995
13.0							1.00000

$\nu = 19$

Q\n	16	17	18	19	20	22	24
0.0	.000000	.000000	.000000	.000000	.000000	.000000	.000000
0.2	.000000	.000000	.000000	.000000	.000000	.000000	.000000
0.4	.000000	.000000	.000000	.000000	.000000	.000000	.000000
0.6	.000000	.000000	.000000	.000000	.000000	.000000	.000000
0.8	.000001	.000000	.000000	.000000	.000000	.000000	.000000
1.0	.000010	.000005	.000003	.000001	.000001	.000000	.000000
1.2	.000099	.000056	.000032	.000018	.000011	.000004	.000001
1.4	.000584	.000370	.000236	.000152	.000098	.000042	.000018
1.6	.002417	.001670	.001161	.000812	.000571	.000287	.000148
1.8	.007604	.005629	.004189	.003132	.002354	.001348	.000786
2.0	.019274	.015083	.011854	.009354	.007412	.004707	.003035
2.2	.041108	.033651	.027642	.022782	.018838	.013005	.009087
2.4	.076261	.064757	.055140	.047079	.040303	.029765	.022200
2.6	.126275	.110488	.096885	.085140	.074976	.058503	.046011
2.8	.190500	.170833	.153454	.138074	.124441	.101572	.083427
3.0	.266213	.243605	.223203	.204771	.188101	.159320	.135604
3.2	.349292	.324995	.302674	.282158	.263285	.229901	.201506
3.4	.435108	.410429	.387415	.365947	.345915	.309743	.278144
3.6	.519336	.495437	.472861	.451538	.431396	.394383	.361305
3.8	.598501	.576270	.555038	.534768	.515420	.479328	.446441
4.0	.670213	.650229	.630961	.612395	.594515	.560726	.529418
4.2	.733166	.715716	.698752	.682276	.666284	.635723	.606995
4.4	.786969	.772103	.757548	.743312	.729402	.702558	.677007
4.6	.831911	.819509	.807292	.795270	.783452	.760454	.738321
4.8	.868725	.858563	.848496	.838539	.828699	.809407	.790662
5.0	.898381	.890180	.882017	.873903	.865850	.849955	.834381
5.2	.921934	.915400	.908869	.902350	.895854	.882957	.870226
5.4	.940415	.935266	.930099	.924924	.919747	.909418	.899153
5.6	.954767	.950747	.946699	.942631	.938549	.930366	.922187
5.8	.965817	.962702	.959556	.956386	.953195	.946772	.940318
6.0	.974263	.971865	.969436	.966982	.964507	.959505	.954455
6.4	.985529	.984129	.982704	.981259	.979794	.976815	.973783
6.8	.991919	.991113	.990290	.989451	.988599	.986856	.985070
7.2	.995501	.995041	.994569	.994088	.993596	.992588	.991549
7.6	.997495	.997233	.996964	.996689	.996408	.995828	.995228
8.0	.998601	.998453	.998300	.998143	.997982	.997649	.997304
8.4	.999216	.999131	.999044	.998954	.998862	.998671	.998472
8.8	.999557	.999509	.999459	.999408	.999355	.999245	.999131
9.2	.999749	.999721	.999692	.999663	.999632	.999569	.999502
9.6	.999856	.999840	.999823	.999806	.999789	.999752	.999713
10.0	.999917	.999908	.999898	.999888	.999878	.999856	.999833
11.0	.999978	.999976	.999973	.999970	.999968	.999962	.999956
12.0	.999994	.999993	.999992	.999992	.999991	.999989	.999987
13.0	1.00000	1.00000	1.00000	1.00000	1.00000	1.00000	1.00000

$\nu = 19$

Q\n	26	28	30	32	34	36	38
0.0	.000000	.000000	.000000	.000000	.000000	.000000	.000000
0.2	.000000	.000000	.000000	.000000	.000000	.000000	.000000
0.4	.000000	.000000	.000000	.000000	.000000	.000000	.000000
0.6	.000000	.000000	.000000	.000000	.000000	.000000	.000000
0.8	.000000	.000000	.000000	.000000	.000000	.000000	.000000
1.0	.000000	.000000	.000000	.000000	.000000	.000000	.000000
1.2	.000000	.000000	.000000	.000000	.000000	.000000	.000000
1.4	.000008	.000004	.000002	.000001	.000000	.000000	.000000
1.6	.000077	.000041	.000022	.000012	.000007	.000004	.000002
1.8	.000466	.000281	.000172	.000106	.000067	.000043	.000027
2.0	.001984	.001314	.000881	.000598	.000410	.000285	.000199
2.2	.006423	.004590	.003313	.002415	.001776	.001318	.000986
2.4	.016713	.012694	.009722	.007504	.005836	.004570	.003603
2.6	.036460	.029097	.023379	.018904	.015379	.012582	.010350
2.8	.068934	.057283	.047860	.040193	.033918	.028755	.024484
3.0	.115963	.099613	.085937	.074442	.064735	.056503	.049490
3.2	.177265	.156488	.138613	.123176	.109796	.098156	.087996
3.4	.250465	.226152	.204734	.185810	.169043	.154144	.140869
3.6	.331694	.305135	.281265	.259763	.240354	.222795	.206876
3.8	.416448	.389064	.364027	.341101	.320075	.300760	.282988
4.0	.500407	.473511	.448557	.425383	.403839	.383786	.365101
4.2	.580006	.554652	.530829	.508434	.487369	.467541	.448861
4.4	.652712	.629628	.607698	.586865	.567070	.548252	.530357
4.6	.717057	.696649	.677076	.658311	.640321	.623075	.606538
4.8	.772488	.754893	.737876	.721429	.705540	.690194	.675373
5.0	.819159	.804308	.789840	.775757	.762059	.748741	.735798
5.2	.857694	.845384	.833313	.821491	.809922	.798609	.787553
5.4	.888986	.878938	.869029	.859269	.849668	.840232	.830964
5.6	.914039	.905944	.897920	.889977	.882127	.874377	.866731
5.8	.933857	.927408	.920984	.914599	.908261	.901978	.895755
6.0	.949376	.944285	.939193	.934112	.929049	.924012	.919006
6.4	.970710	.967607	.964482	.961343	.958194	.955042	.951890
6.8	.983249	.981398	.979524	.977631	.975722	.973802	.971872
7.2	.990484	.989397	.988290	.987167	.986029	.984880	.983721
7.6	.994610	.993976	.993329	.992670	.992000	.991320	.990632
8.0	.996947	.996579	.996203	.995818	.995426	.995026	.994621
8.4	.998266	.998054	.997835	.997611	.997382	.997148	.996910
8.8	.999011	.998888	.998761	.998630	.998497	.998360	.998220
9.2	.999433	.999361	.999287	.999211	.999133	.999052	.998971
9.6	.999673	.999631	.999587	.999543	.999497	.999449	.999401
10.0	.999810	.999785	.999759	.999733	.999706	.999678	.999649
11.0	.999949	.999942	.999935	.999928	.999921	.999913	.999905
12.0	.999986	.999984	.999982	.999980	.999977	.999975	.999973
13.0	1.00000	1.00000	.999995	.999994	.999993	.999993	.999992
14.0			1.00000	1.00000	1.00000	1.00000	1.00000

$\nu = 19$

Q\n	40	50	60	70	80	90	100
0.0	.000000	.000000	.000000	.000000	.000000	.000000	.000000
0.1	.000000	.000000	.000000	.000000	.000000	.000000	.000000
0.2	.000000	.000000	.000000	.000000	.000000	.000000	.000000
0.3	.000000	.000000	.000000	.000000	.000000	.000000	.000000
0.4	.000000	.000000	.000000	.000000	.000000	.000000	.000000
0.5	.000000	.000000	.000000	.000000	.000000	.000000	.000000
0.6	.000000	.000000	.000000	.000000	.000000	.000000	.000000
0.7	.000000	.000000	.000000	.000000	.000000	.000000	.000000
0.8	.000000	.000000	.000000	.000000	.000000	.000000	.000000
0.9	.000000	.000000	.000000	.000000	.000000	.000000	.000000
1.0	.000000	.000000	.000000	.000000	.000000	.000000	.000000
1.1	.000000	.000000	.000000	.000000	.000000	.000000	.000000
1.2	.000000	.000000	.000000	.000000	.000000	.000000	.000000
1.3	.000000	.000000	.000000	.000000	.000000	.000000	.000000
1.4	.000000	.000000	.000000	.000000	.000000	.000000	.000000
1.5	.000000	.000000	.000000	.000000	.000000	.000000	.000000
1.6	.000001	.000000	.000000	.000000	.000000	.000000	.000000
1.7	.000005	.000001	.000000	.000000	.000000	.000000	.000000
1.8	.000018	.000002	.000000	.000000	.000000	.000000	.000000
1.9	.000053	.000009	.000002	.000000	.000000	.000000	.000000
2.0	.000141	.000028	.000007	.000002	.000001	.000000	.000000
2.1	.000338	.000079	.000022	.000007	.000002	.000001	.000000
2.2	.000743	.000200	.000062	.000022	.000008	.000003	.000002
2.3	.001509	.000461	.000160	.000062	.000026	.000012	.000006
2.4	.002859	.000977	.000375	.000158	.000072	.000035	.000018
2.5	.005087	.001922	.000808	.000369	.000181	.000094	.000051
2.6	.008558	.003540	.001612	.000792	.000414	.000228	.000131
2.7	.013691	.006145	.003006	.001576	.000874	.000508	.000307
2.8	.020935	.010113	.005280	.002934	.001716	.001047	.000662
2.9	.030734	.015866	.008784	.005145	.003156	.002012	.001325
3.0	.043493	.023843	.013922	.008552	.005478	.003633	.002482
3.1	.059540	.034470	.021119	.013546	.009022	.006202	.004379
3.2	.079099	.048117	.030799	.020543	.014177	.010067	.007324
3.3	.102268	.065075	.043342	.029958	.021352	.015616	.011674
3.4	.129010	.085525	.059060	.042167	.030950	.023252	.017819
3.5	.159155	.109520	.078166	.057482	.043336	.033365	.026153
3.6	.192413	.136988	.100755	.076118	.058806	.046300	.037049
3.7	.228388	.167725	.126796	.098180	.077564	.062330	.050827
3.8	.266609	.201418	.156134	.123650	.099703	.081635	.067729
3.9	.306551	.237660	.188500	.152389	.125196	.104281	.087897
4.0	.347667	.275976	.223527	.184145	.153901	.130220	.111366
4.1	.389408	.315847	.260774	.218571	.185565	.159292	.138055
4.2	.431248	.356740	.299749	.255243	.219843	.191229	.167775
4.3	.472701	.398125	.339934	.293686	.256318	.225680	.200238
4.4	.513329	.439498	.380809	.333397	.294523	.262227	.235080
4.5	.552759	.480396	.421871	.373866	.333965	.300404	.271874
4.6	.590677	.520409	.462652	.414598	.374146	.339726	.310156
4.7	.626839	.559183	.502728	.455129	.414581	.379706	.349448
4.8	.661058	.596428	.541732	.495038	.454816	.419871	.389273
4.9	.693210	.631917	.579353	.533955	.494439	.459783	.429173

$\nu = 19$

Q\n	40	50	60	70	80	90	100
5.0	.723221	.665480	.615344	.571568	.533089	.499042	.468726
5.1	.751064	.697004	.649515	.607621	.570457	.537300	.507551
5.2	.776752	.726426	.681729	.641917	.606295	.574263	.545317
5.3	.800329	.753724	.711904	.674315	.640407	.609692	.581749
5.4	.821866	.778916	.740000	.704720	.672652	.643401	.616621
5.5	.841452	.802048	.766016	.733087	.702938	.675258	.649765
5.6	.859193	.823190	.789983	.759404	.731216	.705176	.681058
5.7	.875201	.842432	.811959	.783696	.757475	.733111	.710423
5.8	.889597	.859875	.832023	.806014	.781736	.759054	.737826
5.9	.902501	.875631	.850266	.826427	.804047	.783028	.763263
6.0	.914035	.889815	.866793	.845024	.824476	.805082	.786762
6.4	.948742	.933156	.917977	.903314	.889205	.875656	.862653
6.8	.969935	.960218	.950565	.941075	.931800	.922766	.913982
7.2	.982553	.976627	.970643	.964675	.958766	.952942	.947218
7.6	.989937	.986377	.982732	.979053	.975370	.971705	.968070
8.0	.994211	.992092	.989897	.987659	.985399	.983130	.980864
8.4	.996669	.995414	.994102	.992752	.991378	.989989	.988592
8.8	.998078	.997337	.996555	.995744	.994914	.994069	.993215
9.2	.998887	.998449	.997983	.997497	.996996	.996484	.995964
9.6	.999352	.999092	.998814	.998522	.998220	.997910	.997594
10.0	.999620	.999465	.999299	.999124	.998941	.998753	.998561
11.0	.999897	.999854	.999806	.999756	.999704	.999649	.999592
12.0	.999971	.999958	.999944	.999929	.999913	.999897	.999880
13.0	.999991	.999987	.999983	.999978	.999973	.999968	.999963
14.0	1.00000	1.00000	.999995	.999993	.999991	.999990	.999988
15.0			1.00000	1.00000	1.00000	1.00000	1.00000

ν = 20

Q\n	2	3	4	5	6	7	8
0.0	.000000	.000000	.000000	.000000	.000000	.000000	.000000
0.1	.055670	.002752	.000132	.000006	.000000	.000000	.000000
0.2	.111048	.010959	.001044	.000099	.000009	.000001	.000000
0.3	.165849	.024472	.003487	.000492	.000070	.000010	.000001
0.4	.219796	.043047	.008143	.001526	.000286	.000054	.000010
0.5	.272627	.066356	.015604	.003633	.000846	.000198	.000047
0.6	.324098	.093994	.026344	.007310	.002029	.000566	.000159
0.7	.373988	.125495	.040710	.013072	.004198	.001355	.000441
0.8	.422100	.160342	.058906	.021418	.007785	.002843	.001046
0.9	.468265	.197988	.080997	.032790	.013266	.005390	.002205
1.0	.512342	.237865	.106910	.047543	.021120	.009418	.004227
1.1	.554219	.279404	.136446	.065919	.031800	.015392	.007495
1.2	.593814	.322044	.169297	.088034	.045694	.023785	.012448
1.3	.631075	.365248	.205062	.113871	.063093	.035039	.019554
1.4	.665975	.408515	.243276	.143282	.084172	.049537	.029279
1.5	.698514	.451383	.283423	.176001	.108974	.067563	.042045
1.6	.728717	.493440	.324964	.211658	.137410	.089285	.058200
1.7	.756628	.534329	.367360	.249801	.169261	.114735	.077982
1.8	.782311	.573746	.410081	.289923	.204192	.143811	.101506
1.9	.805845	.611445	.452633	.331481	.241778	.176279	.128745
2.0	.827322	.647232	.494560	.373922	.281519	.211791	.159537
2.1	.846844	.680969	.535460	.416706	.322874	.249902	.193591
2.2	.864522	.712563	.574989	.459320	.365279	.290098	.230508
2.3	.880470	.741966	.612862	.501294	.408175	.331824	.269802
2.4	.894805	.769169	.648853	.542213	.451030	.374506	.310929
2.5	.907646	.794198	.682797	.581721	.493348	.417578	.353312
2.6	.919109	.817104	.714582	.619527	.534691	.460504	.396373
2.7	.929310	.837962	.744147	.655402	.574677	.502791	.439551
2.8	.938358	.856865	.771474	.689180	.612996	.544003	.482321
2.9	.946360	.873921	.796583	.720752	.649399	.583769	.524213
3.0	.953416	.889243	.819527	.750062	.683705	.621787	.564820
3.1	.959621	.902953	.840381	.777098	.715792	.657822	.603802
3.2	.965064	.915173	.859244	.801888	.745596	.691704	.640890
3.3	.969825	.926027	.876227	.824491	.773097	.723326	.675882
3.4	.973980	.935633	.891451	.844993	.798319	.752635	.708642
3.5	.977598	.944108	.905042	.863498	.821319	.779625	.739092
3.6	.980742	.951562	.917128	.880123	.842182	.804330	.767207
3.7	.983467	.958100	.927838	.894995	.861013	.826817	.793004
3.8	.985825	.963818	.937297	.908247	.877931	.847178	.816538
3.9	.987862	.968807	.945623	.920009	.893065	.865526	.837892
4.0	.989618	.973149	.952931	.930413	.906547	.881984	.857171
4.1	.991129	.976919	.959328	.939585	.918514	.896684	.874496
4.2	.992428	.980187	.964911	.947646	.929098	.909764	.889997
4.3	.993542	.983012	.969774	.954711	.938429	.921358	.903811
4.4	.994498	.985451	.973999	.960887	.946630	.931602	.916075
4.5	.995315	.987554	.977663	.966270	.953817	.940623	.926926
4.6	.996014	.989362	.980833	.970954	.960099	.948544	.936495
4.7	.996611	.990916	.983571	.975019	.965577	.955481	.944908
4.8	.997120	.992249	.985932	.978541	.970343	.961540	.952285
4.9	.997554	.993391	.987965	.981586	.974481	.966820	.958736

$\nu = 20$

Q\n	2	3	4	5	6	7	8
5.0	.997923	.994369	.989712	.984214	.978066	.971412	.964365
5.1	.998237	.995205	.991213	.986480	.981167	.975396	.969265
5.2	.998505	.995918	.992499	.988429	.983844	.978848	.973522
5.3	.998732	.996528	.993601	.990105	.986153	.981833	.977214
5.4	.998925	.997047	.994544	.991544	.988141	.984410	.980410
5.5	.999088	.997489	.995350	.992777	.989850	.986632	.983172
5.6	.999227	.997866	.996039	.993834	.991318	.988545	.985556
5.7	.999345	.998187	.996627	.994738	.992578	.990190	.987611
5.8	.999445	.998459	.997128	.995512	.993658	.991604	.989380
5.9	.999529	.998691	.997555	.996173	.994583	.992817	.990902
6.0	.999601	.998888	.997919	.996737	.995374	.993858	.992209
6.4	.999794	.999421	.998909	.998279	.997546	.996724	.995825
6.8	.999893	.999698	.999427	.999092	.998699	.998256	.997768
7.2	.999944	.999842	.999698	.999520	.999309	.999071	.998807
7.6	.999971	.999916	.999840	.999745	.999632	.999503	.999360
8.0	.999985	.999956	.999915	.999864	.999803	.999733	.999655
8.4	.999992	.999976	.999954	.999927	.999893	.999856	.999813
8.8	1.00000	.999987	.999975	.999960	.999942	.999921	.999898
9.2		.999993	.999986	.999978	.999968	.999957	.999944
9.6		1.00000	.999993	.999988	.999982	.999976	.999969
10.0			1.00000	.999993	.999990	.999987	.999982
11.0				1.00000	1.00000	1.00000	1.00000

$\nu = 20$

Q\n	9	10	11	12	13	14	15
0.0	.000000	.000000	.000000	.000000	.000000	.000000	.000000
0.1	.000000	.000000	.000000	.000000	.000000	.000000	.000000
0.2	.000000	.000000	.000000	.000000	.000000	.000000	.000000
0.3	.000000	.000000	.000000	.000000	.000000	.000000	.000000
0.4	.000002	.000000	.000000	.000000	.000000	.000000	.000000
0.5	.000011	.000003	.000001	.000000	.000000	.000000	.000000
0.6	.000045	.000013	.000004	.000001	.000000	.000000	.000000
0.7	.000145	.000048	.000016	.000005	.000002	.000001	.000000
0.8	.000389	.000146	.000055	.000021	.000008	.000003	.000001
0.9	.000910	.000379	.000160	.000068	.000029	.000013	.000006
1.0	.001913	.000873	.000402	.000187	.000088	.000042	.000020
1.1	.003677	.001819	.000908	.000457	.000232	.000119	.000062
1.2	.006559	.003484	.001865	.001007	.000549	.000301	.000167
1.3	.010981	.006211	.003540	.002034	.001178	.000687	.000404
1.4	.017405	.010414	.006275	.003809	.002329	.001435	.000890
1.5	.026300	.016549	.010481	.006682	.004290	.002773	.001804
1.6	.038111	.025091	.016616	.011071	.007423	.005008	.003400
1.7	.053216	.036490	.025154	.017436	.012156	.008523	.006010
1.8	.071896	.051141	.036551	.026255	.018957	.013759	.010038
1.9	.094309	.069344	.051204	.037979	.028302	.021190	.015940
2.0	.120477	.091278	.069415	.053000	.040637	.031290	.024195
2.1	.150280	.116986	.091367	.071612	.056338	.044490	.035268
2.2	.183463	.146367	.117104	.093985	.075678	.061144	.049570
2.3	.219655	.179183	.146526	.120146	.098802	.081493	.067421
2.4	.258388	.215075	.179392	.149982	.125710	.105644	.089020
2.5	.299128	.253581	.215341	.183235	.156257	.133559	.114427
2.6	.341298	.294170	.253908	.219529	.190163	.165053	.143555
2.7	.384314	.336265	.294558	.258390	.227025	.199810	.176172
2.8	.427599	.379274	.336711	.299271	.266352	.237400	.211922
2.9	.470613	.422618	.379772	.341587	.307584	.277308	.250341
3.0	.512866	.465745	.423156	.384741	.350131	.318962	.290892
3.1	.553929	.508158	.466312	.428149	.393394	.361766	.332991
3.2	.593441	.549416	.508741	.471264	.436794	.405122	.376036
3.3	.631112	.589151	.550003	.513591	.479792	.448461	.419438
3.4	.666722	.627064	.589729	.554698	.521906	.491257	.462640
3.5	.700120	.662929	.627622	.594226	.562718	.533045	.505135
3.6	.731213	.696586	.663457	.631885	.601882	.573427	.546479
3.7	.759963	.727938	.697076	.667460	.639126	.612078	.586300
3.8	.786379	.756942	.728384	.700802	.674248	.648746	.624298
3.9	.810507	.783604	.757342	.731823	.707113	.683248	.660244
4.0	.832426	.807969	.783955	.760490	.737645	.715467	.693980
4.1	.852237	.830112	.808270	.786816	.765824	.745344	.725409
4.2	.870058	.850134	.830365	.810852	.791669	.772870	.754490
4.3	.886019	.868152	.850340	.832679	.815240	.798077	.781229
4.4	.900255	.884296	.868315	.852402	.836624	.821034	.805672
4.5	.912906	.898702	.884419	.870140	.855929	.841834	.827895
4.6	.924109	.911509	.898789	.886026	.873277	.860589	.847999
4.7	.933996	.922853	.911564	.900196	.888802	.877426	.866102
4.8	.942697	.932871	.922882	.912789	.902642	.892480	.882335
4.9	.950332	.941690	.932876	.923943	.914936	.905889	.896831

$\nu = 20$

Q\n	9	10	11	12	13	14	15
5.0	.957014	.949432	.941675	.933791	.925819	.917790	.909731
5.1	.962849	.956212	.949402	.942461	.935424	.928319	.921170
5.2	.967933	.962134	.956169	.950073	.943877	.937607	.931283
5.3	.972353	.967296	.962081	.956739	.951297	.945777	.940197
5.4	.976189	.971787	.967237	.962565	.957794	.952945	.948034
5.5	.979513	.975687	.971723	.967644	.963471	.959221	.954907
5.6	.982387	.979067	.975619	.972065	.968421	.964702	.960921
5.7	.984870	.981993	.978998	.975905	.972728	.969480	.966172
5.8	.987012	.984521	.981924	.979236	.976470	.973638	.970749
5.9	.988858	.986703	.984453	.982120	.979716	.977250	.974730
6.0	.990446	.988585	.986637	.984615	.982527	.980383	.978189
6.4	.994856	.993827	.992744	.991612	.990438	.989225	.987977
6.8	.997240	.996676	.996079	.995452	.994799	.994121	.993421
7.2	.998520	.998211	.997884	.997539	.997178	.996802	.996413
7.6	.999204	.999036	.998857	.998667	.998468	.998260	.998044
8.0	.999570	.999478	.999380	.999276	.999166	.999051	.998931
8.4	.999766	.999716	.999662	.999604	.999544	.999480	.999414
8.8	.999872	.999844	.999814	.999783	.999749	.999713	.999676
9.2	.999930	.999914	.999897	.999880	.999861	.999841	.999820
9.6	.999961	.999952	.999943	.999933	.999922	.999911	.999899
10.0	.999978	.999973	.999968	.999962	.999956	.999950	.999943
11.0	.999995	.999993	.999992	.999991	.999989	.999987	.999986
12.0	1.00000	1.00000	1.00000	1.00000	1.00000	1.00000	1.00000

$\nu = 20$

Q\n	16	17	18	19	20	22	24
0.0	.000000	.000000	.000000	.000000	.000000	.000000	.000000
0.1	.000000	.000000	.000000	.000000	.000000	.000000	.000000
0.2	.000000	.000000	.000000	.000000	.000000	.000000	.000000
0.3	.000000	.000000	.000000	.000000	.000000	.000000	.000000
0.4	.000000	.000000	.000000	.000000	.000000	.000000	.000000
0.5	.000000	.000000	.000000	.000000	.000000	.000000	.000000
0.6	.000000	.000000	.000000	.000000	.000000	.000000	.000000
0.7	.000000	.000000	.000000	.000000	.000000	.000000	.000000
0.8	.000001	.000000	.000000	.000000	.000000	.000000	.000000
0.9	.000002	.000001	.000000	.000000	.000000	.000000	.000000
1.0	.000010	.000005	.000002	.000001	.000001	.000000	.000000
1.1	.000032	.000017	.000009	.000005	.000003	.000001	.000000
1.2	.000093	.000053	.000030	.000017	.000010	.000003	.000001
1.3	.000240	.000143	.000086	.000052	.000032	.000012	.000005
1.4	.000557	.000350	.000222	.000142	.000091	.000038	.000017
1.5	.001182	.000779	.000517	.000346	.000232	.000107	.000050
1.6	.002323	.001596	.001104	.000767	.000537	.000267	.000136
1.7	.004262	.003039	.002179	.001571	.001138	.000607	.000330
1.8	.007361	.005426	.004019	.002992	.002238	.001269	.000733
1.9	.012047	.009147	.006977	.005345	.004113	.002466	.001502
2.0	.018789	.014652	.011472	.009019	.007119	.004486	.002868
2.1	.028065	.022417	.017972	.014461	.011678	.007694	.005137
2.2	.040324	.032914	.026956	.022149	.018258	.012522	.008692
2.3	.055949	.046569	.038879	.032554	.027337	.019440	.013974
2.4	.075215	.063722	.054130	.046103	.039368	.028924	.021457
2.5	.098270	.084597	.072999	.063140	.054738	.041418	.031613
2.6	.125119	.109281	.095648	.083891	.073730	.057295	.044869
2.7	.155616	.137712	.122094	.108446	.096500	.076819	.061575
2.8	.189479	.169686	.152207	.136749	.123059	.100124	.081964
2.9	.226306	.204865	.185717	.168597	.153271	.127199	.106135
3.0	.265603	.242804	.222233	.203656	.186861	.157887	.134042
3.1	.306808	.282975	.261268	.241482	.223434	.191892	.165492
3.2	.349328	.324800	.302265	.281551	.262498	.228805	.200164
3.3	.392563	.367679	.344634	.323286	.303500	.268125	.237624
3.4	.435934	.411019	.387775	.366088	.345846	.309290	.277355
3.5	.478901	.454256	.431107	.409364	.388940	.351709	.318789
3.6	.520982	.496874	.474087	.452552	.432202	.394788	.361334
3.7	.561760	.538418	.516226	.495136	.475095	.437954	.404402
3.8	.600891	.578504	.557105	.536660	.517134	.480679	.447430
3.9	.638104	.616818	.596371	.576740	.557901	.522490	.489906
4.0	.673198	.653122	.633747	.615062	.597052	.562981	.531373
4.1	.706039	.687245	.669029	.651386	.634311	.601818	.571444
4.2	.736555	.719081	.702075	.685541	.669477	.638740	.609803
4.3	.764723	.748578	.732807	.717418	.702413	.673555	.646205
4.4	.790565	.775736	.761199	.746966	.733042	.706134	.680476
4.5	.814140	.800593	.787269	.774182	.761339	.736410	.712501
4.6	.835535	.823220	.811072	.799103	.787324	.764363	.742224
4.7	.854858	.843715	.832691	.821800	.811052	.790020	.769637
4.8	.872231	.862192	.852232	.842367	.832608	.813438	.794772
4.9	.887788	.878777	.869817	.860919	.852095	.834704	.817696

$\nu = 20$

Q\n	16	17	18	19	20	22	24
5.0	.901664	.893606	.885575	.877581	.869636	.853926	.838498
5.1	.913997	.906816	.899642	.892487	.885360	.871224	.857288
5.2	.924924	.918544	.912156	.905773	.899402	.886729	.874190
5.3	.934575	.928922	.923252	.917575	.911898	.900575	.889332
5.4	.943075	.938081	.933061	.928026	.922982	.912897	.902850
5.5	.950544	.946141	.941708	.937254	.932785	.923828	.914877
5.6	.957090	.953217	.949312	.945381	.941431	.933496	.925544
5.7	.962815	.959415	.955982	.952521	.949038	.942026	.934979
5.8	.967811	.964833	.961821	.958779	.955714	.949531	.943302
5.9	.972165	.969560	.966921	.964254	.961562	.956121	.950626
6.0	.975951	.973676	.971369	.969033	.966673	.961895	.957057
6.4	.986698	.985392	.984061	.982707	.981333	.978533	.975676
6.8	.992701	.991962	.991206	.990435	.989649	.988039	.986386
7.2	.996010	.995596	.995172	.994737	.994292	.993378	.992433
7.6	.997821	.997590	.997352	.997108	.996859	.996343	.995808
8.0	.998807	.998679	.998546	.998410	.998270	.997980	.997678
8.4	.999344	.999273	.999199	.999122	.999044	.998881	.998711
8.8	.999638	.999598	.999556	.999513	.999469	.999377	.999281
9.2	.999798	.999776	.999753	.999728	.999704	.999652	.999597
9.6	.999887	.999874	.999861	.999847	.999833	.999804	.999773
10.0	.999936	.999929	.999921	.999914	.999905	.999889	.999871
11.0	.999984	.999982	.999980	.999978	.999976	.999972	.999967
12.0	1.00000	1.00000	.999995	.999994	.999994	.999993	.999991
13.0			1.00000	1.00000	1.00000	1.00000	1.00000

$\nu = 20$

Q\n	26	28	30	32	34	36	38
0.0	.000000	.000000	.000000	.000000	.000000	.000000	.000000
0.1	.000000	.000000	.000000	.000000	.000000	.000000	.000000
0.2	.000000	.000000	.000000	.000000	.000000	.000000	.000000
0.3	.000000	.000000	.000000	.000000	.000000	.000000	.000000
0.4	.000000	.000000	.000000	.000000	.000000	.000000	.000000
0.5	.000000	.000000	.000000	.000000	.000000	.000000	.000000
0.6	.000000	.000000	.000000	.000000	.000000	.000000	.000000
0.7	.000000	.000000	.000000	.000000	.000000	.000000	.000000
0.8	.000000	.000000	.000000	.000000	.000000	.000000	.000000
0.9	.000000	.000000	.000000	.000000	.000000	.000000	.000000
1.0	.000000	.000000	.000000	.000000	.000000	.000000	.000000
1.1	.000000	.000000	.000000	.000000	.000000	.000000	.000000
1.2	.000000	.000000	.000000	.000000	.000000	.000000	.000000
1.3	.000002	.000001	.000000	.000000	.000000	.000000	.000000
1.4	.000007	.000003	.000002	.000001	.000000	.000000	.000000
1.5	.000024	.000012	.000006	.000003	.000002	.000001	.000000
1.6	.000070	.000037	.000020	.000011	.000006	.000003	.000002
1.7	.000182	.000103	.000059	.000034	.000020	.000012	.000007
1.8	.000430	.000256	.000155	.000095	.000059	.000037	.000024
1.9	.000929	.000583	.000371	.000239	.000156	.000103	.000069
2.0	.001859	.001221	.000812	.000546	.000372	.000255	.000177
2.1	.003473	.002376	.001644	.001149	.000812	.000579	.000416
2.2	.006102	.004330	.003104	.002246	.001641	.001208	.000897
2.3	.010148	.007442	.005507	.004111	.003094	.002347	.001793
2.4	.016065	.012134	.009240	.007092	.005483	.004270	.003347
2.5	.024329	.018870	.014746	.011604	.009193	.007329	.005878
2.6	.035399	.028125	.022495	.018106	.014661	.011940	.009776
2.7	.049682	.040340	.032950	.027067	.022355	.018557	.015480
2.8	.067492	.055888	.046526	.038930	.032732	.027647	.023453
2.9	.089021	.075039	.063555	.054073	.046205	.039643	.034147
3.0	.114322	.097936	.084253	.072775	.063103	.054917	.047960
3.1	.143304	.124575	.108701	.095189	.083643	.073738	.065208
3.2	.175731	.154812	.136834	.121328	.107907	.096249	.086089
3.3	.211246	.188364	.168449	.151062	.135834	.122456	.110668
3.4	.249389	.224833	.203213	.184125	.167226	.152223	.138870
3.5	.289625	.263732	.240690	.220135	.201756	.185282	.170482
3.6	.331380	.304511	.280363	.258617	.238994	.221249	.205170
3.7	.374060	.346586	.321669	.299033	.278433	.259652	.242499
3.8	.417089	.389372	.364023	.340807	.319514	.299954	.281960
3.9	.459918	.432302	.406848	.383360	.361661	.341589	.322998
4.0	.502054	.474850	.449594	.426127	.404301	.383981	.365042
4.1	.543063	.516545	.491760	.468582	.446890	.426573	.407528
4.2	.582581	.556980	.532903	.510251	.488929	.468847	.449919
4.3	.620315	.595819	.572646	.550723	.529976	.510334	.491728
4.4	.656042	.632794	.610683	.589655	.569656	.550630	.532523
4.5	.689608	.667711	.646779	.626776	.607662	.589397	.571938
4.6	.720916	.700435	.680764	.661881	.643758	.626366	.609674
4.7	.749926	.730891	.712530	.694828	.677770	.661335	.645503
4.8	.776641	.759056	.742023	.725536	.709589	.694167	.679257
4.9	.801104	.784947	.769237	.753974	.739157	.724779	.710832

$\nu = 20$

Q\n	26	28	30	32	34	36	38
5.0	.823388	.808618	.794204	.780152	.766465	.753140	.740173
5.1	.843589	.830150	.816990	.804119	.791541	.779260	.767274
5.2	.861820	.849645	.837684	.825949	.814449	.803187	.792165
5.3	.878205	.867219	.856393	.845741	.835273	.824994	.814908
5.4	.892875	.882998	.873238	.863607	.854118	.844777	.835588
5.5	.905964	.897114	.888345	.879671	.871102	.862647	.854311
5.6	.917605	.909699	.901846	.894060	.886350	.878725	.871191
5.7	.927925	.920884	.913873	.906905	.899990	.893138	.886353
5.8	.937050	.930796	.924554	.918336	.912154	.906014	.899924
5.9	.945099	.939556	.934013	.928480	.922968	.917483	.912032
6.0	.952180	.947280	.942368	.937457	.932554	.927668	.922803
6.4	.972773	.969834	.966867	.963880	.960879	.957869	.954853
6.8	.984694	.982972	.981223	.979453	.977664	.975861	.974045
7.2	.991462	.990468	.989455	.988423	.987377	.986317	.985246
7.6	.995255	.994687	.994106	.993512	.992907	.992292	.991668
8.0	.997365	.997042	.996710	.996370	.996023	.995669	.995309
8.4	.998534	.998350	.998162	.997968	.997769	.997566	.997359
8.8	.999181	.999077	.998969	.998859	.998745	.998629	.998510
9.2	.999540	.999481	.999419	.999356	.999291	.999224	.999156
9.6	.999740	.999706	.999671	.999635	.999597	.999559	.999519
10.0	.999852	.999833	.999812	.999791	.999770	.999747	.999724
11.0	.999962	.999957	.999952	.999947	.999941	.999935	.999929
12.0	.999990	.999989	.999987	.999986	.999984	.999983	.999981
13.0	1.00000	1.00000	1.00000	1.00000	1.00000	1.00000	.999995
14.0							1.00000

$\nu = 20$

Q\n	40	50	60	70	80	90	100
0.0	.000000	.000000	.000000	.000000	.000000	.000000	.000000
0.1	.000000	.000000	.000000	.000000	.000000	.000000	.000000
0.2	.000000	.000000	.000000	.000000	.000000	.000000	.000000
0.3	.000000	.000000	.000000	.000000	.000000	.000000	.000000
0.4	.000000	.000000	.000000	.000000	.000000	.000000	.000000
0.5	.000000	.000000	.000000	.000000	.000000	.000000	.000000
0.6	.000000	.000000	.000000	.000000	.000000	.000000	.000000
0.7	.000000	.000000	.000000	.000000	.000000	.000000	.000000
0.8	.000000	.000000	.000000	.000000	.000000	.000000	.000000
0.9	.000000	.000000	.000000	.000000	.000000	.000000	.000000
1.0	.000000	.000000	.000000	.000000	.000000	.000000	.000000
1.1	.000000	.000000	.000000	.000000	.000000	.000000	.000000
1.2	.000000	.000000	.000000	.000000	.000000	.000000	.000000
1.3	.000000	.000000	.000000	.000000	.000000	.000000	.000000
1.4	.000000	.000000	.000000	.000000	.000000	.000000	.000000
1.5	.000000	.000000	.000000	.000000	.000000	.000000	.000000
1.6	.000001	.000000	.000000	.000000	.000000	.000000	.000000
1.7	.000004	.000000	.000000	.000000	.000000	.000000	.000000
1.8	.000015	.000002	.000000	.000000	.000000	.000000	.000000
1.9	.000046	.000007	.000001	.000000	.000000	.000000	.000000
2.0	.000124	.000024	.000005	.000001	.000000	.000000	.000000
2.1	.000302	.000068	.000018	.000005	.000002	.000001	.000000
2.2	.000672	.000175	.000052	.000018	.000007	.000003	.000001
2.3	.001380	.000408	.000138	.000051	.000021	.000009	.000004
2.4	.002640	.000877	.000328	.000135	.000060	.000028	.000014
2.5	.004741	.001746	.000716	.000319	.000153	.000078	.000041
2.6	.008045	.003252	.001447	.000696	.000356	.000193	.000109
2.7	.012972	.005703	.002734	.001406	.000765	.000437	.000260
2.8	.019979	.009473	.004857	.002652	.001525	.000916	.000571
2.9	.029522	.014989	.008165	.004708	.002845	.001788	.001161
3.0	.042024	.022700	.013063	.007912	.005000	.003273	.002208
3.1	.057837	.033046	.019986	.012658	.008329	.005659	.003951
3.2	.077206	.046421	.029372	.019372	.013223	.009292	.006692
3.3	.100250	.063138	.041622	.028481	.020102	.014564	.010789
3.4	.126952	.083401	.057072	.040384	.029384	.021890	.016639
3.5	.157154	.107287	.075959	.055416	.041455	.031677	.024650
3.6	.190570	.134738	.098401	.073819	.056637	.044293	.035213
3.7	.226805	.165563	.124388	.095719	.075159	.060037	.048673
3.8	.265379	.199452	.153777	.121121	.097137	.079113	.065297
3.9	.305756	.235995	.186305	.149897	.122565	.101612	.085254
4.0	.347371	.274707	.221604	.181805	.151314	.127504	.108600
4.1	.389656	.315056	.259226	.216496	.183138	.156640	.135271
4.2	.432066	.356489	.298666	.253540	.217691	.188760	.165089
4.3	.474093	.398455	.339388	.292449	.254549	.223510	.197770
4.4	.515283	.440431	.380851	.332701	.293232	.260462	.232944
4.5	.555244	.481933	.422532	.373767	.333228	.299138	.270175
4.6	.593652	.522531	.463940	.415131	.374019	.339034	.308984
4.7	.630248	.561856	.504633	.456307	.415099	.379641	.348873
4.8	.664843	.599605	.544225	.496852	.455992	.420465	.389343
4.9	.697305	.635540	.582391	.536379	.496265	.461044	.429915

ν = 20

Q\n	40	50	60	70	80	90	100
5.0	.727559	.669485	.618872	.574560	.535537	.500960	.470143
5.1	.755581	.701323	.653468	.611127	.573486	.539846	.509628
5.2	.781384	.730990	.686041	.645875	.609849	.577393	.548022
5.3	.805017	.758466	.716503	.678655	.644423	.613349	.585033
5.4	.826557	.783770	.744816	.709372	.677061	.647521	.620427
5.5	.846099	.806955	.770981	.737978	.707668	.679770	.654024
5.6	.863753	.828095	.795034	.764464	.736193	.710007	.685699
5.7	.879641	.847286	.817037	.788860	.762629	.738187	.715373
5.8	.893888	.864637	.837074	.811220	.787001	.764304	.743010
5.9	.906620	.880265	.855244	.831621	.809359	.788386	.768612
6.0	.917964	.894292	.871659	.850156	.829780	.810485	.792209
6.4	.951836	.936832	.922127	.907846	.894046	.880744	.867936
6.8	.972221	.963021	.953820	.944724	.935793	.927057	.918534
7.2	.984165	.978655	.973051	.967429	.961834	.956297	.950834
7.6	.991037	.987788	.984438	.981036	.977612	.974190	.970782
8.0	.994943	.993047	.991069	.989039	.986978	.984899	.982814
8.4	.997148	.996048	.994889	.993688	.992460	.991212	.989952
8.8	.998388	.997752	.997075	.996369	.995641	.994898	.994143
9.2	.999086	.998717	.998322	.997908	.997478	.997037	.996586
9.6	.999479	.999265	.999034	.998791	.998537	.998275	.998007
10.0	.999701	.999576	.999441	.999298	.999148	.998992	.998832
11.0	.999923	.999890	.999854	.999815	.999774	.999731	.999686
12.0	.999979	.999970	.999960	.999949	.999937	.999925	.999912
13.0	.999994	.999991	.999988	.999985	.999982	.999978	.999974
14.0	1.00000	1.00000	1.00000	1.00000	.999994	.999993	.999992
15.0					1.00000	1.00000	1.00000

$\nu = 24$

Q\n	2	3	4	5	6	7	8
0.0	.000000	.000000	.000000	.000000	.000000	.000000	.000000
0.1	.055786	.002753	.000131	.000006	.000000	.000000	.000000
0.2	.111283	.010961	.001038	.000097	.000009	.000001	.000000
0.3	.166205	.024477	.003468	.000485	.000068	.000009	.000001
0.4	.220277	.043063	.008101	.001504	.000279	.000052	.000010
0.5	.273239	.066393	.015529	.003585	.000825	.000191	.000044
0.6	.324848	.094068	.026231	.007218	.001981	.000545	.000151
0.7	.374881	.125626	.040557	.012920	.004104	.001307	.000419
0.8	.423141	.160556	.058721	.021190	.007623	.002748	.000996
0.9	.469458	.198314	.080795	.032476	.013010	.005222	.002106
1.0	.513690	.238333	.106716	.047142	.020749	.009146	.004049
1.1	.555723	.280047	.136295	.065442	.031298	.014985	.007202
1.2	.595472	.322893	.169232	.087505	.045056	.023215	.012002
1.3	.632882	.366333	.205134	.113329	.062330	.034290	.018921
1.4	.667925	.409861	.243538	.142780	.083313	.048607	.028430
1.5	.700598	.453010	.283931	.175603	.108067	.066471	.040970
1.6	.730922	.495364	.325771	.211436	.136519	.088070	.056907
1.7	.758941	.536555	.368513	.249832	.168466	.113461	.076507
1.8	.784716	.576274	.411622	.290283	.203586	.142563	.099911
1.9	.808325	.614267	.454591	.332241	.241458	.175159	.127118
2.0	.829858	.650334	.496954	.375146	.281581	.210911	.157989
2.1	.849419	.684329	.538298	.418443	.323409	.249379	.192248
2.2	.867116	.716153	.578265	.461606	.366366	.290047	.229503
2.3	.883064	.745755	.616557	.504148	.409878	.332348	.269270
2.4	.897381	.773122	.652940	.545635	.453392	.375692	.310993
2.5	.910187	.798276	.687238	.585697	.496392	.419494	.354081
2.6	.921600	.821269	.719331	.624025	.538417	.463190	.397932
2.7	.931736	.842176	.749153	.660378	.579066	.506265	.441958
2.8	.940707	.861090	.776681	.694579	.618008	.548255	.485605
2.9	.948622	.878121	.801935	.726509	.654979	.588767	.528375
3.0	.955583	.893385	.824966	.756107	.689784	.627477	.569830
3.1	.961685	.907007	.845854	.783359	.722292	.664131	.609607
3.2	.967020	.919114	.864698	.808291	.752432	.698548	.647415
3.3	.971670	.929831	.881614	.830966	.780182	.730611	.683036
3.4	.975713	.939282	.896728	.851472	.805565	.760261	.716322
3.5	.979218	.947588	.910171	.869918	.828643	.787492	.747189
3.6	.982249	.954862	.922079	.886428	.849504	.812339	.775608
3.7	.984864	.961212	.932585	.901138	.868260	.834874	.801599
3.8	.987115	.966738	.941818	.914184	.885039	.855198	.825221
3.9	.989049	.971534	.949905	.925708	.899978	.873430	.846565
4.0	.990706	.975684	.956963	.935847	.913219	.889704	.865744
4.1	.992124	.979266	.963105	.944734	.924907	.904163	.882891
4.2	.993334	.982350	.968433	.952497	.935183	.916953	.898148
4.3	.994365	.984999	.973042	.959257	.944185	.928221	.911662
4.4	.995243	.987270	.977018	.965124	.952043	.938111	.923583
4.5	.995988	.989212	.980441	.970203	.958880	.946759	.934057
4.6	.996620	.990870	.983379	.974586	.964812	.954296	.943226
4.7	.997155	.992282	.985897	.978361	.969942	.960844	.951226
4.8	.997608	.993483	.988049	.981603	.974369	.966517	.958183
4.9	.997990	.994504	.989885	.984382	.978179	.971418	.964215

$\nu = 24$

Q\n	2	3	4	5	6	7	8
5.0	.998313	.995369	.991450	.986759	.981450	.975642	.969431
5.1	.998585	.996101	.992780	.988788	.984252	.979272	.973929
5.2	.998813	.996720	.993909	.990517	.986648	.982387	.977799
5.3	.999006	.997244	.994867	.991988	.988693	.985052	.981121
5.4	.999167	.997685	.995677	.993237	.990435	.987330	.983967
5.5	.999303	.998057	.996363	.994296	.991917	.989272	.986401
5.6	.999417	.998370	.996941	.995194	.993175	.990926	.988477
5.7	.999512	.998633	.997430	.995953	.994243	.992332	.990247
5.8	.999592	.998854	.997841	.996594	.995147	.993525	.991752
5.9	.999659	.999040	.998188	.997136	.995912	.994537	.993031
6.0	.999715	.999196	.998479	.997593	.996558	.995394	.994116
6.4	.999861	.999605	.999249	.998803	.998279	.997685	.997028
6.8	.999932	.999807	.999630	.999407	.999144	.998843	.998509
7.2	.999967	.999905	.999818	.999707	.999575	.999423	.999254
7.6	.999984	.999953	.999910	.999855	.999789	.999712	.999627
8.0	.999992	.999977	.999955	.999928	.999894	.999856	.999813
8.4	1.00000	.999989	.999978	.999964	.999947	.999928	.999906
8.8		.999994	.999989	.999982	.999973	.999963	.999952
9.2		1.00000	.999994	.999991	.999986	.999981	.999976
9.6			1.00000	1.00000	.999993	.999990	.999988
10.0					1.00000	1.00000	.999994
11.0							1.00000

$\nu = 24$

Q\n	9	10	11	12	13	14	15
0.0	.000000	.000000	.000000	.000000	.000000	.000000	.000000
0.1	.000000	.000000	.000000	.000000	.000000	.000000	.000000
0.2	.000000	.000000	.000000	.000000	.000000	.000000	.000000
0.3	.000000	.000000	.000000	.000000	.000000	.000000	.000000
0.4	.000002	.000000	.000000	.000000	.000000	.000000	.000000
0.5	.000010	.000002	.000001	.000000	.000000	.000000	.000000
0.6	.000042	.000012	.000003	.000001	.000000	.000000	.000000
0.7	.000135	.000044	.000014	.000005	.000002	.000001	.000000
0.8	.000363	.000134	.000050	.000019	.000007	.000003	.000001
0.9	.000855	.000350	.000144	.000060	.000025	.000011	.000005
1.0	.001803	.000809	.000366	.000167	.000077	.000036	.000017
1.1	.003481	.001694	.000830	.000410	.000204	.000102	.000052
1.2	.006237	.003261	.001717	.000910	.000486	.000262	.000142
1.3	.010488	.005847	.003280	.001852	.001053	.000603	.000347
1.4	.016697	.009857	.005852	.003496	.002101	.001271	.000774
1.5	.025344	.015750	.009839	.006181	.003905	.002482	.001587
1.6	.036887	.024008	.015700	.010319	.006818	.004530	.003026
1.7	.051728	.035101	.023919	.016374	.011264	.007786	.005409
1.8	.070176	.049447	.034972	.024836	.017715	.012692	.009135
1.9	.092422	.067378	.049283	.036180	.026664	.019730	.014660
2.0	.118515	.089108	.067190	.050827	.038583	.029394	.022477
2.1	.148362	.114712	.088914	.069112	.053885	.042148	.033077
2.2	.181728	.144120	.114534	.091244	.072886	.058387	.046909
2.3	.218253	.177116	.143982	.117292	.095773	.078396	.064338
2.4	.257470	.213351	.177042	.147172	.122587	.102330	.085614
2.5	.298836	.252367	.213363	.180652	.153217	.130191	.110843
2.6	.341757	.293622	.252483	.217367	.187403	.161825	.139976
2.7	.385623	.336521	.293854	.256839	.224752	.196936	.172813
2.8	.429828	.380445	.336874	.298509	.264765	.235096	.209008
2.9	.473801	.424780	.380917	.341765	.306866	.275781	.248098
3.0	.517017	.468942	.425365	.385976	.350434	.318395	.289528
3.1	.559016	.512394	.469628	.430520	.394832	.362306	.332684
3.2	.599408	.554663	.513164	.474808	.439440	.406877	.376927
3.3	.637881	.595349	.555500	.518304	.483673	.451491	.421620
3.4	.674196	.634129	.596234	.560536	.527006	.495576	.466158
3.5	.708186	.670753	.635040	.601112	.568982	.538623	.509986
3.6	.739752	.705050	.671673	.639716	.609221	.580194	.552616
3.7	.768853	.736913	.705961	.676110	.647424	.619931	.593636
3.8	.795498	.766296	.737800	.710132	.683369	.657556	.632714
3.9	.819739	.793207	.767148	.741686	.716908	.692867	.669600
4.0	.841663	.817696	.794013	.770738	.747960	.725739	.704117
4.1	.861382	.839848	.818449	.797305	.776502	.756106	.736160
4.2	.879024	.859773	.840543	.821445	.802563	.783962	.765688
4.3	.894732	.877603	.860409	.843251	.826210	.809348	.792711
4.4	.908656	.893481	.878178	.862840	.847542	.832341	.817284
4.5	.920945	.907555	.893995	.880348	.866681	.853050	.839496
4.6	.931748	.919979	.908012	.895921	.883768	.871602	.859463
4.7	.941211	.930902	.920380	.909711	.898950	.888140	.877320
4.8	.949472	.940471	.931252	.921873	.912381	.902816	.893213
4.9	.956659	.948825	.940774	.932556	.924215	.915785	.907296

$\nu = 24$

Q\n	9	10	11	12	13	14	15
5.0	.962893	.956094	.949084	.941908	.934602	.927199	.919723
5.1	.968287	.962400	.956314	.950066	.943688	.937208	.930648
5.2	.972941	.967857	.962587	.957162	.951610	.945954	.940216
5.3	.976946	.972566	.968013	.963315	.958495	.953574	.948569
5.4	.980387	.976620	.972695	.968636	.964462	.960192	.955839
5.5	.983335	.980103	.976726	.973227	.969621	.965924	.962148
5.6	.985857	.983088	.980189	.977178	.974070	.970876	.967609
5.7	.988011	.985642	.983158	.980572	.977897	.975145	.972324
5.8	.989846	.987823	.985698	.983481	.981184	.978816	.976385
5.9	.991409	.989684	.987867	.985970	.984001	.981967	.979876
6.0	.992737	.991267	.989718	.988096	.986410	.984667	.982871
6.4	.996314	.995549	.994737	.993882	.992989	.992059	.991097
6.8	.998144	.997750	.997330	.996886	.996420	.995933	.995426
7.2	.999068	.998867	.998652	.998424	.998183	.997930	.997667
7.6	.999533	.999431	.999321	.999204	.999080	.998950	.998814
8.0	.999765	.999713	.999657	.999597	.999534	.999467	.999397
8.4	.999882	.999855	.999827	.999796	.999763	.999729	.999693
8.8	.999940	.999926	.999912	.999896	.999879	.999862	.999843
9.2	.999969	.999962	.999955	.999947	.999938	.999929	.999919
9.6	.999984	.999981	.999977	.999972	.999968	.999963	.999958
10.0	.999992	.999990	.999988	.999986	.999983	.999981	.999978
11.0	1.00000	1.00000	1.00000	1.00000	1.00000	1.00000	1.00000

$\nu = 24$

Q\n	16	17	18	19	20	22	24
0.0	.000000	.000000	.000000	.000000	.000000	.000000	.000000
0.1	.000000	.000000	.000000	.000000	.000000	.000000	.000000
0.2	.000000	.000000	.000000	.000000	.000000	.000000	.000000
0.3	.000000	.000000	.000000	.000000	.000000	.000000	.000000
0.4	.000000	.000000	.000000	.000000	.000000	.000000	.000000
0.5	.000000	.000000	.000000	.000000	.000000	.000000	.000000
0.6	.000000	.000000	.000000	.000000	.000000	.000000	.000000
0.7	.000000	.000000	.000000	.000000	.000000	.000000	.000000
0.8	.000000	.000000	.000000	.000000	.000000	.000000	.000000
0.9	.000002	.000001	.000000	.000000	.000000	.000000	.000000
1.0	.000008	.000004	.000002	.000001	.000000	.000000	.000000
1.1	.000026	.000014	.000007	.000004	.000002	.000001	.000000
1.2	.000077	.000043	.000024	.000013	.000007	.000002	.000001
1.3	.000202	.000118	.000069	.000041	.000025	.000009	.000003
1.4	.000474	.000293	.000182	.000113	.000071	.000029	.000012
1.5	.001021	.000660	.000430	.000281	.000185	.000082	.000037
1.6	.002032	.001372	.000932	.000636	.000436	.000209	.000102
1.7	.003777	.002650	.001869	.001324	.000943	.000485	.000254
1.8	.006605	.004797	.003500	.002565	.001888	.001036	.000578
1.9	.010937	.008194	.006164	.004655	.003530	.002053	.001213
2.0	.017251	.013290	.010276	.007975	.006211	.003808	.002367
2.1	.026045	.020576	.016310	.012971	.010350	.006652	.004329
2.2	.037800	.030551	.024766	.020136	.016420	.011013	.007469
2.3	.052941	.043679	.036133	.029971	.024925	.017372	.012230
2.4	.071796	.060350	.050849	.042945	.036355	.026234	.019101
2.5	.094563	.080841	.069256	.059455	.051147	.038086	.028588
2.6	.121292	.105292	.091571	.079785	.069644	.053355	.041168
2.7	.151876	.133686	.117863	.104081	.092060	.072369	.057251
2.8	.186056	.165850	.148043	.132335	.118460	.095325	.077136
2.9	.223439	.201464	.181867	.164376	.148750	.122264	.100986
3.0	.263520	.240082	.218952	.199890	.182681	.153071	.128807
3.1	.305715	.281161	.258802	.238432	.219866	.187475	.160448
3.2	.349395	.324092	.300837	.279460	.259802	.225070	.195604
3.3	.393916	.368233	.344428	.322363	.301908	.265341	.233842
3.4	.438649	.412942	.388928	.366499	.345550	.307695	.274624
3.5	.483004	.457603	.433702	.411222	.390080	.351494	.317345
3.6	.526449	.501647	.478155	.455913	.434862	.396090	.361363
3.7	.568525	.544572	.521745	.500002	.479302	.440850	.406029
3.8	.608849	.585951	.564004	.542983	.522861	.485187	.450721
3.9	.647121	.625437	.604542	.584426	.565072	.528573	.494863
4.0	.683120	.662763	.643050	.623981	.605549	.570551	.537943
4.1	.716698	.697741	.679299	.661380	.643985	.610746	.579524
4.2	.747778	.730255	.713137	.696435	.680154	.648864	.619251
4.3	.776337	.760252	.744477	.729026	.713908	.684693	.656848
4.4	.802406	.787736	.773295	.759100	.745162	.718091	.692120
4.5	.826055	.812755	.799617	.786660	.773896	.748986	.724943
4.6	.847384	.835392	.823509	.811752	.800135	.777364	.755258
4.7	.866518	.855762	.845070	.834461	.823949	.803257	.783064
4.8	.883598	.873995	.864424	.854900	.845437	.826740	.808402
4.9	.898773	.890238	.881709	.873200	.864724	.847917	.831355

ν = 24

Q\n	16	17	18	19	20	22	24
5.0	.912199	.904643	.897075	.889506	.881949	.866913	.852031
5.1	.924028	.917366	.910676	.903971	.897262	.883870	.870561
5.2	.934412	.928558	.922667	.916750	.910817	.898939	.887088
5.3	.943497	.938370	.933199	.927996	.922769	.912273	.901764
5.4	.951419	.946942	.942418	.937857	.933267	.924026	.914742
5.5	.958307	.954408	.950462	.946476	.942458	.934348	.926174
5.6	.964278	.960892	.957459	.953986	.950479	.943383	.936210
5.7	.969443	.966509	.963530	.960511	.957457	.951267	.944991
5.8	.973898	.971362	.968782	.966165	.963513	.958126	.952650
5.9	.977734	.975546	.973317	.971052	.968755	.964078	.959312
6.0	.981029	.979145	.977223	.975267	.973281	.969230	.965092
6.4	.990105	.989085	.988040	.986972	.985882	.983644	.981339
6.8	.994902	.994361	.993804	.993232	.992647	.991440	.990187
7.2	.997393	.997109	.996817	.996516	.996206	.995565	.994896
7.6	.998672	.998524	.998372	.998215	.998053	.997715	.997362
8.0	.999324	.999247	.999168	.999087	.999002	.998826	.998641
8.4	.999655	.999616	.999575	.999532	.999488	.999396	.999299
8.8	.999823	.999803	.999782	.999760	.999737	.999689	.999638
9.2	.999909	.999898	.999887	.999876	.999864	.999839	.999812
9.6	.999953	.999947	.999942	.999936	.999929	.999916	.999902
10.0	.999975	.999972	.999969	.999966	.999963	.999956	.999949
11.0	.999995	.999994	.999994	.999993	.999992	.999991	.999989
12.0	1.00000	1.00000	1.00000	1.00000	1.00000	1.00000	1.00000

$\nu = 24$

Q\n	26	28	30	32	34	36	38
0.0	.000000	.000000	.000000	.000000	.000000	.000000	.000000
0.1	.000000	.000000	.000000	.000000	.000000	.000000	.000000
0.2	.000000	.000000	.000000	.000000	.000000	.000000	.000000
0.3	.000000	.000000	.000000	.000000	.000000	.000000	.000000
0.4	.000000	.000000	.000000	.000000	.000000	.000000	.000000
0.5	.000000	.000000	.000000	.000000	.000000	.000000	.000000
0.6	.000000	.000000	.000000	.000000	.000000	.000000	.000000
0.7	.000000	.000000	.000000	.000000	.000000	.000000	.000000
0.8	.000000	.000000	.000000	.000000	.000000	.000000	.000000
0.9	.000000	.000000	.000000	.000000	.000000	.000000	.000000
1.0	.000000	.000000	.000000	.000000	.000000	.000000	.000000
1.1	.000000	.000000	.000000	.000000	.000000	.000000	.000000
1.2	.000000	.000000	.000000	.000000	.000000	.000000	.000000
1.3	.000001	.000000	.000000	.000000	.000000	.000000	.000000
1.4	.000005	.000002	.000001	.000000	.000000	.000000	.000000
1.5	.000017	.000008	.000004	.000002	.000001	.000000	.000000
1.6	.000050	.000026	.000013	.000007	.000004	.000002	.000001
1.7	.000135	.000073	.000040	.000022	.000013	.000007	.000004
1.8	.000327	.000188	.000110	.000065	.000039	.000024	.000014
1.9	.000726	.000441	.000271	.000169	.000107	.000068	.000044
2.0	.001490	.000950	.000613	.000400	.000264	.000176	.000118
2.1	.002850	.001898	.001278	.000869	.000597	.000414	.000289
2.2	.005120	.003546	.002480	.001750	.001246	.000895	.000648
2.3	.008693	.006236	.004513	.003294	.002423	.001796	.001341
2.4	.014029	.010389	.007754	.005832	.004418	.003370	.002587
2.5	.021626	.016481	.012649	.009775	.007603	.005950	.004684
2.6	.031985	.025016	.019690	.015592	.012420	.009948	.008010
2.7	.045569	.036486	.029379	.023786	.019358	.015833	.013012
2.8	.062757	.051327	.042191	.034850	.028920	.024107	.020180
2.9	.083810	.069879	.058525	.049228	.041579	.035258	.030012
3.0	.108845	.092353	.078670	.067271	.057736	.049727	.042974
3.1	.137820	.118809	.102777	.089208	.077683	.067859	.059456
3.2	.170536	.149146	.130838	.115117	.101576	.089876	.079735
3.3	.206647	.183111	.162688	.144918	.129414	.115850	.103952
3.4	.245685	.220310	.198013	.178375	.161038	.145697	.132090
3.5	.287088	.260238	.236370	.215112	.196141	.179177	.163977
3.6	.330238	.302311	.277219	.254640	.234289	.215913	.199294
3.7	.374486	.345895	.319952	.296384	.274945	.255415	.237597
3.8	.419193	.390343	.363927	.339717	.317507	.297107	.278348
3.9	.463746	.435023	.408501	.383997	.361338	.340369	.320943
4.0	.507590	.479344	.453059	.428589	.405799	.384558	.364747
4.1	.550234	.522772	.497031	.472901	.450274	.429048	.409125
4.2	.591267	.564847	.539915	.516392	.494196	.473248	.453470
4.3	.630358	.605185	.581282	.558594	.537061	.516624	.497223
4.4	.667257	.643487	.620785	.599116	.578438	.558710	.539887
4.5	.701790	.679531	.658156	.637647	.617978	.599121	.581043
4.6	.733855	.713170	.693207	.673958	.655411	.637548	.620349
4.7	.763411	.744325	.725818	.707892	.690544	.673764	.657542
4.8	.790470	.772975	.755935	.739361	.723255	.707615	.692436
4.9	.815087	.799148	.783559	.768336	.753486	.739013	.724915

$\nu = 24$

Q\n	26	28	30	32	34	36	38
5.0	.837353	.822913	.808736	.794840	.781235	.767930	.754926
5.1	.857383	.844369	.831546	.818934	.806544	.794387	.782469
5.2	.875311	.863639	.852100	.840713	.829491	.818447	.807587
5.3	.891283	.880863	.870527	.860296	.850185	.840204	.830363
5.4	.905452	.896187	.886970	.877819	.868750	.859775	.850901
5.5	.917971	.909764	.901578	.893428	.885330	.877294	.869331
5.6	.928990	.921748	.914503	.907273	.900071	.892907	.885791
5.7	.938656	.932286	.925897	.919506	.913124	.906763	.900430
5.8	.947109	.941522	.935906	.930275	.924641	.919011	.913396
5.9	.954478	.949592	.944671	.939725	.934765	.929801	.924839
6.0	.960885	.956624	.952322	.947990	.943638	.939274	.934903
6.4	.978976	.976565	.974112	.971625	.969109	.966568	.964009
6.8	.988895	.987568	.986210	.984825	.983416	.981986	.980537
7.2	.994202	.993486	.992750	.991995	.991224	.990437	.989638
7.6	.996994	.996613	.996219	.995814	.995398	.994973	.994539
8.0	.998447	.998245	.998037	.997821	.997599	.997372	.997138
8.4	.999198	.999092	.998982	.998867	.998750	.998629	.998504
8.8	.999585	.999529	.999471	.999411	.999348	.999284	.999218
9.2	.999784	.999755	.999724	.999692	.999659	.999625	.999590
9.6	.999887	.999872	.999856	.999839	.999821	.999803	.999784
10.0	.999941	.999933	.999924	.999915	.999906	.999896	.999886
11.0	.999988	.999986	.999984	.999982	.999980	.999978	.999976
12.0	1.00000	1.00000	1.00000	1.00000	1.00000	1.00000	.999995
13.0							1.00000

$\nu = 24$

Q\n	40	50	60	70	80	90	100
0.0	.000000	.000000	.000000	.000000	.000000	.000000	.000000
0.1	.000000	.000000	.000000	.000000	.000000	.000000	.000000
0.2	.000000	.000000	.000000	.000000	.000000	.000000	.000000
0.3	.000000	.000000	.000000	.000000	.000000	.000000	.000000
0.4	.000000	.000000	.000000	.000000	.000000	.000000	.000000
0.5	.000000	.000000	.000000	.000000	.000000	.000000	.000000
0.6	.000000	.000000	.000000	.000000	.000000	.000000	.000000
0.7	.000000	.000000	.000000	.000000	.000000	.000000	.000000
0.8	.000000	.000000	.000000	.000000	.000000	.000000	.000000
0.9	.000000	.000000	.000000	.000000	.000000	.000000	.000000
1.0	.000000	.000000	.000000	.000000	.000000	.000000	.000000
1.1	.000000	.000000	.000000	.000000	.000000	.000000	.000000
1.2	.000000	.000000	.000000	.000000	.000000	.000000	.000000
1.3	.000000	.000000	.000000	.000000	.000000	.000000	.000000
1.4	.000000	.000000	.000000	.000000	.000000	.000000	.000000
1.5	.000000	.000000	.000000	.000000	.000000	.000000	.000000
1.6	.000001	.000000	.000000	.000000	.000000	.000000	.000000
1.7	.000002	.000000	.000000	.000000	.000000	.000000	.000000
1.8	.000009	.000001	.000000	.000000	.000000	.000000	.000000
1.9	.000028	.000004	.000001	.000000	.000000	.000000	.000000
2.0	.000080	.000013	.000003	.000001	.000000	.000000	.000000
2.1	.000204	.000040	.000009	.000002	.000001	.000000	.000000
2.2	.000473	.000108	.000029	.000009	.000003	.000001	.000000
2.3	.001008	.000266	.000080	.000027	.000010	.000004	.000002
2.4	.001999	.000599	.000202	.000075	.000030	.000013	.000006
2.5	.003708	.001244	.000465	.000190	.000084	.000039	.000019
2.6	.006483	.002410	.000988	.000439	.000208	.000104	.000055
2.7	.010742	.004381	.001951	.000934	.000475	.000254	.000142
2.8	.016962	.007521	.003609	.001848	.000999	.000565	.000332
2.9	.025640	.012262	.006295	.003426	.001958	.001166	.000719
3.0	.037259	.019081	.010414	.005990	.003600	.002246	.001446
3.1	.052244	.028470	.016424	.009932	.006248	.004065	.002721
3.2	.070920	.040891	.024808	.015700	.010295	.006957	.004825
3.3	.093488	.056741	.036036	.023767	.016183	.011322	.008109
3.4	.119994	.076309	.050524	.034600	.024381	.017605	.012983
3.5	.150330	.099752	.068599	.048617	.035346	.026267	.019894
3.6	.184236	.127077	.090467	.066150	.049485	.037752	.029296
3.7	.221319	.158139	.116188	.087416	.067120	.052448	.041614
3.8	.261076	.192645	.145675	.112496	.088458	.070654	.057210
3.9	.302928	.230181	.178695	.141320	.113569	.092549	.076347
4.0	.346253	.270231	.214882	.173679	.142382	.118180	.099166
4.1	.390412	.312213	.253765	.209229	.174682	.147449	.125675
4.2	.434788	.355507	.294794	.247520	.210128	.180125	.155740
4.3	.478800	.399491	.337370	.288021	.248274	.215853	.189099
4.4	.521925	.443561	.380879	.330147	.288595	.254177	.225374
4.5	.563714	.487158	.424718	.373297	.330516	.294571	.264094
4.6	.603791	.529785	.468316	.416871	.373442	.336465	.304727
4.7	.641862	.571011	.511158	.460303	.416785	.379271	.346702
4.8	.677710	.610487	.552791	.503075	.459988	.422412	.389442
4.9	.711191	.647937	.592838	.544730	.502539	.465345	.432382

ν = 24

Q\n	40	50	60	70	80	90	100
5.0	.742225	.683161	.630995	.584882	.543989	.507572	.474997
5.1	.770792	.716031	.667033	.623219	.583957	.548659	.516808
5.2	.796918	.746480	.700797	.659502	.622135	.588240	.557403
5.3	.820667	.774493	.732192	.693562	.658285	.626018	.596435
5.4	.842137	.800105	.761182	.725296	.692241	.661768	.633626
5.5	.861447	.823385	.787780	.754657	.723898	.695331	.668771
5.6	.878731	.844430	.812037	.781646	.753208	.726612	.701724
5.7	.894133	.863361	.834038	.806307	.780171	.755566	.732403
5.8	.907802	.880310	.853890	.828716	.804828	.782200	.760776
5.9	.919886	.895419	.871718	.848974	.827252	.806555	.786853
6.0	.930533	.908836	.887658	.867199	.847540	.828706	.810685
6.4	.961433	.948420	.935379	.922482	.909824	.897460	.885419
6.8	.979072	.971566	.963881	.956134	.948400	.940726	.933144
7.2	.988825	.984615	.980228	.975737	.971189	.966619	.962049
7.6	.994096	.991780	.989332	.986794	.984193	.981551	.978884
8.0	.996900	.995643	.994298	.992889	.991430	.989936	.988414
8.4	.998377	.997700	.996969	.996195	.995388	.994555	.993701
8.8	.999150	.998787	.998392	.997970	.997528	.997068	.996593
9.2	.999554	.999360	.999147	.998918	.998676	.998423	.998161
9.6	.999765	.999661	.999546	.999422	.999290	.999151	.999007
10.0	.999876	.999820	.999757	.999690	.999618	.999542	.999463
11.0	.999974	.999962	.999948	.999933	.999917	.999900	.999882
12.0	.999994	.999991	.999988	.999985	.999981	.999977	.999973
13.0	1.00000	1.00000	1.00000	1.00000	1.00000	.999995	.999994
14.0						1.00000	1.00000

$\nu = 30$

Q\n	2	3	4	5	6	7	8
0.0	.000000	.000000	.000000	.000000	.000000	.000000	.000000
0.1	.055903	.002753	.000130	.000006	.000000	.000000	.000000
0.2	.111517	.010962	.001033	.000096	.000009	.000001	.000000
0.3	.166561	.024482	.003449	.000478	.000066	.000009	.000001
0.4	.220760	.043078	.008059	.001483	.000271	.000050	.000009
0.5	.273854	.066430	.015455	.003536	.000805	.000183	.000042
0.6	.325600	.094142	.026118	.007126	.001933	.000524	.000143
0.7	.375776	.125758	.040403	.012767	.004010	.001259	.000397
0.8	.424185	.160771	.058533	.020960	.007460	.002654	.000947
0.9	.470656	.198641	.080589	.032159	.012753	.005053	.002007
1.0	.515043	.238804	.106517	.046735	.020375	.008873	.003872
1.1	.557232	.280694	.136138	.064956	.030790	.014575	.006910
1.2	.597136	.323748	.169162	.086965	.044408	.022639	.011556
1.3	.634697	.367427	.205202	.112773	.061552	.033530	.018282
1.4	.669883	.411219	.243798	.142262	.082432	.047658	.027570
1.5	.702691	.454655	.284440	.175187	.107132	.065350	.039873
1.6	.733138	.497308	.326585	.211197	.135595	.086818	.055581
1.7	.761265	.538807	.369680	.249850	.167637	.112141	.074986
1.8	.787132	.578834	.413185	.290636	.202946	.141262	.098256
1.9	.810816	.617127	.456582	.333005	.241108	.173982	.125420
2.0	.832406	.653479	.499393	.376387	.281624	.209976	.156361
2.1	.852003	.687735	.541193	.420215	.323939	.248809	.190822
2.2	.869717	.719794	.581610	.463945	.367468	.289964	.228423
2.3	.885664	.749597	.620334	.507075	.411620	.332862	.268677
2.4	.899961	.777129	.657119	.549153	.455821	.376898	.311021
2.5	.912729	.802408	.691779	.589788	.499533	.421464	.354849
2.6	.924089	.825486	.724187	.628658	.542271	.465971	.399532
2.7	.934156	.846437	.754269	.665505	.583613	.509874	.444454
2.8	.943047	.865357	.781999	.700140	.623205	.552684	.489030
2.9	.950870	.882355	.807395	.732437	.660767	.593979	.532728
3.0	.957731	.897553	.830508	.762326	.696088	.633414	.575082
3.1	.963726	.911078	.851419	.789791	.729028	.670715	.615698
3.2	.968949	.923060	.870232	.814859	.759508	.705686	.654262
3.3	.973483	.933630	.887066	.837592	.787502	.738200	.690539
3.4	.977409	.942915	.902053	.858085	.813036	.768192	.724368
3.5	.980797	.951040	.915331	.876452	.836173	.795654	.755656
3.6	.983713	.958122	.927040	.892824	.857009	.820626	.784372
3.7	.986216	.964273	.937321	.907344	.875663	.843184	.810539
3.8	.988357	.969598	.946310	.920158	.892270	.863437	.834220
3.9	.990186	.974191	.954137	.931414	.906979	.881515	.855517
4.0	.991743	.978140	.960928	.941259	.919943	.897563	.874553
4.1	.993065	.981526	.966798	.949834	.931314	.911736	.891474
4.2	.994186	.984421	.971854	.957273	.941245	.924192	.906434
4.3	.995134	.986889	.976196	.963703	.949882	.935089	.919596
4.4	.995934	.988986	.979912	.969241	.957365	.944580	.931119
4.5	.996608	.990766	.983084	.973995	.963822	.952814	.941165
4.6	.997174	.992271	.985783	.978063	.969376	.959929	.949885
4.7	.997649	.993542	.988074	.981533	.974137	.966055	.957426
4.8	.998046	.994612	.990014	.984485	.978205	.971312	.963922
4.9	.998379	.995511	.991652	.986990	.981670	.975809	.969499

ν = 30

Q\n	2	3	4	5	6	7	8
5.0	.998656	.996266	.993033	.989110	.984615	.979643	.974271
5.1	.998888	.996898	.994194	.990900	.987110	.982903	.978342
5.2	.999080	.997426	.995169	.992407	.989219	.985667	.981805
5.3	.999240	.997867	.995985	.993674	.990997	.988006	.984743
5.4	.999373	.998234	.996668	.994737	.992494	.989979	.987228
5.5	.999483	.998540	.997237	.995627	.993750	.991641	.989326
5.6	.999574	.998793	.997712	.996371	.994804	.993037	.991094
5.7	.999649	.999004	.998108	.996992	.995685	.994207	.992579
5.8	.999711	.999179	.998436	.997509	.996420	.995187	.993824
5.9	.999762	.999323	.998708	.997940	.997034	.996006	.994867
6.0	.999805	.999442	.998934	.998297	.997545	.996689	.995739
6.4	.999911	.999745	.999510	.999212	.998857	.998450	.997996
6.8	.999960	.999884	.999776	.999638	.999473	.999283	.999069
7.2	.999982	.999948	.999898	.999835	.999759	.999671	.999571
7.6	.999992	.999976	.999954	.999925	.999890	.999849	.999803
8.0	1.00000	.999989	.999979	.999966	.999950	.999931	.999910
8.4		1.00000	.999990	.999984	.999977	.999969	.999959
8.8			1.00000	.999993	.999990	.999986	.999981
9.2				1.00000	1.00000	.999993	.999991
9.6						1.00000	1.00000

$\nu = 30$

Q\n	9	10	11	12	13	14	15
0.0	.000000	.000000	.000000	.000000	.000000	.000000	.000000
0.1	.000000	.000000	.000000	.000000	.000000	.000000	.000000
0.2	.000000	.000000	.000000	.000000	.000000	.000000	.000000
0.3	.000000	.000000	.000000	.000000	.000000	.000000	.000000
0.4	.000002	.000000	.000000	.000000	.000000	.000000	.000000
0.5	.000010	.000002	.000001	.000000	.000000	.000000	.000000
0.6	.000039	.000011	.000003	.000001	.000000	.000000	.000000
0.7	.000126	.000040	.000013	.000004	.000001	.000000	.000000
0.8	.000339	.000122	.000044	.000016	.000006	.000002	.000001
0.9	.000801	.000321	.000130	.000053	.000022	.000009	.000004
1.0	.001696	.000747	.000331	.000147	.000066	.000030	.000014
1.1	.003288	.001572	.000755	.000365	.000178	.000087	.000043
1.2	.005917	.003043	.001573	.000817	.000427	.000225	.000119
1.3	.009996	.005486	.003025	.001677	.000934	.000524	.000295
1.4	.015986	.009302	.005435	.003191	.001883	.001117	.000666
1.5	.024376	.014948	.009201	.005688	.003532	.002204	.001382
1.6	.035640	.022914	.014781	.009572	.006225	.004066	.002668
1.7	.050202	.033686	.022670	.015310	.010378	.007063	.004827
1.8	.068402	.047708	.033361	.023400	.016469	.011632	.008246
1.9	.090460	.065345	.047308	.034341	.025003	.018263	.013384
2.0	.116461	.086847	.064884	.048587	.036480	.027467	.020743
2.1	.146341	.112327	.086350	.066512	.051349	.039742	.030840
2.2	.179885	.141745	.111827	.088370	.069971	.055523	.044161
2.3	.216748	.174912	.141282	.114274	.092582	.075148	.061121
2.4	.256464	.211494	.174526	.144176	.119269	.098822	.082024
2.5	.298483	.251038	.211225	.177874	.149959	.126593	.107027
2.6	.342195	.292991	.250918	.215017	.184417	.158346	.136132
2.7	.386960	.336740	.293047	.255127	.222265	.193808	.169169
2.8	.432143	.381636	.336988	.297630	.262999	.232559	.205815
2.9	.477136	.427030	.382083	.341890	.306025	.274065	.245606
3.0	.521378	.472299	.427672	.387238	.350690	.317708	.287974
3.1	.564373	.516864	.473124	.433008	.396315	.362816	.332271
3.2	.605702	.560215	.517854	.478564	.442231	.408705	.377815
3.3	.645022	.601917	.561344	.523322	.487806	.454708	.423917
3.4	.682074	.641615	.603156	.566769	.532462	.500199	.469917
3.5	.716678	.679040	.642935	.608472	.575697	.544616	.515203
3.6	.748725	.714001	.680410	.648083	.617094	.587476	.559236
3.7	.778169	.746383	.715393	.685341	.656320	.628383	.601558
3.8	.805024	.776138	.747771	.720068	.693132	.667028	.641800
3.9	.829348	.803276	.777499	.752161	.727367	.703191	.679684
4.0	.851236	.827854	.804590	.781584	.758938	.736730	.715016
4.1	.870812	.849967	.829106	.808359	.787825	.767581	.747683
4.2	.888220	.869740	.851146	.832555	.814062	.795738	.777642
4.3	.903616	.887319	.870838	.854279	.837728	.821253	.804910
4.4	.917165	.902863	.888331	.873664	.858939	.844218	.829553
4.5	.929031	.916538	.903787	.890863	.877834	.864757	.851679
4.6	.939377	.928510	.917374	.906042	.894573	.883018	.871421
4.7	.948359	.938946	.929261	.919369	.909322	.899165	.888935
4.8	.956127	.948003	.939615	.931017	.922256	.913369	.904389
4.9	.962819	.955833	.948595	.941153	.933544	.925802	.917957

$\nu = 30$

Q\n	9	10	11	12	13	14	15
5.0	.968565	.962577	.956354	.949935	.943353	.936637	.929813
5.1	.973482	.968365	.963032	.957516	.951843	.946040	.940127
5.2	.977676	.973317	.968761	.964035	.959163	.954166	.949063
5.3	.981244	.977541	.973660	.969623	.965452	.961164	.956774
5.4	.984271	.981133	.977835	.974398	.970838	.967169	.963406
5.5	.986832	.984179	.981384	.978465	.975435	.972306	.969089
5.6	.988994	.986756	.984393	.981920	.979347	.976686	.973944
5.7	.990815	.988931	.986938	.984847	.982668	.980410	.978080
5.8	.992346	.990762	.989085	.987321	.985480	.983569	.981593
5.9	.993630	.992302	.990892	.989408	.987855	.986241	.984569
6.0	.994705	.993593	.992410	.991163	.989857	.988496	.987085
6.4	.997498	.996959	.996383	.995771	.995127	.994453	.993750
6.8	.998833	.998577	.998301	.998008	.997697	.997370	.997028
7.2	.999461	.999340	.999210	.999071	.998923	.998767	.998604
7.6	.999752	.999696	.999635	.999570	.999500	.999427	.999349
8.0	.999886	.999860	.999832	.999801	.999769	.999734	.999698
8.4	.999948	.999936	.999923	.999908	.999893	.999877	.999860
8.8	.999976	.999970	.999964	.999958	.999951	.999943	.999935
9.2	.999989	.999986	.999983	.999980	.999977	.999974	.999970
9.6	.999995	.999994	.999992	.999991	.999989	.999988	.999986
10.0	1.00000	1.00000	1.00000	1.00000	.999995	.999994	.999993
11.0					1.00000	1.00000	1.00000

$\nu = 30$

Q\n	16	17	18	19	20	22	24
0.0	.000000	.000000	.000000	.000000	.000000	.000000	.000000
0.1	.000000	.000000	.000000	.000000	.000000	.000000	.000000
0.2	.000000	.000000	.000000	.000000	.000000	.000000	.000000
0.3	.000000	.000000	.000000	.000000	.000000	.000000	.000000
0.4	.000000	.000000	.000000	.000000	.000000	.000000	.000000
0.5	.000000	.000000	.000000	.000000	.000000	.000000	.000000
0.6	.000000	.000000	.000000	.000000	.000000	.000000	.000000
0.7	.000000	.000000	.000000	.000000	.000000	.000000	.000000
0.8	.000000	.000000	.000000	.000000	.000000	.000000	.000000
0.9	.000002	.000001	.000000	.000000	.000000	.000000	.000000
1.0	.000006	.000003	.000001	.000001	.000000	.000000	.000000
1.1	.000021	.000011	.000005	.000003	.000001	.000000	.000000
1.2	.000063	.000034	.000018	.000010	.000005	.000002	.000001
1.3	.000167	.000095	.000055	.000032	.000018	.000006	.000002
1.4	.000399	.000241	.000146	.000089	.000054	.000021	.000008
1.5	.000871	.000552	.000351	.000225	.000144	.000061	.000026
1.6	.001758	.001164	.000775	.000518	.000348	.000159	.000074
1.7	.003312	.002283	.001580	.001098	.000766	.000378	.000189
1.8	.005869	.004192	.003007	.002165	.001564	.000826	.000443
1.9	.009842	.007263	.005379	.003997	.002981	.001675	.000954
2.0	.015713	.011940	.009102	.006961	.005340	.003172	.001907
2.1	.023997	.018726	.014654	.011500	.009050	.005653	.003570
2.2	.035209	.028142	.022551	.018116	.014591	.009537	.006296
2.3	.049819	.040695	.033318	.027339	.022484	.015312	.010521
2.4	.068207	.056827	.047439	.039682	.033260	.023507	.016747
2.5	.090630	.076874	.065318	.055597	.047407	.034653	.025511
2.6	.117193	.101034	.087234	.075435	.065333	.049237	.037340
2.7	.147832	.129345	.113316	.099404	.087319	.067655	.052709
2.8	.182319	.161673	.143522	.127554	.113495	.090175	.071992
2.9	.220273	.197723	.177644	.159758	.143817	.116907	.095429
3.0	.261184	.237052	.215313	.195727	.178073	.147786	.123091
3.1	.304443	.279101	.256028	.235020	.215888	.182575	.154877
3.2	.349383	.323230	.299183	.277077	.256753	.220880	.190512
3.3	.395309	.368750	.344108	.321253	.300058	.262172	.229568
3.4	.441535	.414962	.390102	.366854	.345122	.305824	.271488
3.5	.487414	.461191	.436468	.413175	.391239	.351147	.315625
3.6	.532356	.506806	.482547	.459532	.437709	.397430	.361279
3.7	.575849	.551249	.527738	.505288	.483868	.443970	.407733
3.8	.617469	.594041	.571515	.549878	.529113	.490107	.454291
3.9	.656879	.634796	.613442	.592818	.572919	.535246	.500302
4.0	.693835	.673215	.653172	.633716	.614849	.578872	.545185
4.1	.728176	.709091	.690451	.672270	.654559	.620558	.588444
4.2	.759817	.742297	.725109	.708272	.691798	.659975	.629675
4.3	.788740	.772781	.757057	.741592	.726400	.696883	.668567
4.4	.814986	.800550	.786273	.772176	.758278	.731128	.704901
4.5	.838638	.825667	.812792	.800035	.787414	.762635	.738542
4.6	.859815	.848232	.836696	.825228	.813846	.791395	.769433
4.7	.878664	.868380	.858106	.847860	.837661	.817455	.797578
4.8	.895347	.886265	.877165	.868065	.858980	.840909	.823038
4.9	.910034	.902054	.894036	.885997	.877950	.861882	.845914

$\nu = 30$

Q\n	16	17	18	19	20	22	24
5.0	.922902	.915923	.908893	.901826	.894735	.880526	.866341
5.1	.934124	.928047	.921911	.915728	.909510	.897008	.884474
5.2	.943869	.938599	.933265	.927879	.922452	.911504	.900483
5.3	.952297	.947744	.943127	.938454	.933736	.924191	.914547
5.4	.959559	.955640	.951657	.947619	.943533	.935246	.926842
5.5	.965795	.962432	.959008	.955531	.952006	.944838	.937545
5.6	.971132	.968255	.965321	.962336	.959306	.953128	.946822
5.7	.975685	.973231	.970725	.968171	.965574	.960267	.954834
5.8	.979559	.977472	.975336	.973157	.970938	.966393	.961728
5.9	.982846	.981075	.979261	.977406	.975515	.971634	.967640
6.0	.985628	.984129	.982591	.981016	.979409	.976104	.972694
6.4	.993020	.992265	.991487	.990687	.989866	.988167	.986400
6.8	.996671	.996300	.995917	.995521	.995114	.994266	.993378
7.2	.998432	.998254	.998069	.997877	.997679	.997265	.996829
7.6	.999268	.999183	.999095	.999003	.998908	.998709	.998498
8.0	.999660	.999620	.999578	.999535	.999489	.999395	.999294
8.4	.999842	.999823	.999804	.999783	.999762	.999717	.999669
8.8	.999927	.999918	.999909	.999899	.999889	.999868	.999845
9.2	.999966	.999962	.999957	.999953	.999948	.999938	.999927
9.6	.999984	.999982	.999980	.999978	.999976	.999971	.999966
10.0	.999992	.999992	.999991	.999990	.999989	.999986	.999984
11.0	1.00000	1.00000	1.00000	1.00000	1.00000	1.00000	1.00000

ν = 30

Q\n	26	28	30	32	34	36	38
0.0	.000000	.000000	.000000	.000000	.000000	.000000	.000000
0.1	.000000	.000000	.000000	.000000	.000000	.000000	.000000
0.2	.000000	.000000	.000000	.000000	.000000	.000000	.000000
0.3	.000000	.000000	.000000	.000000	.000000	.000000	.000000
0.4	.000000	.000000	.000000	.000000	.000000	.000000	.000000
0.5	.000000	.000000	.000000	.000000	.000000	.000000	.000000
0.6	.000000	.000000	.000000	.000000	.000000	.000000	.000000
0.7	.000000	.000000	.000000	.000000	.000000	.000000	.000000
0.8	.000000	.000000	.000000	.000000	.000000	.000000	.000000
0.9	.000000	.000000	.000000	.000000	.000000	.000000	.000000
1.0	.000000	.000000	.000000	.000000	.000000	.000000	.000000
1.1	.000000	.000000	.000000	.000000	.000000	.000000	.000000
1.2	.000000	.000000	.000000	.000000	.000000	.000000	.000000
1.3	.000001	.000000	.000000	.000000	.000000	.000000	.000000
1.4	.000003	.000001	.000001	.000000	.000000	.000000	.000000
1.5	.000011	.000005	.000002	.000001	.000000	.000000	.000000
1.6	.000035	.000017	.000008	.000004	.000002	.000001	.000001
1.7	.000096	.000050	.000026	.000014	.000007	.000004	.000002
1.8	.000241	.000133	.000074	.000042	.000024	.000014	.000008
1.9	.000550	.000322	.000190	.000114	.000069	.000042	.000026
2.0	.001161	.000714	.000445	.000280	.000178	.000114	.000074
2.1	.002279	.001470	.000958	.000630	.000418	.000280	.000189
2.2	.004197	.002824	.001917	.001313	.000907	.000632	.000443
2.3	.007292	.005097	.003592	.002552	.001826	.001317	.000956
2.4	.012025	.008699	.006340	.004654	.003439	.002558	.001915
2.5	.018911	.014114	.010604	.008017	.006098	.004667	.003591
2.6	.028492	.021873	.016890	.013116	.010242	.008040	.006343
2.7	.041288	.032516	.025741	.020481	.016375	.013155	.010616
2.8	.057751	.046546	.037688	.030653	.025040	.020540	.016918
2.9	.078223	.064384	.053210	.044149	.036772	.030742	.025794
3.0	.102895	.086323	.072678	.061403	.052054	.044273	.037776
3.1	.131792	.112499	.096328	.082733	.071269	.061571	.053343
3.2	.164759	.142872	.124225	.108298	.094659	.082949	.072867
3.3	.201474	.177227	.156258	.138086	.122303	.108565	.096579
3.4	.241466	.215183	.192140	.171904	.154099	.138404	.124542
3.5	.284144	.256223	.231433	.209393	.189769	.172270	.156640
3.6	.328840	.299723	.273567	.250050	.228882	.209803	.192585
3.7	.374843	.344991	.317888	.293264	.270874	.250496	.231929
3.8	.421436	.391310	.363686	.338347	.315092	.293735	.274105
3.9	.467931	.437968	.410241	.384581	.360829	.338833	.318450
4.0	.513696	.484293	.456853	.431251	.407363	.385070	.364257
4.1	.558173	.529676	.502874	.477676	.453992	.431731	.410804
4.2	.600890	.573589	.547724	.523237	.500063	.478137	.457392
4.3	.641472	.615595	.590912	.567392	.544993	.523669	.503373
4.4	.679636	.655349	.632039	.609692	.588284	.567788	.548172
4.5	.715189	.692604	.670801	.649780	.629533	.610046	.591300
4.6	.748020	.727197	.706984	.687395	.668432	.650089	.632360
4.7	.778093	.759045	.740462	.722365	.704762	.687658	.671051
4.8	.805431	.788134	.771181	.754595	.738392	.722580	.707164
4.9	.830107	.814509	.799153	.784065	.769265	.754765	.740573

$\nu = 30$

Q\n	26	28	30	32	34	36	38
5.0	.852236	.838258	.824441	.810812	.797390	.784192	.771227
5.1	.871959	.859507	.847152	.834918	.822828	.810898	.799139
5.2	.889438	.878406	.867421	.856507	.845684	.834969	.824375
5.3	.904845	.895123	.885408	.875724	.866092	.856526	.847040
5.4	.918360	.909832	.901283	.892736	.884209	.875716	.867271
5.5	.930160	.922712	.915225	.907717	.900206	.892706	.885228
5.6	.940419	.933942	.927412	.920847	.914262	.907669	.901080
5.7	.949301	.943690	.938018	.932301	.926553	.920785	.915006
5.8	.956964	.952120	.947212	.942253	.937255	.932229	.927183
5.9	.963551	.959384	.955151	.950865	.946536	.942174	.937785
6.0	.969195	.965621	.961983	.958291	.954554	.950781	.946978
6.4	.984571	.982688	.980757	.978783	.976771	.974725	.972649
6.8	.992454	.991495	.990507	.989490	.988448	.987382	.986295
7.2	.996372	.995897	.995404	.994894	.994369	.993831	.993279
7.6	.998277	.998045	.997804	.997553	.997295	.997028	.996754
8.0	.999187	.999076	.998959	.998838	.998712	.998582	.998448
8.4	.999618	.999565	.999509	.999451	.999390	.999328	.999263
8.8	.999821	.999796	.999769	.999741	.999712	.999682	.999651
9.2	.999916	.999904	.999891	.999878	.999864	.999850	.999835
9.6	.999960	.999955	.999949	.999942	.999936	.999929	.999921
10.0	.999981	.999979	.999976	.999973	.999969	.999966	.999963
11.0	1.00000	1.00000	1.00000	1.00000	1.00000	.999995	.999994
12.0						1.00000	1.00000

$\nu = 30$

Q\n	40	50	60	70	80	90	100
0.0	.000000	.000000	.000000	.000000	.000000	.000000	.000000
0.1	.000000	.000000	.000000	.000000	.000000	.000000	.000000
0.2	.000000	.000000	.000000	.000000	.000000	.000000	.000000
0.3	.000000	.000000	.000000	.000000	.000000	.000000	.000000
0.4	.000000	.000000	.000000	.000000	.000000	.000000	.000000
0.5	.000000	.000000	.000000	.000000	.000000	.000000	.000000
0.6	.000000	.000000	.000000	.000000	.000000	.000000	.000000
0.7	.000000	.000000	.000000	.000000	.000000	.000000	.000000
0.8	.000000	.000000	.000000	.000000	.000000	.000000	.000000
0.9	.000000	.000000	.000000	.000000	.000000	.000000	.000000
1.0	.000000	.000000	.000000	.000000	.000000	.000000	.000000
1.1	.000000	.000000	.000000	.000000	.000000	.000000	.000000
1.2	.000000	.000000	.000000	.000000	.000000	.000000	.000000
1.3	.000000	.000000	.000000	.000000	.000000	.000000	.000000
1.4	.000000	.000000	.000000	.000000	.000000	.000000	.000000
1.5	.000000	.000000	.000000	.000000	.000000	.000000	.000000
1.6	.000000	.000000	.000000	.000000	.000000	.000000	.000000
1.7	.000001	.000000	.000000	.000000	.000000	.000000	.000000
1.8	.000005	.000000	.000000	.000000	.000000	.000000	.000000
1.9	.000016	.000002	.000000	.000000	.000000	.000000	.000000
2.0	.000048	.000007	.000001	.000000	.000000	.000000	.000000
2.1	.000129	.000021	.000004	.000001	.000000	.000000	.000000
2.2	.000313	.000061	.000014	.000004	.000001	.000000	.000000
2.3	.000699	.000160	.000042	.000012	.000004	.000001	.000001
2.4	.001442	.000380	.000113	.000037	.000013	.000005	.000002
2.5	.002779	.000831	.000277	.000101	.000040	.000017	.000007
2.6	.005029	.001685	.000623	.000250	.000107	.000049	.000023
2.7	.008604	.003197	.001297	.000566	.000263	.000129	.000066
2.8	.013989	.005707	.002519	.001188	.000592	.000310	.000169
2.9	.021717	.009642	.004594	.002322	.001234	.000685	.000395
3.0	.032332	.015500	.007913	.004260	.002400	.001405	.000851
3.1	.046341	.023818	.012947	.007380	.004381	.002693	.001706
3.2	.064164	.035132	.020218	.012138	.007557	.004854	.003204
3.3	.086097	.049931	.030263	.019047	.012382	.008279	.005673
3.4	.112275	.068611	.043592	.028639	.019367	.013429	.009519
3.5	.142656	.091429	.060639	.041427	.029039	.020816	.015218
3.6	.177024	.118483	.081717	.057854	.041904	.030962	.023282
3.7	.214994	.149691	.106989	.078250	.058396	.044358	.034226
3.8	.256045	.184799	.136447	.102800	.078839	.061420	.048519
3.9	.299551	.223393	.169905	.131521	.103413	.082446	.066546
4.0	.344817	.264927	.207015	.164258	.132129	.107590	.088569
4.1	.391125	.308761	.247284	.200689	.164830	.136836	.114694
4.2	.437762	.354196	.290112	.240347	.201194	.170003	.144866
4.3	.484057	.400517	.334827	.282653	.240756	.206749	.178862
4.4	.529403	.447022	.380719	.326948	.282942	.246595	.216308
4.5	.573272	.493055	.427085	.372536	.327100	.288961	.256701
4.6	.615231	.538029	.473251	.418714	.372538	.333190	.299443
4.7	.654937	.581438	.518605	.464810	.418562	.378598	.343876
4.8	.692145	.622871	.562609	.510203	.464505	.424498	.389317
4.9	.726694	.662008	.604815	.554348	.509754	.470235	.435090

ν = 30

Q\n	40	50	60	70	80	90	100
5.0	.758504	.698621	.644867	.596783	.553766	.515210	.480558
5.1	.787561	.732568	.682499	.637138	.596085	.558895	.525142
5.2	.813911	.763783	.717535	.675134	.636342	.600849	.568339
5.3	.837644	.792266	.749877	.710579	.674259	.640718	.609730
5.4	.858884	.818069	.779497	.743362	.709646	.678238	.648984
5.5	.877782	.841290	.806426	.773442	.742391	.713227	.685857
5.6	.894504	.862059	.830740	.800838	.772451	.745583	.720188
5.7	.909226	.880526	.852556	.825619	.799844	.775272	.751891
5.8	.922125	.896861	.872015	.847891	.824637	.802316	.780942
5.9	.933376	.911236	.889276	.867789	.846933	.826785	.807377
6.0	.943151	.923829	.904509	.885469	.866865	.848785	.831271
6.4	.970546	.959734	.948618	.937385	.926156	.915013	.904006
6.8	.985188	.979413	.973341	.967081	.960709	.954277	.947826
7.2	.992714	.989733	.986543	.983199	.979745	.976211	.972621
7.6	.996472	.994972	.993342	.991611	.989801	.987929	.986007
8.0	.998310	.997568	.996752	.995876	.994951	.993985	.992985
8.4	.999196	.998833	.998431	.997994	.997530	.997041	.996531
8.8	.999618	.999443	.999246	.999031	.998800	.998556	.998299
9.2	.999819	.999734	.999638	.999533	.999419	.999298	.999171
9.6	.999914	.999873	.999827	.999775	.999719	.999660	.999596
10.0	.999959	.999939	.999917	.999891	.999864	.999835	.999804
11.0	.999993	.999990	.999986	.999982	.999977	.999972	.999967
12.0	1.00000	1.00000	1.00000	1.00000	1.00000	1.00000	.999994
13.0							1.00000

$\nu = 40$

Q\n	2	3	4	5	6	7	8
0.0	.000000	.000000	.000000	.000000	.000000	.000000	.000000
0.1	.056020	.002753	.000129	.000006	.000000	.000000	.000000
0.2	.111753	.010963	.001027	.000094	.000009	.000001	.000000
0.3	.166919	.024487	.003430	.000471	.000064	.000009	.000001
0.4	.221244	.043094	.008017	.001461	.000264	.000048	.000009
0.5	.274470	.066467	.015379	.003487	.000784	.000176	.000039
0.6	.326354	.094216	.026003	.007034	.001885	.000504	.000135
0.7	.376674	.125890	.040248	.012612	.003917	.001212	.000375
0.8	.425233	.160987	.058343	.020728	.007297	.002560	.000898
0.9	.471857	.198969	.080379	.031837	.012494	.004886	.001910
1.0	.516400	.239277	.106313	.046322	.019996	.008599	.003696
1.1	.558747	.281345	.135977	.064461	.030274	.014162	.006619
1.2	.598807	.324610	.169087	.086412	.043748	.022057	.011109
1.3	.636519	.368530	.205265	.112202	.060757	.032758	.017639
1.4	.671850	.412591	.244056	.141726	.081529	.046691	.026698
1.5	.704793	.456316	.284951	.174753	.106168	.064201	.038755
1.6	.735363	.499275	.327405	.210941	.134638	.085527	.054222
1.7	.763600	.541087	.370862	.249854	.166771	.110773	.073417
1.8	.789560	.581427	.414771	.290984	.202269	.139904	.096538
1.9	.813318	.620025	.458607	.333774	.240726	.172744	.123645
2.0	.834964	.656666	.501879	.377647	.281644	.208982	.154648
2.1	.854597	.691190	.544146	.422022	.324463	.248189	.189310
2.2	.872327	.723487	.585026	.466341	.368586	.289846	.227261
2.3	.888270	.753493	.624195	.510080	.413404	.333366	.268018
2.4	.902545	.781190	.661394	.552770	.458322	.378125	.311011
2.5	.915272	.806595	.696425	.594002	.502778	.423493	.355615
2.6	.926575	.829755	.729154	.633433	.546263	.468853	.401176
2.7	.936570	.850746	.759499	.670791	.588329	.513630	.447047
2.8	.945376	.869665	.787431	.705874	.628601	.557304	.492609
2.9	.953103	.886624	.812965	.738545	.666778	.599425	.537294
3.0	.959859	.901747	.836153	.768728	.702634	.639621	.580600
3.1	.965742	.915164	.857077	.796403	.736016	.677597	.622103
3.2	.970848	.927010	.875844	.821597	.766837	.713142	.661464
3.3	.975263	.937420	.892580	.844374	.795071	.746115	.698425
3.4	.979068	.946526	.907422	.864834	.820742	.776447	.732812
3.5	.982335	.954458	.920514	.883098	.843917	.804129	.764522
3.6	.985132	.961336	.932004	.899304	.864699	.829202	.793525
3.7	.987518	.967277	.942038	.913605	.883217	.851752	.819842
3.8	.989548	.972388	.950761	.926155	.899616	.871896	.843548
3.9	.991269	.976769	.958309	.937113	.914055	.889775	.864753
4.0	.992724	.980510	.964812	.946634	.926699	.905549	.883594
4.1	.993951	.983693	.970392	.954867	.937713	.919385	.900231
4.2	.994982	.986392	.975162	.961954	.947260	.931455	.914835
4.3	.995847	.988673	.979222	.968029	.955494	.941930	.927582
4.4	.996570	.990595	.982667	.973215	.962566	.950976	.938648
4.5	.997173	.992209	.985579	.977625	.968612	.958751	.948208
4.6	.997674	.993561	.988032	.981361	.973761	.965404	.956426
4.7	.998090	.994690	.990092	.984514	.978128	.971072	.963460
4.8	.998435	.995631	.991817	.987167	.981819	.975883	.969452
4.9	.998720	.996412	.993257	.989392	.984926	.979950	.974538

ν = 40

Q\n	2	3	4	5	6	7	8
5.0	.998955	.997059	.994455	.991251	.987534	.983376	.978837
5.1	.999148	.997594	.995450	.992801	.989715	.986251	.982457
5.2	.999306	.998036	.996274	.994089	.991535	.988657	.985495
5.3	.999436	.998399	.996954	.995156	.993047	.990664	.988037
5.4	.999542	.998697	.997515	.996039	.994301	.992332	.990156
5.5	.999629	.998941	.997976	.996766	.995339	.993716	.991918
5.6	.999700	.999141	.998354	.997365	.996194	.994860	.993378
5.7	.999757	.999304	.998664	.997856	.996899	.995804	.994585
5.8	.999804	.999437	.998917	.998259	.997477	.996581	.995581
5.9	.999842	.999545	.999123	.998588	.997951	.997219	.996400
6.0	.999873	.999633	.999291	.998857	.998338	.997741	.997072
6.4	.999947	.999846	.999701	.999515	.999291	.999031	.998739
6.8	.999978	.999936	.999876	.999798	.999703	.999593	.999467
7.2	.999991	.999974	.999949	.999917	.999877	.999831	.999779
7.6	1.00000	.999989	.999979	.999966	.999950	.999931	.999909
8.0		1.00000	.999992	.999986	.999980	.999972	.999963
8.4			1.00000	.999994	.999992	.999989	.999985
8.8				1.00000	1.00000	1.00000	.999994
9.2							1.00000

$\nu = 40$

Q\n	9	10	11	12	13	14	15
0.0	.000000	.000000	.000000	.000000	.000000	.000000	.000000
0.1	.000000	.000000	.000000	.000000	.000000	.000000	.000000
0.2	.000000	.000000	.000000	.000000	.000000	.000000	.000000
0.3	.000000	.000000	.000000	.000000	.000000	.000000	.000000
0.4	.000002	.000000	.000000	.000000	.000000	.000000	.000000
0.5	.000009	.000002	.000000	.000000	.000000	.000000	.000000
0.6	.000036	.000010	.000003	.000001	.000000	.000000	.000000
0.7	.000116	.000036	.000011	.000004	.000001	.000000	.000000
0.8	.000316	.000111	.000039	.000014	.000005	.000002	.000001
0.9	.000748	.000294	.000116	.000046	.000018	.000007	.000003
1.0	.001591	.000687	.000297	.000129	.000057	.000025	.000011
1.1	.003098	.001453	.000684	.000323	.000153	.000073	.000035
1.2	.005600	.002829	.001434	.000729	.000373	.000191	.000099
1.3	.009504	.005130	.002777	.001509	.000823	.000450	.000248
1.4	.015272	.008749	.005025	.002895	.001674	.000971	.000566
1.5	.023397	.014143	.008568	.005204	.003171	.001939	.001190
1.6	.034369	.021807	.013862	.008833	.005644	.003618	.002327
1.7	.048637	.032244	.021409	.014245	.009502	.006356	.004264
1.8	.066568	.045923	.031720	.021949	.015221	.010582	.007376
1.9	.088420	.063242	.045277	.032464	.023321	.016790	.012117
2.0	.114311	.084491	.062492	.046278	.034326	.025510	.018997
2.1	.144208	.109821	.083670	.063807	.048725	.037269	.028558
2.2	.177925	.139230	.108974	.085354	.066926	.052549	.041325
2.3	.215129	.172559	.138412	.111077	.089217	.071740	.057763
2.4	.255361	.209492	.171829	.140976	.115738	.095103	.078234
2.5	.298064	.249581	.208908	.174880	.146459	.122742	.102958
2.6	.342609	.292268	.249196	.212456	.181180	.154587	.131990
2.7	.388329	.336917	.292125	.253232	.219539	.190394	.165205
2.8	.434554	.382851	.337047	.296621	.261032	.229757	.202305
2.9	.480636	.429380	.383270	.341956	.305045	.272135	.242832
3.0	.525975	.475837	.430091	.388531	.350893	.316883	.286203
3.1	.570034	.521599	.476827	.435630	.397850	.363291	.331737
3.2	.612357	.566112	.522846	.482563	.445193	.410621	.378703
3.3	.652574	.608899	.567581	.528692	.492230	.458145	.426353
3.4	.690400	.649574	.610552	.573454	.538328	.505175	.473960
3.5	.725638	.687840	.651368	.616371	.582933	.551091	.520850
3.6	.758169	.723489	.689730	.657058	.625579	.595356	.566421
3.7	.787946	.756396	.725433	.695227	.665899	.637527	.610162
3.8	.814984	.786510	.758353	.730682	.703622	.677261	.651661
3.9	.839350	.813843	.788444	.763312	.738572	.714314	.690606
4.0	.861150	.838463	.815724	.793082	.770655	.748532	.726784
4.1	.880524	.860478	.840265	.820020	.799852	.779847	.760073
4.2	.897631	.880030	.862183	.844209	.826209	.808261	.790432
4.3	.912646	.897283	.881623	.865773	.849820	.833838	.817886
4.4	.925750	.912415	.898756	.884865	.870821	.856688	.842520
4.5	.937123	.925609	.913762	.901661	.889374	.876957	.864460
4.6	.946944	.937052	.926830	.916347	.905660	.894819	.883866
4.7	.955384	.946925	.938150	.929115	.919871	.910460	.900919
4.8	.962604	.955402	.947904	.940157	.932202	.924077	.915812
4.9	.968752	.962647	.956268	.949656	.942844	.935865	.928744

$\nu = 40$

Q\n	9	10	11	12	13	14	15
5.0	.973967	.968812	.963408	.957789	.951983	.946017	.939912
5.1	.978373	.974036	.969476	.964721	.959794	.954717	.949508
5.2	.982082	.978446	.974613	.970604	.966440	.962138	.957713
5.3	.985193	.982155	.978944	.975577	.972071	.968440	.964697
5.4	.987793	.985263	.982582	.979764	.976823	.973770	.970616
5.5	.989960	.987859	.985628	.983277	.980818	.978261	.975613
5.6	.991761	.990021	.988169	.986214	.984165	.982030	.979815
5.7	.993253	.991816	.990283	.988662	.986960	.985183	.983336
5.8	.994485	.993302	.992037	.990696	.989286	.987811	.986276
5.9	.995501	.994528	.993487	.992381	.991216	.989996	.988723
6.0	.996337	.995539	.994683	.993774	.992813	.991806	.990754
6.4	.998414	.998061	.997679	.997271	.996838	.996382	.995902
6.8	.999328	.999176	.999010	.998832	.998643	.998442	.998231
7.2	.999720	.999655	.999585	.999509	.999428	.999342	.999251
7.6	.999885	.999858	.999828	.999797	.999763	.999726	.999688
8.0	.999953	.999942	.999930	.999917	.999902	.999887	.999871
8.4	.999981	.999976	.999971	.999966	.999960	.999954	.999947
8.8	.999992	.999990	.999988	.999986	.999984	.999981	.999979
9.2	1.00000	1.00000	1.00000	.999994	.999993	.999992	.999991
9.6				1.00000	1.00000	1.00000	1.00000

ν = 40

Q\n	16	17	18	19	20	22	24
0.0	.000000	.000000	.000000	.000000	.000000	.000000	.000000
0.1	.000000	.000000	.000000	.000000	.000000	.000000	.000000
0.2	.000000	.000000	.000000	.000000	.000000	.000000	.000000
0.3	.000000	.000000	.000000	.000000	.000000	.000000	.000000
0.4	.000000	.000000	.000000	.000000	.000000	.000000	.000000
0.5	.000000	.000000	.000000	.000000	.000000	.000000	.000000
0.6	.000000	.000000	.000000	.000000	.000000	.000000	.000000
0.7	.000000	.000000	.000000	.000000	.000000	.000000	.000000
0.8	.000000	.000000	.000000	.000000	.000000	.000000	.000000
0.9	.000001	.000000	.000000	.000000	.000000	.000000	.000000
1.0	.000005	.000002	.000001	.000000	.000000	.000000	.000000
1.1	.000017	.000008	.000004	.000002	.000001	.000000	.000000
1.2	.000051	.000027	.000014	.000007	.000004	.000001	.000000
1.3	.000137	.000076	.000042	.000024	.000013	.000004	.000001
1.4	.000331	.000195	.000115	.000068	.000040	.000015	.000005
1.5	.000733	.000453	.000282	.000176	.000110	.000044	.000018
1.6	.001502	.000973	.000632	.000413	.000270	.000117	.000052
1.7	.002870	.001938	.001313	.000893	.000609	.000286	.000136
1.8	.005157	.003616	.002543	.001794	.001269	.000642	.000328
1.9	.008767	.006360	.004626	.003375	.002468	.001332	.000727
2.0	.014180	.010609	.007957	.005983	.004510	.002582	.001494
2.1	.021927	.016871	.013009	.010054	.007787	.004704	.002868
2.2	.032555	.025693	.020316	.016097	.012779	.008105	.005182
2.3	.046578	.037619	.030434	.024665	.020025	.013271	.008861
2.4	.064437	.053147	.043898	.036315	.030088	.020754	.014410
2.5	.086453	.072678	.061175	.051560	.043515	.031126	.022393
2.6	.112792	.096480	.082614	.070820	.060781	.044935	.033387
2.7	.143446	.124652	.108415	.094382	.082248	.062655	.047939
2.8	.178225	.157111	.138597	.122361	.108117	.084638	.066506
2.9	.216766	.193592	.172994	.154687	.138413	.111071	.089415
3.0	.258557	.233665	.211262	.191105	.172969	.141960	.116823
3.1	.302965	.276756	.252897	.231185	.211432	.177113	.148693
3.2	.349281	.322190	.297268	.274352	.253291	.216153	.184794
3.3	.396752	.369227	.343658	.319924	.297904	.258545	.224710
3.4	.444627	.417102	.391305	.367148	.344541	.303626	.267868
3.5	.492189	.465069	.439441	.415248	.392428	.350647	.313577
3.6	.538781	.512426	.487331	.463465	.440787	.398823	.361067
3.7	.583832	.558545	.534300	.511082	.488872	.447367	.409542
3.8	.626862	.602889	.579755	.557461	.536000	.495532	.458212
3.9	.667497	.645022	.623204	.602054	.581578	.542640	.506338
4.0	.705464	.684612	.664256	.644417	.625107	.588104	.553253
4.1	.740585	.721425	.702626	.684211	.666201	.631437	.598388
4.2	.772773	.755327	.738128	.721204	.704575	.672263	.641280
4.3	.802015	.786264	.770669	.755256	.740047	.710314	.681574
4.4	.828364	.814256	.800231	.786314	.772528	.745422	.719026
4.5	.851923	.839382	.826866	.814401	.802008	.777511	.753491
4.6	.872838	.861766	.850678	.839596	.828542	.806582	.784913
4.7	.891278	.881568	.871811	.862028	.852239	.832704	.813312
4.8	.907435	.898970	.890439	.881860	.873250	.855995	.838771
4.9	.921504	.914168	.906753	.899277	.891752	.876612	.861422

$\nu = 40$

Q\n	16	17	18	19	20	22	24
5.0	.933689	.927365	.920956	.914478	.907941	.894740	.881431
5.1	.944184	.938761	.933251	.927667	.922021	.910577	.898988
5.2	.953180	.948550	.943837	.939049	.934197	.924331	.914298
5.3	.960853	.956920	.952906	.948821	.944671	.936209	.927570
5.4	.967371	.964043	.960640	.957169	.953637	.946414	.939013
5.5	.972883	.970078	.967205	.964269	.961275	.955138	.948828
5.6	.977527	.975172	.972755	.970281	.967754	.962561	.957205
5.7	.981425	.979454	.977428	.975351	.973227	.968851	.964324
5.8	.984684	.983041	.981349	.979612	.977832	.974158	.970346
5.9	.987402	.986036	.984627	.983179	.981693	.978618	.975421
6.0	.989661	.988528	.987359	.986155	.984918	.982354	.979681
6.4	.995402	.994880	.994340	.993780	.993203	.991999	.990733
6.8	.998009	.997777	.997536	.997285	.997026	.996481	.995905
7.2	.999155	.999055	.998950	.998841	.998728	.998489	.998234
7.6	.999647	.999605	.999560	.999513	.999465	.999362	.999253
8.0	.999854	.999837	.999818	.999798	.999778	.999735	.999688
8.4	.999940	.999933	.999925	.999917	.999909	.999890	.999871
8.8	.999976	.999973	.999969	.999966	.999963	.999955	.999947
9.2	.999990	.999989	.999988	.999986	.999985	.999982	.999978
9.6	1.00000	1.00000	.999995	.999994	.999994	.999992	.999991
10.0			1.00000	1.00000	1.00000	1.00000	1.00000

$\nu = 40$

Q\n	26	28	30	32	34	36	38
0.0	.000000	.000000	.000000	.000000	.000000	.000000	.000000
0.1	.000000	.000000	.000000	.000000	.000000	.000000	.000000
0.2	.000000	.000000	.000000	.000000	.000000	.000000	.000000
0.3	.000000	.000000	.000000	.000000	.000000	.000000	.000000
0.4	.000000	.000000	.000000	.000000	.000000	.000000	.000000
0.5	.000000	.000000	.000000	.000000	.000000	.000000	.000000
0.6	.000000	.000000	.000000	.000000	.000000	.000000	.000000
0.7	.000000	.000000	.000000	.000000	.000000	.000000	.000000
0.8	.000000	.000000	.000000	.000000	.000000	.000000	.000000
0.9	.000000	.000000	.000000	.000000	.000000	.000000	.000000
1.0	.000000	.000000	.000000	.000000	.000000	.000000	.000000
1.1	.000000	.000000	.000000	.000000	.000000	.000000	.000000
1.2	.000000	.000000	.000000	.000000	.000000	.000000	.000000
1.3	.000000	.000000	.000000	.000000	.000000	.000000	.000000
1.4	.000002	.000001	.000000	.000000	.000000	.000000	.000000
1.5	.000007	.000003	.000001	.000001	.000000	.000000	.000000
1.6	.000023	.000010	.000005	.000002	.000001	.000001	.000000
1.7	.000066	.000032	.000016	.000008	.000004	.000002	.000001
1.8	.000170	.000089	.000047	.000025	.000014	.000008	.000004
1.9	.000401	.000224	.000126	.000072	.000041	.000024	.000014
2.0	.000873	.000515	.000307	.000185	.000112	.000069	.000042
2.1	.001765	.001096	.000686	.000434	.000276	.000177	.000115
2.2	.003341	.002172	.001423	.000940	.000625	.000419	.000283
2.3	.005960	.004038	.002755	.001893	.001310	.000912	.000640
2.4	.010071	.007084	.005015	.003573	.002561	.001847	.001339
2.5	.016204	.011793	.008632	.006354	.004703	.003499	.002617
2.6	.024934	.018717	.014121	.010706	.008157	.006245	.004803
2.7	.036842	.028442	.022055	.017178	.013437	.010555	.008326
2.8	.052460	.041543	.033027	.026358	.021117	.016981	.013706
2.9	.072220	.058530	.047597	.038837	.031796	.026118	.021523
3.0	.096408	.079793	.066237	.055145	.046046	.038559	.032382
3.1	.125131	.105564	.089282	.075704	.064354	.054843	.046855
3.2	.158298	.135884	.116894	.100778	.087074	.075397	.065427
3.3	.195620	.170591	.149034	.130442	.114383	.100489	.088447
3.4	.236630	.209331	.185461	.164568	.146260	.130196	.116082
3.5	.280711	.251577	.225745	.202827	.182478	.164391	.148298
3.6	.327138	.296664	.269296	.244711	.222615	.202742	.184854
3.7	.375124	.343835	.315402	.289566	.266085	.244735	.225313
3.8	.423861	.392283	.363275	.336637	.312176	.289712	.269075
3.9	.472567	.441202	.412099	.385113	.360098	.336911	.315416
4.0	.520515	.489818	.461072	.434176	.409025	.385513	.363535
4.1	.567061	.537428	.509441	.483037	.458146	.434694	.412603
4.2	.611663	.583420	.556535	.530975	.506700	.483660	.461803
4.3	.653888	.627287	.601780	.577358	.554002	.531686	.510376
4.4	.693415	.668636	.644714	.621660	.599471	.578137	.557641
4.5	.730030	.707184	.684990	.663470	.642635	.622487	.603021
4.6	.763616	.742753	.722368	.702489	.683138	.664324	.646052
4.7	.794144	.775261	.756711	.738527	.720735	.703351	.686386
4.8	.821655	.804707	.787973	.771490	.755286	.739379	.723787
4.9	.846251	.831157	.816185	.801369	.786740	.772318	.758122

$\nu = 40$

Q\n	26	28	30	32	34	36	38
5.0	.868077	.854732	.841436	.828225	.815125	.802160	.789348
5.1	.887310	.875591	.863868	.852173	.840533	.828970	.817501
5.2	.904148	.893921	.883653	.873372	.863102	.852865	.842678
5.3	.918798	.909927	.900988	.892008	.883008	.874008	.865023
5.4	.931471	.923819	.916083	.908286	.900448	.892586	.884714
5.5	.942376	.935810	.929151	.922419	.915633	.908805	.901951
5.6	.951712	.946105	.940402	.934621	.928776	.922881	.916948
5.7	.959667	.954900	.950039	.945098	.940091	.935028	.929920
5.8	.966415	.962380	.958255	.954052	.949782	.945455	.941080
5.9	.972115	.968713	.965227	.961667	.958043	.954362	.950631
6.0	.976911	.974054	.971119	.968117	.965053	.961934	.958768
6.4	.989409	.988034	.986610	.985143	.983635	.982089	.980509
6.8	.995299	.994665	.994005	.993321	.992613	.991884	.991135
7.2	.997966	.997683	.997388	.997080	.996760	.996429	.996088
7.6	.999137	.999014	.998885	.998750	.998610	.998464	.998312
8.0	.999639	.999586	.999531	.999473	.999413	.999350	.999285
8.4	.999850	.999828	.999805	.999781	.999755	.999728	.999700
8.8	.999938	.999929	.999920	.999909	.999899	.999887	.999876
9.2	.999975	.999971	.999967	.999963	.999958	.999953	.999949
9.6	.999990	.999988	.999986	.999985	.999983	.999981	.999979
10.0	1.00000	1.00000	.999994	.999994	.999993	.999992	.999991
11.0			1.00000	1.00000	1.00000	1.00000	1.00000

$\nu = 40$

Q\n	40	50	60	70	80	90	100
0.0	.000000	.000000	.000000	.000000	.000000	.000000	.000000
0.1	.000000	.000000	.000000	.000000	.000000	.000000	.000000
0.2	.000000	.000000	.000000	.000000	.000000	.000000	.000000
0.3	.000000	.000000	.000000	.000000	.000000	.000000	.000000
0.4	.000000	.000000	.000000	.000000	.000000	.000000	.000000
0.5	.000000	.000000	.000000	.000000	.000000	.000000	.000000
0.6	.000000	.000000	.000000	.000000	.000000	.000000	.000000
0.7	.000000	.000000	.000000	.000000	.000000	.000000	.000000
0.8	.000000	.000000	.000000	.000000	.000000	.000000	.000000
0.9	.000000	.000000	.000000	.000000	.000000	.000000	.000000
1.0	.000000	.000000	.000000	.000000	.000000	.000000	.000000
1.1	.000000	.000000	.000000	.000000	.000000	.000000	.000000
1.2	.000000	.000000	.000000	.000000	.000000	.000000	.000000
1.3	.000000	.000000	.000000	.000000	.000000	.000000	.000000
1.4	.000000	.000000	.000000	.000000	.000000	.000000	.000000
1.5	.000000	.000000	.000000	.000000	.000000	.000000	.000000
1.6	.000000	.000000	.000000	.000000	.000000	.000000	.000000
1.7	.000001	.000000	.000000	.000000	.000000	.000000	.000000
1.8	.000002	.000000	.000000	.000000	.000000	.000000	.000000
1.9	.000008	.000001	.000000	.000000	.000000	.000000	.000000
2.0	.000026	.000003	.000000	.000000	.000000	.000000	.000000
2.1	.000075	.000010	.000002	.000000	.000000	.000000	.000000
2.2	.000192	.000031	.000006	.000001	.000000	.000000	.000000
2.3	.000451	.000086	.000019	.000005	.000001	.000000	.000000
2.4	.000977	.000218	.000055	.000015	.000005	.000001	.000001
2.5	.001968	.000507	.000145	.000045	.000015	.000006	.000002
2.6	.003711	.001088	.000351	.000123	.000046	.000018	.000008
2.7	.006594	.002175	.000781	.000301	.000124	.000054	.000025
2.8	.011102	.004071	.001610	.000680	.000304	.000143	.000070
2.9	.017793	.007184	.003103	.001421	.000685	.000345	.000181
3.0	.027270	.012016	.005622	.002771	.001430	.000768	.000427
3.1	.040127	.019143	.009629	.005074	.002785	.001584	.000930
3.2	.056896	.029173	.015674	.008775	.005094	.003053	.001882
3.3	.077991	.042700	.024358	.014410	.008803	.005533	.003567
3.4	.103662	.060243	.036289	.022573	.014446	.009481	.006365
3.5	.133962	.082194	.052030	.033875	.022616	.015441	.010755
3.6	.168738	.108771	.072033	.048891	.033924	.024009	.017296
3.7	.207631	.139990	.096599	.068097	.048941	.035791	.026588
3.8	.250107	.175656	.125834	.091823	.068143	.051348	.039230
3.9	.295485	.215372	.159634	.120213	.091860	.071136	.055759
4.0	.342991	.258567	.197686	.153201	.120233	.095459	.076598
4.1	.391797	.304532	.239488	.190511	.153197	.124433	.102005
4.2	.441076	.352473	.284384	.231672	.190477	.157962	.132048
4.3	.490037	.401551	.331608	.276054	.231603	.195745	.166581
4.4	.537963	.450938	.380332	.322906	.275945	.237292	.205257
4.5	.584229	.499850	.429717	.371409	.322756	.281955	.247547
4.6	.628323	.547581	.478953	.420723	.371218	.328978	.292777
4.7	.669847	.593526	.527296	.470029	.420492	.377540	.340174
4.8	.708519	.637194	.574095	.518572	.469762	.426805	.388911
4.9	.744164	.678209	.618808	.565680	.518272	.475966	.438161

ν = 40

Q\n	40	50	60	70	80	90	100
5.0	.776703	.716313	.661011	.610793	.565355	.524279	.487129
5.1	.806143	.751352	.700394	.653465	.610447	.571090	.535093
5.2	.832555	.783268	.736762	.693367	.653105	.615854	.581426
5.3	.856067	.812083	.770018	.730282	.692998	.658141	.625609
5.4	.876844	.837883	.800151	.764098	.729912	.697637	.667241
5.5	.895081	.860807	.827223	.794789	.763731	.734140	.706034
5.6	.910986	.881030	.851353	.822405	.794429	.767548	.741810
5.7	.924775	.898751	.872703	.847057	.822058	.797844	.774487
5.8	.936663	.914182	.891463	.868898	.846724	.825086	.804068
5.9	.946858	.927540	.907841	.888114	.868583	.849389	.830623
6.0	.955560	.939041	.922054	.904911	.887818	.870910	.854277
6.4	.978897	.970439	.961486	.952210	.942733	.933146	.923514
6.8	.990367	.986275	.981844	.977158	.972278	.967252	.962119
7.2	.995736	.993840	.991750	.989503	.987127	.984646	.982078
7.6	.998156	.997307	.996356	.995320	.994212	.993041	.991817
8.0	.999217	.998845	.998425	.997961	.997461	.996927	.996364
8.4	.999671	.999512	.999329	.999127	.998906	.998669	.998417
8.8	.999863	.999796	.999718	.999630	.999535	.999431	.999321
9.2	.999943	.999915	.999882	.999845	.999804	.999759	.999712
9.6	.999977	.999965	.999951	.999935	.999918	.999899	.999878
10.0	.999990	.999985	.999980	.999973	.999966	.999958	.999949
11.0	1.00000	1.00000	1.00000	1.00000	1.00000	1.00000	.999994
12.0							1.00000

$\nu = 60$

Q\n	2	3	4	5	6	7	8
0.0	.000000	.000000	.000000	.000000	.000000	.000000	.000000
0.1	.056137	.002753	.000128	.000006	.000000	.000000	.000000
0.2	.111989	.010964	.001020	.000093	.000008	.000001	.000000
0.3	.167277	.024492	.003410	.000464	.000062	.000008	.000001
0.4	.221729	.043109	.007974	.001440	.000257	.000046	.000008
0.5	.275087	.066504	.015303	.003439	.000763	.000168	.000037
0.6	.327109	.094291	.025887	.006941	.001838	.000483	.000127
0.7	.377574	.126023	.040090	.012457	.003823	.001166	.000354
0.8	.426283	.161204	.058149	.020493	.007133	.002466	.000850
0.9	.473061	.199299	.080165	.031512	.012234	.004718	.001814
1.0	.517762	.239753	.106105	.045903	.019615	.008325	.003522
1.1	.560267	.282000	.135810	.063958	.029752	.013747	.006329
1.2	.600483	.325478	.169006	.085848	.043078	.021469	.010661
1.3	.638348	.369643	.205323	.111616	.059945	.031974	.016990
1.4	.673826	.413975	.244312	.141172	.080603	.045703	.025814
1.5	.706905	.457994	.285463	.174300	.105174	.063023	.037616
1.6	.737599	.501263	.328232	.210668	.133646	.084196	.052828
1.7	.765945	.543394	.372058	.249845	.165867	.109354	.071798
1.8	.791998	.584053	.416382	.291325	.201555	.138488	.094755
1.9	.815831	.622962	.460667	.334548	.240311	.171443	.121791
2.0	.837532	.659898	.504412	.378927	.281642	.207924	.152844
2.1	.857201	.694694	.547162	.423868	.324981	.247514	.187703
2.2	.874946	.727232	.588518	.468796	.369720	.289690	.226010
2.3	.890883	.757445	.628144	.513168	.415233	.333857	.267288
2.4	.905132	.785309	.665768	.556495	.460900	.379375	.310959
2.5	.917816	.810837	.701180	.598346	.506136	.425587	.356379
2.6	.929057	.834077	.734236	.638359	.550404	.471846	.402870
2.7	.938977	.855104	.764848	.676247	.593229	.517546	.449749
2.8	.947693	.874015	.792982	.711790	.634212	.562133	.496360
2.9	.955319	.890926	.818650	.744843	.673029	.605125	.542094
3.0	.961965	.905964	.841903	.775322	.709438	.646121	.586413
3.1	.967732	.919262	.862828	.803202	.743272	.684804	.628857
3.2	.972716	.930960	.881535	.828510	.774437	.720941	.669056
3.3	.977006	.941197	.898154	.851314	.802901	.754382	.706730
3.4	.980686	.950111	.912829	.871719	.828691	.785049	.741688
3.5	.983829	.957836	.925713	.889852	.851879	.812933	.773820
3.6	.986503	.964497	.936960	.905862	.872575	.838080	.803091
3.7	.988770	.970216	.946725	.919910	.890918	.860583	.829529
3.8	.990686	.975103	.955158	.932163	.907065	.880571	.853215
3.9	.992298	.979261	.962404	.942787	.921190	.898200	.874272
4.0	.993650	.982784	.968600	.951949	.933468	.913643	.892856
4.1	.994780	.985756	.973872	.959808	.944078	.927084	.909142
4.2	.995721	.988254	.978338	.966514	.953196	.938710	.923319
4.3	.996503	.990345	.982104	.972208	.960987	.948707	.935581
4.4	.997149	.992089	.985266	.977019	.967611	.957255	.946124
4.5	.997683	.993537	.987910	.981066	.973214	.964523	.955134
4.6	.998121	.994736	.990112	.984455	.977930	.970672	.962793
4.7	.998481	.995725	.991938	.987281	.981882	.975848	.969268
4.8	.998775	.996538	.993447	.989627	.985178	.980183	.974715
4.9	.999014	.997204	.994690	.991568	.987915	.983799	.979274

$\nu = 60$

Q\n	2	3	4	5	6	7	8
5.0	.999209	.997748	.995709	.993166	.990180	.986800	.983072
5.1	.999366	.998191	.996543	.994479	.992045	.989281	.986222
5.2	.999494	.998550	.997222	.995552	.993576	.991324	.988824
5.3	.999597	.998841	.997774	.996426	.994827	.992999	.990963
5.4	.999679	.999076	.998220	.997137	.995847	.994368	.992716
5.5	.999745	.999265	.998581	.997712	.996675	.995482	.994147
5.6	.999798	.999417	.998871	.998176	.997344	.996386	.995310
5.7	.999841	.999538	.999104	.998550	.997885	.997117	.996252
5.8	.999874	.999635	.999291	.998850	.998320	.997706	.997013
5.9	.999901	.999712	.999440	.999090	.998668	.998179	.997626
6.0	.999922	.999773	.999558	.999281	.998947	.998558	.998118
6.4	.999971	.999915	.999833	.999726	.999597	.999446	.999273
6.8	.999989	.999969	.999938	.999899	.999850	.999794	.999728
7.2	1.00000	.999989	.999978	.999964	.999946	.999925	.999901
7.6		1.00000	.999992	.999987	.999981	.999973	.999965
8.0			1.00000	1.00000	.999993	.999991	.999988
8.4					1.00000	1.00000	1.00000

$\nu = 60$

Q\n	9	10	11	12	13	14	15
0.0	.000000	.000000	.000000	.000000	.000000	.000000	.000000
0.1	.000000	.000000	.000000	.000000	.000000	.000000	.000000
0.2	.000000	.000000	.000000	.000000	.000000	.000000	.000000
0.3	.000000	.000000	.000000	.000000	.000000	.000000	.000000
0.4	.000001	.000000	.000000	.000000	.000000	.000000	.000000
0.5	.000008	.000002	.000000	.000000	.000000	.000000	.000000
0.6	.000033	.000009	.000002	.000001	.000000	.000000	.000000
0.7	.000108	.000033	.000010	.000003	.000001	.000000	.000000
0.8	.000293	.000101	.000035	.000012	.000004	.000001	.000001
0.9	.000696	.000268	.000103	.000040	.000015	.000006	.000002
1.0	.001488	.000629	.000266	.000113	.000048	.000020	.000009
1.1	.002910	.001338	.000616	.000284	.000131	.000061	.000028
1.2	.005286	.002620	.001300	.000646	.000322	.000161	.000080
1.3	.009013	.004780	.002536	.001348	.000718	.000383	.000205
1.4	.014554	.008201	.004623	.002609	.001475	.000836	.000474
1.5	.022406	.013337	.007941	.004732	.002824	.001688	.001012
1.6	.033075	.020689	.012942	.008102	.005078	.003188	.002005
1.7	.047031	.030775	.020135	.013180	.008636	.005667	.003724
1.8	.064675	.044090	.030047	.020483	.013974	.009544	.006528
1.9	.086298	.061066	.043189	.030548	.021620	.015316	.010863
2.0	.112058	.082032	.060011	.043898	.032124	.023525	.017245
2.1	.141957	.107186	.080864	.060992	.046012	.034731	.026236
2.2	.175837	.136565	.105962	.082184	.063744	.049459	.038400
2.3	.213386	.170044	.135357	.107688	.085664	.068159	.054255
2.4	.254153	.207330	.168931	.137552	.111972	.091154	.074228
2.5	.297572	.247984	.206394	.171645	.142691	.118611	.098610
2.6	.342997	.291442	.247300	.209661	.177661	.150514	.127517
2.7	.389734	.337049	.291075	.251133	.216542	.186657	.160880
2.8	.437073	.384093	.337047	.295464	.258835	.226654	.198434
2.9	.484322	.431843	.384485	.341958	.303908	.269959	.239734
3.0	.530835	.479582	.432638	.389863	.351037	.315903	.284182
3.1	.576033	.526635	.480768	.438408	.399448	.363729	.331064
3.2	.619418	.572398	.528185	.486844	.448354	.412642	.379594
3.3	.660584	.616350	.574269	.534469	.496997	.461842	.428955
3.4	.699222	.658065	.618488	.580661	.544676	.510571	.478345
3.5	.735113	.697216	.660411	.624889	.590773	.558136	.527010
3.6	.768128	.733575	.699708	.666727	.634772	.603935	.574277
3.7	.798219	.767006	.736152	.705855	.676261	.647475	.619570
3.8	.825404	.797455	.769610	.742057	.714941	.688370	.662426
3.9	.849760	.824941	.800034	.775214	.750616	.726349	.702496
4.0	.871408	.849542	.827451	.805291	.783189	.761246	.739545
4.1	.890507	.871385	.851947	.832329	.812646	.792991	.773441
4.2	.907234	.890632	.873656	.856427	.839045	.821595	.804146
4.3	.921786	.907467	.892748	.877731	.862504	.847140	.831703
4.4	.934362	.922092	.909416	.896421	.883181	.869761	.856216
4.5	.945165	.934714	.923867	.912697	.901268	.889633	.877841
4.6	.954388	.945538	.936314	.926775	.916975	.906959	.896768
4.7	.962219	.954767	.946967	.938871	.930521	.921956	.913210
4.8	.968832	.962589	.956031	.949199	.942128	.934851	.927394
4.9	.974388	.969184	.963699	.957966	.952012	.945865	.939548

$\nu = 60$

Q\n	9	10	11	12	13	14	15
5.0	.979032	.974716	.970151	.965364	.960379	.955217	.949896
5.1	.982897	.979332	.975552	.971576	.967423	.963111	.958655
5.2	.986098	.983167	.980050	.976763	.973321	.969738	.966025
5.3	.988737	.986338	.983779	.981074	.978234	.975271	.972194
5.4	.990905	.988949	.986857	.984640	.982308	.979869	.977330
5.5	.992679	.991089	.989386	.987577	.985670	.983671	.981586
5.6	.994124	.992838	.991456	.989985	.988432	.986801	.985096
5.7	.995298	.994260	.993143	.991952	.990692	.989366	.987978
5.8	.996248	.995413	.994513	.993553	.992534	.991460	.990335
5.9	.997014	.996345	.995622	.994850	.994029	.993163	.992253
6.0	.997629	.997095	.996517	.995897	.995238	.994542	.993810
6.4	.999081	.998869	.998638	.998390	.998124	.997842	.997545
6.8	.999655	.999574	.999486	.999391	.999288	.999179	.999063
7.2	.999874	.999845	.999812	.999776	.999738	.999697	.999654
7.6	.999955	.999945	.999933	.999920	.999906	.999891	.999875
8.0	.999984	.999981	.999976	.999972	.999967	.999962	.999956
8.4	.999995	.999993	.999992	.999990	.999989	.999987	.999985
8.8	1.00000	1.00000	1.00000	1.00000	1.00000	1.00000	.999995
9.2							1.00000

ν = 60

Q\n	16	17	18	19	20	22	24
0.0	.000000	.000000	.000000	.000000	.000000	.000000	.000000
0.1	.000000	.000000	.000000	.000000	.000000	.000000	.000000
0.2	.000000	.000000	.000000	.000000	.000000	.000000	.000000
0.3	.000000	.000000	.000000	.000000	.000000	.000000	.000000
0.4	.000000	.000000	.000000	.000000	.000000	.000000	.000000
0.5	.000000	.000000	.000000	.000000	.000000	.000000	.000000
0.6	.000000	.000000	.000000	.000000	.000000	.000000	.000000
0.7	.000000	.000000	.000000	.000000	.000000	.000000	.000000
0.8	.000000	.000000	.000000	.000000	.000000	.000000	.000000
0.9	.000001	.000000	.000000	.000000	.000000	.000000	.000000
1.0	.000004	.000002	.000001	.000000	.000000	.000000	.000000
1.1	.000013	.000006	.000003	.000001	.000001	.000000	.000000
1.2	.000040	.000020	.000010	.000005	.000003	.000001	.000000
1.3	.000110	.000059	.000032	.000017	.000009	.000003	.000001
1.4	.000270	.000154	.000088	.000051	.000029	.000010	.000003
1.5	.000607	.000366	.000221	.000134	.000081	.000030	.000011
1.6	.001264	.000798	.000505	.000321	.000204	.000083	.000034
1.7	.002452	.001618	.001070	.000709	.000471	.000209	.000094
1.8	.004472	.003069	.002111	.001454	.001004	.000482	.000233
1.9	.007715	.005488	.003911	.002792	.001997	.001028	.000533
2.0	.012657	.009302	.006847	.005048	.003728	.002044	.001129
2.1	.019839	.015020	.011386	.008643	.006571	.003816	.002230
2.2	.029838	.023208	.018071	.014089	.010998	.006729	.004141
2.3	.043216	.034450	.027488	.021956	.017557	.011267	.007267
2.4	.060475	.049302	.040224	.032846	.026847	.017991	.012110
2.5	.082009	.068237	.056812	.047334	.039468	.027513	.019253
2.6	.108057	.091598	.077683	.065920	.055974	.040447	.029321
2.7	.138675	.119561	.103118	.088975	.076811	.057349	.042934
2.8	.173723	.152107	.133210	.116699	.102275	.078668	.060645
2.9	.212866	.189012	.167852	.149093	.132468	.104691	.082887
3.0	.255593	.229864	.206730	.185948	.167287	.135506	.109917
3.1	.301250	.274079	.249346	.226854	.206413	.170987	.141789
3.2	.349077	.320945	.295045	.271226	.249338	.210788	.178330
3.3	.398260	.369662	.343058	.318338	.295390	.254372	.219150
3.4	.447969	.419392	.392551	.367374	.343784	.301037	.263665
3.5	.497404	.469301	.442672	.417476	.393663	.349970	.311133
3.6	.545829	.518603	.492594	.467787	.444156	.400294	.360709
3.7	.592597	.566586	.541552	.517498	.494417	.451119	.411493
3.8	.637170	.612643	.588874	.565880	.543669	.501592	.462585
3.9	.679122	.656277	.633997	.612308	.591228	.550932	.513131
4.0	.718150	.697115	.676479	.656275	.636526	.598459	.562358
4.1	.754059	.734898	.716000	.697398	.679119	.643615	.609604
4.2	.786759	.769481	.752355	.735415	.718689	.685969	.654334
4.3	.816246	.800815	.785449	.770180	.755037	.725218	.696141
4.4	.842594	.828935	.815275	.801645	.788072	.761182	.734754
4.5	.865933	.853944	.841908	.829851	.817799	.793788	.770016
4.6	.886437	.875999	.865480	.854906	.844298	.823055	.801883
4.7	.904314	.895293	.886172	.876972	.867713	.849082	.830397
4.8	.919784	.912044	.904193	.896250	.888231	.872024	.855676
4.9	.933081	.926483	.919772	.912963	.906069	.892079	.877892

$\nu = 60$

Q\n	16	17	18	19	20	22	24
5.0	.944434	.938846	.933147	.927349	.921464	.909475	.897257
5.1	.954068	.949364	.944554	.939648	.934657	.924453	.914006
5.2	.962195	.958257	.954221	.950095	.945888	.937260	.928387
5.3	.969012	.965733	.962365	.958916	.955391	.948138	.940651
5.4	.974700	.971984	.969189	.966320	.963382	.957321	.951042
5.5	.979422	.977183	.974874	.972501	.970066	.965028	.959792
5.6	.983324	.981486	.979589	.977634	.975626	.971461	.967117
5.7	.986532	.985031	.983478	.981876	.980228	.976800	.973215
5.8	.989160	.987939	.986673	.985366	.984018	.981211	.978267
5.9	.991303	.990313	.989286	.988223	.987127	.984838	.982431
6.0	.993043	.992244	.991414	.990554	.989665	.987806	.985847
6.4	.997231	.996903	.996560	.996204	.995834	.995055	.994228
6.8	.998941	.998812	.998677	.998537	.998390	.998080	.997749
7.2	.999608	.999559	.999508	.999455	.999399	.999281	.999154
7.6	.999859	.999841	.999822	.999803	.999782	.999739	.999692
8.0	.999950	.999944	.999937	.999930	.999923	.999907	.999890
8.4	.999983	.999981	.999978	.999976	.999973	.999968	.999962
8.8	.999994	.999993	.999993	.999992	.999991	.999989	.999987
9.2	1.00000	1.00000	1.00000	1.00000	1.00000	1.00000	1.00000

ν = 60

Q\n	26	28	30	32	34	36	38
0.0	.000000	.000000	.000000	.000000	.000000	.000000	.000000
0.1	.000000	.000000	.000000	.000000	.000000	.000000	.000000
0.2	.000000	.000000	.000000	.000000	.000000	.000000	.000000
0.3	.000000	.000000	.000000	.000000	.000000	.000000	.000000
0.4	.000000	.000000	.000000	.000000	.000000	.000000	.000000
0.5	.000000	.000000	.000000	.000000	.000000	.000000	.000000
0.6	.000000	.000000	.000000	.000000	.000000	.000000	.000000
0.7	.000000	.000000	.000000	.000000	.000000	.000000	.000000
0.8	.000000	.000000	.000000	.000000	.000000	.000000	.000000
0.9	.000000	.000000	.000000	.000000	.000000	.000000	.000000
1.0	.000000	.000000	.000000	.000000	.000000	.000000	.000000
1.1	.000000	.000000	.000000	.000000	.000000	.000000	.000000
1.2	.000000	.000000	.000000	.000000	.000000	.000000	.000000
1.3	.000000	.000000	.000000	.000000	.000000	.000000	.000000
1.4	.000001	.000000	.000000	.000000	.000000	.000000	.000000
1.5	.000004	.000002	.000001	.000000	.000000	.000000	.000000
1.6	.000014	.000006	.000003	.000001	.000000	.000000	.000000
1.7	.000043	.000019	.000009	.000004	.000002	.000001	.000000
1.8	.000114	.000056	.000028	.000014	.000007	.000004	.000002
1.9	.000279	.000147	.000078	.000042	.000023	.000012	.000007
2.0	.000628	.000352	.000199	.000113	.000065	.000037	.000022
2.1	.001312	.000777	.000464	.000279	.000168	.000103	.000063
2.2	.002564	.001597	.001001	.000631	.000400	.000256	.000164
2.3	.004712	.003072	.002014	.001327	.000880	.000586	.000393
2.4	.008189	.005565	.003800	.002607	.001798	.001246	.000867
2.5	.013527	.009544	.006763	.004813	.003440	.002470	.001780
2.6	.021331	.015575	.011415	.008398	.006202	.004598	.003421
2.7	.032239	.024284	.018352	.013915	.010586	.008081	.006189
2.8	.046869	.036320	.028224	.021996	.017192	.013477	.010596
2.9	.065760	.052290	.041678	.033303	.026677	.021425	.017250
3.0	.089310	.072702	.059302	.048473	.039707	.032598	.026821
3.1	.117733	.097907	.081555	.068053	.056891	.047649	.039984
3.2	.151022	.128050	.108718	.092440	.078719	.067140	.057357
3.3	.188943	.163050	.140857	.121827	.105502	.091484	.079436
3.4	.231043	.202595	.177796	.156179	.137329	.120885	.106530
3.5	.276681	.246157	.219134	.195217	.174051	.155314	.138721
3.6	.325068	.293029	.264259	.238439	.215275	.194493	.175847
3.7	.375324	.342375	.312398	.285150	.260396	.237914	.217497
3.8	.426532	.393283	.362668	.334512	.308637	.284871	.263048
3.9	.477787	.444822	.414132	.385601	.359103	.334511	.311699
4.0	.528243	.496092	.465855	.437465	.410840	.385894	.362537
4.1	.577148	.546268	.516954	.489176	.462893	.438050	.414589
4.2	.623871	.594631	.566634	.539881	.514358	.490038	.466889
4.3	.667909	.640588	.614221	.588829	.564420	.540990	.518523
4.4	.708894	.683682	.659172	.635400	.612387	.590145	.568675
4.5	.746591	.723594	.701087	.679112	.657702	.636878	.616653
4.6	.780881	.760132	.739697	.719625	.699951	.680705	.661904
4.7	.811750	.793219	.774862	.756730	.738861	.721285	.704026
4.8	.839270	.822876	.806551	.790341	.774285	.758414	.742753
4.9	.863580	.849207	.834823	.820473	.806191	.792009	.777952

$\nu = 60$

Q\n	26	28	30	32	34	36	38
5.0	.884872	.872375	.859813	.847223	.834640	.822091	.809601
5.1	.903369	.892590	.881708	.870758	.859769	.848767	.837774
5.2	.919317	.910088	.900734	.891286	.881769	.872206	.862617
5.3	.932968	.925121	.917139	.909048	.900870	.892625	.884330
5.4	.944575	.937947	.931182	.924302	.917326	.910271	.903150
5.5	.954380	.948816	.943120	.937309	.931399	.925404	.919338
5.6	.962614	.957971	.953203	.948326	.943351	.938292	.933159
5.7	.969489	.965635	.961667	.957598	.953436	.949193	.944878
5.8	.975198	.972016	.968732	.965355	.961894	.958357	.954750
5.9	.979916	.977301	.974597	.971809	.968946	.966014	.963017
6.0	.983794	.981657	.979440	.977151	.974794	.972376	.969900
6.4	.993354	.992437	.991479	.990483	.989450	.988382	.987282
6.8	.997397	.997025	.996635	.996226	.995801	.995358	.994900
7.2	.999018	.998874	.998723	.998563	.998396	.998222	.998041
7.6	.999641	.999588	.999531	.999471	.999408	.999342	.999273
8.0	.999872	.999853	.999832	.999810	.999787	.999763	.999738
8.4	.999955	.999948	.999941	.999933	.999925	.999917	.999908
8.8	.999985	.999982	.999980	.999977	.999974	.999971	.999968
9.2	.999995	.999994	.999993	.999992	.999991	.999990	.999989
9.6	1.00000	1.00000	1.00000	1.00000	1.00000	1.00000	1.00000

$\nu = 60$

Q\n	40	50	60	70	80	90	100
0.0	.000000	.000000	.000000	.000000	.000000	.000000	.000000
0.1	.000000	.000000	.000000	.000000	.000000	.000000	.000000
0.2	.000000	.000000	.000000	.000000	.000000	.000000	.000000
0.3	.000000	.000000	.000000	.000000	.000000	.000000	.000000
0.4	.000000	.000000	.000000	.000000	.000000	.000000	.000000
0.5	.000000	.000000	.000000	.000000	.000000	.000000	.000000
0.6	.000000	.000000	.000000	.000000	.000000	.000000	.000000
0.7	.000000	.000000	.000000	.000000	.000000	.000000	.000000
0.8	.000000	.000000	.000000	.000000	.000000	.000000	.000000
0.9	.000000	.000000	.000000	.000000	.000000	.000000	.000000
1.0	.000000	.000000	.000000	.000000	.000000	.000000	.000000
1.1	.000000	.000000	.000000	.000000	.000000	.000000	.000000
1.2	.000000	.000000	.000000	.000000	.000000	.000000	.000000
1.3	.000000	.000000	.000000	.000000	.000000	.000000	.000000
1.4	.000000	.000000	.000000	.000000	.000000	.000000	.000000
1.5	.000000	.000000	.000000	.000000	.000000	.000000	.000000
1.6	.000000	.000000	.000000	.000000	.000000	.000000	.000000
1.7	.000000	.000000	.000000	.000000	.000000	.000000	.000000
1.8	.000001	.000000	.000000	.000000	.000000	.000000	.000000
1.9	.000004	.000000	.000000	.000000	.000000	.000000	.000000
2.0	.000013	.000001	.000000	.000000	.000000	.000000	.000000
2.1	.000039	.000004	.000000	.000000	.000000	.000000	.000000
2.2	.000106	.000013	.000002	.000000	.000000	.000000	.000000
2.3	.000264	.000039	.000007	.000001	.000000	.000000	.000000
2.4	.000607	.000109	.000022	.000005	.000001	.000000	.000000
2.5	.001289	.000272	.000063	.000016	.000004	.000001	.000000
2.6	.002556	.000627	.000168	.000048	.000015	.000005	.000002
2.7	.004756	.001337	.000406	.000132	.000045	.000017	.000006
2.8	.008355	.002658	.000904	.000327	.000125	.000050	.000021
2.9	.013925	.004955	.001871	.000745	.000312	.000136	.000062
3.0	.022116	.008713	.003616	.001574	.000716	.000338	.000166
3.1	.033616	.014528	.006572	.003101	.001521	.000772	.000405
3.2	.049080	.023075	.011289	.005731	.003010	.001630	.000908
3.3	.069070	.035058	.018417	.009993	.005587	.003209	.001890
3.4	.093987	.051144	.028666	.016525	.009778	.005927	.003672
3.5	.124019	.071896	.042743	.026036	.016224	.010325	.006699
3.6	.159111	.097700	.061281	.039248	.025637	.017056	.011542
3.7	.198955	.128716	.084768	.056824	.038745	.026841	.018872
3.8	.243012	.164852	.113481	.079298	.056221	.040411	.029423
3.9	.290546	.205753	.147450	.106999	.078606	.058431	.043919
4.0	.340678	.250829	.186437	.140013	.106242	.081427	.063006
4.1	.392448	.299296	.229946	.178155	.139221	.109717	.087170
4.2	.444872	.350231	.277264	.220975	.177362	.143364	.116679
4.3	.497003	.402639	.327505	.267791	.220219	.182155	.151536
4.4	.547973	.455515	.379682	.317736	.267106	.225611	.191468
4.5	.597032	.507899	.432769	.369825	.317153	.273017	.235936
4.6	.643564	.558924	.485764	.423024	.369367	.323480	.284178
4.7	.687102	.607852	.537741	.476308	.422706	.375993	.335267
4.8	.727323	.654085	.587889	.528725	.476135	.429502	.388172
4.9	.764040	.697181	.635542	.579431	.528695	.482976	.441837

ν = 60

Q\n	40	50	60	70	80	90	100
5.0	.797190	.736846	.680186	.627726	.579535	.535459	.495239
5.1	.826810	.772922	.721462	.673063	.627948	.586114	.547442
5.2	.853019	.805374	.759157	.715055	.673385	.634250	.597636
5.3	.876000	.834265	.793190	.753464	.715455	.679336	.645165
5.4	.895979	.859739	.823588	.788188	.753922	.721001	.689534
5.5	.913211	.881997	.850470	.819240	.788682	.759026	.730405
5.6	.927960	.901281	.874021	.846727	.819752	.793325	.767594
5.7	.940497	.917857	.894474	.870828	.847240	.823930	.801045
5.8	.951082	.931999	.912091	.891773	.871330	.850962	.830812
5.9	.959963	.943979	.927150	.909825	.892253	.874613	.857038
6.0	.967371	.954063	.939929	.925262	.910275	.895124	.879927
6.4	.986151	.980085	.973452	.966382	.958974	.951306	.943441
6.8	.994427	.991852	.988973	.985840	.982495	.978969	.975292
7.2	.997853	.996820	.995645	.994345	.992937	.991433	.989844
7.6	.999202	.998806	.998349	.997837	.997277	.996671	.996025
8.0	.999712	.999565	.999394	.999201	.998987	.998755	.998504
8.4	.999898	.999846	.999784	.999713	.999634	.999548	.999455
8.8	.999965	.999946	.999924	.999899	.999871	.999840	.999806
9.2	.999988	.999982	.999974	.999965	.999955	.999944	.999932
9.6	1.00000	.999994	.999991	.999988	.999985	.999981	.999977
10.0		1.00000	1.00000	1.00000	.999995	.999993	.999992
11.0					1.00000	1.00000	1.00000

ν = 120

Q\n	2	3	4	5	6	7	8
0.0	.000000	.000000	.000000	.000000	.000000	.000000	.000000
0.1	.056254	.002753	.000128	.000005	.000000	.000000	.000000
0.2	.112226	.010965	.001014	.000091	.000008	.000001	.000000
0.3	.167636	.024497	.003391	.000456	.000060	.000008	.000001
0.4	.222215	.043125	.007931	.001418	.000250	.000043	.000008
0.5	.275706	.066541	.015227	.003390	.000742	.000161	.000035
0.6	.327867	.094365	.025770	.006847	.001790	.000463	.000119
0.7	.378477	.126156	.039931	.012300	.003729	.001119	.000334
0.8	.427336	.161421	.057953	.020256	.006968	.002373	.000803
0.9	.474270	.199631	.079948	.031182	.011972	.004551	.001719
1.0	.519129	.240232	.105892	.045477	.019229	.008051	.003349
1.1	.561793	.282660	.135637	.063444	.029223	.013329	.006040
1.2	.602167	.326353	.168920	.085270	.042396	.020874	.010212
1.3	.640185	.370764	.205377	.111013	.059116	.031177	.016337
1.4	.675809	.415373	.244565	.140600	.079653	.044695	.024919
1.5	.709025	.459691	.285976	.173828	.104150	.061815	.036454
1.6	.739845	.503275	.329066	.210376	.132616	.082823	.051398
1.7	.768301	.545730	.373269	.249822	.164922	.107882	.070127
1.8	.794448	.586713	.418017	.291660	.200800	.137009	.092902
1.9	.818356	.625939	.462764	.335327	.239861	.170074	.119851
2.0	.840111	.663176	.506995	.380228	.281616	.206800	.150944
2.1	.859814	.698248	.550241	.425755	.325493	.246780	.185994
2.2	.877572	.731032	.592088	.471314	.370872	.289494	.224664
2.3	.893501	.761454	.632185	.516345	.417109	.334337	.266481
2.4	.907722	.789484	.670246	.560333	.463562	.380650	.310860
2.5	.920358	.815135	.706049	.602828	.509616	.427751	.357142
2.6	.931535	.838452	.739439	.643447	.554705	.474962	.404619
2.7	.941374	.859509	.770321	.681882	.598327	.521639	.452571
2.8	.949996	.878407	.798655	.717900	.640054	.567192	.500301
2.9	.957517	.895260	.824451	.751342	.679539	.611105	.547156
3.0	.964048	.910201	.847761	.782117	.716520	.652944	.592554
3.1	.969693	.923368	.868673	.810196	.750816	.692364	.635996
3.2	.974550	.934904	.887301	.835604	.782322	.729114	.677079
3.3	.978711	.944955	.903783	.858415	.811006	.763027	.715496
3.4	.982261	.953663	.918269	.878738	.836893	.794021	.751037
3.5	.985275	.961167	.930920	.896709	.860063	.822085	.783583
3.6	.987823	.967598	.941898	.912488	.880633	.847270	.813098
3.7	.989969	.973081	.951367	.926246	.898756	.869679	.839614
3.8	.991767	.977732	.959486	.938162	.914603	.889456	.863225
3.9	.993268	.981658	.966408	.948415	.928360	.906772	.884069
4.0	.994516	.984955	.972274	.957182	.940221	.921819	.902320
4.1	.995549	.987710	.977220	.964632	.950377	.934798	.918175
4.2	.996401	.990001	.981367	.970926	.959018	.945915	.931844
4.3	.997100	.991898	.984825	.976212	.966322	.955373	.943543
4.4	.997672	.993461	.987695	.980626	.972460	.963366	.953486
4.5	.998137	.994743	.990064	.984292	.977587	.970079	.961879
4.6	.998515	.995790	.992010	.987321	.981844	.975681	.968918
4.7	.998821	.996642	.993602	.989810	.985360	.980329	.974784
4.8	.999066	.997331	.994897	.991846	.988248	.984163	.979642
4.9	.999263	.997887	.995945	.993502	.990608	.987308	.983643

$\nu = 120$

Q\n	2	3	4	5	6	7	8
5.0	.999421	.998333	.996791	.994843	.992526	.989874	.986918
5.1	.999546	.998689	.997470	.995923	.994077	.991957	.989585
5.2	.999646	.998973	.998013	.996790	.995326	.993638	.991745
5.3	.999724	.999199	.998445	.997482	.996326	.994989	.993485
5.4	.999786	.999377	.998788	.998033	.997123	.996069	.994880
5.5	.999834	.999517	.999058	.998469	.997756	.996929	.995993
5.6	.999872	.999627	.999271	.998812	.998257	.997610	.996876
5.7	.999902	.999712	.999438	.999082	.998651	.998147	.997575
5.8	.999925	.999779	.999567	.999293	.998959	.998569	.998124
5.9	.999943	.999831	.999669	.999457	.999200	.998898	.998554
6.0	.999956	.999871	.999747	.999585	.999387	.999155	.998890
6.4	.999986	.999958	.999916	.999862	.999796	.999718	.999628
6.8	1.00000	.999987	.999974	.999957	.999935	.999910	.999881
7.2		1.00000	.999992	.999987	.999980	.999973	.999964
7.6			1.00000	1.00000	.999994	.999992	.999989
8.0					1.00000	1.00000	1.00000

ν =120

Q\n	9	10	11	12	13	14	15
0.0	.000000	.000000	.000000	.000000	.000000	.000000	.000000
0.1	.000000	.000000	.000000	.000000	.000000	.000000	.000000
0.2	.000000	.000000	.000000	.000000	.000000	.000000	.000000
0.3	.000000	.000000	.000000	.000000	.000000	.000000	.000000
0.4	.000001	.000000	.000000	.000000	.000000	.000000	.000000
0.5	.000007	.000002	.000000	.000000	.000000	.000000	.000000
0.6	.000031	.000008	.000002	.000001	.000000	.000000	.000000
0.7	.000099	.000029	.000009	.000003	.000001	.000000	.000000
0.8	.000271	.000091	.000031	.000010	.000003	.000001	.000000
0.9	.000647	.000243	.000091	.000034	.000013	.000005	.000002
1.0	.001387	.000573	.000236	.000097	.000040	.000017	.000007
1.1	.002726	.001227	.000551	.000247	.000111	.000050	.000022
1.2	.004974	.002416	.001172	.000568	.000275	.000133	.000065
1.3	.008524	.004435	.002303	.001195	.000619	.000321	.000167
1.4	.013833	.007656	.004230	.002334	.001287	.000710	.000391
1.5	.021404	.012530	.007321	.004272	.002491	.001452	.000847
1.6	.031757	.019561	.012025	.007382	.004528	.002777	.001703
1.7	.045384	.029281	.018851	.012120	.007785	.004998	.003209
1.8	.062718	.042209	.028344	.019005	.012731	.008524	.005706
1.9	.084089	.058813	.041042	.028596	.019904	.013845	.009627
2.0	.109695	.079466	.057436	.041446	.029874	.021517	.015491
2.1	.139577	.104413	.077926	.058060	.043207	.032128	.023877
2.2	.173612	.133737	.102778	.078850	.060416	.046250	.035385
2.3	.211509	.167350	.132099	.104088	.081909	.064394	.050591
2.4	.252827	.204990	.165812	.133880	.107950	.086954	.069991
2.5	.296999	.246230	.203659	.168142	.138626	.114169	.093953
2.6	.343359	.290502	.245209	.206601	.173825	.146087	.122672
2.7	.391180	.337131	.289882	.248803	.213239	.182552	.156143
2.8	.439713	.385368	.336981	.294140	.256376	.223204	.194147
2.9	.488216	.434436	.385734	.341887	.302590	.267500	.236258
3.0	.535993	.483562	.435335	.391242	.351117	.314744	.281871
3.1	.582414	.532014	.484985	.441372	.401125	.364130	.330234
3.2	.626934	.579129	.533926	.491456	.451755	.414794	.380497
3.3	.669108	.624332	.581475	.540722	.502170	.465855	.431765
3.4	.708594	.667155	.627043	.588475	.551591	.516469	.483145
3.5	.745154	.707236	.670150	.634125	.599325	.565857	.533789
3.6	.778648	.744324	.710430	.677195	.644791	.613342	.582936
3.7	.809024	.778270	.747631	.717328	.687530	.658366	.629934
3.8	.836307	.809019	.781612	.754287	.727206	.700496	.674257
3.9	.860587	.836599	.812324	.787944	.763606	.739430	.715513
4.0	.882005	.861104	.839806	.818270	.796628	.774988	.753442
4.1	.900738	.882681	.864163	.845320	.826267	.807102	.787906
4.2	.916992	.901517	.885554	.869216	.852603	.835798	.818875
4.3	.930984	.917825	.904177	.890134	.875779	.861184	.846412
4.4	.942941	.931834	.920256	.908284	.895987	.883426	.870653
4.5	.953084	.943776	.934027	.923902	.913455	.902737	.891792
4.6	.961630	.953883	.945734	.937234	.928428	.919358	.910059
4.7	.968782	.962376	.955611	.948528	.941161	.933545	.925708
4.8	.974730	.969467	.963888	.958025	.951907	.945559	.939006
4.9	.979645	.975347	.970775	.965955	.960909	.955656	.950217

$\nu = 120$

Q\n	9	10	11	12	13	14	15
5.0	.983683	.980194	.976470	.972532	.968397	.964081	.959598
5.1	.986982	.984165	.981150	.977952	.974585	.971062	.967392
5.2	.989661	.987399	.984972	.982391	.979666	.976807	.973823
5.3	.991825	.990018	.988075	.986004	.983811	.981506	.979094
5.4	.993564	.992129	.990581	.988927	.987174	.985325	.983387
5.5	.994955	.993820	.992593	.991280	.989885	.988411	.986863
5.6	.996061	.995168	.994201	.993164	.992059	.990890	.989661
5.7	.996937	.996238	.995479	.994663	.993793	.992872	.991900
5.8	.997628	.997082	.996490	.995852	.995170	.994446	.993682
5.9	.998170	.997746	.997285	.996788	.996257	.995691	.995094
6.0	.998593	.998266	.997909	.997523	.997111	.996671	.996206
6.4	.999526	.999414	.999291	.999157	.999013	.998859	.998696
6.8	.999849	.999812	.999772	.999729	.999681	.999631	.999577
7.2	.999954	.999943	.999930	.999917	.999902	.999887	.999870
7.6	.999987	.999983	.999980	.999976	.999971	.999967	.999962
8.0	1.00000	1.00000	.999994	.999993	.999992	.999991	.999989
8.4			1.00000	1.00000	1.00000	1.00000	1.00000

ν =120

Q\n	16	17	18	19	20	22	24
0.0	.000000	.000000	.000000	.000000	.000000	.000000	.000000
0.1	.000000	.000000	.000000	.000000	.000000	.000000	.000000
0.2	.000000	.000000	.000000	.000000	.000000	.000000	.000000
0.3	.000000	.000000	.000000	.000000	.000000	.000000	.000000
0.4	.000000	.000000	.000000	.000000	.000000	.000000	.000000
0.5	.000000	.000000	.000000	.000000	.000000	.000000	.000000
0.6	.000000	.000000	.000000	.000000	.000000	.000000	.000000
0.7	.000000	.000000	.000000	.000000	.000000	.000000	.000000
0.8	.000000	.000000	.000000	.000000	.000000	.000000	.000000
0.9	.000001	.000000	.000000	.000000	.000000	.000000	.000000
1.0	.000003	.000001	.000000	.000000	.000000	.000000	.000000
1.1	.000010	.000005	.000002	.000001	.000000	.000000	.000000
1.2	.000031	.000015	.000007	.000004	.000002	.000000	.000000
1.3	.000086	.000045	.000023	.000012	.000006	.000002	.000000
1.4	.000216	.000119	.000066	.000036	.000020	.000006	.000002
1.5	.000494	.000288	.000168	.000098	.000058	.000020	.000007
1.6	.001045	.000641	.000394	.000242	.000149	.000057	.000022
1.7	.002060	.001324	.000851	.000547	.000352	.000146	.000061
1.8	.003819	.002557	.001713	.001148	.000770	.000347	.000157
1.9	.006694	.004655	.003238	.002254	.001570	.000763	.000372
2.0	.011151	.008028	.005780	.004164	.003000	.001561	.000815
2.1	.017741	.013181	.009794	.007279	.005412	.002996	.001663
2.2	.027063	.020695	.015826	.012104	.009260	.005426	.003186
2.3	.039729	.031192	.024488	.019226	.015097	.009317	.005759
2.4	.056308	.045286	.036416	.029282	.023547	.015237	.009872
2.5	.077272	.063528	.052216	.042914	.035269	.023830	.016115
2.6	.102946	.086352	.072410	.060709	.050894	.035772	.025158
2.7	.133464	.114021	.097374	.083137	.070971	.051714	.037693
2.8	.168751	.146595	.127294	.110500	.095902	.072215	.054380
2.9	.208509	.183909	.162135	.142889	.125894	.097682	.075776
3.0	.252237	.225577	.201633	.180159	.160923	.128313	.102269
3.1	.299257	.271011	.245300	.221933	.200723	.164068	.134026
3.2	.348760	.319460	.292459	.267619	.244797	.204652	.170962
3.3	.399855	.370056	.342286	.316450	.292448	.249535	.212731
3.4	.451620	.421873	.393862	.367533	.342822	.297978	.258745
3.5	.503158	.473974	.446231	.419907	.394970	.349089	.308210
3.6	.553632	.525466	.498455	.472604	.447903	.401882	.360187
3.7	.602307	.575537	.549659	.524694	.500653	.455338	.413651
3.8	.648569	.623491	.599070	.575338	.552319	.508469	.467558
3.9	.691936	.668761	.646040	.623813	.602110	.560362	.520908
4.0	.732067	.710924	.690066	.669535	.649367	.610223	.572792
4.1	.768750	.749693	.730785	.712069	.693581	.657402	.622429
4.2	.801895	.784914	.767977	.751125	.734392	.701401	.669193
4.3	.831517	.816548	.801546	.786548	.771587	.741882	.712619
4.4	.857716	.844655	.831507	.818306	.805080	.778653	.752400
4.5	.880659	.869373	.857966	.846466	.834899	.811652	.788381
4.6	.900563	.890901	.881098	.871179	.861165	.840932	.820534
4.7	.917677	.909477	.901129	.892653	.884067	.866633	.848944
4.8	.932269	.925367	.918318	.911139	.903844	.888965	.873778
4.9	.944608	.938845	.932941	.926912	.920768	.908183	.895268

$\nu = 120$

Q\n	16	17	18	19	20	22	24
5.0	.954962	.950186	.945281	.940257	.935125	.924571	.913686
5.1	.963587	.959658	.955611	.951457	.947204	.938425	.929329
5.2	.970721	.967510	.964196	.960786	.957286	.950041	.942501
5.3	.976581	.973975	.971279	.968499	.965640	.959703	.953502
5.4	.981365	.979262	.977083	.974832	.972512	.967682	.962618
5.5	.985244	.983558	.981808	.979997	.978127	.974223	.970117
5.6	.988372	.987028	.985631	.984182	.982684	.979549	.976241
5.7	.990880	.989815	.988705	.987553	.986360	.983858	.981210
5.8	.992879	.992039	.991163	.990252	.989307	.987322	.985215
5.9	.994465	.993805	.993117	.992401	.991657	.990090	.988424
6.0	.995715	.995201	.994663	.994102	.993519	.992290	.990979
6.4	.998522	.998340	.998148	.997948	.997739	.997295	.996819
6.8	.999520	.999459	.999395	.999329	.999258	.999109	.998948
7.2	.999852	.999833	.999813	.999792	.999770	.999723	.999672
7.6	.999956	.999951	.999945	.999939	.999932	.999918	.999902
8.0	.999988	.999986	.999984	.999983	.999981	.999977	.999972
8.4	1.00000	1.00000	1.00000	1.00000	.999995	.999994	.999992
8.8					1.00000	1.00000	1.00000

$\nu = 120$

Q\n	26	28	30	32	34	36	38
0.0	.000000	.000000	.000000	.000000	.000000	.000000	.000000
0.1	.000000	.000000	.000000	.000000	.000000	.000000	.000000
0.2	.000000	.000000	.000000	.000000	.000000	.000000	.000000
0.3	.000000	.000000	.000000	.000000	.000000	.000000	.000000
0.4	.000000	.000000	.000000	.000000	.000000	.000000	.000000
0.5	.000000	.000000	.000000	.000000	.000000	.000000	.000000
0.6	.000000	.000000	.000000	.000000	.000000	.000000	.000000
0.7	.000000	.000000	.000000	.000000	.000000	.000000	.000000
0.8	.000000	.000000	.000000	.000000	.000000	.000000	.000000
0.9	.000000	.000000	.000000	.000000	.000000	.000000	.000000
1.0	.000000	.000000	.000000	.000000	.000000	.000000	.000000
1.1	.000000	.000000	.000000	.000000	.000000	.000000	.000000
1.2	.000000	.000000	.000000	.000000	.000000	.000000	.000000
1.3	.000000	.000000	.000000	.000000	.000000	.000000	.000000
1.4	.000001	.000000	.000000	.000000	.000000	.000000	.000000
1.5	.000002	.000001	.000000	.000000	.000000	.000000	.000000
1.6	.000008	.000003	.000001	.000000	.000000	.000000	.000000
1.7	.000026	.000011	.000005	.000002	.000001	.000000	.000000
1.8	.000072	.000033	.000015	.000007	.000003	.000001	.000001
1.9	.000182	.000090	.000044	.000022	.000011	.000005	.000003
2.0	.000426	.000224	.000118	.000063	.000033	.000018	.000010
2.1	.000926	.000517	.000290	.000163	.000092	.000052	.000030
2.2	.001875	.001107	.000655	.000389	.000232	.000139	.000083
2.3	.003568	.002215	.001379	.000861	.000539	.000339	.000213
2.4	.006407	.004166	.002716	.001774	.001162	.000764	.000503
2.5	.010913	.007403	.005031	.003427	.002339	.001600	.001098
2.6	.017711	.012486	.008816	.006236	.004419	.003138	.002233
2.7	.027493	.020074	.014676	.010746	.007880	.005789	.004260
2.8	.040968	.030887	.023310	.017613	.013325	.010096	.007662
2.9	.058794	.045641	.035456	.027570	.021460	.016725	.013051
3.0	.081508	.064979	.051829	.041368	.033046	.026423	.021150
3.1	.109460	.089402	.073042	.059703	.048831	.039968	.032741
3.2	.142761	.119198	.099535	.083139	.069475	.058087	.048598
3.3	.181257	.154398	.131513	.112033	.095463	.081375	.069398
3.4	.224529	.194760	.168905	.146480	.127046	.110215	.095645
3.5	.271913	.239769	.211360	.186289	.164190	.144726	.127593
3.6	.322552	.288677	.258256	.230982	.206563	.184723	.165203
3.7	.375450	.340553	.308751	.279824	.253553	.229723	.208127
3.8	.429549	.394350	.361841	.331878	.304308	.278976	.255724
3.9	.483786	.448979	.416433	.386072	.357802	.331517	.307110
4.0	.537162	.503371	.471419	.441280	.412908	.386244	.361219
4.1	.588785	.556542	.525739	.496388	.468481	.441994	.416892
4.2	.637905	.607633	.578439	.550362	.523421	.497620	.472950
4.3	.683936	.655940	.628709	.602296	.576739	.552061	.528272
4.4	.726457	.700932	.675907	.651445	.627594	.604389	.581853
4.5	.765211	.742246	.719568	.697242	.675321	.653845	.632847
4.6	.800087	.779682	.759398	.739299	.719438	.699857	.680591
4.7	.831099	.813182	.795262	.777399	.759643	.742037	.724615
4.8	.858369	.842808	.827159	.811474	.795799	.780174	.764631
4.9	.882093	.868720	.855202	.841585	.827910	.814211	.800520

ν =120

Q\n	26	28	30	32	34	36	38
5.0	.902528	.891148	.879590	.867894	.856094	.844222	.832304
5.1	.919963	.910368	.900581	.890636	.880561	.870382	.860124
5.2	.934705	.926687	.918475	.910098	.901580	.892942	.884204
5.3	.947065	.940419	.933589	.926596	.919461	.912200	.904830
5.4	.957343	.951879	.946244	.940456	.934531	.928483	.922325
5.5	.965826	.961366	.956754	.952001	.947122	.942127	.937026
5.6	.972775	.969161	.965413	.961541	.957554	.953462	.949272
5.7	.978428	.975520	.972495	.969363	.966130	.962803	.959389
5.8	.982996	.980671	.978247	.975730	.973127	.970441	.967680
5.9	.986664	.984817	.982886	.980878	.978795	.976643	.974425
6.0	.989592	.988133	.986604	.985011	.983356	.981642	.979873
6.4	.996310	.995772	.995204	.994609	.993986	.993337	.992662
6.8	.998775	.998592	.998397	.998191	.997975	.997749	.997513
7.2	.999617	.999558	.999495	.999429	.999359	.999286	.999209
7.6	.999886	.999868	.999849	.999829	.999808	.999785	.999762
8.0	.999968	.999962	.999957	.999951	.999945	.999938	.999932
8.4	.999991	.999990	.999988	.999987	.999985	.999983	.999981
8.8	1.00000	1.00000	1.00000	1.00000	1.00000	1.00000	.999995
9.2							1.00000

$\nu = 120$

Q\n	40	50	60	70	80	90	100
0.0	.000000	.000000	.000000	.000000	.000000	.000000	.000000
0.1	.000000	.000000	.000000	.000000	.000000	.000000	.000000
0.2	.000000	.000000	.000000	.000000	.000000	.000000	.000000
0.3	.000000	.000000	.000000	.000000	.000000	.000000	.000000
0.4	.000000	.000000	.000000	.000000	.000000	.000000	.000000
0.5	.000000	.000000	.000000	.000000	.000000	.000000	.000000
0.6	.000000	.000000	.000000	.000000	.000000	.000000	.000000
0.7	.000000	.000000	.000000	.000000	.000000	.000000	.000000
0.8	.000000	.000000	.000000	.000000	.000000	.000000	.000000
0.9	.000000	.000000	.000000	.000000	.000000	.000000	.000000
1.0	.000000	.000000	.000000	.000000	.000000	.000000	.000000
1.1	.000000	.000000	.000000	.000000	.000000	.000000	.000000
1.2	.000000	.000000	.000000	.000000	.000000	.000000	.000000
1.3	.000000	.000000	.000000	.000000	.000000	.000000	.000000
1.4	.000000	.000000	.000000	.000000	.000000	.000000	.000000
1.5	.000000	.000000	.000000	.000000	.000000	.000000	.000000
1.6	.000000	.000000	.000000	.000000	.000000	.000000	.000000
1.7	.000000	.000000	.000000	.000000	.000000	.000000	.000000
1.8	.000000	.000000	.000000	.000000	.000000	.000000	.000000
1.9	.000001	.000000	.000000	.000000	.000000	.000000	.000000
2.0	.000005	.000000	.000000	.000000	.000000	.000000	.000000
2.1	.000017	.000001	.000000	.000000	.000000	.000000	.000000
2.2	.000050	.000004	.000000	.000000	.000000	.000000	.000000
2.3	.000135	.000014	.000002	.000000	.000000	.000000	.000000
2.4	.000332	.000044	.000006	.000001	.000000	.000000	.000000
2.5	.000755	.000121	.000021	.000004	.000001	.000000	.000000
2.6	.001593	.000304	.000061	.000013	.000003	.000001	.000000
2.7	.003141	.000705	.000166	.000041	.000011	.000003	.000001
2.8	.005823	.001515	.000412	.000117	.000035	.000011	.000003
2.9	.010198	.003036	.000939	.000302	.000101	.000035	.000012
3.0	.016948	.005704	.001984	.000714	.000265	.000102	.000040
3.1	.026846	.010103	.003910	.001558	.000639	.000270	.000117
3.2	.040688	.016950	.007230	.003162	.001418	.000652	.000306
3.3	.059217	.027058	.012609	.006002	.002919	.001450	.000735
3.4	.083033	.041267	.020840	.010715	.005611	.002992	.001624
3.5	.112517	.060355	.032791	.018081	.010127	.005760	.003327
3.6	.147767	.084947	.049317	.028981	.017253	.010408	.006360
3.7	.188570	.115422	.071169	.044309	.027884	.017742	.011415
3.8	.234402	.151856	.098885	.064878	.042938	.028679	.019334
3.9	.284468	.193990	.132715	.091311	.063259	.044154	.031057
4.0	.337759	.241234	.172568	.123948	.089501	.065017	.047529
4.1	.393133	.292713	.217997	.162781	.122034	.091917	.069584
4.2	.449394	.347339	.268226	.207436	.160872	.125205	.097835
4.3	.505374	.403892	.322219	.257185	.205646	.164861	.132569
4.4	.560001	.461114	.378759	.311012	.255628	.210476	.173689
4.5	.612349	.517794	.436545	.367692	.309783	.261270	.220699
4.6	.661669	.572835	.494289	.425895	.366862	.316163	.272738
4.7	.707408	.625308	.550797	.484288	.425505	.373862	.328653
4.8	.749201	.674481	.605030	.541616	.484344	.432974	.387099
4.9	.786863	.719827	.656146	.596783	.542099	.492112	.446652

$\nu = 120$

Q\n	40	50	60	70	80	90	100
5.0	.820365	.761025	.703518	.648888	.597646	.549988	.505917
5.1	.849806	.797934	.746739	.697255	.650069	.605483	.563621
5.2	.875383	.830570	.785597	.741434	.698682	.657697	.618677
5.3	.897366	.859076	.820058	.781185	.743030	.705966	.670228
5.4	.916069	.883691	.850233	.816454	.782878	.749865	.717661
5.5	.931831	.904718	.876339	.847338	.818176	.789185	.760602
5.6	.944994	.922498	.898673	.874054	.849035	.823909	.798895
5.7	.955894	.937390	.917580	.896900	.875680	.854171	.832566
5.8	.964847	.949751	.933428	.916229	.898423	.880221	.861788
5.9	.972144	.959924	.946590	.932418	.917626	.902387	.886839
6.0	.978050	.968230	.957424	.945849	.933677	.921046	.908071
6.4	.991964	.988131	.983796	.979031	.973897	.968446	.962719
6.8	.997267	.995903	.994328	.992564	.990630	.988542	.986313
7.2	.999128	.998678	.998151	.997552	.996887	.996160	.995376
7.6	.999737	.999598	.999433	.999244	.999032	.998798	.998543
8.0	.999924	.999884	.999835	.999779	.999715	.999645	.999568
8.4	.999979	.999968	.999954	.999938	.999920	.999900	.999878
8.8	.999994	.999991	.999988	.999983	.999979	.999973	.999967
9.2	1.00000	1.00000	1.00000	1.00000	.999994	.999993	.999991
9.6					1.00000	1.00000	1.00000

Table B2

PERCENTAGE POINTS OF THE STUDENTIZED RANGE (VALUES OF THE STUDENTIZED RANGE $Q = w/s$ CORRESPONDING TO CUMULATIVE PROBABILITY P FOR SAMPLES OF SIZE n FROM A NORMAL POPULATION, WITH ν DEGREES OF FREEDOM FOR THE INDEPENDENT ESTIMATE s^2 OF THE POPULATION VARIANCE)

P = .001

ν \ n	2	3	4	5	6	7	8	9	10
1	.0022	.0602	.1715	.2834	.3802	.4616	.5302	.5888	.6393
2	.0020	.0602	.1819	.3116	.4284	.5289	.6149	.6890	.7534
3	.0019	.0602	.1866	.3254	.4529	.5642	.6605	.7440	.8170
4	.0019	.0602	.1893	.3336	.4680	.5866	.6898	.7798	.8588
5	.0019	.0603	.1910	.3391	.4783	.6021	.7103	.8053	.8889
6	.0019	.0603	.1923	.3431	.4858	.6135	.7257	.8244	.9116
7	.0018	.0602	.1932	.3461	.4916	.6223	.7376	.8393	.9294
8	.0018	.0602	.1939	.3484	.4961	.6293	.7472	.8514	.9439
9	.0018	.0602	.1945	.3503	.4998	.6350	.7550	.8613	.9558
10	.0018	.0602	.1949	.3518	.5028	.6397	.7615	.8696	.9658
11	.0018	.0602	.1953	.3531	.5053	.6436	.7670	.8766	.9744
12	.0018	.0602	.1956	.3541	.5074	.6471	.7718	.8827	.9818
13	.0018	.0602	.1959	.3550	.5093	.6500	.7759	.8880	.9882
14	.0018	.0602	.1962	.3559	.5109	.6526	.7795	.8927	.9939
15	.0018	.0602	.1964	.3566	.5124	.6549	.7827	.8968	.9989
16	.0018	.0602	.1966	.3572	.5137	.6569	.7855	.9005	1.003
17	.0018	.0602	.1967	.3578	.5148	.6587	.7881	.9038	1.007
18	.0018	.0602	.1969	.3583	.5158	.6604	.7904	.9067	1.011
19	.0018	.0602	.1970	.3587	.5167	.6619	.7925	.9095	1.014
20	.0018	.0602	.1971	.3591	.5176	.6632	.7943	.9119	1.017
24	.0018	.0602	.1975	.3604	.5202	.6675	.8005	.9199	1.027
30	.0018	.0602	.1979	.3618	.5230	.6720	.8068	.9283	1.038
40	.0018	.0602	.1982	.3631	.5258	.6766	.8134	.9370	1.048
60	.0018	.0602	.1986	.3645	.5287	.6813	.8202	.9460	1.060
120	.0018	.0602	.1990	.3660	.5317	.6863	.8274	.9555	1.072
∞	.0018	.0602	.1994	.3674	.5347	.6913	.8348	.9655	1.085

ν \ n	11	12	13	14	15	16	17	18	19
1	.6835	.7226	.7576	.7891	.8177	.8439	.8680	.8903	.9109
2	.8099	.8602	.9052	.9458	.9828	1.016	1.047	1.076	1.103
3	.8813	.9387	.9901	1.036	1.079	1.117	1.154	1.186	1.216
4	.9288	.9912	1.047	1.098	1.145	1.187	1.226	1.262	1.296
5	.9630	1.029	1.089	1.143	1.192	1.238	1.280	1.318	1.354
6	.9891	1.058	1.121	1.178	1.229	1.277	1.321	1.362	1.400
7	1.009	1.082	1.147	1.205	1.259	1.309	1.355	1.397	1.436
8	1.026	1.101	1.167	1.228	1.284	1.335	1.383	1.426	1.467
9	1.040	1.116	1.185	1.247	1.305	1.357	1.405	1.451	1.493
10	1.052	1.129	1.199	1.263	1.322	1.376	1.425	1.472	1.515
11	1.062	1.141	1.212	1.277	1.337	1.392	1.443	1.490	1.534
12	1.071	1.151	1.223	1.290	1.350	1.406	1.458	1.506	1.551
13	1.078	1.159	1.233	1.300	1.362	1.418	1.471	1.520	1.566
14	1.085	1.167	1.241	1.310	1.372	1.429	1.483	1.533	1.579
15	1.091	1.174	1.249	1.318	1.381	1.439	1.494	1.544	1.591
16	1.096	1.180	1.256	1.326	1.389	1.448	1.503	1.554	1.601
17	1.101	1.185	1.262	1.332	1.397	1.456	1.512	1.563	1.611
18	1.105	1.190	1.268	1.339	1.404	1.464	1.520	1.572	1.620
19	1.109	1.195	1.273	1.344	1.410	1.471	1.527	1.579	1.628
20	1.113	1.199	1.277	1.349	1.416	1.476	1.533	1.586	1.636
24	1.124	1.212	1.293	1.367	1.434	1.497	1.555	1.609	1.660
30	1.137	1.227	1.309	1.385	1.454	1.519	1.578	1.634	1.687
40	1.150	1.242	1.326	1.404	1.476	1.542	1.604	1.661	1.715
60	1.163	1.258	1.345	1.424	1.498	1.567	1.631	1.691	1.747
120	1.178	1.275	1.364	1.446	1.523	1.594	1.660	1.722	1.780
∞	1.193	1.293	1.385	1.470	1.549	1.623	1.692	1.757	1.818

P = .001

ν \ n	20	22	24	26	28	30	32	34	36
1	.9303	.9653	.9964	1.023	1.049	1.072	1.093	1.113	1.131
2	1.128	1.173	1.213	1.249	1.282	1.311	1.339	1.364	1.388
3	1.245	1.297	1.344	1.385	1.422	1.457	1.488	1.517	1.544
4	1.327	1.384	1.434	1.480	1.521	1.559	1.593	1.625	1.654
5	1.388	1.449	1.503	1.552	1.596	1.636	1.673	1.707	1.738
6	1.435	1.500	1.557	1.607	1.654	1.697	1.736	1.772	1.805
7	1.474	1.541	1.600	1.654	1.703	1.747	1.787	1.824	1.860
8	1.506	1.575	1.637	1.692	1.743	1.788	1.830	1.869	1.905
9	1.532	1.603	1.668	1.725	1.777	1.823	1.867	1.907	1.945
10	1.555	1.629	1.694	1.753	1.806	1.855	1.900	1.941	1.979
11	1.575	1.650	1.717	1.777	1.832	1.882	1.927	1.969	2.008
12	1.593	1.669	1.738	1.799	1.854	1.905	1.952	1.995	2.035
13	1.608	1.686	1.756	1.818	1.875	1.926	1.974	2.017	2.059
14	1.622	1.702	1.772	1.835	1.893	1.946	1.994	2.038	2.080
15	1.635	1.715	1.786	1.851	1.909	1.962	2.011	2.057	2.099
16	1.646	1.727	1.799	1.865	1.924	1.978	2.028	2.074	2.117
17	1.656	1.738	1.811	1.878	1.938	1.992	2.043	2.089	2.133
18	1.666	1.749	1.822	1.890	1.950	2.005	2.056	2.104	2.147
19	1.674	1.758	1.833	1.900	1.961	2.017	2.069	2.116	2.161
20	1.682	1.766	1.842	1.910	1.972	2.028	2.080	2.128	2.173
24	1.708	1.795	1.873	1.943	2.007	2.065	2.119	2.169	2.215
30	1.736	1.826	1.906	1.979	2.045	2.106	2.162	2.213	2.261
40	1.766	1.859	1.943	2.018	2.087	2.150	2.208	2.262	2.312
60	1.799	1.896	1.983	2.062	2.134	2.200	2.261	2.317	2.370
120	1.835	1.937	2.028	2.110	2.186	2.256	2.320	2.379	2.435
∞	1.876	1.982	2.078	2.165	2.246	2.320	2.388	2.452	2.512

ν \ n	38	40	50	60	70	80	90	100	
1	1.148	1.164	1.231	1.283	1.325	1.361	1.392	1.419	
2	1.409	1.430	1.515	1.582	1.636	1.682	1.722	1.756	
3	1.569	1.592	1.691	1.767	1.830	1.882	1.927	1.966	
4	1.682	1.707	1.815	1.899	1.968	2.025	2.074	2.117	
5	1.768	1.795	1.910	2.001	2.073	2.135	2.188	2.234	
6	1.836	1.865	1.987	2.082	2.159	2.224	2.279	2.328	
7	1.892	1.922	2.050	2.149	2.229	2.297	2.355	2.406	
8	1.939	1.971	2.102	2.205	2.289	2.359	2.420	2.472	
9	1.980	2.012	2.148	2.255	2.341	2.413	2.475	2.529	
10	2.014	2.048	2.188	2.297	2.386	2.460	2.524	2.580	
11	2.045	2.079	2.223	2.335	2.425	2.501	2.567	2.624	
12	2.072	2.107	2.254	2.368	2.461	2.539	2.605	2.664	
13	2.097	2.132	2.282	2.398	2.493	2.572	2.640	2.700	
14	2.119	2.155	2.307	2.425	2.521	2.602	2.671	2.732	
15	2.138	2.175	2.329	2.450	2.548	2.629	2.700	2.762	
16	2.157	2.194	2.350	2.472	2.572	2.655	2.726	2.789	
17	2.173	2.211	2.369	2.493	2.594	2.678	2.750	2.814	
18	2.188	2.226	2.387	2.512	2.614	2.699	2.773	2.837	
19	2.201	2.240	2.403	2.530	2.633	2.719	2.793	2.858	
20	2.215	2.254	2.418	2.546	2.650	2.737	2.812	2.878	
24	2.258	2.298	2.469	2.601	2.709	2.800	2.878	2.946	
30	2.306	2.348	2.525	2.663	2.776	2.870	2.951	3.022	
40	2.359	2.403	2.588	2.733	2.851	2.950	3.035	3.110	
60	2.419	2.465	2.660	2.813	2.938	3.043	3.133	3.212	
120	2.487	2.536	2.744	2.907	3.042	3.155	3.252	3.337	
∞	2.568	2.621	2.846	3.025	3.172	3.297	3.405	3.500	

P = .005

ν\n	2	3	4	5	6	7	8	9	10
1	.0111	.1351	.2975	.4363	.5482	.6391	.7145	.7782	.8331
2	.0100	.1350	.3141	.4761	.6109	.7224	.8158	.8954	.9641
3	.0096	.1349	.3217	.4955	.6427	.7660	.8701	.9592	1.036
4	.0094	.1349	.3261	.5071	.6624	.7935	.9049	1.000	1.083
5	.0093	.1349	.3290	.5149	.6758	.8126	.9293	1.029	1.118
6	.0093	.1349	.3310	.5205	.6856	.8266	.9474	1.051	1.143
7	.0092	.1348	.3325	.5247	.6930	.8374	.9614	1.068	1.163
8	.0092	.1348	.3336	.5280	.6989	.8460	.9727	1.083	1.179
9	.0091	.1348	.3346	.5306	.7036	.8529	.9819	1.094	1.193
10	.0091	.1348	.3353	.5328	.7075	.8587	.9895	1.103	1.203
11	.0091	.1348	.3359	.5346	.7109	.8636	.9960	1.112	1.213
12	.0091	.1348	.3365	.5361	.7137	.8678	1.001	1.118	1.221
13	.0090	.1348	.3369	.5375	.7161	.8714	1.006	1.124	1.228
14	.0090	.1348	.3373	.5386	.7182	.8746	1.010	1.130	1.235
15	.0090	.1348	.3376	.5396	.7201	.8774	1.014	1.134	1.240
16	.0090	.1348	.3379	.5405	.7217	.8799	1.017	1.138	1.245
17	.0090	.1348	.3382	.5413	.7232	.8821	1.020	1.142	1.250
18	.0090	.1348	.3384	.5420	.7245	.8841	1.023	1.146	1.254
19	.0090	.1348	.3387	.5426	.7257	.8859	1.025	1.149	1.257
20	.0090	.1348	.3389	.5432	.7267	.8875	1.028	1.152	1.261
24	.0090	.1348	.3395	.5451	.7302	.8928	1.035	1.161	1.272
30	.0089	.1348	.3401	.5470	.7338	.8982	1.043	1.170	1.283
40	.0089	.1348	.3407	.5489	.7374	.9038	1.050	1.180	1.295
60	.0089	.1348	.3414	.5508	.7412	.9096	1.058	1.190	1.308
120	.0089	.1348	.3420	.5528	.7450	.9156	1.066	1.201	1.321
∞	.0089	.1348	.3427	.5549	.7490	.9218	1.075	1.212	1.335

ν\n	11	12	13	14	15	16	17	18	19
1	.8810	.9234	.9613	.9955	1.026	1.054	1.081	1.105	1.127
2	1.024	1.077	1.125	1.168	1.207	1.243	1.276	1.307	1.335
3	1.104	1.164	1.218	1.267	1.311	1.352	1.390	1.424	1.456
4	1.157	1.222	1.280	1.333	1.381	1.426	1.466	1.504	1.539
5	1.195	1.263	1.326	1.382	1.433	1.479	1.523	1.563	1.600
6	1.223	1.296	1.360	1.418	1.472	1.522	1.567	1.608	1.647
7	1.246	1.321	1.388	1.448	1.504	1.555	1.601	1.645	1.685
8	1.264	1.341	1.410	1.472	1.530	1.582	1.630	1.675	1.717
9	1.280	1.358	1.428	1.493	1.551	1.604	1.654	1.700	1.743
10	1.293	1.372	1.444	1.510	1.569	1.624	1.675	1.722	1.766
11	1.304	1.384	1.457	1.524	1.585	1.641	1.693	1.740	1.785
12	1.313	1.395	1.469	1.537	1.599	1.655	1.708	1.757	1.802
13	1.321	1.404	1.480	1.548	1.610	1.668	1.722	1.771	1.817
14	1.329	1.412	1.489	1.558	1.621	1.680	1.734	1.784	1.830
15	1.335	1.419	1.497	1.567	1.631	1.690	1.744	1.795	1.842
16	1.341	1.426	1.504	1.575	1.639	1.699	1.754	1.805	1.853
17	1.346	1.432	1.511	1.582	1.647	1.707	1.763	1.814	1.863
18	1.351	1.437	1.517	1.588	1.654	1.715	1.771	1.823	1.872
19	1.355	1.442	1.522	1.594	1.660	1.722	1.779	1.831	1.880
20	1.359	1.447	1.527	1.600	1.666	1.728	1.785	1.838	1.888
24	1.371	1.461	1.543	1.617	1.686	1.749	1.807	1.861	1.912
30	1.385	1.477	1.560	1.636	1.706	1.771	1.831	1.887	1.939
40	1.399	1.493	1.578	1.656	1.728	1.794	1.856	1.913	1.967
60	1.413	1.509	1.597	1.677	1.751	1.820	1.883	1.943	1.998
120	1.429	1.528	1.617	1.700	1.776	1.847	1.912	1.974	2.032
∞	1.446	1.547	1.639	1.724	1.803	1.876	1.944	2.008	2.068

P = .005

ν\n	20	22	24	26	28	30	32	34	36
1	1.149	1.187	1.221	1.252	1.280	1.305	1.329	1.351	1.371
2	1.362	1.410	1.453	1.492	1.527	1.559	1.589	1.615	1.641
3	1.487	1.541	1.590	1.634	1.674	1.710	1.743	1.774	1.803
4	1.572	1.631	1.684	1.732	1.775	1.815	1.851	1.884	1.915
5	1.635	1.698	1.755	1.805	1.851	1.893	1.931	1.967	2.000
6	1.684	1.751	1.809	1.862	1.911	1.955	1.995	2.032	2.067
7	1.724	1.793	1.854	1.909	1.959	2.005	2.047	2.086	2.122
8	1.756	1.827	1.891	1.948	1.999	2.046	2.090	2.130	2.167
9	1.783	1.856	1.922	1.980	2.033	2.082	2.126	2.168	2.206
10	1.807	1.882	1.948	2.008	2.062	2.112	2.158	2.200	2.239
11	1.827	1.904	1.972	2.032	2.088	2.139	2.185	2.228	2.268
12	1.845	1.923	1.992	2.054	2.111	2.162	2.209	2.253	2.295
13	1.860	1.939	2.009	2.073	2.130	2.183	2.231	2.276	2.318
14	1.874	1.955	2.026	2.090	2.148	2.201	2.250	2.296	2.338
15	1.887	1.968	2.040	2.105	2.164	2.218	2.268	2.314	2.357
16	1.898	1.980	2.053	2.119	2.179	2.233	2.284	2.330	2.374
17	1.909	1.991	2.065	2.131	2.192	2.247	2.298	2.345	2.389
18	1.918	2.001	2.076	2.143	2.204	2.260	2.311	2.359	2.403
19	1.927	2.010	2.086	2.154	2.215	2.271	2.324	2.372	2.416
20	1.934	2.019	2.095	2.163	2.225	2.282	2.335	2.383	2.428
24	1.960	2.047	2.125	2.196	2.260	2.318	2.372	2.422	2.468
30	1.988	2.078	2.158	2.231	2.297	2.357	2.412	2.464	2.512
40	2.018	2.110	2.194	2.268	2.337	2.399	2.457	2.510	2.560
60	2.051	2.146	2.232	2.310	2.381	2.446	2.506	2.562	2.614
120	2.086	2.186	2.275	2.356	2.431	2.499	2.562	2.620	2.675
∞	2.125	2.229	2.323	2.408	2.487	2.559	2.625	2.688	2.746

ν\n	38	40	50	60	70	80	90	100	
1	1.390	1.407	1.482	1.540	1.588	1.628	1.663	1.693	
2	1.664	1.687	1.780	1.853	1.912	1.962	2.006	2.043	
3	1.829	1.854	1.960	2.042	2.109	2.166	2.215	2.257	
4	1.944	1.972	2.086	2.176	2.248	2.310	2.363	2.409	
5	2.031	2.060	2.182	2.277	2.354	2.419	2.476	2.525	
6	2.100	2.130	2.257	2.357	2.438	2.507	2.566	2.617	
7	2.155	2.187	2.320	2.423	2.508	2.579	2.640	2.694	
8	2.202	2.235	2.372	2.479	2.566	2.639	2.702	2.757	
9	2.242	2.275	2.416	2.526	2.616	2.691	2.756	2.813	
10	2.276	2.310	2.455	2.567	2.659	2.736	2.803	2.861	
11	2.306	2.341	2.489	2.604	2.698	2.776	2.844	2.904	
12	2.332	2.368	2.518	2.636	2.731	2.812	2.881	2.942	
13	2.356	2.393	2.545	2.664	2.762	2.844	2.914	2.975	
14	2.377	2.414	2.569	2.691	2.789	2.872	2.944	3.006	
15	2.397	2.434	2.591	2.714	2.814	2.898	2.971	3.034	
16	2.413	2.452	2.611	2.735	2.837	2.922	2.996	3.059	
17	2.430	2.468	2.629	2.755	2.857	2.944	3.018	3.083	
18	2.444	2.483	2.646	2.773	2.877	2.964	3.039	3.105	
19	2.458	2.497	2.661	2.790	2.895	2.983	3.058	3.125	
20	2.470	2.509	2.675	2.805	2.911	3.000	3.076	3.143	
24	2.511	2.552	2.723	2.857	2.966	3.058	3.137	3.206	
30	2.557	2.599	2.776	2.914	3.028	3.123	3.205	3.277	
40	2.607	2.651	2.835	2.979	3.097	3.197	3.282	3.357	
60	2.663	2.708	2.901	3.053	3.177	3.281	3.371	3.450	
120	2.726	2.774	2.978	3.139	3.270	3.381	3.477	3.562	
∞	2.800	2.851	3.070	3.243	3.385	3.506	3.611	3.703	

P = .01

ν\n	2	3	4	5	6	7	8	9	10
1	.0223	.1919	.3797	.5308	.6498	.7455	.8245	.8912	.9486
2	.0200	.1914	.3994	.5757	.7183	.8348	.9318	1.014	1.084
3	.0193	.1913	.4084	.5976	.7532	.8816	.9892	1.081	1.160
4	.0189	.1912	.4137	.6108	.7747	.9110	1.025	1.124	1.209
5	.0187	.1911	.4172	.6196	.7894	.9315	1.051	1.154	1.244
6	.0185	.1911	.4196	.6260	.8001	.9465	1.070	1.177	1.270
7	.0184	.1911	.4214	.6307	.8083	.9580	1.085	1.195	1.291
8	.0183	.1911	.4228	.6345	.8147	.9672	1.097	1.209	1.307
9	.0182	.1911	.4239	.6375	.8199	.9747	1.106	1.221	1.321
10	.0182	.1910	.4248	.6399	.8242	.9809	1.114	1.230	1.332
11	.0181	.1910	.4256	.6420	.8278	.9861	1.121	1.239	1.342
12	.0181	.1910	.4262	.6437	.8309	.9905	1.127	1.246	1.351
13	.0181	.1910	.4267	.6452	.8335	.9944	1.132	1.253	1.358
14	.0181	.1910	.4272	.6465	.8359	.9978	1.137	1.258	1.365
15	.0180	.1910	.4276	.6476	.8379	1.001	1.141	1.263	1.371
16	.0180	.1910	.4280	.6486	.8397	1.003	1.144	1.267	1.376
17	.0180	.1910	.4283	.6495	.8413	1.005	1.147	1.271	1.380
18	.0180	.1910	.4286	.6503	.8427	1.008	1.150	1.275	1.384
19	.0180	.1910	.4288	.6511	.8440	1.010	1.153	1.278	1.388
20	.0180	.1910	.4291	.6517	.8452	1.011	1.155	1.281	1.392
24	.0179	.1910	.4298	.6538	.8490	1.017	1.163	1.290	1.402
30	.0179	.1910	.4306	.6560	.8529	1.023	1.170	1.300	1.414
40	.0179	.1910	.4313	.6582	.8569	1.028	1.179	1.310	1.426
60	.0178	.1910	.4321	.6604	.8610	1.035	1.187	1.320	1.439
120	.0178	.1909	.4329	.6627	.8652	1.041	1.196	1.331	1.453
∞	.0177	.1909	.4337	.6650	.8695	1.048	1.205	1.343	1.467

ν\n	11	12	13	14	15	16	17	18	19
1	.9988	1.042	1.082	1.119	1.151	1.181	1.209	1.234	1.258
2	1.147	1.202	1.251	1.296	1.337	1.374	1.408	1.440	1.469
3	1.229	1.291	1.347	1.397	1.442	1.484	1.523	1.559	1.592
4	1.284	1.351	1.410	1.464	1.513	1.559	1.600	1.639	1.674
5	1.323	1.393	1.456	1.513	1.565	1.613	1.657	1.698	1.736
6	1.352	1.425	1.491	1.551	1.605	1.655	1.700	1.743	1.783
7	1.376	1.451	1.519	1.580	1.636	1.688	1.736	1.780	1.821
8	1.395	1.472	1.541	1.605	1.662	1.715	1.765	1.810	1.852
9	1.410	1.489	1.560	1.625	1.684	1.738	1.789	1.835	1.878
10	1.423	1.503	1.576	1.642	1.702	1.758	1.809	1.856	1.900
11	1.433	1.515	1.590	1.656	1.718	1.774	1.826	1.875	1.920
12	1.443	1.526	1.601	1.669	1.731	1.789	1.842	1.891	1.936
13	1.452	1.536	1.612	1.680	1.743	1.801	1.855	1.905	1.951
14	1.459	1.544	1.620	1.690	1.754	1.813	1.867	1.917	1.965
15	1.466	1.551	1.628	1.699	1.764	1.823	1.878	1.929	1.977
16	1.472	1.558	1.636	1.707	1.772	1.832	1.887	1.939	1.987
17	1.477	1.564	1.643	1.714	1.780	1.840	1.896	1.948	1.997
18	1.482	1.569	1.648	1.720	1.787	1.848	1.904	1.957	2.005
19	1.486	1.574	1.654	1.726	1.793	1.854	1.911	1.964	2.013
20	1.490	1.579	1.659	1.732	1.799	1.861	1.918	1.971	2.021
24	1.503	1.594	1.675	1.749	1.818	1.881	1.939	1.994	2.045
30	1.516	1.609	1.692	1.768	1.838	1.903	1.963	2.019	2.071
40	1.531	1.625	1.710	1.788	1.860	1.926	1.988	2.045	2.099
60	1.545	1.642	1.729	1.809	1.883	1.951	2.014	2.073	2.128
120	1.561	1.660	1.749	1.831	1.907	1.978	2.043	2.104	2.161
∞	1.578	1.679	1.771	1.856	1.934	2.007	2.074	2.137	2.197

P = .01

ν\n	20	22	24	26	28	30	32	34	36
1	1.280	1.321	1.357	1.390	1.419	1.446	1.471	1.494	1.516
2	1.497	1.547	1.592	1.632	1.669	1.702	1.733	1.761	1.788
3	1.623	1.679	1.730	1.775	1.816	1.853	1.888	1.920	1.950
4	1.708	1.770	1.824	1.872	1.917	1.958	1.995	2.029	2.061
5	1.772	1.836	1.893	1.946	1.993	2.035	2.075	2.111	2.145
6	1.820	1.887	1.948	2.002	2.051	2.096	2.138	2.176	2.211
7	1.859	1.929	1.992	2.048	2.099	2.146	2.188	2.228	2.264
8	1.891	1.964	2.028	2.086	2.138	2.187	2.230	2.271	2.309
9	1.919	1.993	2.059	2.118	2.172	2.221	2.266	2.308	2.347
10	1.942	2.017	2.085	2.145	2.201	2.251	2.297	2.340	2.380
11	1.962	2.038	2.107	2.169	2.225	2.277	2.324	2.368	2.408
12	1.979	2.058	2.127	2.190	2.247	2.299	2.347	2.392	2.433
13	1.995	2.074	2.145	2.209	2.267	2.319	2.369	2.413	2.455
14	2.009	2.089	2.161	2.225	2.284	2.338	2.387	2.432	2.475
15	2.021	2.102	2.175	2.240	2.300	2.354	2.404	2.450	2.493
16	2.032	2.114	2.188	2.254	2.313	2.369	2.419	2.466	2.509
17	2.042	2.125	2.199	2.266	2.326	2.382	2.433	2.480	2.524
18	2.051	2.135	2.210	2.277	2.338	2.395	2.446	2.494	2.538
19	2.060	2.144	2.219	2.287	2.349	2.405	2.458	2.505	2.551
20	2.067	2.152	2.228	2.297	2.359	2.416	2.468	2.517	2.562
24	2.093	2.180	2.258	2.328	2.392	2.450	2.505	2.554	2.601
30	2.120	2.209	2.290	2.362	2.427	2.488	2.543	2.595	2.643
40	2.149	2.241	2.323	2.398	2.466	2.528	2.586	2.640	2.689
60	2.181	2.276	2.361	2.439	2.509	2.574	2.633	2.689	2.740
120	2.215	2.313	2.402	2.483	2.556	2.623	2.686	2.744	2.798
∞	2.253	2.356	2.448	2.532	2.610	2.681	2.746	2.807	2.864

ν\n	38	40	50	60	70	80	90	100	
1	1.536	1.554	1.634	1.696	1.747	1.790	1.827	1.860	
2	1.812	1.836	1.933	2.010	2.072	2.125	2.171	2.211	
3	1.977	2.003	2.113	2.198	2.269	2.327	2.379	2.423	
4	2.091	2.119	2.238	2.330	2.406	2.470	2.524	2.573	
5	2.177	2.207	2.332	2.430	2.510	2.577	2.635	2.686	
6	2.244	2.276	2.406	2.509	2.592	2.663	2.723	2.776	
7	2.299	2.331	2.467	2.573	2.660	2.732	2.796	2.850	
8	2.345	2.378	2.518	2.627	2.716	2.792	2.856	2.913	
9	2.383	2.417	2.561	2.673	2.765	2.842	2.908	2.966	
10	2.417	2.452	2.598	2.713	2.807	2.886	2.953	3.013	
11	2.446	2.482	2.631	2.748	2.843	2.924	2.993	3.054	
12	2.472	2.508	2.660	2.779	2.876	2.958	3.028	3.090	
13	2.494	2.531	2.686	2.807	2.906	2.989	3.060	3.123	
14	2.515	2.552	2.709	2.832	2.932	3.016	3.089	3.152	
15	2.533	2.571	2.730	2.854	2.956	3.041	3.115	3.179	
16	2.550	2.589	2.749	2.875	2.978	3.064	3.138	3.203	
17	2.566	2.604	2.767	2.894	2.997	3.085	3.160	3.226	
18	2.580	2.618	2.783	2.911	3.016	3.104	3.180	3.246	
19	2.593	2.632	2.797	2.927	3.032	3.122	3.198	3.265	
20	2.605	2.644	2.811	2.941	3.048	3.138	3.215	3.283	
24	2.644	2.685	2.857	2.992	3.101	3.194	3.273	3.343	
30	2.688	2.729	2.907	3.046	3.159	3.255	3.337	3.410	
40	2.736	2.779	2.963	3.107	3.225	3.324	3.410	3.485	
60	2.789	2.834	3.026	3.177	3.300	3.404	3.494	3.572	
120	2.849	2.896	3.098	3.257	3.387	3.498	3.593	3.676	
∞	2.918	2.969	3.183	3.354	3.494	3.613	3.716	3.807	

$P = .025$

$\nu \backslash n$	2	3	4	5	6	7	8	9	10
1	.0556	.3070	.5313	.7002	.8301	.9339	1.019	1.091	1.153
2	.0501	.3050	.5537	.7493	.9029	1.026	1.129	1.216	1.291
3	.0481	.3044	.5644	.7737	.9404	1.076	1.189	1.284	1.367
4	.0472	.3040	.5707	.7885	.9636	1.107	1.226	1.328	1.416
5	.0466	.3038	.5748	.7984	.9795	1.128	1.253	1.359	1.451
6	.0463	.3037	.5777	.8056	.9910	1.144	1.272	1.382	1.478
7	.0460	.3036	.5799	.8109	1.000	1.156	1.287	1.401	1.499
8	.0458	.3035	.5815	.8152	1.006	1.166	1.300	1.415	1.515
9	.0456	.3034	.5829	.8185	1.012	1.173	1.310	1.427	1.529
10	.0455	.3034	.5840	.8213	1.017	1.180	1.318	1.437	1.540
11	.0454	.3034	.5849	.8236	1.021	1.185	1.325	1.445	1.550
12	.0453	.3033	.5856	.8256	1.024	1.190	1.331	1.452	1.559
13	.0452	.3033	.5863	.8273	1.027	1.194	1.336	1.458	1.566
14	.0451	.3033	.5868	.8288	1.029	1.198	1.341	1.464	1.572
15	.0451	.3033	.5873	.8300	1.031	1.201	1.345	1.469	1.578
16	.0450	.3033	.5877	.8312	1.033	1.203	1.348	1.473	1.583
17	.0450	.3032	.5881	.8322	1.035	1.206	1.352	1.477	1.588
18	.0450	.3032	.5885	.8331	1.037	1.208	1.354	1.481	1.592
19	.0449	.3032	.5888	.8339	1.038	1.210	1.357	1.484	1.596
20	.0449	.3032	.5891	.8347	1.039	1.212	1.359	1.487	1.599
24	.0448	.3032	.5900	.8370	1.044	1.218	1.367	1.497	1.610
30	.0447	.3031	.5909	.8395	1.048	1.224	1.375	1.506	1.621
40	.0446	.3031	.5918	.8419	1.052	1.230	1.383	1.516	1.633
60	.0445	.3031	.5927	.8445	1.057	1.237	1.392	1.527	1.646
120	.0444	.3030	.5937	.8470	1.061	1.243	1.401	1.538	1.659
∞	.0443	.3031	.5946	.8497	1.066	1.251	1.410	1.550	1.674

$\nu \backslash n$	11	12	13	14	15	16	17	18	19
1	1.208	1.256	1.299	1.338	1.374	1.407	1.437	1.465	1.491
2	1.356	1.415	1.467	1.514	1.557	1.597	1.633	1.667	1.698
3	1.439	1.504	1.562	1.614	1.662	1.706	1.746	1.784	1.818
4	1.494	1.563	1.625	1.681	1.732	1.779	1.822	1.862	1.899
5	1.533	1.605	1.670	1.729	1.782	1.831	1.877	1.919	1.959
6	1.562	1.637	1.704	1.765	1.821	1.872	1.919	1.963	2.004
7	1.585	1.662	1.732	1.795	1.852	1.904	1.953	1.998	2.040
8	1.604	1.682	1.754	1.818	1.877	1.931	1.981	2.027	2.070
9	1.619	1.699	1.772	1.837	1.897	1.953	2.004	2.051	2.095
10	1.632	1.714	1.787	1.854	1.915	1.971	2.023	2.071	2.116
11	1.643	1.726	1.801	1.868	1.930	1.987	2.040	2.089	2.135
12	1.652	1.736	1.811	1.880	1.943	2.001	2.054	2.104	2.151
13	1.660	1.745	1.822	1.891	1.955	2.013	2.067	2.118	2.165
14	1.668	1.754	1.831	1.901	1.965	2.024	2.079	2.130	2.177
15	1.674	1.761	1.838	1.909	1.974	2.034	2.089	2.140	2.188
16	1.680	1.767	1.845	1.917	1.982	2.042	2.098	2.150	2.198
17	1.685	1.773	1.852	1.924	1.990	2.050	2.106	2.159	2.207
18	1.690	1.778	1.857	1.930	1.997	2.057	2.114	2.167	2.216
19	1.694	1.783	1.863	1.936	2.002	2.064	2.121	2.174	2.223
20	1.698	1.787	1.868	1.941	2.008	2.070	2.127	2.181	2.230
24	1.711	1.801	1.883	1.958	2.026	2.090	2.148	2.202	2.253
30	1.724	1.816	1.900	1.976	2.046	2.110	2.170	2.225	2.277
40	1.738	1.832	1.917	1.995	2.066	2.132	2.193	2.250	2.303
60	1.753	1.848	1.935	2.015	2.088	2.155	2.218	2.276	2.331
120	1.768	1.866	1.955	2.036	2.111	2.180	2.245	2.305	2.361
∞	1.784	1.884	1.976	2.059	2.136	2.207	2.274	2.336	2.394

P = .025

ν\n	20	22	24	26	28	30	32	34	36
1	1.515	1.560	1.600	1.635	1.668	1.698	1.725	1.751	1.775
2	1.728	1.782	1.830	1.873	1.912	1.947	1.981	2.011	2.040
3	1.851	1.911	1.963	2.011	2.055	2.094	2.131	2.165	2.196
4	1.934	1.998	2.054	2.106	2.152	2.195	2.234	2.270	2.304
5	1.995	2.062	2.122	2.176	2.224	2.269	2.310	2.348	2.384
6	2.042	2.112	2.174	2.230	2.280	2.327	2.370	2.409	2.446
7	2.080	2.152	2.215	2.273	2.326	2.374	2.418	2.459	2.497
8	2.111	2.184	2.250	2.309	2.363	2.412	2.458	2.500	2.539
9	2.136	2.211	2.279	2.340	2.395	2.445	2.491	2.534	2.574
10	2.159	2.235	2.304	2.365	2.421	2.473	2.520	2.564	2.605
11	2.177	2.255	2.325	2.388	2.445	2.497	2.545	2.590	2.631
12	2.194	2.273	2.344	2.407	2.465	2.518	2.567	2.612	2.654
13	2.208	2.289	2.360	2.425	2.483	2.537	2.587	2.632	2.675
14	2.221	2.302	2.375	2.440	2.499	2.554	2.604	2.650	2.693
15	2.233	2.315	2.388	2.454	2.514	2.569	2.620	2.666	2.710
16	2.243	2.326	2.400	2.466	2.527	2.583	2.634	2.681	2.725
17	2.253	2.336	2.410	2.478	2.539	2.595	2.647	2.694	2.739
18	2.261	2.346	2.421	2.488	2.550	2.606	2.658	2.706	2.751
19	2.269	2.354	2.430	2.498	2.560	2.617	2.669	2.718	2.763
20	2.277	2.362	2.438	2.507	2.569	2.626	2.679	2.728	2.774
24	2.301	2.388	2.465	2.536	2.600	2.658	2.712	2.762	2.809
30	2.326	2.415	2.495	2.567	2.632	2.693	2.748	2.800	2.847
40	2.353	2.444	2.526	2.601	2.668	2.730	2.787	2.840	2.889
60	2.382	2.476	2.561	2.637	2.707	2.771	2.829	2.885	2.935
120	2.414	2.511	2.598	2.677	2.749	2.816	2.877	2.934	2.987
∞	2.449	2.549	2.640	2.722	2.798	2.867	2.931	2.991	3.046

ν\n	38	40	50	60	70	80	90	100	
1	1.798	1.818	1.906	1.976	2.033	2.082	2.123	2.160	
2	2.066	2.092	2.197	2.280	2.348	2.405	2.455	2.499	
3	2.226	2.253	2.370	2.462	2.537	2.600	2.655	2.702	
4	2.335	2.365	2.490	2.587	2.668	2.735	2.794	2.845	
5	2.416	2.448	2.579	2.682	2.766	2.837	2.898	2.952	
6	2.481	2.513	2.649	2.756	2.843	2.917	2.981	3.036	
7	2.532	2.566	2.706	2.816	2.907	2.983	3.048	3.106	
8	2.575	2.609	2.754	2.867	2.959	3.037	3.104	3.164	
9	2.611	2.646	2.794	2.910	3.004	3.084	3.153	3.214	
10	2.642	2.678	2.829	2.947	3.043	3.125	3.195	3.257	
11	2.670	2.706	2.859	2.979	3.078	3.160	3.232	3.294	
12	2.693	2.730	2.886	3.008	3.108	3.192	3.264	3.328	
13	2.715	2.752	2.910	3.033	3.134	3.220	3.293	3.358	
14	2.734	2.772	2.931	3.056	3.159	3.245	3.319	3.385	
15	2.751	2.789	2.950	3.077	3.181	3.268	3.343	3.409	
16	2.766	2.805	2.968	3.096	3.200	3.289	3.365	3.431	
17	2.780	2.819	2.984	3.113	3.219	3.308	3.384	3.451	
18	2.793	2.833	2.999	3.129	3.235	3.325	3.402	3.470	
19	2.805	2.845	3.012	3.143	3.251	3.341	3.419	3.488	
20	2.816	2.856	3.024	3.157	3.265	3.356	3.435	3.503	
24	2.852	2.894	3.066	3.202	3.313	3.406	3.487	3.558	
30	2.892	2.934	3.112	3.251	3.365	3.462	3.545	3.618	
40	2.935	2.979	3.162	3.306	3.424	3.523	3.610	3.685	
60	2.983	3.028	3.218	3.368	3.491	3.594	3.684	3.762	
120	3.037	3.084	3.282	3.438	3.567	3.676	3.770	3.853	
∞	3.098	3.148	3.357	3.523	3.660	3.776	3.876	3.965	

P = .05

ν\n	2	3	4	5	6	7	8	9	10
1	.1113	.4428	.6978	.8828	1.024	1.136	1.228	1.307	1.374
2	.1001	.4370	.7181	.9291	1.092	1.223	1.331	1.423	1.501
3	.0963	.4351	.7285	.9531	1.128	1.270	1.388	1.487	1.574
4	.0944	.4342	.7348	.9679	1.151	1.300	1.423	1.529	1.620
5	.0933	.4336	.7389	.9778	1.167	1.321	1.449	1.558	1.654
6	.0925	.4333	.7419	.9850	1.178	1.336	1.468	1.581	1.678
7	.0920	.4330	.7441	.9905	1.187	1.348	1.483	1.598	1.698
8	.0916	.4328	.7459	.9948	1.194	1.357	1.494	1.612	1.714
9	.0912	.4326	.7472	.9982	1.200	1.365	1.504	1.623	1.727
10	.0909	.4325	.7484	1.001	1.204	1.371	1.512	1.633	1.738
11	.0907	.4324	.7493	1.003	1.208	1.377	1.519	1.640	1.747
12	.0906	.4323	.7501	1.005	1.211	1.381	1.525	1.647	1.755
13	.0904	.4323	.7508	1.007	1.214	1.385	1.530	1.653	1.762
14	.0903	.4322	.7513	1.008	1.216	1.389	1.534	1.659	1.768
15	.0902	.4321	.7519	1.010	1.218	1.392	1.538	1.663	1.773
16	.0901	.4321	.7523	1.011	1.220	1.394	1.541	1.667	1.778
17	.0900	.4321	.7527	1.012	1.222	1.397	1.544	1.671	1.782
18	.0899	.4320	.7531	1.013	1.224	1.399	1.547	1.674	1.786
19	.0899	.4320	.7534	1.013	1.225	1.401	1.550	1.678	1.790
20	.0898	.4320	.7537	1.015	1.227	1.403	1.552	1.680	1.793
24	.0896	.4319	.7546	1.017	1.231	1.409	1.559	1.689	1.803
30	.0894	.4318	.7556	1.019	1.235	1.414	1.567	1.699	1.814
40	.0893	.4317	.7565	1.022	1.239	1.420	1.575	1.708	1.825
60	.0891	.4316	.7575	1.024	1.244	1.427	1.583	1.718	1.837
120	.0889	.4315	.7585	1.027	1.248	1.433	1.592	1.729	1.850
∞	.0887	.4314	.7595	1.030	1.253	1.440	1.600	1.740	1.863

ν\n	11	12	13	14	15	16	17	18	19
1	1.434	1.486	1.534	1.577	1.616	1.651	1.685	1.716	1.744
2	1.571	1.633	1.688	1.738	1.784	1.826	1.865	1.901	1.934
3	1.649	1.716	1.777	1.831	1.881	1.927	1.970	2.009	2.045
4	1.700	1.772	1.835	1.894	1.946	1.995	2.040	2.082	2.120
5	1.737	1.811	1.878	1.938	1.994	2.044	2.091	2.134	2.175
6	1.765	1.841	1.910	1.973	2.029	2.082	2.131	2.176	2.217
7	1.786	1.865	1.936	2.000	2.058	2.112	2.162	2.208	2.251
8	1.804	1.884	1.956	2.021	2.081	2.136	2.187	2.234	2.278
9	1.818	1.900	1.973	2.040	2.101	2.157	2.208	2.256	2.301
10	1.830	1.913	1.988	2.055	2.117	2.174	2.226	2.275	2.321
11	1.840	1.924	2.000	2.068	2.131	2.189	2.242	2.291	2.338
12	1.849	1.934	2.010	2.079	2.143	2.201	2.255	2.305	2.352
13	1.857	1.943	2.019	2.090	2.153	2.212	2.267	2.318	2.365
14	1.864	1.950	2.028	2.098	2.163	2.222	2.277	2.329	2.376
15	1.870	1.957	2.035	2.106	2.171	2.231	2.287	2.339	2.387
16	1.875	1.963	2.042	2.113	2.179	2.239	2.295	2.347	2.396
17	1.880	1.968	2.047	2.120	2.186	2.246	2.303	2.355	2.404
18	1.885	1.973	2.053	2.125	2.192	2.253	2.310	2.362	2.411
19	1.889	1.978	2.057	2.131	2.198	2.259	2.316	2.369	2.418
20	1.893	1.982	2.062	2.135	2.202	2.264	2.322	2.375	2.425
24	1.904	1.995	2.077	2.151	2.219	2.282	2.340	2.395	2.445
30	1.917	2.009	2.092	2.167	2.237	2.301	2.360	2.416	2.467
40	1.930	2.023	2.108	2.185	2.256	2.321	2.382	2.438	2.491
60	1.943	2.038	2.124	2.203	2.275	2.342	2.404	2.462	2.516
120	1.957	2.054	2.142	2.223	2.296	2.365	2.428	2.487	2.543
∞	1.973	2.071	2.161	2.243	2.319	2.389	2.454	2.515	2.572

P = .05

ν\n	20	22	24	26	28	30	32	34	36
1	1.771	1.821	1.865	1.904	1.941	1.974	2.004	2.033	2.059
2	1.966	2.023	2.074	2.121	2.163	2.201	2.237	2.270	2.300
3	2.080	2.142	2.198	2.248	2.294	2.336	2.375	2.411	2.444
4	2.157	2.223	2.283	2.336	2.385	2.429	2.470	2.508	2.543
5	2.213	2.283	2.344	2.400	2.451	2.497	2.540	2.580	2.617
6	2.257	2.328	2.393	2.450	2.502	2.550	2.595	2.635	2.674
7	2.291	2.365	2.430	2.490	2.544	2.593	2.639	2.681	2.720
8	2.320	2.395	2.462	2.523	2.578	2.628	2.675	2.718	2.758
9	2.343	2.420	2.489	2.550	2.607	2.658	2.705	2.749	2.791
10	2.364	2.441	2.511	2.574	2.631	2.683	2.731	2.776	2.818
11	2.381	2.460	2.531	2.595	2.652	2.705	2.754	2.800	2.842
12	2.396	2.476	2.547	2.612	2.671	2.725	2.774	2.820	2.863
13	2.409	2.490	2.563	2.628	2.687	2.742	2.792	2.838	2.881
14	2.421	2.503	2.576	2.642	2.702	2.757	2.807	2.854	2.898
15	2.432	2.514	2.588	2.654	2.715	2.770	2.821	2.869	2.913
16	2.441	2.524	2.599	2.666	2.727	2.783	2.834	2.882	2.927
17	2.450	2.534	2.608	2.676	2.738	2.794	2.846	2.894	2.939
18	2.457	2.542	2.617	2.685	2.747	2.804	2.856	2.905	2.950
19	2.465	2.550	2.625	2.694	2.756	2.813	2.866	2.915	2.960
20	2.471	2.557	2.633	2.702	2.765	2.822	2.875	2.924	2.970
24	2.493	2.580	2.658	2.728	2.792	2.850	2.904	2.955	3.002
30	2.516	2.604	2.684	2.756	2.821	2.881	2.936	2.988	3.036
40	2.540	2.631	2.712	2.786	2.853	2.914	2.971	3.023	3.073
60	2.566	2.659	2.743	2.818	2.887	2.950	3.009	3.063	3.113
120	2.595	2.690	2.776	2.854	2.925	2.990	3.050	3.106	3.158
∞	2.626	2.724	2.813	2.893	2.967	3.034	3.097	3.155	3.210

ν\n	38	40	50	60	70	80	90	100	
1	2.084	2.107	2.206	2.284	2.348	2.402	2.449	2.490	
2	2.329	2.356	2.471	2.560	2.634	2.697	2.751	2.798	
3	2.476	2.505	2.629	2.727	2.807	2.875	2.933	2.985	
4	2.577	2.607	2.739	2.842	2.927	2.999	3.061	3.115	
5	2.651	2.684	2.821	2.929	3.017	3.092	3.156	3.213	
6	2.710	2.743	2.885	2.996	3.088	3.165	3.231	3.290	
7	2.757	2.791	2.937	3.051	3.145	3.224	3.293	3.353	
8	2.796	2.831	2.980	3.097	3.193	3.274	3.344	3.405	
9	2.828	2.865	3.016	3.136	3.233	3.316	3.387	3.450	
10	2.857	2.894	3.048	3.169	3.269	3.352	3.425	3.488	
11	2.881	2.919	3.075	3.198	3.299	3.384	3.458	3.522	
12	2.903	2.941	3.099	3.224	3.326	3.412	3.487	3.552	
13	2.922	2.960	3.121	3.247	3.350	3.437	3.513	3.579	
14	2.939	2.978	3.140	3.267	3.372	3.460	3.536	3.603	
15	2.954	2.993	3.157	3.286	3.391	3.480	3.557	3.625	
16	2.968	3.007	3.173	3.302	3.409	3.499	3.576	3.644	
17	2.981	3.020	3.187	3.318	3.425	3.516	3.594	3.663	
18	2.993	3.032	3.200	3.332	3.440	3.531	3.610	3.679	
19	3.003	3.043	3.212	3.345	3.454	3.545	3.625	3.695	
20	3.013	3.053	3.223	3.357	3.466	3.559	3.639	3.709	
24	3.045	3.086	3.260	3.396	3.509	3.603	3.685	3.756	
30	3.080	3.122	3.300	3.440	3.555	3.652	3.735	3.809	
40	3.119	3.162	3.344	3.488	3.606	3.706	3.792	3.868	
60	3.161	3.205	3.394	3.542	3.664	3.767	3.856	3.934	
120	3.208	3.253	3.449	3.603	3.730	3.838	3.931	4.012	
∞	3.261	3.309	3.513	3.675	3.809	3.922	4.021	4.107	

P = .10

ν\n	2	3	4	5	6	7	8	9	10
1	.2240	.6526	.9446	1.152	1.309	1.435	1.539	1.627	1.704
2	.2010	.6351	.9504	1.179	1.355	1.495	1.611	1.710	1.795
3	.1932	.6294	.9564	1.197	1.383	1.532	1.656	1.761	1.852
4	.1893	.6266	.9606	1.209	1.401	1.557	1.686	1.796	1.891
5	.1870	.6249	.9635	1.217	1.414	1.574	1.707	1.820	1.918
6	.1854	.6238	.9657	1.223	1.424	1.587	1.723	1.839	1.939
7	.1843	.6230	.9673	1.227	1.431	1.597	1.735	1.853	1.956
8	.1835	.6224	.9686	1.231	1.437	1.605	1.745	1.864	1.969
9	.1829	.6220	.9697	1.234	1.442	1.611	1.753	1.874	1.980
10	.1823	.6216	.9705	1.236	1.446	1.617	1.760	1.882	1.989
11	.1819	.6213	.9712	1.238	1.449	1.621	1.766	1.889	1.997
12	.1816	.6211	.9719	1.240	1.452	1.625	1.771	1.895	2.003
13	.1813	.6208	.9724	1.241	1.454	1.628	1.775	1.900	2.009
14	.1810	.6207	.9728	1.242	1.456	1.631	1.779	1.904	2.014
15	.1808	.6205	.9732	1.244	1.458	1.634	1.782	1.908	2.019
16	.1806	.6204	.9736	1.245	1.460	1.636	1.785	1.912	2.023
17	.1805	.6202	.9739	1.245	1.461	1.638	1.788	1.915	2.026
18	.1803	.6201	.9742	1.246	1.463	1.640	1.790	1.918	2.029
19	.1802	.6200	.9745	1.247	1.464	1.642	1.792	1.920	2.032
20	.1800	.6200	.9747	1.248	1.465	1.644	1.794	1.923	2.036
24	.1797	.6197	.9754	1.250	1.469	1.649	1.800	1.931	2.044
30	.1793	.6194	.9762	1.252	1.473	1.654	1.806	1.938	2.053
40	.1789	.6191	.9769	1.254	1.476	1.659	1.814	1.947	2.063
60	.1785	.6189	.9777	1.257	1.480	1.665	1.821	1.955	2.073
120	.1782	.6186	.9785	1.259	1.484	1.670	1.828	1.964	2.083
∞	.1777	.6184	.9794	1.261	1.488	1.676	1.835	1.973	2.094

ν\n	11	12	13	14	15	16	17	18	19
1	1.771	1.831	1.884	1.933	1.978	2.018	2.057	2.092	2.125
2	1.870	1.937	1.997	2.051	2.101	2.147	2.189	2.229	2.265
3	1.933	2.004	2.068	2.126	2.179	2.228	2.273	2.315	2.354
4	1.975	2.049	2.116	2.177	2.232	2.283	2.331	2.375	2.416
5	2.005	2.082	2.151	2.214	2.271	2.324	2.373	2.419	2.461
6	2.028	2.107	2.178	2.242	2.301	2.355	2.405	2.452	2.496
7	2.046	2.126	2.199	2.265	2.325	2.380	2.431	2.479	2.523
8	2.060	2.142	2.216	2.283	2.344	2.401	2.452	2.501	2.546
9	2.072	2.156	2.230	2.298	2.360	2.417	2.470	2.519	2.565
10	2.082	2.167	2.242	2.311	2.374	2.431	2.485	2.535	2.582
11	2.091	2.176	2.252	2.322	2.386	2.444	2.498	2.548	2.595
12	2.099	2.185	2.261	2.331	2.396	2.454	2.509	2.560	2.607
13	2.105	2.192	2.269	2.340	2.404	2.463	2.519	2.570	2.618
14	2.111	2.198	2.276	2.347	2.412	2.472	2.527	2.579	2.627
15	2.116	2.203	2.282	2.353	2.419	2.479	2.535	2.587	2.635
16	2.120	2.209	2.287	2.359	2.425	2.485	2.542	2.595	2.643
17	2.125	2.213	2.292	2.365	2.431	2.491	2.548	2.601	2.650
18	2.128	2.217	2.296	2.369	2.436	2.497	2.554	2.607	2.656
19	2.132	2.221	2.300	2.374	2.440	2.502	2.559	2.612	2.661
20	2.135	2.224	2.304	2.378	2.445	2.506	2.564	2.617	2.667
24	2.145	2.235	2.317	2.391	2.459	2.522	2.580	2.634	2.684
30	2.155	2.247	2.329	2.404	2.473	2.537	2.596	2.651	2.702
40	2.166	2.259	2.343	2.419	2.489	2.553	2.613	2.669	2.721
60	2.178	2.272	2.356	2.434	2.505	2.571	2.632	2.689	2.742
120	2.190	2.285	2.371	2.450	2.522	2.589	2.651	2.709	2.764
∞	2.202	2.299	2.387	2.467	2.541	2.609	2.673	2.732	2.787

P = .10

ν\n	20	22	24	26	28	30	32	34	36
1	2.156	2.212	2.263	2.309	2.351	2.389	2.425	2.458	2.488
2	2.300	2.363	2.419	2.470	2.516	2.559	2.598	2.634	2.668
3	2.391	2.458	2.518	2.573	2.622	2.667	2.709	2.748	2.784
4	2.454	2.524	2.587	2.644	2.695	2.743	2.786	2.827	2.864
5	2.501	2.573	2.638	2.697	2.750	2.799	2.844	2.886	2.925
6	2.536	2.611	2.677	2.738	2.793	2.843	2.889	2.932	2.972
7	2.565	2.641	2.709	2.771	2.827	2.878	2.925	2.969	3.010
8	2.589	2.666	2.735	2.798	2.855	2.907	2.955	3.000	3.041
9	2.608	2.687	2.757	2.821	2.878	2.931	2.980	3.026	3.068
10	2.625	2.704	2.776	2.840	2.898	2.952	3.002	3.048	3.090
11	2.639	2.720	2.792	2.857	2.916	2.970	3.020	3.067	3.110
12	2.651	2.733	2.806	2.871	2.931	2.986	3.037	3.083	3.127
13	2.662	2.745	2.818	2.884	2.945	3.000	3.051	3.098	3.143
14	2.672	2.755	2.829	2.896	2.957	3.013	3.064	3.112	3.156
15	2.681	2.764	2.839	2.906	2.968	3.024	3.075	3.124	3.169
16	2.689	2.773	2.847	2.915	2.977	3.034	3.086	3.134	3.180
17	2.696	2.780	2.855	2.924	2.986	3.043	3.095	3.144	3.190
18	2.702	2.787	2.863	2.931	2.994	3.051	3.104	3.153	3.199
19	2.708	2.794	2.870	2.938	3.001	3.058	3.112	3.161	3.207
20	2.714	2.799	2.876	2.945	3.008	3.066	3.119	3.169	3.215
24	2.732	2.818	2.896	2.966	3.030	3.089	3.143	3.194	3.241
30	2.750	2.839	2.918	2.989	3.054	3.114	3.169	3.220	3.268
40	2.770	2.860	2.940	3.013	3.080	3.141	3.197	3.249	3.298
60	2.792	2.883	2.965	3.040	3.107	3.170	3.227	3.281	3.331
120	2.815	2.908	2.992	3.068	3.138	3.201	3.261	3.315	3.367
∞	2.840	2.935	3.021	3.100	3.171	3.237	3.298	3.354	3.407

ν\n	38	40	50	60	70	80	90	100	
1	2.517	2.544	2.658	2.749	2.824	2.887	2.942	2.990	
2	2.700	2.730	2.856	2.956	3.038	3.108	3.168	3.221	
3	2.818	2.849	2.984	3.090	3.178	3.251	3.315	3.372	
4	2.900	2.933	3.074	3.185	3.276	3.353	3.419	3.478	
5	2.961	2.996	3.141	3.255	3.349	3.429	3.498	3.558	
6	3.010	3.045	3.194	3.311	3.407	3.489	3.560	3.622	
7	3.048	3.084	3.237	3.356	3.455	3.538	3.610	3.674	
8	3.080	3.117	3.272	3.394	3.494	3.579	3.652	3.717	
9	3.107	3.145	3.302	3.426	3.528	3.614	3.688	3.753	
10	3.131	3.168	3.328	3.453	3.556	3.644	3.719	3.785	
11	3.151	3.189	3.350	3.477	3.582	3.670	3.746	3.813	
12	3.169	3.207	3.370	3.498	3.603	3.692	3.770	3.837	
13	3.184	3.223	3.388	3.517	3.623	3.713	3.791	3.859	
14	3.198	3.237	3.403	3.534	3.641	3.732	3.810	3.879	
15	3.211	3.250	3.417	3.549	3.657	3.748	3.827	3.896	
16	3.222	3.262	3.430	3.562	3.671	3.763	3.843	3.913	
17	3.232	3.272	3.442	3.575	3.684	3.777	3.857	3.927	
18	3.241	3.282	3.452	3.586	3.696	3.790	3.870	3.941	
19	3.250	3.291	3.462	3.597	3.707	3.801	3.882	3.953	
20	3.258	3.299	3.471	3.606	3.718	3.812	3.893	3.965	
24	3.285	3.326	3.501	3.639	3.752	3.848	3.931	4.003	
30	3.313	3.355	3.533	3.674	3.789	3.887	3.971	4.046	
40	3.344	3.387	3.569	3.712	3.830	3.930	4.017	4.093	
60	3.377	3.421	3.608	3.755	3.876	3.979	4.068	4.146	
120	3.415	3.460	3.652	3.803	3.928	4.034	4.126	4.207	
∞	3.456	3.503	3.702	3.859	3.989	4.099	4.195	4.279	

P = .20

ν\n	2	3	4	5	6	7	8	9	10
1	.4595	1.011	1.359	1.606	1.793	1.944	2.070	2.176	2.269
2	.4082	.9530	1.309	1.564	1.758	1.914	2.043	2.154	2.249
3	.3913	.9348	1.298	1.558	1.759	1.920	2.053	2.167	2.266
4	.3829	.9259	1.293	1.558	1.763	1.927	2.064	2.181	2.282
5	.3779	.9207	1.291	1.559	1.767	1.934	2.073	2.192	2.295
6	.3745	.9172	1.289	1.561	1.770	1.940	2.081	2.201	2.306
7	.3722	.9147	1.289	1.562	1.773	1.944	2.087	2.208	2.314
8	.3704	.9129	1.288	1.563	1.775	1.948	2.092	2.214	2.321
9	.3690	.9114	1.288	1.563	1.778	1.951	2.096	2.220	2.327
10	.3680	.9103	1.287	1.564	1.779	1.954	2.099	2.224	2.332
11	.3671	.9094	1.287	1.565	1.781	1.956	2.102	2.228	2.337
12	.3663	.9086	1.287	1.565	1.782	1.958	2.105	2.231	2.340
13	.3657	.9079	1.287	1.566	1.783	1.960	2.108	2.234	2.344
14	.3652	.9074	1.287	1.566	1.784	1.961	2.109	2.236	2.347
15	.3647	.9069	1.287	1.567	1.785	1.963	2.111	2.238	2.349
16	.3643	.9064	1.286	1.567	1.786	1.964	2.113	2.240	2.352
17	.3639	.9061	1.286	1.567	1.787	1.965	2.114	2.242	2.354
18	.3636	.9057	1.286	1.568	1.787	1.966	2.116	2.244	2.356
19	.3633	.9054	1.286	1.568	1.788	1.967	2.117	2.245	2.357
20	.3631	.9052	1.286	1.568	1.788	1.968	2.118	2.247	2.359
24	.3623	.9043	1.286	1.569	1.790	1.970	2.121	2.251	2.364
30	.3615	.9035	1.286	1.570	1.792	1.973	2.125	2.256	2.369
40	.3607	.9026	1.285	1.571	1.794	1.976	2.129	2.260	2.375
60	.3599	.9017	1.285	1.571	1.796	1.979	2.133	2.265	2.381
120	.3591	.9009	1.286	1.572	1.798	1.982	2.137	2.271	2.387
∞	.3583	.9001	1.286	1.573	1.800	1.985	2.142	2.276	2.394

ν\n	11	12	13	14	15	16	17	18	19
1	2.351	2.424	2.490	2.549	2.604	2.655	2.701	2.745	2.785
2	2.334	2.409	2.477	2.539	2.595	2.647	2.696	2.741	2.782
3	2.353	2.431	2.501	2.565	2.623	2.677	2.727	2.773	2.816
4	2.371	2.451	2.523	2.588	2.648	2.703	2.754	2.801	2.846
5	2.386	2.467	2.540	2.607	2.668	2.724	2.776	2.824	2.869
6	2.398	2.480	2.555	2.622	2.684	2.741	2.793	2.843	2.889
7	2.407	2.491	2.566	2.635	2.697	2.755	2.808	2.858	2.905
8	2.416	2.500	2.576	2.645	2.708	2.766	2.820	2.871	2.918
9	2.422	2.507	2.584	2.653	2.717	2.776	2.831	2.881	2.929
10	2.428	2.514	2.591	2.661	2.725	2.785	2.839	2.891	2.938
11	2.433	2.519	2.596	2.667	2.732	2.792	2.847	2.898	2.947
12	2.437	2.524	2.602	2.673	2.738	2.798	2.854	2.905	2.954
13	2.441	2.528	2.606	2.678	2.743	2.803	2.859	2.911	2.960
14	2.444	2.532	2.610	2.682	2.748	2.808	2.865	2.917	2.966
15	2.447	2.535	2.614	2.686	2.752	2.813	2.869	2.922	2.971
16	2.450	2.538	2.617	2.689	2.756	2.817	2.873	2.926	2.975
17	2.452	2.541	2.620	2.693	2.759	2.820	2.877	2.930	2.980
18	2.454	2.543	2.623	2.695	2.762	2.824	2.881	2.934	2.983
19	2.456	2.545	2.625	2.698	2.765	2.827	2.884	2.937	2.987
20	2.458	2.547	2.627	2.701	2.768	2.829	2.886	2.940	2.990
24	2.464	2.554	2.635	2.708	2.776	2.838	2.896	2.950	3.000
30	2.470	2.561	2.642	2.717	2.785	2.848	2.906	2.960	3.011
40	2.477	2.568	2.650	2.725	2.794	2.858	2.917	2.972	3.023
60	2.484	2.575	2.659	2.734	2.804	2.868	2.928	2.983	3.035
120	2.490	2.584	2.667	2.744	2.814	2.879	2.940	2.996	3.049
∞	2.498	2.592	2.677	2.754	2.826	2.891	2.953	3.010	3.063

P = .20

ν\n	20	22	24	26	28	30	32	34	36
1	2.824	2.894	2.957	3.014	3.066	3.114	3.157	3.198	3.237
2	2.822	2.894	2.958	3.017	3.070	3.119	3.164	3.207	3.246
3	2.857	2.931	2.998	3.058	3.113	3.163	3.210	3.253	3.294
4	2.887	2.963	3.032	3.093	3.149	3.201	3.249	3.293	3.334
5	2.912	2.989	3.059	3.122	3.179	3.232	3.280	3.326	3.368
6	2.932	3.010	3.081	3.145	3.203	3.257	3.306	3.352	3.394
7	2.948	3.028	3.099	3.164	3.223	3.277	3.327	3.374	3.417
8	2.962	3.042	3.115	3.180	3.240	3.294	3.345	3.391	3.436
9	2.973	3.055	3.128	3.193	3.254	3.309	3.360	3.407	3.451
10	2.983	3.065	3.139	3.205	3.266	3.322	3.373	3.421	3.465
11	2.992	3.074	3.148	3.215	3.276	3.332	3.384	3.432	3.477
12	2.999	3.082	3.157	3.224	3.286	3.342	3.394	3.443	3.488
13	3.006	3.089	3.164	3.232	3.294	3.351	3.403	3.452	3.497
14	3.012	3.096	3.171	3.239	3.301	3.358	3.411	3.460	3.506
15	3.017	3.101	3.177	3.245	3.308	3.365	3.418	3.467	3.513
16	3.022	3.106	3.182	3.251	3.314	3.371	3.424	3.474	3.520
17	3.026	3.111	3.187	3.256	3.319	3.377	3.430	3.480	3.526
18	3.030	3.115	3.192	3.261	3.324	3.382	3.436	3.485	3.532
19	3.033	3.119	3.195	3.265	3.329	3.387	3.440	3.490	3.537
20	3.037	3.123	3.200	3.269	3.333	3.391	3.445	3.495	3.542
24	3.048	3.134	3.211	3.282	3.346	3.405	3.460	3.510	3.558
30	3.059	3.147	3.225	3.296	3.361	3.421	3.476	3.527	3.575
40	3.071	3.160	3.239	3.311	3.377	3.437	3.493	3.545	3.593
60	3.084	3.174	3.254	3.327	3.393	3.455	3.511	3.564	3.613
120	3.098	3.189	3.271	3.345	3.412	3.474	3.532	3.585	3.635
∞	3.113	3.206	3.288	3.364	3.432	3.495	3.554	3.608	3.659

ν\n	38	40	50	60	70	80	90	100
1	3.273	3.306	3.450	3.564	3.657	3.737	3.806	3.867
2	3.282	3.317	3.464	3.580	3.676	3.757	3.828	3.890
3	3.331	3.367	3.518	3.637	3.736	3.819	3.892	3.955
4	3.373	3.409	3.564	3.686	3.787	3.872	3.946	4.011
5	3.407	3.444	3.602	3.726	3.828	3.915	3.991	4.057
6	3.435	3.472	3.632	3.758	3.862	3.950	4.027	4.094
7	3.457	3.495	3.657	3.785	3.891	3.980	4.057	4.125
8	3.477	3.515	3.678	3.808	3.914	4.005	4.083	4.152
9	3.493	3.532	3.697	3.827	3.935	4.026	4.105	4.174
10	3.507	3.546	3.713	3.844	3.953	4.044	4.123	4.194
11	3.519	3.559	3.727	3.859	3.968	4.061	4.141	4.211
12	3.530	3.570	3.739	3.872	3.982	4.075	4.156	4.226
13	3.540	3.580	3.750	3.883	3.994	4.087	4.169	4.240
14	3.548	3.588	3.759	3.894	4.005	4.099	4.181	4.252
15	3.556	3.596	3.768	3.904	4.015	4.109	4.191	4.264
16	3.563	3.604	3.776	3.912	4.024	4.119	4.201	4.274
17	3.569	3.610	3.783	3.920	4.032	4.128	4.210	4.283
18	3.575	3.616	3.790	3.927	4.040	4.136	4.218	4.291
19	3.581	3.622	3.796	3.934	4.047	4.143	4.226	4.299
20	3.586	3.627	3.801	3.940	4.053	4.150	4.233	4.306
24	3.602	3.643	3.820	3.960	4.075	4.172	4.257	4.331
30	3.619	3.662	3.840	3.982	4.098	4.197	4.282	4.357
40	3.638	3.681	3.862	4.006	4.124	4.224	4.310	4.387
60	3.659	3.702	3.887	4.032	4.152	4.254	4.342	4.420
120	3.682	3.726	3.913	4.062	4.184	4.288	4.378	4.457
∞	3.707	3.752	3.943	4.095	4.220	4.327	4.419	4.501

P = .30

ν\n	2	3	4	5	6	7	8	9	10
1	.7206	1.376	1.784	2.073	2.295	2.474	2.623	2.750	2.861
2	.6290	1.249	1.639	1.917	2.130	2.302	2.445	2.567	2.673
3	.5999	1.210	1.598	1.876	2.089	2.261	2.404	2.527	2.633
4	.5857	1.191	1.580	1.858	2.072	2.245	2.389	2.512	2.619
5	.5773	1.180	1.569	1.848	2.063	2.237	2.382	2.505	2.614
6	.5718	1.173	1.562	1.842	2.058	2.233	2.378	2.503	2.611
7	.5679	1.168	1.558	1.838	2.055	2.230	2.376	2.501	2.610
8	.5649	1.164	1.554	1.835	2.053	2.228	2.375	2.501	2.610
9	.5627	1.161	1.552	1.833	2.051	2.227	2.375	2.500	2.610
10	.5609	1.159	1.549	1.831	2.050	2.226	2.374	2.500	2.610
11	.5594	1.157	1.548	1.830	2.049	2.225	2.374	2.500	2.611
12	.5582	1.155	1.546	1.829	2.048	2.225	2.374	2.501	2.611
13	.5571	1.154	1.545	1.828	2.047	2.225	2.374	2.501	2.611
14	.5563	1.153	1.544	1.827	2.047	2.224	2.374	2.501	2.612
15	.5555	1.152	1.543	1.827	2.046	2.224	2.374	2.501	2.612
16	.5548	1.151	1.543	1.826	2.046	2.224	2.374	2.501	2.612
17	.5542	1.150	1.542	1.826	2.046	2.224	2.374	2.502	2.613
18	.5537	1.150	1.541	1.825	2.046	2.224	2.374	2.502	2.613
19	.5532	1.149	1.541	1.825	2.045	2.224	2.374	2.502	2.613
20	.5528	1.148	1.540	1.824	2.045	2.224	2.373	2.502	2.614
24	.5515	1.147	1.538	1.823	2.044	2.224	2.374	2.503	2.615
30	.5502	1.145	1.537	1.822	2.043	2.223	2.374	2.503	2.616
40	.5489	1.143	1.535	1.821	2.043	2.223	2.374	2.504	2.617
60	.5475	1.141	1.534	1.820	2.042	2.223	2.375	2.505	2.619
120	.5462	1.140	1.533	1.819	2.042	2.223	2.376	2.506	2.620
∞	.5449	1.138	1.531	1.818	2.042	2.224	2.377	2.508	2.623

ν\n	11	12	13	14	15	16	17	18	19
1	2.959	3.046	3.126	3.198	3.264	3.325	3.382	3.434	3.483
2	2.767	2.851	2.927	2.995	3.058	3.117	3.171	3.221	3.268
3	2.727	2.811	2.887	2.956	3.019	3.077	3.131	3.182	3.229
4	2.714	2.798	2.874	2.944	3.008	3.066	3.121	3.171	3.219
5	2.708	2.794	2.870	2.940	3.005	3.063	3.118	3.169	3.217
6	2.707	2.792	2.869	2.940	3.004	3.064	3.119	3.170	3.218
7	2.706	2.792	2.870	2.941	3.006	3.065	3.121	3.172	3.221
8	2.707	2.793	2.871	2.942	3.007	3.067	3.123	3.174	3.223
9	2.707	2.794	2.872	2.943	3.009	3.069	3.125	3.177	3.226
10	2.708	2.795	2.873	2.945	3.010	3.071	3.127	3.179	3.228
11	2.708	2.795	2.874	2.946	3.012	3.073	3.129	3.182	3.230
12	2.709	2.796	2.875	2.947	3.013	3.074	3.131	3.183	3.233
13	2.710	2.797	2.876	2.949	3.015	3.076	3.133	3.185	3.235
14	2.710	2.798	2.877	2.950	3.016	3.077	3.134	3.187	3.236
15	2.711	2.799	2.878	2.951	3.017	3.079	3.135	3.188	3.238
16	2.711	2.799	2.879	2.952	3.018	3.080	3.137	3.190	3.240
17	2.712	2.800	2.880	2.953	3.019	3.081	3.138	3.191	3.241
18	2.712	2.801	2.881	2.953	3.020	3.082	3.139	3.192	3.242
19	2.713	2.801	2.881	2.954	3.021	3.083	3.140	3.193	3.243
20	2.713	2.802	2.882	2.954	3.022	3.083	3.141	3.194	3.244
24	2.714	2.803	2.884	2.957	3.024	3.086	3.144	3.198	3.248
30	2.716	2.805	2.886	2.959	3.027	3.090	3.147	3.202	3.252
40	2.718	2.807	2.889	2.963	3.030	3.093	3.152	3.206	3.257
60	2.719	2.810	2.891	2.966	3.034	3.097	3.156	3.210	3.262
120	2.721	2.812	2.894	2.969	3.038	3.102	3.160	3.215	3.267
∞	2.724	2.815	2.898	2.973	3.042	3.106	3.165	3.221	3.273

P = .30

ν\n	20	22	24	26	28	30	32	34	36
1	3.530	3.615	3.691	3.760	3.823	3.881	3.934	3.985	4.031
2	3.312	3.394	3.466	3.533	3.592	3.648	3.699	3.747	3.791
3	3.273	3.354	3.427	3.493	3.553	3.608	3.659	3.707	3.751
4	3.263	3.345	3.418	3.484	3.545	3.600	3.652	3.700	3.744
5	3.262	3.344	3.418	3.484	3.545	3.601	3.653	3.701	3.746
6	3.263	3.346	3.420	3.487	3.548	3.605	3.657	3.705	3.750
7	3.266	3.349	3.424	3.491	3.553	3.609	3.661	3.710	3.755
8	3.269	3.352	3.427	3.495	3.557	3.614	3.667	3.716	3.761
9	3.272	3.356	3.430	3.499	3.561	3.618	3.671	3.720	3.766
10	3.274	3.358	3.434	3.502	3.565	3.622	3.675	3.725	3.771
11	3.277	3.361	3.437	3.506	3.568	3.626	3.679	3.729	3.775
12	3.279	3.364	3.440	3.509	3.571	3.629	3.683	3.732	3.779
13	3.281	3.366	3.442	3.511	3.574	3.632	3.686	3.736	3.782
14	3.283	3.368	3.445	3.514	3.577	3.635	3.689	3.739	3.785
15	3.285	3.370	3.447	3.516	3.580	3.638	3.692	3.742	3.788
16	3.286	3.372	3.449	3.518	3.582	3.640	3.694	3.744	3.791
17	3.288	3.374	3.450	3.520	3.584	3.642	3.696	3.747	3.793
18	3.289	3.375	3.452	3.522	3.586	3.644	3.699	3.749	3.796
19	3.290	3.376	3.454	3.524	3.587	3.646	3.701	3.751	3.798
20	3.291	3.377	3.455	3.525	3.589	3.648	3.702	3.752	3.800
24	3.295	3.382	3.459	3.530	3.595	3.653	3.708	3.759	3.807
30	3.300	3.387	3.465	3.535	3.601	3.660	3.715	3.766	3.814
40	3.304	3.392	3.470	3.542	3.607	3.667	3.722	3.774	3.822
60	3.310	3.398	3.477	3.549	3.614	3.674	3.730	3.782	3.830
120	3.315	3.404	3.483	3.556	3.622	3.683	3.739	3.792	3.841
∞	3.321	3.411	3.491	3.564	3.631	3.692	3.749	3.802	3.851

ν\n	38	40	50	60	70	80	90	100	
1	4.075	4.116	4.291	4.430	4.545	4.642	4.727	4.801	
2	3.833	3.872	4.039	4.171	4.280	4.372	4.453	4.524	
3	3.793	3.832	3.998	4.130	4.239	4.331	4.411	4.482	
4	3.786	3.825	3.993	4.125	4.234	4.327	4.408	4.479	
5	3.788	3.828	3.996	4.129	4.239	4.333	4.414	4.485	
6	3.793	3.833	4.002	4.136	4.247	4.341	4.422	4.494	
7	3.798	3.838	4.009	4.144	4.255	4.349	4.431	4.503	
8	3.804	3.844	4.015	4.151	4.262	4.357	4.439	4.512	
9	3.809	3.849	4.021	4.157	4.270	4.365	4.447	4.520	
10	3.814	3.854	4.027	4.164	4.276	4.372	4.455	4.528	
11	3.818	3.859	4.032	4.169	4.282	4.378	4.461	4.535	
12	3.822	3.863	4.037	4.174	4.288	4.384	4.468	4.541	
13	3.825	3.867	4.041	4.179	4.293	4.390	4.473	4.547	
14	3.829	3.870	4.045	4.183	4.298	4.395	4.478	4.552	
15	3.832	3.873	4.048	4.187	4.302	4.399	4.483	4.557	
16	3.835	3.876	4.052	4.191	4.306	4.403	4.488	4.562	
17	3.838	3.879	4.055	4.195	4.310	4.407	4.492	4.566	
18	3.840	3.881	4.058	4.198	4.313	4.411	4.495	4.570	
19	3.842	3.884	4.060	4.201	4.316	4.414	4.499	4.573	
20	3.844	3.886	4.063	4.203	4.319	4.417	4.502	4.577	
24	3.851	3.893	4.071	4.212	4.328	4.427	4.513	4.588	
30	3.858	3.901	4.080	4.222	4.339	4.439	4.525	4.601	
40	3.867	3.910	4.090	4.233	4.352	4.452	4.538	4.615	
60	3.876	3.919	4.101	4.246	4.365	4.466	4.554	4.631	
120	3.886	3.930	4.113	4.260	4.380	4.482	4.571	4.649	
∞	3.898	3.941	4.127	4.275	4.397	4.500	4.590	4.670	

P = .40

ν\n	2	3	4	5	6	7	8	9	10
1	1.028	1.799	2.280	2.623	2.888	3.102	3.281	3.434	3.568
2	.8729	1.558	1.984	2.288	2.522	2.712	2.870	3.005	3.123
3	.8265	1.488	1.901	2.196	2.423	2.607	2.760	2.891	3.006
4	.8042	1.455	1.862	2.154	2.378	2.559	2.710	2.840	2.954
5	.7912	1.436	1.840	2.129	2.352	2.533	2.683	2.812	2.925
6	.7826	1.423	1.825	2.114	2.336	2.515	2.666	2.794	2.906
7	.7766	1.414	1.815	2.103	2.324	2.503	2.653	2.781	2.894
8	.7721	1.408	1.807	2.094	2.315	2.495	2.644	2.772	2.884
9	.7686	1.402	1.802	2.088	2.309	2.488	2.637	2.765	2.877
10	.7658	1.398	1.797	2.083	2.304	2.482	2.632	2.760	2.872
11	.7636	1.395	1.793	2.079	2.299	2.478	2.627	2.755	2.867
12	.7617	1.392	1.790	2.076	2.296	2.475	2.624	2.752	2.864
13	.7602	1.390	1.787	2.073	2.293	2.472	2.621	2.749	2.860
14	.7588	1.388	1.785	2.070	2.291	2.469	2.618	2.746	2.858
15	.7576	1.386	1.783	2.068	2.288	2.467	2.616	2.744	2.856
16	.7566	1.385	1.781	2.066	2.287	2.465	2.614	2.742	2.854
17	.7557	1.383	1.780	2.065	2.285	2.463	2.612	2.740	2.852
18	.7549	1.382	1.779	2.063	2.283	2.462	2.611	2.739	2.850
19	.7542	1.381	1.777	2.062	2.282	2.460	2.610	2.737	2.849
20	.7536	1.380	1.776	2.061	2.281	2.459	2.608	2.736	2.848
24	.7516	1.377	1.773	2.057	2.277	2.455	2.605	2.733	2.844
30	.7496	1.374	1.770	2.054	2.274	2.452	2.601	2.729	2.840
40	.7476	1.371	1.766	2.050	2.270	2.448	2.597	2.725	2.837
60	.7456	1.368	1.763	2.047	2.267	2.445	2.594	2.722	2.833
120	.7436	1.366	1.760	2.043	2.263	2.441	2.590	2.718	2.830
∞	.7416	1.363	1.757	2.040	2.260	2.438	2.587	2.715	2.826

ν\n	11	12	13	14	15	16	17	18	19
1	3.686	3.792	3.888	3.975	4.055	4.129	4.197	4.261	4.321
2	3.228	3.321	3.406	3.483	3.554	3.619	3.679	3.736	3.789
3	3.107	3.198	3.280	3.354	3.423	3.486	3.545	3.600	3.651
4	3.053	3.143	3.224	3.298	3.366	3.429	3.486	3.540	3.591
5	3.024	3.113	3.193	3.267	3.335	3.396	3.454	3.508	3.558
6	3.005	3.094	3.174	3.248	3.315	3.377	3.434	3.488	3.538
7	2.992	3.081	3.161	3.234	3.302	3.363	3.421	3.475	3.525
8	2.983	3.072	3.152	3.225	3.292	3.353	3.411	3.465	3.515
9	2.976	3.065	3.144	3.217	3.285	3.346	3.403	3.457	3.507
10	2.970	3.059	3.139	3.212	3.279	3.341	3.398	3.452	3.502
11	2.966	3.054	3.134	3.207	3.274	3.336	3.393	3.447	3.497
12	2.962	3.051	3.131	3.203	3.271	3.332	3.390	3.443	3.494
13	2.959	3.048	3.128	3.200	3.268	3.329	3.387	3.440	3.491
14	2.956	3.045	3.125	3.198	3.265	3.327	3.384	3.438	3.488
15	2.954	3.043	3.123	3.196	3.263	3.325	3.382	3.436	3.486
16	2.952	3.041	3.121	3.194	3.261	3.323	3.380	3.434	3.484
17	2.950	3.039	3.119	3.192	3.259	3.321	3.378	3.432	3.482
18	2.949	3.038	3.118	3.191	3.258	3.319	3.377	3.431	3.481
19	2.948	3.036	3.116	3.189	3.257	3.318	3.376	3.429	3.480
20	2.947	3.035	3.115	3.188	3.255	3.317	3.375	3.428	3.478
24	2.943	3.031	3.112	3.185	3.252	3.314	3.371	3.425	3.475
30	2.939	3.028	3.108	3.181	3.248	3.310	3.368	3.421	3.472
40	2.936	3.024	3.105	3.178	3.245	3.307	3.364	3.418	3.468
60	2.932	3.021	3.101	3.174	3.241	3.304	3.361	3.415	3.465
120	2.929	3.017	3.098	3.171	3.238	3.300	3.358	3.412	3.462
∞	2.925	3.014	3.094	3.168	3.235	3.297	3.355	3.409	3.459

P = .40

ν\n	20	22	24	26	28	30	32	34	36
1	4.377	4.480	4.573	4.657	4.734	4.804	4.870	4.931	4.988
2	3.838	3.929	4.011	4.085	4.153	4.216	4.273	4.327	4.377
3	3.699	3.787	3.867	3.938	4.004	4.065	4.120	4.173	4.221
4	3.638	3.726	3.804	3.875	3.940	3.999	4.055	4.106	4.155
5	3.605	3.692	3.770	3.841	3.905	3.965	4.020	4.070	4.118
6	3.585	3.672	3.750	3.820	3.885	3.944	3.998	4.049	4.097
7	3.571	3.658	3.736	3.806	3.870	3.929	3.984	4.035	4.083
8	3.562	3.648	3.726	3.796	3.860	3.919	3.974	4.025	4.072
9	3.554	3.641	3.718	3.788	3.853	3.912	3.966	4.017	4.065
10	3.549	3.635	3.713	3.783	3.847	3.906	3.961	4.012	4.059
11	3.544	3.631	3.708	3.778	3.843	3.902	3.956	4.007	4.055
12	3.540	3.627	3.705	3.775	3.839	3.898	3.953	4.004	4.051
13	3.537	3.624	3.702	3.772	3.836	3.895	3.950	4.001	4.049
14	3.535	3.621	3.699	3.769	3.834	3.893	3.947	3.998	4.046
15	3.533	3.619	3.697	3.767	3.832	3.891	3.945	3.996	4.044
16	3.531	3.617	3.695	3.765	3.830	3.889	3.944	3.995	4.043
17	3.529	3.616	3.694	3.764	3.828	3.888	3.942	3.993	4.041
18	3.528	3.614	3.692	3.762	3.827	3.886	3.941	3.992	4.040
19	3.527	3.613	3.691	3.761	3.826	3.885	3.940	3.991	4.039
20	3.526	3.612	3.690	3.760	3.825	3.884	3.939	3.990	4.038
24	3.522	3.609	3.687	3.757	3.822	3.881	3.936	3.987	4.035
30	3.519	3.606	3.683	3.754	3.819	3.878	3.933	3.984	4.032
40	3.516	3.602	3.680	3.751	3.816	3.875	3.930	3.982	4.029
60	3.513	3.599	3.677	3.748	3.813	3.873	3.928	3.979	4.027
120	3.510	3.596	3.674	3.745	3.810	3.870	3.925	3.977	4.025
∞	3.506	3.594	3.672	3.743	3.808	3.867	3.923	3.974	4.022

ν\n	38	40	50	60	70	80	90	100
1	5.041	5.091	5.305	5.474	5.614	5.734	5.837	5.928
2	4.424	4.468	4.657	4.806	4.930	5.035	5.126	5.207
3	4.267	4.309	4.492	4.637	4.757	4.858	4.947	5.024
4	4.199	4.242	4.422	4.565	4.683	4.784	4.871	4.948
5	4.163	4.205	4.384	4.527	4.644	4.744	4.831	4.907
6	4.142	4.183	4.362	4.504	4.621	4.721	4.807	4.883
7	4.127	4.169	4.347	4.489	4.606	4.705	4.791	4.868
8	4.117	4.158	4.337	4.479	4.595	4.695	4.781	4.857
9	4.109	4.151	4.330	4.471	4.588	4.687	4.774	4.850
10	4.104	4.145	4.324	4.466	4.583	4.682	4.768	4.844
11	4.099	4.141	4.320	4.461	4.578	4.678	4.764	4.840
12	4.096	4.138	4.316	4.458	4.575	4.675	4.761	4.837
13	4.093	4.135	4.314	4.455	4.572	4.672	4.758	4.834
14	4.091	4.133	4.311	4.453	4.570	4.670	4.756	4.832
15	4.089	4.131	4.310	4.451	4.569	4.668	4.755	4.831
16	4.087	4.129	4.308	4.450	4.567	4.667	4.753	4.830
17	4.086	4.128	4.307	4.449	4.566	4.666	4.752	4.828
18	4.084	4.126	4.306	4.448	4.565	4.665	4.751	4.828
19	4.083	4.125	4.305	4.447	4.564	4.664	4.751	4.827
20	4.082	4.124	4.304	4.446	4.563	4.663	4.750	4.826
24	4.079	4.122	4.301	4.444	4.561	4.661	4.748	4.825
30	4.077	4.119	4.299	4.442	4.559	4.660	4.747	4.823
40	4.074	4.117	4.297	4.440	4.558	4.658	4.746	4.823
60	4.072	4.114	4.295	4.438	4.557	4.657	4.745	4.822
120	4.070	4.112	4.293	4.437	4.556	4.657	4.744	4.822
∞	4.067	4.110	4.291	4.435	4.554	4.655	4.743	4.821

P = .50

$\nu \backslash n$	2	3	4	5	6	7	8	9	10
1	1.414	2.338	2.918	3.335	3.658	3.920	4.139	4.327	4.491
2	1.155	1.908	2.377	2.713	2.973	3.184	3.361	3.513	3.645
3	1.082	1.791	2.230	2.545	2.789	2.987	3.152	3.294	3.418
4	1.048	1.737	2.163	2.468	2.704	2.895	3.055	3.193	3.313
5	1.028	1.705	2.124	2.423	2.655	2.843	3.000	3.135	3.253
6	1.015	1.685	2.098	2.394	2.623	2.809	2.964	3.097	3.214
7	1.006	1.670	2.080	2.375	2.601	2.785	2.938	3.070	3.186
8	.9990	1.659	2.067	2.359	2.584	2.767	2.920	3.051	3.165
9	.9938	1.651	2.057	2.347	2.572	2.753	2.905	3.035	3.149
10	.9897	1.645	2.049	2.338	2.561	2.742	2.893	3.023	3.137
11	.9863	1.639	2.042	2.330	2.553	2.733	2.884	3.014	3.127
12	.9836	1.635	2.037	2.324	2.546	2.726	2.876	3.005	3.118
13	.9812	1.631	2.032	2.319	2.540	2.719	2.870	2.998	3.111
14	.9792	1.628	2.028	2.314	2.535	2.714	2.864	2.993	3.105
15	.9775	1.625	2.025	2.310	2.531	2.709	2.859	2.987	3.099
16	.9760	1.623	2.022	2.307	2.527	2.705	2.855	2.983	3.095
17	.9747	1.621	2.020	2.304	2.524	2.702	2.851	2.979	3.091
18	.9735	1.619	2.018	2.301	2.521	2.699	2.848	2.976	3.087
19	.9724	1.618	2.015	2.299	2.518	2.696	2.845	2.973	3.084
20	.9715	1.616	2.013	2.297	2.516	2.693	2.842	2.970	3.081
24	.9685	1.611	2.007	2.290	2.509	2.685	2.834	2.961	3.071
30	.9656	1.606	2.001	2.284	2.501	2.678	2.825	2.952	3.062
40	.9626	1.602	1.996	2.277	2.494	2.670	2.817	2.943	3.053
60	.9597	1.597	1.990	2.270	2.486	2.662	2.808	2.934	3.043
120	.9568	1.592	1.984	2.264	2.479	2.654	2.799	2.925	3.034
∞	.9539	1.588	1.978	2.257	2.472	2.645	2.791	2.915	3.024

$\nu \backslash n$	11	12	13	14	15	16	17	18	19
1	4.637	4.767	4.885	4.992	5.091	5.182	5.266	5.345	5.420
2	3.762	3.867	3.963	4.049	4.129	4.203	4.271	4.335	4.395
3	3.528	3.626	3.715	3.797	3.871	3.940	4.004	4.064	4.120
4	3.419	3.515	3.601	3.680	3.752	3.819	3.881	3.939	3.993
5	3.357	3.451	3.535	3.613	3.684	3.749	3.811	3.867	3.920
6	3.317	3.409	3.493	3.569	3.639	3.704	3.764	3.820	3.873
7	3.288	3.380	3.463	3.538	3.608	3.672	3.732	3.788	3.840
8	3.267	3.358	3.440	3.515	3.585	3.648	3.708	3.763	3.815
9	3.250	3.341	3.423	3.498	3.567	3.630	3.689	3.744	3.796
10	3.237	3.328	3.410	3.484	3.552	3.616	3.674	3.729	3.781
11	3.227	3.317	3.398	3.472	3.540	3.604	3.662	3.717	3.769
12	3.219	3.308	3.389	3.463	3.531	3.594	3.652	3.706	3.757
13	3.211	3.300	3.381	3.455	3.523	3.585	3.643	3.698	3.749
14	3.204	3.293	3.375	3.448	3.515	3.578	3.636	3.690	3.741
15	3.199	3.288	3.369	3.442	3.509	3.572	3.630	3.684	3.735
16	3.194	3.283	3.364	3.436	3.504	3.567	3.624	3.678	3.729
17	3.190	3.278	3.359	3.432	3.499	3.562	3.620	3.673	3.724
18	3.186	3.274	3.355	3.428	3.495	3.558	3.615	3.669	3.719
19	3.183	3.271	3.352	3.424	3.491	3.554	3.611	3.665	3.715
20	3.179	3.268	3.348	3.421	3.488	3.550	3.608	3.661	3.712
24	3.170	3.258	3.338	3.410	3.477	3.539	3.596	3.650	3.700
30	3.160	3.248	3.327	3.400	3.466	3.528	3.585	3.639	3.688
40	3.150	3.238	3.317	3.389	3.456	3.517	3.574	3.627	3.677
60	3.141	3.228	3.306	3.378	3.444	3.505	3.562	3.615	3.665
120	3.131	3.217	3.296	3.367	3.433	3.494	3.551	3.603	3.653
∞	3.121	3.207	3.285	3.356	3.422	3.482	3.538	3.591	3.640

P = .50

ν\n	20	22	24	26	28	30	32	34	36
1	5.489	5.616	5.731	5.835	5.930	6.017	6.098	6.173	6.244
2	4.451	4.554	4.646	4.730	4.807	4.878	4.943	5.004	5.061
3	4.172	4.269	4.356	4.434	4.507	4.573	4.634	4.691	4.745
4	4.044	4.138	4.222	4.298	4.368	4.432	4.492	4.547	4.599
5	3.970	4.062	4.145	4.220	4.288	4.352	4.410	4.464	4.515
6	3.922	4.014	4.095	4.169	4.237	4.299	4.357	4.411	4.461
7	3.889	3.979	4.060	4.133	4.200	4.262	4.319	4.372	4.422
8	3.864	3.953	4.033	4.106	4.174	4.234	4.291	4.344	4.394
9	3.844	3.933	4.013	4.086	4.152	4.214	4.270	4.323	4.372
10	3.829	3.917	3.997	4.069	4.135	4.196	4.253	4.305	4.354
11	3.816	3.904	3.984	4.056	4.122	4.183	4.239	4.291	4.340
12	3.806	3.894	3.973	4.045	4.110	4.171	4.227	4.279	4.328
13	3.797	3.884	3.964	4.035	4.101	4.162	4.218	4.269	4.318
14	3.789	3.877	3.956	4.027	4.092	4.153	4.209	4.261	4.309
15	3.783	3.870	3.949	4.020	4.085	4.145	4.201	4.253	4.302
16	3.777	3.864	3.942	4.014	4.079	4.139	4.195	4.246	4.295
17	3.772	3.859	3.937	4.009	4.073	4.133	4.189	4.241	4.289
18	3.767	3.854	3.932	4.003	4.069	4.128	4.184	4.236	4.284
19	3.763	3.850	3.928	3.999	4.064	4.124	4.180	4.231	4.279
20	3.759	3.846	3.924	3.995	4.060	4.120	4.175	4.227	4.275
24	3.748	3.834	3.912	3.983	4.048	4.107	4.162	4.214	4.262
30	3.736	3.822	3.899	3.970	4.035	4.094	4.149	4.200	4.248
40	3.724	3.809	3.887	3.957	4.021	4.080	4.135	4.186	4.234
60	3.711	3.797	3.874	3.944	4.008	4.067	4.121	4.172	4.220
120	3.699	3.784	3.861	3.930	3.994	4.053	4.107	4.157	4.204
∞	3.686	3.771	3.847	3.916	3.979	4.037	4.091	4.141	4.188

ν\n	38	40	50	60	70	80	90	100	
1	6.310	6.372	6.637	6.847	7.021	7.169	7.297	7.411	
2	5.115	5.165	5.379	5.550	5.690	5.810	5.914	6.006	
3	4.795	4.842	5.043	5.202	5.335	5.447	5.544	5.630	
4	4.647	4.693	4.888	5.043	5.171	5.280	5.374	5.458	
5	4.563	4.608	4.799	4.951	5.077	5.184	5.277	5.359	
6	4.508	4.552	4.741	4.891	5.016	5.121	5.213	5.294	
7	4.469	4.513	4.700	4.850	4.973	5.078	5.169	5.249	
8	4.440	4.484	4.671	4.819	4.941	5.045	5.136	5.215	
9	4.418	4.462	4.647	4.794	4.916	5.020	5.110	5.189	
10	4.400	4.444	4.629	4.775	4.897	5.000	5.090	5.169	
11	4.386	4.429	4.613	4.760	4.881	4.984	5.073	5.152	
12	4.374	4.417	4.600	4.747	4.867	4.970	5.059	5.138	
13	4.364	4.406	4.590	4.736	4.856	4.959	5.048	5.126	
14	4.355	4.397	4.581	4.726	4.846	4.949	5.037	5.116	
15	4.347	4.390	4.573	4.718	4.838	4.940	5.029	5.107	
16	4.340	4.383	4.566	4.710	4.831	4.932	5.021	5.099	
17	4.334	4.377	4.559	4.704	4.824	4.926	5.014	5.092	
18	4.329	4.372	4.554	4.698	4.818	4.920	5.008	5.086	
19	4.324	4.367	4.549	4.693	4.813	4.914	5.003	5.081	
20	4.320	4.363	4.545	4.689	4.808	4.910	4.998	5.076	
24	4.307	4.349	4.530	4.674	4.793	4.894	4.982	5.060	
30	4.293	4.335	4.515	4.659	4.778	4.878	4.966	5.044	
40	4.279	4.321	4.500	4.644	4.762	4.862	4.950	5.027	
60	4.264	4.306	4.485	4.627	4.745	4.845	4.932	5.009	
120	4.249	4.290	4.469	4.610	4.727	4.827	4.914	4.990	
∞	4.232	4.274	4.450	4.591	4.707	4.806	4.892	4.968	

P = .60

ν\n	2	3	4	5	6	7	8	9	10
1	1.947	3.093	3.821	4.347	4.755	5.087	5.365	5.604	5.813
2	1.500	2.338	2.862	3.241	3.535	3.774	3.975	4.147	4.298
3	1.384	2.145	2.617	2.958	3.222	3.437	3.617	3.772	3.908
4	1.331	2.058	2.506	2.829	3.079	3.282	3.453	3.600	3.729
5	1.301	2.008	2.443	2.755	2.997	3.194	3.359	3.501	3.625
6	1.281	1.976	2.402	2.707	2.944	3.136	3.298	3.437	3.558
7	1.267	1.953	2.373	2.674	2.907	3.096	3.255	3.392	3.511
8	1.257	1.937	2.352	2.649	2.879	3.066	3.223	3.357	3.475
9	1.249	1.924	2.336	2.630	2.858	3.043	3.198	3.331	3.448
10	1.243	1.914	2.323	2.615	2.841	3.024	3.178	3.310	3.426
11	1.238	1.905	2.312	2.603	2.827	3.010	3.162	3.293	3.409
12	1.234	1.899	2.303	2.593	2.815	2.997	3.149	3.279	3.394
13	1.231	1.893	2.296	2.584	2.806	2.987	3.137	3.267	3.381
14	1.228	1.888	2.290	2.576	2.798	2.977	3.128	3.257	3.370
15	1.225	1.884	2.284	2.570	2.791	2.969	3.119	3.248	3.361
16	1.223	1.880	2.280	2.564	2.785	2.963	3.112	3.240	3.353
17	1.221	1.877	2.276	2.560	2.779	2.957	3.106	3.234	3.346
18	1.219	1.874	2.272	2.555	2.774	2.951	3.100	3.227	3.339
19	1.218	1.872	2.269	2.551	2.770	2.946	3.095	3.222	3.333
20	1.217	1.870	2.266	2.548	2.766	2.942	3.090	3.217	3.329
24	1.212	1.862	2.256	2.537	2.753	2.929	3.076	3.202	3.312
30	1.208	1.855	2.247	2.526	2.741	2.915	3.061	3.186	3.295
40	1.203	1.848	2.238	2.515	2.729	2.901	3.046	3.171	3.279
60	1.199	1.840	2.229	2.504	2.717	2.888	3.032	3.155	3.263
120	1.195	1.833	2.220	2.493	2.704	2.875	3.017	3.139	3.246
∞	1.190	1.826	2.210	2.482	2.692	2.861	3.002	3.123	3.229

ν\n	11	12	13	14	15	16	17	18	19
1	5.998	6.164	6.314	6.451	6.576	6.693	6.801	6.901	6.996
2	4.432	4.552	4.661	4.760	4.852	4.936	5.014	5.087	5.156
3	4.028	4.136	4.234	4.324	4.406	4.482	4.552	4.618	4.680
4	3.843	3.945	4.038	4.123	4.201	4.273	4.340	4.402	4.461
5	3.736	3.835	3.925	4.007	4.082	4.152	4.216	4.277	4.333
6	3.666	3.763	3.850	3.931	4.004	4.072	4.136	4.195	4.250
7	3.617	3.712	3.798	3.877	3.949	4.016	4.078	4.137	4.191
8	3.580	3.674	3.759	3.837	3.908	3.974	4.036	4.093	4.147
9	3.552	3.644	3.729	3.806	3.876	3.942	4.003	4.059	4.113
10	3.529	3.621	3.705	3.781	3.851	3.916	3.976	4.032	4.085
11	3.510	3.602	3.685	3.760	3.830	3.895	3.954	4.010	4.063
12	3.495	3.586	3.668	3.743	3.813	3.877	3.936	3.992	4.044
13	3.482	3.572	3.654	3.729	3.798	3.862	3.921	3.976	4.028
14	3.471	3.561	3.642	3.717	3.786	3.849	3.908	3.963	4.014
15	3.461	3.551	3.632	3.706	3.774	3.837	3.896	3.951	4.002
16	3.452	3.542	3.623	3.697	3.765	3.827	3.886	3.941	3.992
17	3.445	3.534	3.615	3.688	3.756	3.819	3.877	3.932	3.983
18	3.438	3.527	3.608	3.681	3.749	3.811	3.869	3.923	3.974
19	3.432	3.521	3.601	3.674	3.742	3.804	3.862	3.916	3.967
20	3.427	3.515	3.595	3.669	3.735	3.798	3.856	3.910	3.960
24	3.410	3.497	3.577	3.649	3.716	3.778	3.835	3.889	3.939
30	3.392	3.480	3.558	3.630	3.696	3.757	3.815	3.868	3.918
40	3.375	3.461	3.539	3.611	3.677	3.737	3.793	3.846	3.895
60	3.358	3.443	3.521	3.591	3.656	3.717	3.773	3.825	3.873
120	3.340	3.425	3.501	3.572	3.636	3.695	3.750	3.802	3.850
∞	3.322	3.406	3.482	3.551	3.615	3.674	3.728	3.779	3.827

P = .60

ν\n	20	22	24	26	28	30	32	34	36
1	7.084	7.247	7.393	7.526	7.648	7.760	7.863	7.959	8.049
2	5.220	5.339	5.445	5.542	5.630	5.712	5.788	5.858	5.923
3	4.738	4.845	4.941	5.028	5.108	5.181	5.249	5.313	5.372
4	4.516	4.617	4.708	4.791	4.866	4.936	5.001	5.061	5.117
5	4.387	4.485	4.573	4.653	4.726	4.794	4.856	4.914	4.969
6	4.302	4.398	4.484	4.563	4.634	4.700	4.761	4.818	4.871
7	4.242	4.337	4.421	4.498	4.569	4.634	4.694	4.750	4.802
8	4.198	4.291	4.374	4.450	4.520	4.584	4.643	4.699	4.751
9	4.163	4.255	4.338	4.413	4.482	4.545	4.604	4.659	4.710
10	4.135	4.226	4.308	4.383	4.451	4.514	4.573	4.627	4.678
11	4.112	4.203	4.284	4.358	4.426	4.489	4.547	4.600	4.651
12	4.093	4.183	4.264	4.338	4.405	4.467	4.525	4.578	4.629
13	4.077	4.166	4.247	4.320	4.388	4.449	4.506	4.560	4.610
14	4.063	4.152	4.232	4.305	4.372	4.433	4.491	4.544	4.593
15	4.051	4.139	4.219	4.292	4.359	4.420	4.477	4.530	4.579
16	4.040	4.129	4.209	4.281	4.347	4.408	4.464	4.517	4.566
17	4.031	4.119	4.198	4.270	4.336	4.397	4.454	4.506	4.555
18	4.022	4.110	4.190	4.261	4.327	4.388	4.444	4.496	4.545
19	4.015	4.102	4.181	4.253	4.319	4.379	4.435	4.488	4.536
20	4.008	4.095	4.174	4.246	4.311	4.372	4.428	4.480	4.529
24	3.986	4.073	4.151	4.222	4.287	4.347	4.402	4.454	4.502
30	3.964	4.050	4.128	4.198	4.262	4.322	4.377	4.428	4.476
40	3.942	4.027	4.104	4.174	4.237	4.296	4.350	4.401	4.449
60	3.919	4.003	4.080	4.148	4.212	4.270	4.324	4.374	4.421
120	3.896	3.979	4.054	4.123	4.185	4.242	4.296	4.345	4.392
∞	3.872	3.954	4.028	4.095	4.157	4.214	4.266	4.315	4.361

ν\n	38	40	50	60	70	80	90	100	
1	8.134	8.213	8.553	8.822	9.045	9.234	9.399	9.544	
2	5.985	6.043	6.290	6.487	6.650	6.788	6.908	7.015	
3	5.427	5.480	5.703	5.881	6.028	6.153	6.261	6.357	
4	5.170	5.220	5.432	5.600	5.740	5.859	5.962	6.053	
5	5.020	5.068	5.274	5.437	5.572	5.687	5.787	5.876	
6	4.921	4.969	5.170	5.330	5.462	5.575	5.672	5.759	
7	4.851	4.898	5.096	5.253	5.383	5.494	5.590	5.676	
8	4.799	4.845	5.040	5.196	5.324	5.434	5.529	5.613	
9	4.758	4.803	4.997	5.151	5.278	5.387	5.481	5.564	
10	4.725	4.771	4.962	5.115	5.241	5.349	5.442	5.525	
11	4.698	4.743	4.933	5.085	5.211	5.318	5.410	5.492	
12	4.676	4.720	4.910	5.060	5.185	5.291	5.384	5.466	
13	4.656	4.700	4.889	5.039	5.163	5.269	5.361	5.442	
14	4.640	4.684	4.872	5.021	5.144	5.249	5.341	5.422	
15	4.625	4.670	4.856	5.005	5.128	5.233	5.324	5.404	
16	4.613	4.656	4.842	4.991	5.114	5.218	5.309	5.389	
17	4.601	4.645	4.830	4.978	5.100	5.205	5.295	5.376	
18	4.592	4.634	4.820	4.967	5.089	5.193	5.283	5.363	
19	4.582	4.626	4.810	4.957	5.079	5.182	5.273	5.352	
20	4.574	4.617	4.801	4.948	5.070	5.173	5.262	5.342	
24	4.548	4.591	4.773	4.919	5.039	5.141	5.231	5.310	
30	4.521	4.563	4.744	4.889	5.008	5.110	5.198	5.276	
40	4.493	4.535	4.715	4.857	4.976	5.077	5.164	5.241	
60	4.465	4.506	4.684	4.825	4.942	5.042	5.128	5.205	
120	4.435	4.476	4.651	4.791	4.906	5.004	5.090	5.165	
∞	4.403	4.444	4.616	4.753	4.867	4.963	5.047	5.121	

P = .70

ν\n	2	3	4	5	6	7	8	9	10
1	2.776	4.293	5.265	5.971	6.520	6.967	7.342	7.664	7.946
2	1.961	2.917	3.521	3.960	4.303	4.582	4.818	5.020	5.197
3	1.768	2.596	3.112	3.487	3.779	4.018	4.218	4.392	4.543
4	1.682	2.454	2.932	3.277	3.547	3.766	3.951	4.111	4.250
5	1.635	2.375	2.830	3.159	3.415	3.624	3.799	3.951	4.083
6	1.604	2.324	2.766	3.083	3.330	3.532	3.701	3.847	3.975
7	1.583	2.289	2.720	3.030	3.271	3.467	3.633	3.775	3.900
8	1.567	2.263	2.687	2.992	3.228	3.420	3.582	3.721	3.843
9	1.555	2.243	2.662	2.962	3.194	3.383	3.543	3.680	3.800
10	1.546	2.228	2.642	2.938	3.167	3.354	3.511	3.647	3.765
11	1.538	2.215	2.625	2.919	3.146	3.331	3.486	3.620	3.737
12	1.532	2.205	2.612	2.903	3.128	3.311	3.465	3.598	3.714
13	1.527	2.196	2.600	2.889	3.113	3.295	3.447	3.579	3.694
14	1.522	2.188	2.591	2.878	3.100	3.280	3.432	3.563	3.677
15	1.518	2.182	2.582	2.868	3.089	3.268	3.419	3.549	3.662
16	1.515	2.176	2.575	2.859	3.079	3.258	3.407	3.536	3.649
17	1.512	2.171	2.569	2.852	3.070	3.248	3.397	3.526	3.638
18	1.509	2.167	2.563	2.845	3.063	3.240	3.388	3.516	3.628
19	1.507	2.163	2.558	2.839	3.056	3.232	3.380	3.508	3.619
20	1.505	2.159	2.553	2.833	3.050	3.226	3.373	3.500	3.611
24	1.498	2.148	2.539	2.816	3.031	3.205	3.350	3.475	3.585
30	1.492	2.137	2.525	2.800	3.012	3.184	3.327	3.451	3.559
40	1.485	2.127	2.511	2.783	2.993	3.162	3.305	3.427	3.533
60	1.479	2.116	2.497	2.766	2.973	3.141	3.282	3.402	3.508
120	1.472	2.105	2.483	2.749	2.954	3.120	3.259	3.378	3.481
∞	1.466	2.095	2.469	2.733	2.936	3.099	3.236	3.353	3.455

ν\n	11	12	13	14	15	16	17	18	19
1	8.196	8.420	8.623	8.808	8.978	9.135	9.281	9.417	9.545
2	5.355	5.496	5.624	5.741	5.849	5.948	6.041	6.127	6.209
3	4.678	4.799	4.908	5.009	5.101	5.186	5.266	5.340	5.410
4	4.374	4.486	4.587	4.680	4.765	4.843	4.917	4.985	5.049
5	4.201	4.307	4.404	4.491	4.572	4.647	4.717	4.782	4.843
6	4.089	4.192	4.284	4.369	4.447	4.520	4.587	4.650	4.709
7	4.010	4.110	4.200	4.283	4.359	4.429	4.495	4.556	4.614
8	3.952	4.049	4.138	4.219	4.293	4.362	4.427	4.487	4.543
9	3.907	4.003	4.090	4.169	4.243	4.311	4.374	4.433	4.488
10	3.871	3.965	4.051	4.130	4.202	4.269	4.331	4.389	4.444
11	3.841	3.935	4.020	4.097	4.169	4.235	4.297	4.354	4.408
12	3.817	3.909	3.994	4.070	4.141	4.207	4.268	4.325	4.378
13	3.796	3.888	3.971	4.047	4.118	4.183	4.243	4.300	4.353
14	3.778	3.869	3.952	4.028	4.098	4.162	4.222	4.278	4.331
15	3.763	3.854	3.936	4.011	4.080	4.144	4.204	4.259	4.312
16	3.750	3.840	3.921	3.996	4.065	4.129	4.188	4.243	4.295
17	3.738	3.827	3.909	3.983	4.051	4.115	4.173	4.228	4.280
18	3.727	3.816	3.897	3.971	4.039	4.102	4.161	4.216	4.267
19	3.718	3.806	3.887	3.961	4.028	4.091	4.150	4.204	4.255
20	3.709	3.798	3.878	3.951	4.019	4.081	4.139	4.194	4.244
24	3.683	3.769	3.849	3.921	3.988	4.049	4.107	4.160	4.211
30	3.655	3.741	3.819	3.891	3.957	4.017	4.074	4.127	4.176
40	3.628	3.713	3.790	3.860	3.925	3.986	4.041	4.093	4.142
60	3.601	3.685	3.760	3.830	3.894	3.953	4.008	4.059	4.107
120	3.573	3.656	3.731	3.799	3.861	3.919	3.973	4.024	4.071
∞	3.546	3.627	3.700	3.767	3.829	3.886	3.939	3.988	4.034

P = .70

ν\n	20	22	24	26	28	30	32	34	36
1	9.665	9.886	10.08	10.26	10.43	10.58	10.72	10.85	10.98
2	6.285	6.425	6.551	6.665	6.770	6.866	6.956	7.039	7.117
3	5.475	5.595	5.703	5.802	5.892	5.975	6.052	6.123	6.191
4	5.110	5.221	5.321	5.412	5.495	5.572	5.643	5.709	5.771
5	4.901	5.007	5.102	5.188	5.267	5.340	5.408	5.471	5.530
6	4.764	4.866	4.958	5.042	5.118	5.189	5.254	5.315	5.372
7	4.668	4.767	4.857	4.938	5.013	5.082	5.146	5.205	5.260
8	4.596	4.693	4.781	4.861	4.934	5.002	5.064	5.122	5.177
9	4.540	4.636	4.722	4.801	4.873	4.939	5.001	5.058	5.112
10	4.495	4.590	4.675	4.753	4.824	4.889	4.950	5.007	5.059
11	4.459	4.552	4.636	4.713	4.783	4.848	4.908	4.964	5.016
12	4.428	4.521	4.604	4.680	4.750	4.814	4.873	4.928	4.980
13	4.402	4.494	4.577	4.652	4.721	4.784	4.843	4.898	4.950
14	4.380	4.471	4.553	4.628	4.696	4.759	4.818	4.872	4.923
15	4.361	4.451	4.533	4.607	4.675	4.737	4.796	4.850	4.900
16	4.344	4.434	4.515	4.588	4.656	4.718	4.776	4.830	4.880
17	4.329	4.418	4.499	4.572	4.639	4.701	4.759	4.812	4.862
18	4.315	4.405	4.485	4.557	4.624	4.686	4.743	4.796	4.846
19	4.303	4.392	4.472	4.544	4.611	4.672	4.729	4.782	4.832
20	4.293	4.381	4.460	4.532	4.599	4.660	4.716	4.769	4.819
24	4.258	4.345	4.423	4.495	4.560	4.620	4.676	4.728	4.777
30	4.223	4.309	4.387	4.456	4.521	4.580	4.635	4.687	4.734
40	4.188	4.272	4.348	4.417	4.481	4.539	4.594	4.644	4.691
60	4.152	4.235	4.310	4.378	4.440	4.497	4.551	4.600	4.647
120	4.115	4.197	4.270	4.337	4.398	4.454	4.507	4.555	4.600
∞	4.078	4.158	4.229	4.295	4.354	4.409	4.460	4.508	4.552

ν\n	38	40	50	60	70	80	90	100	
1	11.09	11.20	11.66	12.02	12.32	12.58	12.80	13.00	
2	7.190	7.259	7.552	7.786	7.980	8.144	8.287	8.413	
3	6.254	6.313	6.566	6.767	6.934	7.076	7.199	7.308	
4	5.829	5.885	6.119	6.305	6.459	6.591	6.706	6.806	
5	5.586	5.638	5.861	6.039	6.186	6.312	6.420	6.517	
6	5.426	5.477	5.692	5.864	6.006	6.128	6.234	6.327	
7	5.313	5.362	5.572	5.740	5.879	5.997	6.100	6.191	
8	5.228	5.276	5.483	5.647	5.783	5.899	6.000	6.089	
9	5.162	5.209	5.412	5.574	5.708	5.823	5.922	6.010	
10	5.109	5.156	5.356	5.516	5.648	5.761	5.859	5.946	
11	5.065	5.112	5.310	5.467	5.598	5.710	5.807	5.893	
12	5.029	5.075	5.271	5.427	5.557	5.667	5.764	5.849	
13	4.998	5.043	5.238	5.393	5.521	5.631	5.726	5.811	
14	4.971	5.017	5.209	5.363	5.491	5.600	5.694	5.778	
15	4.948	4.993	5.185	5.337	5.464	5.572	5.666	5.749	
16	4.927	4.972	5.162	5.315	5.441	5.548	5.642	5.724	
17	4.909	4.953	5.143	5.294	5.420	5.527	5.620	5.702	
18	4.893	4.937	5.126	5.276	5.401	5.508	5.600	5.682	
19	4.878	4.922	5.110	5.260	5.384	5.490	5.583	5.664	
20	4.865	4.909	5.096	5.245	5.369	5.474	5.566	5.647	
24	4.823	4.866	5.050	5.198	5.320	5.424	5.515	5.595	
30	4.780	4.822	5.004	5.149	5.269	5.372	5.461	5.540	
40	4.735	4.777	4.956	5.099	5.217	5.318	5.406	5.484	
60	4.690	4.731	4.907	5.047	5.163	5.262	5.349	5.425	
120	4.643	4.683	4.855	4.993	5.106	5.203	5.288	5.362	
∞	4.594	4.633	4.800	4.934	5.044	5.138	5.220	5.293	

P = .80

ν\n	2	3	4	5	6	7	8	9	10
1	4.353	6.615	8.075	9.138	9.966	10.64	11.21	11.70	12.12
2	2.667	3.820	4.559	5.098	5.521	5.867	6.158	6.409	6.630
3	2.316	3.245	3.833	4.261	4.597	4.872	5.104	5.305	5.481
4	2.168	3.004	3.527	3.907	4.205	4.449	4.655	4.832	4.989
5	2.087	2.872	3.358	3.712	3.988	4.214	4.405	4.570	4.715
6	2.036	2.788	3.252	3.588	3.850	4.065	4.246	4.403	4.540
7	2.001	2.731	3.179	3.503	3.756	3.962	4.136	4.287	4.419
8	1.976	2.689	3.126	3.440	3.686	3.886	4.055	4.201	4.330
9	1.956	2.658	3.085	3.393	3.633	3.828	3.994	4.136	4.261
10	1.941	2.632	3.053	3.355	3.590	3.782	3.944	4.084	4.206
11	1.928	2.612	3.027	3.325	3.557	3.745	3.905	4.042	4.162
12	1.918	2.596	3.006	3.300	3.529	3.715	3.872	4.007	4.126
13	1.910	2.582	2.988	3.279	3.505	3.689	3.844	3.978	4.095
14	1.902	2.570	2.973	3.261	3.485	3.667	3.820	3.953	4.069
15	1.896	2.560	2.960	3.246	3.467	3.648	3.800	3.931	4.046
16	1.891	2.551	2.948	3.232	3.452	3.631	3.782	3.912	4.026
17	1.886	2.543	2.938	3.220	3.439	3.617	3.766	3.895	4.008
18	1.882	2.536	2.930	3.210	3.427	3.604	3.753	3.881	3.993
19	1.878	2.530	2.922	3.200	3.416	3.592	3.740	3.867	3.979
20	1.874	2.524	2.914	3.192	3.407	3.582	3.729	3.855	3.966
24	1.864	2.507	2.892	3.166	3.377	3.549	3.694	3.818	3.927
30	1.853	2.490	2.870	3.140	3.348	3.517	3.659	3.781	3.887
40	1.843	2.473	2.848	3.114	3.318	3.484	3.624	3.743	3.848
60	1.833	2.456	2.826	3.089	3.290	3.452	3.589	3.707	3.809
120	1.822	2.440	2.805	3.063	3.260	3.420	3.554	3.669	3.770
∞	1.812	2.424	2.784	3.037	3.232	3.389	3.520	3.632	3.730

ν\n	11	12	13	14	15	16	17	18	19
1	12.50	12.84	13.14	13.43	13.68	13.93	14.14	14.35	14.54
2	6.826	7.002	7.162	7.308	7.442	7.566	7.682	7.790	7.891
3	5.637	5.778	5.906	6.023	6.131	6.230	6.323	6.410	6.491
4	5.128	5.253	5.367	5.471	5.566	5.655	5.738	5.815	5.888
5	4.844	4.960	5.066	5.162	5.251	5.334	5.411	5.482	5.550
6	4.663	4.773	4.873	4.965	5.049	5.128	5.201	5.269	5.333
7	4.537	4.643	4.739	4.827	4.908	4.984	5.054	5.120	5.181
8	4.444	4.547	4.640	4.726	4.805	4.877	4.945	5.009	5.069
9	4.372	4.473	4.564	4.647	4.724	4.796	4.862	4.924	4.982
10	4.316	4.414	4.503	4.585	4.660	4.730	4.795	4.856	4.913
11	4.270	4.366	4.454	4.534	4.608	4.677	4.741	4.801	4.857
12	4.231	4.327	4.413	4.492	4.565	4.633	4.696	4.755	4.810
13	4.199	4.293	4.379	4.457	4.529	4.596	4.658	4.716	4.770
14	4.172	4.265	4.349	4.426	4.498	4.564	4.625	4.683	4.737
15	4.148	4.240	4.324	4.400	4.471	4.536	4.597	4.654	4.707
16	4.127	4.218	4.301	4.377	4.447	4.512	4.572	4.628	4.681
17	4.109	4.199	4.282	4.357	4.426	4.490	4.550	4.606	4.659
18	4.093	4.182	4.264	4.339	4.407	4.471	4.531	4.586	4.638
19	4.078	4.167	4.248	4.323	4.391	4.454	4.513	4.569	4.620
20	4.065	4.154	4.234	4.308	4.376	4.439	4.498	4.552	4.604
24	4.024	4.111	4.190	4.262	4.329	4.391	4.448	4.502	4.552
30	3.982	4.068	4.145	4.216	4.281	4.342	4.398	4.451	4.500
40	3.941	4.025	4.101	4.170	4.234	4.293	4.348	4.399	4.447
60	3.900	3.982	4.056	4.124	4.186	4.244	4.297	4.347	4.395
120	3.859	3.938	4.011	4.077	4.138	4.194	4.246	4.295	4.341
∞	3.817	3.895	3.966	4.030	4.089	4.144	4.195	4.242	4.287

P = .80

ν\n	20	22	24	26	28	30	32	34	36
1	14.72	15.06	15.36	15.63	15.88	16.11	16.32	16.52	16.71
2	7.986	8.162	8.320	8.463	8.594	8.715	8.827	8.931	9.029
3	6.568	6.709	6.835	6.951	7.057	7.154	7.244	7.328	7.407
4	5.956	6.082	6.195	6.298	6.392	6.479	6.560	6.635	6.706
5	5.613	5.730	5.835	5.931	6.019	6.100	6.175	6.245	6.311
6	5.393	5.504	5.604	5.695	5.779	5.856	5.927	5.994	6.056
7	5.239	5.346	5.442	5.530	5.610	5.684	5.753	5.817	5.877
8	5.125	5.228	5.322	5.407	5.485	5.557	5.624	5.686	5.744
9	5.037	5.138	5.229	5.312	5.388	5.459	5.524	5.585	5.641
10	4.967	5.066	5.155	5.237	5.311	5.380	5.444	5.504	5.559
11	4.910	5.007	5.095	5.175	5.248	5.316	5.379	5.437	5.492
12	4.862	4.958	5.044	5.123	5.196	5.262	5.324	5.382	5.436
13	4.822	4.917	5.002	5.080	5.151	5.217	5.278	5.335	5.388
14	4.787	4.881	4.965	5.042	5.113	5.178	5.238	5.295	5.347
15	4.757	4.850	4.934	5.010	5.080	5.144	5.204	5.260	5.312
16	4.731	4.823	4.906	4.981	5.050	5.114	5.174	5.229	5.281
17	4.708	4.799	4.881	4.956	5.025	5.088	5.147	5.202	5.253
18	4.688	4.778	4.859	4.934	5.002	5.065	5.123	5.177	5.228
19	4.669	4.759	4.840	4.914	4.981	5.044	5.102	5.156	5.206
20	4.652	4.742	4.822	4.895	4.963	5.025	5.082	5.136	5.186
24	4.599	4.687	4.766	4.838	4.904	4.964	5.021	5.073	5.122
30	4.546	4.632	4.710	4.779	4.844	4.903	4.958	5.010	5.058
40	4.493	4.576	4.652	4.720	4.783	4.841	4.895	4.945	4.993
60	4.439	4.520	4.594	4.661	4.722	4.778	4.831	4.880	4.925
120	4.384	4.463	4.535	4.600	4.659	4.714	4.765	4.812	4.857
∞	4.329	4.405	4.475	4.537	4.595	4.648	4.697	4.743	4.786

ν\n	38	40	50	60	70	80	90	100	
1	16.88	17.05	17.74	18.30	18.76	19.15	19.49	19.79	
2	9.121	9.207	9.576	9.869	10.11	10.32	10.50	10.66	
3	7.481	7.551	7.849	8.086	8.283	8.450	8.596	8.725	
4	6.771	6.834	7.100	7.313	7.489	7.639	7.769	7.885	
5	6.372	6.430	6.678	6.877	7.041	7.181	7.303	7.411	
6	6.115	6.170	6.406	6.595	6.751	6.885	7.001	7.103	
7	5.934	5.987	6.214	6.397	6.548	6.676	6.788	6.887	
8	5.799	5.851	6.072	6.249	6.395	6.520	6.629	6.725	
9	5.695	5.745	5.961	6.134	6.277	6.399	6.506	6.600	
10	5.612	5.661	5.873	6.042	6.182	6.302	6.407	6.499	
11	5.544	5.592	5.800	5.967	6.105	6.223	6.326	6.416	
12	5.487	5.535	5.740	5.904	6.040	6.156	6.257	6.347	
13	5.438	5.486	5.689	5.850	5.985	6.100	6.200	6.288	
14	5.397	5.444	5.644	5.804	5.937	6.051	6.150	6.237	
15	5.361	5.407	5.606	5.764	5.896	6.008	6.106	6.193	
16	5.329	5.375	5.572	5.729	5.859	5.971	6.068	6.154	
17	5.301	5.347	5.542	5.698	5.827	5.938	6.034	6.119	
18	5.276	5.321	5.515	5.670	5.798	5.908	6.004	6.089	
19	5.254	5.299	5.491	5.645	5.772	5.881	5.976	6.061	
20	5.233	5.278	5.469	5.622	5.749	5.857	5.951	6.035	
24	5.169	5.212	5.400	5.549	5.674	5.780	5.872	5.954	
30	5.103	5.146	5.329	5.475	5.597	5.701	5.791	5.871	
40	5.037	5.078	5.257	5.399	5.518	5.619	5.708	5.786	
60	4.969	5.009	5.183	5.321	5.437	5.535	5.621	5.697	
120	4.899	4.938	5.106	5.240	5.352	5.447	5.530	5.603	
∞	4.826	4.864	5.026	5.155	5.262	5.353	5.433	5.503	

P = .90

ν\n	2	3	4	5	6	7	8	9	10
1	8.929	13.44	16.36	18.49	20.15	21.51	22.64	23.62	24.48
2	4.130	5.733	6.773	7.538	8.139	8.633	9.049	9.409	9.725
3	3.328	4.467	5.199	5.738	6.162	6.511	6.806	7.062	7.287
4	3.015	3.976	4.586	5.035	5.388	5.679	5.926	6.139	6.327
5	2.850	3.717	4.264	4.664	4.979	5.238	5.458	5.648	5.816
6	2.748	3.559	4.065	4.435	4.726	4.966	5.168	5.344	5.499
7	2.680	3.451	3.931	4.280	4.555	4.780	4.972	5.137	5.283
8	2.630	3.374	3.834	4.169	4.431	4.646	4.829	4.987	5.126
9	2.592	3.316	3.761	4.084	4.337	4.545	4.721	4.873	5.007
10	2.563	3.270	3.704	4.018	4.264	4.465	4.636	4.783	4.913
11	2.540	3.234	3.658	3.965	4.205	4.401	4.568	4.711	4.838
12	2.521	3.204	3.621	3.922	4.156	4.349	4.511	4.652	4.776
13	2.505	3.179	3.589	3.885	4.116	4.305	4.464	4.602	4.724
14	2.491	3.158	3.563	3.854	4.081	4.267	4.424	4.560	4.680
15	2.479	3.140	3.540	3.828	4.052	4.235	4.390	4.524	4.641
16	2.469	3.124	3.520	3.804	4.026	4.207	4.360	4.492	4.608
17	2.460	3.110	3.503	3.784	4.004	4.183	4.334	4.464	4.579
18	2.452	3.098	3.488	3.767	3.984	4.161	4.311	4.440	4.554
19	2.445	3.087	3.474	3.751	3.966	4.142	4.290	4.418	4.531
20	2.439	3.078	3.462	3.736	3.950	4.124	4.271	4.398	4.510
24	2.420	3.047	3.423	3.692	3.900	4.070	4.213	4.336	4.445
30	2.400	3.017	3.386	3.648	3.851	4.016	4.155	4.275	4.381
40	2.381	2.988	3.349	3.605	3.803	3.963	4.099	4.215	4.317
60	2.363	2.959	3.312	3.562	3.755	3.911	4.042	4.155	4.254
120	2.344	2.930	3.276	3.520	3.707	3.859	3.987	4.096	4.191
∞	2.326	2.902	3.240	3.478	3.661	3.808	3.931	4.037	4.129

ν\n	11	12	13	14	15	16	17	18	19
1	25.24	25.92	26.54	27.10	27.62	28.10	28.54	28.96	29.35
2	10.01	10.26	10.49	10.70	10.89	11.07	11.24	11.39	11.54
3	7.487	7.667	7.832	7.982	8.120	8.249	8.368	8.479	8.584
4	6.495	6.645	6.783	6.909	7.025	7.133	7.233	7.327	7.414
5	5.966	6.101	6.223	6.336	6.440	6.536	6.626	6.710	6.789
6	5.637	5.762	5.875	5.979	6.075	6.164	6.247	6.325	6.398
7	5.413	5.530	5.637	5.735	5.826	5.910	5.988	6.061	6.130
8	5.250	5.362	5.464	5.558	5.644	5.724	5.799	5.869	5.935
9	5.127	5.234	5.333	5.423	5.506	5.583	5.655	5.723	5.786
10	5.029	5.134	5.229	5.317	5.397	5.472	5.542	5.607	5.668
11	4.951	5.053	5.146	5.231	5.309	5.382	5.450	5.514	5.573
12	4.886	4.986	5.077	5.160	5.236	5.308	5.374	5.436	5.495
13	4.832	4.930	5.019	5.100	5.176	5.245	5.311	5.372	5.429
14	4.786	4.882	4.970	5.050	5.124	5.192	5.256	5.316	5.373
15	4.746	4.841	4.927	5.006	5.079	5.147	5.209	5.269	5.324
16	4.712	4.805	4.890	4.968	5.040	5.107	5.169	5.227	5.282
17	4.682	4.774	4.858	4.935	5.005	5.071	5.133	5.190	5.244
18	4.655	4.746	4.829	4.905	4.975	5.040	5.101	5.158	5.211
19	4.631	4.721	4.803	4.879	4.948	5.012	5.073	5.129	5.182
20	4.609	4.699	4.780	4.855	4.924	4.987	5.047	5.103	5.155
24	4.541	4.628	4.708	4.780	4.847	4.909	4.966	5.021	5.071
30	4.474	4.559	4.635	4.706	4.770	4.830	4.886	4.939	4.988
40	4.408	4.490	4.564	4.632	4.695	4.752	4.807	4.857	4.905
60	4.342	4.421	4.493	4.558	4.619	4.675	4.727	4.775	4.821
120	4.276	4.353	4.422	4.485	4.543	4.597	4.647	4.694	4.738
∞	4.211	4.285	4.351	4.412	4.468	4.519	4.568	4.612	4.654

P = .90

ν\n	20	22	24	26	28	30	32	34	36
1	29.71	30.39	30.99	31.54	32.04	32.50	32.93	33.33	33.71
2	11.68	11.93	12.16	12.36	12.55	12.73	12.89	13.04	13.18
3	8.683	8.864	9.029	9.177	9.314	9.440	9.557	9.666	9.768
4	7.497	7.650	7.789	7.914	8.029	8.135	8.234	8.326	8.412
5	6.863	7.000	7.123	7.236	7.340	7.435	7.523	7.606	7.683
6	6.467	6.593	6.708	6.812	6.908	6.996	7.078	7.155	7.227
7	6.195	6.315	6.422	6.521	6.611	6.695	6.773	6.845	6.913
8	5.997	6.111	6.214	6.308	6.395	6.475	6.549	6.618	6.683
9	5.846	5.956	6.055	6.146	6.229	6.306	6.378	6.444	6.507
10	5.726	5.833	5.930	6.017	6.098	6.173	6.242	6.307	6.368
11	5.630	5.734	5.828	5.914	5.992	6.065	6.132	6.196	6.255
12	5.550	5.652	5.744	5.827	5.904	5.976	6.042	6.103	6.161
13	5.483	5.583	5.673	5.755	5.830	5.900	5.965	6.025	6.082
14	5.426	5.524	5.612	5.693	5.767	5.836	5.899	5.959	6.014
15	5.376	5.473	5.560	5.639	5.713	5.780	5.843	5.901	5.956
16	5.333	5.428	5.515	5.593	5.665	5.732	5.793	5.851	5.905
17	5.295	5.389	5.474	5.552	5.623	5.689	5.750	5.806	5.860
18	5.262	5.355	5.439	5.515	5.585	5.650	5.711	5.767	5.820
19	5.232	5.324	5.407	5.483	5.552	5.616	5.676	5.732	5.784
20	5.205	5.296	5.378	5.453	5.522	5.586	5.645	5.700	5.752
24	5.119	5.208	5.287	5.360	5.427	5.489	5.546	5.600	5.650
30	5.034	5.120	5.197	5.267	5.332	5.392	5.447	5.499	5.547
40	4.949	5.032	5.107	5.174	5.236	5.294	5.347	5.397	5.444
60	4.864	4.944	5.015	5.081	5.141	5.196	5.247	5.295	5.340
120	4.779	4.856	4.924	4.987	5.044	5.097	5.146	5.192	5.235
∞	4.694	4.767	4.832	4.892	4.947	4.997	5.044	5.087	5.128

ν\n	38	40	50	60	70	80	90	100
1	34.06	34.38	35.79	36.91	37.83	38.62	39.30	39.91
2	13.31	13.44	13.97	14.40	14.75	15.05	15.31	15.54
3	9.864	9.954	10.34	10.65	10.91	11.12	11.31	11.48
4	8.493	8.569	8.896	9.156	9.373	9.557	9.718	9.860
5	7.756	7.825	8.118	8.353	8.548	8.715	8.859	8.988
6	7.294	7.358	7.630	7.848	8.029	8.184	8.319	8.438
7	6.976	7.036	7.294	7.500	7.672	7.818	7.946	8.059
8	6.744	6.801	7.048	7.245	7.409	7.550	7.672	7.780
9	6.566	6.621	6.859	7.050	7.208	7.343	7.461	7.566
10	6.425	6.479	6.709	6.895	7.048	7.180	7.295	7.396
11	6.310	6.363	6.588	6.768	6.918	7.047	7.158	7.258
12	6.215	6.267	6.487	6.663	6.810	6.936	7.045	7.142
13	6.135	6.186	6.402	6.575	6.719	6.842	6.949	7.045
14	6.067	6.116	6.329	6.499	6.641	6.762	6.868	6.961
15	6.008	6.057	6.266	6.433	6.573	6.692	6.796	6.888
16	5.956	6.004	6.210	6.376	6.513	6.631	6.734	6.825
17	5.910	5.958	6.162	6.325	6.461	6.577	6.679	6.769
18	5.870	5.917	6.118	6.280	6.414	6.529	6.630	6.719
19	5.833	5.880	6.079	6.239	6.372	6.486	6.585	6.674
20	5.801	5.847	6.044	6.203	6.335	6.447	6.546	6.633
24	5.697	5.741	5.933	6.086	6.214	6.324	6.419	6.503
30	5.593	5.636	5.821	5.969	6.093	6.198	6.291	6.372
40	5.488	5.529	5.708	5.850	5.969	6.071	6.160	6.238
60	5.382	5.422	5.593	5.730	5.844	5.941	6.026	6.102
120	5.275	5.313	5.476	5.606	5.715	5.808	5.888	5.960
∞	5.166	5.202	5.357	5.480	5.582	5.669	5.745	5.812

P = .95

ν\n	2	3	4	5	6	7	8	9	10
1	17.97	26.98	32.82	37.08	40.41	43.12	45.40	47.36	49.07
2	6.085	8.331	9.798	10.88	11.74	12.44	13.03	13.54	13.99
3	4.501	5.910	6.825	7.502	8.037	8.478	8.853	9.177	9.462
4	3.927	5.040	5.757	6.287	6.707	7.053	7.347	7.602	7.826
5	3.635	4.602	5.218	5.673	6.033	6.330	6.582	6.802	6.995
6	3.461	4.339	4.896	5.305	5.628	5.895	6.122	6.319	6.493
7	3.344	4.165	4.681	5.060	5.359	5.606	5.815	5.998	6.158
8	3.261	4.041	4.529	4.886	5.167	5.399	5.597	5.767	5.918
9	3.199	3.949	4.415	4.756	5.024	5.244	5.432	5.595	5.739
10	3.151	3.877	4.327	4.654	4.912	5.124	5.305	5.461	5.599
11	3.113	3.820	4.256	4.574	4.823	5.028	5.202	5.353	5.487
12	3.082	3.773	4.199	4.508	4.751	4.950	5.119	5.265	5.395
13	3.055	3.735	4.151	4.453	4.690	4.885	5.049	5.192	5.318
14	3.033	3.702	4.111	4.407	4.639	4.829	4.990	5.131	5.254
15	3.014	3.674	4.076	4.367	4.595	4.782	4.940	5.077	5.198
16	2.998	3.649	4.046	4.333	4.557	4.741	4.897	5.031	5.150
17	2.984	3.628	4.020	4.303	4.524	4.705	4.858	4.991	5.108
18	2.971	3.609	3.997	4.277	4.495	4.673	4.824	4.956	5.071
19	2.960	3.593	3.977	4.253	4.469	4.645	4.794	4.924	5.038
20	2.950	3.578	3.958	4.232	4.445	4.620	4.768	4.896	5.008
24	2.919	3.532	3.901	4.166	4.373	4.541	4.684	4.807	4.915
30	2.888	3.486	3.845	4.102	4.302	4.464	4.602	4.720	4.824
40	2.858	3.442	3.791	4.039	4.232	4.389	4.521	4.635	4.735
60	2.829	3.399	3.737	3.977	4.163	4.314	4.441	4.550	4.646
120	2.800	3.356	3.685	3.917	4.096	4.241	4.363	4.468	4.560
∞	2.772	3.314	3.633	3.858	4.030	4.170	4.286	4.387	4.474

ν\n	11	12	13	14	15	16	17	18	19
1	50.59	51.96	53.20	54.33	55.36	56.32	57.22	58.04	58.83
2	14.39	14.75	15.08	15.38	15.65	15.91	16.14	16.37	16.57
3	9.717	9.946	10.15	10.35	10.53	10.69	10.84	10.98	11.11
4	8.027	8.208	8.373	8.525	8.664	8.794	8.914	9.028	9.134
5	7.168	7.324	7.466	7.596	7.717	7.828	7.932	8.030	8.122
6	6.649	6.789	6.917	7.034	7.143	7.244	7.338	7.426	7.508
7	6.302	6.431	6.550	6.658	6.759	6.852	6.939	7.020	7.097
8	6.054	6.175	6.287	6.389	6.483	6.571	6.653	6.729	6.802
9	5.867	5.983	6.089	6.186	6.276	6.359	6.437	6.510	6.579
10	5.722	5.833	5.935	6.028	6.114	6.194	6.269	6.339	6.405
11	5.605	5.713	5.811	5.901	5.984	6.062	6.134	6.202	6.265
12	5.511	5.615	5.710	5.798	5.878	5.953	6.023	6.089	6.151
13	5.431	5.533	5.625	5.711	5.789	5.862	5.931	5.995	6.055
14	5.364	5.463	5.554	5.637	5.714	5.786	5.852	5.915	5.974
15	5.306	5.404	5.493	5.574	5.649	5.720	5.785	5.846	5.904
16	5.256	5.352	5.439	5.520	5.593	5.662	5.727	5.786	5.843
17	5.212	5.307	5.392	5.471	5.544	5.612	5.675	5.734	5.790
18	5.174	5.267	5.352	5.429	5.501	5.568	5.630	5.688	5.743
19	5.140	5.231	5.315	5.391	5.462	5.528	5.589	5.647	5.701
20	5.108	5.199	5.282	5.357	5.427	5.493	5.553	5.610	5.663
24	5.012	5.099	5.179	5.251	5.319	5.381	5.439	5.494	5.545
30	4.917	5.001	5.077	5.147	5.211	5.271	5.327	5.379	5.429
40	4.824	4.904	4.977	5.044	5.106	5.163	5.216	5.266	5.313
60	4.732	4.808	4.878	4.942	5.001	5.056	5.107	5.154	5.199
120	4.641	4.714	4.781	4.842	4.898	4.950	4.998	5.044	5.086
∞	4.552	4.622	4.685	4.743	4.796	4.845	4.891	4.934	4.974

P = .95

ν\n	20	22	24	26	28	30	32	34	36
1	59.56	60.91	62.12	63.22	64.23	65.15	66.01	66.81	67.56
2	16.77	17.13	17.45	17.75	18.02	18.27	18.50	18.72	18.92
3	11.24	11.47	11.68	11.87	12.05	12.21	12.36	12.50	12.63
4	9.233	9.418	9.584	9.736	9.875	10.00	10.12	10.23	10.34
5	8.208	8.368	8.512	8.643	8.764	8.875	8.979	9.075	9.165
6	7.587	7.730	7.861	7.979	8.088	8.189	8.283	8.370	8.452
7	7.170	7.303	7.423	7.533	7.634	7.728	7.814	7.895	7.972
8	6.870	6.995	7.109	7.212	7.307	7.395	7.477	7.554	7.625
9	6.644	6.763	6.871	6.970	7.061	7.145	7.222	7.295	7.363
10	6.467	6.582	6.686	6.781	6.868	6.948	7.023	7.093	7.159
11	6.326	6.436	6.536	6.628	6.712	6.790	6.863	6.930	6.994
12	6.209	6.317	6.414	6.503	6.585	6.660	6.731	6.796	6.858
13	6.112	6.217	6.312	6.398	6.478	6.551	6.620	6.684	6.744
14	6.029	6.132	6.224	6.309	6.387	6.459	6.526	6.588	6.647
15	5.958	6.059	6.149	6.233	6.309	6.379	6.445	6.506	6.564
16	5.897	5.995	6.084	6.166	6.241	6.310	6.374	6.434	6.491
17	5.842	5.940	6.027	6.107	6.181	6.249	6.313	6.372	6.427
18	5.794	5.890	5.977	6.055	6.128	6.195	6.258	6.316	6.371
19	5.752	5.846	5.932	6.009	6.081	6.147	6.209	6.267	6.321
20	5.714	5.807	5.891	5.968	6.039	6.104	6.165	6.222	6.275
24	5.594	5.683	5.764	5.838	5.906	5.968	6.027	6.081	6.132
30	5.475	5.561	5.638	5.709	5.774	5.833	5.889	5.941	5.990
40	5.358	5.439	5.513	5.581	5.642	5.700	5.753	5.803	5.849
60	5.241	5.319	5.389	5.453	5.512	5.566	5.617	5.664	5.708
120	5.126	5.200	5.266	5.327	5.382	5.434	5.481	5.526	5.568
∞	5.012	5.081	5.144	5.201	5.253	5.301	5.346	5.388	5.427

ν\n	38	40	50	60	70	80	90	100	
1	68.26	68.92	71.73	73.97	75.82	77.40	78.77	79.98	
2	19.11	19.28	20.05	20.66	21.16	21.59	21.96	22.29	
3	12.75	12.87	13.36	13.76	14.08	14.36	14.61	14.82	
4	10.44	10.53	10.93	11.24	11.51	11.73	11.92	12.09	
5	9.250	9.330	9.674	9.949	10.18	10.38	10.54	10.69	
6	8.529	8.601	8.913	9.163	9.370	9.548	9.702	9.839	
7	8.043	8.110	8.400	8.632	8.824	8.989	9.133	9.261	
8	7.693	7.756	8.029	8.248	8.430	8.586	8.722	8.843	
9	7.428	7.488	7.749	7.958	8.132	8.281	8.410	8.526	
10	7.220	7.279	7.529	7.730	7.897	8.041	8.166	8.276	
11	7.053	7.110	7.352	7.546	7.708	7.847	7.968	8.075	
12	6.916	6.970	7.205	7.394	7.552	7.687	7.804	7.909	
13	6.800	6.854	7.083	7.267	7.421	7.552	7.667	7.769	
14	6.702	6.754	6.979	7.159	7.309	7.438	7.550	7.650	
15	6.618	6.669	6.888	7.065	7.212	7.339	7.449	7.546	
16	6.544	6.594	6.810	6.984	7.128	7.252	7.360	7.457	
17	6.479	6.529	6.741	6.912	7.054	7.176	7.283	7.377	
18	6.422	6.471	6.680	6.848	6.989	7.109	7.213	7.307	
19	6.371	6.419	6.626	6.792	6.930	7.048	7.152	7.244	
20	6.325	6.373	6.576	6.740	6.877	6.994	7.097	7.187	
24	6.181	6.226	6.421	6.579	6.710	6.822	6.920	7.008	
30	6.037	6.080	6.267	6.417	6.543	6.650	6.744	6.827	
40	5.893	5.934	6.112	6.255	6.375	6.477	6.566	6.645	
60	5.750	5.789	5.958	6.093	6.206	6.303	6.387	6.462	
120	5.607	5.644	5.802	5.929	6.035	6.126	6.205	6.275	
∞	5.463	5.498	5.646	5.764	5.863	5.947	6.020	6.085	

P = .975

ν\n	2	3	4	5	6	7	8	9	10
1	35.99	54.00	65.69	74.22	80.87	86.29	90.85	94.77	98.20
2	8.776	11.94	14.01	15.54	16.75	17.74	18.58	19.31	19.95
3	5.907	7.661	8.808	9.660	10.34	10.89	11.37	11.78	12.14
4	4.943	6.244	7.088	7.716	8.213	8.625	8.976	9.279	9.548
5	4.474	5.558	6.257	6.775	7.186	7.527	7.816	8.068	8.291
6	4.199	5.158	5.772	6.226	6.586	6.884	7.138	7.359	7.554
7	4.018	4.897	5.455	5.868	6.194	6.464	6.695	6.895	7.072
8	3.892	4.714	5.233	5.616	5.919	6.169	6.382	6.568	6.732
9	3.797	4.578	5.069	5.430	5.715	5.950	6.151	6.325	6.479
10	3.725	4.474	4.943	5.287	5.558	5.782	5.972	6.138	6.285
11	3.667	4.391	4.843	5.173	5.433	5.648	5.831	5.989	6.130
12	3.620	4.325	4.762	5.081	5.332	5.540	5.716	5.869	6.004
13	3.582	4.269	4.694	5.004	5.248	5.449	5.620	5.769	5.900
14	3.550	4.222	4.638	4.940	5.178	5.374	5.540	5.684	5.811
15	3.522	4.182	4.589	4.885	5.118	5.309	5.471	5.612	5.737
16	3.498	4.148	4.548	4.838	5.066	5.253	5.412	5.550	5.672
17	3.477	4.118	4.512	4.797	5.020	5.204	5.361	5.496	5.615
18	3.458	4.092	4.480	4.761	4.981	5.162	5.315	5.448	5.565
19	3.442	4.068	4.451	4.728	4.945	5.123	5.275	5.405	5.521
20	3.427	4.047	4.426	4.700	4.914	5.089	5.238	5.368	5.481
24	3.381	3.983	4.347	4.610	4.816	4.984	5.126	5.250	5.358
30	3.337	3.919	4.271	4.523	4.720	4.881	5.017	5.134	5.238
40	3.294	3.858	4.197	4.439	4.627	4.780	4.910	5.022	5.120
60	3.251	3.798	4.124	4.356	4.536	4.682	4.806	4.912	5.006
120	3.210	3.739	4.053	4.276	4.447	4.587	4.704	4.805	4.894
∞	3.170	3.682	3.984	4.197	4.361	4.494	4.605	4.700	4.784

ν\n	11	12	13	14	15	16	17	18	19
1	101.3	104.0	106.5	108.8	110.8	112.7	114.5	116.2	117.7
2	20.52	21.03	21.49	21.91	22.30	22.67	23.01	23.32	23.62
3	12.46	12.75	13.01	13.26	13.48	13.69	13.88	14.06	14.23
4	9.788	10.01	10.20	10.39	10.55	10.71	10.85	10.99	11.11
5	8.490	8.670	8.834	8.984	9.124	9.253	9.374	9.486	9.593
6	7.729	7.887	8.031	8.163	8.286	8.399	8.506	8.605	8.698
7	7.230	7.373	7.504	7.624	7.735	7.839	7.935	8.025	8.111
8	6.879	7.011	7.132	7.244	7.347	7.443	7.532	7.616	7.695
9	6.617	6.742	6.856	6.961	7.058	7.148	7.232	7.311	7.385
10	6.416	6.534	6.643	6.742	6.834	6.920	7.000	7.075	7.146
11	6.256	6.369	6.473	6.568	6.657	6.739	6.815	6.887	6.955
12	6.125	6.235	6.335	6.427	6.512	6.591	6.665	6.734	6.799
13	6.017	6.123	6.220	6.309	6.392	6.468	6.539	6.607	6.670
14	5.926	6.029	6.123	6.210	6.290	6.364	6.434	6.499	6.560
15	5.848	5.949	6.041	6.125	6.203	6.276	6.344	6.407	6.467
16	5.781	5.879	5.969	6.052	6.128	6.199	6.265	6.328	6.386
17	5.722	5.818	5.907	5.987	6.062	6.132	6.197	6.258	6.315
18	5.670	5.765	5.852	5.931	6.004	6.073	6.137	6.197	6.253
19	5.624	5.718	5.803	5.881	5.954	6.020	6.083	6.142	6.198
20	5.583	5.675	5.759	5.836	5.907	5.974	6.036	6.093	6.148
24	5.455	5.543	5.623	5.697	5.764	5.827	5.886	5.941	5.994
30	5.330	5.414	5.490	5.560	5.624	5.684	5.740	5.792	5.841
40	5.208	5.288	5.360	5.426	5.487	5.544	5.597	5.646	5.693
60	5.089	5.164	5.232	5.295	5.352	5.406	5.456	5.503	5.546
120	4.972	5.043	5.107	5.166	5.221	5.271	5.318	5.362	5.403
∞	4.858	4.925	4.985	5.041	5.092	5.139	5.183	5.224	5.262

P = .975

ν\n	20	22	24	26	28	30	32	34	36
1	119.2	121.9	124.3	126.5	128.6	130.4	132.1	133.7	135.2
2	23.89	24.41	24.87	25.29	25.67	26.03	26.35	26.66	26.95
3	14.39	14.69	14.95	15.19	15.41	15.62	15.81	15.99	16.15
4	11.23	11.46	11.66	11.84	12.00	12.16	12.30	12.44	12.56
5	9.693	9.878	10.04	10.20	10.34	10.47	10.59	10.70	10.80
6	8.787	8.949	9.097	9.231	9.355	9.469	9.575	9.674	9.767
7	8.191	8.339	8.473	8.595	8.708	8.812	8.909	8.999	9.084
8	7.769	7.907	8.031	8.145	8.250	8.346	8.436	8.520	8.599
9	7.455	7.585	7.702	7.809	7.908	7.999	8.084	8.163	8.237
10	7.212	7.335	7.447	7.549	7.643	7.729	7.810	7.885	7.956
11	7.019	7.137	7.244	7.341	7.431	7.514	7.592	7.664	7.732
12	6.861	6.974	7.078	7.172	7.258	7.338	7.413	7.483	7.548
13	6.730	6.840	6.939	7.031	7.115	7.192	7.265	7.332	7.396
14	6.619	6.726	6.823	6.911	6.993	7.069	7.139	7.204	7.266
15	6.523	6.628	6.723	6.809	6.889	6.962	7.031	7.095	7.155
16	6.441	6.543	6.636	6.721	6.799	6.870	6.938	7.000	7.059
17	6.370	6.469	6.560	6.644	6.720	6.790	6.856	6.917	6.975
18	6.306	6.404	6.493	6.575	6.650	6.720	6.784	6.844	6.900
19	6.250	6.347	6.434	6.514	6.588	6.656	6.719	6.779	6.835
20	6.200	6.295	6.381	6.460	6.532	6.600	6.662	6.720	6.775
24	6.043	6.133	6.215	6.290	6.359	6.423	6.482	6.538	6.589
30	5.888	5.974	6.052	6.123	6.188	6.248	6.305	6.357	6.406
40	5.737	5.818	5.891	5.958	6.020	6.077	6.130	6.179	6.226
60	5.588	5.664	5.733	5.797	5.854	5.908	5.958	6.004	6.048
120	5.442	5.513	5.578	5.637	5.691	5.741	5.788	5.831	5.872
∞	5.299	5.365	5.425	5.480	5.530	5.577	5.620	5.660	5.698

ν\n	38	40	50	60	70	80	90	100
1	136.6	137.9	143.6	148.1	151.8	154.9	157.7	160.0
2	27.22	27.47	28.55	29.42	30.13	30.74	31.27	31.74
3	16.31	16.46	17.08	17.59	18.00	18.36	18.67	18.95
4	12.68	12.79	13.27	13.65	13.96	14.23	14.47	14.68
5	10.91	11.00	11.40	11.72	11.99	12.21	12.41	12.59
6	9.855	9.938	10.30	10.58	10.81	11.02	11.19	11.35
7	9.164	9.239	9.563	9.822	10.04	10.23	10.38	10.53
8	8.673	8.743	9.044	9.286	9.487	9.660	9.810	9.944
9	8.307	8.373	8.657	8.885	9.076	9.238	9.381	9.507
10	8.023	8.086	8.356	8.574	8.755	8.911	9.046	9.167
11	7.796	7.856	8.116	8.325	8.499	8.648	8.779	8.894
12	7.610	7.668	7.919	8.120	8.289	8.433	8.559	8.671
13	7.455	7.512	7.755	7.950	8.113	8.253	8.375	8.484
14	7.324	7.379	7.615	7.806	7.965	8.101	8.220	8.325
15	7.212	7.265	7.496	7.682	7.837	7.970	8.086	8.189
16	7.115	7.167	7.393	7.574	7.726	7.856	7.969	8.070
17	7.030	7.081	7.302	7.480	7.628	7.756	7.868	7.966
18	6.954	7.005	7.221	7.396	7.543	7.667	7.777	7.874
19	6.887	6.936	7.150	7.322	7.465	7.589	7.696	7.792
20	6.827	6.876	7.086	7.255	7.397	7.518	7.624	7.718
24	6.639	6.685	6.885	7.046	7.180	7.296	7.397	7.486
30	6.453	6.497	6.686	6.839	6.965	7.075	7.171	7.255
40	6.270	6.311	6.489	6.633	6.753	6.855	6.945	7.025
60	6.089	6.127	6.295	6.429	6.540	6.636	6.720	6.795
120	5.910	5.946	6.101	6.225	6.329	6.418	6.495	6.564
∞	5.733	5.766	5.909	6.023	6.118	6.199	6.270	6.333

P = .99

$\nu \backslash n$	2	3	4	5	6	7	8	9	10
1	90.03	135.0	164.3	185.6	202.2	215.8	227.2	237.0	245.6
2	14.04	19.02	22.29	24.72	26.63	28.20	29.53	30.68	31.69
3	8.261	10.62	12.17	13.33	14.24	15.00	15.64	16.20	16.69
4	6.512	8.120	9.173	9.958	10.58	11.10	11.55	11.93	12.27
5	5.702	6.976	7.804	8.421	8.913	9.321	9.669	9.972	10.24
6	5.243	6.331	7.033	7.556	7.973	8.318	8.613	8.869	9.097
7	4.949	5.919	6.543	7.005	7.373	7.679	7.939	8.166	8.368
8	4.746	5.635	6.204	6.625	6.960	7.237	7.474	7.681	7.863
9	4.596	5.428	5.957	6.348	6.658	6.915	7.134	7.325	7.495
10	4.482	5.270	5.769	6.136	6.428	6.669	6.875	7.055	7.213
11	4.392	5.146	5.621	5.970	6.247	6.476	6.672	6.842	6.992
12	4.320	5.046	5.502	5.836	6.101	6.321	6.507	6.670	6.814
13	4.260	4.964	5.404	5.727	5.981	6.192	6.372	6.528	6.667
14	4.210	4.895	5.322	5.634	5.881	6.085	6.258	6.409	6.543
15	4.168	4.836	5.252	5.556	5.796	5.994	6.162	6.309	6.439
16	4.131	4.786	5.192	5.489	5.722	5.915	6.079	6.222	6.349
17	4.099	4.742	5.140	5.430	5.659	5.847	6.007	6.147	6.270
18	4.071	4.703	5.094	5.379	5.603	5.788	5.944	6.081	6.201
19	4.046	4.670	5.054	5.334	5.554	5.735	5.889	6.022	6.141
20	4.024	4.639	5.018	5.294	5.510	5.688	5.839	5.970	6.087
24	3.956	4.546	4.907	5.168	5.374	5.542	5.685	5.809	5.919
30	3.889	4.455	4.799	5.048	5.242	5.401	5.536	5.653	5.756
40	3.825	4.367	4.696	4.931	5.114	5.265	5.392	5.502	5.599
60	3.762	4.282	4.595	4.818	4.991	5.133	5.253	5.356	5.447
120	3.702	4.200	4.497	4.709	4.872	5.005	5.118	5.214	5.299
∞	3.643	4.120	4.403	4.603	4.757	4.882	4.987	5.078	5.157

$\nu \backslash n$	11	12	13	14	15	16	17	18	19
1	253.2	260.0	266.2	271.8	277.0	281.8	286.3	290.4	294.3
2	32.59	33.40	34.13	34.81	35.43	36.00	36.53	37.03	37.50
3	17.13	17.53	17.89	18.22	18.52	18.81	19.07	19.32	19.55
4	12.57	12.84	13.09	13.32	13.53	13.73	13.91	14.08	14.24
5	10.48	10.70	10.89	11.08	11.24	11.40	11.55	11.68	11.81
6	9.301	9.485	9.653	9.808	9.951	10.08	10.21	10.32	10.43
7	8.548	8.711	8.860	8.997	9.124	9.242	9.353	9.456	9.554
8	8.027	8.176	8.312	8.436	8.552	8.659	8.760	8.854	8.943
9	7.647	7.784	7.910	8.025	8.132	8.232	8.325	8.412	8.495
10	7.356	7.485	7.603	7.712	7.812	7.906	7.993	8.076	8.153
11	7.128	7.250	7.362	7.465	7.560	7.649	7.732	7.809	7.883
12	6.943	7.060	7.167	7.265	7.356	7.441	7.520	7.594	7.665
13	6.791	6.903	7.006	7.101	7.188	7.269	7.345	7.417	7.485
14	6.664	6.772	6.871	6.962	7.047	7.126	7.199	7.268	7.333
15	6.555	6.660	6.757	6.845	6.927	7.003	7.074	7.142	7.204
16	6.462	6.564	6.658	6.744	6.823	6.898	6.967	7.032	7.093
17	6.381	6.480	6.572	6.656	6.734	6.806	6.873	6.937	6.997
18	6.310	6.407	6.497	6.579	6.655	6.725	6.792	6.854	6.912
19	6.247	6.342	6.430	6.510	6.585	6.654	6.719	6.780	6.837
20	6.191	6.285	6.371	6.450	6.523	6.591	6.654	6.714	6.771
24	6.017	6.106	6.186	6.261	6.330	6.394	6.453	6.510	6.563
30	5.849	5.932	6.008	6.078	6.143	6.203	6.259	6.311	6.361
40	5.686	5.764	5.835	5.900	5.961	6.017	6.069	6.119	6.165
60	5.528	5.601	5.667	5.728	5.785	5.837	5.886	5.931	5.974
120	5.375	5.443	5.505	5.562	5.614	5.662	5.708	5.750	5.790
∞	5.227	5.290	5.348	5.400	5.448	5.493	5.535	5.574	5.611

P = .99

ν\n	20	22	24	26	28	30	32	34	36
1	298.0	304.7	310.8	316.3	321.3	326.0	330.3	334.3	338.0
2	37.95	38.76	39.49	40.15	40.76	41.32	41.84	42.33	42.78
3	19.77	20.17	20.53	20.86	21.16	21.44	21.70	21.95	22.17
4	14.40	14.68	14.93	15.16	15.37	15.57	15.75	15.92	16.08
5	11.93	12.16	12.36	12.54	12.71	12.87	13.02	13.15	13.28
6	10.54	10.73	10.91	11.06	11.21	11.34	11.47	11.58	11.69
7	9.646	9.815	9.970	10.11	10.24	10.36	10.47	10.58	10.67
8	9.027	9.182	9.322	9.450	9.569	9.678	9.779	9.874	9.964
9	8.573	8.717	8.847	8.966	9.075	9.177	9.271	9.360	9.443
10	8.226	8.361	8.483	8.595	8.698	8.794	8.883	8.966	9.044
11	7.952	8.080	8.196	8.303	8.400	8.491	8.575	8.654	8.728
12	7.731	7.853	7.964	8.066	8.159	8.246	8.327	8.402	8.473
13	7.548	7.665	7.772	7.870	7.960	8.043	8.121	8.193	8.262
14	7.395	7.508	7.611	7.705	7.792	7.873	7.948	8.018	8.084
15	7.264	7.374	7.474	7.566	7.650	7.728	7.800	7.869	7.932
16	7.152	7.258	7.356	7.445	7.527	7.602	7.673	7.739	7.802
17	7.053	7.158	7.253	7.340	7.420	7.493	7.563	7.627	7.687
18	6.968	7.070	7.163	7.247	7.325	7.398	7.465	7.528	7.587
19	6.891	6.992	7.082	7.166	7.242	7.313	7.379	7.440	7.498
20	6.823	6.922	7.011	7.092	7.168	7.237	7.302	7.362	7.419
24	6.612	6.705	6.789	6.865	6.936	7.001	7.062	7.119	7.173
30	6.407	6.494	6.572	6.644	6.710	6.772	6.828	6.881	6.932
40	6.209	6.289	6.362	6.429	6.490	6.547	6.600	6.650	6.697
60	6.015	6.090	6.158	6.220	6.277	6.330	6.378	6.424	6.467
120	5.827	5.897	5.959	6.016	6.069	6.117	6.162	6.204	6.244
∞	5.645	5.709	5.766	5.818	5.866	5.911	5.952	5.990	6.026

ν\n	38	40	50	60	70	80	90	100	
1	341.5	344.8	358.9	370.1	379.4	387.3	394.1	400.1	
2	43.21	43.61	45.33	46.70	47.83	48.80	49.64	50.38	
3	22.39	22.59	23.45	24.13	24.71	25.19	25.62	25.99	
4	16.23	16.37	16.98	17.46	17.86	18.20	18.50	18.77	
5	13.40	13.52	14.00	14.39	14.72	14.99	15.23	15.45	
6	11.80	11.90	12.31	12.65	12.92	13.16	13.37	13.55	
7	10.77	10.85	11.23	11.52	11.77	11.99	12.17	12.34	
8	10.05	10.13	10.47	10.75	10.97	11.17	11.34	11.49	
9	9.521	9.594	9.912	10.17	10.38	10.57	10.73	10.87	
10	9.117	9.187	9.486	9.726	9.927	10.10	10.25	10.39	
11	8.798	8.864	9.148	9.377	9.568	9.732	9.875	10.00	
12	8.539	8.603	8.875	9.094	9.277	9.434	9.571	9.693	
13	8.326	8.387	8.648	8.859	9.035	9.187	9.318	9.436	
14	8.146	8.204	8.457	8.661	8.832	8.978	9.106	9.219	
15	7.992	8.049	8.295	8.492	8.658	8.800	8.924	9.035	
16	7.860	7.916	8.154	8.347	8.507	8.646	8.767	8.874	
17	7.745	7.799	8.031	8.219	8.377	8.511	8.630	8.735	
18	7.643	7.696	7.924	8.107	8.261	8.393	8.508	8.611	
19	7.553	7.605	7.828	8.008	8.159	8.288	8.401	8.502	
20	7.473	7.523	7.742	7.919	8.067	8.194	8.305	8.404	
24	7.223	7.270	7.476	7.642	7.780	7.900	8.004	8.097	
30	6.978	7.023	7.215	7.370	7.500	7.611	7.709	7.796	
40	6.740	6.782	6.960	7.104	7.225	7.328	7.419	7.500	
60	6.507	6.546	6.710	6.843	6.954	7.050	7.133	7.207	
120	6.281	6.316	6.467	6.588	6.689	6.776	6.852	6.919	
∞	6.060	6.092	6.228	6.338	6.429	6.507	6.575	6.636	

P = .995

ν\n	2	3	4	5	6	7	8	9	10
1	180.1	270.1	328.5	371.2	404.4	431.6	454.4	474.0	491.1
2	19.93	26.97	31.60	35.02	37.73	39.95	41.83	43.46	44.89
3	10.55	13.50	15.45	16.91	18.06	19.01	19.83	20.53	21.15
4	7.916	9.814	11.06	11.99	12.74	13.35	13.88	14.33	14.74
5	6.751	8.196	9.141	9.847	10.41	10.88	11.28	11.63	11.93
6	6.105	7.306	8.088	8.670	9.135	9.522	9.852	10.14	10.40
7	5.699	6.750	7.429	7.935	8.339	8.674	8.961	9.211	9.433
8	5.420	6.370	6.981	7.435	7.797	8.097	8.354	8.578	8.777
9	5.218	6.096	6.657	7.074	7.405	7.680	7.915	8.120	8.303
10	5.065	5.888	6.412	6.800	7.109	7.365	7.584	7.775	7.944
11	4.945	5.727	6.222	6.588	6.878	7.119	7.325	7.505	7.664
12	4.849	5.597	6.068	6.416	6.693	6.922	7.118	7.288	7.439
13	4.770	5.490	5.943	6.277	6.541	6.760	6.947	7.111	7.255
14	4.704	5.401	5.838	6.160	6.414	6.626	6.805	6.962	7.101
15	4.647	5.325	5.750	6.061	6.308	6.511	6.685	6.837	6.971
16	4.599	5.261	5.674	5.977	6.216	6.413	6.582	6.729	6.859
17	4.557	5.205	5.608	5.903	6.136	6.329	6.493	6.636	6.763
18	4.521	5.156	5.550	5.839	6.067	6.255	6.415	6.554	6.678
19	4.488	5.113	5.500	5.783	6.005	6.189	6.346	6.482	6.603
20	4.460	5.074	5.455	5.732	5.951	6.131	6.285	6.418	6.537
24	4.371	4.955	5.315	5.577	5.783	5.952	6.096	6.221	6.332
30	4.285	4.841	5.181	5.428	5.621	5.780	5.914	6.031	6.135
40	4.202	4.731	5.053	5.284	5.465	5.614	5.739	5.848	5.944
60	4.122	4.625	4.928	5.146	5.316	5.454	5.571	5.673	5.762
120	4.045	4.523	4.809	5.013	5.172	5.301	5.410	5.504	5.586
∞	3.970	4.424	4.694	4.886	5.033	5.154	5.255	5.341	5.418

ν\n	11	12	13	14	15	16	17	18	19
1	506.3	520.0	532.4	543.6	554.0	563.6	572.5	580.9	588.7
2	46.16	47.31	48.35	49.30	50.17	50.99	51.74	52.45	53.12
3	21.70	22.20	22.66	23.08	23.46	23.82	24.15	24.46	24.76
4	15.10	15.42	15.72	15.99	16.24	16.48	16.70	16.90	17.09
5	12.21	12.46	12.69	12.90	13.09	13.27	13.44	13.60	13.75
6	10.63	10.83	11.02	11.20	11.36	11.51	11.65	11.78	11.90
7	9.632	9.812	9.977	10.13	10.27	10.40	10.52	10.64	10.75
8	8.955	9.117	9.265	9.401	9.527	9.644	9.754	9.857	9.953
9	8.466	8.614	8.749	8.874	8.990	9.097	9.198	9.292	9.381
10	8.096	8.234	8.360	8.476	8.583	8.683	8.777	8.865	8.947
11	7.807	7.937	8.055	8.164	8.265	8.359	8.447	8.530	8.608
12	7.575	7.697	7.810	7.914	8.009	8.099	8.183	8.261	8.335
13	7.384	7.502	7.609	7.708	7.800	7.886	7.965	8.040	8.111
14	7.225	7.338	7.442	7.537	7.625	7.707	7.784	7.856	7.924
15	7.091	7.200	7.300	7.392	7.477	7.556	7.630	7.699	7.765
16	6.976	7.081	7.178	7.267	7.349	7.426	7.498	7.566	7.629
17	6.876	6.979	7.072	7.159	7.239	7.314	7.384	7.449	7.511
18	6.788	6.888	6.980	7.064	7.142	7.215	7.283	7.347	7.407
19	6.711	6.809	6.898	6.981	7.057	7.128	7.195	7.257	7.316
20	6.642	6.738	6.826	6.907	6.981	7.051	7.116	7.177	7.235
24	6.431	6.520	6.602	6.677	6.747	6.812	6.872	6.930	6.983
30	6.227	6.310	6.387	6.456	6.521	6.581	6.638	6.691	6.741
40	6.030	6.108	6.179	6.244	6.304	6.360	6.412	6.461	6.507
60	5.841	5.913	5.979	6.039	6.094	6.146	6.194	6.239	6.281
120	5.660	5.726	5.786	5.842	5.893	5.940	5.984	6.025	6.064
∞	5.485	5.546	5.602	5.652	5.699	5.742	5.783	5.820	5.856

P = .995

ν\n	20	22	24	26	28	30	32	34	36
1	596.0	609.5	621.7	632.6	642.7	652.0	660.6	668.5	676.0
2	53.74	54.89	55.92	56.86	57.73	58.52	59.26	59.95	60.59
3	25.03	25.54	26.00	26.42	26.80	27.15	27.48	27.79	28.07
4	17.28	17.61	17.91	18.19	18.44	18.68	18.89	19.09	19.28
5	13.89	14.14	14.38	14.59	14.79	14.96	15.13	15.29	15.44
6	12.02	12.23	12.43	12.61	12.77	12.92	13.06	13.19	13.32
7	10.85	11.03	11.21	11.36	11.50	11.64	11.76	11.88	11.99
8	10.04	10.22	10.37	10.51	10.64	10.76	10.87	10.97	11.07
9	9.465	9.620	9.761	9.890	10.01	10.12	10.22	10.32	10.41
10	9.026	9.170	9.302	9.422	9.532	9.635	9.730	9.820	9.904
11	8.682	8.818	8.941	9.055	9.159	9.256	9.345	9.430	9.509
12	8.405	8.534	8.652	8.759	8.858	8.950	9.036	9.116	9.191
13	8.178	8.302	8.414	8.516	8.611	8.699	8.781	8.857	8.929
14	7.988	8.107	8.215	8.314	8.404	8.489	8.568	8.641	8.710
15	7.827	7.942	8.046	8.141	8.229	8.311	8.387	8.458	8.524
16	7.689	7.800	7.901	7.994	8.078	8.158	8.231	8.300	8.365
17	7.569	7.677	7.775	7.865	7.948	8.024	8.096	8.163	8.226
18	7.464	7.570	7.665	7.753	7.833	7.908	7.978	8.043	8.104
19	7.372	7.474	7.568	7.653	7.732	7.805	7.873	7.937	7.996
20	7.289	7.390	7.481	7.565	7.642	7.713	7.780	7.842	7.901
24	7.034	7.128	7.213	7.291	7.362	7.429	7.491	7.549	7.603
30	6.788	6.875	6.954	7.026	7.093	7.154	7.212	7.265	7.316
40	6.550	6.631	6.704	6.770	6.832	6.889	6.942	6.991	7.038
60	6.321	6.396	6.462	6.523	6.580	6.632	6.681	6.726	6.769
120	6.101	6.169	6.230	6.286	6.337	6.385	6.428	6.470	6.508
∞	5.889	5.951	6.006	6.057	6.103	6.146	6.186	6.223	6.258

ν\n	38	40	50	60	70	80	90	100	
1	683.0	689.6	717.8	740.2	758.8	774.5	788.2	800.3	
2	61.19	61.76	64.19	66.13	67.74	69.10	70.29	71.35	
3	28.34	28.60	29.68	30.55	31.27	31.88	32.42	32.90	
4	19.46	19.63	20.36	20.93	21.42	21.83	22.18	22.50	
5	15.58	15.71	16.27	16.72	17.09	17.41	17.69	17.94	
6	13.43	13.54	14.02	14.40	14.71	14.98	15.21	15.43	
7	12.09	12.18	12.60	12.93	13.21	13.44	13.65	13.84	
8	11.16	11.25	11.63	11.93	12.18	12.39	12.58	12.75	
9	10.49	10.58	10.92	11.20	11.43	11.63	11.80	11.96	
10	9.983	10.06	10.38	10.64	10.86	11.04	11.20	11.35	
11	9.583	9.654	9.957	10.20	10.41	10.59	10.74	10.88	
12	9.262	9.328	9.617	9.850	10.04	10.21	10.36	10.49	
13	8.997	9.061	9.337	9.560	9.747	9.907	10.05	10.17	
14	8.775	8.837	9.103	9.317	9.497	9.652	9.787	9.907	
15	8.587	8.647	8.904	9.111	9.285	9.434	9.565	9.680	
16	8.425	8.483	8.733	8.933	9.102	9.247	9.373	9.486	
17	8.285	8.341	8.583	8.779	8.943	9.084	9.206	9.316	
18	8.162	8.217	8.452	8.643	8.803	8.940	9.061	9.167	
19	8.053	8.106	8.337	8.523	8.679	8.813	8.931	9.036	
20	7.956	8.008	8.234	8.416	8.569	8.700	8.815	8.917	
24	7.655	7.704	7.914	8.083	8.226	8.348	8.455	8.551	
30	7.364	7.409	7.603	7.760	7.893	8.006	8.105	8.193	
40	7.082	7.123	7.302	7.447	7.568	7.672	7.763	7.845	
60	6.808	6.846	7.010	7.143	7.252	7.347	7.431	7.504	
120	6.545	6.580	6.728	6.846	6.946	7.032	7.107	7.173	
∞	6.291	6.322	6.454	6.561	6.649	6.725	6.792	6.850	

P = .999

ν\n	2	3	4	5	6	7	8	9	10
1	900.3	1351.	1643.	1856.	2022.	2158.	2272.	2370.	2455.
2	44.69	60.42	70.77	78.43	84.49	89.46	93.67	97.30	100.5
3	18.28	23.32	26.65	29.13	31.11	32.74	34.12	35.33	36.39
4	12.18	14.99	16.84	18.23	19.34	20.26	21.04	21.73	22.33
5	9.714	11.67	12.96	13.93	14.71	15.35	15.90	16.38	16.81
6	8.427	9.960	10.97	11.72	12.32	12.83	13.26	13.63	13.97
7	7.648	8.930	9.768	10.40	10.90	11.32	11.68	11.99	12.27
8	7.130	8.250	8.978	9.522	9.958	10.32	10.64	10.91	11.15
9	6.762	7.768	8.419	8.906	9.295	9.619	9.897	10.14	10.36
10	6.487	7.411	8.006	8.450	8.804	9.099	9.352	9.573	9.769
11	6.275	7.136	7.687	8.098	8.426	8.699	8.933	9.138	9.319
12	6.106	6.917	7.436	7.821	8.127	8.383	8.601	8.793	8.962
13	5.970	6.740	7.231	7.595	7.885	8.126	8.333	8.513	8.673
14	5.856	6.594	7.062	7.409	7.685	7.915	8.110	8.282	8.434
15	5.760	6.470	6.920	7.252	7.517	7.736	7.925	8.088	8.234
16	5.678	6.365	6.799	7.119	7.374	7.585	7.766	7.923	8.063
17	5.608	6.275	6.695	7.005	7.250	7.454	7.629	7.781	7.916
18	5.546	6.196	6.604	6.905	7.143	7.341	7.510	7.657	7.788
19	5.492	6.127	6.525	6.817	7.049	7.242	7.405	7.549	7.676
20	5.444	6.065	6.454	6.740	6.966	7.154	7.313	7.453	7.577
24	5.297	5.877	6.238	6.503	6.712	6.884	7.031	7.159	7.272
30	5.156	5.698	6.033	6.278	6.470	6.628	6.763	6.880	6.984
40	5.022	5.528	5.838	6.063	6.240	6.386	6.509	6.616	6.711
60	4.894	5.365	5.653	5.860	6.022	6.155	6.268	6.366	6.451
120	4.771	5.211	5.476	5.667	5.815	5.937	6.039	6.128	6.206
∞	4.654	5.063	5.309	5.484	5.619	5.730	5.823	5.903	5.973

ν\n	11	12	13	14	15	16	17	18	19
1	2532.	2600.	2662.	2718.	2770.	2818.	2863.	2904.	2943.
2	103.3	105.9	108.2	110.4	112.3	114.2	115.9	117.4	118.9
3	37.34	38.20	38.98	39.69	40.35	40.97	41.54	42.07	42.58
4	22.87	23.36	23.81	24.21	24.59	24.94	25.27	25.58	25.87
5	17.18	17.53	17.85	18.13	18.41	18.66	18.89	19.10	19.31
6	14.27	14.54	14.79	15.01	15.22	15.42	15.60	15.78	15.94
7	12.52	12.74	12.95	13.14	13.32	13.48	13.64	13.78	13.92
8	11.36	11.56	11.74	11.91	12.06	12.21	12.34	12.47	12.59
9	10.55	10.73	10.89	11.03	11.18	11.30	11.42	11.54	11.64
10	9.946	10.11	10.25	10.39	10.52	10.64	10.75	10.85	10.95
11	9.482	9.630	9.766	9.892	10.01	10.12	10.22	10.31	10.41
12	9.115	9.254	9.381	9.498	9.606	9.707	9.802	9.891	9.975
13	8.817	8.948	9.068	9.178	9.281	9.376	9.466	9.550	9.629
14	8.571	8.696	8.809	8.914	9.012	9.103	9.188	9.267	9.343
15	8.365	8.483	8.592	8.693	8.786	8.872	8.954	9.030	9.102
16	8.189	8.303	8.407	8.504	8.593	8.676	8.755	8.828	8.897
17	8.037	8.148	8.248	8.342	8.427	8.508	8.583	8.654	8.720
18	7.906	8.012	8.110	8.199	8.283	8.361	8.434	8.502	8.567
19	7.790	7.893	7.988	8.075	8.156	8.232	8.303	8.369	8.432
20	7.688	7.788	7.880	7.966	8.044	8.118	8.186	8.251	8.312
24	7.374	7.467	7.551	7.629	7.701	7.768	7.831	7.890	7.946
30	7.077	7.162	7.239	7.310	7.375	7.437	7.494	7.548	7.599
40	6.796	6.872	6.942	7.007	7.067	7.122	7.174	7.223	7.269
60	6.528	6.598	6.661	6.720	6.774	6.824	6.871	6.914	6.956
120	6.276	6.339	6.396	6.448	6.496	6.542	6.583	6.623	6.660
∞	6.036	6.092	6.144	6.191	6.234	6.274	6.312	6.347	6.380

P = .999

ν\n	20	22	24	26	28	30	32	34	36
1	2980.	3047.	3108.	3163.	3213.	3260.	3303.	3343.	3380.
2	120.3	122.9	125.2	127.3	129.3	131.0	132.7	134.2	135.7
3	43.05	43.92	44.70	45.42	46.07	46.68	47.24	47.77	48.26
4	26.14	26.65	27.10	27.51	27.89	28.24	28.57	28.88	29.16
5	19.51	19.86	20.19	20.48	20.75	21.01	21.24	21.46	21.66
6	16.09	16.38	16.64	16.87	17.08	17.28	17.47	17.64	17.81
7	14.04	14.29	14.50	14.70	14.88	15.05	15.20	15.35	15.49
8	12.70	12.91	13.09	13.26	13.42	13.57	13.71	13.84	13.96
9	11.75	11.93	12.10	12.25	12.39	12.53	12.65	12.77	12.87
10	11.03	11.20	11.36	11.50	11.63	11.75	11.87	11.97	12.07
11	10.49	10.65	10.79	10.92	11.04	11.16	11.26	11.35	11.45
12	10.06	10.20	10.34	10.46	10.57	10.68	10.78	10.87	10.96
13	9.704	9.843	9.969	10.09	10.19	10.29	10.39	10.47	10.55
14	9.414	9.546	9.666	9.776	9.878	9.972	10.06	10.14	10.22
15	9.170	9.296	9.411	9.517	9.613	9.703	9.788	9.867	9.940
16	8.963	9.084	9.194	9.295	9.388	9.475	9.556	9.631	9.702
17	8.784	8.900	9.007	9.104	9.194	9.277	9.355	9.429	9.497
18	8.628	8.741	8.844	8.938	9.025	9.106	9.181	9.251	9.318
19	8.491	8.601	8.701	8.792	8.876	8.955	9.028	9.096	9.161
20	8.370	8.477	8.574	8.663	8.745	8.821	8.892	8.959	9.021
24	7.999	8.097	8.185	8.267	8.342	8.411	8.476	8.537	8.594
30	7.647	7.735	7.816	7.890	7.958	8.021	8.080	8.135	8.188
40	7.312	7.393	7.466	7.533	7.594	7.651	7.704	7.754	7.801
60	6.995	7.067	7.133	7.193	7.248	7.299	7.347	7.392	7.433
120	6.695	6.760	6.818	6.872	6.921	6.966	7.008	7.048	7.085
∞	6.411	6.469	6.520	6.568	6.611	6.651	6.689	6.723	6.756

ν\n	38	40	50	60	70	80	90	100	
1	3415.	3448.	3589.	3701.	3794.	3873.	3941.	4002.	
2	137.0	138.3	143.7	148.0	151.6	154.7	157.4	159.7	
3	48.72	49.16	51.02	52.51	53.75	54.81	55.72	56.53	
4	29.43	29.68	30.78	31.65	32.37	32.98	33.52	34.00	
5	21.86	22.03	22.82	23.45	23.97	24.41	24.80	25.15	
6	17.96	18.10	18.73	19.22	19.64	20.00	20.31	20.58	
7	15.62	15.74	16.27	16.69	17.04	17.35	17.61	17.85	
8	14.07	14.18	14.64	15.01	15.32	15.59	15.82	16.02	
9	12.97	13.07	13.49	13.82	14.10	14.34	14.55	14.74	
10	12.16	12.25	12.63	12.94	13.20	13.42	13.61	13.78	
11	11.53	11.62	11.97	12.25	12.49	12.70	12.88	13.04	
12	11.03	11.11	11.44	11.71	11.94	12.13	12.29	12.45	
13	10.63	10.70	11.01	11.27	11.48	11.66	11.82	11.97	
14	10.30	10.37	10.66	10.91	11.11	11.28	11.43	11.57	
15	10.01	10.08	10.37	10.59	10.79	10.96	11.10	11.23	
16	9.769	9.833	10.11	10.34	10.52	10.68	10.82	10.95	
17	9.562	9.623	9.888	10.10	10.29	10.44	10.58	10.70	
18	9.381	9.440	9.696	9.904	10.08	10.23	10.36	10.48	
19	9.221	9.279	9.528	9.730	9.899	10.04	10.17	10.29	
20	9.081	9.137	9.379	9.575	9.740	9.881	10.01	10.12	
24	8.648	8.700	8.921	9.100	9.250	9.380	9.494	9.596	
30	8.237	8.283	8.484	8.647	8.783	8.901	9.004	9.096	
40	7.845	7.887	8.067	8.214	8.337	8.442	8.535	8.618	
60	7.473	7.510	7.671	7.802	7.911	8.005	8.088	8.161	
120	7.121	7.153	7.296	7.411	7.507	7.590	7.662	7.726	
∞	6.787	6.816	6.941	7.041	7.124	7.196	7.259	7.314	

Table B3

CRITICAL VALUES FOR DUNCAN'S MULTIPLE RANGE TEST

[Values of the Studentized Range $Q = w/s$ Corresponding to Protection Level $P = (1-\alpha)^{p-1}$ (Significance Level α) for Testing p Successive Values out of an Ordered Arrangement of m Means of Samples From a Normal Population, with ν Degrees of Freedom for the Independent Estimate s^2 of Population Variance]

PROTECTION LEVEL P = $(.90)^{p-1}$ SIGNIFICANCE LEVEL α = .10

ν \ p	2	3	4	5	6	7	8	9	10
1	8.929	8.929	8.929	8.929	8.929	8.929	8.929	8.929	8.929
2	4.130	4.130	4.130	4.130	4.130	4.130	4.130	4.130	4.130
3	3.328	3.330	3.330	3.330	3.330	3.330	3.330	3.330	3.330
4	3.015	3.074	3.081	3.081	3.081	3.081	3.081	3.081	3.081
5	2.850	2.934	2.964	2.970	2.970	2.970	2.970	2.970	2.970
6	2.748	2.846	2.890	2.908	2.911	2.911	2.911	2.911	2.911
7	2.680	2.785	2.838	2.864	2.876	2.878	2.878	2.878	2.878
8	2.630	2.742	2.800	2.832	2.849	2.857	2.858	2.858	2.858
9	2.592	2.708	2.771	2.808	2.829	2.840	2.845	2.847	2.847
10	2.563	2.682	2.748	2.788	2.813	2.827	2.835	2.839	2.839
11	2.540	2.660	2.730	2.772	2.799	2.817	2.827	2.833	2.835
12	2.521	2.643	2.714	2.759	2.789	2.808	2.821	2.828	2.832
13	2.505	2.628	2.701	2.748	2.779	2.800	2.815	2.824	2.829
14	2.491	2.616	2.690	2.739	2.771	2.794	2.810	2.820	2.827
15	2.479	2.605	2.681	2.731	2.765	2.789	2.805	2.817	2.825
16	2.469	2.596	2.673	2.723	2.759	2.784	2.802	2.815	2.824
17	2.460	2.588	2.665	2.717	2.753	2.780	2.798	2.812	2.822
18	2.452	2.580	2.659	2.712	2.749	2.776	2.796	2.810	2.821
19	2.445	2.574	2.653	2.707	2.745	2.773	2.793	2.808	2.820
20	2.439	2.568	2.648	2.702	2.741	2.770	2.791	2.807	2.819
24	2.420	2.550	2.632	2.688	2.729	2.760	2.783	2.801	2.816
30	2.400	2.532	2.615	2.674	2.717	2.750	2.776	2.796	2.813
40	2.381	2.514	2.600	2.660	2.705	2.741	2.769	2.791	2.810
60	2.363	2.497	2.584	2.646	2.694	2.731	2.761	2.786	2.807
120	2.344	2.479	2.568	2.632	2.682	2.722	2.754	2.781	2.804
∞	2.326	2.462	2.552	2.619	2.670	2.712	2.746	2.776	2.801

ν \ p	11	12	13	14	15	16	17	18	19
1	8.929	8.929	8.929	8.929	8.929	8.929	8.929	8.929	8.929
2	4.130	4.130	4.130	4.130	4.130	4.130	4.130	4.130	4.130
3	3.330	3.330	3.330	3.330	3.330	3.330	3.330	3.330	3.330
4	3.081	3.081	3.081	3.081	3.081	3.081	3.081	3.081	3.081
5	2.970	2.970	2.970	2.970	2.970	2.970	2.970	2.970	2.970
6	2.911	2.911	2.911	2.911	2.911	2.911	2.911	2.911	2.911
7	2.878	2.878	2.878	2.878	2.878	2.878	2.878	2.878	2.878
8	2.858	2.858	2.858	2.858	2.858	2.858	2.858	2.858	2.858
9	2.847	2.847	2.847	2.847	2.847	2.847	2.847	2.847	2.847
10	2.839	2.839	2.839	2.839	2.839	2.839	2.839	2.839	2.839
11	2.835	2.835	2.835	2.835	2.835	2.835	2.835	2.835	2.835
12	2.833	2.833	2.833	2.833	2.833	2.833	2.833	2.833	2.833
13	2.832	2.832	2.832	2.832	2.832	2.832	2.832	2.832	2.832
14	2.831	2.832	2.833	2.833	2.833	2.833	2.833	2.833	2.833
15	2.830	2.833	2.834	2.834	2.834	2.834	2.834	2.834	2.834
16	2.829	2.833	2.835	2.836	2.836	2.836	2.836	2.836	2.836
17	2.829	2.834	2.836	2.838	2.838	2.838	2.838	2.838	2.838
18	2.828	2.834	2.838	2.840	2.840	2.840	2.840	2.840	2.840
19	2.828	2.834	2.839	2.841	2.842	2.843	2.843	2.843	2.843
20	2.828	2.834	2.839	2.843	2.845	2.845	2.845	2.845	2.845
24	2.827	2.835	2.842	2.848	2.851	2.854	2.856	2.857	2.857
30	2.826	2.837	2.846	2.853	2.859	2.863	2.867	2.869	2.871
40	2.825	2.838	2.849	2.858	2.866	2.873	2.878	2.883	2.887
60	2.825	2.839	2.853	2.864	2.874	2.883	2.890	2.897	2.903
120	2.824	2.842	2.857	2.871	2.883	2.893	2.903	2.912	2.920
∞	2.824	2.844	2.861	2.877	2.892	2.905	2.918	2.929	2.939

PROTECTION LEVEL P = $(.90)^{p-1}$ SIGNIFICANCE LEVEL $\alpha = .10$

ν\p	20	22	24	26	28	30	32	34	36
1	8.929	8.929	8.929	8.929	8.929	8.929	8.929	8.929	8.929
2	4.130	4.130	4.130	4.130	4.130	4.130	4.130	4.130	4.130
3	3.330	3.330	3.330	3.330	3.330	3.330	3.330	3.330	3.330
4	3.081	3.081	3.081	3.081	3.081	3.081	3.081	3.081	3.081
5	2.970	2.970	2.970	2.970	2.970	2.970	2.970	2.970	2.970
6	2.911	2.911	2.911	2.911	2.911	2.911	2.911	2.911	2.911
7	2.878	2.878	2.878	2.878	2.878	2.878	2.878	2.878	2.878
8	2.858	2.858	2.858	2.858	2.858	2.858	2.858	2.858	2.858
9	2.847	2.847	2.847	2.847	2.847	2.847	2.847	2.847	2.847
10	2.839	2.839	2.839	2.839	2.839	2.839	2.839	2.839	2.839
11	2.835	2.835	2.835	2.835	2.835	2.835	2.835	2.835	2.835
12	2.833	2.833	2.833	2.833	2.833	2.833	2.833	2.833	2.833
13	2.832	2.832	2.832	2.832	2.832	2.832	2.832	2.832	2.832
14	2.833	2.833	2.833	2.833	2.833	2.833	2.833	2.833	2.833
15	2.834	2.834	2.834	2.834	2.834	2.834	2.834	2.834	2.834
16	2.836	2.836	2.836	2.836	2.836	2.836	2.836	2.836	2.836
17	2.838	2.838	2.838	2.838	2.838	2.838	2.838	2.838	2.838
18	2.840	2.840	2.840	2.840	2.840	2.840	2.840	2.840	2.840
19	2.843	2.843	2.843	2.843	2.843	2.843	2.843	2.843	2.843
20	2.845	2.845	2.845	2.845	2.845	2.845	2.845	2.845	2.845
24	2.857	2.857	2.857	2.857	2.857	2.857	2.857	2.857	2.857
30	2.873	2.873	2.873	2.873	2.873	2.873	2.873	2.873	2.873
40	2.890	2.894	2.897	2.898	2.898	2.898	2.898	2.898	2.898
60	2.908	2.916	2.923	2.927	2.931	2.933	2.935	2.935	2.936
120	2.928	2.940	2.951	2.960	2.967	2.974	2.979	2.984	2.988
∞	2.949	2.966	2.982	2.995	3.008	3.019	3.029	3.038	3.047

ν\p	38	40	50	60	70	80	90	100	
1	8.929	8.929	8.929	8.929	8.929	8.929	8.929	8.929	
2	4.130	4.130	4.130	4.130	4.130	4.130	4.130	4.130	
3	3.330	3.330	3.330	3.330	3.330	3.330	3.330	3.330	
4	3.081	3.081	3.081	3.081	3.081	3.081	3.081	3.081	
5	2.970	2.970	2.970	2.970	2.970	2.970	2.970	2.970	
6	2.911	2.911	2.911	2.911	2.911	2.911	2.911	2.911	
7	2.878	2.878	2.878	2.878	2.878	2.878	2.878	2.878	
8	2.858	2.858	2.858	2.858	2.858	2.858	2.858	2.858	
9	2.847	2.847	2.847	2.847	2.847	2.847	2.847	2.847	
10	2.839	2.839	2.839	2.839	2.839	2.839	2.839	2.839	
11	2.835	2.835	2.835	2.835	2.835	2.835	2.835	2.835	
12	2.833	2.833	2.833	2.833	2.833	2.833	2.833	2.833	
13	2.832	2.832	2.832	2.832	2.832	2.832	2.832	2.832	
14	2.833	2.833	2.833	2.833	2.833	2.833	2.833	2.833	
15	2.834	2.834	2.834	2.834	2.834	2.834	2.834	2.834	
16	2.836	2.836	2.836	2.836	2.836	2.836	2.836	2.836	
17	2.838	2.838	2.838	2.838	2.838	2.838	2.838	2.838	
18	2.840	2.840	2.840	2.840	2.840	2.840	2.840	2.840	
19	2.843	2.843	2.843	2.843	2.843	2.843	2.843	2.843	
20	2.845	2.845	2.845	2.845	2.845	2.845	2.845	2.845	
24	2.857	2.857	2.857	2.857	2.857	2.857	2.857	2.857	
30	2.873	2.873	2.873	2.873	2.873	2.873	2.873	2.873	
40	2.898	2.898	2.898	2.898	2.898	2.898	2.898	2.898	
60	2.936	2.936	2.936	2.936	2.936	2.936	2.936	2.936	
120	2.991	2.994	3.001	3.001	3.001	3.001	3.001	3.001	
∞	3.054	3.062	3.091	3.113	3.129	3.143	3.154	3.163	

PROTECTION LEVEL P = $(.95)^{p-1}$ SIGNIFICANCE LEVEL $\alpha = .05$

ν \ p	2	3	4	5	6	7	8	9	10
1	17.97	17.97	17.97	17.97	17.97	17.97	17.97	17.97	17.97
2	6.085	6.085	6.085	6.085	6.085	6.085	6.085	6.085	6.085
3	4.501	4.516	4.516	4.516	4.516	4.516	4.516	4.516	4.516
4	3.927	4.013	4.033	4.033	4.033	4.033	4.033	4.033	4.033
5	3.635	3.749	3.797	3.814	3.814	3.814	3.814	3.814	3.814
6	3.461	3.587	3.649	3.680	3.694	3.697	3.697	3.697	3.697
7	3.344	3.477	3.548	3.588	3.611	3.622	3.626	3.626	3.626
8	3.261	3.399	3.475	3.521	3.549	3.566	3.575	3.579	3.579
9	3.199	3.339	3.420	3.470	3.502	3.523	3.536	3.544	3.547
10	3.151	3.293	3.376	3.430	3.465	3.489	3.505	3.516	3.522
11	3.113	3.256	3.342	3.397	3.435	3.462	3.480	3.493	3.501
12	3.082	3.225	3.313	3.370	3.410	3.439	3.459	3.474	3.484
13	3.055	3.200	3.289	3.348	3.389	3.419	3.442	3.458	3.470
14	3.033	3.178	3.268	3.329	3.372	3.403	3.426	3.444	3.457
15	3.014	3.160	3.250	3.312	3.356	3.389	3.413	3.432	3.446
16	2.998	3.144	3.235	3.298	3.343	3.376	3.402	3.422	3.437
17	2.984	3.130	3.222	3.285	3.331	3.366	3.392	3.412	3.429
18	2.971	3.118	3.210	3.274	3.321	3.356	3.383	3.405	3.421
19	2.960	3.107	3.199	3.264	3.311	3.347	3.375	3.397	3.415
20	2.950	3.097	3.190	3.255	3.303	3.339	3.368	3.391	3.409
24	2.919	3.066	3.160	3.226	3.276	3.315	3.345	3.370	3.390
30	2.888	3.035	3.131	3.199	3.250	3.290	3.322	3.349	3.371
40	2.858	3.006	3.102	3.171	3.224	3.266	3.300	3.328	3.352
60	2.829	2.976	3.073	3.143	3.198	3.241	3.277	3.307	3.333
120	2.800	2.947	3.045	3.116	3.172	3.217	3.254	3.287	3.314
∞	2.772	2.918	3.017	3.089	3.146	3.193	3.232	3.265	3.294

ν \ p	11	12	13	14	15	16	17	18	19
1	17.97	17.97	17.97	17.97	17.97	17.97	17.97	17.97	17.97
2	6.085	6.085	6.085	6.085	6.085	6.085	6.085	6.085	6.085
3	4.516	4.516	4.516	4.516	4.516	4.516	4.516	4.516	4.516
4	4.033	4.033	4.033	4.033	4.033	4.033	4.033	4.033	4.033
5	3.814	3.814	3.814	3.814	3.814	3.814	3.814	3.814	3.814
6	3.697	3.697	3.697	3.697	3.697	3.697	3.697	3.697	3.697
7	3.626	3.626	3.626	3.626	3.626	3.626	3.626	3.626	3.626
8	3.579	3.579	3.579	3.579	3.579	3.579	3.579	3.579	3.579
9	3.547	3.547	3.547	3.547	3.547	3.547	3.547	3.547	3.547
10	3.525	3.526	3.526	3.526	3.526	3.526	3.526	3.526	3.526
11	3.506	3.509	3.510	3.510	3.510	3.510	3.510	3.510	3.510
12	3.491	3.496	3.498	3.499	3.499	3.499	3.499	3.499	3.499
13	3.478	3.484	3.488	3.490	3.490	3.490	3.490	3.490	3.490
14	3.467	3.474	3.479	3.482	3.484	3.484	3.485	3.485	3.485
15	3.457	3.465	3.471	3.476	3.478	3.480	3.481	3.481	3.481
16	3.449	3.458	3.465	3.470	3.473	3.477	3.478	3.478	3.478
17	3.441	3.451	3.459	3.465	3.469	3.473	3.475	3.476	3.476
18	3.435	3.445	3.454	3.460	3.465	3.470	3.472	3.474	3.474
19	3.429	3.440	3.449	3.456	3.462	3.467	3.470	3.472	3.473
20	3.424	3.436	3.445	3.453	3.459	3.464	3.467	3.470	3.472
24	3.406	3.420	3.432	3.441	3.449	3.456	3.461	3.465	3.469
30	3.389	3.405	3.418	3.430	3.439	3.447	3.454	3.460	3.466
40	3.373	3.390	3.405	3.418	3.429	3.439	3.448	3.456	3.463
60	3.355	3.374	3.391	3.406	3.419	3.431	3.442	3.451	3.460
120	3.337	3.359	3.377	3.394	3.409	3.423	3.435	3.446	3.457
∞	3.320	3.343	3.363	3.382	3.399	3.414	3.428	3.442	3.454

PROTECTION LEVEL P = $(.95)^{p-1}$ SIGNIFICANCE LEVEL $\alpha = .05$

$\nu \backslash p$	20	22	24	26	28	30	32	34	36
1	17.97	17.97	17.97	17.97	17.97	17.97	17.97	17.97	17.97
2	6.085	6.085	6.085	6.085	6.085	6.085	6.085	6.085	6.085
3	4.516	4.516	4.516	4.516	4.516	4.516	4.516	4.516	4.516
4	4.033	4.033	4.033	4.033	4.033	4.033	4.033	4.033	4.033
5	3.814	3.814	3.814	3.814	3.814	3.814	3.814	3.814	3.814
6	3.697	3.697	3.697	3.697	3.697	3.697	3.697	3.697	3.697
7	3.626	3.626	3.626	3.626	3.626	3.626	3.626	3.626	3.626
8	3.579	3.579	3.579	3.579	3.579	3.579	3.579	3.579	3.579
9	3.547	3.547	3.547	3.547	3.547	3.547	3.547	3.547	3.547
10	3.526	3.526	3.526	3.526	3.526	3.526	3.526	3.526	3.526
11	3.510	3.510	3.510	3.510	3.510	3.510	3.510	3.510	3.510
12	3.499	3.499	3.499	3.499	3.499	3.499	3.499	3.499	3.499
13	3.490	3.490	3.490	3.490	3.490	3.490	3.490	3.490	3.490
14	3.485	3.485	3.485	3.485	3.485	3.485	3.485	3.485	3.485
15	3.481	3.481	3.481	3.481	3.481	3.481	3.481	3.481	3.481
16	3.478	3.478	3.478	3.478	3.478	3.478	3.478	3.478	3.478
17	3.476	3.476	3.476	3.476	3.476	3.476	3.476	3.476	3.476
18	3.474	3.474	3.474	3.474	3.474	3.474	3.474	3.474	3.474
19	3.474	3.474	3.474	3.474	3.474	3.474	3.474	3.474	3.474
20	3.473	3.474	3.474	3.474	3.474	3.474	3.474	3.474	3.474
24	3.471	3.475	3.477	3.477	3.477	3.477	3.477	3.477	3.477
30	3.470	3.477	3.481	3.484	3.486	3.486	3.486	3.486	3.486
40	3.469	3.479	3.486	3.492	3.497	3.500	3.503	3.504	3.504
60	3.467	3.481	3.492	3.501	3.509	3.515	3.521	3.525	3.529
120	3.466	3.483	3.498	3.511	3.522	3.532	3.541	3.548	3.555
∞	3.466	3.486	3.505	3.522	3.536	3.550	3.562	3.574	3.584

$\nu \backslash p$	38	40	50	60	70	80	90	100
1	17.97	17.97	17.97	17.97	17.97	17.97	17.97	17.97
2	6.085	6.085	6.085	6.085	6.085	6.085	6.085	6.085
3	4.516	4.516	4.516	4.516	4.516	4.516	4.516	4.516
4	4.033	4.033	4.033	4.033	4.033	4.033	4.033	4.033
5	3.814	3.814	3.814	3.814	3.814	3.814	3.814	3.814
6	3.697	3.697	3.697	3.697	3.697	3.697	3.697	3.697
7	3.626	3.626	3.626	3.626	3.626	3.626	3.626	3.626
8	3.579	3.579	3.579	3.579	3.579	3.579	3.579	3.579
9	3.547	3.547	3.547	3.547	3.547	3.547	3.547	3.547
10	3.526	3.526	3.526	3.526	3.526	3.526	3.526	3.526
11	3.510	3.510	3.510	3.510	3.510	3.510	3.510	3.510
12	3.499	3.499	3.499	3.499	3.499	3.499	3.499	3.499
13	3.490	3.490	3.490	3.490	3.490	3.490	3.490	3.490
14	3.485	3.485	3.485	3.485	3.485	3.485	3.485	3.485
15	3.481	3.481	3.481	3.481	3.481	3.481	3.481	3.481
16	3.478	3.478	3.478	3.478	3.478	3.478	3.478	3.478
17	3.476	3.476	3.476	3.476	3.476	3.476	3.476	3.476
18	3.474	3.474	3.474	3.474	3.474	3.474	3.474	3.474
19	3.474	3.474	3.474	3.474	3.474	3.474	3.474	3.474
20	3.474	3.474	3.474	3.474	3.474	3.474	3.474	3.474
24	3.477	3.477	3.477	3.477	3.477	3.477	3.477	3.477
30	3.486	3.486	3.486	3.486	3.486	3.486	3.486	3.486
40	3.504	3.504	3.504	3.504	3.504	3.504	3.504	3.504
60	3.531	3.534	3.537	3.537	3.537	3.537	3.537	3.537
120	3.561	3.566	3.585	3.596	3.600	3.601	3.601	3.601
∞	3.594	3.603	3.640	3.668	3.690	3.708	3.722	3.735

PROTECTION LEVEL $P = (.99)^{p-1}$ SIGNIFICANCE LEVEL $\alpha = .01$

ν\p	2	3	4	5	6	7	8	9	10
1	90.03	90.03	90.03	90.03	90.03	90.03	90.03	90.03	90.03
2	14.04	14.04	14.04	14.04	14.04	14.04	14.04	14.04	14.04
3	8.261	8.321	8.321	8.321	8.321	8.321	8.321	8.321	8.321
4	6.512	6.677	6.740	6.756	6.756	6.756	6.756	6.756	6.756
5	5.702	5.893	5.989	6.040	6.065	6.074	6.074	6.074	6.074
6	5.243	5.439	5.549	5.614	5.655	5.680	5.694	5.701	5.703
7	4.949	5.145	5.260	5.334	5.383	5.416	5.439	5.454	5.464
8	4.746	4.939	5.057	5.135	5.189	5.227	5.256	5.276	5.291
9	4.596	4.787	4.906	4.986	5.043	5.086	5.118	5.142	5.160
10	4.482	4.671	4.790	4.871	4.931	4.975	5.010	5.037	5.058
11	4.392	4.579	4.697	4.780	4.841	4.887	4.924	4.952	4.975
12	4.320	4.504	4.622	4.706	4.767	4.815	4.852	4.883	4.907
13	4.260	4.442	4.560	4.644	4.706	4.755	4.793	4.824	4.850
14	4.210	4.391	4.508	4.591	4.654	4.704	4.743	4.775	4.802
15	4.168	4.347	4.463	4.547	4.610	4.660	4.700	4.733	4.760
16	4.131	4.309	4.425	4.509	4.572	4.622	4.663	4.696	4.724
17	4.099	4.275	4.391	4.475	4.539	4.589	4.630	4.664	4.693
18	4.071	4.246	4.362	4.445	4.509	4.560	4.601	4.635	4.664
19	4.046	4.220	4.335	4.419	4.483	4.534	4.575	4.610	4.639
20	4.024	4.197	4.312	4.395	4.459	4.510	4.552	4.587	4.617
24	3.956	4.126	4.239	4.322	4.386	4.437	4.480	4.516	4.546
30	3.889	4.056	4.168	4.250	4.314	4.366	4.409	4.445	4.477
40	3.825	3.988	4.098	4.180	4.244	4.296	4.339	4.376	4.408
60	3.762	3.922	4.031	4.111	4.174	4.226	4.270	4.307	4.340
120	3.702	3.858	3.965	4.044	4.107	4.158	4.202	4.239	4.272
∞	3.643	3.796	3.900	3.978	4.040	4.091	4.135	4.172	4.205

ν\p	11	12	13	14	15	16	17	18	19
1	90.03	90.03	90.03	90.03	90.03	90.03	90.03	90.03	90.03
2	14.04	14.04	14.04	14.04	14.04	14.04	14.04	14.04	14.04
3	8.321	8.321	8.321	8.321	8.321	8.321	8.321	8.321	8.321
4	6.756	6.756	6.756	6.756	6.756	6.756	6.756	6.756	6.756
5	6.074	6.074	6.074	6.074	6.074	6.074	6.074	6.074	6.074
6	5.703	5.703	5.703	5.703	5.703	5.703	5.703	5.703	5.703
7	5.470	5.472	5.472	5.472	5.472	5.472	5.472	5.472	5.472
8	5.302	5.309	5.314	5.316	5.317	5.317	5.317	5.317	5.317
9	5.174	5.185	5.193	5.199	5.203	5.205	5.206	5.206	5.206
10	5.074	5.088	5.098	5.106	5.112	5.117	5.120	5.122	5.124
11	4.994	5.009	5.021	5.031	5.039	5.045	5.050	5.054	5.057
12	4.927	4.944	4.958	4.969	4.978	4.986	4.993	4.998	5.002
13	4.872	4.889	4.904	4.917	4.928	4.937	4.944	4.950	4.956
14	4.824	4.843	4.859	4.872	4.884	4.894	4.902	4.910	4.916
15	4.783	4.803	4.820	4.834	4.846	4.857	4.866	4.874	4.881
16	4.748	4.768	4.786	4.800	4.813	4.825	4.835	4.844	4.851
17	4.717	4.738	4.756	4.771	4.785	4.797	4.807	4.816	4.824
18	4.689	4.711	4.729	4.745	4.759	4.772	4.783	4.792	4.801
19	4.665	4.686	4.705	4.722	4.736	4.749	4.761	4.771	4.780
20	4.642	4.664	4.684	4.701	4.716	4.729	4.741	4.751	4.761
24	4.573	4.596	4.616	4.634	4.651	4.665	4.678	4.690	4.700
30	4.504	4.528	4.550	4.569	4.586	4.601	4.615	4.628	4.640
40	4.436	4.461	4.483	4.503	4.521	4.537	4.553	4.566	4.579
60	4.368	4.394	4.417	4.438	4.456	4.474	4.490	4.504	4.518
120	4.301	4.327	4.351	4.372	4.392	4.410	4.426	4.442	4.456
∞	4.235	4.261	4.285	4.307	4.327	4.345	4.363	4.379	4.394

PROTECTION LEVEL P = $(.99)^{p-1}$ SIGNIFICANCE LEVEL $\alpha = .01$

ν\p	20	22	24	26	28	30	32	34	36
1	90.03	90.03	90.03	90.03	90.03	90.03	90.03	90.03	90.03
2	14.04	14.04	14.04	14.04	14.04	14.04	14.04	14.04	14.04
3	8.321	8.321	8.321	8.321	8.321	8.321	8.321	8.321	8.321
4	6.756	6.756	6.756	6.756	6.756	6.756	6.756	6.756	6.756
5	6.074	6.074	6.074	6.074	6.074	6.074	6.074	6.074	6.074
6	5.703	5.703	5.703	5.703	5.703	5.703	5.703	5.703	5.703
7	5.472	5.472	5.472	5.472	5.472	5.472	5.472	5.472	5.472
8	5.317	5.317	5.317	5.317	5.317	5.317	5.317	5.317	5.317
9	5.206	5.206	5.206	5.206	5.206	5.206	5.206	5.206	5.206
10	5.124	5.124	5.124	5.124	5.124	5.124	5.124	5.124	5.124
11	5.059	5.061	5.061	5.061	5.061	5.061	5.061	5.061	5.061
12	5.006	5.010	5.011	5.011	5.011	5.011	5.011	5.011	5.011
13	4.960	4.966	4.970	4.972	4.972	4.972	4.972	4.972	4.972
14	4.921	4.929	4.935	4.938	4.940	4.940	4.940	4.940	4.940
15	4.887	4.897	4.904	4.909	4.912	4.914	4.914	4.914	4.914
16	4.858	4.869	4.877	4.883	4.887	4.890	4.892	4.892	4.892
17	4.832	4.844	4.853	4.860	4.865	4.869	4.872	4.873	4.874
18	4.808	4.821	4.832	4.839	4.846	4.850	4.854	4.856	4.857
19	4.788	4.802	4.812	4.821	4.828	4.833	4.838	4.841	4.843
20	4.769	4.784	4.795	4.805	4.813	4.818	4.823	4.827	4.830
24	4.710	4.727	4.741	4.752	4.762	4.770	4.777	4.783	4.788
30	4.650	4.669	4.685	4.699	4.711	4.721	4.730	4.738	4.744
40	4.591	4.611	4.630	4.645	4.659	4.671	4.682	4.692	4.700
60	4.530	4.553	4.573	4.591	4.607	4.620	4.633	4.645	4.655
120	4.469	4.494	4.516	4.535	4.552	4.568	4.583	4.596	4.609
∞	4.408	4.434	4.457	4.478	4.497	4.514	4.530	4.545	4.559

ν\p	38	40	50	60	70	80	90	100
1	90.03	90.03	90.03	90.03	90.03	90.03	90.03	90.03
2	14.04	14.04	14.04	14.04	14.04	14.04	14.04	14.04
3	8.321	8.321	8.321	8.321	8.321	8.321	8.321	8.321
4	6.756	6.756	6.756	6.756	6.756	6.756	6.756	6.756
5	6.074	6.074	6.074	6.074	6.074	6.074	6.074	6.074
6	5.703	5.703	5.703	5.703	5.703	5.703	5.703	5.703
7	5.472	5.472	5.472	5.472	5.472	5.472	5.472	5.472
8	5.317	5.317	5.317	5.317	5.317	5.317	5.317	5.317
9	5.206	5.206	5.206	5.206	5.206	5.206	5.206	5.206
10	5.124	5.124	5.124	5.124	5.124	5.124	5.124	5.124
11	5.061	5.061	5.061	5.061	5.061	5.061	5.061	5.061
12	5.011	5.011	5.011	5.011	5.011	5.011	5.011	5.011
13	4.972	4.972	4.972	4.972	4.972	4.972	4.972	4.972
14	4.940	4.940	4.940	4.940	4.940	4.940	4.940	4.940
15	4.914	4.914	4.914	4.914	4.914	4.914	4.914	4.914
16	4.892	4.892	4.892	4.892	4.892	4.892	4.892	4.892
17	4.874	4.874	4.874	4.874	4.874	4.874	4.874	4.874
18	4.858	4.858	4.858	4.858	4.858	4.858	4.858	4.858
19	4.844	4.845	4.845	4.845	4.845	4.845	4.845	4.845
20	4.832	4.833	4.833	4.833	4.833	4.833	4.833	4.833
24	4.791	4.794	4.802	4.802	4.802	4.802	4.802	4.802
30	4.750	4.755	4.772	4.777	4.777	4.777	4.777	4.777
40	4.708	4.715	4.740	4.754	4.761	4.764	4.764	4.764
60	4.665	4.673	4.707	4.730	4.745	4.755	4.761	4.765
120	4.619	4.630	4.673	4.703	4.727	4.745	4.759	4.770
∞	4.572	4.584	4.635	4.675	4.707	4.734	4.756	4.776

PROTECTION LEVEL P = $(.995)^{p-1}$ SIGNIFICANCE LEVEL $\alpha = .005$

ν \ p	2	3	4	5	6	7	8	9	10
1	180.1	180.1	180.1	180.1	180.1	180.1	180.1	180.1	180.1
2	19.93	19.93	19.93	19.93	19.93	19.93	19.93	19.93	19.93
3	10.55	10.63	10.63	10.63	10.63	10.63	10.63	10.63	10.63
4	7.916	8.126	8.210	8.238	8.238	8.238	8.238	8.238	8.238
5	6.751	6.980	7.100	7.167	7.204	7.222	7.228	7.228	7.228
6	6.105	6.334	6.466	6.547	6.600	6.635	6.658	6.672	6.679
7	5.699	5.922	6.057	6.145	6.207	6.250	6.281	6.304	6.320
8	5.420	5.638	5.773	5.864	5.930	5.978	6.014	6.042	6.064
9	5.218	5.430	5.565	5.657	5.725	5.776	5.815	5.846	5.871
10	5.065	5.273	5.405	5.498	5.567	5.620	5.662	5.695	5.722
11	4.945	5.149	5.280	5.372	5.442	5.496	5.539	5.574	5.603
12	4.849	5.048	5.178	5.270	5.341	5.396	5.439	5.475	5.505
13	4.770	4.966	5.094	5.186	5.256	5.312	5.356	5.393	5.424
14	4.704	4.897	5.023	5.116	5.185	5.241	5.286	5.324	5.355
15	4.647	4.838	4.964	5.055	5.125	5.181	5.226	5.264	5.297
16	4.599	4.787	4.912	5.003	5.073	5.129	5.175	5.213	5.245
17	4.557	4.744	4.867	4.958	5.027	5.084	5.130	5.168	5.201
18	4.521	4.705	4.828	4.918	4.987	5.043	5.090	5.129	5.162
19	4.488	4.671	4.793	4.883	4.952	5.008	5.054	5.093	5.127
20	4.460	4.641	4.762	4.851	4.920	4.976	5.022	5.061	5.095
24	4.371	4.547	4.666	4.753	4.822	4.877	4.924	4.963	4.997
30	4.285	4.456	4.572	4.658	4.726	4.781	4.827	4.867	4.901
40	4.202	4.369	4.482	4.566	4.632	4.687	4.733	4.772	4.806
60	4.122	4.284	4.394	4.476	4.541	4.595	4.640	4.679	4.713
120	4.045	4.201	4.308	4.388	4.452	4.505	4.550	4.588	4.622
∞	3.970	4.121	4.225	4.303	4.365	4.417	4.461	4.499	4.532

ν \ p	11	12	13	14	15	16	17	18	19
1	180.1	180.1	180.1	180.1	180.1	180.1	180.1	180.1	180.1
2	19.93	19.93	19.93	19.93	19.93	19.93	19.93	19.93	19.93
3	10.63	10.63	10.63	10.63	10.63	10.63	10.63	10.63	10.63
4	8.238	8.238	8.238	8.238	8.238	8.238	8.238	8.238	8.238
5	7.228	7.228	7.228	7.228	7.228	7.228	7.228	7.228	7.228
6	6.682	6.682	6.682	6.682	6.682	6.682	6.682	6.682	6.682
7	6.331	6.339	6.343	6.345	6.345	6.345	6.345	6.345	6.345
8	6.080	6.092	6.101	6.108	6.113	6.116	6.118	6.119	6.119
9	5.891	5.907	5.920	5.930	5.938	5.944	5.949	5.952	5.955
10	5.744	5.762	5.777	5.790	5.800	5.809	5.816	5.821	5.826
11	5.626	5.646	5.663	5.678	5.690	5.700	5.709	5.716	5.722
12	5.531	5.552	5.570	5.585	5.599	5.610	5.620	5.629	5.636
13	5.450	5.472	5.492	5.508	5.523	5.535	5.546	5.556	5.564
14	5.382	5.405	5.425	5.442	5.458	5.471	5.483	5.494	5.503
15	5.324	5.348	5.368	5.386	5.402	5.416	5.429	5.440	5.450
16	5.273	5.298	5.319	5.338	5.354	5.368	5.381	5.393	5.404
17	5.229	5.254	5.275	5.295	5.311	5.327	5.340	5.352	5.363
18	5.190	5.215	5.237	5.256	5.274	5.289	5.303	5.316	5.327
19	5.156	5.181	5.203	5.222	5.240	5.256	5.270	5.283	5.295
20	5.124	5.150	5.172	5.193	5.210	5.226	5.241	5.254	5.266
24	5.027	5.053	5.076	5.097	5.116	5.133	5.148	5.162	5.175
30	4.931	4.958	4.981	5.003	5.022	5.040	5.056	5.071	5.085
40	4.837	4.864	4.888	4.910	4.930	4.948	4.965	4.980	4.995
60	4.744	4.771	4.796	4.818	4.838	4.857	4.874	4.890	4.905
120	4.652	4.679	4.704	4.726	4.747	4.766	4.784	4.800	4.815
∞	4.562	4.589	4.614	4.636	4.657	4.676	4.694	4.710	4.726

PROTECTION LEVEL P = $(.995)^{p-1}$ SIGNIFICANCE LEVEL $\alpha = .005$

ν\p	20	22	24	26	28	30	32	34	36
1	180.1	180.1	180.1	180.1	180.1	180.1	180.1	180.1	180.1
2	19.93	19.93	19.93	19.93	19.93	19.93	19.93	19.93	19.93
3	10.63	10.63	10.63	10.63	10.63	10.63	10.63	10.63	10.63
4	8.238	8.238	8.238	8.238	8.238	8.238	8.238	8.238	8.238
5	7.228	7.228	7.228	7.228	7.228	7.228	7.228	7.228	7.228
6	6.682	6.682	6.682	6.682	6.682	6.682	6.682	6.682	6.682
7	6.345	6.345	6.345	6.345	6.345	6.345	6.345	6.345	6.345
8	6.119	6.119	6.119	6.119	6.119	6.119	6.119	6.119	6.119
9	5.956	5.957	5.957	5.957	5.957	5.957	5.957	5.957	5.957
10	5.829	5.834	5.836	5.836	5.836	5.836	5.836	5.836	5.836
11	5.727	5.735	5.740	5.743	5.744	5.744	5.744	5.744	5.744
12	5.642	5.653	5.660	5.665	5.668	5.670	5.670	5.670	5.670
13	5.571	5.583	5.593	5.600	5.605	5.608	5.610	5.611	5.611
14	5.511	5.525	5.535	5.544	5.550	5.555	5.559	5.561	5.563
15	5.459	5.474	5.486	5.495	5.503	5.509	5.514	5.518	5.520
16	5.413	5.429	5.442	5.453	5.462	5.469	5.475	5.479	5.483
17	5.373	5.390	5.404	5.416	5.425	5.433	5.440	5.445	5.450
18	5.338	5.355	5.370	5.383	5.393	5.402	5.409	5.415	5.420
19	5.306	5.325	5.340	5.353	5.364	5.374	5.382	5.388	5.395
20	5.277	5.296	5.313	5.326	5.338	5.348	5.357	5.364	5.370
24	5.187	5.209	5.226	5.242	5.255	5.267	5.278	5.287	5.295
30	5.098	5.120	5.140	5.157	5.172	5.186	5.198	5.209	5.218
40	5.008	5.032	5.054	5.072	5.089	5.104	5.118	5.130	5.141
60	4.919	4.944	4.967	4.987	5.005	5.021	5.036	5.050	5.062
120	4.830	4.856	4.880	4.901	4.920	4.937	4.953	4.968	4.982
∞	4.740	4.767	4.792	4.813	4.833	4.852	4.869	4.885	4.899

ν\p	38	40	50	60	70	80	90	100	
1	180.1	180.1	180.1	180.1	180.1	180.1	180.1	180.1	
2	19.93	19.93	19.93	19.93	19.93	19.93	19.93	19.93	
3	10.63	10.63	10.63	10.63	10.63	10.63	10.63	10.63	
4	8.238	8.238	8.238	8.238	8.238	8.238	8.238	8.238	
5	7.228	7.228	7.228	7.228	7.228	7.228	7.228	7.228	
6	6.682	6.682	6.682	6.682	6.682	6.682	6.682	6.682	
7	6.345	6.345	6.345	6.345	6.345	6.345	6.345	6.345	
8	6.119	6.119	6.119	6.119	6.119	6.119	6.119	6.119	
9	5.957	5.957	5.957	5.957	5.957	5.957	5.957	5.957	
10	5.836	5.836	5.836	5.836	5.836	5.836	5.836	5.836	
11	5.744	5.744	5.744	5.744	5.744	5.744	5.744	5.744	
12	5.670	5.670	5.670	5.670	5.670	5.670	5.670	5.670	
13	5.611	5.611	5.611	5.611	5.611	5.611	5.611	5.611	
14	5.563	5.563	5.563	5.563	5.563	5.563	5.563	5.563	
15	5.522	5.523	5.523	5.523	5.523	5.523	5.523	5.523	
16	5.485	5.488	5.489	5.489	5.489	5.489	5.489	5.489	
17	5.453	5.456	5.461	5.461	5.461	5.461	5.461	5.461	
18	5.425	5.428	5.436	5.436	5.436	5.436	5.436	5.436	
19	5.399	5.403	5.414	5.415	5.415	5.415	5.415	5.415	
20	5.376	5.380	5.394	5.397	5.397	5.397	5.397	5.397	
24	5.302	5.308	5.329	5.340	5.343	5.343	5.343	5.343	
30	5.227	5.235	5.264	5.281	5.292	5.297	5.298	5.298	
40	5.151	5.160	5.197	5.221	5.238	5.249	5.257	5.261	
60	5.074	5.084	5.128	5.159	5.182	5.199	5.213	5.223	
120	4.995	5.007	5.056	5.094	5.123	5.146	5.166	5.182	
∞	4.913	4.926	4.981	5.024	5.059	5.088	5.114	5.136	

PROTECTION LEVEL $P = (.999)^{p-1}$ SIGNIFICANCE LEVEL $\alpha = .001$

ν \ p	2	3	4	5	6	7	8	9	10
1	900.3	900.3	900.3	900.3	900.3	900.3	900.3	900.3	900.3
2	44.69	44.69	44.69	44.69	44.69	44.69	44.69	44.69	44.69
3	18.28	18.45	18.45	18.45	18.45	18.45	18.45	18.45	18.45
4	12.18	12.52	12.67	12.73	12.75	12.75	12.75	12.75	12.75
5	9.714	10.05	10.24	10.35	10.42	10.46	10.48	10.49	10.49
6	8.427	8.743	8.932	9.055	9.139	9.198	9.241	9.272	9.294
7	7.648	7.943	8.127	8.252	8.342	8.409	8.460	8.500	8.530
8	7.130	7.407	7.584	7.708	7.799	7.869	7.924	7.968	8.004
9	6.762	7.024	7.195	7.316	7.407	7.478	7.535	7.582	7.619
10	6.487	6.738	6.902	7.021	7.111	7.182	7.240	7.287	7.327
11	6.275	6.516	6.676	6.791	6.880	6.950	7.008	7.056	7.097
12	6.106	6.340	6.494	6.607	6.695	6.765	6.822	6.870	6.911
13	5.970	6.195	6.346	6.457	6.543	6.612	6.670	6.718	6.759
14	5.856	6.075	6.223	6.332	6.416	6.485	6.542	6.590	6.631
15	5.760	5.974	6.119	6.225	6.309	6.377	6.433	6.481	6.522
16	5.678	5.888	6.030	6.135	6.217	6.284	6.340	6.388	6.429
17	5.608	5.813	5.953	6.056	6.138	6.204	6.260	6.307	6.348
18	5.546	5.748	5.886	5.988	6.068	6.134	6.189	6.236	6.277
19	5.492	5.691	5.826	5.927	6.007	6.072	6.127	6.174	6.214
20	5.444	5.640	5.774	5.873	5.952	6.017	6.071	6.117	6.158
24	5.297	5.484	5.612	5.708	5.784	5.846	5.899	5.945	5.984
30	5.156	5.335	5.457	5.549	5.622	5.682	5.734	5.778	5.817
40	5.022	5.191	5.308	5.396	5.466	5.524	5.574	5.617	5.654
60	4.894	5.055	5.166	5.249	5.317	5.372	5.420	5.461	5.498
120	4.771	4.924	5.029	5.109	5.173	5.226	5.271	5.311	5.346
∞	4.654	4.798	4.898	4.974	5.034	5.085	5.128	5.166	5.199

ν \ p	11	12	13	14	15	16	17	18	19
1	900.3	900.3	900.3	900.3	900.3	900.3	900.3	900.3	900.3
2	44.69	44.69	44.69	44.69	44.69	44.69	44.69	44.69	44.69
3	18.45	18.45	18.45	18.45	18.45	18.45	18.45	18.45	18.45
4	12.75	12.75	12.75	12.75	12.75	12.75	12.75	12.75	12.75
5	10.49	10.49	10.49	10.49	10.49	10.49	10.49	10.49	10.49
6	9.309	9.319	9.325	9.328	9.329	9.329	9.329	9.329	9.329
7	8.555	8.574	8.589	8.600	8.609	8.616	8.621	8.624	8.626
8	8.033	8.057	8.078	8.094	8.108	8.119	8.129	8.137	8.143
9	7.652	7.679	7.702	7.722	7.739	7.753	7.766	7.777	7.786
10	7.361	7.390	7.415	7.437	7.456	7.472	7.487	7.500	7.511
11	7.132	7.162	7.188	7.211	7.231	7.250	7.266	7.280	7.293
12	6.947	6.978	7.005	7.029	7.050	7.069	7.086	7.102	7.116
13	6.795	6.826	6.854	6.878	6.900	6.920	6.937	6.954	6.968
14	6.667	6.699	6.727	6.752	6.774	6.794	6.812	6.829	6.844
15	6.558	6.590	6.619	6.644	6.666	6.687	6.706	6.723	6.739
16	6.465	6.497	6.525	6.551	6.574	6.595	6.614	6.631	6.647
17	6.384	6.416	6.444	6.470	6.493	6.514	6.533	6.551	6.567
18	6.313	6.345	6.373	6.399	6.422	6.443	6.462	6.480	6.497
19	6.250	6.281	6.310	6.336	6.359	6.380	6.400	6.418	6.434
20	6.193	6.225	6.254	6.279	6.303	6.324	6.344	6.362	6.379
24	6.020	6.051	6.079	6.105	6.129	6.150	6.170	6.188	6.205
30	5.851	5.882	5.910	5.935	5.958	5.980	6.000	6.018	6.036
40	5.688	5.718	5.745	5.770	5.793	5.814	5.834	5.852	5.869
60	5.530	5.559	5.586	5.610	5.632	5.653	5.672	5.690	5.707
120	5.377	5.405	5.431	5.454	5.476	5.496	5.515	5.532	5.549
∞	5.229	5.256	5.280	5.303	5.324	5.343	5.361	5.378	5.394

PROTECTION LEVEL P = (.999)$^{p-1}$ SIGNIFICANCE LEVEL α = .001

$\nu \backslash p$	20	22	24	26	28	30	32	34	36
1	900.3	900.3	900.3	900.3	900.3	900.3	900.3	900.3	900.3
2	44.69	44.69	44.69	44.69	44.69	44.69	44.69	44.69	44.69
3	18.45	18.45	18.45	18.45	18.45	18.45	18.45	18.45	18.45
4	12.75	12.75	12.75	12.75	12.75	12.75	12.75	12.75	12.75
5	10.49	10.49	10.49	10.49	10.49	10.49	10.49	10.49	10.49
6	9.329	9.329	9.329	9.329	9.329	9.329	9.329	9.329	9.329
7	8.627	8.627	8.627	8.627	8.627	8.627	8.627	8.627	8.627
8	8.149	8.156	8.160	8.161	8.161	8.161	8.161	8.161	8.161
9	7.794	7.808	7.817	7.824	7.828	7.831	7.832	7.832	7.832
10	7.522	7.538	7.552	7.562	7.570	7.577	7.582	7.585	7.587
11	7.304	7.324	7.340	7.354	7.364	7.373	7.380	7.386	7.391
12	7.128	7.150	7.168	7.184	7.196	7.207	7.216	7.223	7.230
13	6.982	7.005	7.025	7.042	7.056	7.068	7.079	7.088	7.096
14	6.858	6.883	6.904	6.922	6.937	6.951	6.962	6.973	6.982
15	6.753	6.778	6.800	6.819	6.836	6.850	6.863	6.874	6.883
16	6.661	6.688	6.711	6.730	6.748	6.763	6.776	6.788	6.799
17	6.582	6.609	6.632	6.653	6.670	6.686	6.701	6.713	6.724
18	6.512	6.539	6.563	6.584	6.602	6.619	6.633	6.647	6.658
19	6.450	6.477	6.501	6.523	6.542	6.559	6.574	6.587	6.600
20	6.394	6.422	6.447	6.468	6.487	6.505	6.520	6.534	6.547
24	6.221	6.250	6.275	6.298	6.318	6.336	6.353	6.368	6.381
30	6.051	6.081	6.106	6.130	6.151	6.169	6.187	6.203	6.217
40	5.885	5.915	5.941	5.964	5.986	6.005	6.023	6.040	6.055
60	5.723	5.752	5.778	5.802	5.823	5.843	5.862	5.878	5.894
120	5.565	5.593	5.619	5.642	5.664	5.683	5.702	5.718	5.734
∞	5.409	5.437	5.462	5.485	5.506	5.525	5.543	5.560	5.576

$\nu \backslash p$	38	40	50	60	70	80	90	100
1	900.3	900.3	900.3	900.3	900.3	900.3	900.3	900.3
2	44.69	44.69	44.69	44.69	44.69	44.69	44.69	44.69
3	18.45	18.45	18.45	18.45	18.45	18.45	18.45	18.45
4	12.75	12.75	12.75	12.75	12.75	12.75	12.75	12.75
5	10.49	10.49	10.49	10.49	10.49	10.49	10.49	10.49
6	9.329	9.329	9.329	9.329	9.329	9.329	9.329	9.329
7	8.627	8.627	8.627	8.627	8.627	8.627	8.627	8.627
8	8.161	8.161	8.161	8.161	8.161	8.161	8.161	8.161
9	7.832	7.832	7.832	7.832	7.832	7.832	7.832	7.832
10	7.588	7.588	7.588	7.588	7.588	7.588	7.588	7.588
11	7.394	7.397	7.400	7.400	7.400	7.400	7.400	7.400
12	7.235	7.239	7.251	7.251	7.251	7.251	7.251	7.251
13	7.102	7.108	7.126	7.132	7.132	7.132	7.132	7.132
14	6.989	6.996	7.019	7.030	7.034	7.034	7.034	7.034
15	6.892	6.900	6.927	6.942	6.949	6.951	6.951	6.951
16	6.808	6.816	6.848	6.865	6.875	6.880	6.881	6.881
17	6.734	6.743	6.777	6.798	6.811	6.818	6.821	6.821
18	6.669	6.679	6.715	6.738	6.753	6.762	6.767	6.770
19	6.611	6.621	6.660	6.685	6.702	6.713	6.719	6.723
20	6.558	6.569	6.610	6.637	6.655	6.668	6.676	6.681
24	6.394	6.405	6.451	6.484	6.507	6.525	6.538	6.547
30	6.231	6.243	6.294	6.331	6.360	6.381	6.399	6.412
40	6.069	6.082	6.137	6.178	6.210	6.236	6.257	6.274
60	5.909	5.922	5.980	6.024	6.059	6.088	6.113	6.134
120	5.749	5.763	5.822	5.868	5.906	5.938	5.965	5.988
∞	5.590	5.604	5.663	5.711	5.750	5.783	5.811	5.837

Table B4

COMPARISON OF TYPE I ERROR RATES FOR MULTIPLE COMPARISON TESTS (SINGLE-CLASSIFICATION EXPERIMENTS)

$\alpha_L =$ Type I error rate for LSD (multiple t) test

$\alpha_W =$ Type I error rate for Tukey's studentized range test

$\alpha_E =$ Type I error rate for Fisher's test

$\alpha_X =$ Type I error rate for Tukey's X procedure

$\alpha_S =$ Type I error rate for Duncan's multiple range test

Tabular Entries of the Form .$(X)Y$ Indicate That There Are X Zeros Between the Decimal Point and the First Significant Digit Y

A. Values of α_L corresponding to $\alpha_W = 0.05, 0.01$ and to $\alpha_E = 0.05, 0.01$

m	$\alpha_L \mid \alpha_W = 0.05$																			$\alpha_L \mid \alpha_E = 0.05$
	N=2	N=3	N=4	N=5	N=6	N=7	N=8	N=9	N=10	N=11	N=13	N=16	N=21	N=25	N=31	N=41	N=61	N=121	N → ∞	ALL N
2	.0500	.0500	.0500	.0500	.0500	.0500	.0500	.0500	.0500	.0500	.0500	.0500	.0500	.0500	.0500	.0500	.0500	.0500	.0500	.0500
3	.0250	.0220	.0210	.0205	.0202	.0200	.0199	.0198	.0197	.0196	.0195	.0194	.0193	.0193	.0193	.0192	.0192	.0191	.0191	.0167
4	.0152	.0126	.0117	.0113	.0111	.0109	.0108	.0107	.0107	.0106	.0105	.0105	.0104	.0104	.0103	.0103	.0103	.0102	.0102	.0083
5	.0102	.0081	.0075	.0072	.0070	.0069	.0068	.0068	.0067	.0067	.0066	.0066	.0065	.0065	.0065	.0064	.0064	.0064	.0064	.0050
6	.0073	.0057	.0052	.0050	.0048	.0048	.0047	.0047	.0046	.0046	.0046	.0045	.0045	.0045	.0044	.0044	.0044	.0044	.0044	.0033
7	.0054	.0042	.0038	.0037	.0036	.0035	.0034	.0034	.0034	.0034	.0033	.0033	.0033	.0033	.0032	.0032	.0032	.0032	.0032	.0024
8	.0042	.0032	.0029	.0028	.0027	.0027	.0026	.0026	.0026	.0026	.0025	.0025	.0025	.0025	.0025	.0025	.0025	.0025	.0024	.0018
9	.0033	.0025	.0023	.0022	.0021	.0021	.0021	.0021	.0020	.0020	.0020	.0020	.0020	.0020	.0020	.0019	.0019	.0019	.0019	.0014
10	.0027	.0020	.0019	.0018	.0017	.0017	.0017	.0017	.0017	.0016	.0016	.0016	.0016	.0016	.0016	.0016	.0016	.0016	.0016	.0011
11	.0022	.0017	.0015	.0015	.0014	.0014	.0014	.0014	.0014	.0014	.0013	.0013	.0013	.0013	.0013	.0013	.0013	.0013	.0013	.0009
12	.0019	.0014	.0013	.0012	.0012	.0012	.0012	.0012	.0011	.0011	.0011	.0011	.0011	.0011	.0011	.0011	.0011	.0011	.0011	.0008
13	.0016	.0012	.0011	.0011	.0010	.0010	.0010	.0010	.0010	.0010	.0010	.0010	.0009	.0009	.0009	.0009	.0009	.0009	.0009	.0006
14	.0014	.0010	.0009	.0009	.0009	.0009	.0009	.0008	.0008	.0008	.0008	.0008	.0008	.0008	.0008	.0008	.0008	.0008	.0008	.0005
15	.0012	.0009	.0008	.0008	.0008	.0008	.0007	.0007	.0007	.0007	.0007	.0007	.0007	.0007	.0007	.0007	.0007	.0007	.0007	.0005
16	.0010	.0008	.0007	.0007	.0007	.0007	.0007	.0007	.0006	.0006	.0006	.0006	.0006	.0006	.0006	.0006	.0006	.0006	.0006	.0004
17	.0009	.0007	.0006	.0006	.0006	.0006	.0006	.0006	.0006	.0006	.0006	.0006	.0006	.0006	.0006	.0005	.0005	.0005	.0005	.0004
18	.0008	.0006	.0006	.0005	.0005	.0005	.0005	.0005	.0005	.0005	.0005	.0005	.0005	.0005	.0005	.0005	.0005	.0005	.0005	.0003
19	.0007	.0006	.0005	.0005	.0005	.0005	.0005	.0005	.0005	.0005	.0005	.0004	.0004	.0004	.0004	.0004	.0004	.0004	.0004	.0003
20	.0006	.0005	.0005	.0004	.0004	.0004	.0004	.0004	.0004	.0004	.0004	.0004	.0004	.0004	.0004	.0004	.0004	.0004	.0004	.0003
22	.0005	.0004	.0004	.0004	.0004	.0004	.0003	.0003	.0003	.0003	.0003	.0003	.0003	.0003	.0003	.0003	.0003	.0003	.0003	.0002
24	.0004	.0003	.0003	.0003	.0003	.0003	.0003	.0003	.0003	.0003	.0003	.0003	.0003	.0003	.0003	.0003	.0003	.0003	.0003	.0002
26	.0004	.0003	.0003	.0003	.0003	.0003	.0002	.0002	.0002	.0002	.0002	.0002	.0002	.0002	.0002	.0002	.0002	.0002	.0002	.0002
28	.0003	.0003	.0002	.0002	.0002	.0002	.0002	.0002	.0002	.0002	.0002	.0002	.0002	.0002	.0002	.0002	.0002	.0002	.0002	.0001
30	.0003	.0002	.0002	.0002	.0002	.0002	.0002	.0002	.0002	.0002	.0002	.0002	.0002	.0002	.0002	.0002	.0002	.0002	.0002	.0001
32	.0002	.0002	.0002	.0002	.0002	.0002	.0002	.0002	.0002	.0002	.0002	.0002	.0002	.0002	.0002	.0002	.0002	.0002	.0002	.0001
34	.0002	.0002	.0002	.0002	.0002	.0001	.0001	.0001	.0001	.0001	.0001	.0001	.0001	.0001	.0001	.0001	.0001	.0001	.0001	.(4)9
36	.0002	.0002	.0001	.0001	.0001	.0001	.0001	.0001	.0001	.0001	.0001	.0001	.0001	.0001	.0001	.0001	.0001	.0001	.0001	.(4)8
38	.0002	.0001	.0001	.0001	.0001	.0001	.0001	.0001	.0001	.0001	.0001	.0001	.0001	.0001	.0001	.0001	.0001	.0001	.0001	.(4)7
40	.0001	.0001	.0001	.0001	.0001	.0001	.0001	.0001	.0001	.0001	.0001	.0001	.0001	.0001	.0001	.0001	.0001	.0001	.0001	.(4)6
50	.(4)9	.(4)8	.(4)7	.(4)7	.(4)7	.(4)7	.(4)7	.(4)7	.(4)7	.(4)7	.(4)7	.(4)7	.(4)7	.(4)7	.(4)7	.(4)7	.(4)7	.(4)7	.(4)7	.(4)4
60	.(4)6	.(4)5	.(4)5	.(4)5	.(4)5	.(4)5	.(4)5	.(4)5	.(4)5	.(4)5	.(4)5	.(4)5	.(4)5	.(4)5	.(4)5	.(4)5	.(4)5	.(4)5	.(4)5	.(4)3
70	.(4)4	.(4)4	.(4)4	.(4)4	.(4)4	.(4)4	.(4)4	.(4)4	.(4)4	.(4)3	.(4)3	.(4)3	.(4)3	.(4)3	.(4)3	.(4)3	.(4)3	.(4)3	.(4)3	.(4)2
80	.(4)3	.(4)3	.(4)3	.(4)3	.(4)3	.(4)3	.(4)3	.(4)3	.(4)3	.(4)3	.(4)3	.(4)3	.(4)3	.(4)3	.(4)3	.(4)3	.(4)3	.(4)3	.(4)3	.(4)2
90	.(4)3	.(4)2	.(4)2	.(4)2	.(4)2	.(4)2	.(4)2	.(4)2	.(4)2	.(4)2	.(4)2	.(4)2	.(4)2	.(4)2	.(4)2	.(4)2	.(4)2	.(4)2	.(4)2	.(4)1
100	.(4)2	.(4)2	.(4)2	.(4)2	.(4)2	.(4)2	.(4)2	.(4)2	.(4)2	.(4)2	.(4)2	.(4)2	.(4)2	.(4)2	.(4)2	.(4)2	.(4)2	.(4)2	.(4)2	.(4)1

m	$\alpha_L \mid \alpha_W = 0.01$																			$\alpha_L \mid \alpha_E = 0.01$
	N=2	N=3	N=4	N=5	N=6	N=7	N=8	N=9	N=10	N=11	N=13	N=16	N=21	N=25	N=31	N=41	N=61	N=121	N → ∞	ALL N
2	.0100	.0100	.0100	.0100	.0100	.0100	.0100	.0100	.0100	.0100	.0100	.0100	.0100	.0100	.0100	.0100	.0100	.0100	.0100	.0100
3	.0049	.0042	.0040	.0039	.0038	.0038	.0037	.0037	.0037	.0037	.0037	.0036	.0036	.0036	.0036	.0036	.0036	.0036	.0036	.0033
4	.0029	.0023	.0021	.0021	.0020	.0020	.0020	.0019	.0019	.0019	.0019	.0019	.0019	.0019	.0019	.0019	.0019	.0019	.0018	.0017
5	.0019	.0015	.0013	.0013	.0012	.0012	.0012	.0012	.0012	.0012	.0012	.0012	.0012	.0012	.0012	.0011	.0011	.0011	.0011	.0010
6	.0013	.0010	.0009	.0009	.0008	.0008	.0008	.0008	.0008	.0008	.0008	.0008	.0008	.0008	.0008	.0008	.0008	.0008	.0008	.0007
7	.0010	.0007	.0007	.0006	.0006	.0006	.0006	.0006	.0006	.0006	.0006	.0006	.0006	.0006	.0006	.0006	.0006	.0006	.0006	.0005
8	.0007	.0006	.0005	.0005	.0005	.0005	.0005	.0004	.0004	.0004	.0004	.0004	.0004	.0004	.0004	.0004	.0004	.0004	.0004	.0004
9	.0006	.0004	.0004	.0004	.0004	.0004	.0004	.0004	.0003	.0003	.0003	.0003	.0003	.0003	.0003	.0003	.0003	.0003	.0003	.0003
10	.0005	.0003	.0003	.0003	.0003	.0003	.0003	.0003	.0003	.0003	.0003	.0003	.0003	.0003	.0003	.0003	.0003	.0003	.0003	.0002
11	.0004	.0003	.0003	.0002	.0002	.0002	.0002	.0002	.0002	.0002	.0002	.0002	.0002	.0002	.0002	.0002	.0002	.0002	.0002	.0002
12	.0003	.0002	.0002	.0002	.0002	.0002	.0002	.0002	.0002	.0002	.0002	.0002	.0002	.0002	.0002	.0002	.0002	.0002	.0002	.0002
13	.0003	.0002	.0002	.0002	.0002	.0002	.0002	.0002	.0002	.0002	.0002	.0002	.0002	.0002	.0002	.0002	.0002	.0002	.0002	.0001
14	.0002	.0002	.0002	.0002	.0001	.0001	.0001	.0001	.0001	.0001	.0001	.0001	.0001	.0001	.0001	.0001	.0001	.0001	.0001	.0001
15	.0002	.0001	.0001	.0001	.0001	.0001	.0001	.0001	.0001	.0001	.0001	.0001	.0001	.0001	.0001	.0001	.0001	.0001	.0001	.0001
16	.0002	.0001	.0001	.0001	.0001	.0001	.0001	.0001	.0001	.0001	.0001	.0001	.0001	.0001	.0001	.0001	.0001	.0001	.0001	.(4)8
17	.0001	.0001	.0001	.0001	.0001	.0001	.0001	.0001	.(4)9	.(4)9	.(4)9	.(4)9	.(4)9	.(4)9	.(4)9	.(4)9	.(4)9	.(4)9	.(4)9	.(4)7
18	.0001	.0001	.(4)9	.(4)9	.(4)9	.(4)9	.(4)9	.(4)9	.(4)8	.(4)8	.(4)8	.(4)8	.(4)8	.(4)8	.(4)8	.(4)8	.(4)8	.(4)8	.(4)8	.(4)7
19	.0001	.(4)9	.(4)8	.(4)8	.(4)8	.(4)8	.(4)8	.(4)8	.(4)8	.(4)8	.(4)8	.(4)7	.(4)7	.(4)7	.(4)7	.(4)7	.(4)7	.(4)7	.(4)7	.(4)6
20	.0001	.(4)8	.(4)8	.(4)7	.(4)7	.(4)7	.(4)7	.(4)7	.(4)7	.(4)7	.(4)7	.(4)7	.(4)7	.(4)7	.(4)7	.(4)7	.(4)7	.(4)7	.(4)7	.(4)5
22	.(4)8	.(4)7	.(4)6	.(4)6	.(4)6	.(4)6	.(4)6	.(4)6	.(4)6	.(4)6	.(4)6	.(4)6	.(4)6	.(4)6	.(4)5	.(4)5	.(4)5	.(4)5	.(4)5	.(4)4
24	.(4)7	.(4)6	.(4)5	.(4)5	.(4)5	.(4)5	.(4)5	.(4)5	.(4)5	.(4)5	.(4)5	.(4)5	.(4)5	.(4)5	.(4)5	.(4)5	.(4)5	.(4)5	.(4)5	.(4)4
26	.(4)6	.(4)5	.(4)4	.(4)4	.(4)4	.(4)4	.(4)4	.(4)4	.(4)4	.(4)4	.(4)4	.(4)4	.(4)4	.(4)4	.(4)4	.(4)4	.(4)4	.(4)4	.(4)4	.(4)3
28	.(4)5	.(4)4	.(4)4	.(4)4	.(4)4	.(4)4	.(4)4	.(4)4	.(4)3	.(4)3	.(4)3	.(4)3	.(4)3	.(4)3	.(4)3	.(4)3	.(4)3	.(4)3	.(4)3	.(4)3
30	.(4)4	.(4)3	.(4)3	.(4)3	.(4)3	.(4)3	.(4)3	.(4)3	.(4)3	.(4)3	.(4)3	.(4)3	.(4)3	.(4)3	.(4)3	.(4)3	.(4)3	.(4)3	.(4)3	.(4)2
32	.(4)4	.(4)3	.(4)3	.(4)3	.(4)3	.(4)3	.(4)3	.(4)3	.(4)3	.(4)3	.(4)3	.(4)3	.(4)3	.(4)3	.(4)3	.(4)3	.(4)3	.(4)3	.(4)3	.(4)2
34	.(4)3	.(4)3	.(4)3	.(4)2	.(4)2	.(4)2	.(4)2	.(4)2	.(4)2	.(4)2	.(4)2	.(4)2	.(4)2	.(4)2	.(4)2	.(4)2	.(4)2	.(4)2	.(4)2	.(4)2
36	.(4)3	.(4)2	.(4)2	.(4)2	.(4)2	.(4)2	.(4)2	.(4)2	.(4)2	.(4)2	.(4)2	.(4)2	.(4)2	.(4)2	.(4)2	.(4)2	.(4)2	.(4)2	.(4)2	.(4)2
38	.(4)3	.(4)2	.(4)2	.(4)2	.(4)2	.(4)2	.(4)2	.(4)2	.(4)2	.(4)2	.(4)2	.(4)2	.(4)2	.(4)2	.(4)2	.(4)2	.(4)2	.(4)2	.(4)2	.(4)1
40	.(4)2	.(4)2	.(4)2	.(4)2	.(4)2	.(4)2	.(4)2	.(4)2	.(4)2	.(4)2	.(4)2	.(4)2	.(4)2	.(4)2	.(4)2	.(4)2	.(4)2	.(4)2	.(4)2	.(4)1
50	.(4)1	.(4)1	.(4)1	.(4)1	.(4)1	.(4)1	.(4)1	.(4)1	.(4)1	.(4)1	.(4)1	.(4)1	.(4)1	.(4)1	.(4)1	.(4)1	.(4)1	.(4)1	.(4)1	.(5)8
60	.(4)1	.(5)9	.(5)8	.(5)8	.(5)8	.(5)8	.(5)8	.(5)8	.(5)8	.(5)8	.(5)8	.(5)8	.(5)8	.(5)8	.(5)8	.(5)8	.(5)8	.(5)8	.(5)7	.(5)6
70	.(5)7	.(5)6	.(5)6	.(5)6	.(5)6	.(5)6	.(5)6	.(5)6	.(5)6	.(5)6	.(5)6	.(5)6	.(5)6	.(5)6	.(5)6	.(5)6	.(5)6	.(5)6	.(5)5	.(5)4
80	.(5)5	.(5)5	.(5)5	.(5)5	.(5)5	.(5)4	.(5)4	.(5)5	.(5)4	.(5)5	.(5)4	.(5)4	.(5)4	.(5)4	.(5)4	.(5)4	.(5)4	.(5)4	.(5)4	.(5)3
90	.(5)4	.(5)4	.(5)4	.(5)4	.(5)4	.(5)4	.(5)4	.(5)4	.(5)4	.(5)4	.(5)4	.(5)4	.(5)4	.(5)4	.(5)4	.(5)4	.(5)4	.(5)4	.(5)3	.(5)2
100	.(5)3	.(5)3	.(5)3	.(5)3	.(5)3	.(5)3	.(5)3	.(5)3	.(5)3	.(5)3	.(5)3	.(5)3	.(5)3	.(5)3	.(5)3	.(5)3	.(5)3	.(5)3	.(5)3	.(5)2

B. Maximum values of α_L corresponding to $\alpha_X = 0.05, 0.01$

	$(\alpha_L)_{max} \vert \alpha_X = 0.05$																		
m	N=2	N=3	N=4	N=5	N=6	N=7	N=8	N=9	N=10	N=11	N=13	N=16	N=21	N=25	N=31	N=41	N=61	N=121	N → ∞
2	.0500	.0500	.0500	.0500	.0500	.0500	.0500	.0500	.0500	.0500	.0500	.0500	.0500	.0500	.0500	.0500	.0500	.0500	.0500
3	.0347	.0330	.0324	.0321	.0320	.0319	.0318	.0317	.0317	.0317	.0316	.0316	.0315	.0315	.0315	.0315	.0315	.0314	.0314
4	.0267	.0249	.0244	.0241	.0240	.0239	.0239	.0238	.0238	.0238	.0237	.0237	.0236	.0236	.0236	.0236	.0236	.0236	.0235
5	.0217	.0201	.0197	.0195	.0194	.0194	.0193	.0193	.0193	.0192	.0192	.0192	.0192	.0191	.0191	.0191	.0191	.0191	.0191
6	.0183	.0170	.0166	.0165	.0164	.0164	.0163	.0163	.0163	.0163	.0163	.0162	.0162	.0162	.0162	.0162	.0162	.0162	.0162
7	.0158	.0148	.0145	.0144	.0143	.0143	.0142	.0142	.0142	.0142	.0142	.0142	.0142	.0141	.0141	.0141	.0141	.0141	.0141
8	.0140	.0131	.0129	.0128	.0127	.0127	.0127	.0127	.0126	.0126	.0126	.0126	.0126	.0126	.0126	.0126	.0126	.0126	.0126
9	.0125	.0118	.0116	.0115	.0115	.0115	.0114	.0114	.0114	.0114	.0114	.0114	.0114	.0114	.0114	.0114	.0114	.0114	.0114
10	.0114	.0107	.0106	.0105	.0105	.0105	.0105	.0104	.0104	.0104	.0104	.0104	.0104	.0104	.0104	.0104	.0104	.0104	.0104
11	.0104	.0099	.0097	.0097	.0097	.0097	.0096	.0096	.0096	.0096	.0096	.0096	.0096	.0096	.0096	.0096	.0096	.0096	.0096
12	.0096	.0092	.0091	.0090	.0090	.0090	.0090	.0090	.0090	.0090	.0090	.0090	.0090	.0090	.0089	.0089	.0089	.0089	.0089
13	.0090	.0085	.0085	.0084	.0084	.0084	.0084	.0084	.0084	.0084	.0084	.0084	.0084	.0084	.0084	.0084	.0084	.0084	.0084
14	.0084	.0080	.0080	.0079	.0079	.0079	.0079	.0079	.0079	.0079	.0079	.0079	.0079	.0079	.0079	.0079	.0079	.0079	.0079
15	.0079	.0076	.0075	.0075	.0075	.0075	.0075	.0075	.0075	.0075	.0075	.0075	.0075	.0075	.0075	.0075	.0075	.0075	.0075
16	.0075	.0072	.0071	.0071	.0071	.0071	.0071	.0071	.0071	.0071	.0071	.0071	.0071	.0071	.0071	.0071	.0071	.0071	.0071
17	.0071	.0068	.0068	.0068	.0067	.0067	.0067	.0067	.0067	.0067	.0067	.0067	.0067	.0067	.0067	.0067	.0067	.0067	.0067
18	.0067	.0065	.0065	.0064	.0064	.0064	.0064	.0064	.0064	.0064	.0064	.0064	.0064	.0064	.0064	.0064	.0064	.0064	.0064
19	.0064	.0062	.0062	.0062	.0062	.0062	.0062	.0062	.0062	.0062	.0062	.0062	.0062	.0062	.0062	.0062	.0062	.0062	.0062
20	.0061	.0060	.0059	.0059	.0059	.0059	.0059	.0059	.0059	.0059	.0059	.0059	.0059	.0059	.0059	.0059	.0059	.0059	.0059
22	.0057	.0055	.0055	.0055	.0055	.0055	.0055	.0055	.0055	.0055	.0055	.0055	.0055	.0055	.0055	.0055	.0055	.0055	.0055
24	.0053	.0051	.0051	.0051	.0051	.0051	.0051	.0051	.0051	.0051	.0051	.0051	.0051	.0051	.0051	.0051	.0051	.0051	.0051
26	.0049	.0048	.0048	.0048	.0048	.0048	.0048	.0048	.0048	.0048	.0048	.0048	.0048	.0048	.0048	.0048	.0048	.0048	.0048
28	.0046	.0045	.0045	.0045	.0045	.0045	.0045	.0045	.0045	.0045	.0045	.0045	.0045	.0045	.0045	.0045	.0045	.0045	.0046
30	.0044	.0043	.0043	.0043	.0043	.0043	.0043	.0043	.0043	.0043	.0043	.0043	.0043	.0043	.0043	.0043	.0043	.0043	.0043
32	.0041	.0041	.0041	.0041	.0041	.0041	.0041	.0041	.0041	.0041	.0041	.0041	.0041	.0041	.0041	.0041	.0041	.0041	.0041
34	.0039	.0039	.0039	.0039	.0039	.0039	.0039	.0039	.0039	.0039	.0039	.0039	.0039	.0039	.0039	.0039	.0039	.0039	.0039
36	.0038	.0037	.0037	.0037	.0037	.0037	.0037	.0037	.0037	.0037	.0037	.0037	.0037	.0037	.0037	.0037	.0037	.0037	.0037
38	.0036	.0036	.0036	.0036	.0036	.0036	.0036	.0036	.0036	.0036	.0036	.0036	.0036	.0036	.0036	.0036	.0036	.0036	.0036
40	.0035	.0034	.0034	.0034	.0034	.0034	.0034	.0034	.0034	.0034	.0034	.0035	.0035	.0035	.0035	.0035	.0035	.0035	.0035
50	.0029	.0029	.0029	.0029	.0029	.0029	.0029	.0029	.0029	.0029	.0029	.0029	.0029	.0029	.0029	.0029	.0029	.0029	.0029
60	.0025	.0025	.0025	.0025	.0025	.0025	.0025	.0025	.0025	.0025	.0025	.0025	.0025	.0025	.0025	.0025	.0025	.0025	.0025
70	.0022	.0022	.0022	.0023	.0023	.0023	.0023	.0023	.0023	.0023	.0023	.0023	.0023	.0023	.0023	.0023	.0023	.0023	.0023
80	.0020	.0020	.0020	.0020	.0020	.0020	.0020	.0020	.0020	.0020	.0020	.0020	.0020	.0020	.0021	.0021	.0021	.0021	.0021
90	.0018	.0019	.0019	.0019	.0019	.0019	.0019	.0019	.0019	.0019	.0019	.0019	.0019	.0019	.0019	.0019	.0019	.0019	.0019
100	.0017	.0017	.0017	.0017	.0017	.0017	.0017	.0017	.0017	.0017	.0017	.0017	.0017	.0017	.0017	.0017	.0017	.0017	.0017

m	$(\alpha_L)_{max} \mid \alpha_X = 0.01$																		
	N=2	N=3	N=4	N=5	N=6	N=7	N=8	N=9	N=10	N=11	N=13	N=16	N=21	N=25	N=31	N=41	N=61	N=121	N → ∞
2	.0100	.0100	.0100	.0100	.0100	.0100	.0100	.0100	.0100	.0100	.0100	.0100	.0100	.0100	.0100	.0100	.0100	.0100	.0100
3	.0069	.0064	.0063	.0062	.0062	.0062	.0061	.0061	.0061	.0061	.0061	.0061	.0061	.0061	.0061	.0061	.0061	.0061	.0061
4	.0052	.0047	.0046	.0046	.0045	.0045	.0045	.0045	.0045	.0045	.0045	.0045	.0045	.0045	.0045	.0045	.0044	.0044	.0044
5	.0041	.0038	.0037	.0036	.0036	.0036	.0036	.0036	.0036	.0036	.0036	.0036	.0036	.0036	.0036	.0036	.0036	.0036	.0036
6	.0034	.0031	.0031	.0030	.0030	.0030	.0030	.0030	.0030	.0030	.0030	.0030	.0030	.0030	.0030	.0030	.0030	.0030	.0030
7	.0029	.0027	.0026	.0026	.0026	.0026	.0025	.0026	.0026	.0026	.0026	.0026	.0026	.0026	.0026	.0026	.0026	.0026	.0026
8	.0025	.0024	.0023	.0023	.0023	.0023	.0023	.0023	.0023	.0023	.0023	.0023	.0023	.0023	.0023	.0023	.0023	.0023	.0023
9	.0023	.0021	.0021	.0021	.0020	.0020	.0020	.0020	.0020	.0020	.0020	.0020	.0020	.0020	.0020	.0020	.0020	.0020	.0020
10	.0020	.0019	.0019	.0019	.0019	.0019	.0019	.0019	.0019	.0019	.0019	.0019	.0019	.0019	.0019	.0019	.0019	.0019	.0019
11	.0018	.0017	.0017	.0017	.0017	.0017	.0017	.0017	.0017	.0017	.0017	.0017	.0017	.0017	.0017	.0017	.0017	.0017	.0017
12	.0017	.0016	.0016	.0016	.0016	.0016	.0016	.0016	.0016	.0016	.0016	.0016	.0016	.0016	.0016	.0016	.0016	.0016	.0016
13	.0016	.0015	.0015	.0015	.0015	.0015	.0015	.0015	.0015	.0015	.0015	.0015	.0015	.0015	.0015	.0015	.0015	.0015	.0015
14	.0015	.0014	.0014	.0014	.0014	.0014	.0014	.0014	.0014	.0014	.0014	.0014	.0014	.0014	.0014	.0014	.0014	.0014	.0014
15	.0014	.0013	.0013	.0013	.0013	.0013	.0013	.0013	.0013	.0013	.0013	.0013	.0013	.0013	.0013	.0013	.0013	.0013	.0013
16	.0013	.0012	.0012	.0012	.0012	.0012	.0012	.0012	.0012	.0012	.0012	.0012	.0012	.0012	.0012	.0012	.0012	.0012	.0012
17	.0012	.0012	.0012	.0012	.0012	.0012	.0012	.0012	.0012	.0012	.0012	.0012	.0012	.0012	.0012	.0012	.0012	.0012	.0012
18	.0011	.0011	.0011	.0011	.0011	.0011	.0011	.0011	.0011	.0011	.0011	.0011	.0011	.0011	.0011	.0011	.0011	.0011	.0011
19	.0011	.0011	.0011	.0011	.0011	.0011	.0011	.0011	.0011	.0011	.0011	.0011	.0011	.0011	.0011	.0011	.0011	.0011	.0011
20	.0010	.0010	.0010	.0010	.0010	.0010	.0010	.0010	.0010	.0010	.0010	.0010	.0010	.0010	.0010	.0010	.0010	.0010	.0010
22	.0009	.0009	.0009	.0009	.0009	.0009	.0009	.0009	.0009	.0009	.0009	.0009	.0009	.0009	.0009	.0009	.0009	.0009	.0009
24	.0009	.0009	.0009	.0009	.0009	.0009	.0009	.0009	.0009	.0009	.0009	.0009	.0009	.0009	.0009	.0009	.0009	.0009	.0009
26	.0008	.0008	.0008	.0008	.0008	.0008	.0008	.0008	.0008	.0008	.0008	.0008	.0008	.0008	.0008	.0008	.0008	.0008	.0008
28	.0008	.0008	.0008	.0008	.0008	.0008	.0008	.0008	.0008	.0008	.0008	.0008	.0008	.0008	.0008	.0008	.0008	.0008	.0008
30	.0007	.0007	.0007	.0007	.0007	.0007	.0007	.0007	.0007	.0007	.0007	.0007	.0007	.0007	.0007	.0007	.0007	.0007	.0007
32	.0007	.0007	.0007	.0007	.0007	.0007	.0007	.0007	.0007	.0007	.0007	.0007	.0007	.0007	.0007	.0007	.0007	.0007	.0007
34	.0006	.0006	.0006	.0006	.0007	.0007	.0007	.0007	.0007	.0007	.0007	.0007	.0007	.0007	.0007	.0007	.0007	.0007	.0007
36	.0006	.0006	.0006	.0006	.0006	.0006	.0006	.0006	.0006	.0006	.0006	.0006	.0006	.0006	.0006	.0006	.0006	.0006	.0006
38	.0006	.0006	.0006	.0006	.0006	.0006	.0006	.0006	.0006	.0006	.0006	.0006	.0006	.0006	.0006	.0006	.0006	.0006	.0006
40	.0006	.0006	.0006	.0006	.0006	.0006	.0006	.0006	.0006	.0006	.0006	.0006	.0006	.0006	.0006	.0006	.0006	.0006	.0006
50	.0005	.0005	.0005	.0005	.0005	.0005	.0005	.0005	.0005	.0005	.0005	.0005	.0005	.0005	.0005	.0005	.0005	.0005	.0005
60	.0004	.0004	.0004	.0004	.0004	.0004	.0004	.0004	.0004	.0004	.0004	.0004	.0004	.0004	.0004	.0004	.0004	.0004	.0004
70	.0004	.0004	.0004	.0004	.0004	.0004	.0004	.0004	.0004	.0004	.0004	.0004	.0004	.0004	.0004	.0004	.0004	.0004	.0004
80	.0003	.0003	.0003	.0003	.0003	.0003	.0003	.0003	.0003	.0003	.0003	.0003	.0003	.0003	.0003	.0003	.0003	.0003	.0003
90	.0003	.0003	.0003	.0003	.0003	.0003	.0003	.0003	.0003	.0003	.0003	.0003	.0003	.0003	.0003	.0003	.0003	.0003	.0003
100	.0003	.0003	.0003	.0003	.0003	.0003	.0003	.0003	.0003	.0003	.0003	.0003	.0003	.0003	.0003	.0003	.0003	.0003	.0003

C. Minimum values of α_l corresponding to $\alpha_S = 0.05, 0.01$

m	$(\alpha_L)_{min} \mid \alpha_S = 0.05$																		
	N=2	N=3	N=4	N=5	N=6	N=7	N=8	N=9	N=10	N=11	N=13	N=16	N=21	N=25	N=31	N=41	N=61	N=121	$N \to \infty$
2	.0500	.0500	.0500	.0500	.0500	.0500	.0500	.0500	.0500	.0500	.0500	.0500	.0500	.0500	.0500	.0500	.0500	.0500	.0500
3	.0496	.0443	.0425	.0416	.0411	.0407	.0405	.0403	.0402	.0401	.0399	.0397	.0395	.0395	.0394	.0393	.0392	.0391	.0391
4	.0463	.0395	.0372	.0361	.0354	.0350	.0347	.0345	.0343	.0341	.0339	.0337	.0335	.0334	.0333	.0332	.0331	.0330	.0329
5	.0429	.0357	.0334	.0322	.0316	.0311	.0308	.0306	.0304	.0302	.0300	.0298	.0296	.0295	.0294	.0293	.0292	.0290	.0289
6	.0400	.0328	.0305	.0294	.0287	.0283	.0279	.0277	.0275	.0274	.0272	.0269	.0267	.0266	.0265	.0264	.0263	.0262	.0261
7	.0375	.0305	.0283	.0272	.0265	.0261	.0258	.0255	.0254	.0252	.0250	.0248	.0246	.0245	.0244	.0243	.0242	.0241	.0240
8	.0354	.0286	.0264	.0254	.0247	.0243	.0240	.0238	.0237	.0235	.0233	.0231	.0229	.0228	.0227	.0226	.0225	.0224	.0223
9	.0335	.0270	.0249	.0239	.0233	.0229	.0226	.0224	.0222	.0221	.0219	.0217	.0215	.0214	.0213	.0212	.0211	.0211	.0210
10	.0320	.0257	.0237	.0227	.0221	.0217	.0214	.0212	.0211	.0209	.0208	.0206	.0204	.0203	.0202	.0201	.0200	.0199	.0198
11	.0306	.0245	.0226	.0216	.0211	.0207	.0205	.0203	.0201	.0200	.0198	.0196	.0194	.0194	.0193	.0192	.0191	.0190	.0189
12	.0294	.0235	.0217	.0208	.0202	.0199	.0196	.0194	.0192	.0191	.0190	.0188	.0186	.0185	.0184	.0183	.0183	.0182	.0181
13	.0283	.0227	.0208	.0200	.0194	.0191	.0189	.0187	.0185	.0184	.0183	.0181	.0179	.0178	.0177	.0177	.0176	.0175	.0174
14	.0274	.0219	.0201	.0193	.0188	.0184	.0182	.0180	.0179	.0178	.0176	.0174	.0173	.0172	.0171	.0170	.0169	.0169	.0168
15	.0266	.0212	.0195	.0187	.0182	.0179	.0176	.0174	.0173	.0172	.0170	.0169	.0167	.0166	.0166	.0165	.0164	.0163	.0162
16	.0257	.0206	.0189	.0181	.0176	.0173	.0171	.0169	.0168	.0167	.0165	.0164	.0162	.0162	.0161	.0160	.0159	.0159	.0158
17	.0250	.0200	.0184	.0176	.0172	.0169	.0166	.0165	.0163	.0162	.0161	.0159	.0158	.0157	.0156	.0156	.0155	.0154	.0154
18	.0244	.0195	.0180	.0172	.0167	.0164	.0162	.0161	.0159	.0158	.0157	.0155	.0154	.0153	.0152	.0152	.0151	.0150	.0149
19	.0239	.0190	.0175	.0168	.0163	.0160	.0158	.0157	.0155	.0155	.0153	.0152	.0150	.0149	.0149	.0148	.0147	.0147	.0146
20	.0233	.0186	.0172	.0164	.0160	.0157	.0155	.0153	.0152	.0151	.0150	.0148	.0147	.0146	.0145	.0145	.0144	.0143	.0143
22	.0224	.0179	.0164	.0158	.0153	.0151	.0149	.0147	.0146	.0145	.0144	.0142	.0141	.0140	.0140	.0139	.0138	.0138	.0137
24	.0215	.0172	.0159	.0152	.0148	.0145	.0143	.0142	.0141	.0140	.0138	.0137	.0136	.0135	.0135	.0134	.0133	.0133	.0132
26	.0208	.0167	.0153	.0147	.0143	.0140	.0138	.0137	.0136	.0135	.0134	.0133	.0131	.0131	.0130	.0129	.0129	.0128	.0128
28	.0202	.0162	.0149	.0143	.0139	.0136	.0134	.0133	.0132	.0131	.0130	.0129	.0128	.0127	.0126	.0126	.0125	.0125	.0124
30	.0196	.0157	.0145	.0139	.0135	.0133	.0131	.0129	.0128	.0128	.0127	.0125	.0124	.0124	.0123	.0122	.0122	.0121	.0121
32	.0191	.0153	.0141	.0135	.0132	.0129	.0128	.0126	.0125	.0125	.0123	.0122	.0121	.0121	.0120	.0119	.0119	.0118	.0118
34	.0186	.0150	.0138	.0132	.0129	.0126	.0125	.0123	.0122	.0122	.0121	.0119	.0118	.0118	.0117	.0117	.0116	.0116	.0115
36	.0182	.0146	.0135	.0129	.0126	.0124	.0122	.0121	.0120	.0119	.0118	.0117	.0116	.0115	.0115	.0114	.0114	.0113	.0113
38	.0179	.0144	.0132	.0127	.0123	.0121	.0120	.0118	.0118	.0117	.0116	.0115	.0114	.0113	.0113	.0112	.0111	.0111	.0110
40	.0175	.0141	.0130	.0124	.0121	.0119	.0117	.0116	.0115	.0115	.0114	.0113	.0112	.0111	.0110	.0110	.0109	.0109	.0108
50	.0161	.0130	.0120	.0115	.0112	.0110	.0109	.0108	.0107	.0106	.0105	.0104	.0103	.0103	.0102	.0102	.0102	.0101	.0101
60	.0151	.0123	.0113	.0108	.0106	.0104	.0102	.0101	.0101	.0100	.0099	.0098	.0098	.0097	.0097	.0096	.0096	.0095	.0095
70	.0142	.0117	.0108	.0103	.0101	.0099	.0098	.0097	.0096	.0096	.0095	.0094	.0093	.0093	.0092	.0092	.0092	.0091	.0091
80	.0136	.0112	.0104	.0099	.0097	.0095	.0094	.0093	.0093	.0092	.0091	.0091	.0090	.0089	.0089	.0089	.0088	.0088	.0087
90	.0131	.0108	.0100	.0096	.0094	.0092	.0091	.0090	.0090	.0089	.0089	.0088	.0087	.0087	.0086	.0086	.0086	.0085	.0085
100	.0127	.0105	.0097	.0093	.0091	.0090	.0089	.0088	.0087	.0087	.0086	.0085	.0085	.0084	.0084	.0084	.0083	.0083	.0083

$(\alpha_L)_{\min} | \alpha_S = 0.01$

m	N=2	N=3	N=4	N=5	N=6	N=7	N=8	N=9	N=10	N=11	N=13	N=16	N=21	N=25	N=31	N=41	N=61	N=121	N → ∞
2	.0100	.0100	.0100	.0100	.0100	.0100	.0100	.0100	.0100	.0100	.0100	.0100	.0100	.0100	.0100	.0100	.0100	.0100	.0100
3	.0098	.0085	.0081	.0079	.0077	.0076	.0076	.0075	.0075	.0075	.0075	.0074	.0074	.0074	.0073	.0073	.0073	.0073	.0073
4	.0089	.0072	.0067	.0065	.0063	.0062	.0062	.0061	.0061	.0061	.0060	.0060	.0059	.0059	.0059	.0059	.0059	.0058	.0058
5	.0079	.0063	.0058	.0055	.0054	.0053	.0053	.0052	.0052	.0051	.0051	.0051	.0050	.0050	.0050	.0050	.0049	.0049	.0049
6	.0071	.0056	.0051	.0049	.0047	.0047	.0046	.0046	.0045	.0045	.0045	.0044	.0044	.0044	.0043	.0043	.0043	.0043	.0043
7	.0065	.0050	.0046	.0044	.0042	.0042	.0041	.0041	.0040	.0040	.0040	.0040	.0039	.0039	.0039	.0039	.0039	.0038	.0038
8	.0059	.0045	.0042	.0040	.0039	.0038	.0037	.0037	.0037	.0036	.0036	.0036	.0036	.0035	.0035	.0035	.0035	.0035	.0035
9	.0054	.0042	.0038	.0036	.0035	.0035	.0034	.0034	.0034	.0034	.0033	.0033	.0033	.0032	.0032	.0032	.0032	.0032	.0032
10	.0050	.0039	.0035	.0034	.0033	.0032	.0032	.0032	.0031	.0031	.0031	.0031	.0030	.0030	.0030	.0030	.0030	.0030	.0029
11	.0047	.0036	.0033	.0032	.0031	.0030	.0030	.0029	.0029	.0029	.0029	.0029	.0028	.0028	.0028	.0028	.0028	.0028	.0027
12	.0044	.0034	.0031	.0030	.0029	.0028	.0028	.0028	.0028	.0027	.0027	.0027	.0027	.0026	.0026	.0026	.0026	.0026	.0026
13	.0042	.0032	.0029	.0028	.0027	.0027	.0026	.0026	.0026	.0026	.0026	.0025	.0025	.0025	.0025	.0025	.0025	.0025	.0024
14	.0039	.0030	.0028	.0027	.0026	.0025	.0025	.0025	.0025	.0025	.0024	.0024	.0024	.0024	.0024	.0024	.0023	.0023	.0023
15	.0037	.0029	.0027	.0025	.0025	.0024	.0024	.0024	.0024	.0023	.0023	.0023	.0023	.0023	.0023	.0022	.0022	.0022	.0022
16	.0036	.0028	.0025	.0024	.0024	.0023	.0023	.0023	.0023	.0022	.0022	.0022	.0022	.0022	.0022	.0022	.0021	.0021	.0021
17	.0034	.0027	.0024	.0023	.0023	.0022	.0022	.0022	.0022	.0021	.0021	.0021	.0021	.0021	.0021	.0021	.0021	.0020	.0020
18	.0033	.0026	.0023	.0022	.0022	.0021	.0021	.0021	.0021	.0021	.0020	.0020	.0020	.0020	.0020	.0020	.0020	.0020	.0020
19	.0031	.0025	.0023	.0022	.0021	.0021	.0020	.0020	.0020	.0020	.0020	.0020	.0019	.0019	.0019	.0019	.0019	.0019	.0019
20	.0030	.0024	.0022	.0021	.0020	.0020	.0020	.0020	.0019	.0019	.0019	.0019	.0019	.0019	.0019	.0019	.0018	.0018	.0018
22	.0028	.0022	.0020	.0020	.0019	.0019	.0018	.0018	.0018	.0018	.0018	.0018	.0018	.0018	.0017	.0017	.0017	.0017	.0017
24	.0026	.0021	.0019	.0018	.0018	.0018	.0017	.0017	.0017	.0017	.0017	.0017	.0017	.0017	.0017	.0016	.0016	.0016	.0016
26	.0025	.0020	.0018	.0018	.0017	.0017	.0017	.0016	.0016	.0016	.0016	.0016	.0016	.0016	.0016	.0016	.0016	.0016	.0015
28	.0024	.0019	.0017	.0017	.0016	.0016	.0016	.0016	.0016	.0016	.0015	.0015	.0015	.0015	.0015	.0015	.0015	.0015	.0015
30	.0023	.0018	.0017	.0016	.0016	.0015	.0015	.0015	.0015	.0015	.0015	.0015	.0014	.0014	.0014	.0014	.0014	.0014	.0014
32	.0022	.0017	.0016	.0015	.0015	.0015	.0015	.0014	.0014	.0014	.0014	.0014	.0014	.0014	.0014	.0014	.0014	.0014	.0014
34	.0021	.0017	.0015	.0015	.0014	.0014	.0014	.0014	.0014	.0014	.0014	.0014	.0013	.0013	.0013	.0013	.0013	.0013	.0013
36	.0020	.0016	.0015	.0014	.0014	.0014	.0014	.0013	.0013	.0013	.0013	.0013	.0013	.0013	.0013	.0013	.0013	.0013	.0013
38	.0019	.0015	.0014	.0014	.0013	.0013	.0013	.0013	.0013	.0013	.0013	.0013	.0013	.0013	.0012	.0012	.0012	.0012	.0012
40	.0019	.0015	.0014	.0013	.0013	.0013	.0013	.0013	.0013	.0012	.0012	.0012	.0012	.0012	.0012	.0012	.0012	.0012	.0012
50	.0016	.0013	.0012	.0012	.0011	.0011	.0011	.0011	.0011	.0011	.0011	.0011	.0011	.0011	.0011	.0011	.0011	.0011	.0010
60	.0014	.0012	.0011	.0011	.0010	.0010	.0010	.0010	.0010	.0010	.0010	.0010	.0010	.0010	.0010	.0010	.0010	.0010	.0009
70	.0013	.0011	.0010	.0010	.0010	.0009	.0009	.0009	.0009	.0009	.0009	.0009	.0009	.0009	.0009	.0009	.0009	.0009	.0009
80	.0012	.0010	.0009	.0009	.0009	.0009	.0009	.0009	.0009	.0009	.0008	.0008	.0008	.0008	.0008	.0008	.0008	.0008	.0008
90	.0011	.0009	.0009	.0009	.0008	.0008	.0008	.0008	.0008	.0008	.0008	.0008	.0008	.0008	.0008	.0008	.0008	.0008	.0008
100	.0011	.0009	.0008	.0008	.0008	.0008	.0008	.0008	.0008	.0008	.0008	.0008	.0007	.0007	.0007	.0007	.0007	.0007	.0007

Table B5

COMPARISON OF TYPE II–III ERROR RATES FOR MULTIPLE COMPARISON TESTS (SINGLE-CLASSIFICATION EXPERIMENTS)

$[\delta = 0.5(0.5)3.0]$

$\beta'_L = \beta_L + \gamma_L$, $\beta'_S = \beta_S + \gamma_S$, $\beta'_X = \beta_X + \gamma_X$, $\beta'_W = \beta_W + \gamma_W$ **are the sums of the error rates of Types II and III for the LSD (multiple** t**) test, Duncan's multiple range test, Tukey's** X **procedure, and Tukey's studentized range test, respectively;** $\delta = (\mu_U - \mu_L)/\sigma$**, where** μ_U **and** μ_L **are defined in Chapter 2, subsection 2.2.7, and** σ **is the common population standard deviation.**

A. Values of $\beta_1' = \beta_L'$, $\beta_2' = (\beta_S')_{\max}$, $\beta_3' = (\beta_X')_{\min}$ and $\beta_4' = \beta_W'$ for $\alpha = 0.05$

N	m	δ=0.5				δ=1.0				δ=1.5			
		β_1'	β_2'	β_3'	β_4'	β_1'	β_2'	β_3'	β_4'	β_1'	β_2'	β_3'	β_4'
2	2	.938	.938	.938	.938	.905	.905	.905	.905	.851	.851	.851	.851
	3	.935	.935	.954	.967	.889	.890	.920	.941	.813	.814	.862	.897
	4	.932	.937	.963	.978	.878	.885	.929	.957	.787	.799	.869	.918
	5	.930	.940	.968	.985	.870	.885	.936	.967	.768	.792	.875	.932
	6	.929	.942	.972	.988	.864	.887	.941	.973	.755	.789	.881	.942
	7	.928	.945	.975	.991	.860	.888	.945	.978	.745	.789	.885	.950
	8	.927	.947	.977	.993	.857	.890	.948	.981	.737	.789	.889	.956
	9	.927	.949	.979	.994	.854	.892	.951	.984	.731	.790	.892	.961
	10	.926	.951	.981	.995	.852	.894	.953	.985	.726	.792	.896	.964
	11	.926	.952	.982	.996	.850	.896	.955	.988	.722	.793	.898	.968
	12	.925	.954	.983	.996	.849	.898	.957	.989	.718	.795	.901	.970
	13	.925	.955	.984	.997	.847	.899	.959	.990	.715	.796	.903	.973
	14	.925	.956	.985	.997	.846	.901	.960	.991	.713	.798	.905	.975
	15	.924	.957	.986	.998	.845	.902	.961	.992	.710	.799	.907	.977
	16	.924	.958	.986	.998	.844	.903	.962	.993	.708	.801	.909	.978
	17	.924	.959	.987	.998	.843	.905	.964	.993	.707	.802	.911	.980
	18	.924	.960	.987	.998	.843	.906	.964	.994	.705	.803	.913	.981
	19	.924	.960	.988	.998	.842	.907	.965	.994	.703	.805	.914	.982
	20	.924	.961	.988	.999	.841	.908	.966	.995	.702	.806	.916	.983
	22	.923	.962	.989	.999	.840	.910	.968	.995	.700	.808	.918	.985
	24	.923	.963	.990	.999	.840	.911	.969	.996	.698	.810	.921	.986
	26	.923	.964	.990	.999	.839	.913	.970	.996	.696	.812	.923	.987
	28	.923	.955	.991	.999	.838	.914	.971	.997	.695	.814	.925	.988
	30	.923	.966	.991	.999	.838	.915	.972	.997	.694	.816	.926	.989
	32	.923	.966	.991	.999	.837	.917	.973	.997	.693	.818	.928	.990
	34	.923	.967	.992	.999	.837	.918	.974	.997	.692	.819	.930	.991
	35	.922	.968	.992	.999	.836	.919	.975	.998	.691	.821	.931	.991
	38	.922	.968	.992	1.000	.836	.920	.975	.998	.690	.822	.932	.992
	40	.922	.969	.993	1.000	.836	.920	.976	.998	.690	.823	.933	.992
	50	.922	.971	.994	1.000	.835	.924	.978	.999	.687	.829	.939	.994
	60	.922	.972	.994	1.000	.834	.927	.980	.999	.686	.833	.943	.995
	70	.922	.973	.995	1.000	.833	.929	.982	.999	.684	.837	.946	.996
	80	.922	.974	.995	1.000	.833	.931	.983	.999	.683	.840	.949	.997
	90	.922	.975	.996	1.000	.833	.933	.984	.999	.683	.843	.951	.997
	100	.921	.976	.996	1.000	.832	.934	.985	1.000	.682	.845	.953	.998

N	m	δ=2.0				δ=2.5				δ=3.0			
		β_1'	β_2'	β_3'	β_4'	β_1'	β_2'	β_3'	β_4'	β_1'	β_2'	β_3'	β_4'
2	2	.782	.782	.782	.782	.700	.700	.700	.700	.613	.613	.613	.613
	3	.711	.713	.781	.833	.592	.594	.682	.751	.467	.470	.571	.655
	4	.664	.680	.782	.858	.523	.542	.671	.776	.381	.401	.544	.674
	5	.632	.664	.784	.876	.477	.514	.665	.794	.328	.364	.528	.689
	6	.609	.655	.787	.889	.446	.497	.662	.808	.293	.342	.518	.701
	7	.592	.650	.790	.899	.424	.487	.661	.820	.269	.328	.511	.712
	8	.579	.647	.793	.908	.407	.481	.661	.830	.252	.318	.507	.722
	9	.569	.646	.796	.915	.394	.476	.662	.839	.239	.312	.504	.731
	10	.560	.645	.799	.921	.383	.473	.663	.847	.229	.307	.503	.740
	11	.554	.645	.802	.926	.375	.471	.665	.855	.220	.304	.502	.747
	12	.548	.646	.805	.931	.368	.471	.666	.861	.214	.301	.502	.754
	13	.543	.646	.807	.935	.362	.470	.668	.867	.208	.300	.502	.761
	14	.539	.647	.809	.939	.357	.470	.670	.872	.203	.298	.502	.767
	15	.535	.648	.812	.942	.353	.470	.672	.877	.199	.297	.503	.773
	16	.532	.650	.814	.945	.349	.470	.674	.881	.196	.297	.504	.779
	17	.529	.651	.816	.948	.346	.470	.676	.886	.193	.296	.505	.784
	18	.527	.652	.818	.950	.343	.471	.678	.889	.190	.296	.506	.789
	19	.524	.653	.820	.952	.340	.471	.680	.893	.188	.296	.507	.794
	20	.522	.654	.822	.954	.338	.472	.681	.896	.186	.296	.508	.798
	22	.519	.656	.826	.958	.334	.473	.685	.902	.182	.296	.511	.806
	24	.516	.658	.829	.961	.330	.475	.688	.908	.179	.296	.513	.814
	26	.514	.660	.832	.964	.327	.476	.692	.912	.177	.297	.516	.820
	28	.511	.662	.835	.966	.325	.477	.695	.917	.175	.298	.519	.827
	30	.510	.664	.837	.968	.323	.479	.698	.920	.173	.298	.521	.832
	32	.508	.666	.840	.970	.321	.480	.701	.924	.171	.299	.524	.838
	34	.507	.668	.842	.972	.320	.482	.703	.927	.170	.300	.526	.843
	36	.505	.669	.844	.973	.318	.483	.706	.930	.169	.301	.529	.847
	38	.504	.671	.846	.974	.317	.484	.709	.933	.168	.301	.531	.851
	40	.503	.672	.848	.976	.316	.485	.711	.935	.167	.302	.533	.855
	50	.499	.679	.857	.980	.311	.492	.722	.945	.163	.307	.544	.872
	60	.497	.684	.864	.984	.309	.496	.731	.952	.161	.310	.554	.885
	70	.495	.689	.869	.986	.307	.502	.739	.958	.159	.314	.562	.896
	80	.494	.693	.874	.988	.305	.506	.746	.962	.158	.317	.570	.904
	90	.493	.697	.878	.989	.304	.509	.752	.965	.157	.320	.577	.911
	100	.492	.699	.882	.990	.303	.512	.757	.969	.156	.322	.583	.917

A. Values of $\beta_1' = \beta_L'$, $\beta_2' = (\beta_S')_{\max}$, $\beta_3' = (\beta_X')_{\min}$ and $\beta_4' = \beta_W'$ for $\alpha = 0.05$

		$\delta = 0.5$				$\delta = 1.0$				$\delta = 1.5$			
N	m	β_1'	β_2'	β_3'	β_4'	β_1'	β_2'	β_3'	β_4'	β_1'	β_2'	β_3'	β_4'
3	2	.923	.923	.923	.923	.841	.841	.841	.841	.707	.707	.707	.707
	3	.918	.927	.944	.961	.821	.836	.869	.904	.660	.683	.736	.797
	4	.916	.931	.954	.975	.809	.838	.884	.932	.633	.678	.753	.840
	5	.914	.936	.961	.983	.801	.842	.895	.947	.617	.678	.766	.867
	6	.913	.939	.966	.987	.796	.846	.903	.957	.606	.680	.777	.886
	7	.912	.942	.969	.990	.792	.850	.909	.964	.598	.684	.786	.900
	8	.911	.945	.972	.992	.789	.854	.915	.970	.592	.687	.793	.911
	9	.911	.947	.974	.993	.787	.857	.919	.974	.587	.691	.800	.920
	10	.910	.949	.976	.994	.785	.860	.923	.977	.583	.694	.805	.927
	11	.910	.950	.977	.995	.784	.862	.926	.980	.580	.697	.810	.933
	12	.910	.952	.978	.996	.783	.865	.929	.982	.578	.700	.815	.938
	13	.909	.953	.979	.996	.782	.867	.931	.983	.576	.703	.819	.943
	14	.909	.954	.980	.997	.781	.869	.933	.985	.574	.706	.823	.947
	15	.909	.955	.981	.997	.780	.871	.935	.986	.572	.708	.827	.950
	16	.909	.956	.982	.997	.779	.873	.937	.987	.571	.710	.830	.953
	17	.909	.957	.983	.998	.778	.874	.939	.988	.569	.713	.833	.956
	18	.908	.958	.983	.998	.778	.876	.940	.989	.568	.715	.836	.958
	19	.908	.959	.984	.998	.777	.878	.942	.990	.567	.717	.838	.960
	20	.908	.959	.984	.998	.777	.879	.943	.990	.566	.719	.841	.962
	22	.908	.961	.985	.998	.776	.881	.946	.992	.565	.722	.846	.966
	24	.908	.962	.986	.999	.775	.883	.948	.993	.563	.725	.850	.969
	26	.908	.963	.987	.999	.775	.885	.949	.993	.562	.728	.853	.971
	28	.908	.963	.987	.999	.774	.887	.951	.994	.561	.731	.857	.973
	30	.907	.964	.988	.999	.774	.889	.953	.994	.560	.733	.860	.975
	32	.907	.965	.988	.999	.774	.890	.954	.995	.560	.735	.863	.977
	34	.907	.965	.989	.999	.773	.891	.955	.995	.559	.737	.865	.978
	36	.907	.966	.989	.999	.773	.893	.956	.996	.559	.740	.868	.979
	38	.907	.967	.990	.999	.773	.894	.958	.996	.558	.741	.870	.981
	40	.907	.967	.990	.999	.773	.895	.959	.996	.558	.743	.872	.982
	50	.907	.969	.991	1.000	.772	.899	.963	.997	.556	.750	.881	.986
	60	.907	.970	.992	1.000	.771	.902	.966	.998	.555	.755	.889	.988
	70	.907	.971	.993	1.000	.771	.905	.968	.998	.554	.760	.894	.990
	80	.907	.972	.993	1.000	.770	.907	.970	.999	.553	.763	.899	.992
	90	.907	.973	.994	1.000	.770	.909	.972	.999	.553	.767	.903	.993
	100	.906	.974	.994	1.000	.770	.911	.973	.999	.552	.770	.907	.993

N	m	δ=2.0				δ=2.5				δ=3.0			
		β_1'	β_2'	β_3'	β_4'	β_1'	β_2'	β_3'	β_4'	β_1'	β_2'	β_3'	β_4'
3	2	.537	.537	.537	.537	.364	.364	.364	.364	.218	.218	.218	.218
	3	.463	.491	.557	.641	.276	.302	.367	.458	.138	.157	.207	.287
	4	.424	.474	.569	.694	.235	.279	.370	.509	.106	.135	.202	.324
	5	.401	.469	.580	.729	.212	.269	.374	.544	.0894	.125	.200	.351
	6	.386	.457	.589	.756	.198	.264	.379	.573	.0797	.119	.200	.373
	7	.375	.468	.597	.776	.188	.262	.383	.595	.0732	.116	.201	.392
	8	.367	.469	.605	.794	.180	.261	.388	.615	.0686	.115	.203	.409
	9	.360	.472	.612	.808	.175	.261	.393	.632	.0652	.114	.204	.424
	10	.355	.474	.618	.820	.171	.262	.397	.647	.0627	.113	.206	.437
	11	.351	.476	.623	.830	.167	.263	.402	.661	.0606	.113	.208	.450
	12	.348	.478	.629	.840	.164	.264	.406	.573	.0590	.113	.210	.462
	13	.345	.481	.634	.848	.162	.265	.410	.684	.0576	.113	.213	.473
	14	.343	.483	.638	.855	.160	.266	.413	.694	.0564	.114	.215	.483
	15	.341	.485	.643	.862	.158	.267	.417	.703	.0554	.114	.217	.492
	16	.339	.487	.647	.868	.156	.268	.421	.712	.0546	.115	.219	.501
	17	.337	.489	.651	.873	.155	.270	.424	.720	.0538	.115	.221	.510
	18	.336	.492	.654	.878	.154	.271	.427	.728	.0532	.115	.223	.518
	19	.335	.494	.658	.883	.153	.272	.431	.735	.0526	.116	.225	.525
	20	.333	.495	.661	.887	.152	.273	.434	.741	.0521	.117	.227	.533
	22	.331	.499	.667	.895	.150	.276	.439	.753	.0512	.117	.230	.546
	24	.330	.502	.673	.901	.149	.278	.445	.764	.0505	.118	.234	.559
	26	.329	.505	.678	.907	.148	.280	.450	.774	.0499	.119	.238	.571
	28	.327	.507	.683	.912	.147	.282	.455	.782	.0494	.120	.241	.581
	30	.326	.510	.687	.917	.146	.284	.459	.790	.0490	.121	.244	.591
	32	.325	.513	.692	.921	.146	.285	.463	.798	.0486	.122	.247	.600
	34	.325	.515	.696	.925	.145	.287	.467	.804	.0483	.123	.250	.609
	36	.324	.517	.699	.928	.144	.289	.471	.811	.0480	.124	.253	.617
	38	.323	.519	.703	.931	.144	.290	.475	.816	.0477	.124	.255	.625
	40	.323	.521	.706	.934	.143	.292	.479	.822	.0475	.125	.258	.632
	50	.321	.528	.720	.945	.142	.297	.494	.844	.0466	.128	.270	.664
	60	.319	.535	.732	.953	.141	.302	.507	.861	.0460	.131	.280	.689
	70	.318	.540	.741	.959	.140	.306	.518	.874	.0456	.133	.289	.709
	80	.317	.544	.749	.964	.139	.310	.528	.884	.0453	.135	.297	.726
	90	.317	.548	.757	.967	.139	.313	.536	.893	.0451	.137	.304	.741
	100	.316	.552	.763	.970	.139	.317	.544	.901	.0449	.139	.311	.754

A. Values of $\beta_1' = \beta_L'$, $\beta_2' = (\beta_S')_{\max}$, $\beta_3' = (\beta_X')_{\min}$ and $\beta_4' = \beta_W'$ for $\alpha = 0.05$

		$\delta=0.5$				$\delta=1.0$				$\delta=1.5$			
N	m	β_1'	β_2'	β_3'	β_4'	β_1'	β_2'	β_3'	β_4'	β_1'	β_2'	β_3'	β_4'
4	2	.908	.908	.908	.908	.777	.777	.777	.777	.570	.570	.570	.570
	3	.903	.915	.933	.954	.755	.779	.815	.863	.526	.559	.612	.689
	4	.900	.922	.945	.970	.744	.786	.837	.900	.504	.561	.637	.749
	5	.898	.927	.953	.979	.737	.793	.851	.922	.490	.566	.656	.788
	6	.897	.931	.958	.984	.732	.799	.862	.937	.481	.571	.670	.815
	7	.896	.934	.962	.988	.729	.805	.871	.947	.475	.577	.682	.836
	8	.896	.937	.965	.990	.726	.810	.877	.954	.470	.582	.692	.852
	9	.895	.940	.968	.992	.724	.814	.883	.960	.466	.587	.701	.865
	10	.895	.942	.970	.993	.722	.818	.888	.965	.463	.591	.709	.876
	11	.894	.944	.972	.994	.721	.821	.893	.968	.460	.596	.716	.885
	12	.894	.945	.973	.995	.720	.825	.896	.971	.458	.600	.722	.893
	13	.894	.947	.974	.995	.719	.827	.900	.974	.457	.603	.728	.900
	14	.894	.948	.975	.996	.718	.830	.903	.976	.455	.607	.733	.906
	15	.894	.949	.977	.996	.717	.832	.906	.978	.454	.610	.738	.912
	15	.893	.950	.977	.997	.717	.835	.908	.980	.453	.613	.742	.917
	17	.893	.951	.978	.997	.716	.837	.911	.981	.452	.615	.746	.921
	18	.893	.952	.979	.997	.716	.839	.913	.982	.451	.618	.750	.925
	19	.893	.953	.980	.997	.715	.840	.915	.984	.450	.620	.754	.928
	20	.893	.954	.980	.998	.715	.842	.916	.985	.449	.623	.757	.932
	22	.893	.955	.981	.998	.714	.845	.920	.986	.448	.627	.763	.937
	24	.893	.956	.982	.998	.713	.848	.923	.988	.447	.631	.769	.942
	26	.893	.957	.983	.998	.713	.850	.925	.989	.446	.634	.774	.946
	28	.892	.958	.984	.999	.713	.852	.928	.990	.445	.637	.779	.950
	30	.892	.959	.985	.999	.712	.854	.930	.991	.445	.640	.783	.953
	32	.892	.960	.985	.999	.712	.856	.932	.991	.444	.643	.787	.956
	34	.892	.961	.986	.999	.712	.857	.933	.992	.444	.645	.791	.958
	36	.892	.961	.986	.999	.711	.859	.935	.993	.443	.648	.794	.960
	38	.892	.962	.987	.999	.711	.860	.936	.993	.443	.650	.797	.962
	40	.892	.962	.987	.999	.711	.862	.938	.994	.443	.652	.800	.964
	50	.892	.964	.989	.999	.710	.867	.944	.995	.441	.660	.813	.971
	60	.892	.966	.990	1.000	.710	.871	.948	.996	.440	.667	.823	.976
	70	.892	.967	.991	1.000	.709	.874	.951	.997	.440	.672	.831	.980
	80	.892	.968	.991	1.000	.709	.877	.954	.997	.439	.676	.838	.982
	90	.891	.969	.992	1.000	.709	.879	.956	.998	.439	.680	.843	.984
	100	.891	.970	.992	1.000	.709	.881	.958	.998	.439	.683	.848	.986

N	m	δ=2.0				δ=2.5				δ=3.0			
		β_1'	β_2'	β_3'	β_4'	β_1'	β_2'	β_3'	β_4'	β_1'	β_2'	β_3'	β_4'
4	2	.343	.343	.343	.343	.164	.164	.164	.164	.0611	.0611	.0611	.0611
	3	.288	.319	.373	.460	.119	.139	.176	.245	.0360	.0448	.0628	.101
	4	.262	.314	.391	.525	.100	.131	.184	.294	.0272	.0396	.0639	.126
	5	.247	.314	.405	.571	.0898	.128	.190	.331	.0228	.0374	.0652	.146
	6	.237	.316	.418	.606	.0835	.128	.196	.360	.0203	.0365	.0668	.163
	7	.231	.319	.428	.634	.0793	.128	.202	.385	.0187	.0361	.0684	.178
	8	.226	.322	.437	.657	.0763	.129	.207	.407	.0175	.0360	.0701	.192
	9	.222	.325	.445	.677	.0739	.130	.212	.427	.0167	.0361	.0718	.204
	10	.219	.328	.453	.694	.0721	.131	.216	.444	.0160	.0363	.0734	.215
	11	.216	.331	.460	.709	.0706	.133	.221	.460	.0155	.0366	.0750	.226
	12	.214	.334	.466	.722	.0695	.134	.225	.474	.0151	.0369	.0765	.236
	13	.212	.337	.472	.734	.0685	.135	.228	.487	.0148	.0372	.0780	.246
	14	.211	.340	.478	.745	.0676	.136	.232	.500	.0145	.0375	.0795	.255
	15	.210	.342	.483	.755	.0669	.137	.236	.511	.0142	.0378	.0810	.263
	16	.209	.344	.488	.764	.0663	.139	.239	.522	.0140	.0382	.0824	.271
	17	.208	.347	.492	.772	.0658	.140	.242	.532	.0139	.0385	.0837	.279
	18	.207	.349	.497	.779	.0653	.141	.245	.541	.0137	.0388	.0850	.286
	19	.206	.351	.501	.786	.0648	.142	.248	.550	.0135	.0391	.0863	.294
	20	.205	.353	.505	.793	.0645	.143	.251	.558	.0134	.0394	.0875	.300
	22	.204	.356	.512	.805	.0638	.145	.256	.574	.0132	.0400	.0900	.313
	24	.203	.360	.519	.815	.0633	.147	.261	.588	.0130	.0406	.0922	.325
	26	.202	.363	.525	.824	.0628	.148	.266	.601	.0129	.0411	.0944	.337
	28	.202	.366	.531	.832	.0624	.150	.270	.612	.0128	.0416	.0965	.347
	30	.201	.368	.536	.840	.0621	.151	.274	.623	.0126	.0421	.0985	.357
	32	.200	.371	.541	.847	.0618	.153	.278	.633	.0126	.0426	.100	.367
	34	.200	.373	.546	.853	.0615	.154	.282	.643	.0125	.0430	.102	.376
	36	.200	.375	.551	.858	.0613	.155	.286	.652	.0124	.0435	.104	.385
	38	.199	.377	.555	.863	.0611	.156	.289	.660	.0123	.0438	.106	.393
	40	.199	.379	.559	.868	.0609	.157	.292	.667	.0123	.0442	.107	.401
	50	.198	.387	.576	.887	.0602	.162	.307	.700	.0121	.0459	.115	.435
	60	.197	.394	.590	.901	.0598	.166	.319	.725	.0119	.0473	.121	.463
	70	.196	.399	.602	.912	.0595	.169	.330	.746	.0118	.0485	.127	.487
	80	.196	.403	.612	.921	.0592	.172	.339	.763	.0117	.0495	.132	.508
	90	.195	.407	.621	.928	.0590	.174	.347	.777	.0117	.0504	.137	.527
	100	.195	.411	.629	.933	.0589	.176	.355	.790	.0116	.0513	.141	.543

A. Values of $\beta_1' = \beta_L'$, $\beta_2' = (\beta_S')_{max}$, $\beta_3' = (\beta_X')_{min}$ and $\beta_4' = \beta_W'$ for $\alpha = 0.05$

N	m	δ=0.5				δ=1.0				δ=1.5			
		β_1'	β_2'	β_3'	β_4'	β_1'	β_2'	β_3'	β_4'	β_1'	β_2'	β_3'	β_4'
5	2	.892	.892	.892	.892	.714	.714	.714	.714	.451	.451	.451	.451
	3	.887	.902	.921	.945	.693	.722	.761	.818	.413	.449	.499	.583
	4	.885	.910	.935	.965	.682	.733	.787	.865	.394	.455	.528	.654
	5	.883	.917	.944	.975	.675	.742	.805	.893	.383	.463	.550	.701
	6	.882	.921	.950	.981	.671	.750	.818	.912	.376	.470	.567	.735
	7	.881	.925	.955	.985	.667	.757	.829	.925	.371	.477	.580	.761
	8	.880	.929	.958	.988	.665	.763	.838	.935	.367	.483	.592	.783
	9	.880	.931	.961	.990	.663	.768	.845	.943	.364	.488	.602	.800
	10	.879	.934	.964	.991	.661	.773	.851	.949	.361	.494	.612	.815
	11	.879	.936	.966	.992	.660	.777	.856	.954	.359	.498	.620	.827
	12	.879	.938	.967	.993	.659	.781	.861	.958	.358	.503	.627	.838
	13	.879	.939	.969	.994	.658	.784	.866	.962	.357	.507	.634	.847
	14	.878	.941	.970	.995	.657	.787	.869	.965	.355	.511	.640	.856
	15	.878	.942	.971	.995	.657	.790	.873	.968	.354	.514	.646	.863
	16	.878	.943	.973	.996	.656	.793	.876	.970	.353	.517	.651	.870
	17	.878	.944	.974	.996	.656	.795	.879	.972	.353	.520	.656	.876
	18	.878	.945	.974	.996	.655	.797	.882	.974	.352	.523	.660	.881
	19	.878	.945	.975	.997	.655	.800	.884	.975	.351	.526	.665	.886
	20	.878	.947	.976	.997	.654	.801	.886	.977	.351	.528	.669	.891
	22	.878	.948	.977	.997	.654	.805	.891	.979	.350	.533	.676	.899
	24	.877	.950	.978	.998	.653	.808	.894	.981	.349	.537	.683	.906
	26	.877	.951	.979	.998	.653	.811	.898	.983	.348	.541	.689	.912
	28	.877	.952	.980	.998	.652	.813	.901	.984	.348	.544	.695	.917
	30	.877	.953	.981	.998	.652	.816	.903	.986	.347	.547	.700	.922
	32	.877	.954	.982	.999	.652	.818	.906	.987	.347	.550	.705	.926
	34	.877	.955	.982	.999	.652	.820	.908	.988	.346	.553	.709	.930
	36	.877	.955	.983	.999	.651	.822	.910	.988	.346	.555	.713	.934
	38	.877	.956	.983	.999	.651	.823	.912	.989	.346	.558	.717	.937
	40	.877	.956	.984	.999	.651	.825	.914	.990	.346	.560	.721	.939
	50	.877	.959	.986	.999	.650	.831	.921	.992	.344	.569	.737	.950
	60	.877	.961	.987	.999	.650	.836	.927	.994	.344	.576	.749	.958
	70	.876	.962	.988	1.000	.649	.840	.931	.995	.343	.582	.759	.964
	80	.876	.963	.989	1.000	.649	.843	.935	.996	.343	.587	.767	.968
	90	.876	.964	.990	1.000	.649	.845	.938	.996	.343	.590	.775	.971
	100	.876	.965	.991	1.000	.649	.847	.941	.997	.342	.594	.781	.974

N	m	δ=2.0				δ=2.5				δ=3.0			
		β'_1	β'_2	β'_3	β'_4	β'_1	β'_2	β'_3	β'_4	β'_1	β'_2	β'_3	β'_4
5	2	.209	.209	.209	.209	.0684	.0684	.0684	.0684	.0153	.0153	.0153	.0153
	3	.173	.199	.239	.313	.0484	.0596	.0785	.119	.00872	.0116	.0171	.0310
	4	.157	.199	.257	.378	.0404	.0575	.0847	.155	.00651	.0106	.0182	.0430
	5	.147	.201	.271	.425	.0362	.0573	.0899	.183	.00546	.0102	.0191	.0532
	6	.142	.205	.283	.462	.0336	.0577	.0945	.207	.00485	.0101	.0201	.0622
	7	.137	.208	.293	.493	.0319	.0585	.0986	.228	.00446	.0101	.0209	.0705
	8	.134	.211	.302	.519	.0306	.0594	.102	.247	.00418	.0102	.0218	.0783
	9	.132	.215	.310	.541	.0297	.0603	.106	.263	.00398	.0104	.0227	.0855
	10	.130	.218	.318	.561	.0289	.0613	.109	.279	.00383	.0105	.0234	.0924
	11	.129	.221	.325	.579	.0284	.0623	.112	.293	.00371	.0107	.0242	.0989
	12	.127	.223	.331	.594	.0279	.0631	.115	.306	.00361	.0108	.0250	.105
	13	.126	.226	.337	.609	.0275	.0640	.118	.318	.00353	.0110	.0257	.111
	14	.126	.228	.342	.622	.0272	.0649	.121	.330	.00346	.0111	.0264	.117
	15	.125	.231	.347	.634	.0269	.0657	.123	.341	.00340	.0113	.0271	.122
	16	.124	.233	.352	.645	.0266	.0665	.126	.351	.00335	.0114	.0277	.128
	17	.124	.235	.356	.655	.0264	.0672	.128	.361	.00331	.0116	.0284	.133
	18	.123	.237	.361	.664	.0262	.0679	.130	.370	.00327	.0117	.0290	.138
	19	.123	.239	.365	.673	.0260	.0686	.132	.379	.00324	.0119	.0296	.143
	20	.122	.240	.369	.682	.0259	.0692	.134	.387	.00321	.0120	.0302	.148
	22	.121	.243	.376	.697	.0256	.0705	.138	.403	.00316	.0122	.0313	.157
	24	.121	.247	.383	.710	.0254	.0716	.142	.417	.00311	.0125	.0324	.165
	26	.120	.249	.389	.722	.0252	.0727	.145	.430	.00308	.0127	.0335	.174
	28	.120	.252	.395	.733	.0251	.0737	.148	.442	.00305	.0129	.0344	.181
	30	.120	.254	.400	.743	.0249	.0747	.152	.454	.00302	.0131	.0354	.189
	32	.119	.256	.405	.752	.0248	.0756	.154	.465	.00300	.0133	.0363	.196
	34	.119	.258	.410	.760	.0247	.0764	.157	.475	.00298	.0135	.0372	.203
	36	.119	.260	.415	.768	.0246	.0772	.160	.485	.00297	.0137	.0381	.209
	38	.119	.262	.419	.775	.0245	.0779	.163	.494	.00295	.0138	.0389	.216
	40	.118	.264	.423	.782	.0245	.0786	.165	.502	.00294	.0140	.0397	.222
	50	.118	.271	.441	.809	.0242	.0816	.176	.539	.00289	.0147	.0434	.249
	60	.117	.277	.455	.829	.0240	.0841	.185	.569	.00285	.0153	.0466	.273
	70	.117	.281	.468	.845	.0239	.0861	.194	.594	.00283	.0157	.0496	.294
	80	.116	.285	.478	.858	.0238	.0878	.201	.615	.00281	.0162	.0522	.313
	90	.116	.288	.488	.869	.0237	.0893	.207	.633	.00280	.0165	.0547	.330
	100	.116	.292	.496	.878	.0237	.0907	.213	.649	.00279	.0169	.0569	.345

A. Values of $\beta_1' = \beta_L'$, $\beta_2' = (\beta_S')_{\max}$, $\beta_3' = (\beta_X')_{\min}$ and $\beta_4' = \beta_W'$ for $\alpha = 0.05$

N	m	$\delta=0.5$				$\delta=1.0$				$\delta=1.5$			
		β_1'	β_2'	β_3'	β_4'	β_1'	β_2'	β_3'	β_4'	β_1'	β_2'	β_3'	β_4'
6	2	.877	.877	.877	.877	.653	.653	.653	.653	.350	.350	.350	.350
	3	.872	.889	.909	.936	.632	.666	.707	.771	.319	.355	.400	.483
	4	.869	.899	.925	.959	.622	.679	.737	.828	.304	.363	.431	.560
	5	.868	.906	.935	.970	.616	.690	.758	.861	.296	.372	.453	.612
	6	.866	.911	.942	.977	.611	.700	.773	.884	.290	.380	.471	.651
	7	.866	.916	.947	.982	.608	.708	.786	.901	.286	.387	.485	.682
	8	.865	.919	.951	.985	.606	.715	.796	.913	.282	.393	.498	.707
	9	.864	.922	.954	.988	.604	.721	.804	.923	.280	.399	.509	.728
	10	.864	.925	.957	.989	.603	.726	.812	.931	.278	.405	.518	.746
	11	.864	.927	.959	.991	.602	.731	.818	.938	.277	.410	.527	.761
	12	.864	.929	.961	.992	.601	.735	.824	.943	.276	.414	.535	.774
	13	.863	.931	.963	.993	.600	.739	.829	.948	.274	.418	.542	.786
	14	.863	.933	.965	.994	.599	.743	.833	.952	.274	.422	.549	.796
	15	.863	.934	.966	.994	.599	.746	.837	.955	.273	.426	.555	.806
	16	.863	.935	.967	.995	.598	.749	.841	.958	.272	.429	.561	.814
	17	.863	.937	.968	.995	.598	.752	.845	.961	.271	.432	.566	.822
	18	.863	.938	.970	.996	.597	.754	.848	.963	.271	.435	.571	.829
	19	.863	.939	.970	.996	.597	.757	.851	.965	.270	.438	.576	.836
	20	.862	.940	.971	.996	.596	.759	.854	.967	.270	.440	.581	.842
	22	.862	.941	.973	.997	.596	.763	.859	.970	.269	.445	.589	.852
	24	.862	.943	.974	.997	.595	.766	.863	.973	.269	.449	.596	.861
	26	.862	.944	.975	.998	.595	.770	.867	.975	.268	.453	.603	.870
	28	.862	.945	.976	.998	.595	.772	.871	.977	.268	.456	.609	.877
	30	.862	.946	.977	.998	.594	.775	.874	.979	.267	.460	.615	.883
	32	.862	.947	.978	.998	.594	.778	.877	.981	.267	.463	.620	.889
	34	.862	.948	.979	.998	.594	.780	.880	.982	.267	.465	.626	.894
	36	.862	.949	.979	.999	.594	.782	.883	.983	.266	.468	.630	.899
	38	.862	.949	.980	.999	.593	.784	.885	.984	.266	.470	.635	.903
	40	.862	.950	.981	.999	.593	.785	.887	.985	.266	.473	.639	.907
	50	.861	.953	.983	.999	.593	.793	.896	.988	.265	.482	.656	.922
	60	.861	.955	.985	.999	.592	.798	.903	.991	.264	.489	.670	.933
	70	.861	.956	.986	.999	.592	.802	.909	.992	.264	.495	.682	.941
	80	.861	.957	.987	1.000	.592	.806	.913	.993	.264	.500	.692	.948
	90	.861	.958	.988	1.000	.592	.808	.917	.994	.264	.504	.701	.953
	100	.861	.959	.988	1.000	.591	.811	.921	.995	.263	.508	.708	.957

N	m	δ=2.0				δ=2.5				δ=3.0			
		β_1'	β_2'	β_3'	β_4'	β_1'	β_2'	β_3'	β_4'	β_1'	β_2'	β_3'	β_4'
6	2	.124	.124	.124	.124	.0270	.0270	.0270	.0270	.00355	.00355	.00355	.00355
	3	.101	.120	.148	.205	.0188	.0243	.0330	.0545	.00198	.00281	.00430	.00868
	4	.0912	.122	.163	.260	.0156	.0239	.0369	.0761	.00147	.00263	.00477	.0132
	5	.0856	.125	.175	.303	.0140	.0242	.0401	.0945	.00123	.00258	.00518	.0174
	6	.0820	.128	.185	.338	.0129	.0247	.0429	.111	.00109	.00260	.00555	.0214
	7	.0796	.131	.194	.368	.0123	.0252	.0454	.125	.00100	.00264	.00591	.0251
	8	.0778	.134	.201	.393	.0118	.0258	.0477	.139	.00094	.00270	.00625	.0287
	9	.0765	.137	.208	.416	.0114	.0264	.0498	.151	.00090	.00275	.00657	.0322
	10	.0754	.139	.215	.435	.0111	.0270	.0519	.163	.00086	.00282	.00688	.0355
	11	.0745	.142	.220	.454	.0109	.0276	.0538	.173	.00083	.00288	.00719	.0388
	12	.0738	.144	.226	.470	.0107	.0281	.0555	.183	.00081	.00293	.00747	.0419
	13	.0732	.146	.231	.485	.0106	.0286	.0573	.193	.00079	.00299	.00776	.0451
	14	.0727	.148	.236	.499	.0104	.0291	.0589	.202	.00078	.00305	.00803	.0481
	15	.0722	.150	.240	.512	.0103	.0296	.0605	.211	.00077	.00311	.00830	.0511
	16	.0718	.152	.244	.524	.0102	.0300	.0620	.219	.00075	.00316	.00856	.0540
	17	.0715	.153	.248	.535	.0102	.0305	.0634	.227	.00074	.00322	.00881	.0568
	18	.0712	.155	.252	.545	.0101	.0309	.0648	.235	.00074	.00326	.00906	.0596
	19	.0709	.156	.256	.555	.0100	.0313	.0661	.242	.00073	.00332	.00929	.0623
	20	.0707	.158	.259	.564	.0100	.0316	.0674	.249	.00072	.00336	.00953	.0649
	22	.0703	.160	.266	.582	.00985	.0323	.0699	.263	.00071	.00345	.0100	.0701
	24	.0699	.163	.272	.597	.00976	.0330	.0722	.275	.00070	.00354	.0104	.0750
	26	.0696	.165	.277	.611	.00969	.0336	.0744	.287	.00069	.00362	.0108	.0799
	28	.0694	.167	.282	.623	.00964	.0342	.0765	.298	.00069	.00369	.0112	.0845
	30	.0692	.169	.287	.635	.00958	.0347	.0785	.308	.00068	.00377	.0116	.0891
	32	.0690	.171	.292	.645	.00954	.0352	.0803	.318	.00068	.00383	.0120	.0934
	34	.0688	.172	.296	.655	.00950	.0357	.0822	.327	.00067	.00390	.0124	.0977
	36	.0687	.174	.300	.665	.00947	.0362	.0839	.336	.00067	.00396	.0127	.102
	38	.0686	.175	.304	.673	.00943	.0366	.0856	.345	.00066	.00402	.0131	.106
	40	.0685	.177	.308	.681	.00941	.0370	.0872	.353	.00066	.00407	.0134	.110
	50	.0680	.183	.324	.715	.00930	.0387	.0944	.388	.00065	.00432	.0149	.128
	60	.0677	.187	.338	.741	.00923	.0401	.101	.418	.00064	.00452	.0163	.144
	70	.0675	.191	.350	.762	.00918	.0413	.106	.443	.00064	.00469	.0176	.159
	80	.0674	.194	.360	.779	.00915	.0422	.111	.465	.00063	.00483	.0187	.172
	90	.0672	.197	.369	.793	.00912	.0431	.116	.484	.00063	.00496	.0198	.185
	100	.0672	.199	.377	.805	.00910	.0439	.120	.501	.00063	.00508	.0208	.196

A. Values of $\beta_1' = \beta_L'$, $\beta_2' = (\beta_S')_{\max}$, $\beta_3' = (\beta_X')_{\min}$ and $\beta_4' = \beta_W'$ for $\alpha = 0.05$

		$\delta = 0.5$				$\delta = 1.0$				$\delta = 1.5$			
N	m	β_1'	β_2'	β_3'	β_4'	β_1'	β_2'	β_3'	β_4'	β_1'	β_2'	β_3'	β_4'
7	2	.862	.862	.862	.862	.594	.594	.594	.594	.269	.269	.269	.269
	3	.856	.876	.897	.927	.575	.612	.653	.724	.244	.276	.316	.394
	4	.854	.887	.914	.952	.565	.627	.687	.788	.232	.285	.345	.471
	5	.852	.894	.925	.966	.559	.639	.710	.827	.225	.294	.367	.526
	6	.851	.900	.933	.974	.555	.650	.727	.854	.220	.302	.385	.568
	7	.850	.905	.939	.979	.552	.659	.741	.874	.217	.309	.399	.601
	8	.850	.909	.943	.983	.550	.667	.752	.889	.215	.316	.412	.629
	9	.849	.913	.947	.985	.549	.673	.762	.901	.213	.321	.423	.652
	10	.849	.916	.950	.987	.547	.679	.770	.910	.212	.327	.433	.672
	11	.848	.918	.953	.989	.546	.684	.778	.918	.210	.331	.442	.690
	12	.848	.920	.955	.990	.545	.689	.784	.925	.209	.336	.449	.705
	13	.848	.922	.957	.991	.545	.693	.790	.931	.209	.340	.457	.719
	14	.848	.924	.959	.992	.544	.697	.795	.936	.208	.343	.464	.731
	15	.848	.925	.960	.993	.543	.701	.800	.940	.207	.347	.470	.742
	16	.847	.927	.962	.994	.543	.704	.804	.944	.207	.350	.476	.752
	17	.847	.928	.963	.994	.542	.707	.808	.947	.206	.353	.481	.762
	18	.847	.930	.964	.995	.542	.710	.812	.950	.206	.356	.487	.770
	19	.847	.931	.965	.995	.542	.713	.816	.953	.205	.359	.492	.778
	20	.847	.932	.966	.995	.541	.715	.819	.955	.205	.361	.496	.785
	22	.847	.934	.968	.996	.541	.719	.825	.960	.204	.365	.505	.798
	24	.847	.935	.970	.997	.540	.723	.830	.963	.204	.370	.512	.809
	26	.847	.937	.971	.997	.540	.727	.835	.966	.204	.373	.520	.820
	28	.847	.938	.972	.997	.540	.730	.839	.969	.203	.377	.526	.828
	30	.846	.939	.973	.998	.539	.733	.843	.971	.203	.380	.532	.836
	32	.846	.940	.974	.998	.539	.736	.846	.973	.203	.383	.538	.844
	34	.846	.941	.975	.998	.539	.738	.850	.975	.202	.386	.543	.850
	36	.846	.942	.976	.998	.539	.740	.853	.976	.202	.388	.548	.856
	38	.846	.943	.976	.998	.539	.742	.855	.978	.202	.390	.553	.862
	40	.846	.943	.977	.998	.538	.744	.858	.979	.202	.393	.557	.867
	50	.846	.946	.980	.999	.538	.752	.869	.984	.201	.402	.576	.887
	60	.846	.948	.982	.999	.537	.758	.877	.987	.201	.409	.591	.902
	70	.846	.950	.983	.999	.537	.763	.884	.989	.201	.415	.604	.913
	80	.846	.951	.984	.999	.537	.767	.889	.990	.200	.419	.615	.921
	90	.846	.952	.985	1.000	.537	.770	.894	.992	.200	.423	.624	.929
	100	.846	.953	.986	1.000	.537	.773	.898	.993	.200	.427	.632	.934

N	m	δ=2.0				δ=2.5				δ=3.0			
		β_1'	β_2'	β_3'	β_4'	β_1'	β_2'	β_3'	β_4'	β_1'	β_2'	β_3'	β_4'
7	2	.0710	.0710	.0710	.0710	.0102	.0102	.0102	.0102	.00078	.00078	.00078	.00078
	3	.0575	.0706	.0886	.130	.00703	.00949	.0133	.0236	.00043	.00064	.00102	.00226
	4	.0518	.0726	.100	.173	.00582	.00952	.0153	.0353	.00032	.00061	.00118	.00376
	5	.0485	.0752	.109	.209	.00519	.00977	.0170	.0460	.00026	.00062	.00131	.00526
	6	.0465	.0777	.117	.239	.00481	.0101	.0185	.0558	.00023	.00063	.00144	.00674
	7	.0450	.0801	.124	.264	.00456	.0104	.0199	.0649	.00022	.00065	.00156	.00821
	8	.0440	.0823	.130	.287	.00437	.0107	.0211	.0734	.00020	.00067	.00167	.00966
	9	.0432	.0844	.135	.308	.00424	.0111	.0223	.0815	.00019	.00069	.00178	.0111
	10	.0426	.0864	.140	.326	.00413	.0114	.0234	.0891	.00018	.00071	.00189	.0125
	11	.0421	.0882	.145	.343	.00405	.0117	.0245	.0965	.00018	.00073	.00199	.0139
	12	.0417	.0899	.149	.359	.00398	.0120	.0255	.103	.00017	.00075	.00209	.0153
	13	.0414	.0915	.153	.373	.00392	.0122	.0264	.110	.00017	.00077	.00219	.0167
	14	.0411	.0930	.157	.387	.00387	.0125	.0273	.117	.00017	.00078	.00228	.0181
	15	.0408	.0944	.161	.399	.00383	.0127	.0282	.123	.00016	.00080	.00237	.0194
	16	.0405	.0957	.164	.411	.00379	.0130	.0290	.129	.00016	.00082	.00246	.0208
	17	.0404	.0969	.167	.422	.00376	.0132	.0298	.135	.00016	.00084	.00255	.0221
	18	.0402	.0981	.170	.433	.00373	.0134	.0306	.140	.00016	.00085	.00263	.0235
	19	.0401	.0993	.173	.442	.00371	.0136	.0314	.146	.00016	.00087	.00271	.0247
	20	.0399	.100	.176	.452	.00369	.0138	.0321	.151	.00015	.00088	.00280	.0260
	22	.0397	.102	.181	.469	.00365	.0141	.0335	.161	.00015	.00091	.00296	.0286
	24	.0395	.104	.186	.485	.00362	.0145	.0349	.171	.00015	.00094	.00311	.0311
	26	.0393	.106	.191	.499	.00359	.0148	.0361	.180	.00015	.00096	.00326	.0335
	28	.0392	.107	.195	.513	.00357	.0151	.0373	.188	.00015	.00099	.00340	.0359
	30	.0391	.109	.199	.525	.00355	.0154	.0385	.196	.00015	.00101	.00354	.0383
	32	.0390	.110	.203	.536	.00354	.0156	.0396	.204	.00014	.00103	.00367	.0405
	34	.0389	.111	.207	.547	.00352	.0159	.0407	.212	.00014	.00105	.00381	.0428
	36	.0388	.113	.210	.557	.00351	.0161	.0417	.219	.00014	.00107	.00394	.0451
	38	.0387	.114	.214	.567	.00350	.0163	.0427	.226	.00014	.00109	.00406	.0472
	40	.0386	.115	.217	.576	.00349	.0166	.0436	.233	.00014	.00111	.00418	.0494
	50	.0384	.119	.231	.613	.00345	.0175	.0480	.263	.00014	.00118	.00475	.0596
	60	.0382	.123	.242	.643	.00342	.0182	.0518	.288	.00014	.00125	.00527	.0690
	70	.0381	.126	.253	.667	.00340	.0188	.0552	.311	.00014	.00130	.00575	.0778
	80	.0380	.128	.261	.687	.00339	.0193	.0582	.331	.00014	.00135	.00620	.0861
	90	.0380	.130	.269	.705	.00338	.0197	.0610	.348	.00014	.00139	.00661	.0938
	100	.0379	.132	.276	.720	.00337	.0202	.0636	.364	.00013	.00143	.00701	.101

A. Values of $\beta_1' = \beta_L'$, $\beta_2' = (\beta_S')_{\max}$, $\beta_3' = (\beta_X')_{\min}$ and $\beta_4' = \beta_W'$ for $\alpha = 0.05$

N	m	$\delta=0.5$				$\delta=1.0$				$\delta=1.5$			
		β_1'	β_2'	β_3'	β_4'	β_1'	β_2'	β_3'	β_4'	β_1'	β_2'	β_3'	β_4'
8	2	.846	.846	.846	.846	.539	.539	.539	.539	.203	.203	.203	.203
	3	.841	.863	.884	.917	.521	.559	.601	.676	.184	.212	.246	.317
	4	.838	.874	.903	.945	.511	.576	.637	.746	.175	.221	.273	.391
	5	.837	.883	.915	.960	.506	.590	.662	.791	.169	.230	.294	.445
	6	.835	.889	.924	.969	.502	.601	.681	.821	.166	.237	.310	.488
	7	.835	.895	.930	.975	.500	.610	.696	.844	.163	.244	.324	.522
	8	.834	.899	.936	.980	.498	.619	.708	.862	.162	.250	.336	.551
	9	.834	.903	.940	.983	.496	.626	.719	.876	.160	.255	.346	.576
	10	.833	.906	.943	.985	.495	.632	.728	.887	.159	.260	.356	.597
	11	.833	.909	.946	.987	.494	.638	.736	.897	.158	.264	.365	.616
	12	.833	.911	.949	.989	.493	.643	.743	.905	.157	.269	.372	.633
	13	.833	.913	.951	.990	.492	.647	.750	.912	.157	.272	.379	.648
	14	.832	.915	.953	.991	.492	.652	.756	.918	.156	.276	.386	.662
	15	.832	.917	.955	.992	.491	.656	.761	.923	.156	.279	.392	.675
	16	.832	.918	.956	.993	.491	.659	.766	.928	.155	.282	.398	.686
	17	.832	.920	.958	.993	.490	.662	.770	.932	.155	.285	.403	.696
	18	.832	.921	.959	.994	.490	.665	.775	.936	.155	.287	.409	.706
	19	.832	.922	.960	.994	.490	.668	.778	.939	.154	.290	.413	.715
	20	.832	.923	.961	.995	.489	.671	.782	.942	.154	.292	.418	.723
	22	.831	.925	.963	.995	.489	.675	.789	.947	.154	.296	.427	.738
	24	.831	.927	.965	.996	.489	.680	.795	.952	.153	.300	.434	.752
	26	.831	.929	.966	.996	.488	.684	.800	.955	.153	.304	.441	.764
	28	.831	.930	.968	.997	.488	.687	.805	.959	.153	.307	.448	.774
	30	.831	.931	.959	.997	.488	.690	.809	.961	.152	.310	.454	.784
	32	.831	.933	.970	.997	.487	.693	.813	.964	.152	.313	.460	.792
	34	.831	.934	.971	.998	.487	.696	.817	.966	.152	.315	.465	.800
	36	.831	.935	.972	.998	.487	.698	.820	.968	.152	.317	.470	.807
	38	.831	.935	.973	.998	.487	.700	.823	.970	.152	.320	.475	.814
	40	.831	.936	.973	.998	.487	.702	.826	.971	.152	.322	.479	.820
	50	.831	.939	.976	.999	.486	.711	.839	.977	.151	.330	.499	.845
	60	.831	.942	.979	.999	.486	.717	.848	.982	.151	.337	.514	.863
	70	.830	.944	.980	.999	.486	.723	.856	.984	.151	.342	.527	.878
	80	.830	.945	.982	.999	.485	.727	.863	.987	.150	.347	.538	.889
	90	.830	.946	.983	.999	.485	.730	.868	.988	.150	.350	.548	.898
	100	.830	.947	.984	1.000	.485	.733	.873	.990	.150	.354	.557	.906

N	m	δ=2.0				δ=2.5				δ=3.0			
		β_1'	β_2'	β_3'	β_4'	β_1'	β_2'	β_3'	β_4'	β_1'	β_2'	β_3'	β_4'
8	2	.0398	.0398	.0398	.0398	.00374	.00374	.00374	.00374	.00016	.00016	.00016	.00016
	3	.0321	.0405	.0519	.0798	.00255	.00357	.00514	.00978	.00009	.00014	.00023	.00055
	4	.0288	.0422	.0600	.112	.00210	.00366	.00612	.0157	.00007	.00014	.00028	.00101
	5	.0269	.0441	.0666	.139	.00187	.00381	.00695	.0213	.00005	.00014	.00032	.00149
	6	.0258	.0460	.0722	.163	.00173	.00397	.00769	.0267	.00005	.00015	.00035	.00199
	7	.0250	.0477	.0771	.184	.00164	.00413	.00837	.0319	.00004	.00015	.00039	.00250
	8	.0244	.0493	.0815	.203	.00158	.00430	.00899	.0369	.00004	.00016	.00042	.00303
	9	.0240	.0508	.0855	.221	.00153	.00445	.00958	.0417	.00004	.00016	.00046	.00356
	10	.0236	.0522	.0893	.237	.00149	.00451	.0101	.0464	.00004	.00017	.00049	.00410
	11	.0233	.0535	.0927	.251	.00146	.00475	.0107	.0510	.00004	.00017	.00052	.00465
	12	.0231	.0547	.0959	.265	.00143	.00489	.0112	.0553	.00004	.00018	.00055	.00520
	13	.0229	.0558	.0990	.278	.00141	.00501	.0117	.0596	.00004	.00019	.00058	.00575
	14	.0227	.0569	.102	.290	.00139	.00514	.0121	.0638	.00003	.00019	.00061	.00631
	15	.0226	.0579	.105	.302	.00138	.00525	.0126	.0678	.00003	.00020	.00064	.00687
	16	.0225	.0589	.107	.312	.00136	.00537	.0130	.0718	.00003	.00020	.00067	.00743
	17	.0223	.0597	.110	.322	.00135	.00547	.0134	.0756	.00003	.00021	.00069	.00798
	18	.0222	.0606	.112	.332	.00134	.00557	.0139	.0794	.00003	.00021	.00072	.00855
	19	.0222	.0614	.114	.341	.00133	.00567	.0143	.0830	.00003	.00022	.00075	.00911
	20	.0221	.0621	.116	.350	.00133	.00576	.0146	.0866	.00003	.00022	.00077	.00967
	22	.0220	.0635	.120	.367	.00131	.00594	.0154	.0936	.00003	.00023	.00082	.0108
	24	.0218	.0649	.124	.382	.00130	.00611	.0161	.100	.00003	.00024	.00087	.0119
	26	.0218	.0661	.128	.396	.00129	.00626	.0168	.107	.00003	.00024	.00092	.0130
	28	.0217	.0672	.131	.409	.00128	.00640	.0174	.113	.00003	.00025	.00097	.0141
	30	.0216	.0682	.134	.421	.00128	.00654	.0180	.119	.00003	.00026	.00101	.0152
	32	.0216	.0692	.137	.432	.00127	.00667	.0186	.124	.00003	.00026	.00106	.0163
	34	.0215	.0701	.140	.443	.00127	.00679	.0192	.130	.00003	.00027	.00110	.0173
	36	.0215	.0710	.143	.453	.00126	.00690	.0198	.135	.00003	.00027	.00115	.0184
	38	.0214	.0718	.146	.463	.00126	.00701	.0203	.140	.00003	.00028	.00119	.0194
	40	.0214	.0725	.148	.472	.00125	.00711	.0208	.145	.00003	.00028	.00123	.0205
	50	.0212	.0757	.159	.511	.00124	.00755	.0232	.168	.00003	.00031	.00142	.0256
	60	.0211	.0783	.169	.542	.00123	.00791	.0254	.188	.00003	.00033	.00160	.0304
	70	.0211	.0803	.177	.568	.00122	.00821	.0273	.206	.00003	.00034	.00177	.0351
	80	.0210	.0821	.184	.590	.00122	.00847	.0290	.223	.00003	.00036	.00192	.0396
	90	.0210	.0835	.191	.609	.00121	.00868	.0307	.237	.00003	.00037	.00207	.0439
	100	.0210	.0849	.197	.626	.00121	.00889	.0322	.251	.00003	.00038	.00221	.0480

A. Values of $\beta_1' = \beta_L'$, $\beta_2' = (\beta_S')_{\max}$, $\beta_3' = (\beta_X')_{\min}$ and $\beta_4' = \beta_W'$ for $\alpha = 0.05$

N	m	$\delta=0.5$				$\delta=1.0$				$\delta=1.5$			
		β_1'	β_2'	β_3'	β_4'	β_1'	β_2'	β_3'	β_4'	β_1'	β_2'	β_3'	β_4'
9	2	.830	.830	.830	.830	.487	.487	.487	.487	.152	.152	.152	.152
	3	.825	.849	.872	.908	.470	.509	.551	.629	.137	.161	.190	.252
	4	.823	.861	.892	.938	.461	.527	.588	.704	.130	.170	.214	.320
	5	.821	.871	.905	.955	.456	.541	.614	.753	.126	.177	.232	.371
	6	.820	.878	.915	.965	.453	.553	.635	.787	.123	.184	.247	.413
	7	.819	.884	.922	.972	.450	.563	.651	.812	.122	.190	.260	.447
	8	.819	.888	.927	.977	.449	.572	.664	.832	.120	.195	.271	.477
	9	.818	.892	.932	.980	.447	.579	.675	.848	.119	.200	.280	.502
	10	.818	.896	.936	.983	.446	.586	.685	.862	.118	.205	.289	.524
	11	.818	.899	.939	.985	.445	.592	.694	.873	.118	.208	.297	.544
	12	.817	.901	.942	.987	.444	.597	.702	.882	.117	.212	.304	.561
	13	.817	.904	.944	.988	.444	.602	.709	.890	.117	.215	.311	.578
	14	.817	.905	.946	.989	.443	.607	.715	.897	.116	.219	.317	.592
	15	.817	.908	.948	.990	.443	.611	.721	.904	.116	.221	.323	.605
	16	.817	.909	.950	.991	.442	.614	.726	.909	.115	.224	.329	.618
	17	.816	.911	.952	.992	.442	.618	.731	.914	.115	.227	.334	.629
	18	.816	.912	.953	.993	.441	.621	.736	.919	.115	.229	.339	.640
	19	.816	.914	.955	.993	.441	.624	.740	.923	.115	.231	.343	.649
	20	.816	.915	.956	.994	.441	.627	.744	.926	.115	.233	.348	.659
	22	.816	.917	.958	.994	.440	.631	.751	.933	.114	.237	.356	.675
	24	.816	.919	.960	.995	.440	.636	.758	.938	.114	.241	.363	.690
	26	.816	.921	.962	.996	.440	.640	.764	.943	.114	.244	.370	.703
	28	.816	.922	.963	.996	.440	.644	.769	.947	.113	.247	.376	.715
	30	.816	.924	.964	.996	.439	.647	.774	.950	.113	.249	.382	.726
	32	.816	.925	.965	.997	.439	.650	.778	.953	.113	.252	.388	.736
	34	.816	.926	.967	.997	.439	.653	.783	.956	.113	.254	.393	.745
	36	.815	.927	.968	.997	.439	.655	.786	.958	.113	.256	.398	.753
	38	.815	.928	.968	.997	.439	.658	.790	.961	.113	.258	.402	.761
	40	.815	.929	.969	.998	.438	.660	.793	.963	.113	.260	.407	.768
	50	.815	.932	.973	.998	.438	.669	.807	.970	.112	.268	.426	.797
	60	.815	.935	.975	.999	.438	.676	.818	.975	.112	.274	.441	.819
	70	.815	.937	.977	.999	.437	.681	.827	.979	.112	.279	.454	.837
	80	.815	.938	.979	.999	.437	.686	.834	.982	.112	.283	.466	.850
	90	.815	.940	.980	.999	.437	.689	.840	.984	.112	.286	.475	.862
	100	.815	.941	.981	.999	.437	.693	.846	.986	.112	.290	.484	.871

N	m	δ=2.0				δ=2.5				δ=3.0			
		β_1'	β_2'	β_3'	β_4'	β_1'	β_2'	β_3'	β_4'	β_1'	β_2'	β_3'	β_4'
9	2	.0219	.0219	.0219	.0219	.00133	.00133	.00133	.00133	.00003	.00003	.00003	.00003
	3	.0175	.0227	.0297	.0479	.00090	.00131	.00193	.00391	.00002	.00003	.00005	.00013
	4	.0157	.0241	.0352	.0705	.00074	.00136	.00237	.00667	.00001	.00003	.00006	.00026
	5	.0147	.0254	.0396	.0905	.00066	.00144	.00274	.00947	.00001	.00003	.00007	.00040
	6	.0140	.0267	.0435	.108	.00061	.00151	.00309	.0123	.00001	.00003	.00008	.00055
	7	.0136	.0278	.0469	.125	.00058	.00159	.00340	.0150	.00001	.00003	.00009	.00072
	8	.0133	.0289	.0500	.140	.00055	.00166	.00369	.0178	.00001	.00004	.00010	.00089
	9	.0130	.0299	.0528	.154	.00054	.00174	.00397	.0205	.00001	.00004	.00011	.00108
	10	.0128	.0309	.0554	.167	.00052	.00181	.00424	.0231	.00001	.00004	.00012	.00127
	11	.0127	.0317	.0579	.179	.00051	.00187	.00449	.0257	.00001	.00004	.00013	.00146
	12	.0126	.0326	.0601	.190	.00050	.00193	.00473	.0283	.00001	.00004	.00014	.00166
	13	.0124	.0333	.0623	.201	.00049	.00199	.00497	.0308	.00001	.00004	.00015	.00186
	14	.0124	.0341	.0644	.212	.00049	.00204	.00520	.0333	.00001	.00004	.00016	.00207
	15	.0123	.0347	.0563	.221	.00048	.00210	.00542	.0357	.00001	.00005	.00016	.00228
	16	.0122	.0354	.0682	.231	.00048	.00215	.00563	.0381	.00001	.00005	.00017	.00249
	17	.0121	.0360	.0700	.239	.00047	.00220	.00584	.0405	.00001	.00005	.00018	.00270
	18	.0121	.0365	.0717	.248	.00047	.00224	.00604	.0429	.00001	.00005	.00019	.00292
	19	.0120	.0371	.0734	.256	.00047	.00229	.00624	.0451	.00001	.00005	.00020	.00314
	20	.0120	.0376	.0750	.264	.00046	.00233	.00643	.0474	.00001	.00005	.00020	.00336
	22	.0119	.0386	.0780	.279	.00046	.00241	.00680	.0518	.00001	.00005	.00022	.00381
	24	.0119	.0395	.0808	.292	.00046	.00249	.00715	.0560	.00001	.00006	.00023	.00426
	26	.0118	.0403	.0834	.305	.00045	.00256	.00749	.0602	.00001	.00006	.00025	.00471
	28	.0118	.0411	.0859	.317	.00045	.00262	.00782	.0642	.00001	.00006	.00026	.00517
	30	.0117	.0418	.0883	.328	.00045	.00269	.00813	.0682	.00001	.00006	.00028	.00563
	32	.0117	.0425	.0905	.339	.00044	.00274	.00844	.0720	.00001	.00006	.00029	.00609
	34	.0117	.0431	.0927	.349	.00044	.00280	.00874	.0757	.00001	.00007	.00030	.00655
	36	.0117	.0437	.0948	.359	.00044	.00285	.00902	.0794	.00001	.00007	.00032	.00702
	38	.0116	.0442	.0967	.367	.00044	.00290	.00930	.0829	.00001	.00007	.00033	.00747
	40	.0116	.0447	.0987	.376	.00044	.00295	.00957	.0863	.00001	.00007	.00034	.00794
	50	.0115	.0469	.107	.414	.00043	.00315	.0108	.102	.00001	.00008	.00040	.0102
	60	.0115	.0487	.114	.445	.00043	.00332	.0119	.117	.00001	.00008	.00046	.0125
	70	.0114	.0502	.121	.471	.00043	.00346	.0130	.130	.00001	.00009	.00051	.0147
	80	.0114	.0514	.126	.494	.00043	.00358	.0139	.143	.00001	.00009	.00056	.0169
	90	.0114	.0524	.132	.514	.00042	.00368	.0148	.154	.00001	.00009	.00061	.0191
	100	.0114	.0534	.136	.531	.00042	.00378	.0156	.165	.00001	.00010	.00066	.0211

A. Values of $\beta_1' = \beta_L'$, $\beta_2' = (\beta_S')_{max}$, $\beta_3' = (\beta_X')_{min}$ and $\beta_4' = \beta_W'$ for $\alpha = 0.05$

		$\delta=0.5$				$\delta=1.0$				$\delta=1.5$			
N	m	β_1'	β_2'	β_3'	β_4'	β_1'	β_2'	β_3'	β_4'	β_1'	β_2'	β_3'	β_4'
10	2	.815	.815	.815	.815	.438	.438	.438	.438	.113	.113	.113	.113
	3	.810	.835	.859	.898	.422	.462	.503	.583	.102	.121	.144	.197
	4	.807	.849	.881	.931	.414	.480	.541	.662	.0962	.129	.165	.258
	5	.806	.858	.895	.949	.410	.495	.568	.714	.0931	.135	.181	.306
	6	.804	.866	.905	.960	.407	.507	.589	.751	.0911	.141	.194	.345
	7	.804	.872	.913	.968	.404	.518	.606	.779	.0897	.147	.206	.378
	8	.803	.877	.919	.973	.403	.526	.620	.801	.0887	.151	.215	.407
	9	.803	.882	.924	.977	.401	.534	.632	.819	.0879	.155	.224	.432
	10	.802	.886	.928	.980	.400	.541	.643	.834	.0872	.159	.232	.454
	11	.802	.889	.932	.983	.400	.547	.652	.847	.0867	.163	.239	.474
	12	.802	.892	.935	.985	.399	.553	.660	.858	.0863	.166	.246	.492
	13	.802	.894	.937	.986	.398	.558	.667	.867	.0859	.169	.252	.508
	14	.801	.896	.940	.988	.398	.562	.674	.875	.0856	.171	.258	.523
	15	.801	.898	.942	.989	.397	.566	.680	.882	.0853	.174	.263	.537
	16	.801	.900	.944	.990	.397	.570	.686	.889	.0851	.176	.268	.550
	17	.801	.902	.946	.991	.397	.574	.691	.895	.0849	.178	.273	.562
	18	.801	.903	.947	.991	.395	.577	.696	.900	.0847	.180	.277	.573
	19	.801	.905	.949	.992	.396	.580	.701	.904	.0845	.182	.282	.583
	20	.801	.906	.950	.992	.396	.583	.705	.909	.0844	.184	.286	.593
	22	.801	.908	.952	.993	.395	.588	.713	.916	.0841	.188	.293	.610
	24	.800	.911	.955	.994	.395	.593	.720	.923	.0839	.191	.300	.626
	26	.800	.912	.956	.995	.395	.597	.727	.928	.0838	.194	.306	.641
	28	.800	.914	.958	.995	.395	.601	.732	.933	.0836	.196	.312	.653
	30	.800	.915	.960	.996	.394	.604	.738	.937	.0835	.199	.318	.665
	32	.800	.917	.961	.996	.394	.607	.742	.941	.0834	.201	.323	.676
	34	.800	.918	.962	.996	.394	.610	.747	.944	.0833	.203	.328	.686
	36	.800	.919	.963	.997	.394	.613	.751	.947	.0832	.205	.333	.695
	38	.800	.920	.964	.997	.394	.616	.755	.950	.0831	.206	.337	.704
	40	.800	.921	.965	.997	.394	.618	.759	.952	.0830	.208	.341	.712
	50	.800	.925	.969	.998	.393	.627	.774	.961	.0827	.215	.359	.745
	60	.800	.928	.972	.998	.393	.635	.786	.968	.0826	.220	.374	.770
	70	.800	.930	.974	.999	.393	.640	.796	.972	.0824	.225	.387	.790
	80	.799	.931	.976	.999	.392	.645	.804	.976	.0823	.228	.398	.807
	90	.799	.933	.977	.999	.392	.649	.811	.979	.0823	.231	.407	.820
	100	.799	.934	.978	.999	.392	.652	.817	.981	.0822	.234	.416	.832

N	m	δ=2.0				δ=2.5				δ=3.0			
		β_1'	β_2'	β_3'	β_4'	β_1'	β_2'	β_3'	β_4'	β_1'	β_2'	β_3'	β_4'
10	2	.0118	.0118	.0118	.0118	.00046	.00046	.00046	.00046	.00001	.00001	.00001	.00001
	3	.00943	.0125	.0167	.0281	.00031	.00047	.00070	.00151		.00001	.00001	.00003
	4	.00842	.0134	.0202	.0434	.00025	.00049	.00089	.00275		.00001	.00001	.00006
	5	.00787	.0143	.0231	.0574	.00023	.00053	.00105	.00407		.00001	.00002	.00010
	6	.00752	.0152	.0257	.0704	.00021	.00056	.00120	.00543		.00001	.00002	.00015
	7	.00728	.0159	.0279	.0825	.00020	.00059	.00134	.00682		.00001	.00002	.00020
	8	.00711	.0166	.0300	.0939	.00019	.00063	.00147	.00823		.00001	.00002	.00025
	9	.00698	.0173	.0319	.105	.00018	.00066	.00160	.00965		.00001	.00003	.00031
	10	.00687	.0179	.0337	.115	.00018	.00069	.00172	.0111		.00001	.00003	.00037
	11	.00679	.0185	.0354	.124	.00017	.00071	.00183	.0125		.00001	.00003	.00043
	12	.00672	.0190	.0369	.133	.00017	.00074	.00194	.0139		.00001	.00003	.00050
	13	.00666	.0195	.0384	.142	.00017	.00077	.00205	.0153		.00001	.00004	.00057
	14	.00661	.0200	.0398	.150	.00017	.00079	.00215	.0167		.00001	.00004	.00064
	15	.00657	.0204	.0412	.158	.00017	.00081	.00226	.0181		.00001	.00004	.00071
	16	.00653	.0209	.0425	.166	.00016	.00084	.00236	.0195		.00001	.00004	.00079
	17	.00650	.0212	.0437	.173	.00016	.00086	.00245	.0208		.00001	.00004	.00087
	18	.00647	.0216	.0450	.180	.00016	.00088	.00255	.0222		.00001	.00005	.00095
	19	.00644	.0220	.0461	.187	.00016	.00090	.00264	.0235		.00001	.00005	.00102
	20	.00642	.0223	.0472	.194	.00016	.00091	.00273	.0249		.00001	.00005	.00110
	22	.00638	.0230	.0493	.206	.00016	.00095	.00290	.0275		.00001	.00006	.00127
	24	.00635	.0236	.0513	.218	.00016	.00098	.00307	.0301		.00001	.00006	.00144
	26	.00632	.0241	.0532	.229	.00015	.00101	.00324	.0326		.00001	.00006	.00161
	28	.00630	.0246	.0550	.239	.00015	.00104	.00339	.0351		.00001	.00007	.00179
	30	.00628	.0251	.0567	.249	.00015	.00107	.00354	.0375		.00001	.00007	.00197
	32	.00626	.0255	.0583	.259	.00015	.00110	.00369	.0399		.00001	.00008	.00215
	34	.00625	.0259	.0599	.268	.00015	.00112	.00384	.0423		.00002	.00008	.00233
	36	.00623	.0263	.0614	.276	.00015	.00114	.00398	.0446		.00002	.00008	.00252
	38	.00622	.0267	.0628	.284	.00015	.00117	.00411	.0469		.00002	.00009	.00271
	40	.00621	.0270	.0642	.292	.00015	.00119	.00424	.0491		.00002	.00009	.00290
	50	.00617	.0285	.0704	.327	.00015	.00128	.00486	.0598		.00002	.00011	.00385
	60	.00614	.0297	.0757	.356	.00015	.00135	.00542	.0696		.00002	.00013	.00482
	70	.00612	.0307	.0805	.381	.00015	.00141	.00594	.0788		.00002	.00014	.00581
	80	.00610	.0315	.0847	.403	.00015	.00147	.00642	.0874		.00002	.00016	.00679
	90	.00609	.0322	.0886	.422	.00015	.00151	.00687	.0954		.00002	.00017	.00777
	100	.00608	.0328	.0921	.440	.00014	.00155	.00729	.103		.00002	.00019	.00874

A. Values of $\beta_1' = \beta_L'$, $\beta_2' = (\beta_S')_{\max}$, $\beta_3' = (\beta_X')_{\min}$ and $\beta_4' = \beta_W'$ for $\alpha = 0.05$

		$\delta=0.5$				$\delta=1.0$				$\delta=1.5$			
N	m	β_1'	β_2'	β_3'	β_4'	β_1'	β_2'	β_3'	β_4'	β_1'	β_2'	β_3'	β_4'
11	2	.799	.799	.799	.799	.393	.393	.393	.393	.0831	.0831	.0831	.0831
	3	.794	.821	.846	.887	.378	.417	.458	.537	.0745	.0903	.109	.153
	4	.792	.835	.869	.923	.371	.436	.496	.620	.0705	.0969	.127	.207
	5	.790	.846	.885	.943	.367	.451	.524	.675	.0682	.102	.140	.250
	6	.789	.854	.896	.955	.364	.464	.545	.714	.0667	.108	.151	.286
	7	.788	.861	.904	.964	.362	.474	.563	.745	.0656	.112	.161	.316
	8	.788	.866	.910	.970	.361	.483	.577	.769	.0649	.116	.170	.343
	9	.787	.871	.916	.974	.359	.491	.589	.789	.0643	.119	.177	.367
	10	.787	.875	.920	.977	.358	.498	.600	.805	.0638	.123	.184	.389
	11	.787	.878	.924	.980	.358	.504	.610	.819	.0634	.125	.191	.408
	12	.786	.882	.927	.982	.357	.510	.618	.831	.0631	.128	.196	.426
	13	.786	.884	.930	.984	.356	.515	.626	.842	.0628	.131	.202	.442
	14	.785	.887	.933	.986	.356	.519	.633	.851	.0626	.133	.207	.457
	15	.786	.889	.935	.987	.356	.524	.640	.859	.0624	.135	.212	.471
	16	.786	.891	.937	.988	.355	.528	.646	.867	.0622	.137	.216	.484
	17	.786	.892	.939	.989	.355	.531	.652	.873	.0620	.139	.221	.496
	18	.785	.894	.941	.990	.355	.534	.657	.879	.0619	.141	.225	.507
	19	.785	.896	.943	.991	.354	.538	.662	.884	.0618	.143	.228	.518
	20	.785	.897	.944	.991	.354	.541	.666	.889	.0617	.144	.232	.527
	22	.785	.900	.947	.992	.354	.546	.674	.898	.0615	.147	.239	.546
	24	.785	.902	.949	.993	.354	.551	.682	.905	.0613	.150	.245	.562
	26	.785	.904	.951	.994	.353	.555	.689	.912	.0612	.152	.251	.577
	28	.785	.905	.953	.995	.353	.559	.695	.917	.0611	.154	.256	.591
	30	.785	.907	.954	.995	.353	.562	.700	.922	.0610	.156	.261	.603
	32	.785	.908	.956	.995	.353	.566	.706	.927	.0609	.158	.266	.615
	34	.785	.910	.957	.996	.353	.569	.711	.931	.0608	.160	.271	.626
	36	.785	.911	.959	.996	.352	.571	.715	.934	.0608	.162	.275	.636
	38	.784	.912	.960	.996	.352	.574	.719	.937	.0607	.163	.279	.645
	40	.784	.913	.961	.997	.352	.576	.723	.940	.0607	.165	.283	.653
	50	.784	.917	.965	.998	.352	.586	.740	.951	.0605	.171	.300	.690
	60	.784	.920	.968	.998	.351	.593	.753	.959	.0603	.175	.314	.718
	70	.784	.922	.970	.999	.351	.599	.763	.965	.0602	.179	.326	.740
	80	.784	.924	.972	.999	.351	.604	.772	.969	.0602	.182	.336	.758
	90	.784	.926	.974	.999	.351	.608	.779	.972	.0601	.185	.345	.774
	100	.784	.927	.975	.999	.351	.612	.786	.975	.0601	.187	.353	.787

N	m	δ=2.0				δ=2.5				δ=3.0			
		β_1'	β_2'	β_3'	β_4'	β_1'	β_2'	β_3'	β_4'	β_1'	β_2'	β_3'	β_4'
11	2	.00629	.00629	.00629.	.00629	.00016	.00016	.00016	.00016				
	3	.00500	.00680	.00923	.0162	.00010	.00016	.00025	.00057				.00001
	4	.00446	.00739	.0114	.0262	.00009	.00018	.00033	.00110				.00001
	5	.00416	.00795	.0133	.0356	.00008	.00019	.00039	.00169				.00002
	6	.00398	.00848	.0149	.0447	.00007	.00020	.00046	.00233				.00004
	7	.00385	.00895	.0163	.0534	.00007	.00022	.00051	.00300				.00005
	8	.00375	.00940	.0177	.0616	.00006	.00023	.00057	.00369			.00001	.00007
	9	.00368	.00983	.0189	.0695	.00006	.00024	.00062	.00440			.00001	.00008
	10	.00363	.0102	.0201	.0771	.00006	.00026	.00068	.00512			.00001	.00010
	11	.00358	.0106	.0212	.0843	.00006	.00027	.00073	.00585			.00001	.00012
	12	.00354	.0109	.0222	.0912	.00006	.00028	.00077	.00658			.00001	.00014
	13	.00351	.0112	.0232	.0979	.00006	.00029	.00082	.00733			.00001	.00017
	14	.00349	.0115	.0242	.104	.00006	.00030	.00087	.00808			.00001	.00019
	15	.00346	.0118	.0251	.111	.00006	.00031	.00091	.00882			.00001	.00021
	16	.00345	.0121	.0260	.117	.00005	.00032	.00096	.00957			.00001	.00024
	17	.00343	.0123	.0268	.122	.00005	.00033	.00100	.0103			.00001	.00026
	18	.00341	.0126	.0276	.128	.00005	.00033	.00104	.0111			.00001	.00029
	19	.00340	.0128	.0284	.134	.00005	.00034	.00109	.0118			.00001	.00032
	20	.00339	.0130	.0291	.139	.00005	.00035	.00113	.0126			.00001	.00035
	22	.00337	.0134	.0306	.149	.00005	.00036	.00121	.0141			.00001	.00040
	24	.00335	.0138	.0320	.159	.00005	.00038	.00128	.0155			.00001	.00046
	26	.00333	.0142	.0333	.168	.00005	.00039	.00136	.0170			.00002	.00052
	28	.00332	.0145	.0345	.177	.00005	.00040	.00143	.0185			.00002	.00059
	30	.00331	.0148	.0357	.185	.00005	.00042	.00150	.0199			.00002	.00065
	32	.00330	.0151	.0368	.193	.00005	.00043	.00157	.0213			.00002	.00072
	34	.00329	.0153	.0379	.200	.00005	.00044	.00163	.0228			.00002	.00079
	36	.00329	.0156	.0389	.208	.00005	.00045	.00170	.0242			.00002	.00086
	38	.00328	.0158	.0399	.215	.00005	.00046	.00176	.0255			.00002	.00093
	40	.00327	.0160	.0409	.222	.00005	.00046	.00183	.0269			.00002	.00100
	50	.00325	.0170	.0453	.252	.00005	.00050	.00212	.0335			.00003	.00137
	60	.00324	.0178	.0491	.278	.00005	.00053	.00239	.0398			.00003	.00176
	70	.00323	.0184	.0525	.301	.00005	.00056	.00264	.0458			.00004	.00217
	80	.00322	.0189	.0556	.321	.00005	.00058	.00287	.0514		.00001	.00004	.00258
	90	.00321	.0194	.0584	.339	.00005	.00060	.00309	.0568		.00001	.00005	.00299
	100	.00321	.0198	.0610	.355	.00005	.00062	.00330	.0620		.00001	.00005	.00341

A. Values of $\beta_1' = \beta_L'$, $\beta_2' = (\beta_S')_{max}$, $\beta_3' = (\beta_X')_{min}$ and $\beta_4' = \beta_W'$ for $\alpha = 0.05$

		δ=0.5				δ=1.0				δ=1.5			
N	m	β_1'	β_2'	β_3'	β_4'	β_1'	β_2'	β_3'	β_4'	β_1'	β_2'	β_3'	β_4'
13	2	.768	.768	.768	.768	.313	.313	.313	.313	.0439	.0439	.0439	.0439
	3	.763	.793	.819	.866	.301	.338	.375	.453	.0392	.0490	.0605	.0897
	4	.761	.809	.846	.907	.295	.356	.413	.538	.0370	.0534	.0722	.128
	5	.759	.821	.863	.930	.292	.371	.440	.596	.0357	.0572	.0815	.161
	6	.758	.830	.876	.945	.289	.383	.462	.640	.0349	.0606	.0895	.189
	7	.757	.838	.885	.955	.288	.394	.480	.674	.0344	.0636	.0963	.214
	8	.757	.844	.892	.962	.286	.402	.494	.701	.0339	.0662	.102	.237
	9	.756	.849	.899	.967	.285	.410	.507	.724	.0336	.0687	.108	.258
	10	.756	.853	.904	.971	.285	.417	.519	.743	.0334	.0709	.113	.276
	11	.756	.857	.908	.975	.284	.423	.529	.760	.0332	.0728	.118	.293
	12	.755	.861	.912	.977	.283	.429	.538	.774	.0330	.0748	.122	.309
	13	.755	.864	.915	.980	.283	.434	.546	.787	.0328	.0764	.126	.324
	14	.755	.866	.919	.982	.283	.439	.553	.798	.0327	.0781	.130	.338
	15	.755	.869	.921	.983	.282	.443	.560	.808	.0326	.0795	.133	.351
	16	.755	.871	.924	.985	.282	.447	.567	.817	.0325	.0809	.137	.363
	17	.755	.873	.926	.986	.282	.450	.573	.825	.0324	.0822	.140	.374
	18	.755	.875	.928	.987	.282	.454	.578	.833	.0324	.0835	.143	.385
	19	.754	.877	.930	.988	.281	.457	.583	.839	.0323	.0846	.146	.395
	20	.754	.878	.932	.989	.281	.460	.588	.846	.0322	.0857	.149	.405
	22	.754	.881	.935	.990	.281	.465	.597	.857	.0321	.0877	.154	.423
	24	.754	.883	.937	.991	.281	.470	.605	.866	.0321	.0896	.159	.439
	26	.754	.886	.940	.992	.280	.475	.613	.874	.0320	.0914	.163	.455
	28	.754	.888	.942	.993	.280	.478	.619	.881	.0319	.0929	.168	.468
	30	.754	.889	.944	.993	.280	.482	.625	.888	.0319	.0944	.172	.481
	32	.754	.891	.945	.994	.280	.485	.631	.894	.0318	.0957	.175	.493
	34	.754	.893	.947	.994	.280	.488	.637	.899	.0318	.0970	.179	.505
	36	.754	.894	.949	.995	.280	.491	.641	.904	.0318	.0981	.182	.515
	38	.754	.895	.950	.995	.280	.494	.646	.908	.0317	.0992	.186	.525
	40	.754	.896	.951	.996	.280	.496	.650	.912	.0317	.100	.189	.534
	50	.753	.901	.956	.997	.279	.506	.669	.927	.0316	.105	.202	.574
	60	.753	.904	.960	.997	.279	.514	.683	.938	.0315	.108	.214	.606
	70	.753	.907	.963	.998	.279	.520	.695	.946	.0315	.111	.224	.632
	80	.753	.909	.965	.998	.279	.525	.705	.952	.0314	.113	.232	.653
	90	.753	.911	.967	.999	.279	.529	.714	.957	.0314	.115	.240	.672
	100	.753	.912	.969	.999	.278	.532	.722	.961	.0314	.117	.247	.688

N	m	$\delta=2.0$ β_1'	β_2'	β_3'	β_4'	$\delta=2.5$ β_1'	β_2'	β_3'	β_4'	$\delta=3.0$ β_1'	β_2'	β_3'	β_4'
13	2	.00172	.00172	.00172	.00172	.00002	.00002	.00002	.00002				
	3	.00135	.00193	.00270	.00515	.00001	.00002	.00003	.00008				
	4	.00120	.00214	.00348	.00903	.00001	.00002	.00004	.00016				
	5	.00112	.00234	.00415	.0130	.00001	.00002	.00005	.00027				
	6	.00107	.00254	.00477	.0171	.00001	.00003	.00006	.00040				
	7	.00104	.00271	.00532	.0211	.00001	.00003	.00007	.00053				
	8	.00101	.00287	.00585	.0250	.00001	.00003	.00008	.00068				
	9	.00099	.00303	.00634	.0289	.00001	.00003	.00009	.00084				.00001
	10	.00097	.00317	.00680	.0328	.00001	.00003	.00010	.00100				.00001
	11	.00096	.00330	.00724	.0365	.00001	.00003	.00011	.00117				.00001
	12	.00095	.00343	.00766	.0401	.00001	.00004	.00011	.00135				.00001
	13	.00094	.00354	.00807	.0438	.00001	.00004	.00012	.00154				.00001
	14	.00094	.00366	.00846	.0473	.00001	.00004	.00013	.00172				.00001
	15	.00093	.00376	.00884	.0507	.00001	.00004	.00014	.00192				.00002
	16	.00092	.00386	.00920	.0541	.00001	.00004	.00015	.00211				.00002
	17	.00092	.00395	.00955	.0574	.00001	.00004	.00016	.00231				.00002
	18	.00092	.00405	.00990	.0607	.00001	.00005	.00016	.00251				.00002
	19	.00091	.00413	.0102	.0639	.00001	.00005	.00017	.00272				.00003
	20	.00091	.00422	.0105	.0670	.00001	.00005	.00018	.00292				.00003
	22	.00090	.00437	.0112	.0731	.00001	.00005	.00019	.00334				.00004
	24	.00090	.00451	.0118	.0789	.00001	.00005	.00021	.00377				.00004
	26	.00089	.00465	.0123	.0846	.00001	.00005	.00022	.00420				.00005
	28	.00089	.00477	.0129	.0900	.00001	.00006	.00023	.00463				.00006
	30	.00089	.00489	.0134	.0953	.00001	.00006	.00025	.00507				.00006
	32	.00089	.00500	.0139	.100	.00001	.00006	.00026	.00551				.00007
	34	.00088	.00510	.0144	.105	.00001	.00006	.00027	.00595				.00008
	36	.00088	.00520	.0148	.110	.00001	.00006	.00029	.00640				.00009
	38	.00088	.00529	.0153	.115	.00001	.00006	.00030	.00684				.00010
	40	.00088	.00538	.0157	.119	.00001	.00007	.00031	.00729				.00010
	50	.00087	.00575	.0177	.140	.00001	.00007	.00037	.00950				.00015
	60	.00087	.00606	.0195	.159	.00001	.00008	.00043	.0117				.00020
	70	.00086	.00630	.0211	.176	.00001	.00008	.00048	.0139				.00026
	80	.00086	.00652	.0226	.191	.00001	.00009	.00053	.0160				.00032
	90	.00086	.00659	.0239	.205	.00001	.00009	.00058	.0181				.00038
	100	.00086	.00686	.0252	.217	.00001	.00009	.00062	.0202				.00045

A. Values of $\beta_1' = \beta_L'$, $\beta_2' = (\beta_S')_{\max}$, $\beta_3' = (\beta_X')_{\min}$ and $\beta_4' = \beta_W'$ for $\alpha = 0.05$

		$\delta = 0.5$				$\delta = 1.0$				$\delta = 1.5$			
N	m	β_1'	β_2'	β_3'	β_4'	β_1'	β_2'	β_3'	β_4'	β_1'	β_2'	β_3'	β_4'
16	2	.722	.722	.722	.722	.219	.219	.219	.219	.0160	.0160	.0160	.0160
	3	.717	.750	.780	.833	.210	.241	.272	.343	.0142	.0186	.0237	.0379
	4	.715	.769	.810	.882	.205	.257	.307	.424	.0134	.0207	.0295	.0587
	5	.713	.782	.830	.909	.203	.271	.332	.483	.0130	.0226	.0342	.0778
	6	.712	.793	.844	.927	.201	.282	.352	.529	.0126	.0243	.0383	.0954
	7	.711	.801	.855	.940	.200	.291	.369	.556	.0124	.0258	.0419	.112
	8	.711	.808	.864	.949	.199	.299	.383	.597	.0123	.0271	.0452	.127
	9	.710	.815	.871	.956	.198	.307	.396	.623	.0122	.0284	.0483	.141
	10	.710	.820	.877	.961	.198	.313	.407	.645	.0121	.0295	.0511	.154
	11	.710	.824	.883	.965	.197	.319	.417	.664	.0120	.0305	.0537	.167
	12	.710	.828	.887	.969	.197	.324	.425	.681	.0119	.0314	.0561	.178
	13	.709	.831	.891	.972	.196	.328	.434	.697	.0119	.0323	.0584	.189
	14	.709	.835	.895	.974	.196	.333	.441	.710	.0118	.0331	.0606	.200
	15	.709	.837	.898	.976	.196	.337	.448	.722	.0118	.0339	.0626	.210
	15	.709	.840	.901	.978	.196	.340	.455	.733	.0117	.0346	.0646	.220
	17	.709	.842	.904	.980	.196	.344	.461	.744	.0117	.0353	.0665	.229
	18	.709	.844	.907	.981	.195	.347	.466	.753	.0117	.0359	.0683	.238
	19	.709	.846	.909	.983	.195	.350	.472	.761	.0117	.0366	.0700	.246
	20	.709	.848	.911	.984	.195	.353	.477	.769	.0116	.0371	.0717	.254
	22	.708	.852	.915	.986	.195	.358	.486	.784	.0116	.0382	.0748	.269
	24	.708	.855	.918	.987	.195	.362	.494	.796	.0116	.0392	.0777	.283
	26	.708	.857	.921	.988	.195	.367	.502	.807	.0115	.0401	.0805	.296
	28	.708	.859	.924	.989	.194	.370	.509	.817	.0115	.0409	.0831	.308
	30	.708	.862	.926	.990	.194	.374	.516	.825	.0115	.0417	.0856	.320
	32	.708	.863	.928	.991	.194	.377	.522	.833	.0115	.0424	.0879	.331
	34	.708	.865	.930	.992	.194	.380	.527	.840	.0115	.0431	.0902	.341
	36	.708	.867	.932	.992	.194	.382	.533	.847	.0115	.0437	.0923	.351
	38	.708	.868	.934	.993	.194	.385	.538	.853	.0114	.0443	.0943	.360
	40	.708	.869	.935	.993	.194	.387	.542	.858	.0114	.0449	.0963	.369
	50	.708	.875	.941	.995	.194	.397	.562	.880	.0114	.0472	.105	.408
	60	.708	.879	.946	.996	.193	.404	.578	.895	.0114	.0491	.112	.440
	70	.708	.882	.950	.997	.193	.410	.591	.907	.0113	.0506	.119	.467
	80	.707	.884	.953	.997	.193	.415	.603	.917	.0113	.0519	.125	.490
	90	.707	.886	.955	.998	.193	.419	.612	.924	.0113	.0530	.130	.510
	100	.707	.888	.957	.998	.193	.423	.621	.931	.0113	.0539	.135	.528

N	m	δ=2.0				δ=2.5				δ=3.0			
		β_1'	β_2'	β_3'	β_4'	β_1'	β_2'	β_3'	β_4'	β_1'	β_2'	β_3'	β_4'
16	2	.00023	.00023	.00023	.00023								
	3	.00018	.00027	.00039	.00083								
	4	.00016	.00031	.00054	.00164				.00001				
	5	.00015	.00034	.00066	.00257				.00001				
	6	.00014	.00038	.00078	.00358				.00002				
	7	.00013	.00041	.00090	.00463				.00003				
	8	.00013	.00044	.00101	.00573				.00005				
	9	.00013	.00047	.00111	.00686				.00006				
	10	.00013	.00050	.00121	.00801				.00007				
	11	.00012	.00053	.00131	.00915			.00001	.00009				
	12	.00012	.00055	.00140	.0103			.00001	.00010				
	13	.00012	.00057	.00149	.0115			.00001	.00012				
	14	.00012	.00060	.00158	.0127			.00001	.00014				
	15	.00012	.00062	.00166	.0138			.00001	.00016				
	16	.00012	.00064	.00175	.0150			.00001	.00018				
	17	.00012	.00065	.00183	.0162			.00001	.00020				
	18	.00012	.00067	.00191	.0173			.00001	.00022				
	19	.00012	.00069	.00198	.0185			.00001	.00025				
	20	.00012	.00071	.00206	.0196			.00001	.00027				
	22	.00012	.00074	.00221	.0219			.00001	.00032				
	24	.00012	.00077	.00235	.0241			.00001	.00037				
	26	.00012	.00079	.00249	.0264			.00001	.00042				
	28	.00011	.00082	.00262	.0285			.00001	.00047				
	30	.00011	.00084	.00275	.0307			.00001	.00053				
	32	.00011	.00087	.00287	.0328			.00002	.00059				
	34	.00011	.00089	.00300	.0349			.00002	.00065				
	36	.00011	.00091	.00312	.0370			.00002	.00071				
	38	.00011	.00093	.00323	.0390			.00002	.00077				
	40	.00011	.00094	.00334	.0410			.00002	.00083				
	50	.00011	.00102	.00387	.0506			.00002	.00116				
	60	.00011	.00109	.00435	.0594			.00003	.00150				.00001
	70	.00011	.00114	.00479	.0678			.00003	.00186				.00001
	80	.00011	.00119	.00520	.0757			.00004	.00223				.00001
	90	.00011	.00123	.00558	.0831			.00004	.00260				.00001
	100	.00011	.00126	.00594	.0901			.00004	.00298				.00002

A. Values of $\beta_1'=\beta_L'$, $\beta_2'=(\beta_S')_{\max}$, $\beta_3'=(\beta_X')_{\min}$ and $\beta_4'=\beta_W'$ for $\alpha=0.05$

		δ=0.5				δ=1.0				δ=1.5			
N	m	β_1'	β_2'	β_3'	β_4'	β_1'	β_2'	β_3'	β_4'	β_1'	β_2'	β_3'	β_4'
21	2	.647	.647	.647	.647	.115	.115	.115	.115	.00271	.00271	.00271	.00271
	3	.643	.680	.713	.775	.110	.130	.152	.204	.00239	.00332	.00446	.00799
	4	.640	.701	.748	.835	.107	.143	.177	.270	.00225	.00385	.00589	.0140
	5	.639	.717	.772	.871	.106	.152	.197	.323	.00216	.00431	.00713	.0202
	6	.638	.730	.789	.894	.105	.161	.213	.365	.00211	.00473	.00825	.0264
	7	.637	.740	.802	.911	.104	.168	.226	.401	.00207	.00511	.00927	.0325
	8	.636	.748	.813	.923	.104	.174	.238	.432	.00204	.00545	.0102	.0385
	9	.636	.755	.822	.933	.103	.179	.248	.459	.00202	.00577	.0111	.0444
	10	.636	.761	.830	.940	.103	.184	.257	.483	.00201	.00606	.0119	.0501
	11	.636	.766	.837	.946	.103	.189	.265	.504	.00199	.00633	.0127	.0557
	12	.635	.771	.843	.951	.103	.193	.273	.522	.00198	.00659	.0135	.0611
	13	.635	.775	.848	.956	.102	.196	.280	.540	.00197	.00682	.0142	.0663
	14	.635	.779	.852	.959	.102	.200	.287	.555	.00196	.00704	.0149	.0715
	15	.635	.782	.857	.962	.102	.203	.293	.570	.00196	.00725	.0156	.0764
	16	.635	.785	.860	.965	.102	.206	.298	.583	.00195	.00745	.0162	.0813
	17	.635	.788	.864	.968	.102	.208	.304	.595	.00195	.00763	.0168	.0860
	18	.634	.791	.867	.970	.102	.211	.309	.506	.00194	.00781	.0174	.0906
	19	.634	.793	.870	.972	.102	.213	.314	.617	.00194	.00798	.0180	.0951
	20	.634	.796	.873	.973	.102	.215	.318	.627	.00193	.00815	.0185	.100
	22	.634	.799	.878	.976	.101	.219	.327	.645	.00193	.00844	.0196	.108
	24	.634	.803	.882	.978	.101	.223	.334	.660	.00192	.00873	.0206	.116
	26	.634	.806	.886	.980	.101	.226	.341	.675	.00192	.00899	.0216	.124
	28	.534	.809	.889	.982	.101	.229	.348	.688	.00191	.00921	.0225	.131
	30	.634	.812	.893	.984	.101	.232	.354	.599	.00191	.00944	.0233	.138
	32	.634	.814	.895	.985	.101	.235	.360	.710	.00191	.00965	.0242	.145
	34	.634	.816	.898	.986	.101	.237	.365	.720	.00190	.00985	.0250	.152
	36	.634	.818	.900	.987	.101	.239	.370	.729	.00190	.0100	.0258	.158
	38	.634	.820	.903	.988	.101	.241	.375	.737	.00190	.0102	.0265	.164
	40	.534	.821	.905	.988	.101	.243	.379	.745	.00190	.0104	.0272	.170
	50	.633	.828	.913	.991	.101	.251	.399	.777	.00189	.0111	.0305	.197
	60	.633	.833	.919	.993	.101	.257	.415	.800	.00189	.0116	.0334	.220
	70	.633	.837	.924	.994	.101	.262	.428	.819	.00188	.0121	.0360	.241
	80	.633	.840	.929	.995	.101	.266	.439	.834	.00188	.0125	.0383	.260
	90	.633	.842	.932	.996	.101	.270	.449	.847	.00188	.0128	.0405	.276
	100	.633	.845	.935	.996	.100	.273	.458	.857	.00188	.0131	.0425	.291

N	m	δ=2.0				δ=2.5				δ=3.0			
		β_1'	β_2'	β_3'	β_4'	β_1'	β_2'	β_3'	β_4'	β_1'	β_2'	β_3'	β_4'
21	2	.00001	.00001	.00001	.00001								
	3	.00001	.00001	.00001	.00003								
	4		.00001	.00002	.00008								
	5		.00001	.00003	.00014								
	6		.00001	.00003	.00021								
	7		.00001	.00004	.00029								
	8		.00002	.00004	.00038								
	9		.00002	.00005	.00048								
	10		.00002	.00006	.00059								
	11		.00002	.00006	.00070								
	12		.00002	.00007	.00082								
	13		.00002	.00007	.00095								
	14		.00002	.00008	.00108								
	15		.00002	.00008	.00121								
	15		.00003	.00009	.00134								
	17		.00003	.00009	.00148								
	18		.00003	.00010	.00162								
	19		.00003	.00010	.00177								
	20		.00003	.00011	.00192								
	22		.00003	.00012	.00221								
	24		.00003	.00013	.00252				.00001				
	26		.00003	.00014	.00284				.00001				
	28		.00004	.00015	.00315				.00001				
	30		.00004	.00016	.00348				.00001				
	32		.00004	.00017	.00380				.00001				
	34		.00004	.00017	.00414				.00001				
	36		.00004	.00018	.00447				.00001				
	38		.00004	.00019	.00480				.00001				
	40		.00004	.00020	.00514				.00001				
	50		.00005	.00024	.00683				.00002				
	60		.00005	.00028	.00852				.00003				
	70		.00005	.00032	.0102				.00004				
	80		.00006	.00035	.0119				.00005				
	90		.00006	.00039	.0135				.00007				
	100		.00006	.00042	.0152				.00008				

A. Values of $\beta_1' = \beta_L'$, $\beta_2' = (\beta_S')_{\max}$, $\beta_3' = (\beta_X')_{\min}$ and $\beta_4' = \beta_W'$ for $\alpha = 0.05$

N	m	δ=0.5				δ=1.0				δ=1.5			
		β_1'	β_2'	β_3'	β_4'	β_1'	β_2'	β_3'	β_4'	β_1'	β_2'	β_3'	β_4'
25	2	.590	.590	.590	.590	.0663	.0663	.0663	.0663	.00061	.00061	.00061	.00061
	3	.585	.625	.659	.727	.0633	.0773	.0921	.130	.00054	.00078	.00108	.00211
	4	.583	.648	.698	.796	.0618	.0859	.110	.181	.00050	.00093	.00150	.00405
	5	.582	.665	.724	.837	.0609	.0928	.125	.224	.00048	.00106	.00187	.00622
	6	.581	.679	.743	.864	.0603	.0988	.137	.260	.00047	.00118	.00222	.00853
	7	.580	.690	.758	.884	.0599	.104	.147	.292	.00046	.00129	.00254	.0109
	8	.580	.699	.771	.899	.0596	.108	.156	.319	.00046	.00139	.00284	.0134
	9	.579	.707	.781	.911	.0594	.112	.164	.344	.00045	.00149	.00314	.0158
	10	.579	.713	.790	.920	.0592	.116	.171	.366	.00045	.00158	.00341	.0183
	11	.579	.719	.797	.928	.0591	.119	.178	.387	.00044	.00166	.00368	.0207
	12	.578	.724	.804	.935	.0590	.122	.184	.405	.00044	.00174	.00393	.0232
	13	.578	.729	.810	.940	.0588	.125	.190	.422	.00044	.00181	.00418	.0256
	14	.578	.733	.816	.945	.0588	.128	.195	.437	.00044	.00188	.00442	.0280
	15	.578	.737	.820	.949	.0587	.130	.200	.452	.00044	.00194	.00465	.0304
	16	.578	.740	.825	.952	.0586	.132	.204	.465	.00043	.00200	.00487	.0327
	17	.578	.743	.829	.955	.0585	.134	.209	.477	.00043	.00206	.00509	.0350
	18	.578	.746	.833	.958	.0585	.136	.213	.489	.00043	.00212	.00530	.0374
	19	.578	.749	.836	.960	.0584	.138	.217	.500	.00043	.00217	.00550	.0396
	20	.578	.752	.839	.963	.0584	.139	.221	.511	.00043	.00222	.00570	.0419
	22	.577	.756	.845	.966	.0583	.143	.228	.530	.00043	.00231	.00609	.0462
	24	.577	.760	.850	.970	.0583	.145	.234	.547	.00043	.00241	.00646	.0505
	26	.577	.764	.855	.972	.0582	.148	.240	.562	.00043	.00249	.00681	.0547
	28	.577	.767	.859	.975	.0582	.150	.246	.576	.00043	.00256	.00715	.0587
	30	.577	.770	.863	.976	.0581	.152	.251	.589	.00042	.00264	.00747	.0626
	32	.577	.772	.866	.978	.0581	.154	.256	.601	.00042	.00270	.00779	.0665
	34	.577	.775	.869	.980	.0581	.156	.261	.613	.00042	.00277	.00810	.0703
	36	.577	.777	.872	.981	.0580	.158	.265	.623	.00042	.00282	.00840	.0740
	38	.577	.779	.875	.982	.0580	.160	.269	.632	.00042	.00288	.00868	.0775
	40	.577	.781	.877	.983	.0580	.161	.273	.542	.00042	.00294	.00896	.0810
	50	.577	.788	.887	.987	.0579	.167	.290	.679	.00042	.00317	.0103	.0974
	60	.577	.794	.895	.990	.0579	.172	.304	.708	.00042	.00335	.0114	.112
	70	.577	.798	.901	.991	.0578	.176	.317	.731	.00042	.00351	.0125	.126
	80	.577	.802	.906	.993	.0578	.179	.327	.750	.00042	.00364	.0134	.138
	90	.576	.805	.910	.994	.0578	.182	.336	.766	.00042	.00374	.0143	.150
	100	.576	.807	.914	.994	.0577	.184	.345	.780	.00042	.00385	.0152	.161

N	m	δ=2.0				δ=2.5				δ=3.0			
		β_1'	β_2'	β_3'	β_4'	β_1'	β_2'	β_3'	β_4'	β_1'	β_2'	β_3'	β_4'
25	2												
	3												
	4				.00001								
	5				.00001								
	6				.00002								
	7				.00003								
	8				.00004								
	9				.00005								
	10				.00006								
	11				.00008								
	12			.00001	.00009								
	13			.00001	.00011								
	14			.00001	.00012								
	15			.00001	.00014								
	16			.00001	.00016								
	17			.00001	.00018								
	18			.00001	.00020								
	19			.00001	.00022								
	20			.00001	.00025								
	22			.00001	.00029								
	24			.00001	.00034								
	26			.00001	.00039								
	28			.00001	.00044								
	30			.00001	.00050								
	32			.00001	.00055								
	34			.00002	.00061								
	36			.00002	.00067								
	38			.00002	.00073								
	40			.00002	.00079								
	50			.00002	.00111								
	60			.00003	.00145								
	70			.00003	.00181								
	80			.00003	.00217								
	90			.00004	.00254								
	100			.00004	.00292								

A. Values of $\beta'_1 = \beta'_L$, $\beta'_2 = (\beta'_S)_{\max}$, $\beta'_3 = (\beta'_X)_{\min}$ and $\beta'_4 = \beta'_W$ for $\alpha = 0.05$

		$\delta=0.5$				$\delta=1.0$				$\delta=1.5$			
N	m	β'_1	β'_2	β'_3	β'_4	β'_1	β'_2	β'_3	β'_4	β'_1	β'_2	β'_3	β'_4
31	2	.509	.509	.509	.509	.0279	.0279	.0279	.0279	.00006	.00006	.00006	.00006
	3	.505	.546	.582	.656	.0265	.0336	.0414	.0622	.00005	.00008	.00012	.00026
	4	.503	.571	.624	.733	.0259	.0383	.0514	.0937	.00005	.00010	.00017	.00056
	5	.502	.589	.653	.782	.0255	.0421	.0596	.122	.00005	.00012	.00023	.00094
	6	.501	.604	.674	.815	.0252	.0454	.0667	.147	.00005	.00013	.00028	.00138
	7	.500	.616	.691	.840	.0251	.0483	.0728	.170	.00004	.00015	.00033	.00186
	8	.500	.626	.705	.859	.0249	.0508	.0783	.191	.00004	.00016	.00037	.00238
	9	.499	.634	.717	.874	.0248	.0531	.0834	.210	.00004	.00018	.00042	.00293
	10	.499	.642	.727	.886	.0247	.0552	.0879	.228	.00004	.00019	.00046	.00349
	11	.499	.648	.736	.896	.0247	.0570	.0921	.244	.00004	.00020	.00051	.00408
	12	.499	.654	.744	.905	.0246	.0588	.0961	.260	.00004	.00021	.00055	.00468
	13	.499	.659	.751	.912	.0246	.0603	.100	.274	.00004	.00022	.00059	.00530
	14	.498	.664	.757	.918	.0245	.0619	.103	.287	.00004	.00023	.00063	.00592
	15	.498	.668	.763	.924	.0245	.0632	.106	.300	.00004	.00024	.00067	.00655
	16	.498	.672	.768	.929	.0245	.0645	.110	.312	.00004	.00025	.00071	.00719
	17	.498	.675	.773	.933	.0244	.0657	.112	.323	.00004	.00026	.00075	.00783
	18	.498	.679	.777	.937	.0244	.0669	.115	.334	.00004	.00027	.00079	.00848
	19	.498	.682	.781	.940	.0244	.0679	.118	.344	.00004	.00028	.00082	.00913
	20	.498	.684	.785	.943	.0244	.0690	.121	.353	.00004	.00028	.00086	.00978
	22	.498	.689	.792	.948	.0244	.0708	.125	.371	.00004	.00030	.00093	.0111
	24	.498	.694	.798	.953	.0243	.0725	.130	.388	.00004	.00031	.00100	.0124
	26	.498	.698	.804	.957	.0243	.0741	.134	.403	.00004	.00032	.00107	.0137
	28	.498	.701	.809	.960	.0243	.0755	.138	.417	.00004	.00034	.00113	.0150
	30	.497	.705	.813	.963	.0243	.0768	.142	.430	.00004	.00035	.00119	.0163
	32	.497	.708	.818	.965	.0242	.0780	.145	.442	.00004	.00036	.00125	.0176
	34	.497	.711	.821	.968	.0242	.0792	.148	.454	.00004	.00037	.00131	.0189
	36	.497	.713	.825	.969	.0242	.0802	.151	.465	.00004	.00038	.00137	.0201
	38	.497	.715	.828	.971	.0242	.0813	.154	.474	.00004	.00039	.00143	.0214
	40	.497	.717	.831	.973	.0242	.0822	.157	.484	.00004	.00039	.00149	.0226
	50	.497	.726	.844	.979	.0242	.0861	.170	.525	.00004	.00043	.00175	.0287
	60	.497	.733	.854	.983	.0241	.0892	.180	.558	.00004	.00046	.00199	.0345
	70	.497	.738	.861	.985	.0241	.0917	.190	.585	.00004	.00049	.00222	.0401
	80	.497	.742	.868	.987	.0241	.0937	.198	.608	.00004	.00051	.00243	.0454
	90	.497	.745	.873	.989	.0241	.0954	.205	.627	.00004	.00053	.00262	.0504
	100	.497	.748	.878	.990	.0241	.0969	.211	.644	.00004	.00054	.00281	.0553

		δ = 2.0				δ = 2.5				δ = 3.0			
N	m	β_1'	β_2'	β_3'	β_4'	β_1'	β_2'	β_3'	β_4'	β_1'	β_2'	β_3'	β_4'
31	2												
	3												
	4												
	5												
	6												
	7												
	8												
	9												
	10												
	11												
	12												
	13												
	14												
	15												
	16				.00001								
	17				.00001								
	18				.00001								
	19				.00001								
	20				.00001								
	22				.00001								
	24				.00001								
	26				.00002								
	28				.00002								
	30				.00002								
	32				.00002								
	34				.00003								
	36				.00003								
	38				.00003								
	40				.00004								
	50				.00006								
	60				.00008								
	70				.00010								
	80				.00013								
	90				.00016								
	100				.00018								

A. Values of $\beta_1' = \beta_L'$, $\beta_2' = (\beta_S')_{\max}$, $\beta_3' = (\beta_X')_{\min}$ and $\beta_4' = \beta_W'$ for $\alpha = 0.05$

		$\delta=0.5$				$\delta=1.0$				$\delta=1.5$			
N	m	β_1'	β_2'	β_3'	β_4'	β_1'	β_2'	β_3'	β_4'	β_1'	β_2'	β_3'	β_4'
41	2	.391	.391	.391	.391	.00599	.00599	.00599	.00599				
	3	.388	.427	.464	.541	.00568	.00763	.00983	.0164				.00001
	4	.386	.453	.507	.627	.00554	.00900	.0130	.0277				.00002
	5	.385	.472	.538	.685	.00545	.0102	.0157	.0391			.00001	.00003
	6	.384	.487	.561	.726	.00539	.0112	.0180	.0501			.00001	.00005
	7	.384	.500	.580	.757	.00535	.0121	.0202	.0608			.00001	.00007
	8	.383	.510	.596	.782	.00532	.0129	.0222	.0710			.00001	.00010
	9	.383	.519	.609	.802	.00530	.0136	.0240	.0809			.00001	.00013
	10	.383	.527	.621	.819	.00528	.0143	.0257	.0902			.00001	.00017
	11	.383	.534	.631	.833	.00527	.0150	.0274	.0992			.00001	.00020
	12	.382	.540	.640	.845	.00526	.0155	.0289	.108		.00001	.00002	.00024
	13	.382	.546	.648	.855	.00525	.0161	.0303	.116		.00001	.00002	.00028
	14	.382	.551	.656	.864	.00524	.0166	.0317	.124		.00001	.00002	.00033
	15	.382	.556	.662	.872	.00523	.0171	.0330	.132		.00001	.00002	.00037
	16	.382	.560	.668	.879	.00522	.0175	.0342	.139		.00001	.00002	.00042
	17	.382	.563	.674	.885	.00522	.0179	.0355	.146		.00001	.00002	.00047
	18	.382	.567	.680	.891	.00521	.0183	.0366	.153		.00001	.00003	.00052
	19	.382	.571	.685	.896	.00521	.0187	.0377	.160		.00001	.00003	.00058
	20	.382	.574	.689	.901	.00520	.0191	.0388	.166		.00001	.00003	.00063
	22	.382	.579	.698	.909	.00519	.0197	.0408	.179		.00001	.00003	.00075
	24	.382	.584	.705	.916	.00519	.0203	.0428	.190		.00001	.00003	.00086
	26	.381	.589	.712	.922	.00518	.0209	.0446	.201		.00001	.00004	.00099
	28	.381	.593	.718	.927	.00518	.0214	.0463	.211		.00001	.00004	.00111
	30	.381	.596	.724	.932	.00517	.0219	.0479	.221		.00001	.00004	.00124
	32	.381	.600	.729	.936	.00517	.0223	.0495	.230		.00001	.00005	.00137
	34	.381	.603	.734	.939	.00517	.0227	.0510	.239		.00001	.00005	.00151
	36	.381	.606	.738	.943	.00517	.0231	.0524	.248		.00001	.00005	.00165
	38	.381	.608	.743	.945	.00516	.0235	.0537	.256		.00001	.00005	.00178
	40	.381	.611	.746	.948	.00516	.0238	.0551	.264		.00001	.00006	.00193
	50	.381	.621	.763	.958	.00515	.0253	.0610	.299		.00001	.00007	.00266
	60	.381	.628	.775	.965	.00515	.0265	.0661	.328		.00001	.00008	.00341
	70	.381	.634	.786	.970	.00514	.0274	.0707	.353		.00001	.00009	.00418
	80	.381	.639	.794	.974	.00514	.0282	.0747	.375		.00002	.00011	.00496
	90	.381	.642	.801	.977	.00514	.0289	.0784	.395		.00002	.00012	.00574
	100	.381	.646	.808	.979	.00514	.0295	.0818	.413		.00002	.00013	.00653

A. Values of $\beta_1' = \beta_L'$, $\beta_2' = (\beta_S')_{max}$, $\beta_3' = (\beta_X')_{min}$ and $\beta_4' = \beta_W'$ for $\alpha = 0.05$

N	m	$\delta=0.5$				$\delta=1.0$				$\delta=1.5$			
		β_1'	β_2'	β_3'	β_4'	β_1'	β_2'	β_3'	β_4'	β_1'	β_2'	β_3'	β_4'
61	2	.218	.218	.218	.218	.00022	.00022	.00022	.00022				
	3	.216	.247	.277	.345	.00021	.00030	.00043	.00085				
	4	.215	.268	.315	.430	.00020	.00038	.00062	.00176				
	5	.214	.285	.343	.492	.00020	.00045	.00081	.00286				
	6	.214	.298	.365	.540	.00019	.00052	.00098	.00409				
	7	.213	.309	.383	.579	.00019	.00057	.00115	.00541				
	8	.213	.318	.399	.610	.00019	.00063	.00131	.00679				
	9	.213	.327	.412	.637	.00019	.00068	.00146	.00823				
	10	.213	.334	.424	.660	.00019	.00073	.00161	.00968				
	11	.213	.340	.434	.679	.00019	.00077	.00175	.0112				
	12	.213	.346	.444	.697	.00019	.00081	.00189	.0127				
	13	.212	.351	.453	.712	.00019	.00085	.00203	.0142				
	14	.212	.356	.461	.726	.00019	.00089	.00216	.0157				
	15	.212	.361	.468	.738	.00019	.00092	.00228	.0172				
	16	.212	.364	.475	.749	.00019	.00096	.00241	.0187				
	17	.212	.368	.481	.759	.00019	.00099	.00253	.0202				
	18	.212	.372	.487	.768	.00019	.00102	.00265	.0217				
	19	.212	.375	.493	.777	.00019	.00105	.00276	.0232				
	20	.212	.378	.498	.785	.00019	.00108	.00287	.0246				
	22	.212	.383	.508	.799	.00019	.00113	.00309	.0275				
	24	.212	.388	.516	.811	.00019	.00118	.00330	.0304				
	26	.212	.393	.524	.821	.00019	.00122	.00350	.0333				
	28	.212	.397	.532	.831	.00019	.00126	.00370	.0360				
	30	.212	.400	.538	.839	.00019	.00130	.00388	.0388				
	32	.212	.404	.545	.847	.00019	.00134	.00407	.0415				
	34	.212	.407	.550	.854	.00019	.00137	.00425	.0441				
	36	.212	.410	.556	.860	.00019	.00141	.00442	.0467				
	38	.212	.412	.561	.865	.00019	.00144	.00458	.0493				.00001
	40	.212	.415	.566	.871	.00019	.00147	.00475	.0518				.00001
	50	.212	.425	.586	.891	.00018	.00159	.00551	.0637				.00001
	60	.212	.433	.602	.906	.00018	.00170	.00619	.0747				.00001
	70	.212	.439	.615	.917	.00018	.00178	.00682	.0850				.00002
	80	.212	.444	.627	.926	.00018	.00186	.00740	.0945				.00002
	90	.212	.448	.636	.933	.00018	.00191	.00794	.103				.00003
	100	.212	.451	.645	.939	.00018	.00197	.00845	.112				.00004

A. Values of $\beta_1' = \beta_L'$, $\beta_2' = (\beta_S')_{\max}$, $\beta_3' = (\beta_X')_{\min}$ and $\beta_4' = \beta_W'$ for $\alpha = 0.05$

N	m	δ=0.5				δ=1.0				δ=1.5			
		β_1'	β_2'	β_3'	β_4'	β_1'	β_2'	β_3'	β_4'	β_1'	β_2'	β_3'	β_4'
121	2	.0278	.0278	.0278	.0278								
	3	.0275	.0348	.0423	.0628								
	4	.0274	.0403	.0532	.0955								
	5	.0273	.0447	.0622	.125								
	6	.0272	.0485	.0699	.152								
	7	.0271	.0519	.0767	.176								
	8	.0271	.0548	.0827	.198								
	9	.0271	.0574	.0881	.218								
	10	.0271	.0597	.0931	.236								
	11	.0270	.0619	.0977	.253								
	12	.0270	.0639	.102	.269								
	13	.0270	.0656	.106	.284								
	14	.0270	.0673	.110	.298				.00001				
	15	.0270	.0689	.113	.311				.00001				
	16	.0270	.0703	.117	.323				.00001				
	17	.0270	.0716	.120	.335				.00001				
	18	.0270	.0729	.123	.346				.00001				
	19	.0270	.0741	.126	.357				.00001				
	20	.0270	.0753	.128	.367				.00001				
	22	.0270	.0773	.134	.385				.00001				
	24	.0269	.0792	.138	.402				.00002				
	25	.0269	.0810	.143	.418				.00002				
	28	.0269	.0825	.147	.432				.00002				
	30	.0269	.0840	.151	.445				.00003				
	32	.0269	.0853	.155	.458				.00003				
	34	.0269	.0866	.158	.470				.00004				
	36	.0269	.0877	.161	.480				.00004				
	38	.0269	.0888	.165	.491				.00005				
	40	.0269	.0898	.168	.500				.00005				
	50	.0269	.0941	.181	.542				.00008				
	60	.0269	.0975	.192	.575				.00011				
	70	.0269	.100	.202	.602				.00014				
	80	.0269	.102	.210	.625				.00018				
	90	.0269	.104	.218	.644				.00022				
	100	.0269	.106	.225	.661				.00026				

B. Values of $\beta_1' = \beta_L'$, $\beta_2' = (\beta_S')_{\max}$, $\beta_3' = (\beta_X')_{\min}$ and $\beta_4' = \beta_W'$ for $\alpha = 0.01$

		$\delta = 0.5$				$\delta = 1.0$				$\delta = 1.5$			
N	m	β_1'	β_2'	β_3'	β_4'	β_1'	β_2'	β_3'	β_4'	β_1'	β_2'	β_3'	β_4'
2	2	.988	.988	.988	.988	.980	.980	.980	.980	.968	.968	.968	.968
	3	.986	.987	.991	.993	.975	.976	.983	.988	.955	.956	.968	.977
	4	.986	.987	.992	.996	.971	.974	.984	.991	.943	.949	.969	.982
	5	.985	.988	.994	.997	.968	.974	.986	.993	.934	.945	.969	.985
	6	.984	.989	.994	.998	.965	.974	.987	.994	.925	.943	.969	.987
	7	.984	.989	.995	.998	.963	.974	.987	.995	.919	.942	.970	.988
	8	.983	.990	.995	.999	.961	.975	.988	.996	.913	.942	.971	.990
	9	.983	.990	.996	.999	.959	.976	.989	.997	.909	.942	.971	.991
	10	.983	.991	.996	.999	.958	.976	.989	.997	.905	.942	.972	.992
	11	.983	.991	.996	.999	.957	.977	.989	.997	.901	.943	.972	.992
	12	.983	.992	.997	.999	.956	.977	.990	.998	.898	.943	.972	.993
	13	.982	.992	.997	.999	.955	.978	.990	.998	.896	.944	.973	.993
	14	.982	.992	.997	.999	.954	.978	.991	.998	.894	.944	.973	.994
	15	.982	.993	.997	1.000	.953	.979	.991	.998	.892	.945	.974	.994
	16	.982	.993	.997	1.000	.953	.979	.991	.998	.890	.945	.974	.995
	17	.982	.993	.997	1.000	.952	.980	.991	.999	.888	.946	.975	.995
	18	.982	.993	.997	1.000	.952	.980	.992	.999	.887	.946	.975	.995
	19	.982	.994	.998	1.000	.951	.980	.992	.999	.885	.947	.975	.996
	20	.982	.994	.998	1.000	.951	.981	.992	.999	.884	.948	.976	.996
	22	.981	.994	.998	1.000	.950	.981	.992	.999	.882	.949	.976	.996
	24	.981	.994	.998	1.000	.950	.982	.993	.999	.880	.950	.977	.997
	26	.981	.995	.998	1.000	.949	.982	.993	.999	.879	.950	.977	.997
	28	.981	.995	.998	1.000	.949	.983	.993	.999	.878	.951	.978	.997
	30	.981	.995	.998	1.000	.948	.983	.993	.999	.876	.952	.978	.997
	32	.981	.995	.998	1.000	.948	.984	.993	.999	.875	.953	.979	.998
	34	.981	.995	.998	1.000	.948	.984	.994	.999	.875	.954	.979	.998
	36	.981	.995	.998	1.000	.947	.984	.994	1.000	.874	.954	.980	.998
	38	.981	.996	.998	1.000	.947	.985	.994	1.000	.873	.955	.980	.998
	40	.981	.996	.999	1.000	.947	.985	.994	1.000	.872	.956	.980	.998
	50	.981	.996	.999	1.000	.946	.986	.995	1.000	.870	.958	.982	.999
	60	.981	.997	.999	1.000	.945	.987	.995	1.000	.868	.960	.983	.999
	70	.980	.997	.999	1.000	.945	.988	.996	1.000	.867	.962	.984	.999
	80	.980	.997	.999	1.000	.945	.988	.996	1.000	.866	.963	.985	.999
	90	.980	.997	.999	1.000	.944	.989	.996	1.000	.865	.964	.985	.999
	100	.980	.997	.999	1.000	.944	.989	.996	1.000	.864	.965	.986	.999

N	m	δ=2.0				δ=2.5				δ=3.0			
		β_1'	β_2'	β_3'	β_4'	β_1'	β_2'	β_3'	β_4'	β_1'	β_2'	β_3'	β_4'
2	2	.951	.951	.951	.951	.930	.930	.930	.930	.905	.905	.905	.905
	3	.924	.926	.946	.961	.882	.884	.915	.938	.829	.831	.875	.907
	4	.899	.909	.942	.966	.836	.851	.903	.941	.755	.775	.850	.905
	5	.877	.898	.940	.969	.796	.827	.894	.943	.692	.734	.829	.904
	6	.860	.891	.938	.972	.764	.811	.887	.945	.643	.705	.813	.904
	7	.845	.886	.937	.974	.738	.799	.882	.947	.604	.683	.800	.904
	8	.833	.883	.936	.976	.717	.791	.878	.949	.573	.668	.790	.905
	9	.823	.881	.936	.977	.699	.784	.874	.951	.548	.656	.782	.906
	10	.814	.879	.935	.979	.684	.780	.872	.953	.527	.646	.776	.907
	11	.807	.879	.935	.980	.671	.776	.870	.955	.510	.639	.770	.909
	12	.800	.878	.935	.981	.661	.774	.869	.956	.495	.633	.766	.910
	13	.795	.878	.936	.982	.651	.772	.868	.958	.483	.628	.762	.911
	14	.790	.878	.936	.983	.643	.771	.867	.959	.472	.625	.759	.913
	15	.785	.878	.936	.984	.636	.770	.866	.960	.463	.622	.757	.914
	16	.782	.879	.936	.985	.630	.769	.866	.961	.455	.620	.755	.916
	17	.778	.879	.937	.985	.624	.768	.865	.963	.448	.618	.753	.917
	18	.775	.879	.937	.986	.619	.768	.865	.964	.441	.616	.752	.918
	19	.772	.880	.937	.987	.615	.768	.865	.965	.436	.615	.750	.920
	20	.770	.880	.938	.987	.611	.768	.865	.966	.430	.614	.749	.921
	22	.766	.881	.939	.988	.604	.768	.865	.967	.422	.613	.748	.924
	24	.762	.883	.939	.989	.598	.769	.866	.969	.414	.612	.747	.926
	26	.759	.884	.940	.990	.593	.770	.866	.970	.408	.612	.747	.928
	28	.756	.885	.941	.990	.588	.771	.867	.972	.403	.612	.746	.930
	30	.753	.886	.941	.991	.584	.772	.867	.973	.398	.612	.746	.932
	32	.751	.887	.942	.991	.581	.773	.868	.974	.394	.612	.747	.934
	34	.749	.888	.943	.992	.578	.774	.869	.975	.391	.613	.747	.936
	36	.748	.889	.943	.992	.576	.775	.870	.976	.388	.613	.747	.938
	38	.746	.890	.944	.992	.573	.776	.870	.977	.385	.614	.748	.939
	40	.745	.891	.945	.993	.571	.777	.871	.977	.382	.615	.749	.941
	50	.740	.895	.947	.994	.563	.782	.875	.981	.373	.619	.752	.947
	60	.736	.899	.950	.995	.558	.787	.879	.983	.366	.624	.756	.952
	70	.733	.901	.952	.996	.554	.790	.882	.985	.362	.628	.760	.956
	80	.732	.904	.954	.996	.551	.794	.885	.987	.359	.632	.764	.960
	90	.730	.906	.955	.997	.549	.797	.888	.988	.356	.635	.768	.963
	100	.729	.908	.956	.997	.547	.800	.890	.989	.354	.638	.772	.965

B. Values of $\beta_1' = \beta_L'$, $\beta_2' = (\beta_S')_{\max}$, $\beta_3' = (\beta_X')_{\min}$ and $\beta_4' = \beta_W'$ for $\alpha = 0.01$

N	m	δ=0.5 β_1'	δ=0.5 β_2'	δ=0.5 β_3'	δ=0.5 β_4'	δ=1.0 β_1'	δ=1.0 β_2'	δ=1.0 β_3'	δ=1.0 β_4'	δ=1.5 β_1'	δ=1.5 β_2'	δ=1.5 β_3'	δ=1.5 β_4'
3	2	.983	.983	.983	.983	.960	.960	.960	.960	.916	.916	.916	.916
	3	.981	.984	.988	.992	.950	.956	.966	.976	.884	.898	.918	.941
	4	.980	.985	.990	.995	.943	.956	.969	.983	.863	.891	.920	.953
	5	.979	.986	.991	.996	.938	.957	.972	.987	.848	.888	.922	.961
	6	.978	.987	.992	.997	.934	.958	.973	.989	.837	.888	.924	.966
	7	.978	.988	.993	.998	.932	.959	.975	.991	.829	.888	.925	.970
	8	.978	.989	.994	.998	.929	.961	.976	.993	.822	.889	.927	.973
	9	.977	.989	.994	.999	.928	.962	.977	.994	.817	.890	.929	.976
	10	.977	.990	.995	.999	.926	.963	.978	.994	.813	.892	.931	.978
	11	.977	.990	.995	.999	.925	.964	.979	.995	.809	.893	.932	.980
	12	.977	.991	.995	.999	.924	.965	.980	.995	.806	.894	.933	.981
	13	.977	.991	.996	.999	.923	.966	.981	.996	.804	.896	.935	.983
	14	.976	.992	.996	.999	.922	.966	.981	.996	.801	.897	.936	.984
	15	.976	.992	.996	.999	.922	.967	.982	.997	.799	.899	.937	.985
	16	.976	.992	.996	.999	.921	.968	.982	.997	.798	.900	.938	.986
	17	.976	.992	.996	1.000	.921	.968	.983	.997	.796	.901	.939	.987
	18	.976	.993	.996	1.000	.920	.969	.983	.997	.795	.902	.940	.987
	19	.976	.993	.997	1.000	.920	.970	.984	.998	.793	.903	.941	.988
	20	.976	.993	.997	1.000	.919	.970	.984	.998	.792	.904	.942	.989
	22	.976	.993	.997	1.000	.919	.971	.985	.998	.790	.906	.944	.990
	24	.976	.994	.997	1.000	.918	.972	.985	.998	.789	.908	.945	.990
	26	.976	.994	.997	1.000	.918	.973	.986	.998	.787	.910	.946	.991
	28	.975	.994	.997	1.000	.917	.974	.986	.999	.786	.911	.948	.992
	30	.975	.994	.997	1.000	.917	.974	.987	.999	.785	.913	.949	.992
	32	.975	.994	.998	1.000	.917	.975	.987	.999	.784	.914	.950	.993
	34	.975	.995	.998	1.000	.916	.975	.987	.999	.783	.915	.951	.993
	36	.975	.995	.998	1.000	.916	.976	.988	.999	.783	.917	.952	.994
	38	.975	.995	.998	1.000	.916	.976	.988	.999	.782	.918	.953	.994
	40	.975	.995	.998	1.000	.916	.977	.988	.999	.781	.919	.953	.994
	50	.975	.996	.998	1.000	.915	.978	.990	.999	.779	.923	.957	.996
	60	.975	.996	.998	1.000	.914	.980	.990	.999	.778	.926	.960	.996
	70	.975	.996	.998	1.000	.914	.981	.991	1.000	.777	.929	.962	.997
	80	.975	.996	.999	1.000	.914	.982	.992	1.000	.776	.931	.964	.997
	90	.975	.997	.999	1.000	.913	.982	.992	1.000	.775	.933	.965	.998
	100	.975	.997	.999	1.000	.913	.983	.993	1.000	.775	.935	.967	.998

N	m	δ=2.0				δ=2.5				δ=3.0			
		β'_1	β'_2	β'_3	β'_4	β'_1	β'_2	β'_3	β'_4	β'_1	β'_2	β'_3	β'_4
3	2	.843	.843	.843	.843	.743	.743	.743	.743	.622	.622	.622	.622
	3	.775	.798	.833	.876	.627	.658	.708	.774	.460	.496	.556	.641
	4	.730	.776	.827	.892	.554	.615	.687	.789	.369	.433	.517	.647
	5	.699	.764	.824	.903	.507	.590	.675	.800	.314	.398	.492	.652
	6	.676	.758	.824	.911	.474	.576	.667	.809	.280	.377	.476	.658
	7	.660	.755	.824	.918	.451	.567	.663	.817	.256	.363	.465	.664
	8	.647	.754	.824	.924	.433	.562	.660	.825	.238	.354	.458	.670
	9	.637	.754	.826	.929	.419	.558	.658	.831	.225	.348	.452	.676
	10	.628	.754	.827	.933	.408	.556	.658	.838	.215	.344	.449	.682
	11	.622	.755	.828	.937	.400	.555	.658	.843	.207	.341	.446	.688
	12	.616	.756	.830	.940	.392	.555	.658	.848	.200	.338	.445	.694
	13	.611	.757	.831	.943	.386	.555	.658	.853	.195	.337	.444	.699
	14	.607	.759	.833	.946	.381	.555	.659	.858	.190	.336	.443	.704
	15	.603	.760	.834	.948	.376	.556	.660	.862	.186	.336	.443	.709
	16	.600	.761	.836	.950	.372	.557	.661	.866	.183	.335	.443	.714
	17	.597	.763	.837	.952	.368	.558	.663	.869	.180	.336	.443	.719
	18	.594	.764	.839	.954	.365	.559	.664	.873	.177	.336	.443	.723
	19	.592	.766	.840	.956	.363	.560	.665	.876	.175	.336	.444	.728
	20	.590	.767	.841	.957	.360	.561	.667	.879	.172	.337	.445	.732
	22	.587	.770	.844	.960	.356	.563	.669	.884	.169	.337	.446	.739
	24	.584	.773	.847	.963	.352	.566	.672	.889	.166	.339	.448	.747
	26	.581	.775	.849	.965	.349	.568	.675	.894	.163	.340	.450	.754
	28	.579	.777	.851	.967	.346	.571	.677	.898	.161	.342	.452	.760
	30	.577	.779	.853	.969	.344	.573	.680	.902	.160	.343	.454	.766
	32	.575	.782	.855	.970	.342	.575	.682	.905	.158	.345	.456	.771
	34	.574	.784	.857	.972	.340	.577	.685	.909	.157	.346	.458	.776
	36	.573	.785	.859	.973	.339	.579	.687	.912	.155	.348	.460	.781
	38	.571	.787	.860	.974	.338	.581	.689	.914	.154	.349	.462	.786
	40	.570	.789	.862	.975	.336	.583	.692	.917	.153	.351	.465	.791
	50	.566	.796	.869	.979	.332	.592	.701	.928	.150	.358	.474	.810
	60	.564	.802	.875	.982	.329	.599	.710	.936	.148	.364	.483	.825
	70	.562	.807	.880	.985	.327	.605	.718	.942	.146	.369	.491	.837
	80	.560	.811	.884	.986	.325	.611	.724	.947	.145	.374	.498	.848
	90	.559	.815	.888	.988	.324	.615	.730	.952	.144	.378	.505	.857
	100	.558	.818	.891	.989	.323	.620	.735	.955	.143	.382	.511	.865

B. Values of $\beta_1' = \beta_L'$, $\beta_2' = (\beta_S')_{\max}$, $\beta_3' = (\beta_X')_{\min}$ and $\beta_4' = \beta_W'$ for $\alpha = 0.01$

		$\delta = 0.5$				$\delta = 1.0$				$\delta = 1.5$			
N	m	β_1'	β_2'	β_3'	β_4'	β_1'	β_2'	β_3'	β_4'	β_1'	β_2'	β_3'	β_4'
4	2	.978	.978	.978	.978	.934	.934	.934	.934	.839	.839	.839	.839
	3	.976	.980	.984	.989	.920	.932	.944	.961	.796	.821	.847	.887
	4	.974	.982	.987	.993	.911	.933	.949	.972	.770	.816	.853	.909
	5	.973	.983	.989	.995	.905	.935	.953	.978	.753	.816	.858	.923
	6	.973	.985	.990	.997	.901	.937	.956	.982	.741	.817	.862	.933
	7	.972	.986	.991	.997	.898	.940	.959	.985	.732	.819	.866	.941
	8	.972	.986	.992	.998	.896	.942	.961	.987	.726	.822	.870	.947
	9	.971	.987	.992	.998	.894	.943	.963	.989	.720	.824	.873	.952
	10	.971	.988	.993	.998	.892	.945	.964	.990	.716	.827	.876	.956
	11	.971	.988	.993	.999	.891	.947	.966	.991	.712	.830	.879	.959
	12	.971	.989	.994	.999	.890	.948	.967	.992	.709	.832	.881	.962
	13	.971	.989	.994	.999	.889	.949	.968	.993	.707	.834	.884	.964
	14	.970	.990	.994	.999	.888	.951	.969	.993	.705	.837	.886	.967
	15	.970	.990	.995	.999	.887	.952	.970	.994	.703	.839	.888	.969
	16	.970	.990	.995	.999	.887	.953	.971	.994	.701	.841	.890	.970
	17	.970	.991	.995	.999	.886	.954	.972	.995	.700	.843	.892	.972
	18	.970	.991	.995	.999	.886	.954	.972	.995	.698	.844	.893	.973
	19	.970	.991	.995	.999	.885	.955	.973	.996	.697	.846	.895	.975
	20	.970	.991	.995	1.000	.885	.956	.974	.996	.696	.848	.896	.976
	22	.970	.992	.996	1.000	.884	.957	.975	.996	.694	.851	.899	.978
	24	.970	.992	.996	1.000	.884	.959	.976	.997	.693	.853	.902	.980
	26	.970	.992	.996	1.000	.883	.960	.976	.997	.691	.856	.904	.981
	28	.970	.993	.996	1.000	.883	.961	.977	.997	.690	.858	.906	.982
	30	.970	.993	.996	1.000	.883	.962	.978	.997	.689	.860	.908	.984
	32	.969	.993	.997	1.000	.882	.962	.979	.998	.688	.862	.910	.985
	34	.969	.993	.997	1.000	.882	.963	.979	.998	.688	.864	.911	.985
	36	.969	.994	.997	1.000	.882	.964	.980	.998	.687	.866	.913	.986
	38	.969	.994	.997	1.000	.881	.964	.980	.998	.686	.867	.914	.987
	40	.969	.994	.997	1.000	.881	.965	.981	.998	.686	.869	.916	.988
	50	.969	.994	.997	1.000	.880	.968	.983	.999	.684	.875	.922	.990
	60	.969	.995	.998	1.000	.880	.969	.984	.999	.682	.880	.926	.992
	70	.969	.995	.998	1.000	.880	.971	.985	.999	.681	.884	.930	.993
	80	.969	.995	.998	1.000	.879	.972	.986	.999	.681	.887	.933	.994
	90	.969	.996	.998	1.000	.879	.973	.987	.999	.680	.890	.936	.995
	100	.969	.996	.998	1.000	.879	.974	.987	1.000	.680	.892	.938	.995

		δ = 2.0				δ = 2.5				δ = 3.0			
N	m	β_1'	β_2'	β_3'	β_4'	β_1'	β_2'	β_3'	β_4'	β_1'	β_2'	β_3'	β_4'
4	2	.687	.687	.687	.687	.498	.498	.498	.498	.312	.312	.312	.312
	3	.601	.639	.680	.748	.379	.420	.468	.554	.193	.226	.267	.348
	4	.553	.620	.678	.779	.320	.388	.454	.582	.144	.192	.244	.364
	5	.523	.612	.679	.800	.286	.372	.446	.603	.118	.175	.232	.377
	6	.503	.609	.681	.816	.264	.364	.442	.620	.103	.166	.224	.388
	7	.488	.608	.684	.829	.249	.359	.441	.635	.0928	.160	.220	.399
	8	.477	.609	.687	.840	.238	.357	.441	.648	.0858	.157	.217	.408
	9	.469	.611	.690	.850	.230	.356	.442	.660	.0806	.155	.216	.418
	10	.452	.613	.693	.858	.223	.356	.443	.671	.0766	.153	.215	.427
	11	.456	.615	.697	.865	.218	.357	.445	.681	.0736	.153	.215	.436
	12	.451	.618	.700	.872	.213	.358	.447	.690	.0711	.153	.215	.444
	13	.447	.620	.703	.877	.210	.359	.449	.698	.0690	.153	.216	.451
	14	.444	.622	.706	.882	.206	.361	.451	.706	.0672	.153	.216	.459
	15	.441	.625	.709	.887	.204	.362	.454	.713	.0658	.153	.217	.466
	16	.439	.627	.711	.891	.201	.364	.456	.720	.0645	.154	.218	.473
	17	.436	.629	.714	.895	.199	.365	.458	.726	.0634	.154	.219	.479
	18	.434	.631	.716	.899	.198	.367	.460	.732	.0624	.155	.220	.485
	19	.432	.634	.719	.902	.196	.368	.462	.738	.0615	.156	.221	.491
	20	.431	.636	.721	.905	.194	.370	.464	.743	.0608	.156	.223	.497
	22	.428	.640	.725	.911	.192	.373	.469	.753	.0595	.158	.225	.508
	24	.426	.643	.729	.916	.190	.376	.473	.762	.0584	.159	.227	.519
	26	.424	.647	.733	.920	.188	.379	.477	.770	.0576	.160	.230	.528
	28	.422	.650	.737	.924	.187	.382	.480	.778	.0568	.162	.232	.537
	30	.421	.653	.740	.928	.186	.384	.484	.784	.0562	.163	.234	.546
	32	.419	.656	.743	.931	.185	.387	.487	.791	.0556	.165	.237	.553
	34	.418	.659	.746	.934	.184	.390	.490	.797	.0551	.166	.239	.561
	36	.417	.661	.749	.937	.183	.392	.494	.802	.0547	.167	.241	.568
	38	.416	.664	.752	.939	.182	.394	.497	.807	.0543	.169	.243	.575
	40	.416	.666	.754	.941	.181	.396	.500	.812	.0540	.170	.245	.581
	50	.413	.676	.766	.950	.179	.406	.513	.832	.0527	.176	.254	.610
	60	.411	.684	.775	.957	.177	.414	.524	.848	.0518	.180	.263	.633
	70	.409	.691	.782	.962	.176	.421	.534	.860	.0513	.184	.270	.653
	80	.408	.696	.789	.966	.175	.426	.542	.871	.0508	.188	.277	.670
	90	.407	.701	.795	.969	.174	.431	.550	.879	.0505	.191	.283	.684
	100	.406	.705	.800	.972	.174	.436	.557	.887	.0502	.194	.289	.697

B. Values of $\beta_1' = \beta_L'$, $\beta_2' = (\beta_S')_{\max}$, $\beta_3' = (\beta_X')_{\min}$ and $\beta_4' = \beta_W'$ for $\alpha = 0.01$

		$\delta = 0.5$				$\delta = 1.0$				$\delta = 1.5$			
N	m	β_1'	β_2'	β_3'	β_4'	β_1'	β_2'	β_3'	β_4'	β_1'	β_2'	β_3'	β_4'
5	2	.973	.973	.973	.973	.903	.903	.903	.903	.750	.750	.750	.750
	3	.970	.975	.980	.987	.885	.903	.917	.941	.700	.734	.765	.819
	4	.968	.978	.984	.992	.876	.906	.926	.957	.672	.732	.775	.852
	5	.967	.980	.986	.994	.869	.910	.932	.967	.655	.734	.783	.874
	6	.967	.981	.987	.996	.865	.913	.936	.973	.643	.738	.790	.889
	7	.966	.983	.989	.997	.861	.916	.940	.977	.635	.742	.796	.901
	8	.966	.984	.990	.997	.859	.919	.943	.980	.628	.746	.801	.910
	9	.965	.985	.990	.998	.857	.922	.945	.983	.623	.750	.806	.917
	10	.965	.985	.991	.998	.855	.924	.948	.985	.619	.753	.811	.924
	11	.965	.986	.992	.998	.854	.926	.950	.986	.615	.757	.815	.929
	12	.965	.987	.992	.999	.853	.928	.951	.987	.613	.760	.818	.934
	13	.964	.987	.992	.999	.852	.930	.953	.989	.610	.764	.822	.938
	14	.964	.988	.993	.999	.851	.931	.954	.989	.608	.767	.825	.942
	15	.964	.988	.993	.999	.850	.933	.956	.990	.606	.769	.828	.945
	16	.964	.988	.993	.999	.850	.934	.957	.991	.605	.772	.831	.948
	17	.964	.989	.994	.999	.849	.935	.958	.992	.603	.774	.833	.950
	18	.964	.989	.994	.999	.849	.937	.959	.992	.602	.777	.836	.952
	19	.964	.989	.994	.999	.848	.938	.960	.993	.601	.779	.838	.955
	20	.964	.990	.994	.999	.848	.939	.961	.993	.600	.781	.840	.957
	22	.964	.990	.994	.999	.847	.940	.962	.994	.598	.785	.844	.960
	24	.954	.990	.995	1.000	.847	.942	.964	.994	.597	.789	.848	.963
	26	.964	.991	.995	1.000	.846	.944	.965	.995	.596	.792	.851	.965
	28	.963	.991	.995	1.000	.846	.945	.966	.995	.595	.795	.854	.968
	30	.963	.991	.995	1.000	.845	.946	.967	.996	.594	.798	.857	.970
	32	.963	.992	.996	1.000	.845	.947	.968	.996	.593	.800	.859	.971
	34	.963	.992	.996	1.000	.845	.948	.969	.996	.592	.803	.862	.973
	36	.963	.992	.996	1.000	.844	.949	.970	.997	.592	.805	.864	.974
	38	.963	.992	.996	1.000	.844	.950	.970	.997	.591	.807	.866	.975
	40	.963	.992	.996	1.000	.844	.951	.971	.997	.591	.809	.868	.977
	50	.963	.993	.997	1.000	.843	.954	.974	.998	.589	.817	.877	.981
	60	.963	.994	.997	1.000	.843	.957	.976	.998	.587	.824	.883	.984
	70	.963	.994	.997	1.000	.842	.958	.977	.999	.586	.829	.889	.986
	80	.963	.994	.998	1.000	.842	.960	.979	.999	.586	.833	.893	.988
	90	.963	.995	.998	1.000	.842	.961	.980	.999	.585	.837	.897	.989
	100	.963	.995	.998	1.000	.842	.962	.981	.999	.585	.840	.901	.990

N	m	$\delta=2.0$ β'_1	β'_2	β'_3	β'_4	$\delta=2.5$ β'_1	β'_2	β'_3	β'_4	$\delta=3.0$ β'_1	β'_2	β'_3	β'_4
5	2	.523	.523	.523	.523	.292	.292	.292	.292	.126	.126	.126	.126
	3	.440	.483	.524	.604	.206	.241	.276	.353	.0688	.0867	.107	.156
	4	.398	.470	.527	.647	.169	.222	.269	.386	.0487	.0730	.0977	.171
	5	.373	.466	.531	.677	.148	.213	.267	.411	.0391	.0666	.0932	.183
	6	.357	.465	.536	.700	.136	.210	.267	.432	.0336	.0634	.0909	.194
	7	.345	.467	.541	.718	.127	.208	.268	.450	.0301	.0616	.0898	.204
	8	.337	.469	.546	.734	.121	.208	.269	.466	.0277	.0607	.0894	.213
	9	.330	.472	.551	.748	.117	.208	.271	.480	.0259	.0602	.0895	.221
	10	.325	.475	.555	.760	.113	.209	.274	.493	.0246	.0601	.0898	.229
	11	.320	.478	.560	.771	.110	.211	.276	.505	.0236	.0602	.0904	.237
	12	.317	.482	.564	.780	.108	.212	.279	.516	.0227	.0604	.0910	.245
	13	.314	.485	.568	.789	.106	.214	.281	.526	.0220	.0607	.0917	.252
	14	.311	.488	.572	.796	.104	.215	.283	.536	.0214	.0611	.0925	.258
	15	.309	.490	.575	.803	.103	.217	.286	.545	.0209	.0614	.0933	.265
	16	.307	.493	.579	.810	.101	.218	.288	.553	.0205	.0619	.0942	.271
	17	.305	.496	.582	.816	.100	.220	.291	.561	.0202	.0624	.0951	.277
	18	.304	.499	.585	.821	.0994	.221	.293	.569	.0198	.0628	.0959	.283
	19	.303	.501	.589	.827	.0985	.223	.295	.576	.0196	.0633	.0968	.289
	20	.301	.504	.592	.832	.0978	.224	.297	.583	.0193	.0637	.0977	.294
	22	.299	.508	.597	.840	.0965	.227	.302	.596	.0189	.0647	.0995	.305
	24	.298	.513	.602	.848	.0954	.230	.306	.607	.0186	.0657	.101	.314
	26	.296	.517	.607	.855	.0945	.233	.310	.618	.0183	.0666	.103	.323
	28	.295	.520	.612	.861	.0938	.235	.313	.628	.0180	.0675	.104	.332
	30	.294	.524	.616	.867	.0931	.238	.317	.637	.0178	.0684	.106	.340
	32	.293	.527	.620	.872	.0925	.240	.320	.645	.0176	.0693	.108	.348
	34	.292	.530	.624	.877	.0920	.242	.323	.653	.0175	.0700	.109	.356
	36	.291	.533	.627	.881	.0916	.244	.327	.661	.0173	.0709	.111	.363
	38	.291	.536	.631	.885	.0912	.246	.330	.668	.0172	.0716	.112	.370
	40	.290	.539	.634	.889	.0909	.248	.332	.675	.0171	.0723	.113	.377
	50	.288	.550	.648	.904	.0895	.256	.345	.703	.0167	.0757	.120	.406
	60	.286	.559	.660	.915	.0886	.263	.356	.726	.0164	.0785	.125	.431
	70	.285	.567	.670	.924	.0880	.269	.366	.744	.0162	.0810	.130	.452
	80	.284	.573	.678	.931	.0875	.274	.374	.759	.0161	.0832	.135	.471
	90	.284	.578	.685	.936	.0872	.279	.382	.772	.0160	.0851	.139	.487
	100	.283	.583	.692	.941	.0869	.283	.389	.784	.0159	.0869	.143	.502

B. Values of $\beta_1' = \beta_L'$, $\beta_2' = (\beta_S')_{\max}$, $\beta_3' = (\beta_X')_{\min}$ and $\beta_4' = \beta_W'$ for $\alpha = 0.01$

		$\delta=0.5$				$\delta=1.0$				$\delta=1.5$			
N	m	β_1'	β_2'	β_3'	β_4'	β_1'	β_2'	β_3'	β_4'	β_1'	β_2'	β_3'	β_4'
6	2	.967	.967	.967	.967	.868	.868	.868	.868	.655	.655	.655	.655
	3	.964	.971	.976	.984	.848	.871	.888	.918	.603	.644	.677	.741
	4	.962	.974	.980	.990	.837	.876	.899	.940	.576	.645	.691	.785
	5	.961	.976	.983	.993	.831	.881	.907	.952	.559	.649	.702	.814
	6	.960	.978	.985	.995	.826	.886	.913	.961	.548	.654	.711	.835
	7	.960	.979	.986	.996	.823	.890	.918	.967	.540	.660	.719	.851
	8	.959	.981	.987	.996	.820	.894	.922	.971	.534	.665	.726	.864
	9	.959	.982	.988	.997	.818	.897	.925	.974	.529	.670	.733	.874
	10	.959	.983	.989	.998	.816	.900	.928	.977	.526	.675	.738	.883
	11	.958	.983	.989	.998	.815	.903	.931	.980	.522	.679	.743	.891
	12	.958	.984	.990	.998	.814	.905	.933	.981	.520	.683	.748	.897
	13	.958	.985	.991	.998	.813	.907	.935	.983	.518	.687	.752	.903
	14	.958	.985	.991	.999	.812	.909	.937	.984	.516	.691	.757	.908
	15	.958	.986	.991	.999	.811	.911	.939	.985	.514	.694	.760	.913
	16	.958	.986	.992	.999	.810	.913	.940	.986	.513	.698	.764	.917
	17	.958	.986	.992	.999	.810	.914	.942	.987	.511	.700	.767	.921
	18	.958	.987	.992	.999	.809	.916	.943	.988	.510	.703	.770	.924
	19	.957	.987	.992	.999	.809	.917	.944	.989	.509	.706	.773	.927
	20	.957	.987	.993	.999	.809	.918	.945	.990	.508	.709	.776	.930
	22	.957	.988	.993	.999	.808	.921	.947	.991	.507	.713	.781	.935
	24	.957	.988	.993	.999	.807	.923	.949	.992	.506	.718	.786	.940
	26	.957	.989	.994	.999	.807	.925	.951	.992	.504	.722	.790	.943
	28	.957	.989	.994	1.000	.806	.926	.952	.993	.504	.725	.794	.947
	30	.957	.990	.994	1.000	.806	.928	.954	.993	.503	.729	.797	.950
	32	.957	.990	.995	1.000	.806	.929	.955	.994	.502	.732	.801	.952
	34	.957	.990	.995	1.000	.805	.931	.956	.994	.501	.735	.804	.955
	36	.957	.990	.995	1.000	.805	.932	.957	.995	.501	.737	.807	.957
	38	.957	.991	.995	1.000	.805	.933	.958	.995	.500	.740	.810	.959
	40	.957	.991	.995	1.000	.805	.934	.959	.995	.500	.742	.812	.961
	50	.957	.992	.996	1.000	.804	.938	.963	.996	.498	.752	.823	.968
	60	.957	.992	.996	1.000	.803	.941	.965	.997	.497	.760	.832	.972
	70	.956	.993	.997	1.000	.803	.944	.968	.998	.496	.766	.839	.976
	80	.956	.993	.997	1.000	.803	.946	.970	.998	.496	.772	.845	.979
	90	.956	.993	.997	1.000	.802	.947	.971	.998	.495	.776	.850	.981
	100	.956	.994	.997	1.000	.802	.949	.972	.999	.495	.780	.855	.983

N	m	δ = 2.0				δ = 2.5				δ = 3.0			
		β_1'	β_2'	β_3'	β_4'	β_1'	β_2'	β_3'	β_4'	β_1'	β_2'	β_3'	β_4'
6	2	.377	.377	.377	.377	.155	.155	.155	.155	.0436	.0436	.0436	.0436
	3	.308	.349	.385	.464	.104	.127	.149	.205	.0218	.0294	.0375	.0603
	4	.275	.341	.391	.513	.0829	.117	.147	.235	.0149	.0247	.0346	.0702
	5	.256	.340	.397	.548	.0721	.114	.147	.258	.0118	.0228	.0334	.0782
	6	.243	.341	.404	.575	.0655	.112	.149	.277	.0101	.0218	.0329	.0852
	7	.235	.344	.410	.598	.0611	.112	.150	.294	.00896	.0214	.0329	.0917
	8	.229	.347	.416	.617	.0580	.113	.152	.309	.00821	.0212	.0330	.0978
	9	.224	.350	.421	.634	.0557	.114	.155	.323	.00767	.0212	.0333	.104
	10	.220	.354	.427	.649	.0538	.115	.157	.336	.00726	.0213	.0337	.109
	11	.217	.357	.432	.662	.0524	.116	.159	.347	.00693	.0214	.0341	.114
	12	.214	.361	.436	.674	.0512	.117	.161	.358	.00667	.0216	.0345	.119
	13	.212	.364	.441	.685	.0502	.118	.163	.368	.00647	.0218	.0350	.124
	14	.210	.367	.445	.695	.0494	.120	.166	.378	.00629	.0221	.0355	.129
	15	.209	.370	.449	.704	.0487	.121	.168	.387	.00615	.0223	.0361	.134
	16	.207	.373	.453	.712	.0481	.122	.170	.396	.00602	.0225	.0365	.138
	17	.206	.376	.457	.720	.0476	.123	.172	.404	.00591	.0228	.0371	.143
	18	.205	.379	.460	.727	.0471	.125	.174	.412	.00582	.0230	.0376	.147
	19	.204	.381	.463	.734	.0467	.126	.175	.419	.00573	.0233	.0381	.151
	20	.203	.384	.467	.741	.0463	.127	.177	.426	.00566	.0235	.0385	.155
	22	.202	.388	.473	.752	.0457	.129	.181	.440	.00553	.0240	.0395	.162
	24	.200	.393	.478	.763	.0452	.131	.184	.452	.00542	.0245	.0404	.169
	26	.199	.397	.484	.772	.0447	.133	.187	.463	.00534	.0250	.0414	.176
	28	.199	.400	.489	.781	.0443	.135	.190	.474	.00526	.0254	.0423	.183
	30	.198	.404	.493	.788	.0440	.137	.193	.484	.00520	.0259	.0431	.189
	32	.197	.407	.498	.795	.0437	.139	.196	.493	.00515	.0263	.0440	.195
	34	.197	.411	.502	.802	.0435	.140	.199	.502	.00510	.0267	.0448	.201
	36	.196	.414	.506	.808	.0433	.142	.201	.511	.00506	.0271	.0456	.207
	38	.196	.416	.510	.814	.0431	.143	.204	.519	.00502	.0274	.0464	.212
	40	.195	.419	.513	.819	.0429	.145	.206	.526	.00499	.0278	.0471	.218
	50	.194	.430	.529	.841	.0423	.151	.217	.559	.00486	.0295	.0506	.241
	60	.192	.440	.542	.857	.0418	.156	.226	.585	.00478	.0309	.0537	.262
	70	.192	.447	.552	.870	.0415	.161	.234	.607	.00473	.0321	.0565	.280
	80	.191	.454	.562	.880	.0413	.165	.241	.626	.00468	.0332	.0591	.297
	90	.191	.459	.570	.889	.0411	.168	.247	.542	.00465	.0342	.0615	.312
	100	.190	.464	.578	.896	.0410	.171	.253	.657	.00462	.0350	.0637	.325

B. Values of $\beta_1' = \beta_L'$, $\beta_2' = (\beta_S')_{\max}$, $\beta_3' = (\beta_X')_{\min}$ and $\beta_4' = \beta_W'$ for $\alpha = 0.01$

		$\delta=0.5$				$\delta=1.0$				$\delta=1.5$			
N	m	β_1'	β_2'	β_3'	β_4'	β_1'	β_2'	β_3'	β_4'	β_1'	β_2'	β_3'	β_4'
7	2	.961	.961	.961	.961	.830	.830	.830	.830	.561	.561	.561	.561
	3	.957	.965	.971	.980	.809	.836	.855	.892	.511	.554	.588	.660
	4	.955	.969	.976	.988	.797	.843	.869	.919	.485	.558	.605	.712
	5	.954	.972	.979	.991	.790	.850	.879	.936	.470	.564	.619	.747
	6	.954	.974	.982	.993	.785	.856	.887	.946	.460	.571	.630	.773
	7	.953	.976	.983	.995	.782	.861	.893	.954	.453	.578	.639	.793
	8	.953	.977	.985	.996	.779	.865	.898	.960	.447	.584	.648	.809
	9	.952	.978	.986	.996	.777	.870	.902	.965	.443	.589	.655	.823
	10	.952	.979	.987	.997	.775	.873	.906	.968	.439	.595	.662	.834
	11	.952	.980	.987	.997	.774	.876	.909	.971	.437	.600	.668	.844
	12	.951	.981	.988	.998	.773	.879	.912	.974	.434	.605	.674	.853
	13	.951	.982	.989	.998	.772	.882	.915	.976	.432	.609	.679	.861
	14	.951	.982	.989	.998	.771	.884	.917	.978	.431	.613	.684	.867
	15	.951	.983	.989	.998	.770	.887	.919	.979	.429	.617	.688	.873
	16	.951	.983	.990	.998	.770	.889	.921	.981	.428	.621	.692	.879
	17	.951	.984	.990	.999	.769	.891	.923	.982	.427	.624	.696	.884
	18	.951	.984	.991	.999	.769	.892	.925	.983	.426	.627	.700	.888
	19	.951	.985	.991	.999	.768	.894	.926	.984	.425	.630	.703	.893
	20	.951	.985	.991	.999	.768	.896	.927	.985	.424	.633	.706	.896
	22	.951	.986	.992	.999	.767	.899	.930	.986	.423	.639	.713	.904
	24	.950	.986	.992	.999	.766	.901	.932	.988	.422	.644	.718	.909
	26	.950	.987	.992	.999	.765	.903	.935	.989	.421	.648	.723	.915
	28	.950	.987	.993	.999	.765	.905	.936	.990	.420	.652	.728	.919
	30	.950	.988	.993	.999	.765	.907	.938	.990	.419	.656	.732	.923
	32	.950	.988	.993	.999	.765	.909	.940	.991	.418	.659	.736	.927
	34	.950	.988	.994	1.000	.764	.910	.941	.992	.418	.663	.740	.931
	36	.950	.989	.994	1.000	.764	.912	.943	.992	.417	.666	.743	.934
	38	.950	.989	.994	1.000	.764	.913	.944	.993	.417	.668	.747	.936
	40	.950	.989	.994	1.000	.764	.914	.945	.993	.417	.671	.750	.939
	50	.950	.990	.995	1.000	.763	.920	.950	.995	.415	.683	.763	.949
	60	.950	.991	.995	1.000	.762	.923	.953	.996	.414	.691	.773	.956
	70	.950	.991	.996	1.000	.762	.926	.956	.996	.413	.699	.782	.961
	80	.950	.992	.996	1.000	.762	.929	.958	.997	.413	.705	.789	.966
	90	.950	.992	.996	1.000	.761	.931	.960	.997	.412	.710	.796	.969
	100	.950	.992	.997	1.000	.761	.933	.962	.998	.412	.714	.801	.972

N	m	$\delta=2.0$ β_1'	β_2'	β_3'	β_4'	$\delta=2.5$ β_1'	β_2'	β_3'	β_4'	$\delta=3.0$ β_1'	β_2'	β_3'	β_4'
7	2	.261	.261	.261	.261	.0765	.0765	.0765	.0765	.0135	.0135	.0135	.0135
	3	.207	.242	.271	.342	.0489	.0626	.0755	.111	.00635	.00906	.0119	.0210
	4	.183	.238	.279	.391	.0385	.0583	.0756	.133	.00425	.00769	.0112	.0259
	5	.169	.239	.286	.427	.0331	.0569	.0765	.151	.00331	.00714	.0110	.0301
	6	.161	.241	.293	.455	.0300	.0567	.0779	.166	.00280	.00691	.0109	.0338
	7	.155	.244	.299	.480	.0279	.0571	.0795	.179	.00249	.00683	.0110	.0373
	8	.150	.248	.305	.501	.0264	.0577	.0812	.192	.00227	.00682	.0112	.0407
	9	.147	.251	.311	.519	.0253	.0584	.0829	.203	.00212	.00686	.0114	.0438
	10	.144	.254	.316	.535	.0244	.0593	.0845	.214	.00200	.00694	.0116	.0469
	11	.142	.258	.321	.550	.0237	.0601	.0862	.223	.00191	.00702	.0118	.0499
	12	.140	.261	.326	.563	.0232	.0611	.0879	.233	.00184	.00712	.0121	.0528
	13	.139	.264	.330	.575	.0227	.0620	.0895	.242	.00178	.00723	.0123	.0556
	14	.138	.267	.334	.587	.0223	.0629	.0910	.250	.00173	.00734	.0125	.0584
	15	.136	.270	.338	.597	.0220	.0637	.0925	.258	.00169	.00745	.0128	.0611
	16	.136	.273	.342	.607	.0217	.0646	.0940	.265	.00165	.00756	.0130	.0636
	17	.135	.275	.346	.616	.0215	.0654	.0954	.273	.00162	.00767	.0133	.0662
	18	.134	.278	.349	.624	.0213	.0662	.0968	.279	.00159	.00779	.0135	.0687
	19	.133	.280	.352	.632	.0211	.0670	.0981	.286	.00157	.00789	.0137	.0712
	20	.133	.282	.355	.640	.0209	.0677	.0994	.292	.00155	.00800	.0139	.0735
	22	.132	.287	.361	.654	.0206	.0693	.102	.305	.00151	.00822	.0144	.0783
	24	.131	.291	.367	.666	.0203	.0707	.104	.316	.00148	.00843	.0148	.0827
	26	.130	.294	.372	.677	.0201	.0720	.107	.326	.00146	.00863	.0153	.0870
	28	.130	.298	.377	.688	.0200	.0732	.109	.337	.00144	.00881	.0157	.0913
	30	.129	.301	.382	.697	.0198	.0744	.111	.346	.00142	.00900	.0161	.0953
	32	.129	.304	.386	.706	.0197	.0756	.113	.355	.00141	.00918	.0165	.0992
	34	.128	.307	.390	.714	.0196	.0767	.115	.363	.00139	.00935	.0169	.103
	36	.128	.310	.394	.721	.0195	.0778	.117	.371	.00138	.00953	.0172	.107
	38	.128	.312	.398	.728	.0194	.0787	.118	.379	.00137	.00968	.0176	.110
	40	.127	.315	.401	.735	.0193	.0797	.120	.386	.00136	.00984	.0180	.114
	50	.126	.326	.417	.762	.0190	.0839	.128	.418	.00133	.0105	.0196	.130
	60	.125	.334	.430	.784	.0188	.0874	.135	.445	.00130	.0112	.0211	.145
	70	.125	.341	.441	.801	.0187	.0905	.141	.468	.00129	.0117	.0224	.158
	80	.125	.348	.450	.815	.0185	.0931	.146	.488	.00128	.0122	.0237	.170
	90	.124	.353	.459	.826	.0185	.0954	.151	.505	.00127	.0126	.0248	.181
	100	.124	.358	.466	.836	.0184	.0975	.155	.521	.00126	.0130	.0259	.191

B. Values of $\beta_1' = \beta_L'$, $\beta_2' = (\beta_S')_{\max}$, $\beta_3' = (\beta_X')_{\min}$ and $\beta_4' = \beta_W'$ for $\alpha = 0.01$

		$\delta=0.5$				$\delta=1.0$				$\delta=1.5$			
N	m	β_1'	β_2'	β_3'	β_4'	β_1'	β_2'	β_3'	β_4'	β_1'	β_2'	β_3'	β_4'
∞	2	.954	.954	.954	.954	.790	.790	.790	.790	.472	.472	.472	.472
	3	.951	.960	.966	.977	.768	.798	.820	.863	.426	.470	.503	.578
	4	.949	.964	.972	.985	.756	.808	.837	.896	.403	.476	.522	.636
	5	.947	.967	.976	.989	.749	.816	.849	.916	.389	.483	.537	.676
	6	.947	.970	.978	.992	.744	.823	.858	.930	.380	.491	.550	.706
	7	.946	.972	.980	.994	.740	.830	.865	.940	.374	.498	.560	.730
	8	.946	.974	.982	.995	.737	.835	.871	.947	.369	.505	.569	.749
	9	.945	.975	.983	.996	.735	.840	.877	.953	.365	.511	.578	.765
	10	.945	.976	.984	.996	.733	.844	.881	.957	.362	.517	.585	.779
	11	.945	.977	.985	.997	.732	.848	.885	.961	.360	.522	.592	.791
	12	.945	.978	.986	.997	.731	.851	.889	.965	.358	.527	.598	.802
	13	.944	.979	.986	.997	.730	.854	.892	.967	.356	.532	.604	.811
	14	.944	.980	.987	.998	.729	.857	.895	.970	.355	.537	.609	.819
	15	.944	.980	.987	.998	.728	.860	.897	.972	.353	.541	.614	.827
	16	.944	.981	.988	.998	.728	.862	.899	.974	.352	.545	.619	.834
	17	.944	.981	.988	.998	.727	.865	.902	.975	.351	.548	.623	.840
	18	.944	.982	.989	.998	.727	.867	.904	.977	.350	.552	.627	.846
	19	.944	.982	.989	.999	.726	.869	.906	.978	.350	.555	.631	.851
	20	.944	.983	.989	.999	.726	.870	.907	.979	.349	.558	.635	.856
	22	.944	.983	.990	.999	.725	.874	.911	.981	.348	.564	.641	.865
	24	.943	.984	.990	.999	.724	.877	.913	.983	.347	.569	.648	.873
	26	.943	.985	.991	.999	.724	.879	.916	.984	.346	.574	.653	.879
	28	.943	.985	.991	.999	.723	.882	.918	.985	.345	.578	.658	.886
	30	.943	.985	.992	.999	.723	.884	.920	.986	.345	.582	.663	.891
	32	.943	.986	.992	.999	.723	.886	.922	.987	.344	.586	.668	.896
	34	.943	.986	.992	.999	.722	.888	.924	.988	.344	.589	.672	.900
	36	.943	.987	.993	.999	.722	.890	.926	.989	.343	.593	.676	.904
	38	.943	.987	.993	1.000	.722	.891	.927	.990	.343	.596	.680	.908
	40	.943	.987	.993	1.000	.722	.893	.929	.990	.342	.599	.683	.911
	50	.943	.988	.994	1.000	.721	.899	.935	.992	.341	.611	.698	.925
	60	.943	.989	.994	1.000	.720	.903	.939	.994	.340	.621	.710	.935
	70	.943	.990	.995	1.000	.720	.907	.943	.995	.340	.629	.720	.942
	80	.943	.990	.995	1.000	.720	.910	.945	.996	.339	.635	.728	.948
	90	.943	.991	.996	1.000	.720	.912	.948	.996	.339	.641	.736	.953
	100	.943	.991	.996	1.000	.719	.915	.950	.997	.338	.646	.742	.956

N	m	δ=2.0				δ=2.5				δ=3.0			
		β_1'	β_2'	β_3'	β_4'	β_1'	β_2'	β_3'	β_4'	β_1'	β_2'	β_3'	β_4'
8	2	.174	.174	.174	.174	.0356	.0356	.0356	.0356	.00386	.00386	.00386	.00386
	3	.135	.162	.185	.243	.0220	.0293	.0361	.0564	.00173	.00260	.00351	.00672
	4	.118	.161	.193	.287	.0170	.0276	.0367	.0710	.00113	.00223	.00337	.00881
	5	.109	.162	.200	.321	.0146	.0271	.0377	.0831	.00088	.00209	.00335	.0106
	6	.103	.165	.206	.348	.0131	.0272	.0387	.0935	.00074	.00204	.00338	.0123
	7	.0990	.168	.212	.372	.0122	.0276	.0399	.103	.00065	.00204	.00344	.0140
	8	.0960	.171	.217	.393	.0115	.0281	.0410	.112	.00059	.00205	.00352	.0155
	9	.0937	.174	.222	.411	.0110	.0286	.0422	.120	.00055	.00208	.00361	.0170
	10	.0920	.177	.227	.427	.0106	.0292	.0433	.128	.00052	.00211	.00371	.0185
	11	.0906	.180	.231	.442	.0103	.0297	.0444	.136	.00050	.00215	.00381	.0200
	12	.0894	.183	.235	.456	.0101	.0303	.0455	.143	.00048	.00219	.00391	.0215
	13	.0884	.186	.239	.469	.00986	.0309	.0465	.149	.00046	.00224	.00402	.0229
	14	.0876	.188	.243	.480	.00968	.0314	.0475	.156	.00045	.00228	.00412	.0243
	15	.0869	.191	.247	.491	.00954	.0319	.0485	.162	.00044	.00233	.00422	.0256
	16	.0862	.193	.250	.501	.00941	.0325	.0494	.168	.00043	.00237	.00431	.0269
	17	.0857	.195	.253	.511	.00930	.0330	.0503	.174	.00042	.00241	.00441	.0283
	18	.0852	.197	.256	.520	.00920	.0335	.0512	.179	.00041	.00246	.00451	.0296
	19	.0848	.199	.259	.529	.00911	.0340	.0521	.185	.00041	.00250	.00461	.0309
	20	.0844	.201	.262	.537	.00904	.0344	.0530	.190	.00040	.00254	.00470	.0321
	22	.0837	.205	.268	.552	.00890	.0353	.0546	.200	.00039	.00262	.00489	.0347
	24	.0832	.209	.273	.565	.00880	.0362	.0562	.209	.00038	.00271	.00507	.0371
	26	.0827	.212	.277	.578	.00870	.0370	.0576	.217	.00038	.00278	.00525	.0394
	28	.0823	.215	.282	.589	.00863	.0378	.0591	.226	.00037	.00285	.00542	.0418
	30	.0819	.218	.286	.600	.00856	.0385	.0604	.234	.00037	.00292	.00559	.0440
	32	.0816	.220	.290	.609	.00850	.0392	.0617	.241	.00036	.00299	.00575	.0463
	34	.0814	.223	.294	.618	.00845	.0399	.0630	.248	.00036	.00306	.00591	.0484
	36	.0811	.225	.297	.627	.00841	.0405	.0642	.255	.00036	.00313	.00606	.0506
	38	.0809	.227	.301	.635	.00837	.0411	.0654	.262	.00035	.00318	.00621	.0526
	40	.0807	.229	.304	.643	.00833	.0417	.0665	.268	.00035	.00325	.00636	.0547
	50	.0800	.239	.318	.674	.00820	.0443	.0717	.297	.00034	.00352	.00705	.0643
	60	.0796	.246	.330	.700	.00811	.0465	.0762	.321	.00034	.00376	.00768	.0731
	70	.0792	.253	.341	.720	.00804	.0484	.0802	.342	.00033	.00397	.00825	.0813
	80	.0790	.258	.350	.737	.00800	.0501	.0838	.361	.00033	.00416	.00879	.0889
	90	.0788	.263	.358	.751	.00796	.0515	.0871	.377	.00033	.00432	.00929	.0961
	100	.0786	.267	.365	.764	.00793	.0528	.0901	.392	.00033	.00447	.00976	.103

B. Values of $\beta_1' = \beta_L'$, $\beta_2' = (\beta_S')_{\max}$, $\beta_3' = (\beta_X')_{\min}$ and $\beta_4' = \beta_W'$ for $\alpha = 0.01$

N	m	$\delta=0.5$ β_1'	β_2'	β_3'	β_4'	$\delta=1.0$ β_1'	β_2'	β_3'	β_4'	$\delta=1.5$ β_1'	β_2'	β_3'	β_4'
9	2	.947	.947	.947	.947	.749	.749	.749	.749	.392	.392	.392	.392
	3	.944	.954	.951	.973	.726	.760	.783	.832	.350	.392	.424	.499
	4	.942	.959	.967	.983	.713	.771	.803	.871	.330	.400	.444	.561
	5	.940	.963	.972	.988	.706	.781	.817	.895	.318	.408	.460	.604
	6	.939	.966	.975	.991	.701	.789	.827	.911	.310	.416	.473	.636
	7	.939	.968	.977	.992	.697	.796	.836	.923	.304	.424	.484	.663
	8	.938	.970	.979	.994	.695	.803	.843	.932	.300	.431	.494	.685
	9	.938	.971	.980	.995	.693	.808	.849	.939	.297	.437	.503	.703
	10	.938	.973	.981	.996	.691	.813	.854	.945	.295	.443	.510	.719
	11	.937	.974	.982	.996	.690	.817	.859	.950	.293	.449	.518	.733
	12	.937	.975	.983	.997	.688	.821	.863	.954	.291	.454	.524	.745
	13	.937	.976	.984	.997	.687	.825	.867	.957	.289	.459	.530	.756
	14	.937	.976	.985	.997	.687	.828	.870	.960	.288	.463	.536	.766
	15	.937	.977	.985	.998	.686	.831	.873	.963	.287	.468	.541	.775
	16	.937	.978	.986	.998	.685	.834	.876	.965	.286	.472	.546	.783
	17	.937	.978	.986	.998	.685	.836	.878	.967	.285	.475	.550	.791
	18	.937	.979	.987	.998	.684	.839	.881	.969	.285	.479	.555	.798
	19	.936	.979	.987	.998	.684	.841	.883	.971	.284	.482	.559	.804
	20	.936	.980	.988	.998	.683	.843	.885	.972	.283	.485	.563	.810
	22	.936	.981	.988	.999	.683	.847	.889	.975	.282	.491	.570	.821
	24	.936	.981	.989	.999	.682	.851	.892	.977	.282	.497	.577	.830
	26	.936	.982	.989	.999	.681	.854	.895	.979	.281	.502	.583	.838
	28	.936	.983	.990	.999	.681	.856	.898	.980	.280	.506	.588	.846
	30	.936	.983	.990	.999	.681	.859	.900	.982	.280	.510	.593	.852
	32	.935	.984	.991	.999	.680	.861	.903	.983	.279	.514	.598	.858
	34	.936	.984	.991	.999	.680	.863	.905	.984	.279	.518	.603	.864
	36	.935	.984	.991	.999	.680	.865	.907	.985	.278	.521	.607	.869
	38	.936	.985	.991	.999	.680	.867	.909	.985	.278	.524	.611	.874
	40	.936	.985	.992	.999	.679	.869	.910	.986	.278	.527	.615	.878
	50	.936	.986	.993	1.000	.679	.876	.917	.989	.277	.540	.631	.895
	60	.935	.987	.993	1.000	.678	.881	.923	.991	.276	.550	.644	.908
	70	.935	.988	.994	1.000	.678	.885	.927	.993	.275	.559	.655	.917
	80	.935	.989	.994	1.000	.677	.889	.931	.994	.275	.565	.664	.925
	90	.935	.989	.995	1.000	.677	.892	.934	.994	.275	.571	.673	.931
	100	.935	.989	.995	1.000	.677	.894	.936	.995	.274	.576	.680	.937

N	m	δ=2.0				δ=2.5				δ=3.0			
		β_1'	β_2'	β_3'	β_4'	β_1'	β_2'	β_3'	β_4'	β_1'	β_2'	β_3'	β_4'
9	2	.112	.112	.112	.112	.0158	.0158	.0158	.0158	.00103	.00103	.00103	.00103
	3	.0858	.106	.122	.168	.00947	.0131	.0165	.0273	.00044	.00070	.00097	.00201
	4	.0745	.106	.129	.205	.00726	.0125	.0171	.0360	.00029	.00061	.00095	.00279
	5	.0684	.108	.135	.234	.00618	.0124	.0177	.0435	.00022	.00058	.00096	.00350
	6	.0645	.110	.141	.259	.00554	.0125	.0184	.0502	.00018	.00057	.00098	.00419
	7	.0618	.113	.145	.280	.00512	.0128	.0191	.0565	.00016	.00057	.00101	.00486
	8	.0599	.115	.150	.299	.00483	.0131	.0199	.0624	.00015	.00058	.00105	.00552
	9	.0584	.118	.154	.316	.00462	.0134	.0205	.0680	.00014	.00059	.00108	.00617
	10	.0573	.120	.158	.331	.00445	.0137	.0212	.0733	.00013	.00061	.00112	.00682
	11	.0564	.123	.162	.346	.00432	.0141	.0219	.0784	.00012	.00062	.00116	.00747
	12	.0556	.125	.165	.359	.00421	.0144	.0225	.0833	.00012	.00064	.00120	.00811
	13	.0550	.127	.169	.371	.00412	.0147	.0231	.0879	.00011	.00065	.00123	.00874
	14	.0544	.129	.172	.382	.00405	.0150	.0237	.0925	.00011	.00067	.00127	.00937
	15	.0540	.131	.175	.393	.00399	.0153	.0243	.0968	.00011	.00069	.00131	.0100
	16	.0536	.133	.178	.403	.00393	.0156	.0249	.101	.00011	.00070	.00135	.0106
	17	.0532	.135	.181	.412	.00388	.0159	.0254	.105	.00010	.00072	.00138	.0112
	18	.0529	.137	.183	.421	.00384	.0162	.0259	.109	.00010	.00073	.00142	.0118
	19	.0526	.138	.186	.430	.00381	.0165	.0265	.113	.00010	.00075	.00146	.0125
	20	.0524	.140	.188	.438	.00377	.0167	.0270	.117	.00010	.00076	.00149	.0131
	22	.0519	.143	.193	.453	.00372	.0173	.0280	.124	.00010	.00079	.00156	.0143
	24	.0516	.146	.197	.467	.00367	.0178	.0289	.131	.00009	.00082	.00163	.0154
	26	.0513	.148	.201	.479	.00363	.0182	.0298	.138	.00009	.00085	.00169	.0166
	28	.0510	.151	.205	.491	.00360	.0187	.0306	.144	.00009	.00087	.00176	.0178
	30	.0508	.153	.208	.502	.00357	.0191	.0315	.150	.00009	.00090	.00182	.0189
	32	.0506	.155	.212	.512	.00355	.0195	.0323	.156	.00009	.00092	.00188	.0200
	34	.0505	.157	.215	.522	.00352	.0198	.0330	.162	.00009	.00094	.00194	.0211
	36	.0503	.159	.218	.531	.00350	.0202	.0338	.167	.00009	.00097	.00200	.0222
	38	.0502	.161	.221	.539	.00349	.0206	.0345	.172	.00009	.00099	.00206	.0233
	40	.0500	.163	.224	.547	.00347	.0209	.0352	.177	.00009	.00101	.00212	.0244
	50	.0496	.170	.236	.582	.00341	.0224	.0383	.200	.00008	.00111	.00238	.0295
	60	.0493	.177	.247	.609	.00338	.0237	.0411	.220	.00008	.00119	.00262	.0343
	70	.0491	.182	.256	.632	.00335	.0248	.0436	.238	.00008	.00127	.00285	.0389
	80	.0489	.186	.264	.651	.00333	.0258	.0459	.254	.00008	.00134	.00306	.0432
	90	.0488	.190	.271	.668	.00331	.0266	.0480	.268	.00008	.00139	.00326	.0474
	100	.0487	.194	.278	.683	.00330	.0274	.0500	.282	.00008	.00145	.00345	.0514

B. Values of $\beta_1' = \beta_L'$, $\beta_2' = (\beta_S')_{\max}$, $\beta_3' = (\beta_X')_{\min}$ and $\beta_4' = \beta_W'$ for $\alpha = 0.01$

		$\delta=0.5$				$\delta=1.0$				$\delta=1.5$			
N	m	β_1'	β_2'	β_3'	β_4'	β_1'	β_2'	β_3'	β_4'	β_1'	β_2'	β_3'	β_4'
10	2	.940	.940	.940	.940	.706	.706	.706	.706	.320	.320	.320	.320
	3	.936	.948	.955	.969	.683	.720	.745	.799	.284	.324	.353	.425
	4	.934	.954	.963	.980	.671	.733	.767	.844	.267	.331	.373	.488
	5	.933	.958	.968	.986	.663	.744	.783	.871	.257	.340	.389	.532
	6	.932	.961	.971	.989	.658	.753	.795	.890	.250	.348	.402	.567
	7	.931	.963	.973	.991	.655	.761	.804	.904	.245	.356	.413	.595
	8	.931	.966	.976	.993	.652	.769	.812	.915	.242	.363	.423	.619
	9	.931	.967	.977	.994	.650	.775	.819	.923	.239	.369	.432	.638
	10	.930	.969	.978	.995	.648	.780	.825	.930	.237	.375	.440	.656
	11	.930	.970	.980	.995	.647	.785	.831	.936	.235	.381	.447	.671
	12	.930	.971	.981	.996	.646	.789	.835	.941	.234	.386	.453	.685
	13	.930	.972	.981	.996	.645	.794	.839	.945	.233	.391	.459	.697
	14	.929	.973	.982	.997	.644	.797	.843	.949	.232	.395	.465	.708
	15	.929	.974	.983	.997	.643	.801	.847	.952	.231	.399	.471	.719
	16	.929	.975	.984	.997	.643	.804	.850	.955	.230	.403	.475	.728
	17	.929	.975	.984	.998	.642	.807	.853	.958	.229	.407	.480	.737
	18	.929	.976	.985	.998	.642	.809	.856	.960	.229	.411	.485	.744
	19	.929	.977	.985	.998	.641	.812	.858	.962	.228	.414	.489	.752
	20	.929	.977	.986	.998	.641	.814	.861	.964	.228	.417	.493	.759
	22	.929	.978	.986	.998	.640	.818	.865	.967	.227	.423	.500	.771
	24	.929	.979	.987	.999	.640	.822	.869	.970	.226	.428	.507	.782
	26	.929	.979	.988	.999	.639	.826	.872	.972	.225	.433	.513	.792
	28	.928	.980	.988	.999	.639	.829	.876	.974	.225	.437	.519	.800
	30	.928	.981	.989	.999	.638	.832	.879	.976	.224	.442	.525	.808
	32	.928	.981	.989	.999	.638	.834	.881	.977	.224	.446	.530	.816
	34	.928	.982	.989	.999	.638	.837	.884	.979	.224	.449	.534	.822
	36	.928	.982	.990	.999	.637	.839	.886	.980	.223	.453	.539	.828
	38	.928	.982	.990	.999	.637	.841	.888	.981	.223	.456	.543	.834
	40	.928	.983	.990	.999	.637	.843	.890	.982	.223	.459	.547	.839
	50	.928	.984	.991	1.000	.636	.851	.898	.986	.222	.472	.564	.860
	60	.928	.985	.992	1.000	.636	.857	.905	.988	.221	.482	.578	.076
	70	.928	.986	.993	1.000	.635	.862	.910	.990	.221	.490	.589	.888
	80	.928	.987	.993	1.000	.635	.866	.914	.991	.221	.497	.599	.898
	90	.928	.987	.994	1.000	.535	.869	.917	.992	.220	.503	.608	.906
	100	.928	.988	.994	1.000	.635	.872	.920	.993	.220	.509	.616	.912

N	m	$\delta=2.0$				$\delta=2.5$				$\delta=3.0$			
		β_1'	β_2'	β_3'	β_4'	β_1'	β_2'	β_3'	β_4'	β_1'	β_2'	β_3'	β_4'
10	2	.0705	.0705	.0705	.0705	.00671	.00671	.00671	.00671	.00026	.00026	.00026	.00026
	3	.0532	.0672	.0788	.112	.00394	.00565	.00724	.0127	.00011	.00018	.00026	.00057
	4	.0459	.0678	.0845	.142	.00299	.00543	.00764	.0175	.00007	.00016	.00026	.00083
	5	.0419	.0695	.0893	.166	.00253	.00545	.00804	.0218	.00005	.00015	.00026	.00109
	6	.0395	.0715	.0935	.187	.00226	.00556	.00844	.0258	.00004	.00015	.00027	.00134
	7	.0378	.0735	.0974	.205	.00209	.00571	.00884	.0296	.00004	.00015	.00028	.00159
	8	.0366	.0757	.101	.221	.00197	.00589	.00925	.0332	.00004	.00016	.00030	.00185
	9	.0356	.0776	.104	.236	.00188	.00606	.00963	.0367	.00003	.00016	.00031	.00210
	10	.0349	.0795	.108	.250	.00181	.00624	.0100	.0400	.00003	.00017	.00032	.00236
	11	.0343	.0814	.111	.263	.00175	.00642	.0104	.0433	.00003	.00017	.00033	.00262
	12	.0339	.0831	.113	.274	.00171	.00659	.0107	.0464	.00003	.00018	.00035	.00288
	13	.0335	.0848	.116	.285	.00167	.00677	.0111	.0495	.00003	.00018	.00036	.00314
	14	.0331	.0864	.119	.296	.00164	.00694	.0114	.0525	.00003	.00019	.00037	.00340
	15	.0328	.0880	.121	.306	.00162	.00711	.0117	.0553	.00003	.00019	.00039	.00366
	16	.0326	.0894	.123	.315	.00159	.00726	.0120	.0581	.00003	.00020	.00040	.00392
	17	.0324	.0908	.125	.324	.00157	.00741	.0123	.0610	.00002	.00020	.00041	.00419
	18	.0322	.0922	.128	.332	.00156	.00757	.0126	.0636	.00002	.00021	.00042	.00446
	19	.0320	.0934	.130	.340	.00154	.00771	.0129	.0663	.00002	.00021	.00044	.00472
	20	.0318	.0946	.132	.348	.00153	.00785	.0132	.0688	.00002	.00022	.00045	.00498
	22	.0316	.0970	.135	.362	.00150	.00813	.0138	.0739	.00002	.00023	.00047	.00551
	24	.0313	.0992	.139	.375	.00149	.00840	.0143	.0787	.00002	.00024	.00050	.00603
	26	.0312	.101	.142	.388	.00147	.00864	.0148	.0833	.00002	.00024	.00052	.00656
	28	.0310	.103	.145	.399	.00146	.00887	.0153	.0878	.00002	.00025	.00054	.00708
	30	.0309	.105	.148	.410	.00144	.00909	.0158	.0921	.00002	.00026	.00056	.00760
	32	.0307	.107	.151	.420	.00143	.00931	.0162	.0963	.00002	.00027	.00059	.00812
	34	.0306	.108	.154	.429	.00142	.00952	.0166	.100	.00002	.00028	.00061	.00863
	36	.0305	.110	.156	.438	.00142	.00972	.0171	.104	.00002	.00028	.00063	.00915
	38	.0305	.111	.158	.447	.00141	.00990	.0175	.108	.00002	.00029	.00065	.00966
	40	.0304	.113	.161	.455	.00140	.0101	.0179	.112	.00002	.00030	.00067	.0102
	50	.0301	.119	.171	.490	.00138	.0109	.0197	.129	.00002	.00033	.00076	.0126
	60	.0299	.123	.180	.518	.00136	.0116	.0213	.144	.00002	.00036	.00085	.0150
	70	.0298	.128	.188	.542	.00135	.0122	.0228	.158	.00002	.00038	.00093	.0174
	80	.0297	.131	.194	.563	.00134	.0127	.0242	.171	.00002	.00041	.00101	.0196
	90	.0296	.134	.201	.581	.00134	.0132	.0254	.182	.00002	.00043	.00108	.0218
	100	.0295	.137	.206	.596	.00133	.0136	.0266	.193	.00002	.00045	.00115	.0239

B. Values of $\beta_1' = \beta_L'$, $\beta_2' = (\beta_S')_{\max}$, $\beta_3' = (\beta_X')_{\min}$ and $\beta_4' = \beta_W'$ for $\alpha = 0.01$

		$\delta=0.5$				$\delta=1.0$				$\delta=1.5$			
N	m	β_1'	β_2'	β_3'	β_4'	β_1'	β_2'	β_3'	β_4'	β_1'	β_2'	β_3'	β_4'
11	2	.933	.933	.933	.933	.664	.664	.664	.664	.259	.259	.259	.259
	3	.929	.942	.950	.965	.640	.680	.706	.765	.228	.264	.290	.357
	4	.927	.948	.958	.977	.628	.694	.731	.815	.213	.272	.310	.419
	5	.925	.953	.963	.983	.621	.707	.748	.846	.205	.280	.325	.464
	6	.924	.956	.967	.987	.616	.717	.761	.867	.199	.288	.337	.499
	7	.924	.959	.970	.990	.613	.726	.772	.883	.195	.295	.348	.528
	8	.923	.961	.972	.991	.610	.734	.781	.896	.193	.302	.358	.552
	9	.923	.963	.974	.993	.608	.740	.788	.906	.190	.308	.366	.573
	10	.923	.965	.975	.994	.606	.746	.795	.914	.189	.314	.374	.592
	11	.922	.966	.977	.995	.605	.752	.801	.921	.187	.319	.381	.608
	12	.922	.967	.978	.995	.604	.756	.806	.927	.186	.324	.388	.623
	13	.922	.969	.979	.996	.603	.761	.811	.932	.185	.329	.394	.636
	14	.922	.970	.980	.996	.602	.765	.815	.936	.184	.333	.399	.649
	15	.922	.971	.980	.997	.601	.769	.819	.940	.183	.337	.405	.660
	16	.921	.971	.981	.997	.601	.772	.822	.943	.183	.341	.410	.670
	17	.921	.972	.982	.997	.600	.775	.826	.946	.182	.345	.414	.679
	18	.921	.973	.982	.997	.600	.778	.829	.949	.182	.348	.419	.688
	19	.921	.973	.983	.998	.599	.781	.832	.952	.181	.351	.423	.696
	20	.921	.974	.983	.998	.599	.783	.835	.954	.181	.354	.427	.704
	22	.921	.975	.984	.998	.598	.788	.840	.958	.180	.360	.434	.718
	24	.921	.976	.985	.998	.598	.793	.844	.961	.180	.365	.441	.730
	26	.921	.977	.986	.998	.597	.796	.848	.964	.179	.370	.447	.741
	28	.921	.977	.986	.999	.597	.800	.851	.967	.179	.374	.453	.751
	30	.921	.978	.987	.999	.596	.803	.855	.969	.178	.378	.458	.760
	32	.921	.979	.987	.999	.596	.806	.858	.971	.178	.382	.463	.768
	34	.921	.979	.988	.999	.596	.808	.861	.972	.178	.385	.468	.776
	36	.920	.980	.988	.999	.596	.811	.863	.974	.177	.389	.473	.783
	38	.920	.980	.988	.999	.595	.813	.866	.975	.177	.392	.477	.789
	40	.920	.980	.989	.999	.595	.815	.868	.976	.177	.395	.481	.795
	50	.920	.982	.990	.999	.594	.824	.877	.981	.176	.407	.498	.820
	60	.920	.983	.991	1.000	.594	.831	.884	.984	.176	.417	.512	.839
	70	.920	.984	.992	1.000	.593	.837	.890	.987	.175	.426	.524	.853
	80	.920	.985	.992	1.000	.593	.841	.895	.988	.175	.433	.535	.865
	90	.920	.985	.993	1.000	.593	.845	.899	.990	.175	.438	.543	.875
	100	.920	.986	.993	1.000	.593	.848	.903	.991	.175	.444	.552	.883

N	m	δ=2.0				δ=2.5				δ=3.0			
		β_1'	β_2'	β_3'	β_4'	β_1'	β_2'	β_3'	β_4'	β_1'	β_2'	β_3'	β_4'
11	2	.0433	.0433	.0433	.0433	.00276	.00276	.00276	.00276	.00006	.00006	.00006	.00006
	3	.0322	.0418	.0496	.0734	.00159	.00236	.00307	.00566	.00003	.00004	.00006	.00015
	4	.0277	.0425	.0540	.0962	.00120	.00229	.00330	.00820	.00002	.00004	.00007	.00024
	5	.0252	.0439	.0576	.115	.00101	.00232	.00352	.0105	.00001	.00004	.00007	.00032
	6	.0237	.0455	.0608	.131	.00090	.00239	.00374	.0127	.00001	.00004	.00007	.00041
	7	.0226	.0470	.0638	.146	.00083	.00247	.00395	.0149	.00001	.00004	.00008	.00050
	8	.0219	.0486	.0666	.160	.00078	.00256	.00416	.0170	.00001	.00004	.00008	.00059
	9	.0213	.0501	.0692	.172	.00074	.00265	.00436	.0190	.00001	.00004	.00008	.00068
	10	.0209	.0515	.0715	.184	.00072	.00275	.00456	.0210	.00001	.00004	.00009	.00078
	11	.0205	.0528	.0738	.195	.00069	.00284	.00475	.0230	.00001	.00005	.00009	.00087
	12	.0202	.0541	.0759	.205	.00068	.00292	.00493	.0249	.00001	.00005	.00010	.00097
	13	.0200	.0554	.0780	.214	.00066	.00302	.00511	.0267	.00001	.00005	.00010	.00107
	14	.0198	.0566	.0799	.224	.00065	.00310	.00529	.0286	.00001	.00005	.00011	.00117
	15	.0196	.0577	.0818	.232	.00064	.00318	.00546	.0304	.00001	.00005	.00011	.00127
	16	.0194	.0588	.0835	.240	.00063	.00326	.00562	.0321	.00001	.00005	.00011	.00137
	17	.0193	.0598	.0852	.248	.00062	.00334	.00579	.0339	.00001	.00005	.00012	.00148
	18	.0192	.0608	.0869	.256	.00061	.00342	.00595	.0356	.00001	.00006	.00012	.00159
	19	.0191	.0618	.0885	.263	.00061	.00349	.00610	.0373	.00001	.00006	.00013	.00169
	20	.0190	.0627	.0899	.270	.00060	.00356	.00625	.0389	.00001	.00006	.00013	.00180
	22	.0188	.0645	.0929	.283	.00059	.00370	.00655	.0422	.00001	.00006	.00014	.00201
	24	.0187	.0661	.0955	.295	.00059	.00384	.00683	.0453	.00001	.00007	.00014	.00223
	26	.0186	.0676	.0981	.306	.00058	.00396	.00710	.0484	.00001	.00007	.00015	.00245
	28	.0185	.0690	.101	.317	.00057	.00408	.00736	.0514		.00007	.00016	.00267
	30	.0184	.0703	.103	.327	.00057	.00419	.00761	.0543		.00007	.00017	.00289
	32	.0183	.0716	.105	.336	.00056	.00431	.00786	.0571		.00008	.00017	.00311
	34	.0183	.0728	.107	.345	.00056	.00441	.00809	.0598		.00008	.00018	.00333
	36	.0182	.0740	.109	.353	.00056	.00452	.00832	.0625		.00008	.00019	.00356
	38	.0181	.0750	.111	.361	.00055	.00461	.00855	.0652		.00008	.00019	.00378
	40	.0181	.0761	.113	.369	.00055	.00471	.00876	.0677		.00008	.00020	.00400
	50	.0179	.0807	.121	.403	.00054	.00513	.00977	.0797		.00009	.00023	.00511
	60	.0178	.0844	.128	.431	.00054	.00549	.0107	.0907		.00010	.00026	.00622
	70	.0177	.0876	.134	.455	.00053	.00581	.0115	.101		.00011	.00029	.00731
	80	.0177	.0904	.140	.475	.00053	.00609	.0123	.110		.00012	.00032	.00839
	90	.0176	.0928	.145	.494	.00053	.00634	.0130	.119		.00013	.00034	.00945
	100	.0176	.0949	.149	.510	.00052	.00657	.0136	.127		.00013	.00037	.0105

B. Values of $\beta_1' = \beta_L'$, $\beta_2' = (\beta_S')_{\max}$, $\beta_3' = (\beta_X')_{\min}$ and $\beta_4' = \beta_W'$ for $\alpha = 0.01$

		δ=0.5				δ=1.0				δ=1.5			
N	m	β_1'	β_2'	β_3'	β_4'	β_1'	β_2'	β_3'	β_4'	β_1'	β_2'	β_3'	β_4'
13	2	.917	.917	.917	.917	.580	.580	.580	.580	.164	.164	.164	.164
	3	.913	.928	.937	.956	.557	.600	.628	.693	.142	.169	.189	.244
	4	.911	.936	.947	.971	.546	.617	.655	.752	.132	.177	.206	.299
	5	.909	.941	.954	.979	.538	.631	.675	.790	.127	.184	.219	.340
	6	.908	.946	.958	.983	.534	.642	.690	.816	.123	.191	.230	.374
	7	.908	.949	.962	.986	.531	.653	.703	.837	.121	.198	.240	.402
	8	.907	.952	.965	.989	.528	.661	.713	.853	.119	.203	.248	.427
	9	.907	.954	.967	.990	.526	.669	.722	.866	.117	.208	.256	.448
	10	.906	.956	.969	.992	.525	.676	.730	.876	.116	.213	.263	.467
	11	.906	.958	.970	.993	.523	.682	.737	.885	.115	.218	.269	.484
	12	.906	.959	.972	.994	.522	.688	.743	.893	.114	.222	.275	.500
	13	.906	.961	.973	.994	.521	.693	.749	.900	.114	.226	.280	.514
	14	.906	.962	.974	.995	.521	.697	.754	.906	.113	.230	.285	.527
	15	.905	.963	.975	.995	.520	.702	.759	.911	.113	.233	.290	.539
	16	.905	.964	.976	.996	.519	.706	.763	.916	.112	.236	.294	.550
	17	.905	.965	.977	.996	.519	.709	.767	.920	.112	.239	.299	.561
	18	.905	.966	.977	.996	.518	.713	.771	.924	.111	.242	.303	.571
	19	.905	.967	.978	.997	.518	.716	.775	.927	.111	.245	.307	.580
	20	.905	.967	.979	.997	.518	.719	.778	.930	.111	.248	.310	.588
	22	.905	.969	.980	.997	.517	.725	.784	.936	.110	.253	.317	.604
	24	.905	.970	.981	.998	.516	.730	.789	.940	.110	.257	.323	.619
	26	.905	.971	.981	.998	.516	.734	.794	.944	.110	.261	.329	.631
	28	.904	.971	.982	.998	.516	.738	.798	.948	.110	.265	.334	.643
	30	.904	.972	.983	.998	.515	.742	.802	.951	.109	.268	.339	.654
	32	.904	.973	.983	.998	.515	.745	.806	.954	.109	.272	.344	.664
	34	.904	.974	.984	.999	.515	.748	.810	.956	.109	.275	.348	.673
	36	.904	.974	.984	.999	.515	.751	.813	.958	.109	.278	.353	.682
	38	.904	.975	.985	.999	.514	.754	.816	.960	.109	.281	.357	.690
	40	.904	.975	.985	.999	.514	.756	.819	.962	.108	.283	.361	.697
	50	.904	.977	.987	.999	.513	.767	.830	.969	.108	.294	.377	.728
	60	.904	.979	.988	.999	.513	.775	.839	.974	.108	.303	.391	.752
	70	.904	.980	.989	.999	.513	.782	.847	.978	.107	.311	.402	.771
	80	.904	.981	.990	1.000	.512	.787	.853	.980	.107	.317	.412	.787
	90	.904	.981	.990	1.000	.512	.791	.858	.983	.107	.323	.421	.800
	100	.904	.982	.991	1.000	.512	.795	.863	.984	.107	.327	.429	.811

N	m	δ=2.0				δ=2.5				δ=3.0			
		β_1'	β_2'	β_3'	β_4'	β_1'	β_2'	β_3'	β_4'	β_1'	β_2'	β_3'	β_4'
13	2	.0155	.0155	.0155	.0155	.00043	.00043	.00043	.00043				
	3	.0112	.0153	.0186	.0295	.00024	.00038	.00051	.00103				.00001
	4	.00956	.0158	.0208	.0413	.00018	.00038	.00057	.00163				.00002
	5	.00865	.0166	.0226	.0517	.00015	.00039	.00062	.00223				.00002
	6	.00811	.0174	.0243	.0611	.00013	.00041	.00067	.00282				.00003
	7	.00774	.0182	.0258	.0699	.00012	.00043	.00072	.00342				.00004
	8	.00747	.0190	.0273	.0782	.00011	.00045	.00077	.00403			.00001	.00005
	9	.00727	.0197	.0286	.0858	.00011	.00047	.00082	.00463			.00001	.00006
	10	.00711	.0204	.0298	.0931	.00010	.00049	.00087	.00523			.00001	.00007
	11	.00698	.0211	.0310	.100	.00010	.00051	.00091	.00584			.00001	.00008
	12	.00688	.0217	.0321	.107	.00010	.00053	.00096	.00645			.00001	.00010
	13	.00679	.0223	.0332	.113	.00010	.00055	.00100	.00706			.00001	.00011
	14	.00672	.0229	.0342	.119	.00009	.00057	.00104	.00766			.00001	.00012
	15	.00665	.0235	.0352	.125	.00009	.00059	.00109	.00825			.00001	.00013
	16	.00660	.0240	.0361	.131	.00009	.00061	.00113	.00885			.00001	.00015
	17	.00655	.0245	.0370	.136	.00009	.00062	.00117	.00945			.00001	.00016
	18	.00651	.0250	.0379	.142	.00009	.00064	.00121	.0100			.00001	.00017
	19	.00647	.0255	.0387	.147	.00009	.00066	.00124	.0106			.00001	.00019
	20	.00643	.0260	.0396	.152	.00009	.00067	.00128	.0112			.00001	.00020
	22	.00638	.0268	.0411	.161	.00009	.00071	.00135	.0124			.00001	.00023
	24	.00633	.0277	.0426	.170	.00008	.00074	.00142	.0135			.00001	.00026
	26	.00629	.0284	.0440	.178	.00008	.00077	.00149	.0147			.00001	.00029
	28	.00625	.0292	.0453	.186	.00008	.00079	.00156	.0158			.00001	.00033
	30	.00622	.0298	.0466	.194	.00008	.00082	.00162	.0169		.00001	.00001	.00036
	32	.00620	.0305	.0478	.201	.00008	.00085	.00169	.0180		.00001	.00001	.00039
	34	.00617	.0311	.0490	.208	.00008	.00087	.00175	.0191		.00001	.00001	.00043
	36	.00615	.0317	.0501	.215	.00008	.00089	.00181	.0202		.00001	.00001	.00046
	38	.00613	.0323	.0512	.221	.00008	.00092	.00187	.0212		.00001	.00002	.00050
	40	.00612	.0328	.0522	.228	.00008	.00094	.00192	.0223		.00001	.00002	.00054
	50	.00605	.0352	.0569	.255	.00008	.00104	.00219	.0273		.00001	.00002	.00072
	60	.00602	.0372	.0610	.279	.00008	.00113	.00243	.0321		.00001	.00002	.00091
	70	.00599	.0389	.0646	.300	.00008	.00121	.00266	.0366		.00001	.00002	.00111
	80	.00597	.0404	.0679	.318	.00008	.00127	.00287	.0409		.00001	.00003	.00131
	90	.00595	.0416	.0708	.335	.00008	.00133	.00307	.0450		.00001	.00003	.00152
	100	.00594	.0428	.0736	.350	.00008	.00139	.00326	.0490		.00001	.00003	.00173

B. Values of $\beta_1' = \beta_L'$, $\beta_2' = (\beta_S')_{\max}$, $\beta_3' = (\beta_X')_{\min}$ and $\beta_4' = \beta_W'$ for $\alpha = 0.01$

N	m	δ=0.5				δ=1.0				δ=1.5			
		β_1'	β_2'	β_3'	β_4'	β_1'	β_2'	β_3'	β_4'	β_1'	β_2'	β_3'	β_4'
16	2	.892	.892	.892	.892	.462	.462	.462	.462	.0766	.0766	.0766	.0766
	3	.887	.906	.917	.940	.441	.485	.513	.584	.0658	.0816	.0934	.128
	4	.885	.916	.930	.960	.431	.504	.544	.652	.0608	.0871	.105	.167
	5	.883	.923	.938	.970	.425	.519	.566	.697	.0580	.0921	.114	.199
	6	.883	.928	.944	.976	.421	.532	.583	.731	.0562	.0967	.121	.225
	7	.882	.933	.948	.981	.418	.544	.597	.756	.0549	.101	.128	.249
	8	.881	.935	.952	.984	.416	.553	.609	.777	.0540	.105	.134	.269
	9	.881	.939	.955	.986	.414	.562	.620	.794	.0533	.108	.139	.288
	10	.880	.942	.957	.988	.413	.570	.629	.808	.0527	.112	.144	.305
	11	.880	.944	.959	.989	.411	.576	.637	.821	.0522	.115	.149	.320
	12	.880	.946	.961	.991	.411	.583	.644	.831	.0518	.117	.153	.335
	13	.880	.948	.963	.991	.410	.588	.651	.841	.0515	.120	.157	.348
	14	.880	.949	.964	.992	.409	.594	.657	.849	.0513	.123	.161	.360
	15	.879	.950	.965	.993	.409	.599	.663	.856	.0510	.125	.164	.372
	16	.879	.952	.967	.994	.408	.603	.668	.863	.0508	.127	.167	.383
	17	.879	.953	.968	.994	.408	.607	.673	.869	.0506	.129	.170	.393
	18	.879	.954	.969	.994	.407	.611	.677	.874	.0505	.132	.173	.403
	19	.879	.955	.969	.995	.407	.615	.681	.879	.0503	.133	.176	.412
	20	.879	.956	.970	.995	.406	.618	.685	.884	.0502	.135	.179	.421
	22	.879	.957	.972	.996	.406	.625	.693	.892	.0500	.139	.184	.437
	24	.879	.959	.973	.996	.405	.630	.699	.899	.0498	.142	.189	.452
	26	.879	.960	.974	.997	.405	.635	.705	.905	.0496	.145	.193	.465
	28	.878	.961	.975	.997	.405	.640	.710	.911	.0495	.147	.198	.478
	30	.878	.962	.976	.997	.404	.644	.715	.915	.0494	.150	.201	.490
	32	.878	.963	.977	.997	.404	.648	.720	.920	.0493	.152	.205	.500
	34	.878	.964	.977	.998	.404	.652	.724	.923	.0492	.155	.209	.510
	36	.878	.965	.978	.998	.404	.655	.728	.927	.0491	.157	.212	.520
	38	.878	.965	.979	.998	.404	.658	.732	.930	.0490	.159	.215	.529
	40	.878	.966	.979	.998	.403	.661	.735	.933	.0490	.161	.218	.538
	50	.878	.969	.981	.999	.403	.674	.750	.944	.0487	.169	.231	.574
	60	.878	.970	.983	.999	.402	.684	.762	.952	.0486	.176	.243	.603
	70	.878	.972	.984	.999	.402	.691	.771	.958	.0485	.181	.252	.626
	80	.878	.973	.985	.999	.402	.698	.779	.963	.0484	.186	.261	.646
	90	.878	.974	.986	.999	.402	.703	.786	.966	.0483	.190	.268	.663
	100	.878	.975	.987	.999	.402	.708	.792	.969	.0483	.194	.275	.678

N	m	δ = 2.0				δ = 2.5				δ = 3.0			
		β_1'	β_2'	β_3'	β_4'	β_1'	β_2'	β_3'	β_4'	β_1'	β_2'	β_3'	β_4'
16	2	.00292	.00292	.00292	.00292	.00002	.00002	.00002	.00002				
	3	.00207	.00299	.00378	.00661	.00001	.00002	.00003	.00007				
	4	.00174	.00320	.00440	.0102	.00001	.00002	.00003	.00012				
	5	.00157	.00343	.00494	.0136	.00001	.00002	.00004	.00018				
	6	.00146	.00366	.00543	.0169	.00001	.00002	.00004	.00024				
	7	.00139	.00388	.00588	.0201	.00001	.00003	.00005	.00031				
	8	.00134	.00411	.00630	.0232	.00001	.00003	.00005	.00038				
	9	.00130	.00431	.00670	.0262	.00001	.00003	.00006	.00045				
	10	.00127	.00451	.00708	.0292	.00001	.00003	.00006	.00053				
	11	.00125	.00470	.00745	.0321		.00003	.00006	.00061				
	12	.00123	.00489	.00779	.0349		.00003	.00007	.00069				
	13	.00121	.00507	.00813	.0377		.00004	.00007	.00077				
	14	.00120	.00523	.00845	.0404		.00004	.00008	.00086				
	15	.00119	.00540	.00875	.0430		.00004	.00008	.00094				
	16	.00118	.00555	.00905	.0455		.00004	.00008	.00103				
	17	.00117	.00570	.00934	.0481		.00004	.00009	.00112				
	18	.00116	.00585	.00962	.0505		.00004	.00009	.00121				
	19	.00115	.00599	.00990	.0530		.00005	.00010	.00130				.00001
	20	.00115	.00613	.0102	.0553		.00005	.00010	.00139				.00001
	22	.00114	.00639	.0107	.0600		.00005	.00011	.00158				.00001
	24	.00113	.00664	.0112	.0644		.00005	.00011	.00177				.00001
	26	.00112	.00687	.0116	.0686		.00005	.00012	.00196				.00001
	28	.00111	.00708	.0121	.0728		.00006	.00013	.00215				.00001
	30	.00111	.00729	.0125	.0768		.00006	.00013	.00235				.00001
	32	.00110	.00749	.0129	.0807		.00006	.00014	.00255				.00001
	34	.00110	.00768	.0133	.0845		.00006	.00015	.00274				.00001
	36	.00109	.00786	.0137	.0882		.00007	.00015	.00294				.00002
	38	.00109	.00804	.0141	.0918		.00007	.00016	.00314				.00002
	40	.00109	.00820	.0144	.0953		.00007	.00016	.00334				.00002
	50	.00108	.00895	.0161	.111		.00008	.00019	.00434				.00003
	60	.00107	.00958	.0176	.126		.00009	.00022	.00534				.00004
	70	.00106	.0101	.0189	.139		.00009	.00024	.00634				.00005
	80	.00106	.0106	.0201	.151		.00010	.00027	.00732				.00006
	90	.00106	.0110	.0212	.162		.00011	.00029	.00830				.00007
	100	.00105	.0114	.0223	.172		.00011	.00031	.00927				.00008

B. Values of $\beta_1' = \beta_L'$, $\beta_2' = (\beta_S')_{\max}$, $\beta_3' = (\beta_X')_{\min}$ and $\beta_4' = \beta_W'$ for $\alpha = 0.01$

		$\delta=0.5$				$\delta=1.0$				$\delta=1.5$			
N	m	β_1'	β_2'	β_3'	β_4'	β_1'	β_2'	β_3'	β_4'	β_1'	β_2'	β_3'	β_4'
21	2	.847	.847	.847	.847	.298	.298	.298	.298	.0188	.0188	.0188	.0188
	3	.841	.866	.880	.911	.283	.321	.346	.414	.0158	.0210	.0248	.0377
	4	.839	.879	.897	.938	.275	.340	.377	.486	.0145	.0231	.0292	.0543
	5	.837	.888	.908	.953	.271	.355	.399	.537	.0138	.0251	.0328	.0691
	6	.836	.895	.916	.962	.268	.368	.416	.576	.0133	.0269	.0358	.0825
	7	.835	.901	.922	.969	.266	.379	.431	.608	.0130	.0285	.0386	.0949
	8	.835	.906	.927	.973	.264	.389	.444	.634	.0128	.0300	.0411	.106
	9	.834	.910	.931	.977	.263	.398	.455	.656	.0126	.0314	.0434	.117
	10	.834	.914	.935	.980	.262	.405	.464	.675	.0124	.0328	.0455	.127
	11	.834	.917	.938	.982	.261	.412	.473	.692	.0123	.0340	.0475	.137
	12	.833	.919	.940	.984	.261	.419	.481	.706	.0122	.0351	.0494	.146
	13	.833	.922	.942	.985	.260	.425	.488	.719	.0121	.0363	.0512	.155
	14	.833	.924	.944	.987	.259	.430	.495	.731	.0121	.0373	.0529	.163
	15	.833	.926	.946	.988	.259	.435	.501	.741	.0120	.0383	.0544	.170
	16	.833	.927	.948	.989	.259	.440	.507	.751	.0119	.0392	.0560	.178
	17	.832	.929	.949	.989	.258	.444	.512	.760	.0119	.0401	.0574	.185
	18	.832	.930	.951	.990	.258	.448	.517	.768	.0119	.0409	.0588	.192
	19	.832	.932	.952	.991	.258	.452	.522	.775	.0118	.0418	.0602	.199
	20	.832	.933	.953	.991	.258	.455	.526	.782	.0118	.0425	.0614	.205
	22	.832	.935	.955	.992	.257	.462	.535	.795	.0117	.0440	.0639	.217
	24	.832	.937	.957	.993	.257	.468	.542	.805	.0117	.0454	.0652	.228
	26	.832	.939	.959	.994	.257	.474	.549	.815	.0116	.0467	.0684	.239
	28	.832	.941	.960	.994	.256	.479	.555	.824	.0116	.0478	.0704	.249
	30	.832	.942	.961	.995	.256	.483	.561	.831	.0116	.0489	.0724	.258
	32	.831	.943	.963	.995	.256	.488	.567	.838	.0115	.0500	.0742	.267
	34	.831	.944	.964	.996	.256	.491	.572	.845	.0115	.0510	.0760	.276
	36	.831	.945	.965	.996	.256	.495	.576	.850	.0115	.0520	.0776	.284
	38	.831	.946	.965	.996	.256	.499	.581	.856	.0115	.0528	.0793	.292
	40	.831	.947	.956	.996	.255	.502	.585	.861	.0115	.0537	.0808	.299
	50	.831	.951	.970	.997	.255	.516	.603	.880	.0114	.0575	.0878	.332
	60	.831	.954	.972	.998	.255	.527	.617	.895	.0114	.0606	.0937	.359
	70	.831	.956	.974	.998	.254	.535	.629	.906	.0113	.0632	.0989	.383
	80	.831	.958	.976	.999	.254	.543	.639	.915	.0113	.0655	.104	.403
	90	.831	.959	.977	.999	.254	.549	.648	.922	.0113	.0674	.108	.421
	100	.831	.960	.978	.999	.254	.554	.655	.928	.0113	.0692	.112	.438

N	m	δ=2.0				δ=2.5				δ=3.0			
		β'_1	β'_2	β'_3	β'_4	β'_1	β'_2	β'_3	β'_4	β'_1	β'_2	β'_3	β'_4
21	2	.00014	.00014	.00014	.00014								
	3	.00010	.00016	.00021	.00042								
	4	.00008	.00018	.00026	.00075								
	5	.00007	.00020	.00031	.00111								
	6	.00007	.00022	.00035	.00149								
	7	.00006	.00023	.00039	.00189								
	8	.00006	.00025	.00043	.00230								
	9	.00006	.00027	.00047	.00272				.00001				
	10	.00006	.00029	.00050	.00315				.00001				
	11	.00006	.00030	.00054	.00358				.00001				
	12	.00006	.00032	.00057	.00402				.00001				
	13	.00006	.00033	.00060	.00446				.00001				
	14	.00006	.00035	.00063	.00491				.00001				
	15	.00005	.00036	.00067	.00535				.00002				
	16	.00005	.00038	.00070	.00579				.00002				
	17	.00005	.00039	.00073	.00625				.00002				
	18	.00005	.00041	.00075	.00669				.00002				
	19	.00005	.00042	.00078	.00714				.00003				
	20	.00005	.00043	.00081	.00758				.00003				
	22	.00005	.00045	.00087	.00848				.00003				
	24	.00005	.00048	.00092	.00936				.00004				
	26	.00005	.00050	.00097	.0102				.00004				
	28	.00005	.00052	.00102	.0111				.00005				
	30	.00005	.00054	.00107	.0120				.00006				
	32	.00005	.00056	.00111	.0129				.00006				
	34	.00005	.00058	.00116	.0137				.00007				
	36	.00005	.00060	.00120	.0146				.00007				
	38	.00005	.00061	.00125	.0154				.00008				
	40	.00005	.00063	.00129	.0163				.00009				
	50	.00005	.00071	.00149	.0203				.00013				
	60	.00005	.00077	.00167	.0242				.00017				
	70	.00005	.00083	.00184	.0279				.00021				
	80	.00005	.00088	.00200	.0315				.00026				
	90	.00005	.00093	.00215	.0349				.00030				
	100	.00005	.00097	.00229	.0382				.00035				

B. Values of $\beta_1' = \beta_L'$, $\beta_2' = (\beta_S')_{\max}$, $\beta_3' = (\beta_X')_{\min}$ and $\beta_4' = \beta_W'$ for $\alpha = 0.01$

N	m	δ=0.5				δ=1.0				δ=1.5			
		β_1'	β_2'	β_3'	β_4'	β_1'	β_2'	β_3'	β_4'	β_1'	β_2'	β_3'	β_4'
25	2	.808	.808	.808	.808	.201	.201	.201	.201	.00554	.00554	.00554	.00554
	3	.802	.830	.847	.884	.190	.222	.242	.301	.00462	.00640	.00778	.0127
	4	.799	.845	.867	.917	.185	.238	.269	.368	.00421	.00724	.00948	.0197
	5	.797	.857	.881	.936	.181	.251	.288	.418	.00399	.00800	.0109	.0264
	6	.796	.866	.890	.948	.179	.263	.304	.457	.00384	.00871	.0122	.0329
	7	.796	.873	.898	.956	.178	.272	.318	.490	.00374	.00936	.0133	.0390
	8	.795	.879	.904	.963	.177	.281	.330	.517	.00367	.0100	.0144	.0450
	9	.794	.884	.909	.967	.176	.289	.340	.541	.00361	.0105	.0153	.0507
	10	.794	.888	.913	.971	.175	.296	.349	.562	.00357	.0111	.0163	.0562
	11	.794	.892	.917	.974	.174	.302	.357	.580	.00353	.0116	.0171	.0614
	12	.793	.895	.920	.977	.174	.308	.365	.596	.00350	.0121	.0179	.0665
	13	.793	.898	.923	.979	.173	.313	.372	.611	.00348	.0125	.0187	.0715
	14	.793	.900	.926	.981	.173	.318	.378	.625	.00346	.0129	.0195	.0762
	15	.793	.903	.928	.982	.173	.323	.384	.637	.00344	.0133	.0202	.0808
	16	.793	.905	.930	.983	.173	.327	.390	.648	.00342	.0137	.0209	.0852
	17	.793	.907	.932	.985	.172	.331	.395	.658	.00341	.0141	.0215	.0896
	18	.793	.909	.934	.986	.172	.335	.400	.668	.00340	.0145	.0222	.0938
	19	.792	.910	.935	.987	.172	.339	.404	.677	.00339	.0148	.0228	.0980
	20	.792	.912	.937	.987	.172	.342	.409	.685	.00338	.0151	.0234	.102
	22	.792	.915	.939	.989	.171	.348	.417	.700	.00336	.0158	.0245	.110
	24	.792	.917	.942	.990	.171	.354	.424	.714	.00335	.0164	.0256	.117
	26	.792	.919	.944	.991	.171	.359	.431	.726	.00333	.0169	.0266	.124
	28	.792	.921	.945	.992	.171	.364	.437	.735	.00332	.0174	.0276	.130
	30	.792	.923	.947	.992	.171	.368	.443	.746	.00331	.0179	.0285	.137
	32	.792	.924	.949	.993	.171	.372	.449	.755	.00331	.0184	.0294	.143
	34	.792	.926	.950	.993	.170	.376	.454	.763	.00330	.0188	.0302	.149
	36	.792	.927	.951	.994	.170	.379	.459	.771	.00329	.0193	.0310	.155
	38	.791	.928	.952	.994	.170	.383	.463	.778	.00329	.0197	.0318	.160
	40	.791	.930	.954	.995	.170	.386	.467	.784	.00328	.0200	.0326	.165
	50	.791	.934	.958	.996	.170	.399	.486	.811	.00327	.0217	.0360	.189
	60	.791	.938	.961	.997	.170	.410	.501	.831	.00325	.0231	.0390	.210
	70	.791	.940	.964	.997	.170	.418	.513	.846	.00324	.0244	.0417	.229
	80	.791	.943	.966	.998	.169	.426	.524	.859	.00324	.0254	.0441	.245
	90	.791	.944	.968	.998	.169	.431	.533	.869	.00323	.0263	.0463	.260
	100	.791	.946	.969	.998	.169	.437	.541	.878	.00323	.0271	.0483	.274

N	m	δ=2.0				δ=2.5				δ=3.0			
		β_1'	β_2'	β_3'	β_4'	β_1'	β_2'	β_3'	β_4'	β_1'	β_2'	β_3'	β_4'
25	2	.00001	.00001	.00001	.00001								
	3	.00001	.00001	.00002	.00004								
	4	.00001	.00001	.00002	.00008								
	5	.00001	.00002	.00003	.00012								
	6	.00001	.00002	.00003	.00018								
	7		.00002	.00004	.00023								
	8		.00002	.00004	.00030								
	9		.00002	.00005	.00036								
	10		.00003	.00005	.00043								
	11		.00003	.00005	.00051								
	12		.00003	.00006	.00058								
	13		.00003	.00006	.00066								
	14		.00003	.00007	.00074								
	15		.00004	.00007	.00082								
	16		.00004	.00007	.00090								
	17		.00004	.00008	.00099								
	18		.00004	.00008	.00107								
	19		.00004	.00009	.00116								
	20		.00004	.00009	.00125								
	22		.00005	.00010	.00143								
	24		.00005	.00010	.00161								
	26		.00005	.00011	.00180								
	28		.00005	.00012	.00199								
	30		.00006	.00012	.00218								
	32		.00006	.00013	.00237								
	34		.00006	.00014	.00256								
	36		.00006	.00014	.00276								
	38		.00007	.00015	.00296								
	40		.00007	.00016	.00315								
	50		.00008	.00018	.00414				.00001				
	60		.00009	.00021	.00514				.00001				
	70		.00009	.00024	.00612				.00001				
	80		.00010	.00026	.00711				.00001				
	90		.00011	.00028	.00808				.00002				
	100		.00011	.00031	.00905				.00002				

B. Values of $\beta_1' = \beta_L'$, $\beta_2' = (\beta_S')_{\max}$, $\beta_3' = (\beta_X')_{\min}$ and $\beta_4' = \beta_W'$ for $\alpha = 0.01$

N	m	$\delta=0.5$				$\delta=1.0$				$\delta=1.5$			
		β_1'	β_2'	β_3'	β_4'	β_1'	β_2'	β_3'	β_4'	β_1'	β_2'	β_3'	β_4'
31	2	.746	.746	.746	.746	.105	.105	.105	.105	.00078	.00078	.00078	.00078
	3	.740	.774	.793	.838	.0989	.120	.133	.175	.00064	.00095	.00120	.00216
	4	.737	.793	.818	.881	.0957	.131	.152	.227	.00058	.00112	.00153	.00372
	5	.735	.807	.835	.906	.0939	.141	.167	.269	.00055	.00127	.00183	.00539
	6	.734	.817	.847	.922	.0927	.149	.179	.303	.00053	.00141	.00210	.00709
	7	.733	.826	.857	.934	.0918	.156	.189	.332	.00051	.00154	.00235	.00881
	8	.733	.833	.865	.943	.0912	.163	.198	.358	.00050	.00167	.00258	.0106
	9	.732	.839	.871	.950	.0907	.168	.207	.381	.00050	.00179	.00281	.0123
	10	.732	.845	.877	.955	.0903	.174	.214	.401	.00049	.00190	.00302	.0140
	11	.732	.849	.882	.959	.0900	.178	.220	.419	.00048	.00201	.00322	.0157
	12	.731	.853	.886	.963	.0897	.183	.226	.436	.00048	.00211	.00341	.0174
	13	.731	.857	.889	.966	.0895	.187	.232	.451	.00048	.00221	.00360	.0191
	14	.731	.860	.893	.969	.0893	.191	.237	.465	.00047	.00231	.00378	.0207
	15	.731	.863	.896	.971	.0891	.194	.242	.478	.00047	.00240	.00395	.0224
	16	.731	.866	.898	.973	.0890	.198	.247	.490	.00047	.00248	.00412	.0240
	17	.730	.869	.901	.975	.0888	.201	.251	.501	.00047	.00257	.00428	.0256
	18	.730	.871	.903	.976	.0887	.204	.255	.512	.00046	.00265	.00444	.0272
	19	.730	.873	.905	.978	.0886	.206	.259	.522	.00046	.00273	.00459	.0287
	20	.730	.875	.907	.979	.0885	.209	.263	.531	.00046	.00280	.00474	.0302
	22	.730	.879	.911	.981	.0883	.214	.270	.548	.00046	.00295	.00503	.0333
	24	.730	.882	.914	.983	.0882	.219	.276	.564	.00046	.00309	.00530	.0362
	26	.730	.885	.917	.984	.0881	.223	.282	.578	.00046	.00321	.00557	.0391
	28	.730	.887	.919	.986	.0880	.227	.287	.591	.00045	.00334	.00582	.0419
	30	.729	.890	.922	.987	.0879	.230	.293	.602	.00045	.00345	.00607	.0446
	32	.729	.892	.924	.988	.0878	.233	.297	.613	.00045	.00356	.00630	.0473
	34	.729	.894	.926	.989	.0878	.236	.302	.623	.00045	.00367	.00653	.0499
	36	.729	.895	.927	.989	.0877	.239	.306	.633	.00045	.00377	.00675	.0525
	38	.729	.897	.929	.990	.0877	.242	.310	.641	.00045	.00386	.00697	.0550
	40	.729	.898	.930	.990	.0876	.245	.314	.650	.00045	.00396	.00718	.0574
	50	.729	.905	.937	.993	.0875	.256	.331	.684	.00045	.00437	.00813	.0689
	60	.729	.909	.941	.994	.0873	.265	.344	.710	.00044	.00473	.00900	.0795
	70	.729	.913	.945	.995	.0873	.272	.356	.732	.00044	.00504	.00977	.0891
	80	.729	.916	.948	.996	.0872	.278	.366	.749	.00044	.00531	.0105	.0981
	90	.729	.918	.950	.996	.0871	.283	.375	.764	.00044	.00554	.0112	.106
	100	.729	.920	.952	.997	.0871	.288	.383	.777	.00044	.00576	.0118	.114

N	m	$\delta=2.0$				$\delta=2.5$				$\delta=3.0$			
		β_1'	β_2'	β_3'	β_4'	β_1'	β_2'	β_3'	β_4'	β_1'	β_2'	β_3'	β_4'
31	2												
	3												
	4												
	5												
	6				.00001								
	7				.00001								
	8				.00001								
	9				.00001								
	10				.00002								
	11				.00002								
	12				.00002								
	13				.00003								
	14				.00003								
	15				.00004								
	16				.00004								
	17				.00005								
	18				.00005								
	19				.00006								
	20				.00006								
	22				.00008								
	24				.00009								
	26				.00010								
	28				.00011								
	30				.00013								
	32				.00014								
	34				.00016								
	36				.00017								
	38				.00019								
	40			.00001	.00020								
	50			.00001	.00028								
	60			.00001	.00037								
	70			.00001	.00047								
	80			.00001	.00056								
	90			.00001	.00066								
	100			.00001	.00077								

B. Values of $\beta_1' = \beta_L'$, $\beta_2' = (\beta_S')_{\max}$, $\beta_3' = (\beta_X')_{\min}$ and $\beta_4' = \beta_W'$ for $\alpha = 0.01$

		$\delta=0.5$				$\delta=1.0$				$\delta=1.5$			
N	m	β_1'	β_2'	β_3'	β_4'	β_1'	β_2'	β_3'	β_4'	β_1'	β_2'	β_3'	β_4'
41	2	.640	.640	.640	.640	.0317	.0317	.0317	.0317	.00002	.00002	.00002	.00002
	3	.634	.674	.697	.754	.0295	.0377	.0434	.0623	.00002	.00003	.00004	.00009
	4	.631	.698	.729	.811	.0284	.0428	.0520	.0888	.00002	.00004	.00006	.00017
	5	.630	.715	.750	.846	.0278	.0471	.0589	.112	.00002	.00005	.00007	.00028
	6	.629	.729	.766	.869	.0274	.0509	.0648	.133	.00002	.00005	.00009	.00040
	7	.628	.739	.779	.887	.0271	.0542	.0699	.151	.00001	.00006	.00010	.00054
	8	.627	.749	.789	.900	.0269	.0573	.0745	.169	.00001	.00007	.00011	.00068
	9	.627	.757	.798	.911	.0268	.0600	.0787	.184	.00001	.00007	.00012	.00084
	10	.626	.764	.806	.919	.0266	.0626	.0825	.199	.00001	.00008	.00014	.00100
	11	.626	.770	.812	.926	.0265	.0650	.0860	.212	.00001	.00008	.00015	.00116
	12	.626	.775	.818	.932	.0264	.0671	.0893	.225	.00001	.00009	.00016	.00133
	13	.625	.780	.823	.937	.0264	.0692	.0924	.237	.00001	.00009	.00017	.00151
	14	.625	.784	.827	.941	.0263	.0711	.0952	.248	.00001	.00010	.00018	.00169
	15	.625	.788	.832	.945	.0262	.0729	.0979	.258	.00001	.00010	.00019	.00187
	16	.625	.792	.835	.949	.0262	.0746	.101	.268	.00001	.00011	.00021	.00206
	17	.625	.795	.839	.952	.0262	.0762	.103	.277	.00001	.00011	.00022	.00225
	18	.625	.798	.842	.954	.0261	.0778	.105	.286	.00001	.00012	.00023	.00244
	19	.624	.801	.845	.957	.0261	.0792	.108	.295	.00001	.00012	.00024	.00263
	20	.624	.804	.848	.959	.0261	.0806	.110	.303	.00001	.00013	.00025	.00282
	22	.624	.809	.853	.963	.0260	.0832	.114	.319	.00001	.00014	.00027	.00322
	24	.624	.813	.858	.966	.0260	.0856	.118	.333	.00001	.00014	.00029	.00361
	26	.624	.817	.862	.968	.0259	.0879	.121	.346	.00001	.00015	.00030	.00401
	28	.624	.821	.865	.971	.0259	.0899	.124	.358	.00001	.00016	.00032	.00441
	30	.624	.824	.869	.973	.0259	.0918	.127	.370	.00001	.00017	.00034	.00482
	32	.624	.826	.872	.974	.0258	.0936	.130	.380	.00001	.00017	.00036	.00522
	34	.624	.829	.874	.976	.0258	.0953	.133	.390	.00001	.00018	.00037	.00562
	36	.624	.832	.877	.977	.0258	.0969	.136	.400	.00001	.00019	.00039	.00603
	38	.623	.834	.879	.979	.0258	.0984	.138	.409	.00001	.00019	.00041	.00644
	40	.623	.836	.882	.980	.0258	.100	.141	.418	.00001	.00020	.00042	.00684
	50	.623	.845	.891	.984	.0257	.106	.151	.455	.00001	.00023	.00050	.00884
	60	.623	.851	.898	.987	.0257	.111	.160	.485	.00001	.00025	.00057	.0108
	70	.623	.856	.903	.989	.0256	.115	.168	.510	.00001	.00027	.00064	.0127
	80	.623	.861	.908	.990	.0256	.119	.175	.532	.00001	.00029	.00070	.0146
	90	.623	.864	.912	.992	.0256	.122	.181	.551	.00001	.00031	.00076	.0165
	100	.623	.867	.915	.992	.0256	.125	.187	.568	.00001	.00032	.00081	.0183

		$\delta=2.0$				$\delta=2.5$				$\delta=3.0$			
N	m	β_1'	β_2'	β_3'	β_4'	β_1'	β_2'	β_3'	β_4'	β_1'	β_2'	β_3'	β_4'
41	2												
	3												
	4												
	5												
	6												
	7												
	8												
	9												
	10												
	11												
	12												
	13												
	14												
	15												
	16												
	17												
	18												
	19												
	20												
	22												
	24												
	26												
	28												
	30												
	32												
	34												
	36												
	38												
	40												
	50												
	60												
	70												
	80												
	90				.00001								
	100				.00001								

B. Values of $\beta_1' = \beta_L'$, $\beta_2' = (\beta_S')_{\max}$, $\beta_3' = (\beta_X')_{\min}$ and $\beta_4' = \beta_W'$ for $\alpha = 0.01$

		$\delta=0.5$				$\delta=1.0$				$\delta=1.5$			
N	m	β_1'	β_2'	β_3'	β_4'	β_1'	β_2'	β_3'	β_4'	β_1'	β_2'	β_3'	β_4'
61	2	.442	.442	.442	.442	.00206	.00206	.00206	.00206				
	3	.437	.480	.505	.573	.00189	.00268	.00326	.00546				
	4	.434	.507	.542	.647	.00182	.00324	.00425	.00926				
	5	.433	.527	.569	.697	.00177	.00373	.00512	.0132				
	6	.432	.543	.589	.733	.00174	.00418	.00589	.0171				
	7	.431	.557	.606	.761	.00172	.00459	.00660	.0210				
	8	.430	.568	.619	.783	.00171	.00498	.00726	.0249				
	9	.430	.578	.631	.801	.00170	.00534	.00787	.0287				
	10	.430	.587	.641	.816	.00169	.00568	.00845	.0324				
	11	.429	.595	.650	.828	.00168	.00600	.00900	.0360				
	12	.429	.602	.658	.839	.00167	.00630	.00952	.0395				
	13	.429	.608	.665	.849	.00167	.00658	.0100	.0430				
	14	.429	.614	.672	.857	.00166	.00686	.0105	.0463				
	15	.429	.619	.678	.865	.00166	.00712	.0109	.0496				.00001
	16	.428	.624	.683	.871	.00166	.00736	.0114	.0528				.00001
	17	.428	.628	.688	.877	.00165	.00760	.0118	.0560				.00001
	18	.428	.633	.693	.883	.00165	.00783	.0122	.0591				.00001
	19	.428	.636	.698	.888	.00165	.00805	.0126	.0621				.00001
	20	.428	.640	.702	.892	.00165	.00826	.0130	.0650				.00001
	22	.428	.647	.709	.900	.00164	.00866	.0137	.0708				.00001
	24	.428	.653	.716	.907	.00164	.00904	.0144	.0763				.00001
	26	.428	.658	.722	.913	.00164	.00939	.0151	.0815				.00002
	28	.428	.663	.728	.918	.00163	.00972	.0157	.0867				.00002
	30	.427	.667	.733	.923	.00163	.0100	.0164	.0917				.00002
	32	.427	.671	.737	.927	.00163	.0103	.0169	.0964				.00002
	34	.427	.675	.742	.930	.00163	.0106	.0175	.101				.00003
	36	.427	.678	.746	.934	.00163	.0109	.0180	.105				.00003
	38	.427	.682	.750	.937	.00163	.0111	.0186	.110				.00003
	40	.427	.685	.753	.940	.00163	.0114	.0191	.114				.00004
	50	.427	.697	.768	.950	.00162	.0125	.0213	.133				.00005
	60	.427	.707	.779	.958	.00162	.0134	.0234	.151				.00007
	70	.427	.715	.789	.963	.00162	.0142	.0252	.166				.00010
	80	.427	.721	.797	.967	.00162	.0149	.0268	.180				.00012
	90	.427	.726	.803	.971	.00161	.0154	.0283	.193				.00014
	100	.427	.731	.809	.973	.00161	.0160	.0297	.204				.00017

B. Values of $\beta_1' = \beta_L'$, $\beta_2' = (\beta_S')_{\max}$, $\beta_3' = (\beta_X')_{\min}$ and $\beta_4' = \beta_W'$ for $\alpha = 0.01$

		$\delta = 0.5$				$\delta = 1.0$				$\delta = 1.5$			
N	m	β_1'	β_2'	β_3'	β_4'	β_1'	β_2'	β_3'	β_4'	β_1'	β_2'	β_3'	β_4'
121	2	.0992	.0992	.0992	.0992								
	3	.0977	.118	.130	.170								
	4	.0969	.132	.152	.225								
	5	.0964	.144	.169	.268								
	6	.0961	.153	.182	.305				.00001				
	7	.0959	.162	.194	.336				.00001				
	8	.0957	.169	.204	.363				.00001				
	9	.0956	.176	.213	.387				.00002				
	10	.0955	.181	.221	.408				.00002				
	11	.0954	.187	.228	.427				.00002				
	12	.0953	.192	.235	.444				.00003				
	13	.0953	.196	.241	.460				.00003				
	14	.0952	.201	.246	.475				.00004				
	15	.0952	.204	.252	.488				.00005				
	16	.0951	.208	.257	.501				.00005				
	17	.0951	.212	.261	.513				.00006				
	18	.0951	.215	.266	.523				.00007				
	19	.0951	.218	.270	.534				.00007				
	20	.0950	.221	.274	.543				.00008				
	22	.0950	.226	.281	.561				.00010				
	24	.0950	.231	.288	.577				.00011				
	26	.0949	.236	.294	.591				.00013				
	28	.0949	.240	.300	.604			.00001	.00015				
	30	.0949	.243	.306	.616			.00001	.00017				
	32	.0949	.247	.311	.627			.00001	.00018				
	34	.0948	.250	.315	.637			.00001	.00020				
	36	.0948	.253	.320	.646			.00001	.00022				
	38	.0948	.256	.324	.655			.00001	.00025				
	40	.0948	.259	.328	.663			.00001	.00027				
	50	.0948	.271	.346	.698			.00001	.00038				
	60	.0947	.280	.360	.724			.00001	.00050				
	70	.0947	.288	.372	.745			.00001	.00062				
	80	.0947	.294	.382	.762			.00001	.00075				
	90	.0947	.299	.392	.777		.00001	.00002	.00089				
	100	.0947	.304	.400	.790		.00001	.00002	.00103				

Table B6

SAMPLE SIZE FOR MULTIPLE COMPARISON TESTS WITH PRESCRIBED ERROR RATES (SINGLE-CLASSIFICATION EXPERIMENTS)

$[\delta = 0.5(0.5)3.0]$

α and β' are respectively the Type I error rate and the sum of the error rates of Types II and III for the test under consideration; N_L, N_S, N_X, and N_W are respectively the minimum sample sizes required so that α and β' will not exceed the prescribed values for the LSD (multiple t) test, Duncan's multiple range test, Tukey's X procedure, and Tukey's studentized range test; $\delta = (\mu_U - \mu_L)/\delta$, where μ_U and μ_L are defined in Chapter 2, subsection 2.2.7, and σ is the common population standard deviation.

A. $\alpha = 0.05$, $B' = 0.10$

m	N_L					
	$\delta = 0.5$	$\delta = 1.0$	$\delta = 1.5$	$\delta = 2.0$	$\delta = 2.5$	$\delta = 3.0$
2	86	23	11	7	5	4
3	85	22	11	7	5	4
4	85	22	10	6	5	4
5	85	22	10	6	4	3
6	85	22	10	6	4	3
7	85	22	10	6	4	3
8	85	22	10	6	4	3
9	85	22	10	6	4	3
10	85	22	10	6	4	3
11	85	22	10	6	4	3
12	85	22	10	6	4	3
13	85	22	10	6	4	3
14	85	22	10	6	4	3
15	85	22	10	6	4	3
16	85	22	10	6	4	3
17	85	22	10	6	4	3
18	85	22	10	6	4	3
19	85	22	10	6	4	3
20	85	22	10	6	4	3
22	85	22	10	6	4	3
24	85	22	10	6	4	3
26	85	22	10	6	4	3
28	85	22	10	6	4	3
30	85	22	10	6	4	3
32	85	22	10	6	4	3
34	85	22	10	6	4	3
36	85	22	10	6	4	3
38	85	22	10	6	4	3
40	85	22	10	6	4	3
50	85	22	10	6	4	3
60	85	22	10	6	4	3
70	85	22	10	6	4	3
80	85	22	10	6	4	3
90	85	22	10	6	4	3
100	85	22	10	6	4	3

m	$(N_S)_{max}$					
	$\delta = 0.5$	$\delta = 1.0$	$\delta = 1.5$	$\delta = 2.0$	$\delta = 2.5$	$\delta = 3.0$
2	86	23	11	7	5	4
3	91	24	11	7	5	4
4	94	24	11	7	5	4
5	97	25	12	7	5	4
6	99	25	12	7	5	4
7	101	26	12	7	5	4
8	102	26	12	7	5	4
9	104	26	12	7	5	4
10	105	27	12	7	5	4
11	106	27	12	7	5	4
12	107	27	12	7	5	4
13	108	27	13	7	5	4
14	109	28	13	7	5	4
15	109	28	13	7	5	4
16	110	28	13	7	5	4
17	110	28	13	7	5	4
18	111	28	13	7	5	4
19	111	28	13	7	5	4
20	112	28	13	8	5	4
22	113	29	13	8	5	4
24	114	29	13	8	5	4
26	114	29	13	8	5	4
28	115	29	13	8	5	4
30	116	29	13	8	5	4
32	116	29	13	8	5	4
34	117	30	13	8	5	4
36	117	30	13	8	5	4
38	117	30	13	8	5	4
40	118	30	14	8	5	4
50	119	30	14	8	5	4
60	121	30	14	8	5	4
70	122	31	14	8	5	4
80	122	31	14	8	5	4
90	123	31	14	8	5	4
100	124	31	14	8	5	4

m	$(N_x)_{min}$ $\delta=0.5$	$\delta=1.0$	$\delta=1.5$	$\delta=2.0$	$\delta=2.5$	$\delta=3.0$
2	86	23	11	7	5	4
3	96	25	12	7	5	4
4	102	26	12	8	5	4
5	106	27	13	8	5	4
6	110	28	13	8	5	4
7	113	29	13	8	5	4
8	115	29	14	8	6	4
9	117	30	14	8	6	4
10	119	30	14	8	6	4
11	121	31	14	8	6	4
12	122	31	14	8	6	4
13	124	31	14	8	6	4
14	125	32	15	9	6	4
15	126	32	15	9	6	4
16	127	32	15	9	6	4
17	128	33	15	9	6	4
18	129	33	15	9	6	4
19	130	33	15	9	6	4
20	131	33	15	9	6	4
22	132	34	15	9	6	4
24	134	34	15	9	6	4
26	135	34	16	9	6	4
28	136	35	16	9	6	4
30	137	35	16	9	6	4
32	139	35	16	9	6	5
34	140	35	16	9	6	5
36	140	36	16	9	6	5
38	141	36	16	9	6	5
40	142	36	16	9	6	5
50	146	37	17	10	6	5
60	148	38	17	10	7	5
70	151	38	17	10	7	5
80	153	39	17	10	7	5
90	155	39	18	10	7	5
100	156	40	18	10	7	5

m	N_w $\delta=0.5$	$\delta=1.0$	$\delta=1.5$	$\delta=2.0$	$\delta=2.5$	$\delta=3.0$
2	86	23	11	7	5	4
3	106	28	13	8	6	5
4	120	31	14	9	6	5
5	130	33	15	9	6	5
6	138	35	16	10	7	5
7	144	37	17	10	7	5
8	150	38	18	10	7	5
9	155	39	18	11	7	5
10	159	40	19	11	7	5
11	163	41	19	11	7	5
12	166	42	19	11	8	6
13	170	43	20	11	8	6
14	173	44	20	12	8	6
15	176	45	20	12	8	6
16	178	45	21	12	8	6
17	181	46	21	12	8	6
18	183	46	21	12	8	6
19	185	47	21	12	8	6
20	187	47	21	12	8	6
22	191	48	22	13	8	6
24	194	49	22	13	9	6
26	197	50	23	13	9	6
28	200	51	23	13	9	6
30	203	51	23	13	9	6
32	206	52	23	14	9	6
34	208	53	24	14	9	6
36	210	53	24	14	9	7
38	212	54	24	14	9	7
40	214	54	24	14	9	7
50	223	56	25	15	10	7
60	230	58	26	15	10	7
70	236	60	27	15	10	7
80	241	61	27	16	10	7
90	246	62	28	16	10	7
100	250	63	28	16	11	8

B. $\alpha = 0.05$, $\beta' = 0.05$

m	N_L					
	$\delta = 0.5$	$\delta = 1.0$	$\delta = 1.5$	$\delta = 2.0$	$\delta = 2.5$	$\delta = 3.0$
2	105	27	13	8	6	5
3	105	27	13	8	5	4
4	105	27	13	8	5	4
5	105	27	12	7	5	4
6	105	27	12	7	5	4
7	105	27	12	7	5	4
8	105	27	12	7	5	4
9	105	27	12	7	5	4
10	105	27	12	7	5	4
11	105	27	12	7	5	4
12	105	27	12	7	5	4
13	105	27	12	7	5	4
14	105	27	12	7	5	4
15	105	27	12	7	5	4
16	105	27	12	7	5	4
17	105	27	12	7	5	4
18	105	27	12	7	5	4
19	105	27	12	7	5	4
20	105	27	12	7	5	4
22	105	27	12	7	5	4
24	105	27	12	7	5	4
26	105	27	12	7	5	3
28	105	27	12	7	5	3
30	105	27	12	7	5	3
32	105	27	12	7	5	3
34	105	27	12	7	5	3
36	105	27	12	7	5	3
38	105	27	12	7	5	3
40	105	27	12	7	5	3
50	105	27	12	7	5	3
60	104	27	12	7	5	3
70	104	27	12	7	5	3
80	104	27	12	7	5	3
90	104	27	12	7	5	3
100	104	27	12	7	5	3

m	$(N_S)_{max}$					
	$\delta = 0.5$	$\delta = 1.0$	$\delta = 1.5$	$\delta = 2.0$	$\delta = 2.5$	$\delta = 3.0$
2	105	27	13	8	6	5
3	111	29	13	8	6	4
4	115	30	14	8	6	4
5	118	30	14	8	6	4
6	121	31	14	8	6	4
7	123	31	14	8	6	4
8	124	32	14	8	6	4
9	126	32	15	9	6	4
10	127	32	15	9	6	4
11	128	33	15	9	6	4
12	129	33	15	9	6	4
13	130	33	15	9	6	4
14	131	33	15	9	6	4
15	132	33	15	9	6	4
16	132	34	15	9	6	4
17	133	34	15	9	6	4
18	134	34	15	9	6	4
19	134	34	15	9	6	4
20	135	34	15	9	6	4
22	136	34	16	9	6	4
24	137	35	16	9	6	4
26	137	35	16	9	6	4
28	138	35	16	9	6	4
30	139	35	16	9	6	4
32	139	35	16	9	6	4
34	140	35	16	9	6	4
36	140	35	16	9	6	4
38	141	36	16	9	6	4
40	141	36	16	9	6	4
50	143	36	16	9	6	4
60	144	36	16	9	6	4
70	145	37	17	10	6	4
80	146	37	17	10	6	4
90	147	37	17	10	6	5
100	147	37	17	10	6	5

m	$(N_X)_{min}$ $\delta=0.5$	$\delta=1.0$	$\delta=1.5$	$\delta=2.0$	$\delta=2.5$	$\delta=3.0$
2	105	27	13	8	6	5
3	117	30	14	9	6	5
4	123	32	15	9	6	5
5	128	33	15	9	6	5
6	132	34	16	9	6	5
7	135	35	16	9	6	5
8	138	35	16	9	6	5
9	140	36	16	10	6	5
10	142	36	17	10	7	5
11	144	37	17	10	7	5
12	146	37	17	10	7	5
13	147	37	17	10	7	5
14	149	38	17	10	7	5
15	150	38	17	10	7	5
16	151	38	17	10	7	5
17	152	39	18	10	7	5
18	153	39	18	10	7	5
19	154	39	18	10	7	5
20	155	39	18	10	7	5
22	157	40	18	10	7	5
24	159	40	18	11	7	5
26	160	41	18	11	7	5
28	161	41	19	11	7	5
30	163	41	19	11	7	5
32	164	41	19	11	7	5
34	165	42	19	11	7	5
36	166	42	19	11	7	5
38	167	42	19	11	7	5
40	168	42	19	11	7	5
50	171	43	20	11	7	5
60	175	44	20	11	8	5
70	177	45	20	12	8	5
80	179	45	20	12	8	6
90	181	46	21	12	8	6
100	183	46	21	12	8	6

m	N_W $\delta=0.5$	$\delta=1.0$	$\delta=1.5$	$\delta=2.0$	$\delta=2.5$	$\delta=3.0$
2	105	27	13	8	6	5
3	129	33	16	9	7	5
4	143	37	17	10	7	5
5	154	39	18	11	7	6
6	163	42	19	11	8	6
7	170	43	20	12	8	6
8	176	45	20	12	8	6
9	181	46	21	12	8	6
10	186	47	22	13	8	6
11	190	48	22	13	9	6
12	194	49	22	13	9	6
13	197	50	23	13	9	6
14	201	51	23	13	9	6
15	204	52	23	14	9	7
16	207	52	24	14	9	7
17	209	53	24	14	9	7
18	212	54	24	14	9	7
19	214	54	24	14	9	7
20	216	55	25	14	9	7
22	220	56	25	14	10	7
24	224	57	26	15	10	7
26	227	57	26	15	10	7
28	230	58	26	15	10	7
30	233	59	27	15	10	7
32	236	60	27	15	10	7
34	239	60	27	16	10	7
36	241	61	27	16	10	7
38	243	61	28	16	10	7
40	246	62	28	16	10	7
50	255	64	29	17	11	8
60	262	66	30	17	11	8
70	269	68	30	17	11	8
80	274	69	31	18	12	8
90	279	70	32	18	12	8
100	284	71	32	18	12	8

C. $\alpha = 0.01$, $\beta' = 0.10$

m	N_L					
	$\delta = 0.5$	$\delta = 1.0$	$\delta = 1.5$	$\delta = 2.0$	$\delta = 2.5$	$\delta = 3.0$
2	121	32	15	10	7	6
3	121	31	15	9	7	5
4	120	31	15	9	6	5
5	120	31	14	9	6	5
6	120	31	14	9	6	5
7	120	31	14	8	6	4
8	120	31	14	8	6	4
9	120	31	14	8	6	4
10	120	31	14	8	6	4
11	120	31	14	8	6	4
12	120	31	14	8	6	4
13	120	31	14	8	6	4
14	120	31	14	8	6	4
15	120	30	14	8	6	4
16	120	30	14	8	6	4
17	120	30	14	8	6	4
18	120	30	14	8	5	4
19	120	30	14	8	5	4
20	120	30	14	8	5	4
22	120	30	14	8	5	4
24	120	30	14	8	5	4
26	120	30	14	8	5	4
28	120	30	14	8	5	4
30	120	30	14	8	5	4
32	120	30	14	8	5	4
34	120	30	14	8	5	4
36	120	30	14	8	5	4
38	120	30	14	8	5	4
40	120	30	14	8	5	4
50	120	30	14	8	5	4
60	120	30	14	8	5	4
70	120	30	14	8	5	4
80	120	30	14	8	5	4
90	120	30	14	8	5	4
100	120	30	14	8	5	4

m	$(N_S)_{max}$					
	$\delta = 0.5$	$\delta = 1.0$	$\delta = 1.5$	$\delta = 2.0$	$\delta = 2.5$	$\delta = 3.0$
2	121	32	15	10	7	6
3	127	33	16	10	7	5
4	132	34	16	10	7	5
5	135	35	16	10	7	5
6	138	35	16	10	7	5
7	140	36	17	10	7	5
8	142	36	17	10	7	5
9	144	37	17	10	7	5
10	146	37	17	10	7	5
11	147	37	17	10	7	5
12	148	38	17	10	7	5
13	149	38	17	10	7	5
14	151	38	17	10	7	5
15	152	38	18	10	7	5
16	152	39	18	10	7	5
17	153	39	18	10	7	5
18	154	39	18	10	7	5
19	155	39	18	10	7	5
20	155	39	18	10	7	5
22	157	40	18	10	7	5
24	158	40	18	10	7	5
26	159	40	18	11	7	5
28	160	40	18	11	7	5
30	161	41	18	11	7	5
32	162	41	18	11	7	5
34	162	41	19	11	7	5
36	163	41	19	11	7	5
38	164	41	19	11	7	5
40	164	41	19	11	7	5
50	167	42	19	11	7	5
60	169	43	19	11	7	5
70	171	43	19	11	7	5
80	172	43	20	11	7	5
90	173	44	20	11	7	5
100	174	44	20	11	7	5

m	$(N_X)_{min}$ $\delta=0.5$	$\delta=1.0$	$\delta=1.5$	$\delta=2.0$	$\delta=2.5$	$\delta=3.0$
2	121	32	15	10	7	6
3	131	34	16	10	7	6
4	138	36	17	10	7	5
5	142	37	17	10	7	5
6	146	37	17	10	7	5
7	149	38	18	10	7	5
8	151	39	18	11	7	5
9	153	39	18	11	7	5
10	155	40	18	11	7	5
11	157	40	18	11	7	5
12	159	40	18	11	7	5
13	160	41	19	11	7	5
14	161	41	19	11	7	5
15	163	41	19	11	7	5
16	164	42	19	11	7	5
17	165	42	19	11	7	5
18	166	42	19	11	7	5
19	167	42	19	11	7	5
20	168	42	19	11	7	5
22	169	43	19	11	8	5
24	171	43	20	11	8	6
26	172	44	20	11	8	6
28	173	44	20	12	8	6
30	174	44	20	12	8	6
32	175	44	20	12	8	6
34	176	45	20	12	8	6
36	177	45	20	12	8	6
38	178	45	20	12	8	6
40	179	45	20	12	8	6
50	183	46	21	12	8	6
60	186	47	21	12	8	6
70	188	48	21	12	8	6
80	190	48	22	12	8	6
90	192	48	22	13	8	6
100	194	49	22	13	8	6

m	N_W $\delta=0.5$	$\delta=1.0$	$\delta=1.5$	$\delta=2.0$	$\delta=2.5$	$\delta=3.0$
2	121	32	15	10	7	6
3	143	37	18	11	8	6
4	156	40	19	11	8	6
5	166	43	20	12	8	6
6	174	45	21	12	8	6
7	181	46	21	13	9	6
8	186	47	22	13	9	6
a	191	49	22	13	9	7
10	195	50	23	13	9	7
11	199	51	23	14	9	7
12	203	52	23	14	9	7
13	206	52	24	14	9	7
14	209	53	24	14	9	7
15	212	54	24	14	9	7
16	214	54	25	14	10	7
17	217	55	25	14	10	7
18	219	55	25	15	10	7
19	221	56	25	15	10	7
20	223	56	26	15	10	7
22	227	57	26	15	10	7
24	231	58	26	15	10	7
26	234	59	27	15	10	7
28	237	60	27	16	10	7
30	239	60	27	16	10	7
32	242	61	28	16	10	7
34	244	62	28	16	11	8
36	246	62	28	16	11	8
38	249	63	28	16	11	8
40	251	63	28	16	11	8
50	259	65	29	17	11	8
60	266	67	30	17	11	8
70	272	69	31	18	12	8
80	277	70	31	18	12	8
90	282	71	32	18	12	8
100	286	72	32	18	12	9

D. $\alpha=0.01$, $\beta'=0.05$

m	N_L						m	$(N_S)_{max}$					
	$\delta=0.5$	$\delta=1.0$	$\delta=1.5$	$\delta=2.0$	$\delta=2.5$	$\delta=3.0$		$\delta=0.5$	$\delta=1.0$	$\delta=1.5$	$\delta=2.0$	$\delta=2.5$	$\delta=3.0$
2	145	38	18	11	8	6	2	145	38	18	11	8	6
3	144	37	18	11	7	6	3	152	39	18	11	8	6
4	144	37	17	10	7	5	4	156	40	19	11	8	6
5	144	37	17	10	7	5	5	160	41	19	11	8	6
6	144	37	17	10	7	5	6	163	42	19	11	8	6
7	144	37	17	10	7	5	7	166	42	19	11	8	6
8	143	37	17	10	7	5	8	168	43	20	11	8	6
9	143	37	17	10	7	5	9	170	43	20	12	8	6
10	143	36	17	10	7	5	10	171	44	20	12	8	6
11	143	36	17	10	7	5	11	173	44	20	12	8	6
12	143	36	17	10	7	5	12	174	44	20	12	8	6
13	143	36	17	10	7	5	13	176	44	20	12	8	6
14	143	36	17	10	6	5	14	177	45	20	12	8	6
15	143	36	17	10	6	5	15	178	45	20	12	8	6
16	143	36	17	10	6	5	16	179	45	21	12	8	6
17	143	36	17	10	6	5	17	180	45	21	12	8	6
18	143	36	17	10	6	5	18	181	46	21	12	8	6
19	143	36	17	10	6	5	19	181	46	21	12	8	6
20	143	36	17	10	6	5	20	182	46	21	12	8	6
22	143	36	16	10	6	5	22	183	46	21	12	8	6
24	143	36	16	10	6	5	24	185	47	21	12	8	6
26	143	36	16	10	6	5	26	186	47	21	12	8	6
28	143	36	16	10	6	5	28	187	47	21	12	8	6
30	143	36	16	10	6	5	30	188	47	21	12	8	6
32	143	36	16	10	6	5	32	189	48	21	12	8	6
34	143	36	16	10	6	5	34	189	48	22	12	8	6
36	143	36	16	10	6	5	36	190	48	22	12	8	6
38	143	36	16	10	6	5	38	191	48	22	12	8	6
40	143	36	16	10	6	5	40	192	48	22	13	8	6
50	143	36	16	9	6	5	50	194	49	22	13	8	6
60	143	36	16	9	6	5	60	197	50	22	13	8	6
70	143	36	16	9	6	5	70	198	50	23	13	8	6
80	143	36	16	9	6	5	80	200	50	23	13	9	6
90	143	36	16	9	6	5	90	201	51	23	13	9	6
100	143	36	16	9	6	5	100	202	51	23	13	9	6

m	$(N_x)_{min}$ $\delta=0.5$	$\delta=1.0$	$\delta=1.5$	$\delta=2.0$	$\delta=2.5$	$\delta=3.0$
2	145	38	18	11	8	6
3	156	40	19	11	8	6
4	163	42	19	12	8	6
5	168	43	20	12	8	6
6	172	44	20	12	8	6
7	175	45	20	12	8	6
8	178	45	21	12	8	6
9	180	46	21	12	8	6
10	182	46	21	12	8	6
11	184	47	21	12	8	6
12	185	47	21	12	8	6
13	187	47	22	13	8	6
14	188	48	22	13	8	6
15	190	48	22	13	8	6
16	191	48	22	13	8	6
17	192	49	22	13	9	6
18	193	49	22	13	9	6
19	194	49	22	13	9	6
20	195	49	22	13	9	6
22	197	50	23	13	9	6
24	198	50	23	13	9	6
26	200	51	23	13	9	6
28	201	51	23	13	9	6
30	203	51	23	13	9	6
32	204	51	23	13	9	6
34	205	52	23	13	9	6
36	206	52	23	14	9	6
38	207	52	24	14	9	6
40	208	52	24	14	9	6
50	212	53	24	14	9	7
60	215	54	24	14	9	7
70	217	55	25	14	9	7
80	220	55	25	14	9	7
90	222	56	25	14	9	7
100	224	56	25	15	9	7

m	N_W $\delta=0.5$	$\delta=1.0$	$\delta=1.5$	$\delta=2.0$	$\delta=2.5$	$\delta=3.0$
2	145	38	18	11	8	6
3	168	43	20	12	9	7
4	183	47	22	13	9	7
5	194	50	23	14	9	7
6	202	52	24	14	10	7
7	209	53	24	14	10	7
8	215	55	25	15	10	7
9	220	56	26	15	10	7
10	225	57	26	15	10	7
11	229	58	26	15	10	7
12	233	59	27	16	10	8
13	237	60	27	16	10	8
14	240	61	28	16	11	8
15	243	61	28	16	11	8
16	246	62	28	16	11	8
17	248	63	28	16	11	8
18	251	63	29	17	11	8
19	253	64	29	17	11	8
20	255	64	29	17	11	8
22	259	65	30	17	11	8
24	263	66	30	17	11	8
26	266	67	30	17	11	8
28	269	68	31	18	12	8
30	272	69	31	18	12	8
32	275	69	31	18	12	8
34	277	70	31	18	12	8
36	280	70	32	18	12	9
38	282	71	32	18	12	9
40	284	72	32	18	12	9
50	293	74	33	19	12	9
60	301	76	34	19	13	9
70	307	77	35	20	13	9
80	313	79	35	20	13	9
90	318	80	36	20	13	9
100	322	81	36	21	13	10

Table B7

TABLES FOR ANALYSIS OF VARIANCE BASED ON (STUDENTIZED) RANGE

[Pearson and Hartley (1966), Table 30, p. 201]

A. Scale factor, c, and equivalent degrees of freedom, ν, appropriate to a simple classification into k groups of n observations

	k													
	1		2		3		4		5		10		d_n	C.D.
n	ν	c	ν	c	ν	c	ν	c	ν	c	ν	c		
2	1.0	1.41	1.9	1.28	2.8	1.23	3.7	1.21	4.6	1.19	9.0	1.16	1.13	0.88
3	2.0	1.91	3.8	1.81	5.7	1.77	7.5	1.75	9.3	1.74	18.4	1.72	1.69	1.82
4	2.9	2.24	5.7	2.15	8.4	2.12	11.2	2.11	13.9	2.10	27.6	2.08	2.06	2.74
5	3.8	2.48	7.5	2.40	11.1	2.38	14.7	2.37	18.4	2.36	36.5	2.34	2.33	3.62
6	4.7	2.67	9.2	2.60	13.6	2.58	18.1	2.57	22.6	2.56	44.9	2.55	2.53	4.47
7	5.5	2.83	10.8	2.77	16.0	2.75	21.3	2.74	26.6	2.73	52.9	2.72	2.70	5.27
8	6.3	2.96	12.3	2.91	18.3	2.89	24.4	2.88	30.4	2.87	60.6	2.86	2.85	6.03
9	7.0	3.08	13.8	3.02	20.5	3.01	27.3	3.00	34.0	2.99	67.8	2.98	2.97	6.76
10	7.7	3.18	15.1	3.13	22.6	3.11	30.1	3.10	37.5	3.10	74.8	3.09	3.08	7.45

B. Scale factor, c, and equivalent degrees of freedom, ν, for analysis of double classification, with k blocks and n treatments

	n															
	2		3		4		5		6		7		8		9	
k	ν	c	ν	c	ν	c	ν	c	ν	c	ν	c	ν	c	ν	c
2	1.0	1.00	2.0	1.35	2.9	1.58	3.8	1.75	4.7	1.89	5.5	2.00	6.3	2.10	7.0	2.18
3	1.9	1.05	3.7	1.48	5.6	1.76	7.4	1.96	9.3	2.12	11.3	2.26	13.4	2.37	15.7	2.46
4	2.7	1.07	5.4	1.54	8.2	1.84	11.0	2.06	13.9	2.23	16.9	2.38	20.1	2.50	23.6	2.60
5	3.6	1.08	7.2	1.57	10.9	1.88	14.6	2.12	18.5	2.30	22.4	2.45	26.6	2.57	31.1	2.68
6	4.5	1.09	8.9	1.59	13.6	1.91	18.2	2.15	23.0	2.34	27.9	2.49	33.0	2.62	38.3	2.73
7	5.4	1.09	10.7	1.61	16.3	1.93	21.8	2.18	27.6	2.37	33.3	2.52	39.3	2.65	45.4	2.76
8	6.3	1.10	12.5	1.62	19.0	1.95	25.4	2.20	32.1	2.39	38.7	2.55	45.6	2.68	52.5	2.79
9	7.1	1.10	14.3	1.63	21.7	1.96	29.0	2.21	36.6	2.41	44.0	2.57	51.8	2.70	59.6	2.81
10	8.1	1.10	16.1	1.63	24.4	1.97	32.6	2.22	41.0	2.42	49.3	2.58	57.9	2.71	66.6	2.83
20	16.7	1.11	33.9	1.66	51.5	2.02	68.8	2.28	86.0	2.48	103	2.64	119	2.78	134	2.90
d_n		1.13		1.69		2.06		2.33		2.53		2.70		2.85		2.97
C.D.	0.87		1.80		2.71		3.62		4.50		5.33		6.10		6.79	

C.D. = constant difference.

Table B8

5% AND 1% CRITICAL VALUES FOR THE DISCORDANCY TEST OF A LOWER AND UPPER OUTLIER-PAIR BASED ON THE INTERNALLY STUDENTIZED RANGE T FOR A SAMPLE OF SIZE n

n	5%	1%
3	2.00	2.00
4	2.43	2.45
5	2.75	2.80
6	3.01	3.10
7	3.22	3.34
8	3.40	3.54
9	3.55	3.72
10	3.69	3.87
12	3.91	4.13
14	4.09	4.34
16	4.24	4.52
18	4.37	4.67
20	4.49	4.80
30	4.89	5.26
40	5.16	5.56
50	5.35	5.77
60	5.51	5.94
100	5.90	6.36
200	6.39	6.84
500	6.94	7.42
1000	7.33	7.80

Author Index

Armitage, John V. v

Balaam, L. N. 45
Balakrishnan, N. vii, 14, 18, 20-24, 56
Barnett, Vic 52, 53
Beyer, William H. 26, 33, 38, 45
Blanch, Gertrude v
Braun, Henry I. 34, 47
Buenaventura, Angeles, R. 3, 12, 13

Carmer, S. G. 45
Carter, Nancy J. 45, 46
Chen, M. J. 52, 53
Childs, Aaron 23, 24, 56
Clemm, Donald S. v-vii, 5, 7, 9, 13, 14, 25, 56, 272
Cournot, A. A. 35, 45

David, Herbert A. 15, 18, 48, 51-53, 272
Davis, Owen L. 49, 51
Dixon, Wilfrid J. 3, 12, 13, 18, 52, 53
Duncan, David B. v, 25, 26, 30-33, 37, 38, 40, 42, 44, 45, 567, 575, 645
Dunnett, Charles W. 46

Fettis, Henry E. 4, 13, 44, 46
Fieller, N. R. J. 52, 53
Fisher, Ronald A. 36, 42, 46, 48, 51, 567

Greenberg, Bernard G. 53
Grubbs, Frank E. 14, 18
Guthrie, Eugene H. v, 5, 7, 9, 13, 25, 272

Harter, H. Leon v, vii, 5, 7, 9, 13, 14, 18, 20, 21, 25, 26, 33, 35, 45, 46, 56, 272
Hartley, H. O. v, 10, 11, 13-15, 18, 19, 25-27, 33, 38, 46, 48, 49, 51-53, 272, 655
Hochberg, Yosef 35, 46
Hsu, Jason C. 35, 46

Jennett, W. J. 15
Johnson, Norman L. 22-24

Kendall, Maurice G. 4, 13
Keuls, M. 26, 31-33, 36, 37, 40, 42, 45, 46
Kotz, Samuel 22-24
Krishnaiah, P. R. 46

Lewis, Toby 52, 53
Link, Richard F. 3-5, 13
Lund, J. R. 30, 31, 33
Lund, R. E. 30, 31, 33

Massey, Frank J., Jr. 3, 12, 13, 18
Mathis, John E. vii
May, Joyce M. 25, 26, 33
May, Thomas E. 45, 46
McKay, A. T. 14, 18, 25, 33
Merrington, Maxine 10, 11, 13
Miller, Rupert G., Jr. 35, 45, 46
Moore, P. G. 52, 53
Mosteller, Frederick 3, 13

Newman, D. 25, 26, 31-33, 36, 37, 40, 42, 45, 46

Owen, Donald B. 43, 46

Patnaik, P. B. 15, 18, 48, 51
Pearson, Egon S. 10, 11, 13-15, 18, 19, 25-27, 33, 38, 46, 48, 51-53, 272, 655
Pearson, Karl 11, 13
Pillai, K. C. Sreedharan 3, 13

Rider, Paul R. 3, 13
Rodgers, J. W. 15, 19
Royston, J. P. 31, 33

Sarhan, Ahmed E. 53

Schwertman, Neil C. 45, 46
Shapiro, Samuel S. 52, 53
Shewhart, W. A. 14, 19
Snedecor, George W. 49, 51
Stephens, Michael A. 52, 53
"Student" 14, 19, 26, 36, 46
Swanson, M. B. 45

Tamhane, Ajit C. 35, 46
Teichroew, Daniel v, 17, 19
Thompson, Catherine M. 10, 11, 13
Thompson, G. W. 52, 53
Tippett, L. H. C. 14, 19
Tukey, John W. v, 26, 34-37, 40-43, 46, 47, 567, 575, 645

Weaver, Chalmers L. 14, 18
Wilk, Martin B. 52, 53
Wine, R. Lowell 42, 47

Young, D. H. 22, 24

Subject Index

Alternative hypothesis 10, 11, 18
Analysis of variance 15, 31, 35-37, 48, 49, 655
Asymptotic formula 5, 7
Average quality 20

Binary bits 4, 16
Binary form 4, 5, 7, 9, 10

Chi-square distribution 18, 48
Confidence limits 36
Confidence procedures 1, 35, 36
  Simultaneous 30
Control charts 20, 21, 265
  $\bar{X}$ 20, 265, 266
  R 20, 21, 265, 266
  Standard deviation 20
Control limits 14, 20, 21
  Lower 20, 21
  Upper 20, 21
Critical region 18
Critical values 1, 2, 4, 9, 10, 12, 15, 24-26, 30, 31, 43-45, 267, 269, 555, 657
  for discordancy test 657
  for Duncan's multiple range test 2, 25, 26, 30, 31, 44, 45, 555
  for F' test 1, 4, 9, 10
  for LSD test 43
  Studentized range 2
Cumulants 14
Cumulative distribution function 1, 3, 5-7, 10, 11, 43, 57
  of F 10
  of noncentral t 43
  of range 1
  of ratio of two ranges 1, 3, 5, 7, 11, 57

Decimal form 4, 7, 9-11, 16
Degrees of freedom 2, 25, 27, 29, 31, 32, 36, 37, 39, 44, 48, 49, 52, 273, 515, 555, 656
Discordancy tests 52, 53, 657
  Critical values for 657
Dispersion 1, 14
Double classification experiment 48, 49, 656
Double exponential distribution 45
Duncan's multiple range test 26, 30-33, 37, 40, 42, 44, 45, 555, 567, 575, 645
  Critical values for 26, 30, 31, 44, 555

Error rates 2,2 6, 35, 39, 45, 645
  Comparisonwise 45
  Experimentwise 45
Experimental design 39, 42
Exponential distribution 3

F distribution 2, 48-50
Fisher's test 36, 42, 567
Five-point formula 16
Fixed range test 35, 36, 42, 43
F test 1-4, 9, 10, 12, 35, 115
F' test 1, 3, 4, 9, 10, 12, 115

Gamma function 43

Incomplete beta function 3, 10, 11
Infinite double series 3
Interpolation 1, 6, 9-11, 16, 26, 28-30, 32, 44
  Error 29
  Harmonic 11, 26
  Inverse 1, 9, 16, 26, 28-30
  Lagrangian 26
  Linear 6
  Linear harmonic 29, 30, 32, 44
  Linear inverse 29
  Ninth-degree 9

Sixteenth-degree 11

Level of significance 2, 9, 24, 30-33, 35, 37, 39, 43, 44, 49, 50, 555
Logistic distribution 45
LSD (multiple t) test 35, 36, 39, 40, 43, 45, 567, 575, 645
Lund and Lund algorithm 30

Mean 20
Pooled 20
Mean sqaure 2, 39
between classes 2
Error 2, 39
for error 2
Median 1
Method of least squares 28
Mid-range 1
Moment constants 14
Moment 1, 14, 17, 261
Fourth 14, 17
of the range 1, 14, 17, 261
Third 14, 17
Monte Carlo studies 45
Multinomial distribution 22-24
Multiple comparison tests 2, 15, 17, 26, 31, 32, 35, 37, 38, 40, 42, 43, 45, 567, 575, 645
Duncan's 26, 31-33, 37, 40, 42, 45, 567, 575, 645
Error rates for 35
Fisher's 36, 42, 567
Newman-Keuls's 26, 31-33, 36, 37, 40
Sample sizes for 35
Tukey's 26, 35-37, 40, 42, 43, 45, 567, 575, 645
Multiple range test 35-37, 39, 40, 42, 43, 645
Power study of 42
Multivariate hypergeometric distribution 22, 23
Multivariate normal distribution 23

Newman-Keuls test 26, 31-33, 36, 37, 40, 42, 45
Noncentral t distribution 43
Cumulative distribution of 43
Noncentrality parameter 43
Normal approximation 23
Normal population (distribution) 1, 3-5, 10, 12, 14-18, 20, 23, 24, 27, 29, 31, 43, 45, 48, 52, 57, 109, 125, 257, 261, 273, 515, 555
Null distribution 52
Null hypothesis 9-11, 23, 24, 48
Numerical integration 4-8, 17, 26, 28, 44

One-sided tests 10
One-way classification experiment 48
Order statistic 1, 17, 22, 23
Expected values of 17
Outlier 52
Discordancy tests for 52, 53
Critical values for 657
Outlier-testing 52, 53

Pearson curves 14
Percentage points 1-5, 9-11, 14, 16, 17, 24-26, 29-31, 44, 48, 52, 56, 109, 257, 515
Lower 3, 14, 25, 26, 52
of externally studentized range 52
of F 10, 11, 48
of ratio of two ranges 3-5, 9-11, 109
of standardized range 52
of studentized range 1, 2, 9, 17, 29-31, 44, 515
Upper 3, 14, 24-26, 52
Polynomial approximation 28
Power 1, 4, 9-12, 18, 52, 115
of F test 1, 4, 9-11, 115
of F' test 1, 4, 9-11, 115
of multiple range tests 42
Probability density function 1, 3-7
of range 1, 4-6
of ratio of two ranges 1, 3, 5, 7
Probability integral 1, 2, 14-17, 25-30, 125, 273
of the range 1, 14-16, 25-27, 30, 125
of the studentized range 1, 2, 14, 15, 17, 25-29, 273
Probability mass function 22
Process variability 20

q distribution 49
Quadrature 25, 26
Quasi-range 1, 56

Randomized block experiment 39, 42, 49
Randomized experiment 48

Range 1-3, 5, 9, 10, 12, 14-18, 20, 22, 23, 25-27, 31, 35, 39, 42, 48-50, 52, 55, 125, 257, 261
  Expected value of 20
  Mid- 1
  Moments of 1, 14, 17, 261
  Percentage points of 14, 16, 25, 257
  Probability integral of 1, 14-16, 25-27, 125
  Quasi- 1, 56
  Standardized 4, 5, 52
    Percentage points of 52
Rectangular distribution 3, 45 (*see also* Uniform distribution)
Replicated experiments 1
  Analysis of 1
Root-mean-square estimate 1
Rounding error 4, 11, 16

Sample sizes 35, 42, 45, 645
Seven-point formula 5, 7, 8, 16, 17, 28
Significance tests 1, 36
Simpson's rule 4
Single-classification experiment 1, 37, 39, 42, 48, 567, 575, 645, 656
Size of the test 4, 9
Standard deviation 1, 9, 14, 17, 18, 25, 27, 29, 40, 48, 52, 575, 645
Standard error 2, 31, 32, 36, 38
  of the mean 2, 31, 32, 36, 38
Statistical quality control 1, 14
Studentized maximum modulus 1
Studentized range 1, 2, 5, 14, 15, 17, 25-32, 35, 37, 38, 44, 45, 48-50, 53, 271, 273, 515, 555, 575, 645, 655
  Externally 52, 53
    Percentage points of 52
  Internally 52, 53, 657
  Percentage points of 17, 29-31, 38, 44, 515
  Probability integral of 1, 14, 15, 17, 25-29, 273
  Upper quantiles of 30, 36
Student *t* distribution 25, 36, 38
Sum of squares 2
  Error 2
  Total 2

t test 35, 36, 567, 575, 645
  Multiple 36, 567, 575, 645
Tests of homogeneity 22, 23
Tests of hypotheses 1, 18
Test statistic 22, 23
Tolerance 5, 9, 11, 29
Trapezoidal rule 4, 17, 44
Truncation error 8, 9, 16
Tukey's test 26, 36, 37, 40, 42, 43, 45, 567, 575, 645
Two-sided tests 10
Type I error 2, 12, 18, 35, 36, 39, 41, 567, 645
Type II error 12, 40, 41, 575, 645
Type III error, 40, 41, 575, 645

Uniform distribution 3, 45 (*see also* Rectangular distribution)
Uniformly most powerful test 10

Variance 1, 9, 10, 12, 15, 17, 31, 38, 48, 52, 273, 515, 555